PAI
TEXTBOOK OF PEDIATRICS

PAI
TEXTBOOK OF PEDIATRICS

Editor-in-Chief
Anoop Verma
MD FIAP FIAMS FCGP FPNC FPAI
Senior Pediatric Consultant and Director
Swapnil Institute of Child Health
Raipur, Chhattisgarh, India
National Secretary General, Pediatric Association of India (since 2018)
National Executive Board Member, IAP 2000, 2005, 2012, 2014, 2015
National Vice President, IAP 2005
National Chairperson, Academy of Pediatric Neurology (2008–2012)
Central Working Committee Member, IMA HQ 2007, 2009, 2011, 2012
CG State President, IAP 2006
CG State President, IMA 2007

Executive Editor
KP Sarbhai
MD FPAI FCGP FPNC
Chief Pediatrician
Sarbhai Nursing Home and Research Center
Raipur, Chhattisgarh, India
Past National Chairperson, Academy of Pediatric Neurology

Forewords
Gadadhar Sarangi
BC Chhaparwal
Nimain Mohanty

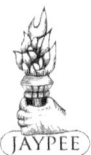

JAYPEE BROTHERS MEDICAL PUBLISHERS
The Health Sciences Publisher
New Delhi | London

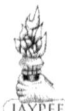 **Jaypee Brothers Medical Publishers (P) Ltd**

Headquarters

Jaypee Brothers Medical Publishers (P) Ltd
EMCA House, 23/23-B
Ansari Road, Daryaganj
New Delhi 110 002, India
Landline: +91-11-23272143, +91-11-23272703
+91-11-23282021, +91-11-23245672
Email: jaypee@jaypeebrothers.com

Corporate Office

Jaypee Brothers Medical Publishers (P) Ltd
4838/24, Ansari Road, Daryaganj
New Delhi 110 002, India
Phone: +91-11-43574357
Fax: +91-11-43574314
Email: jaypee@jaypeebrothers.com

Overseas Office

JP Medical Ltd
83 Victoria Street, London
SW1H 0HW (UK)
Phone: +44 20 3170 8910
Fax: +44 (0)20 3008 6180
Email: info@jpmedpub.com

Website: www.jaypeebrothers.com
Website: www.jaypeedigital.com

© 2022, Jaypee Brothers Medical Publishers

The views and opinions expressed in this book are solely those of the original contributor(s)/author(s) and do not necessarily represent those of editor(s) of the book.

All rights reserved. No part of this publication may be reproduced, stored or transmitted in any form or by any means, electronic, mechanical, photocopying, recording or otherwise, without the prior permission in writing of the publishers.

All brand names and product names used in this book are trade names, service marks, trademarks or registered trademarks of their respective owners. The publisher is not associated with any product or vendor mentioned in this book.

Medical knowledge and practice change constantly. This book is designed to provide accurate, authoritative information about the subject matter in question. However, readers are advised to check the most current information available on procedures included and check information from the manufacturer of each product to be administered, to verify the recommended dose, formula, method and duration of administration, adverse effects and contraindications. It is the responsibility of the practitioner to take all appropriate safety precautions. Neither the publisher nor the author(s)/editor(s) assume any liability for any injury and/or damage to persons or property arising from or related to use of material in this book.

This book is sold on the understanding that the publisher is not engaged in providing professional medical services. If such advice or services are required, the services of a competent medical professional should be sought.

Every effort has been made where necessary to contact holders of copyright to obtain permission to reproduce copyright material. If any have been inadvertently overlooked, the publisher will be pleased to make the necessary arrangements at the first opportunity. The **CD/ DVD-ROM** (if any) provided in the sealed envelope with this book is complimentary and free of cost. **Not meant for sale.**

Inquiries for bulk sales may be solicited at: jaypee@jaypeebrothers.com

PAI Textbook of Pediatrics

First Edition: **2022**

ISBN: 978-93-90595-89-1

Editorial Board

EDITOR-IN-CHIEF
Dr Anoop Verma

EXECUTIVE EDITOR
Dr KP Sarbhai

SECTION EDITORS

Nutritional Diseases: **Dr AK Rawat**

Neonatology: **Dr Sharja Phuljhele**

Vaccinology: **Dr KP Sarbhai**

Infectious Diseases: **(Col) DY Shrikhande**

Gastroenterology: **Dr Rimjhim Shrivastava**

Hematology–Oncology: **Dr Kiran Makhija**

Respiratory System: **Dr Atanu Bhadra**

Neurology: **Dr Anoop Verma**

Cardiology: **Dr Asok Kumar Dutta**

Nephrology: **Dr Renu Kale**

Endocrinology: **Dr Hari R Mangtani**

Rheumatology: **Dr Vijay Kamale**

Genetic Disorders: **Dr Amar Verma**

Dermatology: **Dr Vijay P Makhija**

Miscellaneous: **Dr Onkar Khandwal**

Contributors

Aabha Nagral MD DNB (Gastroenterology)
Certificate of Sponsored Training in
Liver Transplantation
Royal College of Physicians, England, UK
Consultant Gastroenterologist
Apollo and Jaslok Hospitals
Mumbai, Maharashtra, India

AK Ganju MD Fellow Hematology (USA)
Consultant Hematologist
Ganju Hematology Clinic and Hospital
Nagpur, Maharashtra, India

AK Rawat MD FPAI
Former Dean
Head and Professor
Department of Pediatrics
Medical College
Sagar, Madhya Pradesh, India

Akash Lalwani MD DCH FNIAP
Senior Resident
Department of Pediatrics
Pt JNM Medical College
Raipur, Chhattisgarh, India

Alka Srivastava MRCPCH DCH
Consultant Pediatrician
Allahabad Child Developmental Center
Prayagraj, Uttar Pradesh, India

Alok Kumar MD
Senior Resident
PDCC (Pediatric Gastroenterology)
Era's Lucknow Medical College and Hospital
Lucknow, Uttar Pradesh, India

Amar Verma MBBS (Gold Medalist) MD
DCH PhD (Medicine)
Professor
Department of Pediatrics and Neonatology
Deputy Director
Department of Genetic Diseases Research
Rajendra Institute of Medical Sciences
Ranchi, Jharkhand, India

Amish Udani DCH DNB (Pediatrics)
Postgraduate Fellowship in Pediatric Nephrology
Consultant Pediatric Nephrologist
BJ Wadia Hospital for Children
Lokmanya Tilak Municipal Medical College
and General Hospital
Mumbai, Maharashtra, India

Anil K Goel
MD (Ped) ACEE (Ped Emergency Med)
Professor and Head
Department of Pediatrics and Pediatric
Emergency
All India Institute of Medical Sciences
Raipur, Chhattisgarh, India

Anindya Kundu DCH MD (Cal)
Freelance Pediatric Practitioner
Kolkata, West Bengal, India

Anita Verma MBBS (Hons) MD
(Pharmacology and Therapeutics)
Former Professor
GD Medical College (West Bengal)
Ranchi, Jharkhand, India

Anoop Kumar
MBBS DCH MD FIAP (PDFPN) FCGP FIAMS
Pediatric Neurologist and Neurophysiologist
Gen-Next Neurocare Center
Aligarh, Uttar Pradesh, India

Anoop Verma
MD FIAP FIAMS FCGP FPNC FPAI
Senior Pediatric Consultant and Director
Swapnil Institute of Child Health
Raipur, Chhattisgarh, India
National Secretary General, Pediatric
Association of India (since 2018)
National Executive Board Member, IAP 2000,
2005, 2012, 2014, 2015
National Vice President, IAP 2005
National Chairperson, Academy of Pediatric
Neurology (2008–2012)
Central Working Committee Member, IMA
HQ 2007, 2009, 2011, 2012
CG State President, IAP 2006
CG State President, IMA 2007

Anupa Prasad MD Fellowship in Genetics
Associate Professor (Biochemistry)
Rajendra Institute of Medical Sciences
Ranchi, Jharkhand, India

Aradhana Mishra
DCH Fellow in Pediatric Oncology
Consultant Pediatric Oncologist
Ashish Hospital
Jabalpur, Madhya Pradesh, India

Arpana Verma MD
Senior Resident
Department of Obstetrics and Gynecology
All India Institute of Medical Sciences
Raipur, Chhattisgarh, India

Arun Agrawal
MD (Pediatrics) FIAP MNAMS FIAMS FPAI FPNC
Director
Chandra Laxmi Group of Hospital
Ghaziabad, Uttar Pradesh, India
Honorary Professor of IMA

Arun Agrawalla MD
Consultant
Ekta Institute of Child Health
Raipur, Chhattisgarh, India

(Surgeon Captain) Ashok Bhandari
MBBS MD (PGIMER Chandigarh)
Senior Adviser and Professor
Head
Department of Pediatrics
Command Hospital (Central Command)
Lucknow, Uttar Pradesh, India

Ashutosh V Yajurvedi
DCH Fellow Neonatology
Consultant Pediatrician
Yajurvedi Hospital
Solapur, Maharashtra, India

Ashwani Agrawal DCH
Senior Pediatrician
Agrawal Child Clinic
Raipur, Chhattisgarh, India

Asok Kumar Datta MD FIAP FPAI
Professor and Head
Department of Pediatrics
Burdwan Medical College
Burdwan, West Bengal, India

Atanu Bhadra MBBS DCH
Medical Superintendent
ESI Hospital
Asansol, West Bengal, India

Atish N Bakane DCH DNB (Ped) FNB
Pediatric Hemato-oncology
Consultant Pediatric Hematology
Oncology and BMT
Center for Bone Marrow Transplant and
Cellular Therapy
Indraprastha Apollo Hospital
New Delhi, India

Atul Kulkarni MD
Assistant Professor
Ashwini Medical College
Medical Director
Ashwini Hospital
Solapur, Maharashtra, India

Basundhara Bhattacharya MBBS
Junior Resident
IPGMER and SSKM Hospital
Kolkata, West Bengal, India

Bhaswati C Acharyya DCH MD (Ped)
DNB (Ped) DNB (Gastro) MRCPCH (UK)
Consultant Pediatric Gastroenterologist and
Hepatologist
AMRI Hospitals, Kolkata
Associate Professor
Institute of Child Health
Kolkata, West Bengal, India

Bonny Sen MBBS
Junior Resident
Government Medical College
Kolkata, West Bengal, India

Debapriya Roy MBBS MD (Pediatrics)
Professor
Department of Pediatrics
Government Medical College
Kolkata, West Bengal, India

Dinesh Bhurani MD DM Clinical
Hematology (Vellore) FRCPA (Australia)
Director
Department of Hemato-Oncology Services
and Bone Marrow Transplant
Rajiv Gandhi Cancer Institute and Research
Centre
New Delhi, India

Ganesh Ramaswamy
MBBS DNB MNAMS MRCPCH (UK) PhD
Senior Consultant Pediatrician
Rainbow Children's Hospital
Chennai, Tamil Nadu, India

(Col) DY Shrikhande MD
Professor and Head
Department of Pediatrics
Rural Medical College
Ahmednagar, Maharashtra, India

Gaurav Kharya MD DM
Clinical Lead
Center for Bone Marrow Transplant and
Cellular Therapy
Senior Consultant
Pediatric Hematology Oncology and
Immunology
Indraprastha Apollo Hospital
New Delhi, India

Gautam Ray MD (Ped) DM (Gastro)
Assistant Professor
Division of Pediatric Gastroenterology
School of Digestive and Liver Diseases
IPGMER and SSKM Hospital
Kolkata, West Bengal, India

Hari R Mangtani DCH DNB PDCC
(Pediatric Endocrinology) (Liverpool UK)
Consultant Endocrinologist
Pearl Endocrine Clinic
Nagpur, Maharashtra, India

Hemant Kumar
MBBS (Hon) DCH MD DNB (Ped)
Professor
Department of Pediatrics
Patna Medical College and Hospital
Patna, Bihar, India

Inder Nathani MD
Consultant
Ekta Institute of Child Health
Raipur, Chhattisgarh, India

Indranil Halder DCH MD (Resp Medicine)
FCCP FICP European Diploma in Adult
Respiratory Medicine
Associate Professor
Department of Pulmonary Medicine
College of Medicine and JNM Hospital
Nadia, West Bengal, India

Jessica Hlawndo MD
Senior Resident
Department of Pediatrics
Atal Bihari Vajpayee Institute of Medical
Sciences and Dr RML Hospital
New Delhi, India

Jijo Joseph John MD (Ped) DAA FPRD
Associate Professor
Believers Church Medical College Hospital
Thiruvalla, Kerala, India

Jyotish Patel MD (Ped)
Sickle Cell Treatment and Research Centre
Shishudeep Multispecialty Hospital
Surat, Gujarat, India

Kalpana Dutta MD
Professor
Department of Pediatrics
Government Medical College
Kolkata, West Bengal, India

Kamirul Islam MD
Senior Resident
Department of Pediatrics
Burdwan Medical College
Burwan, West Bengal, India

Kanak Ramnani
DNB Fellowship in Pediatric Neurology
Assistant Professor
Department of Pediatrics
Pt JNM Medical College
Raipur, Chhattisgarh, India

Kinshuk Sarbhai MD
Resident
Department of Pulmonary Medicine
Kalinga Institute of Medical Sciences
Bhubaneswar, Odisha, India

Kiran Makhija MD
Consultant Pediatrician
Makhija Hospital
Raipur, Chhattisgarh, India

KP Sarbhai MD FPAI FCGP FPNC
Chief Pediatrician
Sarbhai Nursing Home and Research Center
Raipur, Chhattisgarh, India
Past National Chairperson
Academy of Pediatric Neurology

Kripasindhu Chatterjee MD FIAP
Associate Professor
Department of Pediatrics
Gouri Devi Institute of Medical Sciences and
Hospital
Durgapur, West Bengal, India

Madhu Sinha MD
Senior Pediatric Consultant
Mohit Immunization and Child Care Clinic
Patna, Bihar, India

Mahipal Khandelwal MBBS DNB IPNA
(Fellow in Pediatric Nephrology)
Consultant Nephrologist
BT Savani Hospital
Rajkot, Gujarat, India

Malathi Sathiyasekaran
MD DCH DM MNAMS
Senior Consultant Pediatric
Gastroenterologist
Rainbow Children's Hospital
Chennai, Tamil Nadu, India

Manika Verma
MBBS (RIMS) DNB (Radiotherapy)
Senior Resident (Academic)
Department of Medical Oncology and
Radiotherapy
All India Institute of Medical Sciences
Patna, Bihar, India

Neelam Verma MS MD DCh PhD FIAP FPAI
WHO Fellow
Professor and Former Head
Department of Pediatrics
Patna Medical College
Patna, Bihar, India

Neeraj Sehgal MD
Assistant Professor
Department of Pediatrics
Government Medical College
Amritsar, Punjab, India

Nilam Thaker MD IPNA FELLOWSHIP
Endocrinologist
Department of Endocrinology
All India Institute of Medical Sciences
Ahmedabad, Gujarat, India

Nilay Mozarkar DNB Pediatrics
In-Charge of SNCU, DEIC
District Hospital
Raipur, Chhattisgarh, India

Nimain Mohanty MD DCH
Former Professor
Department of Pediatrics
MGM Medical College
Navi Mumbai, Maharashtra, India

Nitin Kadam MD
Director
MGM Medical College
Navi Mumbai, Maharashtra, India

Nitin Sharma
MS MCh (Pediatric Surgery) FMAS FISPU
Associate Profesor
Department of Surgery
DK Superspecialty Postgraduate Institute
and Research Center
Raipur, Chhattisgarh, India

Nurul Islam MBBS MD (Pediatrics) FNB
(Pediatric Cardiology)
Consultant Pediatric Cardiologist
Health World Hospital, Durgapur
Ramakrishna Mission Seva Pratisthan
Kolkata, West Bengal, India

Onkar Khandwal MD
Professor
Department of Pediatrics
Pt JNM Medical College
Raipur, Chhattisgarh, India

Prachi Bichpuria MD
Assistant Professor
Department of Pediatrics
Pt JNM Medical College
Raipur, Chhattisgarh, India

Prachi Chaudhary MD (Pediatrics)
Associate Professor
Pediatrics and Consultant Physician BMT
MGM Medical College
Indore, Madhya Pradesh, India

Prakash G Mathew MBBS
PG2 Pediatrics
All India Institute of Medical Sciences
Raipur, Chhattisgarh, India

Pranati Sharma
MBBS MS FAGE MCh (Neurosurgery)
Assistant Professor
Department of Neurosurgery
All India Institute of Medical Sciences
Rishikesh, Uttarakhand, India

Prankur Pandey MD
Assistant Professor
Department of Pediatrics
Pt JNM Medical College
Raipur, Chhattisgarh, India

Prasanth KS DCH DNB (Pediatrics) DM (Gastro)
Consultant Pediatric Gastroenterologist
SAT Hospital and
Assistant Professor
Department of Gastroenterology
Government Medical College
Thiruvananthapuram, Kerala, India

Puja Dhupar MD DNB
Pediatric Intensivist and Neonatologist
Petals Children Hospital
Raipur, Chhattisgarh, India

Rachita Sarangi MD (Pediatrics)
Professor
Department of Pediatrics
Institute of Medical Sciences and SUM
Hospital (Siksha 'O' Anusandhan)
Bhubaneswar, Odisha, India

Raghvendra Singh DNB (Pediatrics)
Consultant
Ekta Institute of Child health
Raipur, Chhattisgarh, India

Rahul Sinha DM (Pediatric Neurology)
Senior Resident
Department of Pediatrics
All India Institute of Medical Sciences
New Delhi, India

Rajiv Kumar Gupta MS
Professor
Department of Ophthalmology
Rajendra Institute of Medical Sciences
Ranchi, Jharkhand, India

Rakesh Singh MD CFIN
Fellowship in Neonatology
Consultant Neonatologist and Pediatrician
Ram Krishna Care Hospital
Raipur, Chhattisgarh, India

(Col Retd) Rama Krishnan Sanjeev
MBBS MD (Pediatrics) (AFMC, Pune)
Associate Professor (Pediatrics)
Rural Medical College
Pravara Institute of Medical Sciences (DU)
Ahmednagar, Maharashtra, India

Raman Shrivastava DNB (Orthopedics)
MNAMS (Fellow Pediatric Orthopedic)
Consultant Pediatric Orthopedic Sugeon
DK Superspecialty Postgraduate Institute
and Research Center
Raipur, Chhattisgarh, India

Ravi Kant Narayan MBBS MD
Senior Resident
Department of Anatomy
All India Institute of Medical Sciences
Patna, Bihar, India

Ravinder Makkar MD (Medicine) MBA
Medical Director
Sanofi Genzyme India
New Delhi, India

Reena Karkhele
MD (Fellowship in Rheumatology)
Associate Professor
MGM Medical College
Navi Mumbai, Maharashtra, India

Renu Kale MBBS MD FISPN (Fellow of Indian
Society of Pediatric Nephrology)
Associate Professor
Raipur Institute of Medical Sciences
Raipur, Chhattisgarh, India

Reny Joseph MD (Ped) DCH
Consultant Pediatrician
MGM Muthoot Hospital
Pathanamthitta, Kerala, India

Rimjhim Shrivastava
MBBS PGDMCH DNB (Ped)
Pediatric Gastroenterologist and Hepatologist
Consultant Gastroenterologist
Raipur, Chhattisgarh, India

Rohan Karkra MBBS
Resident
Department of Gastroenterology
JSS Medical College
Mysuru, Karnataka, India

Ruchi Parikh
DNB (Fellowship in Pediatric Endocrinology)
Consultant Endrocrinologist
NH SRCC Children Hospital
Mumbai, Maharashtra, India

SA Krishna MD FIAP
Professor and Head
Department of Pediatrics
Nalanda Medical College
Patna, Bihar, India

Sakshi Karkra MD (Pediatrics) Fellowship
in Pediatric Gastroenterology, Hepatology & Liver
transplantation
Head
Pediatric Gastroenterology
Hepatology and Liver Transplantation
Artemis Hospital
Gurugram, Haryana, India

Saman Beg MD
Senior Resident
PDCC (Pediatric Gastroenterology)
Era's Lucknow Medical College and Hospital
Lucknow, Uttar Pradesh, India

(Sqn Ldr) Sangeetha Balasubramani
MBBS DCH DNB (Ped)
Professor
Department of Pediatrics
Command Hospital Air Force
Bengaluru, Karnataka, India

Sanjeev Joshi MD
Director
Criticare and Joshi Hospital
Yavatmal, Maharashtra, India

Sarita Agrawal MD
Professor and Head
Department of Obstetrics and Gynecology
Associate Dean, Student Welfare
All India Institute of Medical Sciences
Raipur, Chhattisgarh, India

Saurabh Gupta MD
Resident
Department of Pulmonary Medicine
Kalinga Institute of Medical Sciences
Bhubaneswar, Odisha, India

Saurabh Uppal MD MRCPCH (Fellowship in
Pediatric Endocrinology)
Consultant Endocrinologist
Endo-kidz Clinics
Jalandhar, Punjab, India

SBP Singh MD
Consultant Pediatrician
Child Care Clinic
Begusarai, Bihar, India

Seema Jain DNB Fellow in Pediatric
Nephrology Post-doctoral Fellowship in Dialysis
Medicine
Senior Pediatrician
District Hospital
Durg, Chhattisgarh, India

Seema Shah MD
Assistant Professor
Department of Biochemistry
All India Institute of Medical Sciences
Raipur, Chhattisgarh, India

(Gp Capt) Shamsher S Dalal MBBS
MD (Ped) DM (Neonatology)
Professor
Department of Pediatrics
Command Hospital Air Force
Bengaluru, Karnataka, India

Shantanu Verma MD Fellowship in
Neonatology
Director and Consultant Neonatologist
Swapnil Institute of Child Health
Raipur, Chhattisgarh, India

Sharja Phuljhele MD
Professor and Head
Department of Pediatrics
Pt JNM Medical College
Raipur, Chhattisgarh, India

Shashank Kumar MBBS
Junior Resident
Department of Pediatrics
Patna Medical College
Patna, Bihar, India

Sheffali Gulati MD DM
Chief
Child Neurology Division
Center of Excellence and
Advanced Research on Childhood
Neurodevelopmental Disorders
Department of Pediatrics
All India Institute of Medical Sciences
New Delhi, India

Shilpa Bhargava MBBS DCH
Registrar
Department of Pediatrics
Pt JNM Medical College
Raipur, Chhattisgarh, India

Shrish Bhatnagar MD
Head
Department of Pediatrics
Pediatric Gastroenterology
Era's Lucknow Medical College and Hospital
Lucknow, Uttar Pradesh, India

Sibabrata Patnaik MD
Associate Professor
Department of Pediatrics
Pediatric Intensivist
Kalinga Institute of Medical Sciences
Bhubaneswar, Odisha, India

Smita Malhotra MD
Consultant Pediatric Gastroenterologist and Hepatologist
Indraprastha Apollo Hospital
New Delhi, India

Somdipa Pal MD
Senior Resident
Department of Pediatrics
Atal Bihari Vajpayee Institute of Medical Sciences and Dr RML Hospital
New Delhi, India

Sonali Singh DM (Pediatric Neurology)
Senior Resident
Department of Pediatrics
All India Institute of Medical Sciences
New Delhi, India

Soutrik Seth MD PDT DM (Neonatology)
Department of Neonatology
IPGMER and SSKM Hospital
Kolkata, West Bengal, India

Subroto Chakrabartty MD
Professor
Department of Pediatrics
The Institute of Child Health
Kolkata, West Bengal, India

Sudip Saha MD (Pediatrics)
Professor
Department of Pediatrics
College of Obstetrics, Gynecology and Child Health
Kolkata, West Bengal, India

Suman Mittal MD DM
Medical Oncologist
Mittal Institute of Medical Sciences
Raipur, Chhattisgarh, India

Suman Sudha Tirkey MD
Assistant Professor and Head
Department of Pediatrics
Government Medical College
Ambikapur, Chhattisgarh, India

Sunil Bhat MD FPHO FRAH
Director and Head
Pediatric Hematology and Oncology and BMT
Narayana Health City
Bengaluru, Karnataka, India

Sunil Jondhale MD
Associate Professor
Department of Pediatrics
All India Institute of Medical Sciences
Raipur, Chhattisgarh, India

Supratim Datta MD
Professor and Head
Department of Pediatrics
IPGMER and SSKM Hospital
Kolkata, West Bengal, India

Suresh Natarajan
MBBS DNB MNAMS MRCPCH (UK) PhD DAA
Senior Consultant Pediatrician
Rainbow Children's Hospital
Chennai, Tamil Nadu, India

Swapan Kumar Ray MBBS DCH DNB MNAMS
Professor
Department of Pediatrics
MGM Medical College and Lions Seva Kendra Hospital
Kishanganj, Bihar, India

Swati Kanodia MD PGDD (Fellowship in Pediatric Endocrinology)
Consultant Endocrinologist
BL Kapoor Superspecialty Hospital
New Delhi, India

Swati Yadav MD (Pediatrics)
Associate Professor
Department of Pediatrics
Chhattisgarh Institute of Medical Sciences
Bilaspur, Chhattisgarh, India

Tapas Som MD DM (Neonatology)
Associate Professor
Department of Neonatology
All India Institute of Medical Sciences
Bhubaneswar, Odisha, India

Taraknath Ghosh MBBS MD (Ped)
Professor
Department of Pediatrics
NICU In-charge
Burdwan Medical College
Burdwan, West Bengal, India

TP Yadav MD
Professor
Department of Pediatrics
Atal Bihari Vajpayee Institute of Medical Sciences and Dr RML Hospital
New Delhi, India

Tripty Naik MD
Assistant Professor
Department of Pediatrics
All India Institute of Medical Sciences
Raipur, Chhattisgarh, India

Tushar Jagzape
MD (Pediatrics) DIP (Allergy & Asthma) MPhil HPE GSMS-FAIMER Fellow 2015
Additional Professor
Department of Pediatrics
All India Institute of Medical Sciences
Raipur, Chhattisgarh, India

Vasant Khalatkar
MD (Pediatrics) FIAP PD Diploma in Pediatric Infectious
Guide for DCH
Consultant Pediatrician
Colors Children Hospital
Nagpur, Maharashtra, India

Vibhor Borkar MD PDCC DM (Pediatric Gastroenterology)
Consultant Gastroenterologist
NH SRCC Children Hospital
Mumbai, Maharashtra, India

Vijay Kamale MD DCH
Professor and Head
Department of Pediatrics
MGM Medical College
Navi Mumbai, Maharashtra, India

Vijay P Makhija MD DNB
Consultant Pediatrician
Makhija Children Hospital
Raipur, Chhattisgarh, India

Vikas Goel MD DM (Hematology)
Consultant Hematologist
Sanjeevani CBCC Cancer Hospital
Raipur, Chhattisgarh, India

Vineet Wankhede DCH DND PDFPN
Consultant Pediatric Neurologist
Healthcity Children Hospital
Nagpur, Maharashtra, India

Vishal MD (Ped)
Assistant Professor
Department of Pediatrics
Hazaribagh Medical College
Hazaribagh, Jharkhand, India

Vishnu Biradar
MD PDCC Fellowship in Pediatric Liver Transplant
Gastroenterologist
Surya Mother and Child Care Superspecialty Hospital
Pune, Maharashtra, India

Yogesh Waikar
MBBS MD DNB MNAMS Fellow in Pediatric Gastroenterology and Liver Transplant
Consultant Gastroenterologist
Superspecialty GI Kids Clinics and Imaging Center
Nagpur, Maharashtra, India

Foreword

The book is the outcome of the sincere and the undaunted effort of many a members of Pediatric Association of India (PAI). Apart from the regular journal, it is the first publication of PAI for young pediatricians and pediatrics practitioners of the country. It is a useful book of its own standing which is rare in the table top for ready reference. The efforts of Dr Anoop Verma and his team is praise worthy. The Chhattisgarh Branch of PAI as a whole with all the PAI members deserve praise for this maiden venture.

The book will be useful for general practitioners and pediatricians in the management of day-to-day pediatrics problems encountered in office practice. The treatment instructions along with the available common market preparation will make therapy a beautiful hand on experience. The clinical presentation of the diseases in short, the appropriate investigations and therapy at large will help the practitioners, students as well as pediatrics fraternity.

It is a long-cherished ambition, which came true. What has been decided in the birthday of PAI at IMA House, New Delhi materialized after a long gap of 9 years. It is expected that many such will roll out in the pipeline in the days to come. The wonderful book in the present shape and the effort of many a pediatricians and super specialists in pediatrics. Hope it will cater for the very purpose, it is created.

Gadadhar Sarangi
MD MNAMS FICMCH FIAP FPAI
Founder Secretary and Patron
Pediatric Association of India

Foreword

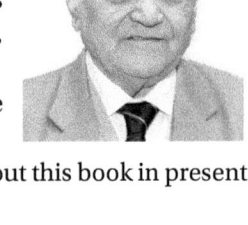

It is a matter of great pleasure and utmost satisfaction to me that Pediatric Association of India (PAI) is progressing ahead day-by-day and is fulfilling its goal to help the pediatricians in their office practice.

With this target in mind, this tabletop quick clinical reckoner is being published, which will be an extremely useful guide to practicing general pediatricians, undergraduate and postgraduate students and general practitioners who can refer the concerned chapter for a quick overview of the topic, relevant investigations and management protocol.

My sincere compliments to all the authors for their sincere efforts to disseminate the knowledge by contributing chapters for this prestigious publication.

I congratulate the whole editorial board led by Dr Anoop Verma, for their untiring effort to bring out this book in present shape.

I am sure that this book will be popular amongst the practicing pediatricians and will contribute in rational management of diseases in office practice.

BC Chhaparwal MD FIAP FPAI
National President, 2020
Pediatric Association of India

Foreword

I have immense pleasure in wring this forward for the reference book in pediatrics, carefully compiled by our seasoned stalwarts of the Pediatric Association of India.

The book is a unique venture to not only serve as a desk reference for every pediatrician in the developing world, but also as a textbook for the budding pediatricians and general practitioners alike. Experienced teachers and seasoned practicing pediatricians have put in their best effort in the most brilliant manner, covering most of the clinical conditions peculiar to the region, not adequately covered in western textbooks.

Very carefully designed sub-specialty chapters presented in this book in a lucid but structured manner, will go a long way in fulfilling the long unmet need of our undergraduate and postgraduate students in so far as the competence-based pediatric education is concerned. No doubt, the book is bound to help producing most competent pediatricians for the service of our society in general and the sick tiny-tots in particular.

Nimain Mohanty
MD (PGI, CHG) PGPN FPAI
Professor Emeritus Pediatrics
MGM Institute of Health Sciences
Navi Mumbai, Maharashtra, India

Preface

"I never did anything worth by an accident, nor did any of my inventions come by accident."
–Thomas A Edison

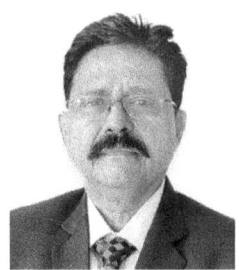

There is felt the need for a handbook, which can be readily used as an instant reference in a busy clinic or hospital. Pediatric Association of India (PAI) recognized this necessity for long, and brought the best brain with their experience and vision to give the best in this book.

The book is focused on the need of common pediatricians, undergraduates, postgraduates, specialists and super-specialists. The chapters written are well thought of and planned to include the common clinical conditions seen in office practice.

It is a basic fact in medicine that more you see, more you learn and the more you are compelled to search, gradually your brain accumulate rich clinical acumen. Chance favors the prepared mind and referring the text of this book is making use of good chance in right perspective.

"To indulge in a large number of investigation, or to repeat and extend them without good reason, is both crude medicine and distasteful."
–John Apley

This book focuses more on using relevant investigations more precisely. Reaching the diagnosis on clinical ladder one must make use of desired investigations listed in each chapter. The practice of extensive and irrelevant investigations is to be discouraged.

"The young physician starts life with twenty drugs for each disease, and the old physician ends life with one drug for twenty diseases. Remember how much you do not know. Do not pour strange medicines into your patients."
–Sir William Osler

The adage is very apt, and this must be a lesson to all who are practicing medicine. The concept of having "prescription assistance" after many chapters is a new idea to assist the treating physician to quickly search the market preparation that saves time and improves the confidence of treating physician and quality of prescription.

We must remember a famous quote by Dr Meharban Singh. "It is unfortunate fact that most people in the world are now suffering from drugs and not from the disease. Because no drug is indeed entirely safe but most disease is either mild or self-limiting".

Hope the readers of this book will enjoy the essence and the style of the book to improve their personal practice for the benefit of the patient.

Anoop Verma

Acknowledgments

I am extremely thankful to Pediatric Association of India (PAI) and the stalwarts Dr Gadadhar Sarangi, Dr Chourjeet Singh, Dr Nimain Mohanty, and Dr SA Krishna along with the Executive Board of Pediatric Association of India, for honoring and showing faith on me to bring forth the difficult task, of publishing the book with a new concept.

I am grateful to the National President of PAI, Dr BC Chhaparwal for rendering help and guidance all throughout the publication.

I have no words to convey my deep sense of gratitude to a wonderful person Dr KP Sarbhai, Executive Editor, for his tireless support in planning, execution and repeated checking of the manuscript to give to the present shape.

The Section Editors were the soul of this book. The mammoth task of, to check and to make a faultless manuscript, was a no simple job. I convey my sincere thanks to all, namely, Dr AK Rawat, Dr Sharja Phuljhele, Col DY Shrikhande, Dr Rimjhim Shrivastava, Dr Kiran Makhija, Dr Atanu Bhadra, Dr Asok Kumar Dutta, Dr Renu Kale, Dr Hari R Mangtani, Dr Vijay Kamale, Dr Amar Verma, Dr Vijay P Makhija, Dr Onkar Khandwal.

The Pediatric Association of India and the Editorial Board personally wish to convey our sincere condolences to Col DY Shrikhande, who was one of the most active Senior Executive Board Member, and one of the Section Editor in the book, and the present shape of the chapter was his imagination, unfortunately he left us untimely for his heavenly abode.

In the mid of the book publication our Chief Advisor and Founder Secretary of PAI, Dr Gadadhar Sarangi left us for his heavenly abode. We convey our sincere tribute to the divine soul.

The contributors are the main brain behind each article. I convey my sincere thanks to all, for being so responsive and were on toes till completion of the manuscript.

I acknowledge the help of my wife, Mrs Rashmi Verma; son, Dr Shantanu Verma; and daughter-in-law, Dr Souyma Verma, for their constant help and encouragement all through out the project.

My due regards of Shri Jitendra P Vij (Group Chairman), Mr Ankit Vij (Managing Director) of M/s Jaypee Brothers Medical Publisher (P) Ltd, New Delhi, India, for all assistance required for the publication. Ms Ruby Sharma and Dr Rajul Jain (Senior Development Editor) deserve special mention for their special efforts and support.

Contents

SECTION 1: TRIAGE

1. **Stabilization of a Sick Child in Emergency....3**
   AK Rawat

SECTION 2: NUTRITIONAL DISEASES

2. **Nutritional Rickets 7**
   Anoop Verma
3. **Scurvy 10**
   Anoop Verma
4. **Vitamin A Deficiency 12**
   Anoop Verma
5. **Zinc Deficiency in Children 14**
   Anoop Verma
6. **Food Allergies 16**
   Tushar Jagzape
7. **Food Poisoning 20**
   Tushar Jagzape
8. **Failure to Thrive 25**
   SA Krishna
9. **Worm Infestation 27**
   SA Krishna, Madhu Sinha

SECTION 3: NEONATOLOGY

10. **Care of Normal Newborn....................31**
    Akash Lalwani
11. **Minor Developmental Peculiarities of Newborn 33**
    Sharja Phuljhele
12. **Common Neonatal Problems.............36**
    Sharja Phuljhele
13. **Common Feeding Problem 39**
    Shilpa Bhargava
14. **Crying Infant 43**
    Prachi Bichpuria
15. **Neonatal Sepsis....................................46**
    Anil K Goel, Seema Shah, Prakash G Mathew
16. **Neonatal Hypoglycemia 51**
    Hari R Mangtani
17. **Neonatal Hypothermia 56**
    Swati Yadav
18. **Therapeutic Hypothermia 58**
    Puja Dhupar
19. **Neonate Born of Mother with Chronic Systemic Disorder 62**
    Rakesh Singh
20. **Neonate Born of Mother with Maternal Infection 65**
    Rakesh Singh
21. **Neonatal Follow-up for Normal Newborn and Young Children 74**
    Suman Sudha Tirkey
22. **Follow-up of High-risk Newborn 78**
    Puja Dhupar
23. **Neonatal Thrombocytopenia................84**
    Shantanu Verma
24. **Neonatal Dermatosis 87**
    Prankur Pandey
25. **Newborn Screening Program 91**
    Kanak Ramnani

SECTION 4: VACCINOLOGY

26. **DPT/DT, DTaP/Tdap** 95
    KP Sarbhai

27. **Rotavirus Vaccine** 96
    KP Sarbhai

28. **Pneumonia Vaccine** 100
    KP Sarbhai

29. **Typhoid Vaccine** 104
    KP Sarbhai

30. **Hepatitis A Vaccine** 106
    KP Sarbhai

31. **Human Papillomavirus Vaccine** 109
    KP Sarbhai

32. **Influenza Vaccine** 112
    KP Sarbhai

33. **Rabies Vaccine** 116
    KP Sarbhai

34. **Japanese Encephalitis Vaccine** 120
    KP Sarbhai

35. **Varicella Vaccine** 123
    KP Sarbhai

36. **Meningococcal Vaccine** 127
    KP Sarbhai

SECTION 5: INFECTIOUS DISEASES

37. **Diphtheria** 131
    SBP Singh

38. **Tetanus** 134
    SBP Singh

39. **Pertussis** 138
    Raghvendra Singh

40. **Enteric Fever** 140
    Ashwani Agrawal

41. **Measles** 143
    Ashwani Agrawal

42. **Mumps** 146
    Arun Agrawalla

43. **Rubella** 148
    Arun Agrawalla

44. **Varicella and Herpes Zoster** 150
    Inder Nathani

45. **Leptospirosis** 153
    Inder Nathani

46. **TORCH Infections** 156
    Sangeetha Balasubramani, Shamsher S Dalal

47. **Rickettsial Diseases** 161
    Atul Kulkarni, Ashutosh V Yajurvedi

48. **Malaria** 166
    AK Rawat

49. **Tuberculosis** 168
    DY Shrikhande

50. **Leprosy** 173
    Vijay P Makhija

51. **Dengue** 176
    Neelam Verma

52. **Re-emerging Infections in Pediatrics** 180
    Ashok Bhandari

53. **COVID-19** 184
    Rama Krishnan Sanjeev

SECTION 6: GASTROENTEROLOGY

54. **Chronic Pain Abdomen in Children** 191
    Smita Malhotra

55. **Chronic Constipation** 195
    Bhaswati C Acharyya

56. Recurrent Vomiting in Infants and Children.. 197
    Vibhor Borkar

57. Celiac Disease in Children 201
    Vibhor Borkar

58. Gallstones in Children 203
    Aabha Nagral

59. Upper Gastrointestinal Bleeding in Children 206
    Shrish Bhatnagar, Saman Beg

60. Lower Gastrointestinal Bleed 210
    Gautam Ray

61. Acute Pancreatitis in Children 213
    Rimjhim Shrivastava

62. Ascites 216
    Yogesh Waikar

63. Cholestasis in Newborns and Infants 220
    Rimjhim Shrivastava

64. Abnormal Liver Function Tests 223
    Malathi Sathiyasekaran, Suresh Natarajan

65. Asymptomatic Hepatomegaly 227
    Sakshi Karkra, Rohan Karkra

66. Acute Viral Hepatitis 231
    Gautam Ray

67. Acute Liver Failure 233
    Sakshi Karkra, Rohan Karkra

68. Chronic Hepatitis B 238
    Shrish Bhatnagar, Alok Kumar

69. Metabolic Liver Disease in Children 241
    Malathi Sathiyasekaran, Ganesh Ramaswamy

70. Liver Mass on Imaging in Children 246
    Bhaswati C Acharyya

71. Liver Transplantation 249
    Prasanth KS

72. Foreign Body Ingestion in Children 253
    Vishnu Biradar

SECTION 7 — HEMATOLOGY–ONCOLOGY

73. ABC of CBC 259
    Prachi Chaudhary

74. Approach to Normocytic Anemia 264
    Atish N Bakane, Gaurav Kharya

75. Iron Deficiency Anemia 270
    Tripty Naik

76. Megaloblastic Anemia 273
    Nilay Mozarkar

77. Sickle Cell Disorders 277
    Jyotish Patel

78. Thalassemia 281
    Sunil Bhat

79. Aplastic Anemia in Children 284
    Sunil Jondhale

80. Leukemias in Children 288
    Suman Mittal

81. Lymphoma in Children 291
    Vikas Goel

82. Immune Thrombocytopenia in Children 293
    AK Ganju

83. Hemophilia 297
    Aradhana Mishra

84. Hematopoietic Stem Cell Transplantation 300
    Dinesh Bhurani

85. Blood Component Therapy 303
    Kiran Makhija

SECTION 8 — RESPIRATORY SYSTEM

86. Common Cold 309
    Subroto Chakrabartty

87. Allergic Rhinitis 310
    Subroto Chakrabartty

88. **Rhinosinusitis in Children** 312
    Anindya Kundu

89. **Croup and Epiglottitis** 315
    Raghvendra Singh

90. **Acute Bronchiolitis** 318
    Kripasindhu Chatterjee

91. **Wheezing in Children** 323
    Atanu Bhadra

92. **Community-acquired Pneumonia** 327
    Indranil Halder

93. **Pleural Effusion** 332
    Swapan Kumar Ray

94. **Empyema Thoracis** 334
    Swapan Kumar Ray

95. **Lung Abscess** 336
    Swapan Kumar Ray

96. **Pneumothorax** 338
    Kinshuk Sarbhai, Saurabh Gupta

97. **Hydrocarbon Aspiration** 342
    Taraknath Ghosh

98. **Foreign Body in Lungs** 344
    Saurabh Gupta, Kinshuk Sarbhai

SECTION 9 — NEUROLOGY

99. **Cerebral Palsy** 349
    Sheffali Gulati, Rahul Sinha, Sonali Singh

100. **Autism Spectrum Disorder** 356
    Alka Srivastava

101. **Febrile Seizure** 361
    Anoop Verma, Vasant Khalatkar

102. **Childhood Absence Epilepsy** 363
    Sanjeev Joshi

103. **Childhood Epilepsy with Centrotemporal Spikes** 366
    Sanjeev Joshi

104. **Juvenile Myoclonic Epilepsy** 369
    Anoop Kumar

105. **West Syndrome** 371
    Anoop Kumar

106. **Breath-holding Spells** 374
    Sanjeev Joshi

107. **Neurotuberculosis** 376
    Vineet Wankhede

108. **Neurocysticercosis** 380
    Anoop Verma, Arun Agrawal, Pranati Sharma

109. **Headache in Children** 385
    Anoop Verma

110. **Acute Rheumatic Chorea** 389
    Anoop Verma, Onkar Khandwal

111. **Neuro-Wilson's Disease** 391
    Vineet Wankhede

112. **Ataxia** 396
    KP Sarbhai

113. **Duchene Muscular Dystrophy** 400
    Kanak Ramnani

114. **Spinal Muscular Dystrophy** 403
    Kanak Ramnani

115. **Benign Acute Childhood Myositis** 405
    Anoop Verma

116. **Bell's Palsy** 406
    Anoop Verma

117. **Traumatic Brain Injury** 408
    Anil K Goel

SECTION 10 — CARDIOLOGY

118. **Approach to a Neonate with Congenital Heart Disease** 415
    Tapas Som

119. **Approach to a Child with Cyanotic Heart Disease** 420
    Kamirul Islam

120. **Ventricular Septal Defect** 425
Rachita Sarangi

121. **Atrial Septal Defect** 429
Taraknath Ghosh

122. **Patent Ductus Arteriosus** 432
*Supratim Datta, Basundhara Bhattacharya,
Debapriya Roy*

123. **Endocardial Cushion Defect** 435
*Kalpana Dutta, Basundhara Bhattacharya,
Bonny Sen*

124. **Tetrology of Fallot** 440
Hemant Kumar

125. **Transposition of Great Arteries** 445
Nurul Islam

126. **Complex Congenital Heart Disease** 451
Asok Kumar Datta

127. **Kawasaki Disease
(Cardiac Manifestation)** 453
Asok Kumar Datta

128. **Anomalous Left Coronary Artery
Originating from Pulmonary Artery** 455
Soutrik Seth

129. **Myocardial Disease** 459
Asok Kumar Datta

130. **Pericardial Disease** 461
Asok Kumar Datta

131. **Pulmonary Hypertension** 462
Asok Kumar Datta

132. **Cardiac Failure** 463
Sibabrata Patnaik

133. **Cardiomyopathy in Children** 469
Sudip Saha

134. **Cardiac Arrhythmias** 472
Soutrik Seth

135. **Infective Endocarditis** 486
Asok Kumar Datta

SECTION 11 — NEPHROLOGY

136. **Urinary Tract Infection** 491
Hemant Kumar, Shashank Kumar

137. **Nephrotic Syndrome** 496
Renu Kale

138. **Hematuria in Children** 501
Seema Jain

139. **Renal Stones** 505
Nilam Thaker

140. **Hypertension in Pediatrics** 509
Amish Udani

141. **Voiding Disorders in Children** 513
Mahipal Khandelwal

SECTION 12 — ENDOCRINOLOGY

142. **Childhood Hypothyroidism** 521
Saurabh Uppal, Neeraj Sehgal

143. **Childhood Obesity** 524
Ruchi Parikh

144. **Type 1 Diabetes** 529
Saurabh Uppal

145. **Precocious Puberty** 534
Swati Kanodia

146. **Disorders of Sex Development** 538
Ruchi Parikh

SECTION 13: RHEUMATOLOGY

147. Laboratory Tests in Pediatric Rheumatology. 545
 Reena Karkhele, Vijay Kamale

148. Juvenile Idiopathic Arthritis 548
 Reena Karkhele, Vijay Kamale

149. Pediatric Systemic Lupus Erythematosus 554
 Jijo Joseph John, Reny Joseph

150. Lupus Nephritis 558
 Jijo Joseph John, Reny Joseph

151. Rheumatic Fever 561
 Vijay Kamale, Nitin Kadam

152. Juvenile Dermatomyositis 566
 TP Yadav, Somdipa Pal

153. Henoch–Schönlein Purpura 568
 TP Yadav, Jessica Hlawndo

154. Kawasaki Disease 570
 Vijay Kamale, Nimain Mohanty

SECTION 14: GENETIC DISORDERS

155. Genetic Counceling 577
 Amar Verma, Anita Verma

156. Common Chromosomal Disorders 580
 Manika Verma, Anita Verma, Amar Verma

157. Dysmorphic Child 587
 Anoop Verma

158. Karyotyping 591
 Amar Verma, Anita Verma

159. Inborn Errors of Metabolism 594
 Anupa Prasad

160. Prenatal Screening and Diagnosis of Congenital Disorders 599
 Sarita Agrawal, Arpana Verma

161. Lysosomal Storage Diseases in India 606
 Ravinder Makkar

SECTION 15: DERMATOLOGY

162. Urticaria and Angioedema 615
 Vijay P Makhija

163. Papular Urticaria 617
 Vijay P Makhija

164. Atopic Dermatitis 618
 Vijay P Makhija

165. Pityriasis Versicolor 621
 Vijay P Makhija

166. Tinea Infections 622
 Vijay P Makhija

167. Scabies 624
 Vijay P Makhija

168. Impetigo 626
 Vijay P Makhija

169. Acne Vulgaris 627
 Vijay P Makhija

170. Stevens–Johnson Syndrome 629
 Anoop Verma

171. Hand, Foot, and Mouth 632
 Anoop Verma

SECTION 16: MISCELLANEOUS

172. **Common Ophthalmic Problems in Children** 637
    Rajiv Kumar Gupta, Vishal

173. **Common Orthopedic Problems in Children** 644
    Raman Shrivastava

174. **Common Pediatric and Neonatal Surgical Problems** 648
    Nitin Sharma

175. **How to Read X-ray Chest? (Step-by-Step Guide)** 656
    Amar Verma, Ravi Kant Narayan, Anita Verma

    Index 661

SECTION 1: Triage

1. Stabilization of a Sick Child in Emergency

CHAPTER 1

Stabilization of a Sick Child in Emergency

AK Rawat

As soon as a sick child arrives in the emergency room, the immediate aim is to identify and treat any life-threatening condition to save life and prevent further deterioration. The process should be quick, sequential, and systematically performed in such a way that several signs are assessed and managed simultaneously by a team. The approach is simple ABCDs in this sequence.

STEP A: EXCLUDE CERVICAL SPINE INJURY AND MAINTAIN TEMPERATURE

Check: Airway and breathing.
- *If obstructed breathing due to complete obstruction by a foreign body is suspected. Begin:*
  - *Infants:* Back slaps and chest thrusts
  - *Post infancy:* Heimlich maneuver
- *Not breathing and gasping and central pulse is felt*
  - *Action:* Open airway and start bag and mask ventilation.
- *Not breathing/gasping and no central pulse is felt*
  - *Action:*
    - Start cardiopulmonary resuscitation (CPR)
    - Chest compression
    - Open airway
    - Start bag and mask ventilation.
    - Attach monitors and automated external defibrillator (AED)
    - Collect blood sample
    - Secure intravenous (IV) line
- *Central cyanosis*
  - *Action:*
    - Ensure airways are open
    - Give oxygen.
    - Attach monitors.
- *Severe respiratory distress identified with any one of the following signs:*
  - Labored or very fast breathing
  - Use of accessory muscles of respiration
  - Severe lower chest in-drawing
  - Head nodding with each breath
  - Inability to feed because of respiratory problem
  - Abnormal respiratory noises, e.g., stridor, grunting, marked wheezing
  - $SPO_2 < 90\%$
  - *Action:*
    - Ensure position and airways are open.
    - Give oxygen.
    - Start specific treatment, e.g., bronchodilators.

STEP B: CIRCULATION

- Assess for shock.
- Cold hands
- Capillary refill time (CRT) ≥ 3 seconds
- Weak and fast pulse
  (In infants >160 per minute; post infancy >140 per minute)
  - *Action*
    - Stop bleeding if any
    - Position head at level
    - Give oxygen
    - Keep warm
    - Secure IV line
    - Attach monitors
- *If not SAM (identified by visible severe wasting or bilateral pitting edema if Anthropometry could not done):* Normal saline (NS) bolus and continuous monitoring
- *If severe acute malnutrition (SAM):*
  - Give IV glucose
  - IV 0.45% saline + 5% dextrose 15 mL/kg in 1 hour
  - Assess continuously for volume overload after 1 hour decide further treatment.

STEP C: COMA/CONVULSION

Action:
- Ensure airways are open.
- Position to prevent aspiration.
- Give oxygen.
- Attach monitors.
- Secure IV line, collect sample.
- Correct hypoglycemia.
- Give anticonvulsants if seizures continue.

STEP D: DEHYDRATION

Severe in a case of acute watery diarrhea.

Any two signs:
1. Lethargy
2. Sunken eyes
3. Very slow skin pinch

- *If child is not SAM*: Secure IV line and begin rapid infusion of NS/Ringer's lactate (RL) according to plan C
- *If child is SAM:*
  - No IV fluids unless shock is present
  - Give ORS orally/through nasogastric tube (NGT)

Further management after initial stabilization will depend on response to initial treatment, result of findings on monitors, investigation and imaging study results with continuous monitoring and modifying treatment accordingly.

SUGGESTED READING

1. Guidelines: Updates on paediatric emergency triage, assessment and treatment: care of critically ill children, 2016. WHO Library Cataloguing-in-Publication Data, ISBN 978 92 4 151021 9.
2. Kliegman RM, St Geme J. Emergency medicine and critical care. In: Wright JL, Krug SE (eds). Nelson TB of Pediatrics, 21st edition. Philadelphia: Elsevier; 2019.

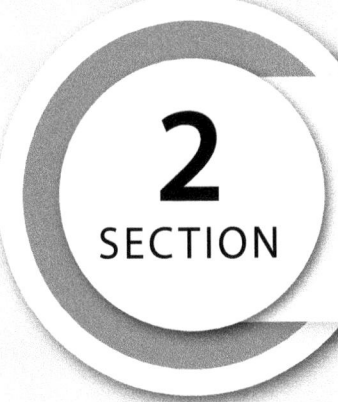

SECTION 2: Nutritional Diseases

2. Nutritional Rickets
3. Scurvy
4. Vitamin A Deficiency
5. Zinc Deficiency in Children
6. Food Allergies
7. Food Poisoning
8. Failure to Thrive
9. Worm Infestation

CHAPTER 2: Nutritional Rickets

Anoop Verma

INTRODUCTION

Nutritional rickets (NR) is the most common form of growing bone disease, caused by vitamin D deficiency (VDD) and calcium deficiency. The prevalence of VDD rickets in developing countries are prolong breast-feeding, poor vitamin D (VD) supplementation, inadequate exposure to sun, sociocultural practices, dark-colored skin, diet low in calcium and high phosphates, excessive covering of body by cloths, and genetic factors. It is a fact that only around 10% of VD is derived from diet and >90% are formed in the skin.

Rickets is a disease of growing bones; therefore, features are seen early in growing bones. In malnutrition and hypothyroidism, the growth rate is slow; therefore, the bony changes are less evident.

CLINICAL FEATURES

Clinical features specific to change in bony tissues—*craniotabes* is seen in infant older than 2-3 months. There is ping-pong sensa-tion on pressing the skull bone due to thinning of outer table, especially over posterior parietal and occipital bone. *Frontal bossing* and *caput quadratum* (hot cross bun appearance) are due to thickening of parietal and frontal bones. Anterior fontanelle closure is delayed, enlargement of wrist, rachitic rosary, delayed teething, and enamel hypoplasia. "O" and "X" types of leg deformity are seen. "O" deformity is *Genu varum* (Femoral intercondylar distance of >5 cm) in infant and "X" deformity is *Genu vulgus* type of leg deformity is seen in later age. *Double malleolus* sign is seen when child starts putting weight on legs. Chest deformity in the form of Harrison sulcus, pectus carinatum, kyphosis, and narrow pelvis can be associated.

Clinical features not specific to change in bony tissues are hypocalcemic seizures, hypotonia, constipation, proximal myopathy, anemia, pancytopenia, heart failure, benign intracranial hypertension, short stature (low height-for-age).

DIAGNOSIS

Diagnosis of NR is established by a thorough history and physical examination, and it is confirmed by laboratory and radiological findings.

- *Laboratory investigation* (**Table 1**):
  - *Calcium*: In mild VDD rickets, the calcium is typically mildly low (7-8 mg/dL), normally it is 8-10 mg/dL but in severe cases the calcium may be much lower resulting in symptoms of hypocalcemia.
  - Phosphorus levels are normal to low (normal level 3.8-6.0 mg/dL). Rickets associated with hypophosphatemic rickets have profoundly low levels of phosphorus (<1.5 mg/dL). This is usually due to renal wasting of phosphorus.

TABLE 1: Laboratory diagnosis according to etiology of rickets.

Type of rickets	Calcium	PO_4	ALP	PTH	VD	Urine phosphorus	Bicarbonates
Nutritional	Low/Normal	Low	High	High	Low	Low	Normal
Familial Hypophosphatemic	Normal	Very low	High	Normal	Normal 25OHD Low 1, 25OHD	High	Normal
RTA	Normal	Low	High	Normal		High	Low urine pH
VDDR 1	Low/Normal	Low	High	High	High 25OHD Low 1, 25OHD	Low	Normal
VDDR 2	Low	Low	High	High	High 25OHD 1,25OHD		Normal

(ALP: alkaline phosphatase; PO_4: phosphates; PTH: parathyroid hormone; RTA: renal tubular acidosis; VD: vitamin D; VDDR: vitamin D-dependent rickets)

- *Magnesium*: Hypomagnesemia is frequently seen when calcium levels are low.
- *Alkaline phosphatase (ALP)*: ALP is an excellent marker of disease activity. In normal child, ALP levels are high up to 500 IU/L, as compared to adult; in nutritional rickets ALP is very high—1,500 IU/L, but in severe malnutrition, ALP may be normal, despite low level of VD.
- *VD metabolites*: Both 25(OH)D3 and 1,25(OH)2D3 can be estimated but the level of 25(OH)D3 is estimated for practical purpose, as it is more stable and present in bigger amount in serum; the level below 20 ng/mL is considered hypovitaminosis.
- *Parathyroid hormone (PTH) level*: PTH level is not required in routine NR cases. It is higher in NR.
- *Renal function test*: Serum creatinine, urinary calcium, pH, and amino acids can be used to exclude or diagnose Fanconi syndrome and proximal renal tubular acidosis.
- *Radiographs*: X-ray wrist: The earliest findings radiologically are seen in distal ulnar region in infants. *X-ray knee joint* is advised to see the lower and upper metaphyses of the knees in grown-up children. There is, to begin with, a "radiolucent" line resulting from accumulation of the uncalcified osteoid between the epiphysis and metaphysis causing its widening. The widening, cupping, and fraying of the metaphysis, giving rise to a brush-like appearance, along with osteopenia are typical radiological findings in classical cases.

A *Milkman pseudofracture*, also known as *looser's zone*, is a radiolucent pseudofracture 2–5 mm wide and have sclerotic borders characteristically seen in osteomalacia. They are bilateral and symmetric, and are perpendicular to the cortical margins of bones. Common sites are femoral neck, medial part of femoral shaft, immediately under lesser, trochanter, on pubic, and ischial rami. Pathologic fractures may be present.

TREATMENT

Basic Principle:
- Rickets is not a medical emergency therefore slow correction is always better.
- Oral vitamin D restores the serum VD concentrations equally better than the intramuscular (IM) route.
- Vitamin D can be advised with a meal or on an empty stomach as absorption is independent of meals.
- Calcium supplementation in a physiological dose results in rapid bone mineralization.

Vitamin D and calcium administration: VD supplementation is done on daily dose schedule or weekly large dose schedule. *VD (cholecalciferol)* preparations are available in the market in various forms. There is high variability of the content of cholecalciferol in the Indian market that has to be taken care of while selecting the proper preparation.

Calcium preparations are available in the Indian market as calcium carbonate, gluconate, and citrate. Calcium carbonate is the cheapest with highest elemental calcium of 40% then rest and it should be the preparation of choice. Calcium preparations are to be taken after food and in divided doses.

For 1 month to 1 year of age:
- Daily dose of VD: 2,000 IU + calcium 500 mg/d × 3 months
- Weekly dose of VD: 60,000 IU once week orally × 6 weeks + calcium 500 mg/d × 6 weeks, followed by maintenance dose of VD 400 IU/d + calcium
- 250–500 mg/d total of 6 weeks (total of 3 months).

For 1 year to 18 years of age:
- Daily dose of VD: 3,000–6,000 IU + calcium 600–800 mg/d × 3 months
- Weekly dose of VD: 60,000 IU once week orally × 6 weeks + calcium 600–800 mg/d × 6 weeks, followed by maintenance dose of VD 600 IU/d + calcium 600–800 mg/d total of 6 weeks (total of 3 months).

Follow-up

- It takes a minimum of *3 months of treatment* for VD and calcium deficiency to show improvement. *Repeat X-ray after 3 months* shows evidence of healing as a *line of preparatory calcification or proximal zone of calcification (PZC)*, at the distal end of osteoid. Further increase in calcification is an indication of progressive healing.
- If there is no evidence of healing at the end of 3 months, think of nonnutritional cause of rickets or resistant rickets. But a second trial of 6 lakh doses of VD is tried, as above, before labeling it to be a case of resistant rickets.
- The biochemical healing is revealed by normalization of serum calcium and phosphorus level, which normally takes 3–4 weeks. ALP levels take several months to normalize.
- Bony deformities may take years to show some improvement.
- After healing, the physiological dose of VD should be continued as per age.

Rickets mimic: There are few conditions which have similar presentation as of rickets but with subtle differences, and have different treatment options.
- *Metaphyseal dysplasia*: The presentation is similar to rickets but the growth plate is not wide and there is differential involvement of the bone, femur shows change but tibia is not affected. Serum calcium, PO_4, and serum ALP are normal.
- *Hypophosphatasia*: Clinical presentation is similar to rickets, but X-ray long bone reveals tongue-like radiolucency projecting from growth plate to metaphysis whereas in rickets, the metaphysis is uniformly wide. Serum ALP is less; calcium and PO_4 are normal.
- *Mucopolysaccharidosis*: It has unique phenotype with corneal clouding.

PRESCRIPTION ASSISTANCE

Vitamin D Preparations

Contents	Trade name	Availability (drops/syrup/tablets/injection)
Vitamin D injection	Arachitol injection	Arachitol injection (1 mL/600,000 IU)
Vitamin D sachet	Calshine, Vitanova, D3 Must, Calcirol	60,000 IU
Vitamin D tablets	D3 Must, 60 K	
Vitamin A D capsules		
Vitamin D drops	Vitanova, Calshine P, Supra D3, D3 Must Forte, Arbivit-3	800 IU/mL

Calcium with Vitamin D Preparations

Trade name	Calcium	Vitamin D
Syrup Ostocalcium (calcium phosphate)	82 mg/5 mL	200 IU
Tablet Ostocalcium (calcium phosphate)	323 mg	400 IU
Syrup Corallium D3 (coral calcium)	200 mg/5 mL	125 IU
Tablet Corallium D3 (coral calcium)	500 mg	500 IU
Syrup Calcinol (calcium carbonate)	750 mg/5 mL	
Syrup Boomcal (calcium carbonate)	215 mg/5 mL	200 IU
Tablet Boomcal (calcium carbonate)	625 mg	400 IU
Syrup Caldikind (calcium carbonate)	250 mg/5 mL	125 IU
Tablet Caldikind (calcium carbonate)	500 mg	
Syrup Calcimax (calcium carbonate)	625 mg	200 IU
Tablet Caldikind 250 (calcium carbonate)	250 mg	200 IU
Tablet Caldikind 500 (calcium carbonate)	500 mg	200 IU

SUGGESTED READING

1. Indian Academy of Pediatrics 'Guideline for Vitamin D and Calcium in Children' Committee; Khadilkar A, Khadilkar V, Chinnappa J, Rathi N, Khadgawat R, Balasubramanian S, et al. Prevention and treatment of vitamin D and calcium deficiency in children and adolescents: Indian Academy of Pediatrics (IAP) Guidelines. Indian Pediatr. 2017;54(7):567-73.
2. Khadilkar AV. Vitamin D deficiency in Indian adolescents. Indian Pediatr. 2010;47(9):755-6.
3. Özkan B. Nutritional rickets. J Clin Res Pediatr Endocrinol. 2010;2(4):137-43.

3 Scurvy

Anoop Verma

INTRODUCTON

Scurvy is a rare disease in clinical practice caused by deficiency of vitamin C. Vitamin C is a water-soluble vitamin and converts proline to hydroxyproline, which is an important constituent of collagen. It is responsible for collagen synthesis; its deficiency causes deficient production of osteoid which is responsible for the characteristic findings seen on X-ray. Vitamin C also plays an important role as a cofactor, enzyme complement, cosubstrate, reducing agent, and an antioxidant in several important biochemical reactions. Therefore, vegetables, fresh fruits, or dietary supplements are essential as a rich source of vitamin C. The *recommended daily allowance* (RDA) of vitamin C is 15–45 mg for age 1–13 years and 65–75 mg for age 14–18 years.

CLINICAL PRESENTATION

Scurvy presents as a spectrum of sign and symptoms, but may cause confusion when the presentation is isolated or noncontiguous. The initial features are nonspecific such as irritability, loss of appetite, low grade fever and the dermatological features such as petechiae, ecchymoses, hyperkeratosis, and cork screw hairs are late manifestations. There is swelling of knee and ankle due to hemorrhages beneath the periosteum and the joints.

The fractures around growth plate can cause extreme bone and joints pains.

The infant often sleeps with hip and knee semiflexed; this presentation is called *"pseudoparalysis."* The child is frequently irritable and does not like handling, due to *pain and tenderness* of the limb. The child shows a paradoxical behavior and cries even on mothers lap. A *"scorbutic beading"* is seen at the costochondral junctions due to subluxation of joint.

Iron deficiency anemia is common in scurvy, and is secondary to a combination of bleeding, and decreased absorption of iron from gut. The hemorrhagic manifestations seen are petechiae, purpura and ecchymoses, epistaxis, and the characteristic perifollicular hemorrhages.

A practical mnemonic for remembering manifestation of scurvy is four "*H*"—(1) hemorrhagic signs, (2) hyperkeratosis, (3) hematologic abnormalities, and (4) hypochondriasis.

Vitamin C deficiency coexists with other nutritional deficiencies such as thiamine, pyridoxine, cobalamin, and vitamin D.

INVESTIGATIONS

The presence of classical features and high index of suspicion gives you clues for the diagnosis of scurvy. The important investigations is radiological mainly and the biochemical assessment rarely.

*Radiological clues in scurvy (**Fig. 1**):*
- X-ray distal end of long bones, e.g., knees and ankle are ideally indicated.
- The presence of *generalized osteopenia* and the classical *"ground-glass"* appearance is by virtue of deficient osteoid matrix and loss of trabeculae.
- Bones become fragile and fracture are easily seen which often heal with abundant callus formation.
- The *"penciling of the cortex"* of diaphysis and epiphysis is due to thin and sharply contrasted cortex as compared to medullary region.

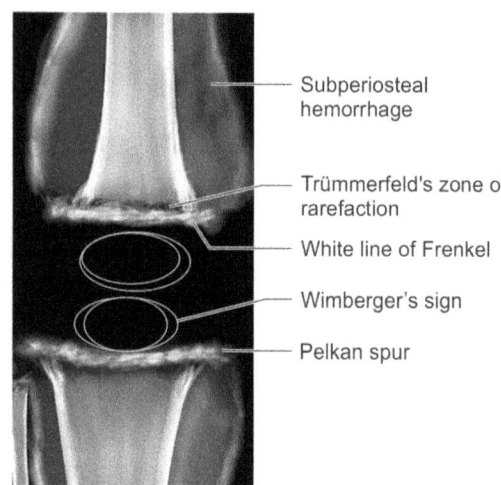

Fig. 1: Radiological clues in scurvy.

PRESCRIPTION ASSISTANCE

Pharmacological name	Market preparation	Availability (drops/syrup/tablets/injection)	Dosages
Vitamin C	Limcee, Celin, Redoxon, Suckcee, Cecon, Zu C	Tablet Limcee, Celin, Redoxon 500 mg, tablet Suckcee, Limcee chewable 200 mg, Cecon drops 100 mg/mL, Zu-C chewable tablets	Doses: See the text

- An irregular but thickened *"white line of Frenkel"* appears at the metaphysis, representing the zone of well-calcified cartilage.
- The late but specific radiological finding of scurvy is a zone of rarefaction known as *"Trümmerfeld zone of rarefaction"* beneath Frenkel line in the metaphysis.
- The presence of *"Pelkan spur"* at the periphery zone of metaphysical calcification, is seen during healing fractures of the Trümmerfeld zone.
- *"Wimberger ring sign"* is a circular, white opaque shadow seen in the growth center around the epiphysis.
- *"Subperiosteal hemorrhages"* are seen during the healing phase of scurvy.

Ultrasound helps in detecting bony irregularity, bulky subcutaneous plane, intramedullary or periosteal mass, and subperiosteal hemorrhagic collections.

Magnetic resonance imaging is only done to rule out malignancy, especially leukemia where the areas of hemorrhage within bones at the site of fracture and in the periosteum are seen.

Biochemical Estimation

- *Plasma level of vitamin C*: Low plasma ascorbate concentration of <0.2 mg/dL, usually is considered deficient. But the result varies if recent supplementation of vitamin C is given.
- *Vitamin C level in the buffy-coat of the leukocytes* is a better estimate of the vitamin body stores. Leukocyte concentrations of ≤10 µg/10^8 WBCs are considered deficient and indicate latent scurvy. This is a costly procedure and is not available freely.
- *Urinary excretion of vitamin C* after parenteral ascorbic acid infusion of 100 mg, around 80% should be excreted within 5 hours if the body stores are not deficient.

TREATMENT

- No standard treatment protocol is available as the disease is rare. In children, scurvy is treated with 100 mg of ascorbic acid given 3 times daily for a week, then 100 mg daily for several weeks until tissue saturation is normal. The regimen may be administered intramuscularly, intravenously, or orally.

- *Effects of vitamin C supplementation*:
  - The spontaneous bleeding and constitutional symptoms are first to recover in days, while ecchymoses and abnormal bones are resolved late, in weeks.
  - Calcification of subperiosteal hematoma occurs quickly by virtue of two mechanisms: (1) Formation of subperiosteal bone beneath the elevated periosteal sleeve and the underlying protruding shaft undergoes rapid resorption and gets aligned with long axis of bone. (2) The epiphysis becomes centered on the widened metaphyses.
- *Splintage* and *vitamin C supplementation* is required for displaced epiphysis and the procedure like a closed or open surgical reduction is rarely required.
- Remodeling of bone in a child is complete without residual deformity or growth disturbance.

Overdoses of Vitamin C

A dose of over 2,000 mg per day in males and females aged 19 years and above may produce gastrointestinal side effect. Avoid more than 400 mg of vitamin C in children from 1 to 3 years, 650 mg between 4 and 8 years, 1,200 mg between 9 and 13 years, 1,800 mg between 14 and 18 years of age. Prolong use of high doses may induces renal stone, bony spur formation, and nutritional imbalance (as high dose reduces the absorption of vitamin B_{12} and copper).

DIFFERENTIAL DIAGNOSIS

The close diagnosis of scurvy is pseudoparalysis mimickers such as osteomyelitis, syphilis, arthritis, and child abuse. The other differentials are hematological and soft-tissue malignancies, Henoch–Schönlein purpura, systemic lupus erythematosus (SLE), and platelet dysfunction.

SUGGESTED READING

1. Chambial S, Dwivedi S, Shukla KK, John PJ, Sharma P. Vitamin C in disease prevention and cure: an overview. Indian J Clin Biochem. 2013;28:314-28.
2. Shah D, Sachdev H. Vitamin C (ascorbic acid). In: Behrman R, Kliegman R, Stanton B, (eds). Nelson Textbook of Pediatrics, 19th edition. Philadelphia: Elsevier Science; 2012. pp. 198-200.
3. Weinstein M, Babyn P, Zlotkin S. An orange a day keeps the doctor away: scurvy in the year 2000. Pediatrics. 2001;108:E55.

4 CHAPTER

Vitamin A Deficiency

Anoop Verma

INTRODUCTION

Vitamin A deficiency (VAD) is the leading cause of preventable blindness seen in children. Vitamin A (VA) is responsible for the formation of rhodopsin. VA maintains epithelial tissues integrity and is important for lysosome stability and glycoprotein synthesis. Children are prone to VAD due to decreased dietary intake and poor absorption leading to depleted VA stores in the body. The high prevalence of infectious diseases such as measles, diarrhea, respiratory infections, and lack of education are contributing factors for VAD.

The dietary sources of VA are milk, egg, fish liver oils. Beta carotene, which is a precursor of VA is found in yellow fruits and vegetables, e.g., papaya, mango, carrot, and green leafy vegetable. VAD is less seen below 6 months of age due to rich liver storage during the early months and milk being the rich source of VA.

WHO CLASSIFICATION: MAJOR SIGNS AND SYMPTOMS OF VAD

	Primary signs	Secondary signs
X1A	Conjunctival xerosis	XN: Night blindness
X1B	Bitot's spot	XF: Fundal changes
X2A	Corneal xerosis	XS: Corneal scarring
X2B	Keratomalacia	
X3A	Corneal ulceration < (1/3)	
X3B	Corneal ulceration > (1/3)	

- *XN (Night blindness)*: Night blindness is the earliest manifestation of VAD. Children are unable to move as the night sets in, and prefer to sit in a secure corner, often unable to search food or toys. Night blindness responds fast, and takes usually 24–48 hours, to VA therapy.
- *Conjunctival xerosis*: Conjunctiva becomes dry, wrinkled, and smoky. There is transformation of normal columnar epithelium to the stratified squamous type, in VAD histologically. This results in loss of goblet cells and formation of agranular cell layer and keratinization.
- *X1B*: Bitot's spots are patches of bulbar conjunctival xerosis seen in the temporal quadrant, as an isolated oval or triangular patch adjacent to the limbus in the interpalpebral fissure. It is almost always bilateral. It has foamy or cheesy appearance due to accumulation of saprophytic bacteria and keratin. Bitot's spots are readily recognized and serve as a useful clinical criterion for assessing the VA status of the population.

Bitot's spots should not be confused with pinguecula or pterygium, which are more often nasal than temporal and limited largely to adults. Pinguecula is an elevated, fatty, yellowish lesion whereas, pterygium is fleshy and actually invades the cornea.

Bitot's spot is sometimes seen in the absence of active VAD in school-growing children. Careful history of previous bouts of night blindness or xerophthalmia must be asked; this lesion is inactive Bitot's spot. To differentiate active and inactive Bitot's spot, one has to observe their response to VA therapy. Active conjunctival xerosis and Bitot's spots begin to resolve within 2–5 days and most will disappear within 2 weeks.

- *X2*: Corneal xerosis—Corneal changes begin early in VAD, long before they can be seen with the naked eye. The cornea develops into classical xerosis, with a hazy, lusterless, dry appearance, first observable near the inferior limbus. Many children with night blindness have characteristic superficial punctuate lesions of the inferonasal aspects of the cornea, which stain brightly with fluorescein. Early diagnosis is only possible through a slit-lamp examination. In follow-up, corneal xerosis responds within 2–5 days to VA therapy, with the cornea regaining its normal appearance in 1–2 weeks.
- *X3 A-X3 B*: Corneal ulceration/keratomalacia involving less than one third of the corneal surface (X3A) generally spares the central pupillary zone, and prompt therapy preserves useful vision. More widespread involvement (X3B), especially generalized liquefactive necrosis usually results in perforation, extrusion of intraocular contents, and loss of the globe. Prompt therapy may still save the other eye and the child's life.

PRESCRIPTION ASSISTANCE

TABLE 1: Laboratory diagnosis according to etiology of rickets.

Pharmacological name	Market preparation	Availability (drops/syrup/tablets/injection)	Dosages
Vitamin A	Aquasol, Vitamin A cap (USV), Rovigon tablet	Cap Aquasol 50,000 IU, and injection 100,000 IU in 2 mL	*Doses:* See the text Vitamin A supplementation
Vitamin A	Aquasol, Vitamin A Cap (USV), Rovigon tablet, Lukvit drops, Arovit tablet	Cap Aquasol 50,000 IU, and injection 100,000 IU in 2 mL Vitamin A cap (USV), Rovigon (Vitamin A 10,000 IU + Vitamin E 25 mg) Lukvit Drops 1 lakh U/mL	*Doses:* See the text Vitamin A supplementation By Lukvit A

- *XS corneal scaring*: The after effect of VAD include opacities or scars of varying densities leading to loss of intraocular contents, phthisis bulbi, and a scarred shrunken globe.
- *XF*: Xerophthalmic fundus—The small white retinal lesions described in some cases of VAD are of investigational interest only. They may be accompanied by constriction of the visual fields and will largely disappear within 2–4 months in response to VA therapy.

DIAGNOSIS

- The clinical recognition is very important. Follow the *WHO clinical classification* of VAD and grade them accordingly.
- *Serum retinol* measurements <20 µg/dL is indicative of VAD.
  It must be adjusted to C-reactive protein (CRP) levels for subclinical infections, otherwise it can overestimate VAD burden. It may not be an operationally feasible indicator for community use.
- Staining of eye with 1% *Rose Bengal*
- *Pupillary reflexes*: Early sign can be picked up by flashing light to the pupil and covering other, the degree of impairment of PR can be estimated.
- *Dark adaptometry* is a simple tool for VAD.

PREVENTION

The Government of India is running Vitamin A Prophylaxis Program; according to this program, children between 9 months and 5 years are given nine mega doses of VA at 6-month interval. The first two doses coincide with MMR vaccination and DPT first booster in a dose of 1 mL for infants and 2 mL after 1 year. VA supplementation causes considerable reduction in child mortality.

TREATMENT OF VITAMIN A DEFICIENCY

Oil miscible vitamin A	<1 year (IU)	>1 year (IU)
Immediately (D1)	1 lakh	2 lakh
Next day (D2)	1 lakh	2 lakh
After 2–4 weeks (D14–21)	1 lakh	2 lakh
Severe PEM (repeat monthly till PEM resolves)	1 lakh	2 lakh

(PEM: protein-energy malnutrition)
Parenteral doses: in persisting vomiting and severe malabsorption
Source: Elizabeth KE. Nutrition and Development, 4th edition.

In keratomalacia, atropinization and ophthalmic consultations are needed. Water-soluble preparation such as aquasol is given 5,000 IU/kg/d, intramuscular for 5 days followed by oral therapy. The another way is to give 5,000 IU/kg/d for 5 days followed by 25,000 IU/d till recovery (Nelson Textbook of Pediatrics).

SUGGESTED READING

1. Elizabeth KE. Nutrition and Development, 4th edition. Hyderabad: Paras Medical Publishers.
2. Imdad A, Herzer K, Mayo-Wilson E, Yakoob MY, Bhutta ZA. Vitamin A supplementation for preventing morbidity and mortality in children from 6 months to 5 years of age. Cochrane Database Syst Rev. 2010;(12):CD008524.
3. World Health Organization. (2011). WHO Guideline: Vitamin A supplementation for infants and children 6–59 months of age. [online] Available from: http://www.who.int/nutrition/publications/micronutrients/guidelines/vas_6to59_months/en/. [Last accessed May, 2021].

CHAPTER 5: Zinc Deficiency in Children

Anoop Verma

INTRODUCTION

Zinc is one of the trace elements and is required for the development of normal growth in infants and children. Zinc acts as cofactor in various enzymes. The body organs which are rich in zinc are eyes, liver, kidney, prostate, bones, and muscles.

SOURCES OF ZINC

Diet rich in phytate such as cereal decreases the absorption of zinc. Eggs, liver, cheese, nuts, oysters, grapes, and grains are rich sources of zinc.

Recommended daily allowance of zinc is 2-3 mg in infants, 3-8 mg in children 1-9 years of age, and 11 mg in children > 14 years of age **(Table 1)**. Nursing and pregnancy increase zinc needs due to increased requirements.

CAUSES OF ZINC DEFICIENCY

It is more commonly seen in people of developing countries where consumption of phytates are high. Phytate inhibits the absorption of zinc. The diseases which reduce the absorption of zinc are chronic diarrhea, malabsorption syndrome, cirrhosis of liver, celiac disease, and Crohn's disease.

CLINICAL MANIFESTATION OF ZINC DEFICIENCY

Mild deficiency presents with poor appetite, weight loss, altered taste and smell sensation, and enhanced susceptibility to infections. Zinc deficiency also leads to moderate-to-severe growth retardation, hypogonadism, skin changes, diarrhea, and acrodermatitis enteropathica (AE). The zinc deficiency induces thymic atrophy and reduces the level of serum thymulin, which can be used as early marker of the deficiency. The excess of zinc can reduce the level of iron and copper, hence can be used in Wilson's disease. The normal serum level of zinc is 60-150 mg/dL. Zinc is neither conserved in body nor there is tissue reserve, so its level depends on regular zinc supplementation.

ASSESSMENT OF ZINC STATUS

- There is no single parameter, in clinical practice to identify the zinc deficiency with certainty.
- The clinical signs and symptoms of zinc deficiency merges with other nutrient deficiency and systemic diseases.
- The first clinical observation of zinc deficiency is change in the velocity of growth with faltering of height and weight measurement.
- *Estimation of plasma zinc level*: It is presumed that low level is indicative of zinc deficiency state.
- The World Health Organization (WHO) uses "zinc-phytate ratio" as qualitative index of bioavailability of zinc, in a reference diet, and also help in calculating the recommended daily zinc intake.

TABLE 1: Recommended daily allowance of zinc.

Age	Male	Female	Pregnancy	Lactation
0–6 months	2 mg	2 mg		
7–12 months	3 mg	3 mg		
1–3 years	3 mg	3 mg		
4–8 years	5 mg	5 mg		
9–13 years	8 mg	8 mg		
14–18 years	11 mg	9 mg	12 mg	13 mg
19+ years	11 mg	8 mg	11 mg	12 mg

PRESCRIPTION ASSISTANCE

Pharmacological name	Market preparation	Availability dosages (drops/syrup/tablets/injection)	
Zinc acetate	Cool-Z, Zn20	Syrup Zn20, 20 mg/5 mL, Tablet 20 mg, Syrup Cool-Z, Syrup Zincris 20 mg/5 mL	See the text
Zinc gluconate	Zinconia, Livzinc	Syrup Zinconia 20 mg/5 mL, Tablet 50 mg	
Zinc sulfate	Live zinc 20,	Syrup Live Zinc 20 mg/5 mL	

BOX 1: Dose schedule of zinc in diarrhea.

Children from 3 to 6 months: 10 mg per day

Children above 6 months: 20 mg per day

Duration of treatment:
- Acute diarrhea—14 days
- Persistent diarrhea—4 weeks

Recommendations below 3 months must await further research due to lack of adequate data till date

Role of Zinc in Diarrhea

Zinc is used in the treatment of diarrhea. It reduces the quantity of stool and duration of diarrhea, when administered with ORS, in patient with acute watery diarrhea, in children aged 3–36 months **(Box 1)**.

Role of Zinc in Celiac Disease

- Small intestine maintains the zinc homeostasis. In celiac disease, the proximal small intestine is at fault, and contributes lot to the deficiency of zinc in celiac patients.
- Factors responsible for deficiency of zinc in celiac disease are: There is loss of fat and phosphate with insoluble zinc complexes, with massive loss of intestinal fluid. Injury to the intestinal epithelium further hampers the absorption of zinc.
- Zinc preparation is given in a patient of CD for 2–4 weeks.

Role of Zinc in Respiratory System

- Zinc supplements enhances the immune mechanism to protect against the cold and upper respiratory infections.
- Studies from India and Vietnam revealed that large reduction of cases, around 41%, of acute lower respiratory infection (ALRI).
- In a randomized controlled trial (RCT) from Bangladesh, zinc supplementation has protective effect against pneumonia, severe pneumonia, suppurative otitis media, and it also mortality due to pneumonia.

Role of Zinc in Malaria

The zinc is essential for important lymphocytic functions which are implicated in resistance to *Plasmodium falciparum* parasite. The vital lymphocytic functions are production of immunoglobulin, interferons, and tumor necrosis factor and increase in the microbiological activities of macrophages. Zinc supplementation reduces the morbidity due of *P. falciparum* but not with other species of *Plasmodium*.

ACRODERMATITIS ENTEROPATHICA

- Acrodermatitis enteropathica (AE) is characterized by periorificial dermatitis, alopecia, and diarrhea.
- *There are two types of (AE)*: (1) Autosomal recessive in nature caused by mutations in the *SLC39A4* gene on chromosome *8q24.3*, which codes for the zinc transporter protein *ZIP4*. (2) Acquired: It occurs due to low nutritional intake or decreased peripheral release of zinc from the blood.
- The diagnosis is by estimation of low plasma zinc.
- *Treatment*: Zinc sulfate 50–150 mg/day (elemental zinc 1–2 mg/kg/day).

Overdoses of zinc preparations: If the zinc salt is taken >100–300 mg/day, it can induce toxicity. If the dose exceeds 2 g/day, it may lead to GI upset and convulsions. Chronic usage can lead to lethargy, anemia, and neurological deterioration as it reduces the copper level.

PREPARATIONS AVAILABLE

Among the commercially available preparations, most of the preparations contain zinc sulfate. This is the cheapest salt available but this preparation is not easily absorbed and causes stomach upset. Zinc citrate is another option available with better tolerance. All the zinc preparations must be taken with juice or water or after meals. Always avoid taking zinc with iron and calcium preparations. *Zinc sulfate 4.4 mg = 1 mg elemental zinc; zinc acetate is* equivalent to elemental zinc 20 mg/5 mL.

SUGGESTED READING

1. Elizabeth KE. Nutrition and Development, 4th edition. Delhi: Paras Medical Publisher.
2. Lazzerini M, Wanzira H. Oral zinc for treating diarrhoea in children. Cochrane Database Syst Rev. 2016;12(12):CD005436.
3. Rawal P, Thapa BR. Zinc in child health: a mineral that means a lot. IJPP. 2011;13(1):57-64.

6 Food Allergies

Tushar Jagzape

INTRODUCTION

- Food allergy is one of the most common causes of severe anaphylaxis all over the world. As defined by an expert panel of the National Institute of Allergy and Infectious Diseases, food allergy is an adverse health effect arising from a specific immune response that occurs reproducibly on exposure to a given food.
- The exact prevalence of food allergies is not known. Many studies indicate that the prevalence of food allergy is increasing worldwide.
- Approximately 3.5–8% of children are having food allergies.
- Food allergy is not equivalent to food intolerance.
- Any abnormal clinical response to ingestion of food is described broadly as adverse food reactions which comprise food intolerance and food allergy **(Flowchart 1)**.

PATHOPHYSIOLOGY

- The immune mechanism involved in food allergies is both IgE mediated and non-IgE medicated. Some allergies have a mixed mechanism.
- IgE-mediated immune mechanism involves inflammation which is induced by cellular components and mediated by eosinophils and T-cells.
- It is possible to identify these patients with the help of in vivo and in vitro detection of specific IgE.
- T-cell-dependent immune mechanism is responsible for food allergies such as celiac disease and probably in food protein-induced enterocolitis.
- The first contact with an allergen leading to an allergic immune response is known as allergic sensitization. The subsequent exposure which leads to clinical symptoms is known as secondary immune response.
- An individual can get sensitized through respiratory, cutaneous, or oral route. Most of the symptoms in

Flowchart 1: Adverse food reactions.

patients with IgE-mediated reaction are due to release of preformed inflammatory mediators, e.g., histamine due to activation and degranulation of basophils and mast cells.
- These cells are activated due to crosslinking of IgE via high-affinity receptor, Fcε RI due to food allergen. The mast cells and basophils also synthesize and release other inflammatory mediators such as leukotrienes, proteases, inflammatory cytokines, e.g., IL 4, and other chemotactic molecules.
- Symptoms can be local or systemic based on the ability of allergen to breech the mucosal barrier. The role of late-phase response is not clear in food allergies, but it might be responsible for diseases such as eosinophilic esophagitis.
- The delayed type reaction which can occur after 24–48 hours of contact with the allergen resembles type IV hypersensitivity reactions.
- Based on route of sensitization the food allergens are divided into two classes:
  - *Class 1*: These allergens cause sensitization via oral route, e.g., milk, egg, peanut
  - *Class 2*: These allergens cause sensitization via the respiratory tract, e.g., major birch pollen allergen Bet v1.

EPIDEMIOLOGY

- The exact incidence of food allergies has not been fully established but prevalence is considered to be increasing. There are discrepancies in the studies due to self-reporting versus proven food allergies.
- Infants and toddlers have highest prevalence of food allergy (6–8%) which decrease with age to around 4% among adults. Though there are no studies of food allergies in India, the EuroPrevall study reported a rate of 1.2% of specific IgE (sIgE) among the South Indian adults.
- Food allergy is responsible for the maximum number of anaphylaxis reactions in children. Eggs, tree nuts, peanuts, wheat, milk, soy, fish, and shellfish are responsible for 90% of the food allergies, the so called "The Big 8" of food allergies.

CLINICAL FEATURES

- As mentioned in the pathophysiology, the clinical symptoms could be immediate due to IgE-mediated mechanism or delayed due T-cell involvement.
- The common symptoms are:
  - Urticarial rash, flushing of skin, pruritus, and angioedema.
  - In respiratory system, the patient can have cough, hoarseness due to laryngeal and/or pharyngeal edema.
  - Gastrointestinal symptoms (GI) symptoms may be seen in food allergy which include pain in abdomen, distension of abdomen, flatulence, nausea, vomiting, loss of appetite, colitis, and diarrhea.
  - Neurological manifestation could be anxiety, irritability, confusion, and loss of consciousness.
  - The patient can present with anaphylactic shock, vascular collapse, tachycardia, or cardiac dysrhythmia when cardiovascular system (CVS) is involved.
- Some of the respiratory allergens have similarity with food allergens. Sensitization to these respiratory allergens cause a cross-reactive immune response, e.g., sensitization to the major birch pollen allergen, Bet v1 cross-react with antigen in food such as apples, carrots, nuts, and celery. So when a person who is sensitized to Bet v1 ingest apple, carrots, or nuts, he/she develops an IgE-mediated local allergic reaction in the form of local itching, swelling of lips, or tongue. Systemic reactions do not occur commonly as the Bet v1-related plant food allergen are digested in the GI tracts. But rarely if large amount of plant food allergens are ingested during exercise, then systemic reactions can occur.
- T-cell mediated clinical features are mostly delayed and of chronic nature and present as atopic dermatitis, bronchial asthma, rhinoconjunctivitis, chronic diarrhea. When predominantly eosinophils are involved in chronic inflammation, eosinophilic esophagitis or gastroenteritis may be the presentation.
- Cow's milk protein allergy (CMPA) is common in children, but the exact burden of this entity in Indian children is not known. The symptoms are similar to other food allergies due to IgE-mediated or non-IgE-mediated mechanism. Poddar U et al. in their study found that CMPA was responsible for around 30% cases of chronic diarrhea.

INVESTIGATIONS

- The diagnosis of food allergies and for that matter, any allergic disorder is based on thorough clinical history. Investigations will only help to corroborate clinical history.
- Once a food allergy is diagnosed, then it is important to identify the food responsible.
- Short listing of the food items for testing can be obtained by case histories and symptom diary.
- For IgE-mediated allergies, identification of specific IgE by in vivo, i.e., skin prick test (SPT) or by serological tests can be done **(Fig. 1)**.

Allergy skin testing can be divided into two main groups:
1. *Epicutaneous test*: Prick skin testing, puncture skin test.
2. *Intradermal skin test*: The latter is associated with more risk, hence not routinely done. SPT do not have a high positive predictive value (around 50%), but negative predictive value of >95% make them very useful. The patient is more likely to react to food allergen if the wheal size on SPT is larger.

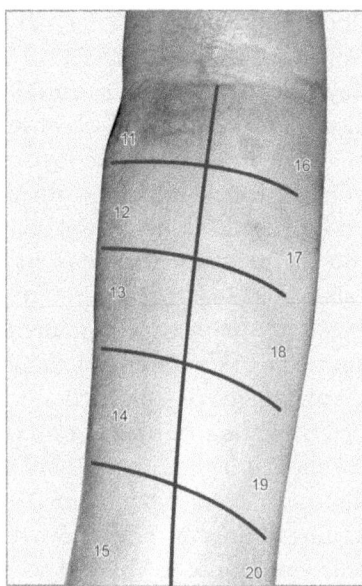

Fig. 1: Showing the allergy skin prick test (SPT). Antigen in number 11 is showing a positive test (induration). Number 20 is histamine (positive control).

- In vitro tests to measure the serum sIgE are an alternative to SPT. There are various tests available commercially, e.g., fluorescence enzyme immunoassay (FEIA-CAP), radioallergosorbent test (RAST), chemiluminescent ImmunoCAP. The test results are not affected by medications but they are difficult to interpret as the predictive values changes for the food. Total serum IgE estimation is not indicated for evaluation of food allergy. Presence of specific IgE is not sufficient to label a patient as having a food allergy as this is not always associated with symptoms.
- For non-IgE mediated disorders such as atopic dermatitis, food protein-induced enterocolitis and eosinophilic esophagitis atopy patch test have been used. The atopy patch test is more specific but less sensitive as compared to SPT. Examination of the biopsy specimen obtained through endoscopy is an important investigation for non-IgE-mediated disorders. There is no role of measuring allergen-specific IgG.
- Double-blind placebo-controlled (DBPC) oral food challenge test is considered as the gold standard for diagnosis of food allergy but it is associated with risk of severe anaphylaxis. To reduce the risk, open challenge or single-blind (patient) oral food challenge is being used. The suspected food allergen is given to the patient under strict monitoring in gradually increasing doses. The patient is generally put on an elimination diet before going for the oral challenge test.
- Never methods such as in vitro multiplex allergen tests are being employed at many places. A new technique called component-resolved diagnostics (CRD) has been established to differentiate between true allergy and sensitization.

MANAGEMENT

Emergency Management

As mentioned earlier, food allergy is one of the most common causes of anaphylaxis; it should be managed as per the standard treatment of anaphylaxis. Injectable adrenaline is the drug of choice.

Antihistamines are used as adjuvants. Steroids for late phase reactions. The patients/parents should be educated about identifying severe reaction and using injectable epinephrine. Though prefilled adrenaline injections are not available in India, an alternative of using prefilled 1-mL syringes/insulin syringe stored in a dark box like a spectacle case is being used in India. The parents/patients should be counseled about the disease, avoidance of food and prehospital treatment.

Avoidance of Allergenic Food

Once identified, the food allergen should be avoided but it is many times not possible to identify the hidden allergen. The exposure may occur at home or outside the home. Sometimes exposure through skin also has been associated with reactions but most of the severe reactions occur after ingestion.

Allergen Immunotherapy

Allergen immunotherapy is the only disease-modifying therapy available for allergic diseases. It is nothing but administration of increasing dose of allergen extract to lessen the symptoms due to causative allergen. Though currently it has only been approved for allergic rhinoconjunctivitis and allergic asthma. Studies have confirmed the effectivity of sublingual immunotherapy in patients of hazelnut allergy. Some other studies have also found it to be useful in milk, egg, and fish allergy.

Primary Prevention

Delaying the introduction of allergen or removal of allergen from the mother's diet during pregnancy and promote breastfeeding was used as an approach to prevent food allergies in children. The impact of these interventions has not been that encouraging. The American Academy of Pediatrics no longer recommends avoidance of any food during pregnancy and do not specifically recommend on food reintroduction besides breastfeeding and no solids until 4 months of age.

KEY MESSAGES

- Food allergies are common in pediatric age group and the prevalence is steadily increasing.
- The most common food allergens are milk, egg, wheat, fish, tree nuts, soy, peanut, and shell fish.

- The allergy could be IgE or non-IgE mediated. The clinical features range from skin manifestations to gastroenteritis to anaphylaxis.
- Proper history and investigations to evaluate presence of sIgE such as SPT are important for the diagnosis.
- Oral food challenge test is most specific.
- Avoidance of food is currently the only treatment.
- Immunotherapy is showing promising results.

SUGGESTED READING

1. Boyce JA, Assa'ad A, Burks AW, Jones SM, Sampson HA, Wood RA, et al. Guidelines for the diagnosis and management of food allergy in the United States: summary of the NIAID-Sponsored Expert Panel Report. Nutr Res. 2011; 31(1):61-75.
2. Burney PG, Potts J, Kummeling I, Mills ENC, Clausen M, Dubakiene R, et al. The prevalence and distribution of food sensitization in European adults. Allergy. 2014;69(3):365-71.
3. Cianoferonia A, Spergel JM. Food allergy: review, classification and diagnosis. Allergol Int. 2009;58(4):457-66.
4. Enrique E, Malek T, Pineda F, Palacios R, Bartra J, Tella R, et al. Sublingual immunotherapy for hazelnut food allergy: a follow-up study. Ann Allergy Asthma Immunol. 2008;100(3):283-4.
5. Enrique E, Pineda F, Malek T, Bartra J, Basagaña M, Tella R, et al. Sublingual immunotherapy for hazelnut food allergy: a randomized, double-blind, placebo-controlled study with a standardized hazelnut extract. J Allergy Clin Immunol. 2005;116(5):1073-9.
6. Foong RX, du Toit G, Fox AT. Asthma, food allergy, and how they relate to each other. Front Pediatr. 2017;5:89.
7. Han Y, Kim J, Ahn K. Food allergy. Korean J Pediatr. 2012;55:153-8.
8. Lieberman JA, Sicherer SH. Diagnosis of food allergy: epicutaneous skin tests, in vitro tests, and oral food challenge. Curr Allergy Asthma Rep. 2011;11(1):58-64.
9. Longo G, Berti I, Burks AW, Krauss B, Barbi E. IgE-mediated food allergy in children. Lancet. 2013;382(9905):1656-64.
10. Mahesh PA, Wong GW, Ogorodova L, Potts J, Leung TF, Fedorova O, et al. Prevalence of food sensitization and probable food allergy among adults in India: the EuroPrevall INCO study. Allergy. 2016;71(7):1010-9.
11. Patriarca G, Nucera E, Pollastrini E, Roncallo C, De Pasquale T, Lombardo C, et al. Oral specific desensitization in food-allergic children. Dig Dis Sci. 2007;52(7):1662-72.
12. Poddar Yachha SK, Krishnani N, Srivastava A. Cow's milk protein allergy: an entity for recognition in developing countries. J Gastroenterol Hepatol. 2010;25(1):178-82.
13. Robison RG. Food allergy: Diagnosis, management and emerging therapies. Indian J Med Res. 2014;139(6):805-13.
14. Sicherer SH, Sampson HA. Food allergy: epidemiology, pathogenesis, diagnosis and treatment. Clinical review in allergy and immunology. J Allergy Clin Immunol. 2014; 133(2):291-307; quiz 308.
15. Valenta R, Hochwallner H, Linhart B, Pahr S. Food allergies: the basics. Gastroenterology. 2015;148(6):1120-31.e4.
16. Vedanthan PK. Allergy skin testing. In: Vedanthan PK, Nelson H, Agashe SN, Mahesh PA, Katial R (eds). Textbook of Allergy for the Clinician, 1st edition. USA: CRC Press; 2014. pp. 36-46.
17. Vijayan A. Food allergen: a growing problem. RRJFPDT. 2016:4(3).

7 Food Poisoning

Tushar Jagzape

INTRODUCTION

Foodborne diseases (FBD) or foodborne illnesses are a broad term which is used to describe clinical conditions which can occur after ingestion of food contaminated with infectious organisms or noninfectious substances and includes toxin-mediated food poisoning; gastroenteritis following ingestion of chemicals or preformed toxins; and bacterial, viral, or parasitic infections. In general, food poisoning is the term commonly used to describe disease due to ingestion of bacterial contaminated food or bacterial toxins. In this section, we will primarily focus on bacterial food poisoning.

EPIDEMIOLOGY

- The exact incidence is very difficult to calculate. Foodborne illnesses are common worldwide but more common in developing countries.
- As per the American estimates, every sixth individual is affected annually by foodborne illness.
- The most common bacterial pathogens as per the Centers for Disease Control and Prevention (CDC) estimates are *Campylobacter, Escherichia coli* O157, *Salmonella, Shigella,* and *Yersinia enterocolitica.*
- These organisms caused approximately 291,162 illnesses in children < 5 years in a year.
- Children are more affected in comparison to adults. A large proportion of childhood deaths are accounted by diarrheal disorders.

ETIOLOGY AND PATHOPHYSIOLOGY

- The pathogenesis is different for different organisms.
- Based on the pathophysiology, the etiology can classically be categorized into invasive or inflammatory and noninvasive or noninflammatory.
- Etiological agents causing inflammatory damage where leukocytes are seen in stools are: *Campylobacter,* enteroinvasive *E. coli* (EIEC), *Salmonella, Shigella, Vibrio parahaemolyticus,* and *Yersinia*; these cause disease by invasion of intestinal tissue **(Flowchart 1)**.
- The organisms which do not cause much inflammation as is evident from absence of fecal leukocytes are: *Bacillus cereus, Staphylococcus aureus, Clostridium botulinum, C. perfringens, V. cholerae,* enterotoxigenic *E. coli* (ETEC), and enterohemorrhagic *E. coli* (EHEC); these organisms act through toxin **(Flowchart 1)**.

CLINICAL FEATURES (TABLE 1)

The prominent symptoms and signs are related to gastrointestinal system and include:
- Nausea and vomiting

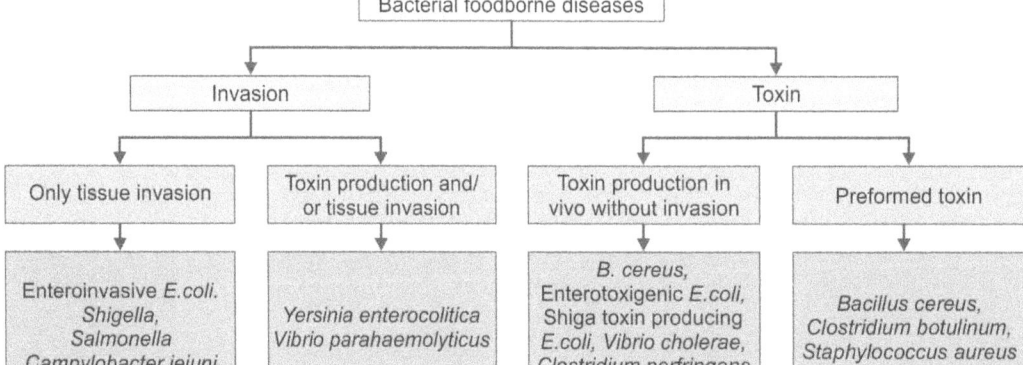

Flowchart 1: Pathogenic mechanisms in bacterial foodborne diseases.

TABLE 1: Summary of common causes, clinical features and treatment of food poisoning.

Incubation period	Mechanism	Organisms	Clinical features	Source	Treatment
Short incubation period (1–6 hours)	Preformed toxins/noninvasive	*Staphylococcus aureus*	Profuse vomiting associated with nausea and abdominal cramps, diarrhea may be present. Fever uncommon	Meat, cream pastries, and mayonnaise	Usually resolves in 24 hours
		Bacillus cereus	• *Emetic form*: Vomiting and abdominal cramps • Diarrhea in 1/3rd and fever uncommon	Stale rice, meats, gravy, vanilla and sauces, stews	Usually resolves in 12 hours
Moderate incubation period (8–16 hours)	In vivo production of toxins; noninvasive	*B. cereus*	• Diarrheal form—diarrhea and abdominal cramps • Occasionally vomiting. Fever not common	Fried rice	Resolves in by 24 hours
		Clostridium perfringens	• Severe crampy abdominal pain, watery diarrhea • Vomiting and fever unlikely	Cooked meat/poultry stored without refrigeration	Resolves within 24 hours
Long incubation period (>16 years)	Some toxin mediated, some invasive				
	Toxin-producing organisms	*Clostridium botulinum*	Diarrhea followed by or accompanied with paralysis. Cranial nerve palsies, descending paralysis Fever is usually absent	Home-canned foods, honey	Severity related to quantity of toxin ingested
Period (>16 years)	Some invasive				
		Enterotoxigenic *Escherichia coli* (ETEC)	Most common cause of travelers diarrhea abdominal cramps, copious diarrhea, uncommonly accompanied with vomiting and fever	Contaminated salad, ice, or water	3–4 days
		Enterohemorrhagic *E. coli* (EHEC)	• Severe abdominal cramps and watery diarrhea, dysentery. No fever • May lead to hemolytic uremic hemolytic uremic syndrome	• Unpasteurized milk or juice • Contaminated beef	
		Vibrio cholerae	Diarrhea, nausea and vomiting, hemolytic uremic syndrome	Contaminated food or water	Up to 1 week
		V. cholerae	• Diarrhea, nausea and vomiting, abdominal cramps, muscle cramps and dehydration of varying severity • No fever	Contaminated food or water	Up to 1 week
	Invasive organisms	*Salmonella*—nontyphoidal strains	• Nausea, vomiting, diarrhea and abdominal cramps • Fever can be present. May cause dysentery	Poultry, meat, and dairy products	
		Shigella	• Bacillary dysentery—diarrhea with blood in stools, mucus and pain • Tenesmus, small volume, stool, toxemia occasionally causing seizures in children	Contaminated food or water or person to person	Resolves in few days
		Campylobacter jejuni	Prodrome of fever, headache, and myalgia	• Undercooked meat, poultry, unpasteurized dairy products • Seizures in children	Resolves by 7 days

Contd...

Contd...

Incubation period	Mechanism	Organisms	Clinical features	Source	Treatment
		C. jejuni	Prodrome of fever, headache, and myalgia • *Intestinal phase*: Diarrhea along with fever, malaise and abdominal pain • Diarrhea could be mild to profuse and bloody	Undercooked meat, poultry, unpasteurized dairy products and drinking from fresh water streams	Resolves by 7 days
		Yersinia enterocolitica and Y. pseudotuberculosis	Fever, diarrhea, and abdominal pain, mesenteric adenitis mimicking appendicitis	Contaminated food or water	1–3 weeks
		Enteroinvasive E. coli (EIEC)	High incidence of fever and bloody diarrhea	Contaminated food or water	

- Profuse watery diarrhea
- Dehydration
- Bloody diarrhea
- Pain in abdomen of varying severity and cramps.

Other systemic symptoms are:
- Fever, myalgia, oliguria, lymphadenopathy, and neurological symptoms such as motor weakness, visual disturbances, cranial nerve involvement, and paresthesia
- The child can have neck stiffness and meningeal signs. The child can also present with urticaria, anaphylaxis, and autonomic disturbances such as flushing, hypotension, dizziness, and headache.

DIFFERENTIAL DIAGNOSIS

- Infection caused by different organisms such as other bacterial and viral pathogens.
- In case of dysentery, other causes of blood in stool such as inflammatory bowel disease, polyps, or other hematogenous malformations and intussusception should be considered.
- In case of botulism, other causes of paralysis such as Guillain–Barré syndrome, poliomyelitis, and tick paralysis can be thought of.

INVESTIGATIONS

- Investigations are not routinely required for diagnosis and treatment purpose.
- Stool routine microscopy and culture may be indicated only in case of severe or persistent cases and mostly in cases of bloody diarrhea. The culture positivity rate for stool is around 40%.
- In presence of travel history, stool for ova and cyst examination may be indicated.
- In case of patients who are having high-grade fever and severe symptoms suggestive of bacteremia, blood culture can be requested.
- For assessment of other organ dysfunction and hydration status serum electrolytes, serum creatinine and blood urea levels are required.
- In suspected cases of bacteremia and hemolytic uremic syndrome, complete blood count (CBC) and peripheral blood smear are indicated.
- For epidemiological purpose of suspected food poisoning, testing of food or vomitus for toxin may be done.

MANAGEMENT (TABLE 2)

- Most of the cases of food poisoning are self-limiting and need only supportive therapy in the form of hydration and maintenance of electrolyte balance. Oral rehydration therapy as per the Integrated Management of Newborn and Childhood Illness (IMNCI) guidelines should be used.
- Antimicrobials are not indicated when the infection is due to the following organisms: Enterohemorrhagic and enteroinvasive *E. coli*, *B. cereus*, *S. aureus*, *V. parahaemolyticus*, *Yersinia*, and *C. perfringens*.
- On the other hand, there are no antivirals for viral gastroenteritis.
- Protozoal agents are susceptible to many available antimicrobials.
- In patients suffering from travelers' diarrhea due to enterotoxigenic *E. coli*, use of antibiotics are not routinely recommended. But patients who have dysentery or associated fever, the duration of illness may be reduced by use of antibiotics. Antibiotics which have been found useful includes quinolone, azithromycin or rifaximin, and trimethoprim-sulfamethoxazole (TMP-SMX).
- In case of cholera, fluid replacement is of outmost importance. Antibiotics are indicated for reducing the duration of illness and shedding of bacteria. Doxycycline, azithromycin, or erythromycin are recommended.
- Though shigellosis is a self-limited illness, use of azithromycin and third-generation cephalosporin (cefixime and cefpodoxime) and ciprofloxacin may reduce the transmission and duration of disease.
- Similarly, for *Salmonella* infection (gastroenteritis), antibiotics are only indicated if bacteremia occurs.

TABLE 2: Summary of antimicrobial for common pathogens.

Name of the organism	Drug of choice	Second drug
Enterotoxigenic Escherichia coli	• Ciprofloxacin: 15–30 mg/kg/24 h divided q 12 h PO or IV • Rifaximin 200 mg three times daily × 3 days (12 years and above)	• Azithromycin 10 mg/kg od 3–5 days • TMP/SMX: 6–8 mg/kg/day of TMP divided bd if sensitive × 3 days
Vibrio cholerae	• Doxycycline: 2–4 mg/kg PO single dose • Azithromycin: 20 mg/kg as a single dose (maximum 1 g)	• Erythromycin: 12.5 mg/kg/dose 4 times a day × 3 days (500 mg max per dose) • Ciprofloxacin: 20 mg/kg PO single dose
Salmonella gastroenteritis	Not usually recommended	• Cefixime: 15 mg/kg/day for 7–10 days or • Ceftriaxone: 75 mg/kg/day once daily × 7 days • Azithromycin: 8–10 mg/kg/day × 7 days
Shigella	• Cefixime: 8 mg/kg/24 h divided q 12–24 h PO, 3–5 days • Cefpodoxime: Children: 10 mg/kg/24 h divided q 12 h PO • Azithromycin: 12 mg/kg 1st day followed by 6 mg/kg/day for 4 days	• Ciprofloxacin 500 mg bd × 3 days or Levofloxacin 500 mg od × 3 days • Ceftriaxone: 50 mg/kg/24 h as a single dose IV/IM • TMP/SMX: 6–8 mg/kg/day divided of TMP bd × 3 days (If sensitive)
Campylobacter diarrhea	• Not usually required • Ciprofloxacin: 15–30 mg/kg/24 h divided q 12 h PO or IV; 3–5 days	Azithromycin: 10 mg/kg/day 3–5 days
Giardia lamblia	• Metronidazole: 15 mg/kg/day PO in three doses × 5 days • Tinidazole: 50 mg/kg/day PO (maximum 2 g) once	• Nitazoxanide: 1–3 years: 100 mg PO every 12 h × 3 days • 4–11 years: 200 mg PO every 12 h × 3 days • >11 years: 500 mg orally 12 h × 3 days • Albendazole: 10–15 mg/kg (maximum 400 mg) orally once daily for 5 days
Entamoeba histolytica	Metronidazole: 35–50 mg/kg/day PO in 3 divided doses × 7–10 days followed by Paromomycin: 25–35 mg/kg/day PO in 3 divided doses × 7 days or Iodoquinol: 30–40 mg/kg/day PO in three doses × 20 day	• Tinidazole: 50 mg/kg/day PO (maximum 2 g) × 3–5 days

(IV: intravenous; IM: intramuscular; PO: per oral; TMP/SMX: trimethoprim-sulfamethoxazole)

For *Salmonella* enteric fever, oral cefixime is the drug of choice. Azithromycin is the other effective oral drug.

- *Campylobacter* infections with severe manifestations may benefit from use of macrolide, especially erythromycin, a quinolone, or a parenteral aminoglycoside. Azithromycin is possibly useful.
- For rotavirus, Norwalk and other feco-oral route borne viral infections, supportive care is indicated.
- Botulism needs supportive treatment, except in case of an infant where antitoxin is indicated.
- Metronidazole/tinidazoles are useful in treatment of giardiasis and amebiasis. Nitazoxanide is broad antidiarrheal drug useful for giardia and cryptosporidiosis.
- Zinc is recommended for children younger than 5 years of age once the vomiting subsides. It can be used for both watery and bloody diarrhea. Zinc supplementation at dose of 20 mg per day for children above 6 months and 10 mg per day for children below 6 months for 14 days shortens the duration of diarrhea and subsequent diarrhea episodes. This effect is more pronounced in children with zinc deficiency.
- Vitamin A supplementation has no role in acute diarrhea; it has a significant impact on morality associated with diarrheal diseases.
- Current data do not support folic acid and/or vitamin D supplementation for diarrhea.
- Similarly, there is no concrete evidence of utility of any specific probiotic preparation in treatment of food poisoning. Addition of *Lactobacillus* GG to oral rehydration solution (ORS) was found to be effective in a clinical trial for pediatric infectious diarrhea. But at present, they are not universally recommended for want of robust data.
- Other drugs such as antimotility, antispasmodic, and antisecretory agents are better avoided in pediatric age group.
- *Prevention of food poisoning*: Improvement in practices of food handling.

SUGGESTED READING

1. Bhutta ZA. Acute gastroenteritis in children. In: Kliegman RM, Stanton BF, Schor NF, St Geme JW, (eds). Nelsons Textbook of Pediatrics, 1st South Asia Edition. Elsevier; 2016;1854-75.
2. Fort GG. Food poisoning, bacterial. Ferri`s Clinical Advisor. 2020, 563-7.e1 (www.cliniclakey.com, accessed on 16th May 2020)
3. Guarino A, Albano F, Ashkenazi S, et al. European Society for Paediatric Gastroenterology, Hepatology, and Nutrition/European Society for Paediatric Infectious Diseases evidence-based guidelines for the management of acute gastroenteritis in children in Europe. J Pediatr Gastroenterol Nutr. 2008;46(Suppl 2):S81-122.
4. Lazzerini M, Wanzira H. Oral zinc for treating diarrhoea in children. Cochrane Database of Systematic Reviews. 12:CD005436.
5. Lopez AL. Cholera. In: Kliegman RM, Stanton BF, Schor NF, St Geme JW, (eds). Nelsons Textbook of Pediatrics, 1st South Asia Edition. Elsevier; 2016.1400.
6. Mandell GL et al. Principles and Practice of Infectious Diseases, 6th edition. Philadelphia, 2005, Churchill Livingstone.
7. Mayo-Wilson E, Imdad A, Herzer K, et al. Vitamin A supplements for preventing mortality, illness, and blindness in children aged under 5: systematic review and meta-analysis. BMJ. 2011;343:d5094.
8. Roy SK, Raqib R, Khatun W, Azim T, Chowdhury R, Fuchs GJ, et al. Zinc supplementation in the management of shigellosis in malnourished children in Bangladesh. Eur J Clin Nutr. 2008;62:849-55.
9. Schleiss MR. Principles of antiparastitic therapy. In: Kliegman RM, Stanton BF, Schor NF, St Geme JW, (eds). Nelsons Textbook of Pediatrics, 1st South Asia Edition. 2016; pp. 1673-87.
10. Singhal T, Lodha R, Kabra SK. Infections and infestation. In: Paul VK, Bagga A, (eds). Ghai Essential Pediatrics, 8th edition. CBS Publisher and Distributors Pvt Ltd. pp. 209-77.
11. Sood SK. Pediatric Food Poisoning. Available on: www.Emedicine.medscape.com last access on 12th May 2020
12. Steiner T. Treating foodborne illness. Infect Dis Clin N Am. 2013;27:555.
13. Szajewska H, Mrukowicz JZ. Probiotics in the treatment and prevention of acute infectious diarrhea in infants and children: a systematic review of published randomized, double-blind, placebo-controlled trials. J Pediatr Gastroenterol Nutr. 2001;33(Suppl 2):S17-25.

CHAPTER 8: Failure to Thrive

SA Krishna

INTRODUCTON

The term "failure to thrive" (FTT) was mentioned as early as 1915 by an American pediatrician, Dr Henry Dight Chaplin.

- Failure to thrive is when there is a failure to grow at the expected rate, i.e., growth falls away from standardized weight or height centile.
- Weight is the most sensitive indicator in infants and young children, while height is a better indicator in older child. Under stress, head circumference growth is more preserved than linear growth which is more than the weight.
- *Causes*:
  - Organic causes
  - *Nonorganic causes*: These are also an important entity. Social, psychological, and environmental factors are responsible for nonorganic FTT.

INVESTIGATIONS

Organic Causes

- *Basic investigations*: Complete blood count (CBC), erythrocyte sedimentation rate (ESR), C-reactive protein (CRP), R/E urine, C/S of urine, liver function test (LFT), serum creatinine, serum calcium, phosphorus.
- Immunoglobulins, celiac antibody screening.
- *In severe faltering of growth*: Inborn errors of metabolism (IEM) screening, karyotyping, serum lead, abdominal ultrasonography (USG), upper gastrointestinal (GI) endoscopy, small intestinal biopsy, chest X-ray (CXR), bone age, skeletal survey, head computed tomography (CT)/magnetic resonance imaging (MRI), ECG, R/E stool, especially for occult blood.

MANAGEMENT: MULTIDISCIPLINARY APPROACH

- An appropriate feeding atmosphere at home is a prerequisite for children with FTT.
- *If nonorganic cause*: Advice is needed from a pediatric dietitian. If the condition resolves in the next few weeks, positive reinforcement is needed. Subsequent growth should be supervised as an outpatient.
- Indications of hospitalization and its management:
  - Include severe malnutrition, suspected child abuse, or failure of outpatient management.
  - Admitted patients should undergo basic investigations and their response should be observed and adequate dietary input should be supervised.
  - Evaluation of parent child feeding interaction should be done.
  - *Diet therapy*: A diet that is relatively energy rich may promote catch up that is paralleled by central fat accretion while a diet that better meets protein requirements may be paralleled by increased lean mass accretion; so focus has changed from supplementing only energy to providing adequate energy and protein; 8.9–11.5% of energy should be supplied as protein. The requirements set should be practically achievable for the parent and child; supplement should be accepted by the child.
  - The route of feeding is related to the child's ability to achieve the energy requirements.
  - If nutritional requirements are not met orally, then enteral feeding must be considered; if still not met, then parenteral nutrition is recommended.
- *In severe malnutrition*:
  - Child should be refed carefully, with an incremental increase in calories for the fear of refeeding syndrome.
  - The hallmark of refeeding syndrome is the development of severe hypophosphatemia during the first week of starting to reefed, producing weakness, rhabdomyolysis, arrhythmias, seizures altered consciousness, or sudden death.
  - Phosphate levels should be monitored during refeeding and administered if low.
  - Minimal catch-up growth should generally be two to three times the average weight gain for the corrected age.

- Multivitamin supplements should be given to all children to meet the recommended dietary allowance (RDA) as their deficiencies coexist.
- Adequate growth in hospital suggests a nonorganic cause.
- If FTT occurs again at home after improvement in hospital, then the need of social services is there for family assessment and proper intervention.
- If FTT continues in hospital in spite of adequate dietary input, occult organic disease is most likely and extensive investigation is warranted. Associated comorbidities such as developmental delay and cerebral palsy should be identified and managed accordingly.

FOLLOW-UP

- Careful monitoring of growth parameters and overall development is warranted.
- Weekly growth checks using same clinic scale until sustained growth is documented for months. Home visit service should be provided.
- Child's clinical course should be closely documented.

PROGNOSIS

The prognosis depends on the severity of FTT:
- Prognosis is good in mild FTT.
- FTT early in life is concerning whatever the cause may be, as the maximal brain growth occurs in first 6 months of life. It has been shown to be associated with deficits in IQ in later life.
- Early FTT is also associated with dyslipidemia, hypertension, and glucose intolerance for cardiovascular disease as an adult.
- Severe FTT, irrespective of cause, may be associated with later developmental and behavioral impairment.

SUGGESTED READING

1. Kliegman R. Nelsons Textbook of Pediatrics, First South Asian edition. India: Elsevier; 2016.
2. Pataki C, Sirotnak AP. Medspace. Updated on Nov 05, 2018.
3. Tasker RC, McClure RJ, Acerini CL. Oxford Handbook of Paediatrics, 2nd edition. UK: Oxford University Press; 2013.
4. Venkateshwar V, Raghu Raman TS. Failure to thrive. Med J Armed Forces India. 2000;56(3): 219-24.

Worm Infestation

SA Krishna, Madhu Sinha

INTRODUCTION

Helminthiasis or worm infestation is any macroparasitic disease of humans and other animals in which a part of the body is infected with parasitic worms known as Helminthes. It continues to be among the common diseases affecting children from low- and middle-income countries.

Major groups of worm infestations of public health importance include Nematodes (*Ascaris* or roundworm, *Enterobiasis* or pinworm, *Ancylostoma* or hookworm and *Trichuris* or whipworm and threadworm, etc.), Cestodes (Tapeworm), and Trematodes (Flukes, uncommon in children).

SYMPTOMS

- Most of these infections are mild and remain unnoticed.
- Moderate-to-heavy infestations produce symptoms such as loss of appetite, nausea, vomiting, abdominal pain, perianal itching, growth faltering anemia, and malnutrition. Pulmonary symptoms such as cough and breathlessness and seizures are also observed.

MODES OF TRANSMISSION

The simplest is by accidental ingestion of infective eggs (*Ascaris, Echinococcus, Enterobius, Trichuris*) or larvae (some hookworms). Other worms have larvae that actively penetrate the skin (hookworms, schistosomes, *Strongyloides*). In several cases, infection requires an intermediate host vector; in some cases, the larvae are contained in the tissues of the intermediate host and are taken in when a human eats that host (*Clonorchis* in fish, tapeworms in meat and fish, *Trichinella* in meat).

DIAGNOSIS

These infestations pose difficulty in diagnosis due to lack of trained personnel and technology and also due to intermittent shedding of eggs and larvae.

- *Conventional methods*:
  - Stool examination for adult worms and their segments and microscopy for different ova and cyst anal swab are done.
  - Stool culture is mainly used for isolating *Strongyloides stercoralis* which is viviparous Hookworm is artificially cultured in laboratory to produce rhabditiform larvae.
  - *Hemogram*: It is done for eosinophilia, mainly associated with ascariasis, trichuriasis, strongyloidiasis, and Hookworm infestation. Low hemoglobin and low ferritin are observed.
  - Occult blood test in stool is done in the case of chronic Hookworm infestation.
- *Serology-based assays*:
  - Mainly in situations where fecal samples are not available
  - Antigen detection assay and antibody detection assay
  - *Drawback*: Invasive and persistence of infection even after infection is over.
- *Molecular-based approaches*: Rapid detection and accurate quantification of helminthic eggs.
- *Radiological findings*:
  - In ascariasis, worm intestinal tracks may be visualized. This may be particularly obvious when 2 worms are lying parallel, like "trolley car lines". Appendicitis and cholecystitis can also be seen. In hookworm infection, intestinal hypermotility, proximal jejunal dilatation, coarsening of the mucosal folds are seen.
  - *Contrast-enhanced computed tomography (CECT) head*: For ring enhancing lesion with or without perilesional edema in case of neurocysticercosis.

TREATMENT

Treatment of Neurocysticercosis

- *Antiparasitic drugs*: The use of these drugs is controversial. Parenchymal lesions resolve spontaneously with or without antiparasitic drugs. Subarachnoid shows better results with treatment.
  - *Albendazole*: Drug of choice—
    Dose: 15 mg/kg/d PO divided in two doses for 7 days
  - *Praziquantel*: 50–100 mg/kg/d in three divided doses for 28 days

TABLE 1: Helminths treatment—alternative drugs.

Ascaris	Albendazole 400 mg	• Piperazine citrate 15 mg/kg 12 hourly for 3 days • Ivermectin 200 µg/kg/d OD for 1–2 days orally once • Mebendazole 100 mg bid orally for 3 days or 500 mg once • Pyrantel pamoate 11 mg/kg once
Strongyloides	Ivermectin	• 200 µg/kg/day • Thiabendazole 50 mg/kg bid orally for 2 days Albendazole 400 mg once for 2 days
Enterobius	Pyrantel pamoate	• Ivermectin doses same • Mebendazole same doses • Albendazole same doses
Trichuris	Mebendazole	• Albendazole 400 mg once for 3 days • Ivermectin for 3 days (same doses) repeated after 2 weeks for 1–2 days
Hookworm	Albendazole	Pyrantel pamoate for 3 days (same doses) Mebendazole
Hymenolepis nana	Praziquantel 25 mg/kg orally	Albendazole for 3 days, Nitazoxanide 7.5 mg/kg bid orally for 3 days
Trichinella	Mebendazole 200–400 mg orally for 3 days, then 400–500 mg Tid for 10 days	Steroids for severe symptoms (doses same) once
Taeniasis	Praziquantel 5–10 mg/kg	Niclosamide 50 mg/kg orally once

- *Steroids*:
  - Prednisolone—2 mg/kg/d or oral dexamethasone—0.15 mg/kg/d concurrent with albendazole or starting albendazole on the 3rd day of corticosteroids
- *Anticonvulsants*:
  - Most associated seizures are readily controlled with standard anticonvulsants. Monotherapy is done with first-line anticonvulsant drug.
  - Carbamazepine and phenytoin are usually preferred. Antiepileptic drug can be withdrawn after 1 year of seizure free period if the lesion disappears and the EEG gets normal.
- *Broad-spectrum anthelmintics*: Albendazole and mebendazole:
  - First-line treatment of intestinal roundworm and tapeworm
  - *Pyrantel pamoate praziquantel*: Effective against *Taenia* and schistosomiasis
  - *Ivermectin*: Effective against adult and larval forms
  - *Artemisinin*: Emerging as drug of choice for trematodes
- *Helminths treatment—alternative drugs* **(Table 1)**
- *Surgical treatment*: Intestinal obstruction for removing worms from the biliary tree.
- *Preventive measures*:
  - Proper disposal of feces
  - *Personal protection*: Food, water, skin
  - *Personal hygiene*:
    - Washing hands after defecation
    - Nail cutting
    - Daily bathing
    - Avoiding scratching perianal region
- *Preventive chemotherapy*:
  - Deworming using Albendazole (400 mg) or Mebendazole (500 mg) is recommended as a public health intervention to all.
  - Young children 12–23 months of age, preschool children between 1 and 4 years of age, and school-age children 5–12 years living in areas where the baseline prevalence of any soil transmitted infection is 20% or more among children.
  - Deworming is to be done annually or biannually where the baseline prevalence is more than 50%.

KEY MESSAGES

- Helminthiasis continues to be common in children of low and middle income countries.
- Only moderate-to-heavy infestations produce symptoms.
- Lack of trained personnel and technology pose difficulty in diagnosis.
- Albendazole and mebendazole are the first line of treatment.
- Antiparasitic drugs are not always indicated in management of neurocysticercosis.

SUGGESTED READING

1. Bharti B, Bharti S, Khurana S. Worm infestation: diagnosis, treatment and prevention. Indian J Pediatr. 2018;85(11): 1017-24.
2. Helminthic infestations in children. [online] Available from: https://www.vims.ac.in/education/pdf/Helminthic-infestations-in-children.pdf. [Last accessed March, 2021).
3. Khurana S, Sethi S. Laboratory diagnosis of soil transmitted helminthiasis. Trop Parasitol. 2017;7(2):86-91.
4. Ndao M. Diagnosis of parasitic diseases: old and new approaches. Interdiscip Perspect Infect Dis. 2009;2009:278246.
5. World Health Organization. (2015). Investing to overcome the global impact of neglected tropical diseases. Third WHO Report on neglected diseases. [online] Available from: https://www.who.int/neglected_diseases/9789241564861/en/. [Last accessed March, 2021).

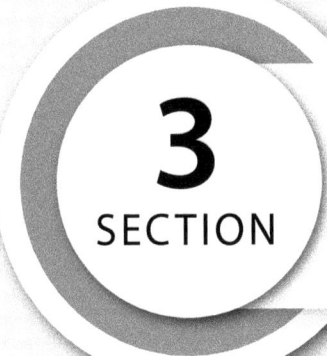

SECTION 3: Neonatology

10. Care of Normal Newborn
11. Minor Developmental Peculiarities of Newborn
12. Common Neonatal Problems
13. Common Feeding Problem
14. Crying Infant
15. Neonatal Sepsis
16. Neonatal Hypoglycemia
17. Neonatal Hypothermia
18. Therapeutic Hypothermia
19. Neonate Born of Mother with Chronic Systemic Disorder
20. Neonate Born of Mother with Maternal Infection
21. Neonatal Follow-up for Normal Newborn and Young Children
22. Follow-up of High-risk Newborn
23. Neonatal Thrombocytopenia
24. Neonatal Dermatosis
25. Newborn Screening Program

CHAPTER 10: Care of Normal Newborn

Akash Lalwani

GENERAL CONSIDERATION

A normal newborn is one who weighs >2,500 g, breathes normally and regularly, has warm trunk and soles (T: 36.5–37.4°C), pink in color (no central cyanosis), spontaneous body movements (active), and sucks actively on breast.

Basic needs at birth for the first few weeks of life are: Warmth, normal breathing, mother's milk, and protection from infection.

Warm Chain during Delivery

- Ensure the delivery room is warm (25°C) with no draughts.
- Dry the baby immediately; remove the wet cloth.
- Wrap the baby with clean dry cloth.
- Keep the baby close to the mother (ideally skin-to-skin) to stimulate early breastfeeding.
- Postpone bathing/sponging for 24 hours.

Warm Chain after Delivery

- Keep the baby clothed and wrapped with the head covered.
- Minimize bathing, especially in cool weather or for small babies.
- Keep the baby close to the mother.
- Use kangaroo mother care (KMC) for stable low birth weight (LBW) babies and for rewarming stable bigger babies.

In normothermic baby, both abdomen and feet are warm to touch; in a baby with cold stress, abdomen is warm but feet are cold to touch; in baby with moderate-to-severe hypothermia, both abdomen and feet are cold to touch. Heat loss occurs via four processes: (1) Radiation, (2) conduction, (3) convection, and (4) evaporation.

Method of Caring of LBW Babies

- Low birth weight babies account for nearly 40% of our institutional deliveries.
- Conventional care of LBW babies is expensive. KMC is an alternative, inexpensive, and baby- and mother-friendly method of care for the LBW babies.
- The infant is placed between mother's breasts in direct skin-to-skin contact and will be discharged on exclusive breastfeeding.

Kangaroo mother care is useful in caring of LBW infants below 2,000 g. It is a way to humanize high technology.

KMC has been shown to have benefits on:
- Breastfeeding
- Thermal control and metabolism
- Growth
- Satisfaction of senses of the baby
- Other effects.

Kangaroo mother care can be initiated in a baby who is otherwise stable but may still be on intravenous fluids, tube feeding, and/or oxygen.

Ensure that baby's neck is not too flexed or too extended, breathing is normal, feet and hands are warm during KMC.

When mother is not available, other family member such as grandmother, father or other relative can provide KMC.

Follow-up visit: The smaller the baby at discharge, the earlier and more frequent follow-up visits would be needed.
- One follow-up visit every 2 weeks period till weight of the baby is 3 kg.
- Thereafter one follow-up per month till 6 months of age.
- One follow-up every 3 months till 1 year of age.

Clean Chain

- Clean attendant's hands (washed with soap). Clean delivery surface.
- Clean cord-cutting instrument (i.e., razor, blade). Clean string to tie cord.
- Clean cloth to wrap the baby. Clean cloth to wrap the mother.

Tips for Infection Prevention

- All caregivers should wash hands before handling the baby.
- Feed only breast milk.
- Keep the cord clean and dry; do not apply anything.

- Use a clean cloth as a diaper/napkin.
- Wash your hands after changing diaper/napkin. Keep the baby clothed.
- Prevention of infection is more cost effective than treating infection in neonates.
- Person with active infection should not allowed to entry into the baby care area.
- 2-minute, hand washing (6 steps) to be done before entering the unit.
- 20-second hand washing to be done before and after touching babies.

Initiate breastfeeding within half an hour after birth. Exclusive breastfeeding should be given for the first 6 months of life; complimentary food should be started after 6 months of age.

Cord Care

- Put ties (using a sterile tie) tightly around cord at 2 cm and 5 cm from the abdomen.
- Cut between the ties with a sterile instrument (e.g., blade).
- Observe oozing of blood. If blood oozes, place a second tie between the skin and first tie.
- Do not apply any substance to the stump.
- Do not bind or bandage the stump.
- Leave the stump uncovered.

Eye Care

- Clean eyes immediately after birth with swab soaked in sterile water using separate swab for each eye. Clean from medial to lateral side.
- Give prophylactic eye drops within 1 hour of birth as per the hospital policy.
- Putting anything else in baby's eyes can cause infection.

Baby Bath

- First bath to be postponed for at least 24 hours or longer.
- At birth, the baby should be cleared off blood and meconium but not vernix.
- Bath them using lukewarm water only. Unmedicated soap should not be used.

Baby Massage

- Massage can be given from 3 to 4 weeks of life.
- Use nonirritating oil such as coconut oil. Do not use mustard oil.
- Massage improves the circulation in skin and muscles, gives comfort to child, and increases maternal bonding.

COMMON NEONATAL PROBLEMS

- Nasal block causes noisy breathing with excessive crying.
- Evening colic is associated with distended abdomen and inconsolable crying.
- Gastroesophageal reflux causes vomiting and crying.
- *Gastrocolic reflex*: Passage of stool after feeds.

Stools and Urine

- Most babies pass meconium by 24 hours.
- Most babies pass urine by 48 hours.
- Babies pass black tarry stools in first 2–3 days, then greenish stools for 1–2 days and then normal yellow stools.
- Babies usually pass urine 6–12 times a day.

Cephalohematoma

Fluctuant swelling, does not cross sutures, resolves spontaneously in few weeks.

Caput Succedaneum

Nonfluctuant, pitting swelling, not limited by sutures, resolves spontaneously in few days.

Subconjunctival Hemorrhage

It is a common finding in some babies; blood gets resolved spontaneously.

Vaginal Bleeding and Discharge

Menstrual-like bleeding or vaginal discharge occurs in one-fourth female babies on 3rd to 5th day. Bleeding or discharge lasts for 2–4 days. No treatment is required.

Nasolacrimal Duct Blockage

Wetness or watering from one or both eyes, eyes not congested.

Treatment: Lacrimal sac massage—15–20 times/day.

Mastitis Neonatorum

Engorgement of breasts on 3rd to 4th day. It lasts for few days or weeks. Squeezing should be avoided.

Neonatal Jaundice

- Most of the newborns develop yellow color of their skin (jaundice) after the first day.
- It appears on 2nd day, reaches a peak on 4th or 5th day and then disappears by 10th to 14th day.
- This is called physiological jaundice and usually it is self-limiting.

SUGGESTED READING

1. Singh M. Care of the Newborn, 8th edition. New Delhi: CBS Publishers Pvt Ltd; 2017.
2. Singh M. The Art and Science of Baby and Child Care, 4th edition. New Delhi: CBS Publishers Pvt Ltd; 2015.

11 Minor Developmental Peculiarities of Newborn

Sharja Phuljhele

INTRODUCTION

Minor developmental peculiarities of a newborn infant are very benign clinical conditions which hardly require any treatment. These are as given in the following text.

VOMITING

- Vomit on first day is due to irritation of stomach by swallowing of amniotic fluid.
- Vomiting soon after feed is due to faulty technique of feeding.
- The proper advice regarding feeding and burping must be imparted to all mothers.
- If vomiting persists for longer, it leads to some other conditions.

FAILURE TO PASS MECONIUM AND URINE

- Healthy babies must void within 24 hours of age.
- The babies pass black stools during first 2–3 days of life, followed by greenish stools for next 1–2 days.
- The nonpassage of meconium should be informed to the physician or other healthcare professionals.

CONSTIPATION

- Babies on cow's milk formula are often constipated due to hard-casein curds.
- Constipation is best managed by giving frequent breastfeeding.
- The laxatives should be avoided.

DIARRHEA

- The breastfeed babies develop increased frequency of stools if the mother is taking ampicillin, cephalosporins, tetracyclines, certain laxatives and following excessive consumption of foods with high organic acid content such as oranges, cherries, tomatoes, and chilies.
- The intake of large quantities of glucose, water, and honey by the baby may result in diarrhea.
- Diarrhea may also occur due to overfeeding or serious underfeeding.

PHYSIOLOGICAL JAUNDICE

- Physiological jaundice appears on the second day of birth reaches peak on the fourth or fifth day and disappears by 8–10 days.
- The best management for physiological jaundice is exposing the baby to sunlight for about 10–20 minutes. If necessary, phototherapy can be given.
- While exposing the baby to sunlight, baby's eyes and perineal area should be covered.

HICCUPS AND SNEEZING

- Hiccups are produced by spasmodic contractions of diaphragm and are characterized by sudden, noisy and jerky retractions of suprasternal notch and xiphisternal region. It occurs usually immediately after a feed due to distension of stomach and irritation of diaphragm.
- Sneezing occurs due to irritation of the nostrils by secretions. It should be sucked out by mucus sucker or using catheter.

FEVER

- During summer months when environmental temperature goes above 39°C, some healthy newborn babies may develop fever on the second or third day of life.
- The baby should be dressed with light and loose cotton clothes and the environment kept cool in summer.

EXCESSIVE CRYING

- The babies usually cry when they are hungry or discomfort.
- This may be due to unpleasant sensation of full bladder before passing urine, painful evacuation or hard stools or mere soiling by urine and stools.
- The insect bites should also be kept in mind as an important cause of night crying.

ORAL THRUSH

- The infection most commonly occurs during passage of the baby through infected birth canal.

- Infected feeding bottle, contaminated breast nipples, and prolonged antibiotic therapy may also result in candidiasis.
- The oral lesions are characterized by discrete white patches or spots over the buccal mucosa and gums.
- The baby may be able to suck normally but swallowing may be difficult due to posterior oropharyngeal white patches.
- Oral application of 0.5% solution of gentian violet after each feed gives prompt response in most cases.

EXCESSIVE SLEEPINESS

- Some babies may keep their eyes closed most of the time during the first 48 hours.
- During first few days, many infants go to sleep after taking only few sucks on the bottle or breast.
- The baby should be kept arouse during feed by tickling on the soles and behind the ears.
- Heavy maternal sedation during labor may be associated with excessive sleepiness in the baby for the first 48 hours.

MASTITIS NEONATORUM

- The enlargement of breasts occurs in full-term babies of both sexes on third or fourth day and may last for few days or even weeks.
- Lack of inactivation of progesterone and estrogen after birth due to immaturity of neonatal liver, leads to further rise in their levels thus resulting in hypertrophy of breasts.
- The local massage and fomentation should be curbed and mother reassured.

VAGINAL BLEEDING

- The development of menstrual-like withdrawal bleeding may occur in above one fourth of female babies after 3-5 days of birth.
- The bleeding is mild and lasts for 2-4 days. The local aseptic cleaning of genitals is advised.

CAPUT SUCCEDANEUM

- It is a boggy, diffuse, edematous swelling of soft tissues of scalp over the presenting part. The swelling is present at birth and its size and severity is related to the duration of labor.
- The swelling is pitting, nonfluctuant and not limited by sutures unlike cephal hematoma. It disappears spontaneously over next few days.

CEPHAL HEMATOMA

- It is subperiosteal collection of blood secondary to injury during delivery. The swelling appears after 2-3 days of birth. It is a fluctuant swelling and does not cross the suture line.
- It resolves spontaneously after a few days or weeks. Incision or aspiration is contraindicated unless it gets infected.

ASYMMETRIC HEAD SHAPE

Occiput or one of the parietal areas may become flat and bald. If head size is normal, there is no cause for concern. Proper positioning of head with support of soft pillows, to ensure that the prominent part of the head touches the cot, leads to gradual rounding of the head shape.

CRANIOTABES

Softening of skull bone which can be pressed like a table tennis ball is called craniotabes. Localized craniotabes may be normally seen due to in-utero pressure of the skull against mother's pubic bone.

SORE BUTTOCKS AND NAPKIN RASHES

- Use of nylon or watertight plastic napkins and delay in changing the napkins cause redness, induration, and excoriation due to ammoniacal dermatitis.
- The bottom should be cleaned gently with wet cotton and kept dry and exposed to air.
- Application of soothing ointment or coconut oil provides relief.

ERYTHEMATOXICUM

- It is erythematous rash with central pallor (wheal-like) appearing on the second or third day in term babies.
- The rash starts on the face and spreads to the trunk and extremities in about 24 hours.
- It disappears spontaneously after 2-3 days without any specific treatment.

HARLEQUIN COLOR CHANGE

The baby suddenly becomes blanched and pale on one half of the body while the other half remains pink. The episodes of color change last for a few minutes and occur in normal babies due to unexplained vasomotor phenomenon.

STORK BITES (SALMON PATCHES OR NEVUS SIMPLEX)

These are discrete pinkish-gray sparse capillary hemangiomata commonly located at nape of the neck, upper eyelids, forehead, and root of the nose. They invariably disappear after a few months.

SUBCONJUNCTIVAL HEMORRHAGE

Semilunar arcs of subconjunctival hemorrhage located at the outer canthus is a common finding in normal babies. The blood gets resorbed after a few days without leaving any pigmentation.

SUBCUTANEOUS FAT NECROSIS

- During early newborn period, some babies develop subcutaneous fat necrosis as localized areas of induration without any inflammatory signs over the buttocks, back, cheeks, or limbs.
- There is no clinical significance and the condition resolves spontaneously.

TONGUE TIE

- It may be either in the form of thin broad membrane or thick fibrous frenulum under the tongue with an orchard the tip of the tongue due to traction.
- Tongue tie interferes with sucking or delay the development of speech. The genuine tongue tie may be snipped after 3 months if it is a source of anxiety to the parents.

ACNE NEONATORUM

- Typical acne lesions may be seen over the forehead, nose, and cheeks at birth in term babies.
- They occur due to transplacental passage of maternal androgens to the fetus.
The skin lesions gradually diminish in size and disappear spontaneously within the next few days.

CONGENITAL TEETH

- The eruption of one or more lower incisor teeth before or soon after birth is seen in one in 4,000 babies.
- The teeth may become loose and interfere with breast-feeding. There is a risk of spontaneous dislodgement with aspiration. It is advised to get the natal teeth extracted.

CONGENITAL HYDROCELE

A small sac containing fluid may be noticed in one of the scrotal sacs at birth or during first week of life. It disappears spontaneously during first 3 months of life.

BOWED LEGS

In normal babies, when legs are extended, they form a concavity inward due to genu varus giving an appearance of bowed legs. It is not suggestive of rickets or bony deformity. After first birthday, bowing of legs is replaced by physiological knock knees.

UMBILICAL HERNIA

- When the cord has fallen off, umbilical hernia may manifest after the age of 2 weeks or later. It may be associated with divarication of recti. Most of these disappear spontaneously by 6 months to 1 year.
- Application of coin and bandage over the hernia is not recommended, as it may further weaken the anterior abdominal wall.
- Any associated conditions such as increased intra-abdominal pressure such as excessive crying, constipation, and persistent cough, should be identified and managed appropriately.

SUGGESTED READING

1. Singh M. Care of the Newborn, 8th edition. New Delhi: CBS Publishers Pvt Ltd; 2017.
2. Singh M. The Art and Science of Baby and Child Care, 4th edition. New Delhi: CBS Publishers Pvt Ltd; 2015.

CHAPTER 12: Common Neonatal Problems

Sharja Phuljhele

INTRODUCTION

Common neonatal problems are a unique spectrum encountered in a neonate. A large proportion of these are developmental and physiological, which require reassurance alone. They do not require investigations of any sort which may even prove detrimental. While, there are a few subtle signs which are the manifestations of serious underlying conditions, which require early diagnosis and treatment to reduce mortality and morbidity. Thus, the role of investigations and management of these problems is of paramount importance in the treatment and prognosis of certain common neonatal problems.

A GUIDE TO THE COMMON NEONATAL PROBLEMS SWELLING AND HEAD DEFORMITY

Most common causes for a baby presenting with swelling and deformity of the head are caput succedaneum, cephalhematoma, and subgaleal collection. A *"Caput succedaneum"* occurs due to injury to the scalp during delivery and is characterized by pitting edema of the scalp. This remains external to the periosteum and crosses suture lines of the skull bones, unlike *cephalhematoma,* where there is sub-periosteal collection of blood. These conditions are self-resolving, requiring nointervention and just need reassurance to the parents and attenders. However, conditions such as *subgaleal hemorrhages* are rare but potentially lethal. Early recognition and management in the form of massive blood transfusion is found to be of use.

MASTITIS NEONATORUM

"Mastitis neonatorum" is a condition which causes engorgement of breast due to the presence of maternal hormones. It is seen in both sexes and resolve in a few weeks. There is a need of reassurance alone.

MONGOLIAN SPOT

"Mongolian spot" is a bluish discoloration over the back and buttock or small "hemangioma" requiring reassurance alone.

UMBILICAL SWELLING

The causes for swelling at the umbilicus are umbilical hernia and umbilical granuloma:
- *Umbilical hernia* is generally small, and occasionally a large swelling around the umbilicus, which increases over a few weeks to months before disappearing on its own. However, surgical intervention might be necessary if it increases after 1 year of age or fails to disappear by 4 years of age.
- *Umbilical granuloma* manifests as a small flesh, like pale nodule at the base of umbilicus with persistent discharge. Management includes cauterization with silver nitrate or the application of common salt, which may have to be repeated every 3–4 days still the base is dry.

SWELLING IN GENITAL AREA

- The common causes of swelling in the genital area in a baby are hydrocele, scrotal swelling and inguinal hernia.
- Most of these swellings can be diagnosed clinically but ultrasonography helps us to identify torsion testis which is a surgical emergency. Hence, the investigation of choice is sonography and color Doppler sonography. It is a safe, fast, and effective tool to examine the scrotum and its contents. When the sonographic findings are equivocal, magnetic resonance imaging is employed.
- *Hydrocele* is a very common scrotal swelling, and often spontaneously resolves in the first year. However, if a communicating scrotal or spermatic cord hydrocele persists beyond 12–18 months, it is typically repaired surgically.
- *Neonatal testicular torsion:* The management remains controversial and depends on whether the testicular torsion occurred in the prenatal or postnatal setting. In prenatally torsed testis, often the only treatment offered is reassurance. Postnatal torsion is generally regarded as a surgical emergency and immediate surgery to salvage the affected testis and orchiopexy on the contralateral testis is performed.

- *Inguinal hernias* are common in boys, especially in premature neonates.

  Bowel enters the scrotal sac via a patent processus vaginalis, more commonly on the right side. It needs semiurgent surgery usually performed to prevent the theoretical risk of incarceration.

ICTERUS

Between 60 and 80% of healthy infants are expected to present with idiopathic neonatal jaundice. Neonatal jaundice is the discoloration of skin and sclera color to yellowish in a newborn by bilirubin, normally due to delayed maturity of hepatic enzymes. It usually occurs after 2-3 days of birth and disappears within 7-10 days. Most of these need reassurance alone. However, appearance of jaundice within 24 hours and that lasting for >2 weeks is considered pathological jaundice and mandates further investigation. Caution should be taken in case of low birthweight baby and G6PD deficiency.

RASH

The most common innocuous rash in the neonatal period is erythematoxicum and miliria.
- *"Erythema toxicum"* is characterized by a reddish flat rash over the face and trunk. It has an unknown etiology and appears on the 2nd to 3rd day of life and resolves spontaneously within the next 2-3 days. This needs reassurance alone.
- *"Miliaria"* is a condition where eruptions are seen in intertriginous areas, face, scalp as a result of obstructed sweat glands. These should be differentiated from other conditions such as neonatal acne, seborrheic dermatitis and melanosis which require specific treatment.

VAGINAL BLEEDING

Vaginal bleeding is rare and occurs as a result of maternal hormone withdrawal in female babies and requires reassurance alone.

REGURGITATION

Regurgitation in infants is physiological and most are happy and healthy even if they frequently spit up or vomit (*"Happy Spitters"*), and babies usually outgrow GER (gastroesophageal reflux) by their first birthday. These patients have no underlying predisposing factors or conditions, growth and development are normal, and pharmacologic treatment is typically not necessary. These "Happy Spitters" should be differentiated from pathological gastroesophageal reflux disease or GERD, who frequently experience complications, requiring careful evaluation and treatment.

BREAST MILK DIARRHEA

Frequent passage of semi-liquid stools up to 20-25/day, is erroneously termed as "breast milk diarrhea." If the baby has adequate weight gain and frequent urination, it requires reassurance alone. Likewise, infrequent stooling in the absence of inadequate weight gain needs no intervention.

CRYING INFANT

Crying is part of the normal development of a baby and is a form of communication with their caregivers. It is nonspecific, caused by different stimuli, such as hunger, manifestation of discomfort or pain or simply the baby's need to approach the caregiver for emotional comfort and safety.

Occasional crying for no obvious reason in the evening is termed as "evening colic" and is managed by sedatives.

ABNORMAL MOVEMENTS

Some babies usually make abnormal movements and noises while asleep.

Jitteriness, startle response, benign nocturnal myoclonus and Moro reflex which are benign conditions, may be confused as convulsions. Video recording and EEG are sometimes necessary in case of doubtful abnormal movements or subtle convulsions.

CRYING BEFORE MICTURITION

Due to unpleasant sensation of full bladder or passage of hard stools, babies often cry just before micturition or defecation. This requires reassurance alone.

EPIPHORA

Persistent watering from one or both eyes in the absence of congestion might be due to blockage of nasolacrimal duct. The area between the eye and the root of the nose is firmly massaged with the help of a finger and thumb, with inner pressure exerted from above downward along the lateral margin of the nose. This is done 15-20 times, at least three times a day and is continued for 1-2 months or till watering disappears. If the duct remains closed after 5-6 months, probing and syringing through the punctum is done.

FREQUENT STOOLS

Babies are known to pass stools right after feeding due to exaggerated gastrocolic reflex and it is considered a normal behavior. The condition requires reassurance alone.

CLUMSY BABY

Babies keep their eyes closed for most of the times during the first 48 hours of birth. In the initial few days, infants go to sleep after only a few sucks of breastfeeding and they should be kept awake by tickling their toes or behind the ears. Heavy maternal sedation during labor, likewise barbiturates, bromides, and opioid intake in nursing mothers is usually associated with excessive sleepiness. In a previously active and alert baby, lethargy and lack of interest in feeds is an important and serious sign of systemic disease.

CRADLE CAP

It might be a case of cradle cap characterized by crusting over the scalp, which may lead to development of seborrheic dermatitis during early infancy.

Shampoo with savlon or cetrimide can be applied over the scalp. This is followed by gradual resolution.

NATAL VERSUS NEONATAL TEETH

This is a rare condition when the baby has teeth at birth (natal teeth) or they erupt within 30 days of birth (neonatal teeth). They often represent primary dentition, but are smaller, conical, yellowish with poor/absent root formation. They are usually asymptomatic requiring no intervention; however, difficulty and discomfort during suckling, sublingual ulceration, and laceration over mother's breast mandates extraction of teeth.

PHYSIOLOGICAL EXFOLIATION

This is usually seen in post-term babies, who present with dry skin and exaggerated transverse skin creases. This can be managed by application of paraffin, olive oil and glycerine.

SNEEZES, YAWNS, AND HICCUPS

The above are normal responses in a newborn. Hiccups tend to occur usually after feeds, due to a distended stomach and irritation of diaphragm. Sneezing is usually due to irritation of nostrils due to secretions. Most healthy babies yawn before and after sleep.

INFREQUENT STOOLS

Often the babies on cow's milk and formula feeds are constipated. If the baby passes stools at a gap of 2–3 days, the parents may be reassured. But, if the infrequency of passing stools is greater than 5 days, the clinician should arouse suspicion toward the diagnosis of Hirschsprung's disease.

Most of the complaints that are encountered in neonates are usually brought to the notice by keen observation by mothers, who stay worried because of minor peculiarities. Many of these conditions are developmental and physiological variations and require reassurance and proper advice alone. Thus, a proper understanding of the most common neonatal problems is essential to differentiate between minor variations and subtle signs of serious systemic pathologies.

SUGGESTED READING

1. Amir LH. Management of common lactation and breastfeeding problem In: Jatoi I, Kaufmann M (eds). Management of Breast Diseases. Berlin, Heidelberg: Springer; 2016.
2. Martin RJ, Fanaroff AA. Fanaroff and Martin's Neonatal Perinatal Medicine Diseases of the Fetus and Infant, 11th edition. Netherlands: Elsevier; 2019.
3. Meek JY. New Mother's Guide to Breastfeeding. USA: American Academy of Pediatrics; 2017.
4. Singh M. Care of the Newborn, 8th edition. New Delhi: CBS Publishers Pvt Ltd; 2017.
5. Singh M. The Art and Science of Baby and Child Care, 4th edition. New Delhi: CBS Publishers Pvt Ltd; 2015.
6. World Health Organization. WHO global strategy on infant and young child feeding. Geneva: World Health Organization; 2009.

13 CHAPTER: Common Feeding Problem

Shilpa Bhargava

INTRODUCTION

The act of breastfeeding, one of nature's most rewarding and beneficial processes, can sometimes seem intimidating, especially during first few weeks of motherhood. Breastfeeding is a natural act, as well as a learned behavior which both the mother and the baby have to learn.

"I think my baby is not getting enough milk" is one of the most common problems with which the mother steps in the OPD.

Apart from this, there are many more problems which hinder the breastfeeding and create discomfort to mother and baby and become a reason to terminate breastfeeding or switch over to top feed.

To get rid of common feeding problem, the mainstay is still a good position and attachment of breastfeed baby. The solution of common problems of feeding is not so uncommon. Let's have a look at some of them.

REGURGITATION

Most healthy babies regurgitate some curdled milk after some feed but gain weight satisfactorily, the reason being the swallowed air during feeding causes distension and discomfort.

Solution:
- Burping after every feed.
- Put the baby to bed in the right lateral position with head ends lightly raised.

ENGORGEMENT OF BREAST

The breast becomes heavy, swollen, hard, red and painful on third or fourth day after delivery.

It becomes engorged because of infrequent and ineffective feeding.

Solution:
- Best treatment is early and frequent feeding.
- Analgesic to relieve pain.
- Congestion is relieved by expressing milk between feeding either manually or by breast pump and by warm compresses.
- *In severe engorgement*: Cold compresses between feeding, and gel packs/ice packs are used for relief is comfortable and reduces welling.
- Chilled cabbage leaves with hole in the center can be placed over breast to relieve pain and swelling.
- Engorgement can lead to plugged duct or mastitis if not treated.

SORE OR CRACKED NIPPLE

It may be caused by:
- Poor attachment—most common cause
- Wrong nursing position
- Not taking care of nipples.

Solution:
- Continue breastfeeding.
- Apply "hind milk" after nursing. It contains fat and anti-infective substance which acts as a emollient and helps in healing.
- In dry climate, emollient creams, i.e., (ultrapurified medical-grade lanolin) over nipples in between feeds can help.
- Usage of nursing bra with a breast shell to avoid pressure over tender nipple.
- Avoid frequent washing of breast with soap to prevent dryness.
- Avoid plastic breast shield and plastic-lined nursing pads, as it can hold in moisture.

FLAT/RETRACTED NIPPLE

- Flat nipples may be almost indistinguishable from areola or protrude only slightly with stimulation.
- Inverted nipple retracts inward, rather than becoming erect when the areola is compressed.
- Proper latch on is difficult.
- May lead to complications such as engorgement and sore nipple.

Solution:
- In case of flat nipples, a nipple shield may be helpful in getting proper latch on nipple rolling for nipple protrusion, have no effect.

- Manual/electric breast pumps can be used to draw nipple out before breastfeeding.
- Syringing is the most useful method to treat inverted/flat nipple.
- Compress the areola to make nipple as erect as possible before feeding.

LATCHING PAIN

Pain in breast is experienced during feeding due to poor attachment.

Solution: Proper position and good attachment.

CLOGGED DUCTS

Sometimes a tender localized lump in one breast with redness may appear discomfort during breastfeeding. This lump may result of a clogged milk duct which can be due to infrequent feeds, poor attachment, tight clothing, and sore nipple.

Solution:
- Encourage frequent feeding.
- Ensure good attachment **(Box 1)**.
- Different feeding position to allow better drainage of affected area.
- Application of warm moist towels on the affected breast, followed by gentle massage.
- Before each feed, gently massage the breast from outside toward nipple.
- If not treated well may lead to breast infection.

MASTITIS

It is bacterial infection of breast tissue. The causes are:
- Insufficient drainage of breast
- Infrequent feeding or long gap between feeds
- Poor attachment
- Unrelieved engorgement
- Tight clothing
- It is usually caused by milk stasis, which results in noninfective inflammation and if the stasis persists, it becomes infected.

Usually affect only a part of one breast unlike engorgement where whole of both breasts are affected.

> **BOX 1:** Key points of proper nursing position and good attachment.
>
> - *Key points of proper nursing position*:
>   - The baby's head and body should be in a straight line.
>   - His face should face the breast, with his nose opposite to the nipple.
>   - His mother should hold his body close to hers.
> - *Key points of good attachment*:
>   - Baby's chin is close to the breast.
>   - Baby's mouth is wide open.
>   - Lower lip is turned everted.
>   - Much of the areola is inside the baby's mouth.

Symptoms

It causes flu-like symptoms of fever, chills, headache, nausea, and malaise along with local breast symptoms of redness, tenderness, swelling, heat, and pain.

Treatment
- Continue breastfeeding
- Milk removal (by feeding or pumping)
- Warm compresses
- Antibiotics such as amoxicillin
- Rest, plenty of fluids and analgesics.

LEAKING BREAST

While feeding from one breast, the milk from other breast drips or leaks or when something stimulate letdown reflex like another baby crying. It is very common and usually settles down within first 4–6 weeks.

Solution:
- Counseling of mother
- Washable nursing pads are advisable
- Frequent feeding.

STRONG LETDOWN REFLEX

It causes a rush of milk along with oversupply of milk.

Infant tries to gulp down milk very fast, sometimes results in choking, coughing, or sputtering.

Solution:
- Ask mother to hold the nipple between index and middle finger to reduce the force of milk ejection by light compression on milk ducts.
- Break off the latch and allow the baby to come on and off the breast at will to avoid choking, sputtering, and coughing.
- Nurse the infant in a semiupright position.

Solution:
- Breastfeed on one side for each feeding.
- Gradually increase the time/feeding.
- Express milk manually to relieve pressure before breastfeed.
- To prevent aggressive sucking, feed the baby before he becomes overly hungry.

SLEEPY BABY

- Typically occurs in first week of life
- Misleads the mother to assume that baby has had satisfied feeds
- To ensure an adequate milk supply, baby should be aroused during the feeds or for feeds if the interval between the two feeds is longer than 3 hours.

Solution: To wake up a sleepy baby:

- Stimulate him by rubbing his back or placing on the bare chest.
- Tickle the soles.
- If falls asleep latching, compress the breast to ensure more milk flow or gently rub on pinna to arouse the baby.

ORAL THRUSH

- White spots inside cheeks and over the tongue look like milk curd.
- Caused by fungus *Candida albicans*, which often follows the use of antibiotics in the baby or in the mother.
- It may result in difficulty in breastfeeding.

Management:
- *Gentian violet paint*: Apply 0.25% to baby's mouth daily for 5 days or until 3 days after lesion heals.
- *Nystatin suspension (100,000 IU/mL)*: Apply 1 mL by dropper by baby's mouth four times daily after breastfeeds for 7 days.

NIPPLE CONFUSION

- It starts when the baby is offered one to two bottle feeds along with breastfeeds.
- Mechanisms for sucking from breast and rubber teat of feeding bottle are different. Bottle feeding is easier as the baby can readily get the milk by pressing the soft rubber teat, while breastfeeding requires considerable effort and coordination.
- When the baby is offered both the options, he refuses to breastfeed as it needs more effort and start sucking and biting at nipple with unsatisfactory effort. This is due to "nipple confusion."
- To avoid it, bottle feeding should be discouraged.

NOT ENOUGH MILK

The most common complaint of mothers: A practical approach if mother says that she does not have enough milk would be as following:
- Decide whether the baby is getting enough milk or not
- To evaluate reasons of not enough milk
- Management of underlying cause.

To decide that the baby is getting sufficient milk, ask the mother about:
- Weight gain of baby
- Urine output
- Breastfeeding frequency.

Perceived insufficiency: If a baby is gaining weight according to the expected growth velocity and is passing dilute urine six or more times in 24 hours, then milk intake is adequate. It is only the mother's presumption of not having enough milk. This condition is called perceived insufficiency.

Situations which make a mother to think that her breast milk is insufficient are:
- A crying baby not to be satisfied with feeds
- Baby's demand to feed very often and for a long time
- The breast is feeling soft
- Not being able to express her milk.

Management
- Counseling and reassurance
- *Low breast milk intake*: Two reliable signs indicating not enough milk:
  1. Poor weight gain
  2. Low urine output
  Reasons for baby not getting enough milk are summarized in **Table 1**.

To evaluate the cause for low milk supply:
- Take proper history and observe breastfeeding.
- Newborn examination regarding the growth parameters, complete general examination, oromotor dysfunction, etc.
- Maternal examination, particularly local examination of breast.
- Look for mother's confidence, motivation, and knowledge regarding breastfeeding.
- Evaluate other factors such as stress, overwork, fatigue, or medication.

MANAGEMENT

Most milk insufficiency is due to unrealistic expectation and mismanagement of breastfeeding. Approximately only <2%

TABLE 1: Reasons for baby not getting enough milk.

Breastfeeding factors	Mother: Psychological factors	Mother: Physical conditions
Delayed start	Lack of confidence	Contraceptive pills
Infrequent feeds	Depression	Severe malnutrition
No night feeds	Worry, stress	Alcohol
Short feeds		Smoking
Poor attachments		Pituitary failure (rare)
Bottles, pacifiers		Poor breast development (rare)
Prelacteal feeds		

of mothers have true milk insufficiency. Most of the reasons can be allayed by taking simple measures such as:
- Proper technique of breastfeeding.
- Good attachment and nursing position.
- Frequent feeding.
- Encourage night feed.
- No prelacteals and supplements, only exclusive breastfeeding.
- Counsel mother for feeding from one breast for 12–15 minutes, so the baby gets fore and hind milk both, resulting in proper growth.
- Encourage mother to take rest and stay relaxed.
- Elicit family support to her.
- Boosting up her confidence.
- Avoid smoking and alcohol and take care of nutrition.
- *Role of galactogogues*: These are substan-ces credited to enhance milk production. Best form of lactogogue is suckling at the breast; in ayurvedic system, large number of food items, herbs such as fenugreek seeds, fennel, Tulsi seeds, alfalfa, etc., are considered as galactogogues and are also available in form of capsules, granules, and powder. Its role is not fully proven. Effect is mainly psychological. Drugs such as metoclopramide also have been tried as galactogogues.

CONCLUSION

If we practitioner really want to help mothers to establish breastfeeding, the best way is to teach proper technique of breastfeeding. Listen and answer queries and worries satisfactorily. Repeated counseling sessions in follow-up will help to establish art of breastfeeding and to combat common feeding problems.

KEY MESSAGES

- Breastfeeding is a natural act but also a learned behavior.
- Problems related to breastfeeding are common and treatable.
- Proper attachment or "latchment" is indeed the key for successful feeding.
- Most problems can be corrected by proper feeding technique.
- Counseling plays an important role.

SUGGESTED READING

1. Amir LH, Livingstone VH. Management of common lactation and breastfeeding problem. Management of breast disease. 2016:81-104.
2. Meek JY, Yu W. New Mother's Guide to Breastfeeding, 3rd edition. USA: Bantam; 2017.
3. Shelov SP, Altmann TR. Caring for Your Baby and Young Child: The Complete and Authoritative Guide, 7th edition. USA: Bantam; 2019.
4. Singh M. Care of the Newborn, 8th edition. New Delhi: CBS Publishers; 2017.
5. Singh M. The Art and Science of Baby and Child Care, 4th edition. New Delhi: CBS Publishers; 2015.
6. World Health Organization. (2009). WHO global strategy on infant and young child feeding. [online] Available from: https://www.who.int/whosis/whostat/2009/en/. [Last accessed May, 2021].

CHAPTER 14: Crying Infant

Prachi Bichpuria

INTRODUCTION

- Infants cannot speak and cry is their only language to express their needs and draw attention. Newborns are transitioning from life in the womb to the external environment.
- Infants cry as a response to an internal or external stimulus and is a form of basic instinctive communication. On any given day, a newborn might cry for up to 2 hours or even longer. Up to 27% of parents describe problems with infant crying in the first 4 months and up to 38% identify a problem with their infant crying within the first year.
- Parents can be concerned about the amount of time that their infant cries, how the infant can be consoled, and disrupted sleeping patterns.
- A cry that starts slowly and builds up to a loud rhythm usually indicates a hunger cry, while a cry of pain might be a sudden, long, high-pitched shriek. Picking upon any patterns can help better respond to baby's cries.

DECODING THE TEARS

- Periodic crying in infants is most commonly due to hunger, thirst, wet nappies, and boredom. An intelligent mother can differentiate whether baby is crying due to hunger, discomfort, or mere sleepiness.
- Many babies cry before passing urine, become quiet while passing urine and again start crying. It is normal and should not be considered as a sign of discomfort.
- Most infants cry while falling asleep. Babies may cry due to fatigue or overstimulation. Some babies are happy-go-lucky while others are sensitive, very demanding and easily frustrated. Babies also cry when they are cold or overclothed.
- Excessive cry and irritability may be due to teething, blocked nose, bodyache, viral infections, otitis media, infection in any part of the body or unrecognized injury like pulled elbow or shoulder. Most babies are comforted when picked up and cuddled but if they become more uncomfortable on picking up, it indicates painful condition involving limbs, joints or bones. Babies with diarrhea cry out of thirst rather than intestinal colic.
- Many babies develop excessive and inconsolable cry after receiving the shot of DTwP (diphtheria, tetanus toxoids and whole-cell pertussis); these babies should not be given whole-cell pertussis vaccine, instead vaccination should be completed with acellular pertussis vaccine (DTaP) or dual antigen (DT).
- Inconsolable cry when associated with swelling of one testis suggests torsion of testis and is an emergency. When cry is inconsolable in presence of fever and refusal to feeds, it suggests serious condition of the baby.
  Crying and fussiness while feeding is suggestive of teething, nose block, thrush and aphthous ulcers.
- Always search for "Red Flag" in a crying infant (**Box 1**). The presence of any of the symptoms to do thorough examination and refer to pediatric hospital for workup and admission.

BOX 1: Red flag signs in excessively crying infant.
- Fever high-grade
- Off feeds and lethargy
- Abnormal activity
- Sweating, poor weight gain
- Suspicious trauma, unexplained bruising
- Tachycardia > 180/min
- Passing blood in stool
- Vomiting which is bilious
- AF full and tense
- Not moving a limb

TYPES OF CRIES

Hunger Cry

It is feed time. Baby starts crying slowly in rhythmic and repetitive manner which builds up a loud rhythm if not attended to. Baby becomes quiet while and after the feed.

Cry of Discomfort

- Baby with wet nappy strains and becomes restless with wriggling movements of legs. Change of nappy provides immediate relief.
- Tired, sleepy, and bored baby.
- Cry starts as grizzle which then increases in intensity. It is usually associated with yawning and rubbing of eyes and baby slowly dozes off to sleep.

Cry of Pain

The cry is intense, high pitched, and persistent and baby is inconsolable. It may be temporarily relieved on picking up and cuddling. If it worsens on picking up, it suggests painful condition of limbs, joints, or bones.

Colicky Baby

The episodes of colic are common in the evening or night. The baby screams loudly and draws legs toward abdomen writhing in pain. Rocking, patting, and placing the baby on tummy may provide relief.

Night Crying

During the first few weeks of life, most babies sleep during the day and are awake and playful during the night. This is probably due to continuation of their in utero pattern of activity. Infants are not aware of the day and night and even physiological whimpering due to hunger and wet napkin appears too loud and disturbing to the tired parents during the night. Gastroesophageal reflux disease (GERD) is an important cause of night crying. Excessive crying may occur due to cold, overclothing or insect bite. Night crying may also occur due to pinworms, nappy rash, and blocked nose.

Infantile Colic

- The conventional definition of colic given by *Wessel's* "Rule of three." *(Any healthy baby with crying spells that occur for at least 3 hours a day, three times in a week for 3 consecutive weeks. They thrive well and are healthy). Recently a modified Wessel's Rule of three has been described*:
  1. Paroxysm of irritability, fussing, or crying that occurs without a cause.
  2. Episodes lasting 3 or more hours per day and occurring at least 3 days per week for at least 1 week.
  3. Absence of failure to thrive.
- It is the most common cause of unexplained crying in infants between 2 and 8 weeks of age. The spells occur every day at the same time in a clockwise manner. The infant cries loudly and pulls his legs over the abdomen, gurgling sound may be felt by placing hands over the abdomen and infant may pass flatus to get temporary relief.
- Excessive crying leads to further swallowing of air which initiates *colic-crying-colic cycle*. This episode lasts for 2–3 hours until infant is tired and falls asleep. This crying spells usually disappears by 12 weeks of age. The frequency seems equal in breastfed and bottle-fed babies.
- The exact cause of evening colic is not known but may be due to intestinal colic, milk allergy, over sensitive or overactive baby, excessive stimulation by parents or grandparents, parental anxiety and emotional tension at home.

MANAGING TRICKS

- Whenever baby cries check whether he is hungry or nappy is wet.
- Infant should be picked up and hand can be gently rubbed over his head or tummy. Cuddling with gentle rhythmic rocking movements helps. Some parents are hesitant to console a crying infant out of fear of spoiling the baby. It is important to remember that baby cannot be spoilt with love and care during the first 6 months of life, so one has to be compassionate and caring while consoling a crying infant.
- One has to make sure baby is not cold or overclothed or crying as a result of insect bite or out of pain and discomfort.
- *Paracetamol* can be safely given to relief the discomfort due to teething, inflammatory painful condition or unrecognized trauma.
- Application of *soothing cream or coconut oil* over the anus is useful in relieving perianal itching.
- Infant with evening colic will get temporary relief by rhythmic rocking, gentle massage over abdomen, placing him on his tummy over the lap, cycling movements of legs, singing or talking softly or by taking the baby for a walk on stroller or going for drive in a car.
- *Antispasmodic drops*: The *Simethicone drops* (40 mg) or *Fennel oil* (0.0007 mL) has often being prescribed by practitioner. However the studies on simethicone has shown no proven benefit. *Dicyclomine* drops are contraindicated in infants below 6 months of age. Recently *Lactobacillus reuteri* when given for 21 days, has shown significant reduction of crying episode. The use of *proton pump inhibitors* must be discouraged unless there is evidence of GER.
- There is no need to change the type or mode of feeding but attempts should be made to reduce the environmental stress and decrease the stimulation of the infant.
- Those who realize that an infant can be in a situation where abuse is a possibility, support can be offered to give a parent or caregiver a break when needed.
- Crying is a normal behavior in infants and will subside at some point. Parents can be encouraged to take a calming break if needed while the baby is safe in the crib.

SUGGESTED READING

1. Biagioli E, Tarasco V, Lingua C, Moja L, Savino F. Pain-relieving agents for infantile colic. Cochrane Database Syst Rev. 2016;9(9): CD009999.
2. Cook F, Seymour M, Giallo R, Cann W, Nicholson JM, Green J et al. Comparison of methods for recruiting and engaging parents in online interventions: study protocol for the cry baby infant sleep and settling program. BMC Pediatrics. 2015;(1):174.
3. Ismail J, Nallasamy K. Crying infant. Indian J Pediatr. 2017; 84(10):777-81.
4. Johnson JD, Cocker K, Chang E. Infantile colic: recognition and treatment. American Family Physician. 2015;92(7):577-82.
5. Kaley F, Reid V, Flynn E. The psychology of infant colic: a review of current research. Infant Ment Health J. 2011;32(5):526-41.
6. Kliegman RM, St. Geme J. Nelsons Textbook of Pediatrics, 21st edition. US: Elsevier; 2019.
7. Singh M. Care of the Newborn, revised 8th edition. New Delhi: CBS Publishers; 2017.
8. Singh M. The Art and Science of Baby and Child Care, 4th edition. New Delhi: CBS Publishers; 2015.

15 CHAPTER

Neonatal Sepsis

Anil K Goel, Seema Shah, Prakash G Mathew

INTRODUCTION

Neonatal sepsis is one of the leading causes of neonatal mortality and morbidity among term and preterm infants in low- and middle-income countries due to poor hygiene and suboptimal practices for infection control. Although improvements in neonatal intensive care has decreased the impact of early-onset sepsis in term infants, preterm infants remain at high risk for both early-onset sepsis and its sequelae. Sepsis-related mortality is largely preventable with timely recognition, rational antimicrobial therapy, and aggressive supportive care.

Epidemiology

Estimating the burden of neonatal infections in developing countries is difficult because of factors such as more number of home deliveries and hospital-based statistics does not represent a true burden of sepsis in the community.

Population-based studies from developing countries have reported clinical sepsis rates ranging from 49 to 170 per 1,000 live births. The neonatal mortality rate in India is 23 per 100 live births and neonatal sepsis is the third leading cause of neonatal mortality, next to prematurity and perinatal complications.

The proportion of early-onset sepsis in India ranges from 10.4 to 85.0%. The incidence of culture-positive sepsis ranged from 16 to 54%.

Definition

Neonatal sepsis is a clinical syndrome characterized by signs and symptoms of infection with or without accompanying bacteremia in the neonatal period.

It encompasses various systemic infections of newborn such as septicemia, meningitis, pneumonia, and urinary tract infections.

Local infections, i.e., superficial infections such as conjunctivitis and oral thrush are not usually included under neonatal sepsis.

Classification of Sepsis in Nutshell

Neonatal sepsis can be classified into two major categories, early onset sepsis and late onset sepsis, depending upon the onset of symptoms. **Table 1** provides points of differentiation among them.

TABLE 1: Classification of neonatal sepsis and its differentiation.

	Early-onset sepsis	Late-onset sepsis
Onset	Within 72 hours of life	After 72 hours to 28 days of life, but young infants up to 120 days of life should be screened and managed as per LONS guidelines unless proved otherwise
Source	Vertical transmission via maternal genital tract	Hospital or community
Presentation	Respiratory/pneumonia	Septicemia/meningitis/pneumonia
Etiology	Group B *Streptococcus*, *Escherichia coli*	CONS, *Klebsiella*
Indian set up	• *Staphylococcus aureus* • *Klebsiella* spp. • *E. coli* • *Pseudomonas aeruginosa* • *Listeria monocytogenes*	• *S. aureus* • Nonhemolytic *Streptococcus* • *Klebsiella* spp. • *E. coli* • *P. aeruginosa* • Untyped gram-negative • Nonfermenting • Gram-negative

(LONS: late-onset neonatal sepsis ; CONS: coagulase-negative *Staphylococcus*)

RISK FACTORS

Early-onset Sepsis

Perinatal factors:
- Preterm premature rupture of membranes
- Prolonged rupture of membranes (>18 hours)
- Prolonged duration of labor (>18 hours)
- More than or equal to three per vaginal examinations
- *Chorioamnionitis*: Intrapartum temperature >100.4°F with any two features (fetal tachycardia/foul smelling/ liquor/uterine tenderness/maternal TLC >15,000)
- Maternal fever during delivery (higher than 38°C)

Other possible associations:
- Prematurity (gestational age less than 37 weeks)
- Low birth weight (<2,500 g)
- Perinatal asphyxia (APGAR <4 at 1 minute)
- Discarding of colostrum and use of prelacteal feeds
- Intrapartum antibiotic administration
- Immunodeficiency states
- Inborn errors of metabolism (IEM, e.g., galactosemia).

Late-onset Sepsis

- Low birth weight
- Breakage of natural barriers (skin and mucosa)
- Prolonged use of an indwelling catheter
- Invasive procedures (e.g., endotracheal intubation)
- Skin integrity breach, e.g., needle pricks or intravenous (IV) fluids
- Necrotizing enterocolitis
- Prolonged use of antibiotics.

Risk Factors for Nosocomial Infection

- Neonatal intensive care unit (NICU) setting
- Not receiving maternal breast milk
- Prolong use and unhygienic indwelling catheter
- Total parenteral nutrition
- Surgical problems and complications.

WHEN TO SUSPECT NEONATAL SEPSIS IN A NEONATE IN AN EMERGENCY ROOM?

Based on history:
- Possible risk factors and associations
- History of colostrum discard and use of prelacteal feeding
- Temperature instability such as fever or marbling of skin in the absence of hypothermia
- The definite focus of infection, e.g., branding, oozing umbilicus, or cellulitis
- Respiratory distress after 3 days of life
- Low leukocyte count at admission.

Detailed history including chief complaints and possible risk factors associated with sepsis have to be elicited as signs and symptoms are often subtle and nonspecific; hence, a high index of suspicion is required for early diagnosis of neonatal sepsis.

Based on physical findings:
- Abnormal breathing pattern as evident by mother or emergency physician, e.g., shallow breathing, increased or decreased rate breathing, increased efforts, or gasping respiration.
- Abnormal behavior as evident by high-pitched cry, irritability, seizures, lethargic, hypotonia, the mother feels that her kid is not doing well, bulging anterior fontanel.
- Abnormal circulation as evident by tachycardia, hypotension, prolonged capillary refill time, pallor, cyanosis, or mottling of the skin, petechiae.
- Nonspecific features include temperature instability (fever or hypothermia), refusal or poor feeding, vomiting, diarrhea, jaundice, abdominal distension, bleeding or pus from the umbilicus (periumbilical erythema/ tenderness), sclerema.

Red flags: Elicit focused history and perform a careful assessment for sources of bacteremia (the focus of infection) that includes meningitis, urinary tract infection, omphalitis, draining ears, discharging eyes, or skin infection to decide the possible organism and subsequent choice and duration of antibiotics.

CONDITIONS THAT MIMICS SEPSIS

Early-onset and late-onset sepsis mimics are given in **Tables 2 and 3**, respectively.

INVESTIGATIONS

Sepsis Screen

Components	Abnormal value
Absolute neutrophilic count	Low value 1,800/mm^3 (refer Manroe chart for term and Mouzinho's chart for VLBW infants)
Immature total neutrophilic count	>0.2
Micro-ESR	>15 mm in 1" hour
CRP	>1 mg/dL

- *C-reactive protein (CRP)*: It may not be elevated in early stages of infection due to the time taken for its synthesis in the liver and eventual appearance in the blood.
- *Procalcitonin (PCT)*: Plasma PCT levels increase 3–4 hours after exposure to bacterial agents and within 6–24 hours it reaches peak values. After 24 hours of age it then decreases and reaches normal values of below 0.5 ng/mL by 48–72 hours of age. No definite age-matched control values are available. At a cut-off value of 0.5 ng/mL for PCT and 10 mg/L for CRP, the sensitivity of PCT was found to be higher (77.5%) than that of CRP (66.3%) whereas specificity was 79.4% for PCT and 76.4% for CRP.

TABLE 2: Differential diagnosis of early onset sepsis.

Transient tachypnea of the newborn	Respiratory distress syndrome	Intracranial hemorrhage	Congenital cyanotic heart disease
• Near-term neonate, tachypnea with minimal or no respiratory distress • Improvement within 12–24 hours on minimal oxygen requirement (<40%), CXR reveals hyperinflation with patchy atelectasis	• Premature and low birth weight infants • Manifests immediately after birth, tachypnea with signs of respiratory distress, improvement gradually in 3 days with specific therapy	• Usually in preterm infants, less likely by trauma or asphyxia • Presentation with apnea, bradycardia, and seizures • History of assisted delivery • Intracranial USG is helpful	• Tachypnea, tachycardia, low saturation • Cyanosis, hyperoxia tests used to distinguish cyanotic heart disease from others

(CXR: chest X-ray; USG: ultrasonography)

TABLE 3: Differential diagnosis of late onset sepsis.

Necrotizing enterocolitis	Metabolic disease	Bowel obstruction
• Premature babies • Nonspecific symptoms mimicking sepsis • Abdominal distension, vomiting, frank or occult blood in stools • Faulty feeding practices and infection may be the reason	• Family history of unexplained sibling death • Consanguinity • *Screening*: Serum ammonia, metabolic acidosis (lactic) sugar and urinary ketones	• Vomiting and lump after feeding • Congenital hypertrophic pyloric stenosis • To rule out Down syndrome association, USG is helpful

(USG: ultrasonography)

TABLE 4: Normal CSF analysis in neonates.

CSF components	Term neonates	Preterm
Cells/mm^3	8 (0–30)	5 (0–44)
PMN (%)	60	8 (0–66)
CSF protein (mg/dL)	90 (20–170)	148 (54–370)
CSF glucose (mg/dL)	52 (34–119)	67 (33–217)
CSF/blood glucose (%)	51 (44–248)	

(CSF: cerebrospinal fluid; PMN: polymorphonuclear neutrophils)

- *Blood culture*: It is still a gold standard for diagnosis of sepsis. The possibly paired sample will be of more utility, but it has its own limitation. A significant number of kids with bacteremia may have sterile blood culture (BACTEC method), and other tissue fluid analysis such as cerebrospinal fluid (CSF) (normal values **Table 4**) and urine may help in arriving at a bacteriological diagnosis.
- *Radiology*: Chest X-ray, abdominal X-ray, and neuroimaging may act as an adjunct to the primary survey in diagnosing and managing complications.
- *Urinary culture*: It may have utilities in late-onset sepsis. Sometimes the presentation is occult and present with conjugate jaundice.
- Newer biomarkers include presepsin, hepcidin, CD64, IL-6 (interleukin 6), soluble TNF (tumor necrosis factor) receptor, E-selectin, ICAM (intercellular adhesion molecule 1).

Newer Diagnostic Techniques

- *Automated blood culture systems*: Matrix-assisted laser desorption ionization time-of-flight (MALDI-TOF) mass spectroscopy can identify organisms in blood cultures much earlier.
- Multiplex polymerase chain reaction (PCR) can detect the identity of the bacteria or fungi, as well as the presence of antimicrobial resistance genes within hours of identification of the pathogen.
- PCR can be performed on blood and other body fluids directly without the need to first culture causative organisms.
- Quantitative real-time amplification systems (q PCR).

Red Flags

Serial measurements of CRP combined with other acute phase reactants such as PCT, IL-6, and IL-8 may improve the diagnostic accuracy in suspected individuals.

MANAGEMENT

Sepsis management starts with prophylactic measures that need to be taken in utero.

Neonates after initial stabilization and routine evaluation should be assessed for sepsis correlated with a history of risk factors for early-onset sepsis. An easy algorithm is seen in **Flowchart 1**.

CHAPTER 15 | Neonatal Sepsis

Flowchart 1: Antibiotic use for sepsis in neonates and children.

Sources: Fuchs A, Bielicki J, Mathur S, Sharland M, Van Den Anker JN. Antibiotic use for sepsis in neonates and children: 2016 evidence update. WHO reviews. 2016.
Wallen LD, Ferrieri P. Newborn sepsis and meningitis. Avery's Diseases of the Newborn, 10th edition. Canada: Elsevier; 2018. pp. 553-65.
(CBC: complete blood count; WBC: white blood cell)

TABLE 5: Choice of empirical antibiotics.

Clinical situation	Septicemia/pneumonia	Meningitis
Community-acquired; resistant strains unlikely	Ampicillin or penicillin and gentamicin (first line)	Cefotaxime and gentamicin
Hospital-acquired or when there is a low-to-moderate probability of resistant strains	Ampicillin or cloxacillin and amikacin (second line)	Cefotaxime and amikacin
Hospital-acquired sepsis or when there is a high probability of resistant strains	Cefotaxime and amikacin (third line)	Cefotaxime and amikacin

Sources: Adapted from Paul VK. Ghai Essential Pediatrics, 9th edition. New Delhi: CBS Publishers Pvt. Limited; 2019.

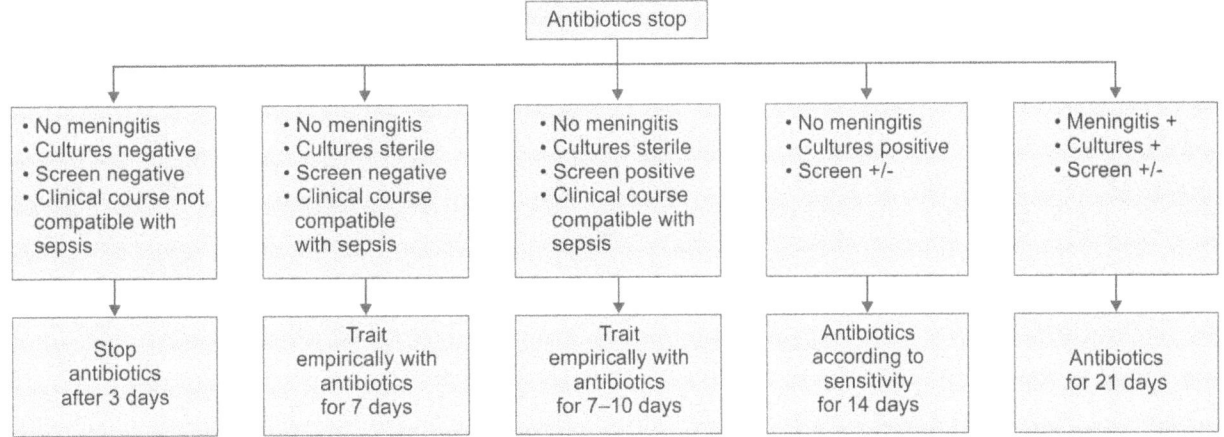

Flowchart 2: When to stop antibiotics?

Source: Adapted from Paul VK. Ghai Essential Pediatrics, 9th edition. New Delhi: CBS Publishers Pvt Limited; 2019.

KEY MESSAGES

- Prevention is the best way to decrease the incidence of sepsis in newborn.
- Clinical presentation may be subtle and nonspecific. Abnormal appearance, behavior, or circulation raises suspicion of sepsis in the presence of risk factors.
- A full diagnostic evaluation including CBC, blood, CSF, and urine culture is mandatory for diagnosis besides history and physical findings.
- Procalcitonin (PCT) is more specific than CRP for bacterial infections and rises more rapidly in response to infection than CRP.
- Blood culture is the definitive and gold standard for diagnosis.
- A specific and adequate duration of antibiotics is essential for better results **(Table 5)**.
- One should select, start, and continue antibiotic as per the own institute antibiotic policy, and to stop antibiotics follow the standard protocol **(Flowchart 2)**.
- Neonatal sepsis is fatal if untreated; mortality is as high as 20–30% in premature infants and 2–3% in full-term infants.

SUGGESTED READING

1. Agarwal R. Newborn infants. Essential Pediatrics, 9th edition. 2019, New Delhi: CBS Publishers & Distributors; 2019. pp. 161-2.
2. Ershad M, Mostafa A, Cruz MD, Vearrier D. Neonatal sepsis. Curr Emerg Hosp Med Rep. 2019;7(3):83-90.
3. Ganatra HA, Zaidi AKM. Neonatal infections in the developing world. Semin Perinatol. 2010;34:416-25.
4. Pavan Kumar DV, Mohan J, Rakesh PS, Prasad J, Joseph L. Bacteriological profile of neonatal sepsis in a secondary care hospital in rural Tamil Nadu, Southern India. J Family Med Prim Care. 2017;6:735-8.
5. Sgro M, Yudin MH, Lee S, Sankaran K, Tran D, Campbell D. Early-onset neonatal sepsis: it is not only group B Streptococcus. Paediatr Child Health. 2011;16(5):269.
6. Shah S, Goel AK, Garg R, Padhy M, Gupta A, Procalcitonin and C-reactive protein in early diagnosis of neonatal sepsis. Indian Journal of Medical Specialties. 2014;5(1).
7. Wallen LD, Ferrieri P. Newborn sepsis and meningitis. Avery's Diseases of the Newborn, 10th edition. Canada: Elsevier; 2018. pp. 553-65.
8. Zea-Vera A, Ochoa TJ. Challenges in the diagnosis and management of neonatal sepsis. J Trop Pediatr. 2015;61(1):1-13.

16 Neonatal Hypoglycemia

Hari R Mangtani

INTRODUCTION

Glucose is the key fuel for cerebral metabolism, particularly in the neonate. Neonatal hypoglycemia thus can lead to development of severe encephalopathy and an irreversible brain damage leading to neurological sequelae. To maintain the plasma glucose (PG) levels to normal, an elaborate defense mechanism has evolved involving substrate availability along with hormonal and enzyme activities. Thus, to arrive at an appropriate diagnosis of neonatal hypoglycemia and its management, requires understanding of the mechanism that maintains the PG levels within a narrow normal range.

PHYSIOLOGY

In utero, the mother and the fetus behave as a single pool for glucose. The fetus gets unrestricted supply of glucose from the mother and thus the glucose concentration in the fetus is similar to the glucose concentration in the mother's blood. However, the fetal pancreas is responsive to the glucose concentrations and secrete proportionate insulin in response. At birth, the supply of glucose is stopped and the neonate, facilitated by the hormonal changes (decrease in plasma insulin and increase in glucagon levels) and enzyme activity (increase glycogenolysis, gluconeogenesis), adapts to the extrauterine environment of self-dependence on supply of glucose for metabolic and energy needs.

DEFENSE MECHANISM AGAINST HYPOGLYCEMIA

In the postabsorptive state, the PG concentration is maintained by a highly integrated neuroendocrine and metabolic defense mechanism. The first defense is suppression of insulin. Further fall in PG concentration leads to secretion of glucagon and activation of the sympathoadrenal system increasing the epinephrine concentration. This activates glycogenolysis and mobilization of glucose stored in the liver along with gluconeogenesis. With prolonged fasting, the plasma cortisol and growth hormone levels also rise. Adipose tissue lipolysis releases glycerol and free fatty acids (FFA). Glycerol participates in gluconeogenesis and FFA replaces glucose as energy substrate in skeletal and heart muscle. FFA is converted to beta-hydroxybutyrate (BOHB) and acetoacetate in liver (ketogenesis). BOHB is the predominant ketoacid and partly supports the brain's energy need. This defense mechanism in neonate is similar to that in older children and adults, except that the PG levels fall rapidly with earlier exhaustion of glycogen reserve and hyperketonemia developing sooner. This occurs because of their disproportionately larger brain size relative to body mass and a higher glucose utilization rate per kilogram of body weight compared to older children and adults. The disruption of this endocrine and metabolic adaptation leads to majority of cases of neonatal hypoglycemia.

DEFINITION OF HYPOGLYCEMIA

Clinical hypoglycemia is defined as a PG concentration below a certain threshold that leads to development of signs and symptoms of impaired brain function. This can be recognized easily in adults and older children (Whipple's triad) but difficult to demonstrate in neonates. A specific PG level cannot be used to define hypoglycemia as the neuroglycopenic symptoms occur over a range of PG concentration, and is also altered by the presence of alternative fuel (ketones) and occurrence of antecedent hypoglycemia. Moreover, the extent of brain injury is also dependent on the degree and duration of hypoglycemia than a specific PG level. Thus, there has been a lack of consensus regarding the cutoff PG level to define neonatal hypoglycemia. However, for the practical purposes a cutoff of around 50 mg/dL along with the symptoms consistent with hypoglycemia can be used as a level to define hypoglycemia, particularly in first 48–72 hours of life after which a higher cutoff of 65–70 mg/dL is suggested to be used to define hypoglycemia.

SYMPTOMS OF HYPOGLYCEMIA

- Changes in levels of consciousness, irritability, and lethargy
- Apnea and cyanotic spells

- Coma
- Feeding poorly
- Hypothermia
- Hypotonia and limpness
- Tremor/seizures.

ETIOPATHOGENESIS

During the first 48 hours of life, a neonate goes through a phase of "transitional" hypoglycemia during which the PG levels fall immediately after birth and reach a level below those in older infants and children. This hypoglycemia is hypoketonemic and demonstrate inappropriately large glycemic response to glucagon. This suggest that a mild and transient hyperinsulinemia occurs immediately after birth in which there is a lower mean PG threshold for suppression of insulin secretion compared to older children and adults. In the next 48–72 hours, the mean PG levels increase with the maturation of glucose stimulated insulin secretion mechanism and reach a level similar to those in older infants and children. Thus, it appears prudent to delay diagnostic evaluation for suspected persistent hypoglycemic disorder until 48–72 hours of life.

Some neonates can be identified based on clinical features as being high risk of developing hypoglycemia (**Box 1**). This transient hypoglycemia occurring in at-risk newborns might resolve spontaneously within a few days or may persist for a few weeks after birth. The mechanism underlying development of hypoglycemia in these at-risk infants variably includes substrate limitation, immature enzymatic and hormonal response, and dysregulated insulin secretion (referred to as perinatal stress hyperinsulinism).

A subset of neonates developing hypoglycemia early in life might have an underlying persistent hypoglycemic disorder (**Table 1**). It includes most commonly congenital hyperinsulinism (CHI) occurring due to unregulated insulin secretion secondary to mutations in several key enzymes involved in regulation of insulin secretion. Insulin inhibits glucose production by inhibiting glycogenolysis and gluconeogenesis. In addition, it suppresses lipolysis with

BOX 1: Neonates at increased risk of hypoglycemia and require glucose screening.

- Symptoms of hypoglycemia
- Large for gestational age (even without maternal diabetes)
- Perinatal stress [birth asphyxia/ischemia, fetal distress, maternal preeclampsia/eclampsia or hypertension, intrauterine growth restriction (small for gestational age), meconium aspiration syndrome, polycythemia, hypothermia]
- Premature or postmature delivery
- Infant of diabetic mother
- Syndromic features and midline defects
- Family history of genetic form of hypoglycemia

TABLE 1: Causes of neonatal hypoglycemia.

Congenital hyperinsulinism	• Transient (perinatal asphyxia, IUGR, infant of diabetic mother) • Persistent (genetic mutations in enzymes involved in regulation of insulin secretion)
Counter-regulatory hormone deficiency	• Growth hormone deficiency • Adrenal insufficiency • Hypopituitarism
Glycogen storage disorder	• Gliucose-6-phosphatase deficiency • Amylo-1-6-glucosidase deficiency • Glycogen synthase deficiency
Gluconeogenic disorders	• Fructose-1-6-bisphosphatase deficiency • Phosphoenolpyruvate carboxykinase deficiency • Pyruvate carboxylase deficiency
Fatty acid oxidation disorders	• Long-chain acyl-CoA dehydrogenase deficiency • Medium-chain acyl-CoA dehydrogenase deficiency • Short-chain acyl-CoA dehydrogenase deficiency
Defect in ketone body synthesis/utilization	• HMG-CoA lyase deficiency • HMG-CoA synthase deficiency
Carnitine deficiency	• Carnitine palmitoyltransferase deficiency • Carnitine deficiency
Defects in glucose transporter	GLUT-1, GLUT-2, GLUT-3 defect
Other metabolic conditions	• Galactosemia • Tyrosinemia • Fructosemia • Propionic acidemia • Maple syrup urine disease

(IUGR: intrauterine growth restriction; HMG-CoA: 3-hydroxy-3-methylglutaryl-CoA; GLUT: glucose transporter) release of FFA and also ketogenesis, leading to development of hypoketotic hypoglycemia, thereby depriving brain from both glucose and ketone bodies. Thus, there is an increased risk of hypoglycemic brain injury and an increased risk of neurological sequelae.

The counter regulatory hormones such as glucagon, adrenalin, cortisol, and growth hormone are important for uninterrupted supply of glucose to vital organs. A deficiency of cortisol and growth hormone is not uncommon to present as hypoglycemia. Primary adrenal disorder could present with severe hyponatremia, vomiting, shock, atypical genitalia, and hyperpigmentation in addition to hypoglycemia whereas midline defect, jaundice, and microphallus are more commonly seen in congenital hypopituitarism.

Certain inborn errors of metabolism (IEM) can present with hypoglycemia in the neonatal period and can have additional variable signs and symptoms. A disorder in fatty acid oxidation will limit supply of ketones and lead to development of hypoketotic hypoglycemia. Patients with fatty acid oxidation disorder (FAOD) present with acute encephalopathy, cardiomyopathy, rhabdomyolysis, and derangement of liver function.

Glycogen storage disorders are a group of inherited metabolic disorders which may present with neonatal hypoglycemia accompanied by hepatomegaly (except GSD 0). As fatty acid oxidation and ketogenesis are intact, these infants have ketotic hypoglycemia and lactic acidosis. Similar biochemical features can be seen in gluconeogenic disorders occurring due to deficiency of enzymes of gluconeogenic pathway.

WORKUP/INVESTIGATION OF PERSISTENT HYPOGLYCEMIA

History

In a patient of hypoglycemia, a detailed history should include episode's timing and its relationship with food, antenatal history to know pregnancy issues (preeclampsia, intrauterine growth restriction, gestational diabetes), birth history (low birth weight, prematurity, perinatal asphyxia, and fetal distress), family history (consanguinity, infantile deaths), and history of medications such as beta-blockers.

Physical Examination

A thorough physical examination to search for the underlying cause for hypoglycemia is must. It should include looking for evidence of hypopituitarism (micropenis, undescended testis, and cleft lip/palate), adrenal disorder (hyperpigmentation and atypical genitalia), glycogenosis (hepatomegaly), or Beckwith–Wiedemann syndrome (omphalocele, ear crease, large tongue, hemihypertrophy).

Investigations

Unwell infants and high-risk babies (**Box 1**) require PG level monitoring. Checking PG concentration when indicated clinically (lethargy, poor feeding, and apneic spell) or before feed is the standard practice. It is not uncommon to encounter transient hypoglycemia, particularly during the first 48 hours of life. However, presence of persistent hypoglycemia must be excluded in following neonates before discharge:
- Infants with severe symptomatic hypoglycemia
- Requiring intravenous dextrose to maintain their PG levels
- Syndromic characteristics
- Positive clinical features (midline defect and micropenis)
- Positive family history of genetic form of hypoglycemia.

To identify the etiology of hypoglycemia, a "critical sample" should be obtained, at the time of spontaneous presentation, whenever possible, before treatment as it may rapidly alter the levels of hormones (insulin in particular) and metabolic substrates such as FFA and BOHB.

Assay of bicarbonate, blood gas, lactate, and ketone bodies (BOHB) help in distinguishing categories of hypoglycemic disorders (**Flowchart 1**). As BOHB assay is not

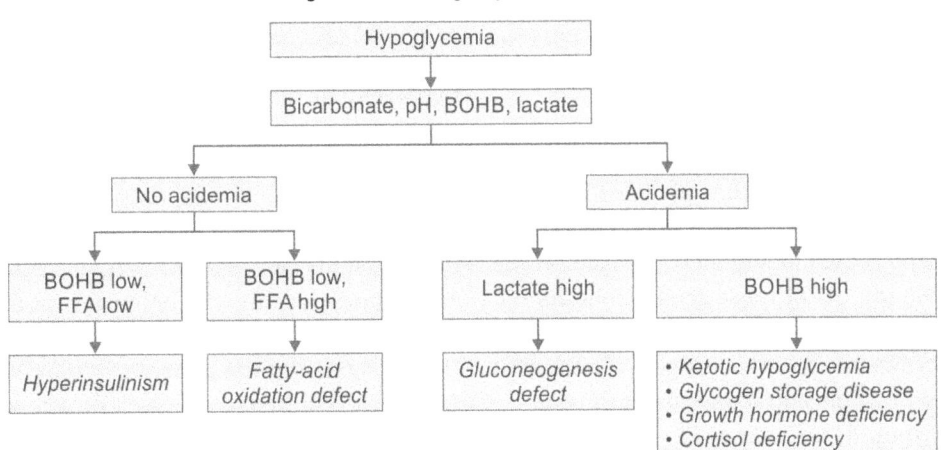

Flowchart 1: Algorithm showing major categories of hypoglycemia.

(BOHB: beta-hydroxybutyrate; FFA: free fatty acid)

readily available one might use the available bedside ketone meter. Urinary ketone levels (first void after episode of hypoglycemia) can also be used as a surrogate for identifying ketogenesis. In the absence of "critical sample", a provocative fast can be performed under guidance of a pediatric endocrinologist as the duration of fast and the specimens to be obtained are tailored based on suspected diagnosis.

Additional blood samples (EDTA and plain; 2–3 mL each) are obtained during hypoglycemia and kept for further testing to identify specific etiology, e.g.:
- Insulin, C-peptide, and FFA for suspected hyperinsulinism
- Plasma total and free carnitine and acylcarnitine profile for suspected FAOD
- Growth hormone and cortisol levels for suspected hypopituitarism.

Further investigations are performed to confirm the likely diagnosis and are planned based on the results of initial workup.

A plasma level of adrenocorticotropin and cortisol is collected simultaneously for a suspected primary adrenal insufficiency. However, the diagnosis of suspected secondary or tertiary adrenal insufficiency requires an adrenocorticotropic hormone (ACTH) stimulation test.

A growth hormone stimulation test may be required to diagnose growth hormone deficiency.

A genetic testing is required to identify specific genes responsible for the development of the inherited forms of CHI and thus to prognosticate and also to plan further therapeutic interventions.

Fatty acid oxidation disorder can be diagnosed by acylcarnitine profile analysis by tandem mass spectrometry (TMS). Urinary organic acid profile can detect increased excretion of dicarboxylic acid and their metabolite. However, it may be normal in between the episodes of hypoglycemia.

A simultaneous measurement of plasma levels of C-peptide along with plasma insulin levels helps to identify Munchausen syndrome by proxy, which demonstrates high plasma levels of insulin with associated low plasma concentration of C-peptide levels.

MANAGEMENT OF NEONATES WITH HYPOGLYCEMIA

The age of neonate along with the suspected etiology is to be considered while setting the goal of therapy. For a high-risk neonate without the suspicion of a congenital hypoglycemia disorder, the suggested goal of treatment is to maintain the PG concentration >50 mg/dL for those aged <48 hours and >60 mg/dL in those aged >48 hours. However, in neonates with suspected hypoglycemia disorder, the goal of treatment should be to maintain PG concentration >70 mg/dL.

Hypoglycemia should be managed as a medical emergency. Mild asymptomatic episodes of hypoglycemia can be managed by increasing the frequency or volume of feed in an otherwise normal neonate tolerating oral or nasogastric feeds. An episode of severe symptomatic hypoglycemia is rapidly reversed with intravenous dextrose. The initial dose is 200 mg/kg using 10% dextrose is followed by a continuous infusion of dextrose-containing fluids with a glucose delivery rate (GDR) of 4–6 mg/kg/min. A specialist (pediatric endocrinologist) should be involved if the patient requires a higher GDR (>8 mg/kg/min), to maintain normal concentrations of PG, which suggests presence of underlying hyperinsulinemia. In such cases, glucagon is expected to raise the PG levels to normal or above within 10–15 minutes of its administration and to maintain that concentration up to 1 hour. The dose of 0.5–1 mg (independent of weight), given intravenous, intramuscular, or subcutaneously, is usually effective in achieving this result. A continuous intravenous infusion of glucagon (5–10 µg/kg/h) could be administered to stabilize PG concentration. The nonspecific treatment with glucocorticoids for hypoglycemia should be discouraged. Similarly, oral dextrose solutions do not provide additional benefit over milk and should not be used.

The long-term therapy is based on the specific etiology in consultation with a specialist. The first-line therapy of CHI is diazoxide (5–20 mg/kg/day q8 hourly) administered orally. As diazoxide causes fluid retention and may cause complications such as hyponatremia, cardiac failure, and sometimes pulmonary hypertension, the treatment with diazoxide involves strict fluid restriction and is usually combine with a thiazide diuretic.

In diazoxide-unresponsive patients, octreotide, a somatostatin analog, can be used. The dose range is 5–40 µg/kg/day q6–8 hourly. The side effects of octreotide include tachyphylaxis, necrotizing enterocolitis, and cholelithiasis. The patients responsive to octreotide treatment could be shifted to once a month intramuscular lanreotide, a long-acting depot preparation of octreotide. Growth suppression also is a side effect of octreotide treatment when used for a long time.

Rapid genetic analysis is required in diazoxide-unresponsive patients, which is helpful in their further management. Patients with a homozygous or compound heterozygous mutations in the *ABCC8* or *KCNJ11* often have a diffuse form of CHI and require a near-total pancreatectomy in medically unresponsive patients. This surgical modality of treatment is associated with long-term complication of diabetes mellitus and exocrine pancreatic insufficiency. On the other hand, patients with heterozygous mutations of *ABCC8* or *KCNJ11* usually have a focal disease and can be cured by focal resection of the pancreatic lesion. An ^{18}F-DOPA PET/CT scan is required to delineate the site of focal lesion in the pancreas before resection, is available only in a few centers in India.

Once the PG concentration of a neonate is controlled by medical therapy, the parents should receive adequate training regarding frequent checking of glucose levels at home and also should have a written plan regarding identification and treatment of an episode of hypoglycemia which may occur at home. The doses of the medications should be adjusted on a regular basis, and any plan to taper or discontinue therapy should be discussed with the specialist.

The long-term therapy of hypopituitarism/hypoadrenalism should include the replacement of deficient hormones including growth hormone, cortisol, thyroxine, and desmopressin. The dose adjustment and long-term follow-up of such patients should be done by an experienced pediatric endocrinologist.

For metabolic disorders, the most important modality of treatment is to avoid prolonged fasting, especially during an illness. Maintaining adequate carbohydrate intake either enterally or parenterally will help maintain PG concentration and suppresses the production of toxic metabolites. However, metabolic defect if diagnosed should be managed in consultation with a physician experienced in managing metabolic disorders.

CONCLUSION

Neonatal hypoglycemia is a common disorder typically seen in at-risk neonates. Usually, it is transient and mild but can be persistent and severe. A detailed history, thorough physical examination, and appropriate investigations including "critical sample" and its interpretation help to pinpoint etiological diagnosis. CHI is a heterogeneous disorder causing recurrent hypoglycemia with a high risk of permanent neurological damage. It may be responsive to medical treatment and the ones who are unresponsive require advance surgical treatment. Other endocrine or metabolic disorders causing hypoglycemia should be diagnosed and managed involving the specialist in that field.

Neonatal Hypothermia

Swati Yadav

INTRODUCTION

A newborn baby is physiologically homeothermic and equipped with a thermostat hypothalamus. During pregnancy, maternal mechanism maintains the intrauterine temperature. From this comfortable environment, baby comes out naked, wet, and partially asphyxiated in the labor room environment. After birth, the newborn must adapt to their environment by metabolic production of heat.

After birth skin temperature falls by 0.3°C and core temperature by 0.1°C. Primary source of heat in the newborn is nonshivering thermogenesis, which involves the utilization of brown adipose tissue.

Normal temperature in newborn is 36.5–37.5°C.

Four mechanisms by which a newborn may lose heat to environment are as follows:
1. Radiation
2. Convection
3. Evaporation
4. Conduction

CAUSES

- *Excessive heat loss due to:*
  - Cold environment
  - Wet or naked body
  - Cold linen
  - During transport and various procedure, blood sampling
  - Bath
- *Poor ability to conserve heat:*
  - Large surface area
  - Poor insulation
  - Paucity of fat
  - Poor muscle tone
- *Poor metabolic heat production:*
  - Deficiency of brown fat
  - Hypoxia
  - Hypoglycemia
  - Central nervous system (CNS) damage due to anoxia, intracranial hemorrhage, and malformation.

RECORDING TEMPERATURE

Axillary temperature is as good as rectal and safer. It is recorded by placing thermometer against roof of axilla, free from moisture. Baby's arm is held close to thermometer in place and reading is taken after 3 minutes.

Rectal temperature: This method is not used routinely. However, it can be used as a guide for temperature in cold sick neonates.

Skin temperature: It is recorded by thermistor. The probe is attached to the skin over upper abdomen. The thermistor records temperature and displays it on the panel.

Hypothermia is skin temperature ≤35.5°C and core temperature <36°C.

Hypothermia has been categorized into:
- *Mild hypothermia (cold stress):* Core temperature—36–36.4°C. Warm trunk and cold extremities. Extremities bluish and cold. Poor weight gain if chronic cold stress.
- *Moderate hypothermia:* Core temperature—32–35.9°C. Cold trunk, cold extremities. Poor sucking, lethargy, week cry, and fast breathing.
- *Severe hypothermia:* Core temperature <32°C. Lethargic, poor perfusion, mottling, fast or slow breathing, and bleeding.

THE CONCEPT OF "WARM CHAIN"

The baby must be kept warm at the place of birth and during transport for special care either from home to hospital or within the hospital. The warm chain is a set of 10 interlinked procedures carried out at birth and later, which will minimize the likelihood of hypothermia in all newborns.

- Warm delivery room (>25°C)
- Warm resuscitation
- Immediate drying
- Skin-to-skin contact between baby and mother
- Breastfeeding
- Bathing and weighing postponed
- Appropriate clothing and bedding

- Mother and baby together
- Warm transportation
- Training/awareness of healthcare providers.

How to prevent hypothermia?

In labor room:
- Baby to be received on prewarmed basinet having a radiant heat source.
- Immediate drying and effective covering with prewarmed blanket.
- Ensure the head is well covered.
- Bath should be given after 12–24 hours, when baby has stabilized his temperature.

In ward:
- Baby should lie next to mother as warm body of mother serve as a biologically controlled incubator.
- Baby should be adequately clothed and head and feet should be covered with cap and socks.
- Bath should be replaced by alternate-day sponging.

In newborn intensive care unit (NICU):
- NICU temperature should 28 ± 2°C.
- Baby < 1,800 g and gestational age < 35 weeks should be kept in open care system.

During transport:
- Baby should be transported in transport incubator.
- Baby should be covered with warm linen.
- Baby should be in skin-to-skin contact with mother.

HOME CARE

- *The kangaroo method (skin-to-skin contact)*: It is one of the most appropriate method to be used in caring for the infant, especially preterm babies, since it:
    - Assists in maintaining temperature of the infant
    - Facilitates breastfeeding
    - Helps to increase duration of breastfeed
    - Improves mother–infant bonding.
- Baby should be kept dried, effectively clothed with woolen cap, socks, and mittens.
- Baby should be kept in warm room.
- Oil massage should be done; it will decrease insensible water loss.
- Bathing should be avoided immediately after birth. Preferably, give bath to normal baby on second day in summer and during winter daily sponging and once a week bath. In small and low birth weight (LBW) baby, postpone till the cord falls or preferably till weight is 2.5 kg.

SUGGESTED READING

1. Avery GB. In: Mullett MD, Seshia MMK, MacDonald MG. Avery's Neonatology: Pathophysiology & Management of the Newborn, 6th edition. Philadelphia: Lippincott Williams & Wilkins; 2005.
2. Singh M. Care of the Newborn, 8th edition. New Delhi: CBS Publishers Pvt. Ltd.; 2017.
3. Stark AR, Hansen AR, Martin C, Eichenwald EC. Chloherty and Stark's manual of Neonatal Care. Philadelphia: Wolters Kluwer; 2016.
4. World Health Organization. NNF Teaching Aids. [online] Available from: https://www.newbornwhocc.org/teaching.html. [Last accessed September, 2021].

18 CHAPTER

Therapeutic Hypothermia

Puja Dhupar

INTRODUCTION

India contributes to the largest neonatal mortality in the world with over 27% of global neonatal mortality being attributed to India. Birth asphyxia complicated by hypoxic-ischemic encephalopathy (HIE) occurs in approximately 1–3/1,000 live births in the developed countries. The rate of HIE is nearly 20-fold higher in low- and middle-income group countries (LMICs). HIE kills nearly a quarter of those afflicted and leads to permanent neurodevelopment sequelae in another 25%.

The current management of birth asphyxia and its sequelae focus on attenuating the multiorgan dysfunction. Therapeutic hypothermia (TH) which has been frequently used in adult cardiac and neurological disorders has been found to be useful in the management of birth asphyxia and resultant neonatal encephalopathy (NE).

DEFINITIONS

Therapeutic hypothermia is a modality of reducing the core body temperature of the asphyxiated neonate (who suffers from moderate-to-severe hypoxic encephalopathy) to 33–34°C for a period close to 72 hours using external devices in a controlled environment under close monitoring followed by slow rewarming (0.2–0.5°C/h).

Neonatal encephalopathy is an abnormal neurological status due to extensive central nervous system (CNS) injury which occurs as a sequence of events (asphyxia being one of them) in a neonate. The neonate with encephalopathy can be categorized into mild, moderate, or severe using the Sarnat and Sarnat classification.

PATHOGENESIS OF NE DUE TO HYPOXIC INJURY TO CNS

The pathogenesis of HIE involves two interdependent processes. (1) Primary energy failure, which is characterized by decrease in the levels of energy-rich substrates such as adenosine triphosphate (ATP) and phosphocreatine. (2) The secondary energy failure causes extensive neuronal injury and is responsible for major clinical manifestations of NE. The aim of any therapy is to prevent the onset of secondary energy failure. It is during the therapeutic window of 6 hours (during the latent phase) between the primary and secondary energy failure that interventions should be directed to contain and reverse the damage caused due to hypoxia and ischemia.

How to recognize a neonate of NE?
- The possibility of a neonate suffering from NE is high if it is born with a cord pH of <7
- A base deficit of at least >12 mEq/L
- There is an evidence of multi-organ dysfunction (renal, cardiac, CNS, etc.)
- Contributing causes such as trauma, metabolic disorders, and structural malformations have been excluded.

Appropriate investigations will confirm the occurrence of asphyxia and assess the severity of multiorgan involvement.

How to confirm birth asphyxia?
An umbilical arterial blood pH < 7 at birth indicates asphyxia along with a history of failure to initiate spontaneous respiratory efforts at birth.

INVESTIGATIONS TO ASSESS MULTI-SYSTEM/ORGAN INVOLVEMENT

Abnormalities of the following investigations suggest multi-organ dysfunction:
- *Brain*: Cranial sonography, computed tomography (CT), magnetic resonance imaging (MRI), electroencephalography (EEG), amplitude-integrated EEG (aEEG)
- *Heart*: Cardiac enzymes [Troponin T, creatine phosphokinase-brain/heart (CPK-MB/BB)], echocardiography, chest X-ray, electrocardiography (ECG)
- *Kidneys*: Urine microscopy, kidney function tests (KFTs), renal Doppler
- *Lungs*: Chest X-ray, arterial blood gases (ABG)
- *Gastrointestinal tract (GIT)*: X-ray abdomen
- *Miscellaneous*: Blood sugar, serum calcium, sepsis screen if needed.

TEMPERATURE MAINTENANCE

- Baby should be placed under a servo-controlled radiant warmer. The temperature should be maintained in normal range of 36.5–37.5°C.
- If a neonate of >36 weeks' gestation with birth asphyxia is brought to the hospital within 6 hours of birth, then TH should be immediately initiated if such a facility is available.

AIRWAY MAINTENANCE

The airway and the breathing should be monitored and any secretions should be removed to ensure a patent airway. If the neonate is having gasping respiration or absence of respiration, immediate assisted ventilation should be provided.

CIRCULATION MAINTENANCE

Efforts should be made to identify features of shock [capillary filling time (CFT) > 3 seconds, hypotension, collapsed inferior vena cava (IVC) on functional echocardiography] and promptly corrected.

FLUIDS AND FEEDS

Intravenous (IV) fluids can be started depending on the clinical condition of the baby. Efforts should be made to initiate enteral feeding as soon as possible in babies who are clinically stable without any evidence of major organ system involvement.

MEDICATIONS

- Vitamin K 1 mg intramuscularly (IM) along with IV 10% calcium gluconate should be administered at a rate of 5 mL/kg/day prophylactically to all neonates. Calcium should be administered under cardiac monitoring.
- Blood sugar should be maintained in the normal euglycemic range. If need arises, a dextrose infusion should be initiated.
- Inotropes such as dobutamine can be considered in case of poor organ perfusion.
- Drugs such as phenobarbitone and phenytoin can be considered in case of seizures.

It is important to remember that drugs such as sodium bicarbonate, respiratory stimulants, atropine, and mannitol have no role in the acute management of birth *asphyxia*.

MONITORING

The following monitoring needs to be done:
- *Temperature*: It should be monitored and maintained in the normal range of 36.5–37.5°C. In cases where TH has been initiated, core body temperature of 33–34°C is maintained for a period of 72 hours.
- *CNS*:
  - The neurological status should be monitored every 8 hours.
  - *Respiratory*: The status should be monitored every 2–3 hours.
- *Cardiovascular system (CVS)*: The CV status assessment should include:
  - Heart rate
  - Color
  - Capillary refill time (CRT)
  - Peripheral pulses
  - Pulse oximetry
  - Noninvasive blood pressure (NIBP).
- *Kidney*:
  - Urine output should be measured daily (it should normally be >1 mL/kg/h after the first 24 hours of life).
  - *Blood sugar*: Monitoring every 6–8 hours during the first 24 hours and later as required.
  - Serum calcium should be monitored.
- *Feed intolerance*: It should be detected/monitored (vomiting, increase in abdominal girth by >2 cm and increased pre-feed aspirate indicates feed intolerance).

MECHANISM OF ACTION OF THERAPEUTIC HYPOTHERMIA

Numerous mechanisms have been suggested which contribute to the beneficial effects of TH. Some of the major mechanisms are as follows:
- Decreased energy utilization
- Suppression of free radical-induced injury
- Decreased severity of secondary energy failure
- Reduction in the extent of brain injury
- Inhibition of inflammation and resultant release of cytokines.

INDICATIONS OF USE OF THERAPEUTIC HYPOTHERMIA

Therapeutic hypothermia should be considered as a treatment of choice for any neonate who fulfils the following criteria:
- Term gestation (>36 weeks)
- Age < 6 hours
- Absence of major congenital anomalies
- *Meeting the following criteria*:
  - *Evidence of perinatal asphyxia*: Umbilical cord pH or ABG in the first hour of life <7 or base excess (BE): 16 mEq/L

    or
  - History of a perinatal acute event (cord prolapse or placental abruption)

    or
  - Apgar score <5 at 10 minutes

- Need for ventilation beyond the 10th minute of life
- Evidence of moderate-to-severe encephalopathy before 6 hours of life (as evidenced by seizures, altered level of consciousness, decreased spontaneous activity, tone abnormalities, abnormal neonatal reflexes, and autonomic system abnormalities).

EQUIPMENT

Currently two types of equipment are available to administer TH.

Recommended TH devices and accessories:
- *Selective head cooling*: Cool cap; not recommended for LMICs
- *Whole-body hypothermia*: Cooling mattress
- Rectal probes.

INEXPENSIVE INNOVATIVE COOLING DEVICES

A number of innovative low-cost devices have been used by units in LMIC's to administer TH. Published randomized controlled trials (RCTs) of these devices have revealed promising results. The safety and efficacy of these devices cannot be established till validation and certification by licensing authorities. Some devices in use are as follows:
- Frozen gel packs (used in immunization clinics)
- Phase-changing material (PCM)
- Water bottles filled with tap water.

TECHNIQUE OF THERAPEUTIC HYPOTHERMIA

Target Temperature

After initiation of cooling, the recommended rectal temperatures in selective head cooling is 34.5°C whereas in whole-body cooling, the temperatures are lowered till 33.5°C.

Duration

The target temperatures should be maintained for 72 hours.

Rewarming

Rewarming should be slow over a 4-hour period wherein the temperature is slowly increased at the rate of 0.5°C per hour till it reaches 36.5°C.

Method

Selective head cooling is administered by a helmet and total-body cooling with a whole-body mattress with servocontrol to adjust the neonate's temperature according to his body temperature. During the process of TH, temperatures should be not be allowed to drop below 33°C. Temperatures lower than this are less neuroprotective and extremely low temperatures are associated with increased incidence of mortality. Extending the duration of cooling to beyond 72 hours with an aim of achieving better neuroprotection is futile; it can be dangerous and is not recommended.

MANAGEMENT OF VITAL FUNCTIONS DURING THERAPEUTIC HYPOTHERMIA

Respiratory System

- Maintain normal blood gases, avoid hyperoxia, hypercarbia, and hypocarbia.
- Maintain normocarbia. Hypothermia decreases the delivery of oxygen to the tissues, try to maintain normal PaO_2 levels of 50–100 mm Hg. Close monitoring of lung compliance is desired during the initiation and rewarming phases of TH.

Circulatory System

Therapeutic hypothermia leads to bradycardia and decreased cardiac output. Monitor the BP, CFT, and urine output closely to detect signs of hypoperfusion early. If facilities exist, then functional echocardiography can be used to monitor superior vena cava (SVC) flow as it reflects cerebral circulation. Adjustments in the dose of inotropes are needed during the rewarming phase when cardiac output and SVC flow increase.

Fluid and Electrolytes

Initial fluid should be 10% dextrose followed by normal maintenance fluid. Close monitoring of the urine output and the weight of the neonate can give an idea of the fluid requirement during TH. Syndrome of inappropriate antidiuretic hormone secretion (SIADH), if detected, needs to be managed. Monitoring of K, Ca, Mg, and glucose is of prime importance during TH.

Nutritional Management

Do not initiate enteral nutrition till the rewarming has been completed as TH can decrease the mesenteric circulation and there are chances of ischemia of the bowel. Alternatively minimal enteral nutrition can be initiated during the TH. Total parenteral nutrition (TPN) should be planned and initiated early to prevent calorie deficit.

Renal System

Detection and management of acute kidney injury is of prime importance.

Hematological System

Address coagulation abnormalities with fresh frozen plasma (FFP) if required and thrombocytopenia with platelet transfusions, if indicated.

Pain Management and Developmentally Supportive Care

Untreated pain has been shown to affect the neurobehavior of the neonate adversely. Efforts should be initiated to control pain effectively using narcotic agents such as morphine or fentanyl. Unit should practice developmentally supportive care (DSC) to optimize neurodevelopmental outcomes.

CLINICAL AND LABORATORY MONITORING DURING THERAPEUTIC HYPOTHERMIA

Careful monitoring is essential to ensure a favorable clinical outcome in neonates initiated on TH. At the outset, a vascular access should be secured by inserting an umbilical venous and arterial line.

Urine output can be monitored using a urinary catheter.

Vital Signs

All vital signs such as core body temperature, heart rate, respiratory rate, BP, CFT, urine output, and SpO_2.

Neurological Examination

It can be carried out using the Dubowitz method and Sarnat staging should be done daily till 7 days after TH.

Cardiovascular System

Daily echocardiography for evaluating cardiac functions is required.

Central Nervous System

Daily cranial ultrasound is required for diagnosis of intracranial bleeds and cerebral Doppler for cerebral blood flow measurements. An EEG can be used if available and MRI for neuroimaging.

Skin

Skin lesions and evidence of subcutaneous fat necrosis should be monitored daily.

Biochemistry: Complete blood count (CBC), liver function test (LFT), KFT, prothrombin time (PT), activated partial thromboplastin time (aPTT).

SIDE EFFECTS OF THERAPEUTIC HYPOTHERMIA

The common side effects observed with TH are as follows: Hypotension, low platelets, clotting abnormalities [increased prothrombin time (PT) and aPTT], electrolyte disturbances, skin burns, and sclerema. Most of the side effects are seen when adherence to the TH protocol is not strictly enforced. Careful monitoring during TH can prevent the occurrence of major side effects.

KEY MESSAGES

- There is no doubt that TH has shown extremely promising results as far as the combined outcomes of mortality and neurodevelopment intactness postasphyxial encephalopathy is concerned.
- The need of the hour is to focus on improving the existing special newborn care unit (SNCU) network and work toward achieving a better regionalization of neonatal care in India. The need is to improve the quality of care in our SNCUs, provide adequate staff, infrastructure, transport linkages, monitoring facilities, and on-site and off-site trainings.
- The clinician at peripheral health facilities and the practitioners should not feel frustrated due to the lack of TH and should make all attempts to prevent HIE by institution of an accurate Neonatal resuscitation program (NRP) as per the standard guidelines.
- The clinician should make all attempts to transport the neonate to the nearest center having facilities for TH by the shortest route and the fastest mode of transport.
- Only providing TH does not end the job as a good follow-up for identification of neurodevelopmental disabilities and institution of early stimulation program with a team of developmental specialists and pediatric neurologists is of prime importance.

SUGGESTED READING

1. Datta V. Therapeutic hypothermia for birth asphyxia in neonates. Indian J Pediatr. 2017;84:219-26.

19 Neonate Born of Mother with Chronic Systemic Disorder

Rakesh Singh

INTRODUCTION

Good maternal health is necessary for the best pregnancy outcome. Women with chronic medical conditions should receive prepregnancy advice before conception to ensure they are on safe and effective treatment. Maternal illnesses often make them unable for optimal adaptations to pregnancy and therefore best pregnancy outcome is compromised. Mother with chronic systemic disorder if not adequately managed during pregnancy then it leads to fetal and infant malnutrition (Barker hypothesis).

In this topic, we will discuss some of the most prevalent maternal illnesses affecting pregnancy and fetal and neonatal health.

HYPERTENSION, PREECLAMPSIA, ECLAMPSIA, AND HELLP SYNDROME

- Preexisting chronic hypertension may become superimposed with pregnancy-induced hypertension (PIH) or pre-eclampsia (PET)—risk of PET is raised.
- *PIH*: BP >140/90 in second half of pregnancy with no proteinuria usually associated with little or no risk to the fetus unless severe.
- Fetal growth assessment (+/– umbilical artery Doppler studies), amniotic fluid measurement, and monitoring for raised maternal liver enzymes, urate, and lactate dehydrogenase (LDH) may be required, as well as monitoring for proteinuria.
- Preeclampsia = hypertension + renal involvement (usually proteinuria).
- Increased risk in primigravida, extremes of maternal age, obesity, maternal illness (diabetes, lupus, hypertension, renal disease) and multiple pregnancy.
- Associated with increased risk of placental failure, intrauterine growth restriction (IUGR), and preterm deliveries varies for mild (5%) to severe (1%) pregnancies. Severity worsen with early onset.
- Severe PET associated with increased risk of abruption.
- Neonates of affected mother may have polycythemia, neutropenia, and thrombocytopenia.
- If severe PET in previous pregnancy, low-dose aspirin from 16 weeks reduces risk of recurrence by 20%.
- Maternal condition improves after delivery of placenta.

Eclampsia

Seizures are associated with hypertension and proteinuria. Risk of fetal hypoxia is high.

HELLP Syndrome

Hemolysis, elevated liver enzymes, low platelet (HELLP) syndrome: Neonates born to mother with hypertension (preexisting, PIH, pre-eclampsia, and HELLP syndrome) may have/or present with:

- IUGR.
- Weight below the 10th percentile significantly increases the risk of mortality and in perinatal mortality.
- High risk of fetal demise/still birth in case of severe preeclampsia/eclampsia.
- In mild cases, the risk of fetal demise is over 50% less than pregnancies with severe preeclampsia.
- Delivery is recommended for all women with severe preeclampsia no later than 34 weeks' gestation and delivery recommended for women who develop preeclampsia regardless of disease severity at 37 weeks.
- Thrombocytopenia generally identified at birth or within first 2–3 days following delivery, with resolution by 10 days of life in most cases.
- 50% incidence of neutropenia.
- There is increased risk for development of bronchopulmonary dysplasia (BPD), even after adjusting for gestational age, birth weight, and other clinical confounders.
- Altered umbilical artery flow may lead to develop necrotizing enterocolitis (NEC), persistent postnatal flow abnormalities in superior mesenteric artery (SMA) which slowly recover over 1 week.
- High risk of preterm deliveries.
- Breastfeeding is safe with most maternal antihypertensives, apart from angiotensin-converting enzymes (ACE) inhibitors (except safe with captopril).

Hydralazine/methyldopa: Good safety profile, few side effects in fetus and neonate.

MATERNAL DIABETES

- Complications of pregnancy due to maternal diabetes
- Risk of fetal/neonatal complications
- Increased with worsening maternal glycemic control
- Risk of congenital malformations is three times more than in nondiabetic women and related to maternal HbA1c at the time of conception (therefore no increased risk in gestational diabetes)
- *Abnormalities include*:
  - Congenital heart disease
  - Sacral agenesis (caudal regression syndrome)
  - Microcolon
  - Renal tract anomalies
  - Neural tube defects
  - Microcephaly
- Increased risk of spontaneous miscarriage
- Increased risk of late intrauterine fetal death
- IUGR is three times more common than in nondiabetic women due to placental dysfunction with small-vessel disease
- Polyhydramnios (due to fetal polyuria)
- Preterm labor
- Macrosomia due to increased fetal insulin (anabolic and growth factor-like effect) increases risk of instrumental or cesarean birth, birth trauma, fetal distress, and neonatal encephalopathy
- Hypoglycemia (due to fetal by hyperinsulinemia) usually resolves within 48 hours
- Surfactant deficiency leads to transient tachypnea of the newborn (TTNB) or respiratory distress syndrome (RDS)-like picture
- Transient hypertrophic cardiomyopathy (septal)
- Polycythemia (increases risk of significant jaundice)
- Other biochemical disturbances (hypocalcemia, hypomagnesemia).

Management of Infants of Diabetic Mothers

- Check antenatal ultrasound scan results and examine carefully for signs of macrosomia, congenital abnormalities [congenital heart defect (CHD), sacral agenesis, microcolon, neural tube defects (NTDs)], signs of respiratory distress, and heart murmurs.
- Routine newborn intensive care unit (NICU) admission is not recommended and babies of women with diabetes should not be separated from their mothers unless there is a clinical complication or there are abnormal clinical signs that warrant admission.
- Monitor babies for hypoglycemia (Starting within 2–4 hours of birth).
- Encourage breastfeeding and start feeds as soon as possible after birth (within 30 minutes):
  - Continue feeds at frequent interval (2–3 hourly) until blood glucose monitoring can be discontinued.
  - If enteral feeding is contraindicated, start intravenous (IV) infusion of 10% dextrose.
  - Check blood sugar before second, third and fourth feeds and until there have been at least two satisfactory measurements (i.e., > 2.6 mmol/L).
- Observe baby for signs of polycythemia and jaundice. Blood tests (Serum bilirubin, full blood count, calcium and magnesium) should be carried out if any clinical signs are present.
- Echocardiogram if heart murmurs or other signs of cardiac disease present [CHD or transient hypertrophic (Septal) cardiomyopathy].
- Discharge can be done after 48 hours of age if blood glucose levels are maintained and tolerating full oral feeds.

MOTHER WITH SYSTEMIC LUPUS ERYTHEMATOSUS

- Systemic lupus erythematosus (SLE) is the most common connective tissue disorder seen among reproductive age group women.
- Patients with SLE have a high prevalence of fetal wastage (recurrent spontaneous abortions), IUGR, preterm delivery, stillbirth, and perinatal death.
- Fetal survival is higher when the disease is in remission.
- Predictors of fetal wastage include active nephritis, hypertension and circulating antiphospholipid antibodies (e.g., lupus anticoagulant or anticardiolipin antibodies), later likely the most important factor associated with pregnancy loss.
- Infants of mothers with SLE are at risk for the neonatal lupus syndrome. This constellation of findings consists of abnormalities in the heart and skin or development of clinical features of SLE and occurs from transplacental passage of maternal antibodies. Congenital complete heart block (third-degree heart block) due to permanent damage to the cardiac conduction system (his bundle fibrosis) by anti-Ro and anti-la antibodies is the most frequently seen heart abnormality.
- Skin is the other major organ system involved in the neonatal lupus syndrome. Cutaneous lesions are frequently widespread macular rashes, although a butterfly rash and discoid lesions are found occasionally. These inflammatory lesions generally appear within the first few weeks of life and disappear spontaneously within 6 months, coexistent with the clearance of maternal auto-antibodies.

- Hematologic manifestations such as anemia and thrombocytopenia, neutropenia and glomerulonephritis, hepatosplenomegaly, and neurologic symptoms are unusual.
- Treatment of symptomatic babies with complete heart block involves management of heart failure with diuretics, isoprenaline infusion to maintain adequate heart rate, and esophageal or transvenous pacing. Permanent epicardial pacing is rarely needed.

MOTHER WITH RENAL DISORDERS

- Mild renal dysfunction typically has little if, any, effect on pregnancy outcome.
- In moderate-to-severe renal insufficiency (e.g., serum creatinine >1.4 mg/dL) adverse pregnancy events are well described. These pregnancies are especially risky. Maternal complications include anemia, vascular accidents, placental abruption, chronic hypertension, PIH, preeclampsia, proteinuria and worsening renal function.
- Perinatal complications such as IUGR, stillbirth, prematurity, polyhydramnios and mid trimester pregnancy loss.
- Dialysis may be used during pregnancies complicated by renal insufficiency. Pregnancy success rates in dialysis patients are at most 52% and outcomes generally are more promising for hemodialysis rather than continuous ambulatory peritoneal dialysis.
- Complications associated with peritoneal dialysis in pregnancy include preterm labor and acute peritonitis. Hemodialysis may be accompanied by hypotension, electrolyte imbalances and preterm labor.
- Pregnancy is no longer an unusual event among women of childbearing age with functioning renal transplants.
- Breastfeeding for transplant recipient mothers remains an area in which recommendations are evolving. The lack of reported adverse effects, together with the documented benefits of breast feeding, outweigh the theoretical risks.

MOTHERS WITH HEART DISEASE

- Maternal cardiac disease may be accompanied by significant maternal and perinatal morbidity and mortality.
- Functional cardiac status before or early in pregnancy is an important prognostic indicator of maternal and fetal outcome.
- As per the New York Heart Association (NYHA) classification, better prognosis is expected during pregnancy for women with class I and II than for those with classes III or IV.
- Fetal risks include premature delivery, IUGR, and stillbirth (especially with maternal cyanotic heart disease).
- The risk of a fetus inheriting polygenic cardiac disease is varied according to the parent's condition, being 3% in conditions such as Tetralogy of Fallot but as high as 10–18% with atrial septal defect (ASD), coarctation of aorta, and aortic stenosis.
- Peripartum cardiomyopathy has been defined clinically as the onset of cardiac failure with no identifiable cause in the last month of pregnancy or within 5 months after delivery, in the absence of heart disease before the last month of pregnancy.
- In most cases of heart diseases such as cardiomyopathy, valvular heart disease (regurgitation) after maternal stabilization, induction and vaginal delivery can be attempted. The advantages of vaginal delivery are minimal blood loss, greater hemodynamic stability, avoidance of surgical stress and less chances of postoperative infection and pulmonary complications.

SUGGESTED READING

1. Singh M. Care of the Newborn, 8th edition. New Delhi: CBS Publishers Pvt Ltd; 2017.

20 Neonate Born of Mother with Maternal Infection

Rakesh Singh

INFANT BORN TO MOTHER WITH HEPATITIS B VIRUS INFECTION

Introduction

Acute viral hepatitis is defined by the following clinical criteria:
- Symptoms consistent with viral hepatitis
- Elevation of serum aminotransaminase levels to >2.5 times the upper limit of normal
- The absence of other causes of live disease.

At least five agents have been identified as causes of viral hepatitis: (1) Hepatitis A virus (HAV), (2) hepatitis B virus (HBV), (3) hepatitis C virus (HCV), (4) hepatitis D virus (HDV), and (5) hepatitis E virus (HEV).

Transmission of HBV occurs by percutaneous or per mucosal routes from infected blood or body fluids. The transmission of HBV from infected mothers to their newborns is thought to result primarily from exposure to maternal blood at the time of delivery. Transplacental transfer accounts for <4% of all cases.

When acute maternal HBV infection occurs during the first and second trimesters of pregnancy, there is generally little risk to the newborns because antigenemia is usually cleared by term and anti-HBV antibodies are present. Acute maternal HBV infection during late pregnancy or near the time of delivery, however, may result in up to 90% transmission rate in the absence of any prophylaxis and is most common in women who have both HBsAg (hepatitis B surface antigen) and HBeAg (hepatitis B e-antigen) detected in blood, indicating high plasma HBV DNA levels.

Risk of Vertical Transmission

- *Mother HBsAg +ve but HBeAg –ve*: 5–20%
- *Mother HBsAg +ve and HBeAg +ve*: 70–90%.

Investigations

Prenatal testing of all pregnant women for HBsAg is recommended.

Follow-up Testing of Vaccinated Newborns

Perform anti-HBs antibodies and HBsAg testing at 9–18 months of age.

Scenario 1: Infant with anti-HBs negative and HBsAg positive has HBV infection and needs follow-up in liver clinic.

Scenario 2: Infant with anti-HBs titers 10 mIU/mL or more and HBsAg negative are immune; no action required.

Scenario 3: Infant with anti-HBs titers <10 mIU/mL and HBsAg negative: no HBV infection but failed to respond to immunization—needs repeat vaccination (three doses).

Management

At birth: Give hepatitis B vaccine along with hepatitis B immunoglobulin (HBIg) (100 IU/0.5 mL) intramuscularly (IM) in different thighs. (Preferably within 12 hours of life but not later than 48–72 hours of birth). Complete HBV immunization as per schedule.

Infant vaccinated with three-dose schedule for Infant < 2 kg: Do not count birth dose and give three more doses.

Infant 2 kg or more: Give a total of three doses counting the birth dose.

Infant vaccinated with four-dose schedule: It remains the same for all babies, irrespective of birth weight.
- HBV infection is not a contraindication to breastfeeding.
- HBV vaccine gives 70–90% of active immunity. HBIg gives additional 10–30% immunity. If HBIg is unaffordable or unavailable; give the vaccine alone.
- 90% infected infants become chronic carriers.
- For mothers with unknown HBsAg status at birth (antenatal testing not done):
  - Perform urgent maternal testing for HBsAg.
  - Give HBV vaccine to the infant within 12 hours of birth.
- *If mother is positive for HBsAg or the maternal results are delayed*: Give HBIg within 12 hours to infant with birth weight <2 kg and within 7 days of life to infants with birth weight >2 kg.

Prevention

- The principal strategy for the prevention of neonatal HBV disease has been to use a combination of passive and active immune prophylaxis for newborns at high risk for infection as well as routine active neonatal immunization to protect against postnatal exposure.
- Prevention of nosocomial spread from HBsAg-positive infants in the nursery is minimized if nursery personnel wear gloves and gowns when caring for infected infants. Immunization of healthcare workers is also strongly recommended.

INFANT BORN OF MOTHER WITH VARICELLA INFECTION

Introduction

The causative agent of varicella (chickenpox) is a DNA virus and a member of the herpes virus family. The same agent is responsible for herpes zoster (shingles), hence, this virus is referred to as varicella zoster virus (VZV). The overall estimated risk of the congenital varicella syndrome following maternal infection is low, with only 0.4% in the first 12 weeks of pregnancy, and 2% from 13 to 20 weeks' gestation. It is primarily seen with gestational varicella but may rarely occur with maternal zoster. Incubation period of varicella is 10–21 days.

Mode of Transmission

The primary mode of transmission of VZV is through respiratory droplets from patients with chickenpox. Spread through contact with vesicular lesions also can occur. Typically, individuals with chickenpox are contagious from 1 to 2 days before and 5 days after the onset of rash. Transplacental transfer of VZV may take place, presumably secondary to maternal viremia, but its frequency is unknown. Varicella occurs in approximately 25% of newborns whose mothers developed varicella within the peripartum period. The onset of disease usually occurs 13–15 days after the onset of maternal rash. The greatest risk of severe infant disease is seen when maternal varicella occurs in the 5 days before or 2 days after delivery. In these cases, there is insufficient time for the fetus to acquire transplacentally derived VZV-specific antibodies. Symptoms generally begin 5–10 days after delivery, and the expected mortality is high, approximately 30%. When in utero transmission of VZV occurs before the peripartum period, then there is no obvious clinical impact in most fetuses; however, congenital varicella syndrome can occur.

Diagnosis

- Infants with congenital varicella resulting from in utero infection occurring before the peripartum period—nothing is required.
- With neonatal disease, the presence of a typical vesicular rash, laboratory confirmation can be made by:
  - Culture of vesicular fluid—sensitivity is not optimal.
  - Demonstration of a four-fold rise in VZV antibody titer by enzyme-linked immunosorbent assay (ELISA).
  - Antigen can also be detected from cells at the base of a vesicle by immunofluorescent antibody or polymerase chain reaction (PCR) detection. It is a highly sensitive, specific, and rapid method and is preferred when vesicles are present.

Treatment

- *If a mother develops chickenpox (rash) between 5 days prior to and 2 days following delivery*: Infant does not have protective antibodies and likelihood of severe neonatal disease is high. Separate mother and baby (isolation) until maternal lesions have dried up and crusted. If baby develops rash, baby to stay with mother. Mother/baby with active vesicles is isolated from other mother and babies.
VZIg is given within 72 hours of exposure (not required if mother has zoster). Dose of VZIg is 62.5 IU IM for infant <2 kg and 125 IU IM for infants > 2 kg. Consider IV acyclovir (60 mg/kg/day) divided every 8 hourly with the appearance of any vesicular lesions in a newborn whether VZIg has been given or not.
If VZIg is unavailable, IVIg at a dose of 400 mg/kg may be given because it will contain anti-VZV antibodies.
Give expresses breast milk (EBM) even if mother–infant dyad is separated. Breastfeeding is allowed once mother is noninfectious.
- If mother develops chickenpox (rash) before 5 days prior to delivery infant has protective antibodies and likelihood of severe disease is low. Do not separate baby from mother; continue breastfeeding. Isolate dyad from other infants. VZIg is not administered. Consider acyclovir if baby develops rash.
- *If mother develops chickenpox (rash) after 2 days of delivery*: Infant does not have protective antibodies but likelihood of severe neonatal disease is low. Separate mother and baby until maternal lesions have dried up and crusted. If baby develops rash—baby to stay with mother. Mother/baby with active vesicles is isolated from other mother and babies. VZIg is not administered. Consider acyclovir if baby develops rash.

Exposure of a hospitalized infant to healthcare provider with chickenpox:

- All exposed susceptible patients should be discharged as soon as possible.
- All exposed susceptible patients who cannot be discharged should be placed in isolation from 8 to 21 days.

- Ascertain gestation of infant and take maternal history of chickenpox:
  - *Infant < 28 weeks*: Give VZIg, regardless of maternal history of varicella.
  - *Infant 28–36 weeks and no maternal history of chickenpox*: Give VZIg.
  - *For healthy term infant (37 weeks or more)*: No need for VZIg.

INFANT BORN TO MOTHER WITH PERINATAL HERPES SIMPLEX VIRUS

Introduction

Herpes simplex virus (HSV), a lifelong infection, is a double-stranded, enveloped DNA virus with two virologically distinct types: HSV-1 and HSV-2. HSV-2 was previously the primary cause of genital lesions, yet HSV-1 has become the predominant virus type in genital lesions of young women. Both types produce clinically indistinguishable neonatal syndromes. The virus can cause localized disease of the infant's skin, eye, or mouth (SEM) or may disseminate by cell-to-cell contiguous spread or viremia. After adsorption and penetration into host cells, viral replication proceeds, resulting in cellular swelling, hemorrhagic necrosis, formation of intranuclear inclusions, cytolysis, and cell death.

Transmission

- Intrapartum transmission is the most common cause of neonatal HSV infection because it is associated with active shedding of virus from the cervix or vulva at the time of delivery. Up to 90% of newborn infections occur as a result of intrapartum transmission. Transmission far more likely in primary than secondary infection as there is no maternal antibody to afford protection.
- *Antenatal transmission*: In utero infection with HSV has been documented but is uncommon. Spontaneous abortion has occurred with primary maternal infection before 20 weeks' gestation.
- *Postnatal transmission*: A small percentage (10%) of neonatal HSV infections result from postnatal HSV exposure. Sources include symptomatic and asymptomatic oropharyngeal shedding by either parent, hospital personnel, or other contacts and maternal breast lesions.

Presentation

- Typically at 7–14 days
- Often initially nonspecific, with irritability, lethargy, fever, or failure to feed
- Consider in any babies with sepsis-like illness, particularly if deranged liver function tests (LFTs) and or coagulation.

The three classical presentations are:
1. *Skin, eye, and mouth disease*: Disease localized to mucous membranes may progress to encephalitis or disseminated disease.
2. *Central nervous system (CNS) disease/encephalitis* can be isolated or occur in association with SEM or disseminated disease. Encephalitis is present in 70% of neonatal herpes. Mortality is 10% with treatment and high rate of neurological impairment at follow-up.
3. *Disseminated disease*: Multiorgan involvement—encephalitis, pneumonitis, hepatitis, disseminated intravascular disease (DIC), keratoconjunctivitis. Frequently no skin lesions are present. Mortality is 60% with treatment.

Management

- Babies born to mothers with active lesions thought to be primary should be advised to have elective cesarean section. Otherwise vaginal delivery is reasonable.
- Breastfeeding is not contraindicated as long as there are no breast lesions.
- *Asymptomatic baby and mother with active lesions*:
  - Send swabs for viral HSV detection from vesicular lesions if present and from conjunctiva, throat, nasopharynx and rectum (HSV surface culture or PCR) and HSV blood PCR.
  - Observe for skin and scalp rashes (especially vesicular lesions), respiratory distress (can cause pneumonitis), seizures, signs of sepsis.
  - HSV surface culture or PCR and HSV blood PCR: Any positive—send cerebrospinal fluid (CSF) cell count, chemistries, HSV PCR, serum alanine aminotransferase (ALT), blood platelets and start IV acyclovir 20 mg/kg dose every 8 hourly. Evaluate newborn at 24 hours—infant asymptomatic, CSF and ALT normal, PCR/culture negative—preemptive therapy for 10 days.
- Babies born to mother without genital lesions or those born by cesarean section may be discharged early but parents should be instructed to look out for any rashes or signs of viremia and to be in follow-up for 6 weeks.
- Babies with suspected herpes simplex infection (maternal primary or nonprimary first infection):
  - After clinical examination obtain, HSV surface culture (or PCR) HSV blood PCR, CSF cell count, chemistries, HSV PCR, serum ALT, blood platelets.
  - *Start IV acyclovir at 20 mg/kg/dose every 8 hourly*: Evaluate newborn at 24 hours—infant asymptomatic, CSF and ALT normal, PCR/culture negative—Preemptive therapy for 10 days.
- *If infant symptomatic or reports/culture positive*: Treat for 14 days for SEM and 21 days for CNS or disseminated disease—repeat CSF, HSV PCR at the end of therapy in CNS disease—if positive then continue acyclovir for 7 more days; if negative then discontinue therapy.

INFANT BORN TO MOTHERS WITH TUBERCULOSIS

Introduction

Tuberculosis (TB) is caused due to infection with *Mycobacterium tuberculosis*.

Neonates are very susceptible to *M. tuberculosis*. Virtually all infections are acquired postnatally from maternal TB, rarely from staff with open TB, less commonly close household contacts. It can be acquired antenatally (congenital TB).

Congenital TB

- Occurs with maternal miliary TB or a recent primary infection.
- 50% of mothers are previously undiagnosed.

Mode of Transmission

- Infection from genital tract is rare, usually results in abortion or stillbirth
- Transplacental
- Hematogenous leads to primary focus in liver
- Via amniotic fluid by ingestion or aspiration.

Presentation

- Asymptomatic at birth, but most have an abnormal chest X-ray (CXR) and are symptomatic by 2-3 weeks.
- Symptomatic at birth, very sick, and may be infectious.

Clinical Features of Congenital TB

Fever, respiratory distress, hepatosplenomegaly, lymphadenopathy, poor feeding, meningitis (present in one third of cases), papules, petechiae, poor weight again.

Diagnosis

- Gastric aspirates for TB GeneXpert, if TB GeneXpert not available then sent for acid-fast bacilli (AFB) staining (only 10% positive).
- CXR
- Mantoux test
- TB PCR (25–83% positive)
- Culture takes 6 weeks
- Lumbar puncture
- Diagnosis often has to rely on making the diagnosis in the mother.

Treatment

Recommended treatment:

- *2HRZE + 4 HR (E)*: Daily doses for isoniazid (INH) 7–15 mg/kg, rifampicin (R) 10–20 mg/kg ethambutol (E) 15–25 mg/kg, pyrazinamide (Z) 30–40 mg/kg.
- May require antitubercular treatment (ATT) for 9–12 months.
- Adjust the dose of ATT drugs at each postnatal visit according to weight.

No need to give pyridoxine routinely. If ethambutol is given in a dose of 20 mg/kg/day or lesser and for 2 months, the risk of optic neuritis is negligible.

Reassure the mother that it is safe to breastfeed her baby. Separation of mother and neonates is necessary only if mother is sick/nonadherent to treatment/sputum positive (open TB).

Treatment approach of a baby with congenital TB is shown in **Flowchart 1**.

Give Bacillus Calmette-Guérin (BCG) at birth as INH does not interfere with BCG uptake.

- Dose of INH 10 mg/kg/day
- Adjust the dose of ATT dugs at each postnatal visit according to weight.
- No need to give pyridoxine routinely.

INFANT WITH MATERNAL TOXOPLASMOSIS

Introduction

Toxoplasma gondii, an obligate intracellular protozoan parasite, is an important human pathogen, especially for the fetus, newborn, and immunocompromised patient.

T. gondii exists in three infectious forms: (1) Tachyzoites, (2) tissue cysts containing bradyzoites, and (3) oocysts containing sporozoites. The tachyzoite is the form responsible for symptoms during acute infection, whereas the tissue cyst is responsible for latent infection. The only definitive host of *T. gondii* is the cat. Intermediate hosts include all warm-blooded animals and human.

Risk of congenital infection rises as pregnancy progresses, but sequelae are more severe with infection early in pregnancy. Overall risk of congenital infection following maternal infection in pregnancy varies from 20 to 50%.

Clinical Manifestations

- Maternal infection is asymptomatic in >90% of women. However, symptoms can include fatigue, painless lymphadenopathy, and chorioretinitis.
- Fetal findings on ultrasound (US) include hydrocephalus, brain, splenic and hepatic calcifications, hepatosplenomegaly, and ascites.
- *Neonatal infection*: Four recognized patterns of presentation for congenital toxoplasmosis:
  1. *Subclinical/asymptomatic infection*: Most infants with congenital toxoplasmosis (70–90%) do not have overt signs of infection at birth. If untreated, a large proportion will later demonstrate visual, CNS deficits, hearing impairment, learning disabilities, or mental retardation several months to year later.

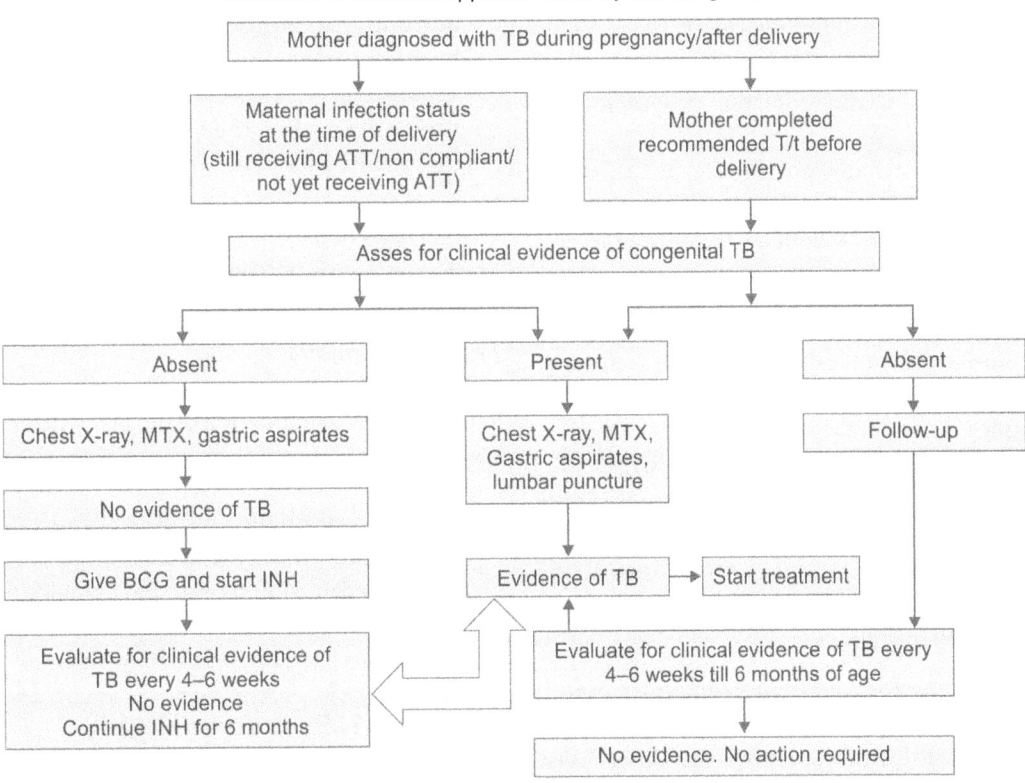

Flowchart 1: Treatment approach of a baby with congenital TB.

(ATT: antitubercular treatment; INH: isoniazid; T/t: treatment; TB: tuberculosis; MTX: mantoux test)

2. *Neonatal symptomatic disease*: Signs of congenital disease at birth include maculopapular rash, lymphadenopathy, hepatosplenomegaly, jaundice, pneumonitis, diarrhea, hypothermia, petechiae, and thrombocytopenia. CNS symptoms include cerebral calcifications, hydrocephalus, seizures, CSF abnormalities meningoencephalitis and chorioretinitis.
3. Delayed onset is most often seen with premature infants and occurs within the first 3 months of age.
4. Sequelae or relapse in infancy through adolescence of a previously untreated infection. Chorioretinitis develops in up to 85% of adolescents/young adults with previously untreated congenital infection.

Diagnosis

- Diagnosis is by a combination of serology, looking for IgM and/or IgA initially, then following IgG through the first year of life. Positive IgM or IgA antibody at least 10 days after birth is diagnostic. A positive IgG at 12 months of age is diagnostic of congenital toxoplasmosis.
- PCR-blood, CSF, and urine should be tested in infants with suspected infection. A positive PCR is diagnostic of infection. When CSF PCR results were combined with IgM and IgA antibody results for diagnosis, sensitivity is increased.
- CSF analysis.
- *Pathologic findings*: *T. gondii*-specific immunoperoxidase staining can be performed on any tissue.
- Ophthalmic examination at birth and every 3 months until 18 months of age followed by every 6–12 months until 18 years old.
- Computed tomography (CT) scan without contrast is the preferred study for brain imaging to look for calcifications, hydrocephalus, and cerebral atrophy.
- *Routine laboratory tests*: Abnormal complete blood count (CBC), liver enzymes and bilirubin levels can also be seen with disseminated disease.
- Screening for hearing loss with otoacoustic emission (OAE) or auditory brainstem response by 3 months of age. Full audiologic evaluation by 24 months of age.

Treatment

Maternal infection with Toxoplasma:
- Gestation <18 weeks: Maternal treatment with spiramycin
- Gestation >18 weeks or positive amniotic fluid PCR or affected fetus

Maternal treatment with pyrimethamine, sulfadiazine and folinic acid: At birth (if mother infected)—perform histopathology of placenta.

Evaluate the newborn:
- Physical examination of newborn (majority are asymptomatic)
- Eye examination for chorioretinitis
- CT scan of brain
- Serology
- Other tests such as CSF analysis.

Normal parameters: Regular follow-up and repeat IgG titer at 12 months of age. If IgG at 12 months negative—infant not infected, no follow-up required.

Abnormal parameters: Congenital infection or symptoms at follow-up.

For congenital infection and if positive IgG at 12 months, i.e., asymptomatic congenital infection—treat infant for 12 months with pyrimethamine, sulfadiazine and folinic acid and regular follow-up.

Dosage:
- Pyrimethamine 2 mg/kg once daily for 2 days, then 1 mg/kg once daily for 6 months, then 1 mg/kg three times a week to complete 1 year of therapy.
- *Sulfadiazine*: 50 mg/kg every 12 hourly for 1 year.
- *Folinic acid*: 10 mg three times a week, administered until 1 week after completing pyrimethamine.
- Prednisone (0.5 mg/kg 12 hourly) may be added if CSF protein exceeds 1 g/dL or active chorioretinitis with lesions very close to macula.

Follow-up: Includes neurologic and ophthalmologic examinations at 3 monthly intervals for first 2 years, 6 monthly intervals in third year and annually thereafter until adolescence.

INFANT BORN TO MOTHER WITH SYPHILIS INFECTION

Introduction

Syphilis is caused by the spirochete, *Treponema pallidum*. It is a sexually transmitted infection (STD). Pregnant women with syphilis can transmit it through the placenta to the fetus or at birth to the neonate. Congenital infection can have severe consequences to the fetus and newborn including perinatal death, premature delivery, low birth weight, congenital anomalies, active congenital syphilis and long-term sequelae such as deafness and neurologic impairment.

Diagnosis of Syphilis

Routine serological testing for syphilis (STS) must be undertaken in all women at first prenatal visit. In high risk cases, it should be repeated at 28 weeks and at delivery. Routine STS in neonates for screening purpose is not useful in view of high false-negative rates.

Serologic tests for syphilis:
- Nontreponemal tests include the rapid plasma reagin (RPR) card test, the Venereal Disease Research Laboratory (VDRL) slide test, the unheated serum reagin (USR), and the toluidine red unheated serum test (TRUST). Nontreponemal tests will be positive in approximately 80% of cases of primary syphilis, nearly 100% cases of secondary syphilis, and 75% cases of latent and tertiary syphilis.
- Treponemal tests include the fluorescent treponemal antibody absorption test (FTA-ABS), *T. pallidum* hemagglutination assay (TPHA) and enzyme immunoassay (EIA). These tests are not used for screening rather they are used to confirm positive nontreponemal tests.

Management

Mother with syphilis (reactive VDRL/RPR and confirmed by reactive TPHA/FTA-ABS).

Evaluate the infant:
- Assess adequacy of maternal treatment.
- Pathologic examination of the placenta or umbilical cord.
- Dark-field microscopy of suspicious lesions or body fluids.
- Clinical examination of infant for evidence of syphilis (nonimmune hydrops, anemia, jaundice, hepatosplenomegaly, rhinitis, skin rash, pseudoparalysis).
- Quantitative VDRL/RPR on infant serum (not cord blood). No need for TPHA/FTA-ABS.

Scenario 1: Proven or Highly Probable Disease

- Physical abnormalities suggestive of congenital syphilis
- VDRL/RPR: 4 × higher titer than the mother's titer
- Positive dark-field test of body fluids.

Additional evaluation:
- CSF (VDRL, cell count, and protein concentration)
- CBC (with differential and platelet count)
- Other tests as clinically indicated [long-bone and CXR, LFTs, neuroimaging, ophthalmologic examination and brainstem evoked response audiometry (BERA)].

Treatment

Penicillin G (1–1.5 lakh units/kg/day) administered as 50,000 units/kg/dose every 12 hourly IV during first 7 days of life and then 8 hourly for a total of 10 days.

Procaine penicillin G: 50,000 units/kg/dose IM in a single dose daily for 10 days.

Scenario 2: Possible Congenital Syphilis

Presence of all three:
1. Normal physical examination
2. VDRL/RPR <4 × of maternal titer
3. *Mother*: Not treated/inadequately treated/treated with nonpenicillin regimen treated <4 weeks before delivery. Additional evaluation as done for scenario 1.

Treatment: As for scenario 1.

If any part of the infants evaluation is abnormal or not interpretable (e.g., CSF sample contaminated with blood), or if follow-up is not certain, then full 10-day course of penicillin-G should be given.

Benzathine penicillin G 50,000 units/kg/dose/IM in a single dose if the complete evaluation is normal and follow-up is certain.

Scenario 3: Congenital Syphilis Less Likely

Presence of all three:
1. Normal physical examination
2. VDRL/RPR <4 × of maternal titers
3. Mother adequately treated during pregnancy and <4 weeks before delivery and does not have any reinfection or relapse.
No additional evaluation is required.

Treatment

No treatment is required if follow-up is certain. Benzathine penicillin G 50,000 units/kg/dose IM in a single dose might be considered, particularly if follow-up is uncertain.

Scenario 4: Congenital Syphilis Unlikely

Presence of all three:
1. Normal physical examination
2. VDRL/RPR titer < 4 × of maternal titer
3. Mother adequately treated before pregnancy and her VDRL/RPR titer remained low and stable before and during pregnancy and at delivery.
No additional evaluation is required.

Treatment: Same as scenario 3.

PERINATAL HUMAN IMMUNODEFICIENCY VIRUS INFECTION

Introduction

The human immunodeficiency virus (HIV) pandemic is one of the most serious health crises the world faces today. The UNAIDS estimated that since 1995 more than 350,000 new HIV infections in children have been prevented due to antiretroviral therapy (ART) for prophylaxis in pregnant women. Most children living with HIV acquire the infection through mother-to-child transmission (MTCT), especially in the perinatal period.

Early diagnosis of HIV infection in a pregnant women followed by counseling optimizes her medical and psychosocial care, and also decreases the incidence of MTCT.

Risk Factors for Perinatal HIV Transmission

- *Maternal factors*: Advanced disease (low CD4 count, high viral load, symptoms of AIDS), primary maternal infection during pregnancy, rupture of membranes for >4 hours, maternal bleeding, mother not on ART, vaginal delivery, other STDs, isolated HIV-1 infection.
- *Fetoplacental factors*: Chorioamnionitis, placenta previa, first of twins, prematurity (increased peripartum transmission).
- *Postnatal factors*: Breastfeeding, higher breast milk virus load, mastitis or nipple lesions, maternal seroconversion during breastfeeding, infant on breastfeeding having thrush at <6 months of age.

Prevention of Perinatal HIV

In absence of any intervention, the risk of perinatal transmission is 15–30%.

Breastfeeding increases the risk by additional 5–20%.

The risk of MTCT can be reduced to under 2% by interventions that include antiretroviral (ARV) prophylaxis given to women during pregnancy and labor and to the infant in the first 6 weeks of life, obstetrical interventions including elective cesarean delivery (prior to the onset of labor and rupture of membranes), and complete avoidance of breastfeeding.

ARV regime for treating infants born to HIV infected women: If mother received ART adequately and regularly in antenatal period:

- *Infant exclusively breastfeeding*: Daily nevirapine (NVP) prophylaxis at birth and continued for 4–6 weeks.
- *Infant on exclusive replacement feeding*: Daily NVP prophylaxis (or twice daily AZT) at birth and continued for 4–6 weeks.

High-risk infant should receive following regimen, irrespective of type of feeding: Two drugs: AZT given twice daily and NVP once daily for first 6 weeks of life irrespective of type of feed followed by either both (AZT and NVP) or NVP alone for an additional 6 weeks (total of 12 weeks) for infants of mother who are receiving ART and are breastfeeding.

High-risk Infants

- Mother receiving <4 weeks of ART at the time of delivery (if viral load testing not available).
- Mother having high viral load as defined by ribonucleic acid >1,000 copies/mL within 4 weeks before delivery.
- Mother acquiring infection during pregnancy or breastfeeding.
- HIV exposure first identified at delivery or in postpartum period in a breast fed infant with a negative HIV test prenatally.

Drug dosages: Used for MTCT:
- *Infant from birth to 6 weeks*:
  - Birth weight <2 kg:
    - NVP 2 mg/kg/dose OD or/and GA >35 weeks (0.2 mL/kg once daily)
    - Zidovudine 4 mg/kg/dose BD or (0.4 mL/kg BD)
  - Birth weight between 2 and 2.5 kg:
    - NVP 10 mg OD (1 mL of syrup OD)
    - Zidovudine 10 mg dose BD (1 mL of syrup BD)

- Birth weight > 2.5 kg.
  - NVP 15 mg OD (1.5 mL of syrup once daily)
  - Zidovudine 15 mg BD (1.5 mL of syrup BD)
- Age >6–12 weeks:
  - NVP 20 mg OD (2 mL syrup OD)
  - Zidovudine dose not established for prophylaxis use treatment dose 60 mg BD (6 mL syrup BD)
  - NVP syrup (1 mL-10 mg); Zidovudine syrup (1 mL-10 mg)
  - NVP first dose to be given within 6–12 hours of delivery.
- Premature infants <35 weeks of GA should be dosed using expert guidance.

Postnatal Diagnosis of HIV Infection

- In children younger than 18 months, diagnosis of HIV infection in based on a positive virological test at 6 weeks for HIV or its components (usually by HIV-DNA PCR) by dry blood spot (DBS). If positive result with DBS, then it is confirmed by a second test on a separate sample with whole blood repeated at the earliest.
- In breastfeeding infants (as they are at constant risk of acquiring HIV infection), virological assays to detect HIV should be conducted at least 6 weeks or more after the complete cessation of breastfeeding.
- Confirmation tests for HIV by antibody tests (three rapid tests) has to be done at 18 months for all babies.
- For breastfeeding infants diagnosed HIV positive, pediatric ART should be started and breastfeeding to be continued ideally until the baby is 2 years old.
- Based on revised World Health Organization (WHO) guidelines, one may perform additional nucleic acid testing (NAT) at birth in order to identify in-utero transmission of infection. Infants who have positive NAT at birth are likely to have infected in utero. In such infant, ART must be started immediately after obtaining blood sample for second test to confirm the infection as these infants will have faster progression of the disease. If the second test is negative, a third NAT should be done before interrupting ART.

Cotrimoxazole Prophylaxis

- Cotrimoxazole prophylaxis is recommended for all HIV-exposed infants under age 18 months starting at 4–6 weeks of age and continued until HIV infection can be excluded.
- In children < 6 months dose is 2.5 mL once daily (syrup trimethoprim 40 mg and sulfamethoxazole 200 mg/5 mL). According to weight:

3–5.9 kg	2.5 mL
6–9.9 kg	5 mL
10–14.9 kg	7.5 mL
15–19.9 kg	10 mL
20–24.9 kg	10 mL

Immunization

- HIV-exposed or infected but asymptomatic children should receive all standard vaccines as per national immunization schedule.
- HIV-infected children with immune suppression or symptoms should receive all standard vaccines except BCG, oral polio vaccine (OPV), and varicella vaccines.
- Consider *Haemophilus influenza* type B (HiB) and pneumococcal vaccines in all HIV-exposed children (irrespective of symptoms or CD4 count).

APPROACH TO AN INFANT WITH SUSPECTED CONGENITAL CYTOMEGALOVIRUS INFECTION

Introduction

Cytomegalovirus (CMV) is a double-stranded enveloped DNA virus. It is a member of the herpes virus family, it is highly species specific. CMV infection in the newborn baby can be congenitally or perinatally/postnatally acquired. CMV is present in saliva, urine, genital secretions, breast milk and blood/blood products of infected persons and can be transmitted by exposure to any of these sources. Perinatal acquisition of CMV usually has no long term implications for the baby.

Clinical Disease (Manifestations)

In congenital infection, it may present at birth or may manifest with symptoms later in infancy. Only very low birthweight (VLBW) preterm infants (<1,500 g) or immunosuppressed infants will have symptomatic disease from peripartum or postnatal CMV acquisition.

- *Congenital symptomatic CMV disease* can present as an acute fulminant infection involving multiple organ systems with as high as 30% mortality.
  Constellation of signs such intrauterine growth restriction (IUGR), jaundice, petechiae or purpura, hepatosplenomegaly, microcephaly, retinitis, pneumonitis and/or "blueberry muffin spots" reflecting extramedullary hematopoiesis.
  Laboratory abnormalities include elevated hepatic transaminases and bilirubin levels (as much as half conjugated), anemia and thrombocytopenia.
- *Asymptomatic congenital infection*: At birth in 5–15% of neonates can manifest as late disease in infancy, throughout the first 2 years of life. Abnormalities include developmental abnormalities, hearing loss, seizures, mental retardation, motor spasticity, and acquired microcephaly.
- Peripartum and postnatally acquired CMV infection may occur from intrapartum exposure to the virus within the maternal genital tract, from exposure to infected breast milk, from exposure to infected blood or blood products

or through urine or saliva. Almost all term infants remain asymptomatic with the exception of severely immune-compromised infants. Hearing testing over the first 2 years of life is done if documented to have acquired CMV.

- **CMV pneumonitis**: It has been associated with pneumonitis occurring primarily in preterm infants < 4 months old. Symptoms include tachypnea, cough, coryza, and nasal congestion. Intercostal retractions, hypoxemia, and apnea may occur. A small number of infants may require respiratory support.
- Transfusion-acquired CMV infection can be prevented by using blood/blood products from CMV-seronegative donors or filtered, leuko-reduced products.

Diagnosis

There are these rapid diagnostic techniques:

- **CMV PCR**: CMV may be detected by PCR in urine, saliva, or blood. Sensitivity and specificity of this test are quite high for saliva and urine but a negative PCR in blood does not rule out infection.
- *Spin-enhanced or "shell vial" culture*: Virus can be isolated from saliva and in high titers from urine. A negative result generally rules out CMV infection, except in infants who may have acquired infection within the prior 2–3 weeks.
- **CMV antigen**: Positive results confirm CMV infection and viremia; however, negative results do not rule out CMV infection.
- **CMV IgG and IgM**: Serum antibody titers to CMV has limited usefulness for the neonate, although negative IgG titers in both maternal and infant sera are sufficient to exclude congenital CMV infection. Infected infants will continue to produce IgG whereas uninfected infants usually show a decline in IgG within 1 month and have no detectable titers by 4–12 months.

Management

Consider congenital CMV infection in the following scenarios:

- *Infant with symptomatic disease*:
  - Infant with abnormal imaging consistent with CMV infection—periventricular calcifications, periventricular leukomalacia (PVL), ventriculomegaly, vasculitis, polymicrogyria.
  - *Abnormal fetal ultrasound*: Echogenic bowel, IUGR, microcephaly or abnormal fetal brain imaging, hepatic calcifications, fetal hydrops or ascites.

- *Infant born to mother with CMV infection during pregnancy*: Perform urine/saliva PCR within first 3 weeks, if negative—congenital infection ruled out, if positive—congenital infection, then perform detailed physical and neurological evaluation, CBC, LFT, hearing and ophthalmology evaluation and USG cranium, CT/MRI (if microcephaly or neurological signs).

If moderate or severe symptomatic infection: Treat infant with oral valganciclovir or IV ganciclovir for 6 months if diagnosed within 1 month of life (efficacy of initiating treatment in >1 month is not known).

If mild symptomatic infection: Follow-up till 2 years, no treatment required. (Majority of infected infant (90%) are asymptomatic at birth. However, 15% will develop long-term sequelae (SNHL) within first 2 years of life mandating regular follow-up with hearing evaluation.

If asymptomatic infection with normal hearing: Follow-up till 2 years, no treatment required.

If asymptomatic infection with isolated SNHL: Treat one-to-one basis after discussion—follow-up till 2 years, no treatment required.

Dose of valganciclovir is 16 mg/kg/dose 12 hourly orally and that of ganciclovir is 6 mg/kg/dose IV 12 hourly. Absolute neutrophil count and aminotransferases need to be monitored during treatment for neutropenia and transaminitis.

SUGGESTED READING

1. Eichenwald EC, Hansen AR, Stark AR, Martin CR. Cloherty and Stark's Manual of Neonatal care, 8th edition. Philadelphia: Lippincott Williams & Wilkins (LWW), 2016.
2. Fox G, Hoque N, Watts T. Oxford Handbook of Neonatology, 2nd edition. USA: Oxford University Press; 2017.
3. MacDonald MG, Mullett MG, Seshia MMK. Avery's Neonatology: Pathophysiology and Management of the Newborn, 6th edition. Philadelphia: Lippincott Williams & Wilkins (LWW); 2005.
4. Paul VK, Bagga A. Ghai Essential Pediatrics, 9th edition. New Delhi: CBS Publishers Pvt Ltd; 2018.
5. Roberton NRC. In: Rennie JM, Roberton NRC. Rennie and Roberton's Textbook of Neonatology, 5th edition. London: Churchill Livingstone; 2014.
6. World Health Organization (WHO). Consolidated guidelines on the use of antiretroviral drugs for treating and preventing HIV infection, 2nd edition. Geneva: WHO; 2016.

21 CHAPTER
Neonatal Follow-up for Normal Newborn and Young Children

Suman Sudha Tirkey

INTRODUCTION

Follow-up or well-child visits for infants and young children up to 5 years of age provide opportunities for physician to screen for medical problem to provide anticipatory guidance and promote good health. There are certain questions at follow-up which has to answered while examinations of normal newborn as why, when, what, and how.

WHY TO EXAMINE?

The timing of initial follow-up care of the newborn after nursery discharge is based on several factors:
- The newborns' gestational age and postnatal age at discharge.
- Whether the newborn is breastfeeding or formula feeding.
- The quality and efficiency of the newborns feeding abilities.
- Presence of risk factors that predispose to complications or hospital admission.
- Birth weight or discharge weight.

For newborn discharged within 48 hours after delivery, the OPD follow-up should be in 48 hours of discharge. If early follow-up cannot be ensured, early discharge should be deferred. For newborns discharged between 48 and 72 hours of age, OPD follow-up should be within 2–3 days of discharge.

The follow-up visit is designed to perform the following functions:
- Assess the infants' general state of health including weight, hydration, and degree of jaundice.
- Identify new problems.
- Review adequacy of oral intake and assess elimination pattern.
- Assess quality of mother–infant bonding.
- Reinforce parental education.
- Provide anticipatory guidance and healthcare maintenance.

WHEN TO EXAMINE?

According to the American Academy of Pediatrics (AAP) recommendations, babies should get checkup at birth, 3–5 days after birth and then at 1, 2, 4, 6, 9, and 12 months.

According to the Indian Academy of Pediatrics (IAP) recommended monitoring should be done at 6, 10, 14 weeks, 6, 9, and 12 months along with immunization contact.

HOW AND WHAT TO EXAMINE?

Most important in the examination of the newborn is observation.

Physical examination of newborn includes:
- Measurements of weight, length, and head circumference which must be compared with standardized growth data.
- *Vitals*: Body temperature heart rate and respiratory rate should be recorded by nurse.
- Observation of respiratory pattern is important.
- Palpation and auscultation of abdomen and chest wall is important.
- Inspection and palpation of umbilicus and umbilical cord should be done.
- Open diaper and examine genitalia and perineum.
- Examination of the hips and lower extremities for the range of motion of hip and perform Barlow and Ortolani maneuver.
- Neonatal reflexes should be examined.
- Feeding should be assessed.
- Status of immunization according to the age.
- If any danger sign encountered in examination of newborn follow-up will be according to the risk involved along with the investigations.

Day-wise Examination of Newborn during Visits

Newborn examination on first day of life:
- Assessment of any difficulty maintaining body temperature and vitals.
- Initiate breastfeeding, support correct attachment and position.

- Make sure the cord is well tied and does not bleed.
- Check for jaundice in any location to rule out pathological jaundice.

Newborn examination on 2nd and 3rd days:
- Newborns that have been infected during birth can show symptoms of infection.
- Weight loss of 5–7% is normal in first days of life but should not exceed 10% of birth weight.
- Watch for physiological jaundice.
- Check for passage of urine and stools.

Newborn examination at 7 days:
- The newborn should start gaining weight and return to his/her birth weight by the 14th day after birth.
- Newborns that have been infected during birth can show symptoms of infection.
- Examine the newborn for jaundice.
- Immunization according to the national guidelines.

The well-child visit allows for comprehensive assessment of a child and the opportunity of further evaluation if abnormalities are detected.

A complete history during the well child includes information about:
- Birth history
- Prior screening
- Diet
- Sleep
- Dental care according to age
- Medical, surgical history if any
- Family and social history if any
- Immunization history at each visit.

Examination:
- A head-to-toe examination including review of growth (in each visit).
- Developmental surveillance in terms of achievement of milestones (in each visit).

Well-child visit provide the opportunity to answer parents or care givers question and to provide age-appropriate guidance.

Well-child visit according to the IAP is with national immunization schedule **(Table 1)**.

DEVELOPMENT AND SURVIEILLANCE

The AAP and IAP recommends early identification and developmental delays. Any areas of concern should be evaluated with a formal developmental screening. A child who does not attain the milestones by he recommended limit is a red flag sign and should be evaluated for cause of developmental delay.

IRON DEFICIENCY

Multiple reports have associated iron deficiency with neurodevelopment. The AAP recommends supplements for preterm infants beginning at 1 month of age and exclusively breastfed term infants at 6 months of age. The AAP recommends measurements of hemoglobin level at 12 months of age.

IMMUNIZATIONS

As per the IAP recommendation well-child visits are along with immunization schedule. Additional vaccines should be necessary based on medical history. Immunization history should be reviewed at each wellness visit.

ANTICIPATORY GUIDANCE

Safety

Infants should not be left alone on any high surface, and stairs should be secured by gates. Young children should be closely supervised at all times. Small objects are a choking hazard, especially for children younger than 3 years. Latex balloons, round objects, food can cause life-threatening airway obstruction. Long strings and cords can cause strangulation.

Dental Care

Infants should never have a bottle in bed and should be weaned by a cup by 12 months of age. Begin brushing teeth at tooth eruption with parents and caregivers supervising brushing until mastery. Assessment of dental health should occur at well-child visit.

Screen Time

Video chatting is acceptable for children <18 months otherwise digital media should be avoided. The AAP recommends screen time of maximum 1 h/day. Longer usage can cause sleep problems, increased risk of obesity, and social emotional delays.

Sleep

To decrease the risk of sudden infant death syndrome (SIDS), the AAP recommends that infant sleep on their backs on a firm mattress for the first year of life with no blankets or other soft objects on the crib. Breastfeeding, pacifier use, and room sharing protect against SIDS. Infant's exposure to tobacco, alcohol, drugs and sleeping in the bed with parents and caregivers increases the risk of SIDS.

Diet and Activity

- The AAP and IAP recommend breastfeeding until at least 6 months of age and ideally for the first 12 months.
- Vitamin D supplements 400 IU for the first year of life in exclusive breastfed babies is recommended to prevent vitamin D deficiency and rickets.
- Weaning should be started at the age of 6 months.
- Drinking juice should be avoided before 1 year of age.

TABLE 1: Well-child visit according to the IAP is with national immunization schedule.

Age	Points of examination to be considered
6 weeks	• Weight, length, and head circumference (HC) measurements, vaccines • *Vision*: Vertical tracking should be achieved at 4–6 weeks
10 weeks	• Weight, length, and HC measurements, vaccines and development • Social smile • No visual fixation or following is the red flag sign – If the child appears to take no notice of the surrounding, blindness can be suspected and the baby should be screened and further evaluated
14 weeks	• Physical examination, growth, vaccines and development • Neck holding • Social smile • Coos (musical vowel sound) • *Hearing*: By 3–4 months, the child turns his head toward the source of the sound
6 months	• Physical examination, growth, vaccines, and history of weaning should be taken and counseling regarding proper weaning should be done • *Development*: Sits in tripod fashion • Recognizes strangers, stranger anxiety • Monosyllables (ba, da, pa) • Not achieving vocalization till 6 months is the red flag sign
9 months	• Physical examination, growth, vaccines and development • Sitting without support • Waves bye-bye • Bisyllable (mama, dada, baba) • Hemoglobin estimation to rule out iron deficiency anemia
12 months	• Physical examination, growth and vaccines • *Development*: Stands without support • One to two words with meaning • *Red flag sign*: Sitting without support not attained by 10 months • Standing with assistance by 12 months • Deworming and continue iron with vitamin D supplements
18 months	• Physical examination, growth, vaccines and development • Runs • Scribbles • Undressing • *Red flag sign*: Hands and knees crawling not attained till 14 months • Standing alone is not attained by 17 months • Walking alone is not achieved by 18 months • Single words by 18 months
5 years	• Physical examination, growth, vaccines and development • Walks up and downward • Can ride tricycle • Hops on one foot • Can copy cross and triangle • Knows full name • Says song or poem • Asks meaning of words

SUGGESTED READING

1. American Academy of Pediatrics Section on breastfeeding and the use of human milk. Pediatrics. 2012;129(3):e827-e41.
2. Baker RD, Greer FR; Committee on Nutrition. Diagnosis and prevention of iron deficiency and iron deficiency anemia in infants and young children. Pediatrics. 2010;126(5):1040-50.
3. Cloherty JP, Eichenwald EC, Stark AR. In: Cloherty JP, Eichenwald EC (eds). Manual of Neonatal Care, 6th edition. Philadelphia: Wolters Kluwer Health; 2011.
4. Committee on injury, Violence, and Poison Prevention. Prevention of choking among children. Pediatrics. 2010;125(3): 601-7.
5. Committee on Practice and Ambulatory Medicine, Bright Futures Periodicity Schedule Workgroup. 2017 Recommendations

for Preventive Pediatric Health Care. Pediatrics. 2017;139(4): e20170254.
6. Council of Communications and Media. Media and Young minds. Pediatrics. 2016; 138(5):e20162591.
7. Council on Children with Disabilities; Section on Developmental Behavioral Pediatrics; Bright Futures Steering Committee; Medical Home Initiatives for Children with Special Needs Project Advisory Committee. infants and children with developmental disorders in the medical home algorithm for developmental surveillance and screening. Pediatrics. 2006;118(1):405-20.
8. Ghai Essential Paediatrics, 8th edition Development; 48-55.
9. Heyman MB, Abrams SA, American Academy of Pediatrics Section on Gastroenterology, Hepatology, and Nutrition; Committee on Nutrition. Fruit juice in infants, children and adolescents: Current recommendations. Pediatrics. 2017;139(6):e20170967.
10. Illingworth RS. The Development of the Infant and the Young Child, 9th edition. USA: Elsevier; 1999.
11. Kendrik D, Young B, Mason-Jones AJ, Ilyas N, Achana FA, Cooper NJ, et al. Home safety education and provision of safety equipment for injury prevention (review). Evid Based Child Health. 2013;8(3):761-939.
12. McInerny TK, Adam HM, Campbell DE, DeWitt TG, Foy JM, Kamat DM. Follow up care of the healthy newborn. In: Taylor A, Parekh J (eds). Textbook of Pediatric Care. Illinois, United States: American Academy of Pediatrics; 2020.
13. Moon RY; Task Force on Sudden Infant Death Syndrome. SIDS and other sleep related infant deaths: Evidence base for 2016 updated recommendation for a safe infant sleeping environment. Pediatrics. 2016; 138(5):e20162940.
14. Section on Oral Health. Maintaining and improving the oral health of young children. Pediatrics. 2014;134(6):1224-9.
15. Taeusch WH, Ballard RA, Gleason CA. In: Smith JB (Ed). Avery's Disease of the Newborn. Initial Evaluation: History and Physical examination of the newborn, 10th edition. USA: Elsevier Saunders; 2017.
16. Turner K. Well-child visits for infants and young children. Am Fam Physician. 201815;98(6):347-53.
17. Wagner CL, Greer FR; American Academy of Pediatrics Section on Breastfeeding; Committee on Nutrition. Prevention of Rickets and Vitamin D Deficiency in infants, children and adolescents. Pediatrics. 2008;122(5)1142-52.
18. World Health Organization. Complete examination of a newborn. [online] Available from: https://www.euro.who.int/__data/assets/pdf_file/0006/146814/EPC_FAC_guide_pt2_mod_1N_7N.pdf. [Last accessed August, 2021].

CHAPTER 22: Follow-up of High-risk Newborn

Puja Dhupar

INTRODUCTION

Improving perinatal and neonatal care has led to increased survival of infants who are at risk for long-term morbidities such as developmental delay, and visual and hearing problems. Moreover, many of these neonates tend to have higher incidence of growth failure and ongoing medical illnesses. A proper and appropriate follow-up program would help in early detection of these problems thus paving way for early intervention.

WHO NEEDS FOLLOW-UP?

All healthcare facilities caring for sick neonates must have follow-up program. It requires establishing multidisciplinary team. The level of follow-up should be based on anticipated severity of risk to neurodevelopment. The at-risk neonates may seem healthy and can be missed on a routine follow-up. At-risk neonates should be identified before discharge from newborn intensive care unit (NICU) and accordingly classify risk factors **(Table 1)**.

WHERE TO FOLLOW AND WHO SHOULD FOLLOW-UP?

Place of follow-up should be easily accessible to parents and should be mentioned in discharge card. Low-risk infants can be followed up at "Well baby clinic". Moderate- and high-risk infants should be followed up in or near facility providing level II and level III NICU care as it requires multidisciplinary approach involving team which includes pediatrician, child psychologist, pediatric neurologist, ophthalmologist, audiologist, occupational therapist, social worker, and dietician all under one roof.

WHEN? TIMING OF FOLLOW-UP VISITS

Initial follow-up visits should be *7–10 days* after the neonatal discharge. This is essential to evaluate how the infant is adapting to the home environment.

A clinic visit at *4 months* corrected age is important to document problems of inadequate catchup. Growth and severe neurologic abnormalities that might require

TABLE 1: Classification of risk factors.

Mild risk	Moderate risk	High risk
• Preterm weight: 1,500–2,500 g • HIE 1 transient • Hypoglycemia • Suspected sepsis • Neonatal jaundice • Needing PT • IVH grade 1	• Babies with weight 1,000–1,500 g • Gestation < 33 weeks • Twins/triplets • Moderate HIE • Hypoglycemia blood sugar < 25 mg/dL • Neonatal sepsis • Hyperbilirubinemia > 20 mg/dL or requirement of exchange transfusion • IVH grade 2 • Suboptimal home environment	• Babies with <1,000 g or gestation < 28 weeks • Major morbidities such as chronic lung disease, IVH, PVL • Severe HIE surgical conditions such as diaphragmatic hernia, TEF • SFD < 3rd centile or LFD > 97th centile • Mechanical ventilation > 24 hours • Persistent prolonged hypoglycemia and hypocalcemia • Seizures • Meningitis • Shock requiring inotropic/vasopressors • Infants born to HIV mother • Twin–twin transfusion • Neonatal bilirubin encephalopathy • Major malformations • IEM or other genetic disorders • Abnormal neurological examination at discharge

(HIE: hypoxic-ischemic encephalopathy; HIV: human immunodeficiency virus; IEM: inborn errors of metabolism; IVH: intraventricular hemorrhage; LFD: large-for-dates; PVL: periventricular leukomalacia; SFD: small-for-dates; TEF: tracheoesophageal fistula)

TABLE 2: High-risk baby follow-up schedule.

Who will follow-up	High-risk team
Where	High-risk clinic
When	†4 months, 8 months, 1 year and yearly till 6 years

†Age: Age used for follow-up is calculated as corrected age. Corrected age is the sum of chronologic age in weeks minus the difference between 40 weeks of gestation and gestational age at birth. The correction is to be considered till 2 years of age.

intervention or physical therapy. *8 months* corrected age is a good time to identify the presence of developing cerebral palsy or other neurologic abnormality. It is also an excellent time for the first developmental assessment (preferably using the Bayley Scales of Infant Development).

By *18–24 months* corrected age, most transient neurologic findings have resolved, and the neurologically abnormal child may show adaptation to neurologic sequelae.

Beyond the age of *3 years*, other tests may be performed. These tests further validate the child's mental abilities. Language may also be measurable at this age.

From *4 years* of age, more subtle neurologic, visuomotor, and behavioral difficulties are measurable. These difficulties affect school performance even in children who have normal intelligence.

Ideally follow-up should continue till late adolescence as many cognitive, learning and behavioral problems more common in at-risk newborn may only become apparent on longer follow-up **(Table 2)**.

POINTS TO REMEMBER

- Correct for gestational age (preterm birth) until at least 2 years of age.
- Many abnormalities are observed during the 3-month postdischarge period of convalescence, most are transient and have little prognostic significance (Do not emphasize too much to parents).
- Be available, honest, and optimistic. After the initial diagnosis of abnormality is made, most children show improvement restitution, and growth.
- The majority of high-risk children do well.
- In some cases, the diagnosis of cerebral palsy, hydrocephalus, or blindness is made during the first year of life. Early intervention and supportive psychological help that can be facilitated by the follow-up clinic are crucial.
- Except when a severe neurologic or sensory disorder persists, ultimate development depends on parental education, social class, the child's genetic potential and the environment.
- The functional capacity attained is more important than the medical diagnosis of abnormality.

WHAT TO LOOK FOR IN FOLLOW-UP?

- Medical examination nutrition, growth, and immunization
- Ophthalmological assessment
- Hearing language and speech **(Flowchart 1)**
- Neurological examination
- Development assessment
- Function
- Behavior cognitive and intelligence status

Medical Examination

Physical examination, nutrition and growth, immunization, unresolved medical issues, laboratory tests (hemoglobin, calcium, phosphate, alkaline phosphate).

Complete physical examination must look for common anticipated medical problems some of which may have impact on developmental outcomes, e.g., hip examination, dysmorphism, signs of intrauterine (IU) infections, neurocutaneous markers.

Head Circumference

Head circumference (OFC) is the most important and simple tool that can predict abnormal brain growth.

- OFC centile < (microcephaly)/> length centile (hydrocephalus).
- Static/dropping centile of OFC in relation to length centile on serial follow-up.
- Growth–weight and length plotted on growth chart and compare centiles.
- Birth weight and discharge weight must be compared. Weight centile must be interpreted against length centile.

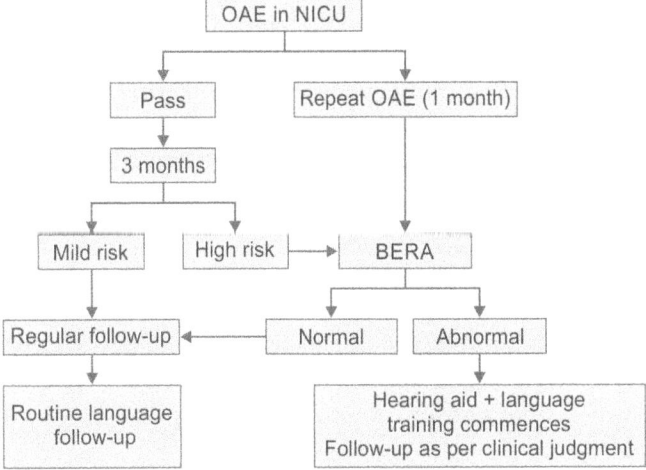

Flowchart 1: Hearing assessment.

(BERA: brainstem-evoked auditory response; OAE: otoacoustic emission; NICU: newborn intensive care unit)

Note: Infants with permanent hearing loss who receive intervention services prior 6 months of age have significantly better language outcomes.

- Poor growth may be a pointer to medical problems (can affect neurodevelopment).
- Poor growth is also often seen in babies with neurodevelopmental disorder (NDD) (as the feeding is not optimal).
- OFC must be recorded and plotted serially every health visit till 2 years of age.
- It must be assessed in context of length of the baby.
- Weight and length must be plotted at every health visit till 6 years of age.

In preterm babies <40 weeks' gestation use IU growth charts Fenton, later postnatal growth charts provided by the Centers for Disease Control and Prevention (CDC) can be used.

Unresolved medical problems must be addressed and medications reviewed:
- Chronic lung disease
- Gastroesophageal reflex disease
- Reactive airway disease.

Postdischarge Nutrition

Human milk fortifier: Preterm and very low birthweight (VLBW) babies continue to grow poorly, postdischarge nutrition remains a major issue during follow-up.

Because of their poor postnatal growth, there is a need for continuation of higher energy intakes. Deficiencies have been described with nutrients such as vitamin A, E, D, iron, zinc, and copper and most of these needs to be supplemented in preterm diet either by fortification or using preterm formula as they are deficient in preterm mature milk.

Recommendation
- Ensure adequate nutrition.
- *Iron*: Start at 4–6 weeks (can start at 2 weeks) till 2 years of age (3 mg/kg/day of elemental iron).
- *Calcium (as phosphate salt)*: Start when on full feeds—150 mg/kg/day of elemental calcium till term. (Monitor Hb, Ca, P, alkaline phosphatase, nearing 40 weeks corrected age).
- Multivitamin supplementation till approximately 3.5 kg.
- *Weaning may be started at 6 months corrected age in preterm babies.*

Immunization

The preterm/VLBW babies should be immunized according to chronological age and as per guidelines for full-term newborn. For hepatitis B, one should wait till the baby is 2,000 g.

Vision Screening

Retinopathy of prematurity (ROP) is emerging as one of the leading causes of preventable childhood blindness in India.

TABLE 3: Milestones for visual assessment.

Check	Vision
0–3 months	• Follows face from side to side • Smiles at your face
3–6 months	• Moves both eyes together • Reaches out for objects

- Screening for ROP should be performed in all preterm neonates who are born <34 weeks' gestation and/or <1,750 g birth weight as well as in babies 34–36 weeks gestation or 1,750–2,000 g birthweight if they have risk factors for ROP.
- The first retinal examination should be performed not later than 4 weeks of age or 30 days of life in infants born ≥ 28 weeks of gestational age. Infants born < 28 weeks or < 1,200 g birth weight should be screened early, by 2–3 weeks of age, to enable early identification of AP-ROP.
- The retinal findings should be classified and documented based on the international classification of retinopathy of prematurity (ICROP) guidelines.
- Follow-up examinations should be based on the retinal findings and should continue until complete vascularization or regressing ROP is documented or until treated based on the early treatment for retinopathy of prematurity (ETROP) guidelines.
- Laser photocoagulation delivered by the indirect ophthalmoscopic device is the mainstay of ROP treatment.
- The responsibility of recognition of infants for screening lies with the pediatrician/neonatologist.
- Communication with the parents regarding timely screening for ROP, seriousness of the issue, possible findings and consequences is extremely important.
- An assessment of refraction and examination for squint, other visual problems must be performed at least at 1 year and yearly thereafter till school age (5 years) **(Table 3)**.

Neurobehavioral and Neurological Assessment

Neurobehavioral assessment and neonatal neurological examination must form a part of routine clinical examination of newborn infant. Although predictive power of isolated neurological signs is not great but certain abnormal findings are associated with greater frequency of abnormal outcomes **(Table 4)**.

Neurological Examination

Infants with mild-to-moderate abnormalities may improve with time. This is known as transient neuromotor dysfunction. Infants with severe early neurological dysfunction is likely to have worst neurodevelopment outcome.

TABLE 4: Abnormal neurological finding and frequency of abnormal outcomes.	
Neurological signs in neonates (mostly term)	Increased risk of cerebral palsy
Abnormal tone limb, neck trunk	12–25 fold
Diminished cry for >1 day	21 fold
Weak or absent suck	14 fold
Need for garage or tube feeding	16–22 fold
Diminished activity >1 day	19 fold

Neuromotor Follow-up (Flowchart 2)

A structured age-appropriate neuromotor assessment should be performed by corrected age at least once during first 6 months, once during second 6 months and once yearly.

Gross motor function classification system: It is used for assessment of severity of motor disability and function after 2 years of age.

Neuroimaging: USG/CT/MRI

Neuroimaging is a very important complement to clinical assessment in the management of preterm and term neonates with encephalopathy.

Problems associated with imaging are the choice of right technique, timing, risk of radiation, need for sophisticated machines and trained manpower, etc.

Recommendations:
- All preterm babies born before 32 weeks and <1,500 g birthweight must undergo screening neurosonograms at 1–2 weeks and 36–40 weeks' corrected age.
- Ultrasounds (USGs) may be performed more often if the preterm baby has a catastrophic event such as seizure, frequent apnea that may reflect intraventricular hemorrhage (IVH).
- With limited facility available, it is advisable to have at least one USG at ~40 weeks of gestation in preterm babies.
- Babies with ventriculomegaly and cystic periventricular leukomalacia (PVL) have a very high incidence of cerebral palsy as compared to those with a normal neurosonogram.
- Magnetic resonance imaging (MRI) is more sensitive in detection of preterm brain injury, but USG has similar specificity in detection of severe lesions. (ventriculomegaly, cystic PVL and grade 3, 4 IVH).
- MRI is the diagnostic imaging modality in all babies with encephalopathy if intracerebral hemorrhage (ICH) is not suspected.
- Computed tomography (CT) is a better method for detection of intracranial calcifications.
- *Limitations:* USG is operator dependent, CT has risk of radiation exposure and MRI requires sedation and monitoring is not possible during the procedure unless monitors that are MRI compatible are available.

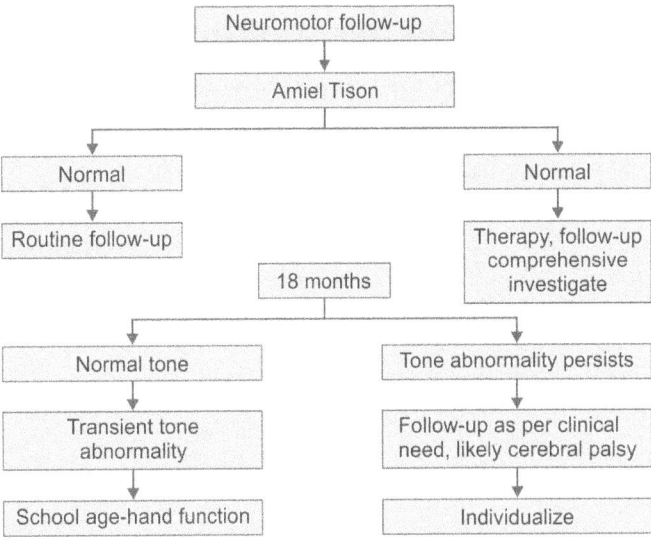

Flowchart 2: Algorithm for neuromotor follow-up.

Note:
- Serial comprehensive assessments by trained observers given an idea whether tone abnormalities are transient or persistent.
- A diagnosis of cerebral palsy is generally evident if the neurological signs persist by 18–24 months.
- Loss of abnormal neurological findings by 12 months is associated with better outcomes.

TABLE 5: Direct observation chart (DOC).	
Check milestone	DOC: If not achieved refer for developmental assessment
• 2 months • 4 months • 8 months • 12 months	• Social smile • Head holding • Sit alone • Stand alone • Make sure the baby can see, hear, and listen

Developmental Assessment

Developmental evaluation is a depth assessment to create a profile of child's strengths and weaknesses to all developmental areas. Its results are used to plan interventions. Various development scales which are commonly used are:
- *Direct observation chart (DOC):* Self-explanatory card that can be sued by parents **(Table 5)**
- Trivandrum development screening chart (TDSC)
- Denver development screening test (DDST)
- Developmental assessment scales for Indian infant (DASII)
- Cognitive developmental follow-up program and algorithm **(Table 6 and Flowchart 3)**.

Language and Speech Assessment

Comprehensive assessment of speech and language must be done between 1 and 2 years of age using Language Evaluation Scale Trivandrum (LEST).

Behavioral

- High incidence of behavioral problems in the high-risk newborn.

Cognitive Development Follow-up (Table 6 and Flowchart 3)

TABLE 6: Cognitive tests.

Cognitive test	DQ	DQ	IQ
Use till	Developmental assessment scales for Indian infant 0-2 ½ years Indian adaptation of Bayley's	• Bayley scale of infant development: III 0-3 ½ years • Revision of Bayley's II	• Wechsler intelligence scale, Stanford–Binet test • Above 2 ½ years
Results	Motor and mental scales	Motor, mental, language, socioemotional adaptive scales	Performance and verbal IQ
When	If fails screen or yearly	If fails screen or yearly	Yearly
Delay	DQ < 70	DQ < 70	IQ < 70, Borderline: 70–85

(DQ: digital intelligence; IQ: intelligence quotient)
Note: In the Indian context, the DASII is the best cognitive developmental assessment tool till 2 ½ years of age.

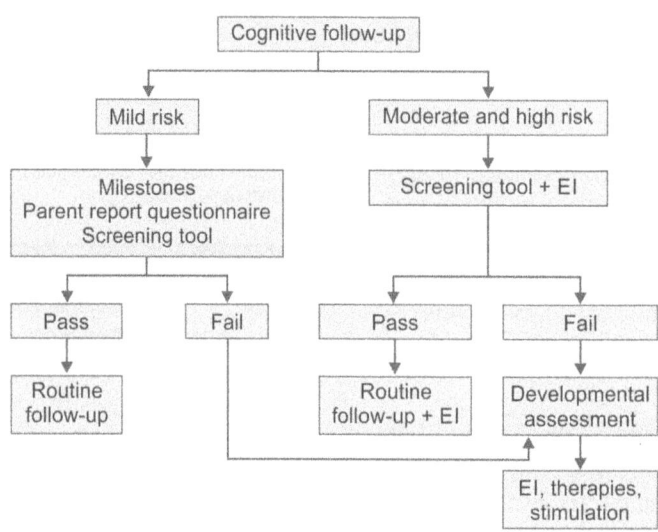

Flowchart 3: Cognitive follow-up algorithm.

(EI: early intervention)
Note: Early Intervention program must be started in the NICU itself once the neonate is medically stable and continued till least 1 year of age.

TABLE 7: Red flags for autism.

Check	Pervasive developmental disorder
12 months	No babbling, pointing, or other gestures
16 months	No single words
24 months	No two-word spontaneous phrases
	Any loss of any language or social skills at any age

- Pediatrician monitoring follow-up must probe for attention issues in social settings and its effect on learning
- With the rise in incidence of autism, administering a simple screen like the M-CHART-R follow-up at 18 months may help identify children with autistic features earlier **(Table 7)**.

HIGH RISK NEWBORN FOLLOW-UP PROTOCOL

Components	1½ Months	2½ Months	3½ Months	6 Months	9 Months	12 Months	18 Months	24 Months
Parental concerns	At every visit							
Medical problems	At every visit							
Vaccination	As per IAP schedule (2012)							
Anthropometry	At every visit ((weight, head circumference, thigh volume)							
Nutrition								
Diet	Exclusive breastfeeding				Weaning		Home diet	

Contd...

Contd...

Components	1½ Months	2½ Months	3½ Months	6 Months	9 Months	12 Months	18 Months	24 Months
MV drops	For preterm only vitamin D for all							
Iron	For preterm only				For term	For preterm	–	Yearly
Calcium/PO_4	For preterm only				For term	–	–	Yearly
Formula shift to term formula at 2.5 kg weight								
Neurological exam	At every visit							
Development test	Screening at each visit		Formal testing		Screening at each visit	Behavioral assessment	–	Formal testing
Eye evaluation	ROP screening at 1 month of age				For vision, squint, optic atrophy	–	–	For vision, squint, optic atrophy
Hearning	OAE at discharge, BERA for testing or confirmation at 3 months. Screen at each visit							
CT or MRI brain	As clinically indicated							
USG brain (!)	(i) At 36–40 weeks corrected age							
Language	–	–	–	–		LEST	–	LEST	–
Conseling	At every visit							
Biochemical screen	–	–	–	–	Hb, urine	–	Hb	Hb, urine, BP

(BERA: brain evoked response auditory; CT: computed tomography; Hb: hemoglobin; LEST: Language Evaluation Scale Trivandrum; MRI: magnetic resonance imaging; OAE; otoacoustic emissions; USG: ultrasonography)

CHAPTER 23: Neonatal Thrombocytopenia

Shantanu Verma

INTRODUCTION

- Thrombocytopenia is extremely common in the newborn intensive care unit (NICU) setting, and can be a marker of underlying disease, and are prone for risk factor for hemorrhage.
- In new born and infants, the normal range for platelet count is 150×10^3 to $450 \times 10^3/\mu L$. Platelet count decreases over the first few days after birth and begin to rise by 1 week of life.
- *Relation of platelet and spontaneous bleed*:
    - The chances of spontaneous bleeding is rare at platelet count of >1 lac.
    - Risk of spontaneous bleeding is minimal to mild at counts of 20×10^3 to $100 \times 10^3/\mu L$.
    - Risk of spontaneous bleeding is moderate if count is between 5×10^3 and $20 \times 10^3/\mu L$.
    - Risk of spontaneous bleeding is severe below counts of $5 \times 10^3/\mu L$.
- The preterm neonates tend to have slightly lower mean platelet counts than term infants and adults, a lower limit of "normal" of $150 \times 10^9/L$ still applies. Around 2% of healthy term infants will fall below this level, with many more sick preterm infants having low counts. Around 20% of neonates <28 weeks gestation develop severe thrombocytopenia ($<50 \times 10^9/L$).

CAUSES

The common causes of thrombocytopenia are different in sick neonate as compared to healthy neonate **(Table 1)**.

Fetal Thrombocytopenia

Fetal thrombocytopenia is mainly due to neonatal alloimmune thrombocytopenia (NAIT), the congenital infection and chromosomal abnormalities are the other principal considerations.

Thrombocytopenia in ill, preterm baby are commonly secondary to sepsis, followed by necrotizing enterocolitis (NEC), birth asphyxia, chronic intrauterine hypoxia, TORCH (toxoplasmosis, other agents, rubella, cytomegalovirus, and herpes simplex) infections, or disseminated intravascular coagulation.

TABLE 1: Causes of neonatal thrombocytopenia.

Type	Ill-appearing, premature		Well-appearing, full term	
	Early onset (<24 h)	Late onset (>72 h)	Early onset (<24 h)	Late onset (>72 h)
Common	• Sepsis • TORCH infection • Birth asphyxia • DIC • NEC	• Sepsis • Thrombosis • DIC • NEC • Drug-induced	• Placental insufficiency • Autoimmune • Alloimmune (NAIT) • Occult infection	• Occult infection • NEC
Rare	*Chromosomal disorders:* • Trisomy 13 • Trisomy 18 • Trisomy 21 • Turner syndrome	• Inborn errors of metabolism • Fanconi anemia	*Inherited syndromes:* • Bernard-Soulier • Wiskott-Aldrich • Thrombocytopenia absent radii • Others vascular tumors • Kasabach-Merritt	• Inborn errors of metabolism • Fanconi anemia

(DIC: disseminated intravascular coagulation; NAIT: neonatal alloimmune thrombocytopenia; NEC: necrotizing enterocolitis; TORCH: toxoplasmosis, other agents, rubella, cytomegalovirus, and herpes simplex)

Early-onset Neonatal Thrombocytopenia

- The typical pattern of low/low-to-normal platelet counts at birth (100–200 × 10^9/L), with levels falling to a nadir of 50–100 × 10^9/L at 4-5 days, and returns to normal by 7-10 days.
- It is seen in placental insufficiencies in preterm babies and in fetal hypoxia.
  These infants show a typical pattern of low/low-to-normal platelet counts at birth (100–200 × 10^9/L), with levels falling to a nadir of 50–100 × 10^9/L at 4-5 days. Counts generally return to normal at 7-10 days.
- There is associated transient neutropenia, nucleated RBC, and polycythemia.
- There is low chance of spontaneous bleed, if platelet count remains above 50 × 10^9/L. These babies grow well.
- *Causes*: In normal term infant, the causes are:
  - NAIT:
    - It has high risk of hemorrhage pronounced thrombocytopenia, with platelets typically below 50 × 10^9/μL.
    - NAIT occurs when the fetus inherits a paternal platelet antigen not carried by the mother; this antigen then becomes a target for maternal antibodies.
      Maternal platelets are normal.
    - NAIT frequently is symptomatic in first pregnancy.
    - There is significant risk of potential morbidity and mortality. Approximately 10-30% of newborns will develop intracranial hemorrhage (ICH), with about half occurring in utero.
    - The neurological sequelae is seen in 10% of affected neonate and death in 20% of affected neonates.
  - Placental insufficiency produces mild-to-moderate thrombocytopenia (50 × 10^3 to 150 × 10^3/μL) which resolves spontaneously within 7-10 days after birth. They presents with small for gestational age, intrauterine growth restriction, or maternal hypertension, diabetes, or preeclampsia.
  - *Neonatal autoimmune thrombocytopenia*:
    - Occurs due to maternal platelet autoantibodies because of maternal immune thrombocytopenia and systemic lupus erythematosus.
    - Two platelet levels normalize at age 10-60 days as maternal autoantibodies are cleared from the baby's circulation.
    - Around 10% of infants will be affected. There is low risk of significant hemorrhage (<1%), but should have cord full blood count done and if low, platelet count monitored during the first 3-5 days. If count falls to <30 × 10^9/L, consider intravenous immunoglobulin therapy.
  - Idiopathic.

Late-onset Neonatal Thrombocytopenia

- Thrombocytopenia after first 3 days of life and is due to sepsis or NEC until proven otherwise.
- Platelet count often drops to 50 × 10^9/L or below. Once the precipitant is controlled levels rise again over 5-7 days. There is significant risk of hemorrhage, though the benefit of transfusing with platelets is not clear.

What are the risk of thrombocytopenia?

- In active bleeding, neonate should be transfused to maintain platelet count above 100 × 10^9/L.
- The strongest predictors for ICH are gestation <28 weeks, early thrombocytopenia, and acute systemic infection or NEC.
- Infants with NAIT should be considered separately as they are at relatively higher risk at the same platelet count when compared to other etiologies.
- No role of prophylactic platelet transfusion on morbidity in neonates.

PLATELET TRANSFUSION GUIDELINE (TABLE 2)

- The transfusions of platelets above 50 × 10^9/L are not necessary.
- A level of 20 × 10^9/L platelet is a safe threshold in absence of other risk for platelet transfusion.
- The Indications of platelet transfusion are: (1) gestation of <28 weeks (2) early-onset severe thrombocytopenia, and (3) NEC.

PRACTICE POINTS

- Consider clinical risk factors in addition to absolute platelet count:
  - Timing of onset (early vs. late)

TABLE 2: Platelet transfusion guidelines.

Platelet count (×10^9)	Indications for transfusion
<20	All neonates
<30	• Neonates <1,000 g and <7 days • Clinically unstable (e.g., fluctuating BP) • Previous major bleeding (e.g., Grade 3-4 intraventricular hemorrhage, pulmonary hemorrhage) • Current minor bleeding • Concurrent coagulopathy requiring surgery or exchange transfusion • Neonatal alloimmune thrombocytopenia (NAIT)
<50	• Major hemorrhage requiring surgery or exchange transfusion • NAIT

- Primary origin (maternal, placental, or neonatal/fetal)
- Individual risk for bleeding (gestational age, postnatal age, NEC/sepsis, surgery, signs of bleeding).

- In a clinically stable, term neonate without NAIT, signs of infection or pre existing IVH the threshold for transfusion of $<20 \times 10^9$/L seems safe.

- Persistent unexplained thrombocytopenia should be investigated for uncommon causes.

SUGGESTED READING

1. Sillers L, Van Slambrouck C, Lapping-Carr G. Neonatal thrombocytopenia: etiology and diagnosis. Pediatr Ann. 2015;44(7): E175-80.

24 Neonatal Dermatosis

Prankur Pandey

INTRODUCTION

- The skin is the first barrier of the newborns to counter various noxious factors of the environment once the baby comes out of the safe and secure intrauterine life to the external world.
- Baby's protective but delicate cover should be disturbed as little as possible. Infant skin has deficient intercellular bridges and greater body surface area-to-weight ratio than adults that facilitates easy absorption and toxicity of topically applied substances, rendering them more susceptible to electrolyte imbalance, fluid imbalance, and thermal instability. Hence, it is imperative to differentiate the innocuous and self-limiting neonatal dermatological condition requiring minimal interventions from pathological dermatoses.

MILIARIA

Miliaria occurs due to obstruction of eccrine ducts. It is of three types:
1. *Miliaria rubra* (prickly heat) is caused by deep intraepidermal obstruction of eccrine ducts followed by an inflammatory response.
2. *Miliaria crystallina* is caused by superficial obstruction resulting in trapping of sweat.
3. *Miliaria pustulosa* variant of miliaria rubra with intense inflammatory response.

Signs and Symptoms

- *Miliaria rubra*: Erythematous papules on forehead, upper trunk, flexural areas, and underclothings.
- *Miliaria crystallina*: Fragile, noninflamed, small vesicles with clear fluid.
- *Miliaria pustulosa*: Pustules with surrounding erythema in a distribution pattern similar to miliaria rubra.

Treatment

- Avoid environmental overheating, bundling of infants, and thick oil-based emollients/oil.
- Cool baths or sponge
- Most of the lesions resolve spontaneously with these measures.

Differentials

Miliaria pustulosa/rubra, staphylococcal folliculitis, miliaria crystallina, neonatal herpes simplex.

When to refer?

Neonate presenting with markedly inflamed lesions and with diagnostic uncertainty.

INFANTILE ACROPUSTULOSIS

Acropustulosis of infancy is an idiopathic noninfective pustulosis occurring between 2 months and 3 years of age. The lesions appear as crops on a weekly or monthly basis and tends to subside by 3-4 years of age.

Signs and Symptoms

- Extremely pruritic, tense vesicopustules on hands and feet, including the palms and soles, and sides of digits occasionally in trunk, proximal extremities and scalp.
- Lesions last for 5-10 days, resolve spontaneously and recur every 2-4 weeks.

Diagnosis

- It is recognized mainly by clinical examination. Staining the vesicular fluid by Wright stain, there is presence of neutrophil and eosinophils.
- Gram stain is negative and on mineral oil preparation, there is no evidence of scabies.

Differentials

- Scabies
- Dyshidrotic eczema.

Treatment

- *Pruritus*: Topical corticosteroid twice daily during flares; oral antihistaminics.
- Severe cases may rarely require Dapsone.

When to refer?
No response to therapy.

INTERTRIGO

Intertrigo is an inflammatory dermatosis confined to the major body folds and provoked by moisture and constant friction between opposing skin surfaces.

Clinical Features

Erythema and superficial skin erosions are present in anterior neck fold, axillae, inguinal creases. Secondary infection with *Candida* species is common leading to bright red erythema and satellite lesions; less frequently *Streptococcus pyogenes* infection can be seen.

Differentials

Seborrheic dermatitis, candidal diaper dermatitis, tinea cruris, and erythrasma.

Treatment

- Absorbent powder to reduce moisture and friction
- *Severe cases*: Low-potency topical corticosteroids
- Topical antifungal and antibiotic if secondarily infected.

TRANSIENT NEONATAL PUSTULAR MELANOSIS

It is a benign self-limiting disease of unknown etiology, although rare but mostly seen in darker skin.

Signs and Symptoms

Present at birth. Pustules with surrounding erythema or ruptured pustules appearing as small hyperpigmented macules with a rim of surrounding scales.

Forehead, chin, neck, and trunk are most commonly and palm and soles are rarely involved. Pustules resolve over several days whereas hyperpigmented macules may take 3-4 months.

Differentials

Miliaria, staphylococcal folliculitis, infantile acropustulosis, congenital candidiasis.

Diagnosis

- *Wright stain*: Neutrophilic predominance; Gram stain—no organisms
- Potassium hydroxide (KOH) mount to exclude congenital candidiasis.

Treatment

No treatment is required. It resolves spontaneously and does not recur.

NEONATAL ACNE

Neonatal acne most commonly affects males and facial area is involved exclusively. It occurs because in first few weeks of life under the influence of maternal androgens, sebaceous glands produce a considerable amount of sebum.

Signs and Symptoms

Presence of comedones and inflammatory papules over cheeks.

Differentials

- Miliaria rubra
- Treatment
- It is self-limiting, and resolves in 2–3 weeks. Oil-based emollients should be avoided.

NEONATAL HERPES SIMPLEX

Infection of the neonate by herpes simplex virus (HSV) is a serious condition with high mortality, resulting from transmission of HSV1 and HSV2 by genital tract secretions during delivery. Pneumonia and/or encephalitis are frequent complications.

Signs and Symptoms

Onset is between 2 and 20 days. Multiple grouped vesicles on erythematous patches distributed randomly over the scalp, face trunk and extremities. The vesicles have a tendency to localize over mucocutaneous junctions. Oral lesions include erosions of the tongue, palate, gingivae, and buccal mucosa.

Diagnosis

- Tzanck smear
- Polymerase chain reaction (PCR).

Treatment

- Isolation of affected neonate.
- Ophthalmic examination and prophylactic topical vidarabine ophthalmic preparation should be used.
- IV acyclovir 30 mg/kg/day in three divided doses for 14–21 days. No role of topical acyclovir.

CUTIS MARMORATA

It is a physiologic response to cooling resulting in dilatation of small venules and capillaries.

Signs and Symptoms

Reticulated bluish mottling of the skin seen on the trunk and extremities, which disappears on rewarming. Tendency may persist for first few months of life. In Down's syndrome, trisomy 18, and Cornelia de Lange syndrome, this may be persistent.

Treatment
Reassurance.

CUTIS MARMORATA ALBA
A white negative pattern of cutis marmorata is cutis marmorata alba which may be created by a transient hypertonia of the deep vasculature. It is a transitory disorder of no clinical significance.

CUTIS MARMORATA TELANGIECTASIA CONGENITA
It manifests shortly after birth. It closely resembles cutis marmorata but it does not resolve on rewarming the neonate.

Signs and Symptoms
Red marbled mottled patches, accentuated by decrease in ambient temperature, may be associated with atrophy or ulceration of the skin, limb hypoplasia, hyperplasia, or vascular abnormalities, e.g., port-wine stain, Sturge-Weber syndrome. Neurological disorders such as macrocephaly, seizures, hydrocephalus, and ocular abnormalities such as glaucoma, retinal pigmentation, and retinal detachment have been associated. Adams–Oliver syndrome is characterized by cutis marmorata telangiectasia congenita with aplasia cut is congenital and distal transverse limb defects.

Treatment
- Resolves spontaneously in first 2–3 years of life.
- Ophthalmologic and neurologic opinion is necessary.

SCLEREMA NEONATORUM
Diffuse fast spreading, wax-like hardening of the skin and subcutaneous tissue in preterm or sick neonates during the first few weeks of life.

Risk Factors
Sepsis, respiratory distress, dehydration, and congenital heart disease.

Signs and Symptoms
Diffuse nonpitting woody induration usually starts on buttocks and legs and progresses to involve all areas, except soles, palms, and genitalia.

Treatment
Treatment of underlying cause.

Prognosis
About 50–70% mortality. Survival if any however, is intact.

ERYTHEMA TOXICUM
It is of unknown etiology and occurs in approximately 50% of newborns; rarely observed in premature infants.

Signs and Symptoms
Discrete, blotchy erythematous macules, each with a central papule, vesicle or pustule. Occasionally the papules, vesicles, or pustules may occur in clusters to form an erythematous plaque. Palms and soles are spared. Usually begins at 24–48 hours after birth, new lesions appear for several days; the process lasts about a week. Rarely lesions may be present at birth or appear as late as 10 days of life.

Differentials
Transient neonatal pustular melanosis, miliaria crystallina, neonatal acne, staphylococcal folliculitis, bullous impetigo, scabies, infantile acropustulosis, HSV, and incontinentia pigmenti.

Diagnosis
- Wright stain of vesicular fluid shows eosinophils.
- Tzanck smear, viral culture, and Gram stain will help in ruling out infectious causes.
- Skin biopsy is rarely needed to exclude incontinentia pigmenti.

Treatment
Self-limiting, no treatment is required.

SUCKLING BLISTER
Sucking blisters on lips of newborns are seen due to vigorous suckling by the fetus in utero. Bullae or erosions may be seen over the dorsal aspect of fingers, thumbs, wrists, and lips.

Differentials
Bullous impetigo, epidermolysis bullosa, and neonatal herpes simplex.

Treatment
Topical antibacterial cream.

SEBACEOUS GLAND HYPERPLASIA
It occurs due to maternal androgen stimulation.

Signs and Symptoms
Pearly-white pinpoint papules over tip of the nose, seen in 2–8 days' old newborns. It usually disappears in few days.

Differentials
Milia: The papules differ from milia which are epidermal inclusion cysts, usually solitary and white in color.

Treatment
Reassurance.

SEBORRHEIC DERMATITIS
Commonly known as Cradle cap because it occurs most commonly over the scalp.

Infantile seborrheic dermatitis (ISD) is a self-limiting condition which probably occurs due to hormonal fluctuations and colonization by *Malassezia furfur*.

Signs and Symptoms
Greasy scaling on a red base involving the scalp and the face may spread to the intertriginous zones, such as the umbilicus and anogenital region. ISD shows a marked predilection for the for so-called "seborrheic" areas where there is a high density of sebaceous glands (i.e., forehead, ears, eyebrows, and nose).

Differentials
Atopic dermatitis: High risk of relapses and the presence of pruritus in atopic patients.

Treatment
Self-limiting, resolves in first few months. Severe cases scales can be removed with a soft brush after shampooing or after applying an emollient with white petrolatum or antifungal.

Shampoos may contain antifungal agents.

NEONATAL IRRITANT DERMATITIS
Irritants in newborns may vary from antiseptic cleansers, lotions, baby wipes causing dermatitis within 24–48 hours of exposure to delicate newborn skin.

Signs and Symptoms
Intense erythema with formation of papules and vesicles over the areas of contact with the irritant. Newborn is restless and irritable as a consequence.

Treatment
- Avoidance of offending agent.
- Clean this skin with lukewarm water.
- *Emollient*: White soft paraffin application two to three times a day for 1–2 weeks.
- Occasionally mild topical steroid such as hydrocortisone may be needed.

UMBILICAL POLYP

Signs and Symptoms
Bright red shiny polypoidal growth over the umbilicus at birth and is the result of a partially patent omphalomesenteric duct. The lesions are usually asymptomatic and secrete serous, mucoid, and rarely serosanguinous exudate.

Polyps may be accompanied by potentially serious internal omphalomesenteric remnant, such as Meckel's diverticulum attached to the umbilicus by obstructing fibrous bands.

Treatment
- Surgical excision is required.
- Underlying urinary tract abnormalities should be ruled out.

UMBILICAL GRANULOMA
It is also known as granuloma pyogenicum of the umbilicus.

Signs and Symptoms
Red raw granulomatous growth over the umbilicus with purulent discharge.

Treatment
Cauterization with silver nitrate solution, 20% KOH.

TIPS FOR CARE OF NEWBORN SKIN
- Double rinse all baby clothes, bedding, blankets, and other washable items before exposing newborn to them.
- For first few months, do your infants wash separate from rest of the family's.
- Contrary to the popular notion, infant does not ordinarily need any lotions, oils, or powders. If skin is very dry, use non perfumed baby, lotion or cream sparingly to the dry areas.
- Massage involved in applying the lotion makes the baby feel good.
- Never use any skin care products that are not specifically made for babies, because they contain perfumes or other chemicals that can irritate infant's skin.
- Only care a baby's nails require is trimming, which can be done by soft baby nail clippers. A good time to trim is just after bath or when the baby is asleep.
- Biting of baby's nails should be avoided in order to trim, to prevent the risk of condition called herpetic whitlow.
- Newborns toenails grow much slowly and are very soft and pliable, they need not be kept short as fingernails.
- Toenails may look ingrown but should not be a cause of concern if skin alongside is not red, inflamed, or hard.

SUGGESTED READING
1. American Academy of Pediatrics. Hannemann RE (Ed). Caring for your baby and young child (American Academy of Pediatrics) the complete and authoritative guide, 7th edition. New York: Random House Publishing Group; 2019.
2. Eichenfield LF, Frieden IJ. Neonatal and Infant Dermatology, 3rd edition. Netherlands: Elsevier; 2014.
3. Paller AS, Mancini AJ. Hurwitz Clinical Pediatric Dermatology, 5th edition. Netherlands: Elsevier; 2015.
4. Singh M. Care of the Newborn, 8th edition. New Delhi: CBS Publishers Pvt Ltd.; 2016.
5. Singh M. The art and science of baby and child care, 4th edition. New Delhi: CBS Publishers Pvt Ltd.; 2015.

25 Newborn Screening Program

Kanak Ramnani

INTRODUCTION

Newborn screening is a public health program designed to screen asymptomatic babies at birth for any inborn errors of metabolism (IEM) before they manifest. Therefore, the blood sample of these babies may be collected any time between 48 and 72 hours of birth and be screened for various diseases. This is the most important preventive public health program already being implemented in majority of the developed countries; but in India there is currently no government-funded program for masses. This is a program and does not complete with one screening test but would be useful to prevent disability and death by early intervention, follow-up and counseling.

India is a vast country with multiple cultures and genetic traits; the incidence of various diseases is different in different states. Therefore, these geographical variations need to be understood before planning the health programs of the country. Similarly, clear guidelines regarding the timing and procedure of sample collection and how to interpret the reports is essential. There is no doubt that newborn screening programs are essential but there are no guidelines regarding which diseases should be covered and no universal program is running in the country. In 2011, National Neonatology Forum (NNF) had advised to include three diseases: (1) Congenital hypothyroidism (CH), (2) congenital adrenal hyperplasia (CAH), and (3) glucose-6-phosphate dehydrogenase (G6PD) deficiency in the screening panel to be screened for all the neonates of India; but it could not be taken up till date. With the huge population load of our country, it has been estimated that every day at least 30 newborns are born with various neonatal disorders; the incidence being around 1:1,000. At present only three states are following neonatal screening programs for all the babies born in the government sector.

What is newborn screening?

A newborn screening test is a simple test performed on newborn babies to check for potentially fatal or harmful disorders which cannot be otherwise detected at birth; these tests look for serious developmental, genetic, and metabolic disorders.

What is the ideal time for sample collection?

Blood spots collected too early or too late may yield false results; sample should be best collected between 24 and 48 hours of age. However, in special circumstances, blood may be drawn earlier or later.

Which diseases can be added in the newborn screening list?

Wilson and Jungner proposed the following criteria for inclusion of a condition in screening:

- Condition should have important health problem/frequency.
- Test should be acceptable to the population (reliable/simple).
- Disease does not manifest at birth/routine examination.
- Treatment will prevent mortality and morbidity.
- Delay in diagnosis will cause irreversible damage.
- Screening is cost effective.

Firstly, there are few challenges in implementation of newborn screening program in India; which includes the awareness and attitude of the healthcare providers and the government officials regarding this matter. Second is the economic feasibility of running the program for the whole country. Third is the counseling of the parents for the effectivity of such tests and the need to deviate from the current practice of not testing; next would be the assessment of the disease burden according to the demographic profile and creating an appropriate battery of tests required and the most important part is the *follow-up* of these patients along with their treatment and genetic counseling. Thus, it is important to teach not only the public but also the medical staff regarding newborn screening.

COMPONENTS OF NEWBORN SCREENING

The American Academy of Pediatrics (AAP) states that newborn screening is a complex system that encompasses five very important components:

1. *Testing of all newborns involves the following*:
    - A blood test that screens for certain metabolic and genetic conditions
    - A pulse oximetry test to rule out critical congenital heart defects
    - A routine hearing test to rule out congenital deafness
2. Timely follow-up of abnormal screening results
3. Diagnostic tests to confirm the results of initial screening blood tests

4. *Management of the disease*: Using multidisciplinary approach
5. Ongoing evaluation of the newborn screening.

For a country like India, a practical approach would be to categorize the condition as following:
- *Category A (all newborns)*: Screening for CH and deafness should be a must.
  CAH and G6PD deficiency may be added in phased manner.
- *Category B (high-risk neonate)*: It is essential if there is history of mental retardation, seizure disorder, critically ill newborn, critically ill newborn, IEM, or consanguinity—phenylketonuria, homocystinuria, alkaptonuria, galactosemia, sickle cell anemia, cystic fibrosis, biotinidase deficiency, maple syrup urine disease (MSUD), and tyrosinemia.
- *Category C*: Expanded Newborn Screening—by tandem mass spectrometry (TMS) screening 30-40 IEM resource-rich settings.
  A special note should be taken for diseases such as hemoglobinopathies that are prevalent in a particular part of the country and they should be added in the screening list of that part of the country.

How is newborn screening done?

The hospital staff would at first fill details and vitals of the newborn in the newborn screening card that consists of special absorbent paper to collect the sample. Then we collect few drops of the neonates blood by heal prick (the medial and lateral part of the heel is preferred) on the absorbent paper which is sent to the laboratory. The sample can be collected by hospital nursery staff, laboratory staff, or outpatient birth providers.

Before filling the card, the expiry date should be well checked. We should avoid touching the areas within the circles on the filter paper section before, during, and after collection of the sample.
- Select puncture site and clean with 70% isopropanol.
- Use a sterile, disposable lancet with 2.0 mm, or, less point.
- Wipe away first blood drop.
- Use second large blood drop to apply to surface of the Food and Drug Administration (FDA)-approved filter paper surface.
- If not completely filled, add a second large drop immediately. Fill, all required circles completely, fill from one side of filter paper only.
- Dry specimen at room temperature 3-4 hours in horizontal position.
- Cord blood should not be used for newborn screening.

Variables Affecting Measurements for Specimens Collected on Filter Paper
- Handling and storage of paper
- Humidity condition of paper
- Volume of blood collected
- Hematocrit level of blood donor
- Absorption time of blood.

Techniques for Blood Tests

Tandem Mass Spectroscopy (MS/MS) for metabolic diseases, isoelectric focusing (IEF) or high-performance liquid chromatography (HPLC) for hemoglobinopathies, and DNA arrays are used in sequencing and labeled bead technologies.

COMMON CONDITIONS

- *Congenital hypothyroidism*: CH is usually sporadic and occurs in 3,000–4,000 infants. The ideal time to obtain blood spot is ideal time to obtain blood spot is 5 days after birth to prevent the false-positive high values due to the physiological neonatal thyroid-stimulating hormone (TSH) surge.
  The cut-off for reporting elevated TSH is above 20-25 mU/mL.
  Levels > 50 mU/mL are usually associated with permanent hypothyroidism and the levels in between need to be reviewed.
- *CAH*: The average incidence of the condition is 1 in 15,000 neonate. Primary markers used for screening for 21OH, 17-hydroxyprogesterone (17OHP) any out of range report needs to be confirmed before labeling the baby as CAH.
- *G6PD deficiency*: G6PD deficiency newborn screening is more important in the northern states of India and can be done by enzyme analysis or primary DNA screening.
- *Hearing assessment*: Currently, hearing screening in newborns is performed via otoacoustic emission (OAE) and automated auditory brainstem response (AABR) testing. OAE has to be performed in infants older than 24 hours with a minimum 34 weeks corrected age. It has to be performed by trained technician; it is a noninvasive procedure, the ear probe is placed in outer ear canal. It is a bedside procedure taking 10-15 minutes.
- *Sickle cell anemia and other hemoglobinopathies*: Over 700 hemoglobin variants may be identified by these methods, and 25-30 are considered clinically significant; newborn screening for sickle cell disease is performed by HPLC testing to determine the presence of abnormal hemoglobins in whole blood. All abnormal newborn screening test results need appropriate confirmatory blood tests including testing the parents and siblings.

SUGGESTED READING

1. Watson MS, Lloyd MA, Mann MY, Rinaldo P, Howell RR. Newborn screening: toward a uniform screening panel and system. Genet Med. 2006;8(Supple 1):1S-252S.

SECTION 4

Vaccinology

26. DPT/DT, DTaP/Tdap
27. Rotavirus Vaccine
28. Pneumonia Vaccine
29. Typhoid Vaccine
30. Hepatitis A Vaccine
31. Human Papaillomavirus Vaccine
32. Influenza Vaccine
33. Rabies Vaccine
34. Japanese Encephalitis Vaccine
35. Varicella Vaccine
36. Meningococcal Vaccine

CHAPTER 26: DPT/DT, DTaP/Tdap

KP Sarbhai

Q1. Why vaccine against diphtheria, pertussis, and tetanus (DPT) have to be used repeatedly?

Ans: Immunity following primary DTP wanes fast; therefore, three primary doses at 1.5, 2.5, and 3.5 months are followed by booster at 1.5 years and then at 4.5 years. Immunity produced by booster at 4.5 years wanes over next 6–12 years. This increases adolescent and adult pertussis cases. Therefore, one booster is needed at 10 years. At 10 years, DPT cannot be used and Tdap (tetanus, diphtheria, and pertussis) vaccine is used.

Q2. Why DPT cannot be used at 10 years' booster?

Ans: Standard strength DTP and DTaP vaccine cannot be used beyond 7 years due to increased reactogenicity.

Use of Td (tetanus and diphtheria)/TT (tetanus toxoid) is also not recommended. Single dose of Tdap, at 10 years to a child vaccinated with DTP in childhood produces immunogenic response similar to three full doses of DTP, but reactogenicity is drastically reduced.

Q3. What brands of Tdap are available in market?

Ans: Boostrix® from GSK and Adacel® from Sanofi. Adacel® contains five pertussis antigens; Boostrix® contains three pertussis antigens.

Recommendation: If any acellular pertussis-containing vaccine is used it must have at least three or more components. Therefore, either of the two vaccines can be used.

Q4. In what other situations Tdap can be used?

Ans:
- If child misses second booster at 5 years of age and now if he is 7 then we cannot give DPT for fear of high reactogenicity, and Tdap is used.
- Healthcare personnel who have not received Tdap vaccine should receive a single dose of Tdap vaccine.
- Adults of 18–64 years who have completed their childhood vaccination schedule, a booster dose of Td vaccine is indicated once every 10 years till the age of 65 years; one dose of Tdap vaccine may be given in place of Td vaccine.
- Immunization of a pregnant lady is an effective approach to protect very young infants and neonates before they receive DPT vaccination. The Indian Academy of Pediatrics (IAP) recommends single dose Tdap during third trimester regardless of number of years from prior Td/Tdap vaccination. Tdap has to be repeated in every pregnancy. If a lady has received Tdap vaccine 1 year prior to pregnancy, still she will have to take it again in third trimester due to rapid waning of immunity.
- Pregnant women who have never received previous vaccination, three doses of Td vaccine is recommended. One of the three doses should be Tdap. Tdap in every pregnancy is mandatory.

All the possible contacts of the newborn child should receive Tdap in advance to avoid infection. This is called Cocooning.

Q5. Is there any recommendation for repeat dose of Tdap?

Ans: There is no data to support the repeated dose of Tdap (Austria is an exception where Tdap is recommended every 10 years). In our country, Tdap is repeated only in each pregnancy.

Q6. What are the contraindications for use of Tdap?

Ans:
- History of (H/o) anaphylaxis to any component, H/o encephalopathy within 7 days of pertussis vaccination.
- Adults with acute illness.
- Unstable neurological conditions (stroke and acute encephalopathies).
- Tdap is to be deferred, until acute illness resolves or Td may be given.

Q7. What is the difference between DTaP and Tdap?

Ans: Diphtheria toxoid in pediatric vaccines is three to five times higher and is denoted as DTaP. It is used in pentavalent and hexavalent vaccine. In adult formulations, diphtheria toxoid is less denoted by Tdap. Amount of TT is equal in each product so it remains "T."

Rotavirus Vaccine

KP Sarbhai

Q1. By what age it is presumed that every child gets rotavirus infection?

Ans: Almost every child is infected by 2 years, irrespective of socioeconomic status. Children aged 6 months to 2 years of age are most vulnerable.

Q2. Which is the major culprit strain of rotavirus?

Ans: G1P8 is major culprit. It is responsible for >60% of cases. Strain G9 is increasing recently and is responsible for >4% cases globally.

Q3. What is the difference between natural rotavirus infection and vaccine-induced infection?

Ans: Rotavirus vaccine (RVV) mimics natural infection. Two natural rotavirus infections confer virtually 100% protection against moderate and severe infection, regardless of the type. So is the case with two/three doses of RVV.

Q4. Which immune mechanism protects children against rotavirus?

Ans: Exact mechanism is not yet known. Rotavirus infection is followed by a complex immune response. IgG, IgM, and IgA antibodies are produced against VP7, VP6, VP4, and NSP4. Intestinal lymphocytes and receptor activation are there.

All these immune components contribute in protection against rotavirus infection.

Q5. When to vaccinate a baby and what is the logic behind?

Ans: Mean age for rotavirus hospitalization is younger in India than in more developed countries. 20% of all rotavirus hospitalizations occur by 3 months, so early protection is needed in India.

Q6. How a newborn is protected from rotavirus infection?

Ans: Higher antibody titer against rotavirus in mother's blood which is transmitted transplacentally. Higher rotavirus antibody level is present in breast milk. If we give vaccine very early, there will be less seroconversion. However, in one study, it has been concluded that maternal serum antibody level does not influence seroconversion. It was also concluded in one study that breastfeeding also does not affect the seroconversion; on the contrary, breastfeeding improves seroconversion. Further there is no significant effect of coadministered oral polio vaccine (OPV) on human rhinovirus (HRV) immune response. We can conclude:

No effect of breast milk on immunogenicity, no effect of maternal Ab on immunogenicity, and no effect of OPV on immunogenicity.

Q7. What is the World Health Organization (WHO) recommendation for RVV doses?

Ans: The WHO recommends that the first dose of RVV be administered as soon as possible at 6 weeks of age along with DPT1 and 2 to ensure induction of protection prior to natural rotaviral infection. RVV at 6 and 10 weeks provides protection against severe rotavirus gastroenteritis (RVGE).

Q8. What are the different RVV available?

Ans:
- *Rotarix (GSK)*: Rotarix is a monovalent, human, live attenuated RVV containing one rotavirus strain of G1P(8) specificity. Rotarix is useful for the prevention of RVGE caused by G1 and non-G1 types (G3, G4, and G9). Administered as a 2-dose series in infants and children (USFDA approval, 2008).
- *RotaTeq (MSD)*: H Fred Clark and Paul Offit are the inventors of RotaTeq. RotaTeq is alive, oral pentavalent vaccine that contains five rotavirus strains produced by reassortment. Parent strains of the reassortants isolated from human and bovine hosts.

Four reassortant rotaviruses are present on the outer capsid, (serotypes G1, G2, G3, or G4) are from the human rotavirus parent strain and their attachment protein VP4 is from the bovine rotavirus parent strain. The fifth reassortant virus expresses the attachment protein VP4, (type P1A), from the human rotavirus parent strain and the outer capsid protein VP7 (serotype G6) from the bovine rotavirus parent strain [United States Food and Drug Administration (USFDA) approval, 2006].

- *Rotavac (Bharat Biotech)*: It is indigenously developed vaccine by Bharat Biotech. It is a monovalent human bovine (116E) live attenuated RVV. It is stable without buffer, sweet in taste. The 116E rotavirus strain developed as part of Indo-US Vaccine action program. It is a naturally occurring reassortant strain G9 P(11) containing 1 bovine rotavirus gene P(11) and 10 human rotavirus genes.
- *Rotasiil (Serum Institute of India)*: It is a pentavalent vaccine. It has five viral strains (human and bovine reassortant strains) of serotype G1, G2, G3, G4, and G9. All these strains constitute *VP7* gene of respective serotype from human strains reasserted with bovine rotavirus. Each strain is propagated in VERO cell individually then all five strains are blended. It protects against any severe rotavirus infection. Vaccine has no preservative. It conforms to the intellectual property (IP) and the WHO requirements.

Q9. How does rotavirus spread?

Ans: Rotavirus spreads via feces through hand-to-mouth contact and can be picked up from surfaces such as toys, hands or dirty nappies. It can also spread through the air by sneezing and coughing. It most often spreads when someone who is infected does not wash hands properly after going to the toilet. Washing hands and keeping surfaces clean can help reduce the spread of the virus but will never completely stop it.

Q10. What if baby spits out the vaccine or vomits immediately after having it?

Ans: The drops will be given again. Do not worry about overdosing. Even if some of the vaccine went in first time, there's no harm in mistakenly having two doses at the same time. Vaccination is a much more effective way to protect babies from getting infected.

Q11. What if baby misses the first dose of rotavirus vaccine?

Ans: They can have it a month later at 3 months of age, but in any case before 14 weeks 6 days of age. If they miss the second dose of RW (normally given at 3 months), still it can be given but all the two/three doses have to be completed before 8 months.

Q12. Why cannot older babies have the rotavirus vaccination?

Ans: Older children have very often already had a rotavirus infection so there is no point in vaccinating them. Also, as they get older, 1 in 1,000 get intussusception.

It is extremely rare before 3 months of age and most of the cases happen between 5 months and a year. There is a very small chance (2 in 100,000) that the first dose of the vaccine might also cause this blockage to develop. To reduce the risk of this happening, the first dose of the vaccine will not be given to babies older than 15 weeks of age. The first dose after 5 months and risk of intussusception is 1/1,000, the first dose before 3 months and risk of intussusception is 2/100,000.

Q13. Which babies should not have the rotavirus vaccine?

Ans: Confirmed anaphylactic reaction to a previous dose of RVV or allergy to any component of RVV. Severe allergy to latex. Babies with "severe combined immunodeficiency" (SCID) a rare genetic disease that makes babies very vulnerable to infection should not get RVV.

Fructose intolerance, glucose–galactose malabsorption or sucrose-isomaltase in sufficiency, which are rare inherited disorders. History of "intussusception" Babies who are mildly ill can get the vaccine. Babies who are moderately or severely ill should wait until they recover. This includes babies with moderate or severe diarrhea or vomiting. HIV/AIDS, long-term steroids, and cancer treatment with X-rays or drugs are few other contraindications.

Q14. Is the rotavirus vaccine made in eggs? Does this affect children with allergies?

Ans: This vaccine is not made in eggs and is perfectly safe for babies with allergies. Any baby with a history of allergy to the vaccine or constituents of the vaccine should not be vaccinated.

Q15. Does the RVV contain thimerosal?

Ans: No. Thimerosal is a mercury-based substance, commonly included as a preservative in vaccines. It has been eliminated from all routine childhood vaccines including rotavirus.

Q16. What if baby is ill on the day the vaccination is due?

Ans: There's no reason to postpone unless baby is seriously ill with a fever or diarrhea and vomiting. If baby is well enough to have the other routine vaccinations, they can have the RVV as well.

Q17. How long the RVV can protect baby?

Ans: It is not yet known, clinical trials have shown two doses or more of the vaccine protect for several years.

Q18. Is it ok to breastfeed baby after the vaccination?

Ans: There are no problems linked with breastfeeding the babies who have recently had the RVV.

Q19. Do mother needs to take special care when changing baby's nappy after rotavirus vaccination?

Ans: Yes. Because the vaccine is given to baby by mouth, it is possible that the virus in the vaccine will pass through baby's gut and be picked up by whoever changes their nappy. The vaccine contains only a weakened form of the rotavirus, so traces of it in a baby's nappy will not harm healthy people, but it could pose a risk for people with a weak immune system (such as anyone taking long-term steroid tablets or having chemotherapy). As a precaution, anyone in close contact with recently vaccinated babies should take special care with personal hygiene, including washing their hands carefully after changing the baby's nappy.

Q20. Will the RVV stop baby getting any sickness and diarrhea?

Ans: No. Rotavirus is not the only cause of sickness and diarrhea in babies, so some may still get unwell. But it prevents dehydrating diarrhea in any case. However, the vaccine will stop about eight out of 10 babies that have the vaccine getting vomiting caused by rotavirus. And the more is the number of babies that have the vaccine, the more difficult it will be for the virus to spread (Herd effect).

Q21. If the baby is premature, when should he/she have the RVV?

Ans: The Advisory Committee on Immunization Practices (ACIP) supports vaccination of preterm infants according to the same schedule and precautions as full-term infants and under the following conditions:

If the infant's chronological age meets the age requirements for RW (e.g., age 6 weeks to 14 weeks 6 days for dose 1), the infant is clinically stable, and the vaccine is administered. Vaccinate preterms with the same schedule.

Q22. What is the age schedule for rotavirus vaccination?

Ans: RotaTeq®, Rotavac, and Rotasiil are administered in a three-dose series, with doses administered at ages 6, 10, and 14 weeks. Rotarix® is administered in a two-dose series, with doses administered at ages 6 and 10 weeks. The minimum age for dose 1 of RVV is 6 weeks; the maximum age for dose 1 is 14 weeks and 6 days. Vaccination should not be initiated for infants aged 15 weeks and 0 days or older because of insufficient data on safety of dose 1 of RVV in older infants. The minimum interval between doses of RVV is 4 weeks; no maximum interval is set. All doses should be administered by age 8 months and 0 days.

Q23. How well does RVV work to prevent rotavirus disease?

Ans: Efficacy studies have demonstrated that RVV is 85–98% protective against severe rotavirus disease, 74–87% protective against rotavirus disease of any severity in the first year after vaccination.

Q24. What is the risk of a vaccine reaction?

Ans: With a vaccine, like any medicine, there is a chance of side effects. These are usually mild and go away on their own. Serious side effects are also possible, but are very rare. Most babies who get RVV do not have any problems with it. But some problems have been associated with RVV:

- *Mild problems*: Babies might become irritable, or have mild, temporary diarrhea or vomiting after getting a dose of RVV.
- *Serious problems*: There is a small risk of intussusceptions from rotavirus vaccination, usually within a week after the first or second vaccine dose. This additional risk is estimated to range from about 1 in 20,000 infants to 1 in 100,000 infants who get RVV. Large prelicensure clinical trials of both RotaTeq and Rotarix did not find an increased risk for intussusception among vaccine recipients.

A large postlicensure study of more than 1.2 million RVV recipients found a very small increased risk of intussusception (1–1.5 additional cases of intussusception per 100,000 vaccinated infants) in the 7–21 days following the first dose. No increased risk of intussusception was found after the second or third doses. It is believe that the benefits of rotavirus vaccination outweigh the risks associated with vaccination and that routine vaccination of infants should continue. Chances of intussusception are 1/100,000 if first dose is given before 3 months. Chances of intussusception are 1/1,000 if the first dose is given after 5 months. Intussusception occurs 7–21 days after the first dose. There is nearly no risk of intussusception after second or third dose.

Q25. Is it possible for adults to contract rotavirus? What are the symptoms in adults?

Ans: Rotavirus infection of adults is usually asymptomatic but may cause diarrheal illness. Outbreaks of diarrheal illness caused by rotavirus have been reported, especially among elderly persons living in retirement communities.

Q26. Can RotaTeq (RV5; Merck) and Rotarix (RV1; GlaxoSmithKline)/Rotasiil vaccines be used interchangeably? If so, what schedule should we follow?

Ans: The ACIP recommends that the RW series be completed with the same product whenever possible. However, vaccination should not be deferred because the product used for a previous dose is not available or is unknown. In these situations, the provider should continue or complete the series with the product available. A total of 3 doses of RVV should be administered. The minimum interval between doses of RVV is 4 weeks. All doses should be administered by age 8 months and 0 days.

Q27. If the first dose of RVV is inadvertently given to a child aged 15 weeks 0 days or older, should the series be continued?

Ans: Infants for whom the first dose of RW was inadvertently administered at age of 15 weeks or older should receive the remaining doses of the series at the routinely recommended intervals. Timing of the first dose does not affect the safety and efficacy of the remaining doses. RW should not be given after age of 8 months 0 days even if the series is incomplete.

Q28. Can rotavirus vaccine be given via G-Tube? If so, is it okay to flush with normal saline or sterile water?

Ans: The manufacturer has not addressed this issue but the CDC considers administration of RVV via gastrostomy tube to be acceptable practice. There should be no problem flushing the tube after vaccine has been administered.

Q29. A child received the first RVV and after a while he got the disease (laboratory confirmed). Should we continue the vaccine?

Ans: Infants who have had RVGE before receiving the full series of rotavirus vaccination should still start or complete the schedule because according to the age and interval recommendations, the initial rotavirus infection might provide only partial protection against subsequent rotavirus disease.

Q30. Can RVV be given to an infant who has an immunosuppressed household contact?

Ans: Having an immunocompromised household contact is not usually areas on for delaying routine vaccination for kids in the household. RVV should be administered to contacts of immunocompromised patients when indicated. All members of the household should wash their hands after changing the diaper of an infant. This minimizes rotavirus transmission from an infant who received RVV.

Q31. Rotarix is a monovalent vaccine which has G1P8 serotypes. Will it work against G2P4 serotype which is not present in the vaccine?

Ans: Data has shown that effectiveness of rotarix G2P4 is as high as against G1P8.

Q32. Does RVV works in malnourished children?

Ans: Vaccine efficacy in well-nourished and malnourished children is nearly equal.

CHAPTER 28

Pneumonia Vaccine

KP Sarbhai

Q1. What is the incidence of pneumonia in our country in under 5?

Ans: It is approximately 23%.

Q2. How can we protect children from pneumonia?

Ans: Exclusive breastfeeding, adequate nutrition, prevent low birth weight, reduced indoor air pollution, and hand washing are few simple and common measures to protect a child.

Q3. How can we prevent pneumonia from developing in children?

Ans:
- Vaccination against pertussis, pneumococci, Hib (*Haemophilus influenzae* type b), and measles
- Prevention of HIV, Cotrimoxazole prophylaxis in a case of HIV
- Zinc supplementation in a case of diarrhea.

Q4. What is noninvasive pneumococcal disease (NIPD)?

Ans: *Streptococcus pneumoniae* normally harbors in nasopharynx as a part of normal flora. When immune system is suppressed due to any reason, pneumococci spread from nasopharynx to adjacent mucosal tissues leading to NIPD because it occurs at sites which are not sterile otherwise such as blood and cerebrospinal fluid (CSF). NIPD includes pneumonia, sinusitis, otitis media (OM), and bronchitis. Noninvasive pneumonia is less dangerous than invasive pneumonia. NIPD is also called as mucosal disease.

Q5. What is invasive pneumococcal disease (IPD)?

Ans: From nasopharynx when immune system is suppressed, they enter bloodstream and invade sterile sites such as meninges, joints, and bones (IPD) when pneumococcal infection reaches blood and CSF, it is called as IPD, because blood, and CSF are normally sterile. Bacteremia, bacteremic pneumonia, and meningitis are included in IPD. Heart valves, bones, joints, and peritoneal cavity receive infection through bloodstream so are included in IPD. Bacteremia is common between 6 months and 2 years. Of all the IPD, 40% have occult or asymptomatic bacteremia and resolves spontaneously without complications. 10% develop meningitis and other complications. Bacteremic pneumonia is potentially life-threatening and causes twice as many deaths as pneumonia without bacteremia. Noninvasive may become invasive at any time.

Q6. What decides the virulence of *Streptococcus pneumoniae*?

Ans: Polysaccharide capsule surrounding the cell wall is responsible for virulence and stimulates protective AB formation. Higher the polysaccharide content, more virulent is the organism. Polysaccharide in capsule is chemically distinct and immunologically specific for each serotype. *S. pneumoniae* is a facultative anaerobe and is able to grow aerobically or anaerobically.

Q7. What are the risk factors for pneumococcal disease to occur?

Ans:
- *Age*: Adults > 65, children <2 years. Median age for PD in children varies. It is 6 months for meningitis, 11.5 months for bacteremia, 14 months for pneumonia and 2nd year of life for OM.
- Daycare attendance is a factor because of airborne spread.
- *Immune status*: Child with three or more episodes of OM within 6 months is at high risk for IPD, HIV, nonfunctional spleen, and nephrotic syndrome on steroids are at high risk.
- *Recent antibiotic use*: Oral antibiotic within last 3 months increases the risk of development of IPD.
- Season plays significant role.
- *Breastfeeding*: Decreases risk of NIPD (OM) in first year of life. Country, poverty, crowding, and exposure to cigarette smoke are additional factors.

Q8. What are the pneumococcal serotypes?

Ans: More than 90 different serotypes or strains are present worldwide. Each serotype has structurally different polysaccharide. Serogroups are designated by numbers, viz., 1, 6, 19, 14. Those with a lower number are more invasive and virulent.

Sometimes designated number may have a letter added to it to emphasize antigenic difference among serotypes, e.g., 6B, 9V.

Q9. Why IPD is more serious in <2 years' age?

Ans: In adults and children >2 years' age, capsule induces an immune response. This is not so in <2 years' age, because in <2 years, immune system is still immature and does not recognize capsular polysaccharide antigen and fails to produce antibodies. As a consequence, pneumococcal infection is more severe in children <2 years' age as the child is not immunologically protected. Infants are born with immature immune system. It does not recognize polysaccharide antigen and its exposure results in production of IgM rather than IgG because response is T-cell independent. IgM protection is short lived and does not give complete immunity. IgG acquired from mother is not long lasting. Exposure to conjugate vaccine stimulates T-cell-dependent response producing more specific IgG antibodies some of which are converted into memory cells. Repeated vaccination produces higher titers. After 2 years' age, infant recognizes polysaccharide antigen and produces T-cell-dependent response but much weaker than conjugate vaccine.

Q10. Why conjugation of Pneumococcal polysaccharide vaccine is needed?

Ans: Polysaccharide vaccines are poorly immunogenic in children <2 years of age and do not stimulate long-term immunological memory. Pneumococci have outer polysaccharide coating. Coating makes it difficult for infants/young child's immature immune system to respond to bacterium. A process of linking the polysaccharide antigen to protein carrier (e.g., Diphtheria or Tetanus) that infant's immune system already recognizes, is done in order to provoke an immune response.

Q11. What are the problems with the use of polysaccharide vaccine?

Ans: PPV23 activates B cells but do not induce immunological memory. It adopts T-cell-independent pathway. Weak and short-lasting IgM immune response is produced. No affinity maturation of IgM and no antibody class switching to IgG. There is a lack of booster effect on revaccination. Limited impact on pneumococcal nasopharyngeal carriage is seen.

Q12. By what mechanism pneumococcal conjugate vaccine (PCV) produces a good immunological response?

Ans: PCV induces a strong immune response and immunological memory by activating B and T cells. Combination of polysaccharide protein antigen-conjugate is captured by B cells and other antigen presenting cells (APC). APC present these antigens to T-helper2 (Th2) cells. Activation of Th2 cells helps B cells to differentiate into memory B cells and plasma cells. This is antibody class switching.

Q13. What are the additional antigens present in PCV13?

Ans: It is 3, 6A and 19A. PCV13 gives direct protection against 6A and 19A while PCV10 gives cross protection for these two antigens. Cross protection is short lived and does not last >2 years. The Advisory Committee on Vaccines & Immunization Practices (ACVIP) believes that the direct protection rendered by the serotype included in a vaccine formulation is definitely superior to any cross protection offered by the unrelated serotypes even of the same group in a PCV formulation.

Q14. Why PCV13 is superior to PCV10?

Ans: PCV10 gives good protection against NIPD (mucosal). PCV13 gives protection against both, IPD and NIPD. For prevention of IPD and acute otitis media (AOM), one needs higher titers of antibodies which is there with PCV13 as compared to PCV10. It also gives better protection against nasopharyngeal carriage.

Q15. What is herd effect and out of the two vaccines, which gives better herd effect?

Ans: Herd effect or herd immunity is indirect protection of unvaccinated persons thereby increasing the prevalence of immunity because use of vaccine prevents circulation of infectious agents in suscepti-ble population. 6B and 19F present in both PCV10 and PCV13 have herd effect, but massive herd effect is seen with 6A and 19A present in PCV13. Herd effect is seen even with a coverage of 35%. Robust herd effect is seen after a mass coverage of 60–70%.

Q16. What is the World Health Organization (WHO) recommendation on use of PCV in children?

Ans: The WHO recommends the inclusion of PCVs in childhood immunization programs worldwide. In particular, countries with high childhood mortality (i.e., under-5 mortality rate of >50 deaths/1,000 births) should make the introduction of these multicomponent PCVs a high priority.

Q17. Compare PCV10 and 13 as for as doses schedule is concerned.

Ans: Single dose of PCV10 after 2 years of age does not give reasonable immune response. It needs two doses, 4 weeks apart to give immune response comparable to full primary series of immunization with booster (3+1). It has been found that three primary doses of PCV10 followed by one booster dose of PCV13 gives far better immunity than 3+1 doses of PCV10 alone.

Q18. Who are the high-risk persons for pneumococcal vaccine?

Ans: Patients with sickle cell disease (SCD), HIV, Cochlear implant, CSF leak are considered as high risk.

Q19. How pneumococcal vaccination is planned in high-risk persons?

Ans:

- Children aged 2–18 years who are at increased risk for PD should receive both PPV23 after PCV as follows:
  - *Children > 2 years*: 1 dose of PPV23 after completing PCV schedule (recommended gap between two vaccines is 8 weeks). Children who have received PPV23 previously should also receive recommended PCV doses.
  - Children (24–71 months) with underlying medical condition, one dose of PCV if three doses were received previously or two doses if fewer than three doses of PCV were received.
  - *Children 6–18 years*: (with SCD, HIV, Cochlear implant, CSF leak) A single dose of PCV to previously unvaccinated child. The second dose of PPV23 should be given after 5 years if necessary in high-risk persons. No more dose is recommended.
- PPV23 is never used alone for prevention of PD in high-risk individuals. When elective splenectomy or cochlear implant is being planned, PCV/PPSV23 vaccine should be completed at least 2 weeks before surgery or immunocompromising therapy. PCV should be given before PSV23 as it facilitates and improves immunogenicity of PSV23. After a course of PCV, a shot of PSV23 is needed to improve the coverage against few more strains.
- Person with functional asplenia are at highest risk for pneumococcal infection because of reduced clearance of encapsulated bacteria from blood stream. They are at increased risk of fulminant pneumococcal sepsis.
- *The IAP recommendation*: Treat prematurity and very low birth weight (VLBW) infants as high risk for pneumococcal vaccination. PCV must be offered to these babies on priority basis.

Q20. What are the advantages of PCV13?

Ans: It offers three additional serotypes 3, 6A, and 19A.

- *Serotype 3*: Frequent cause of IPD and OM. Necrotizing pneumonia and empyema (20%). It is an atypical serotype/abundantly capsulated so it is less sensitive to immune reactions. It has ability to produce biofilms which may induce persistent infection and pose difficulty for eradication.
- *Serotype 6A*: Responsible for significant incidence of PD and AB resistance. 6A in PCV13 induces 100% titer. 6B in PCV7 and PCV10 gives partial cross protection against 6A (Incidence: 16.6%).
- *Serotype 19A*: Important cause of IPD, AOM, mastoiditis, and AB resistance. Leads to invasive disease with high mortality. It is most important differentiator over PCV7 and PCV10.

Q21. Why PCV13 is a better choice over PCV10/PSV23?

Ans: PCV10 is not approved beyond 5 years of age but PCV13 can be used not only beyond 5 years but in fact beyond 50 years of age. Immunocompromised should take PCV13 followed by PSV23 after 2 months. PCV13 can be taken one dose between 50 and 64. The second dose is not required. After the age of 65, only PSV23 can be given, to be repeated after 5 years. PSV23 does not protect against IPD and puts heavy load on immune system. If PSV has been given, detain PCV13 from 2 months to 1 year. Pneumococcal polysaccharide vaccine does not elicit a good immune response because it is T-cell independent. It has no effect on nasopharyngeal carriage and, therefore, herd immunity. It cannot be used in children less than 2 years of age. When polysaccharides are conjugated with a protein, they generate T-cell-dependent immune response, hence can effectively be used in infants and children. <2 years' vaccination with PPV23 leads to a depletion of the existing memory B lymphocyte pool. Also, new memory B lymphocytes is not formed. This leads to hyporesponsiveness on subsequent exposure to antigen, as the immune response may be lower (Clutterbuck et al.). Technically once an adult has taken PCV13, there is no need to take a booster. Booster does not increase the immune response even if given after 1 year. Some boosting will occur if given after 4-year gap. In PCV13, serotype 3 has weakest response and serotype 3 is responsible for necrotizing pneumonia. In PCV10, serotypes 1 and 5 have weakest response. Immunogenicity is same in preterm and term with PCV13.

Q22. What is the impact of pneumococcal vaccination on antibiotic resistance?

Ans: Pneumococcal vaccine and for that matter, all vaccines decrease use of antibiotics thus lower the risk of antibiotic resistance.

Q23. Should PCV be advised to elderly person also?

Ans: There is a huge socioeconomic burden of vaccine-preventable disease in adults. Pneumonia is responsible for 1.6 million deaths annually in children and older adults. Aging immune system and associated risk factors, make elderly vulnerable. Avidity of IgG antibodies become slower with age; this also adds to the risk. Emerging antibiotic resistance trends globally and in India, and it makes the situation far more difficult for elderly.

Q24. Why PPSV23 cannot be used in elderly?

Ans: There are limitations of PPSV23:
- Inconsistent evidence against nonbacteremic CAP
- Questionable protection against IPD in high-risk groups
- Revaccination gives hyporesponsiveness and increased reactogenicity. Waning of immune response over 5-year period is seen.

Q25. What are the recent updates in pneumococcal vaccines?

Ans: In countries where PCV (10/13) are in regular use, there is an increase in IPD cases due to serotypes not covered by these vaccines such as 22F, 33F, 15B/C, and 11A. In Europe and US22F, 15A (11%), 23A (8%), 35B (8%), and 6C (5%) account for 32% cases of IPD. To combat this situational 5-valent PCV is being developed which includes serotype 22F and 33F. 20-valent pneumococcal vaccine is also under trial which includes all the strains of PCV13 and 7 additional serotypes, viz., 8, 10A, 11A, 12F, 15BC, 22F, and 33F. Together the 20 serotypes will protect majority of PD prevalent presently globally. Six of these seven serotypes (8, 10A, 11A, 15BC, 22F, 33F) are associated with high case fatality rate. Four of these serotypes (11A, 15BC, 22F, 33F) are associated with antibiotic resistance and meningitis. The vaccine manufacturing companies are trying to develop serotype-independent pneumococcal vaccine which includes common protein.

Q26. Is there any Indian company trying to develop PCV?

Ans: The Serum Institute of India is developing a 10-valent vaccine focusing on the serotypes prevalent in India, Asia, Africa, Latin America, and Caribbean.

29 Typhoid Vaccine

KP Sarbhai

Q1. Why there is a vaccine for typhoid and not for paratyphoid?

Ans: Initially there was a combination of typhoid, paratyphoid A, and paratyphoid B (TAB) vaccine. Then it was found that paratyphoid is a less common cause of enteric fever and the vaccine for paratyphoid has poor protection and more adverse effects. Hence, TAB vaccine was changed to TA vaccine and later to T vaccine, i.e., *Salmonella typhi* vaccine. Acetone-inactivated vaccine is considered as better than phenol-killed vaccine (efficacy 79–88% and 51–66%, respectively).

Q2. What is the status of oral typhoid vaccine?

Ans: It is not available in India anymore.

Q3. What is the status of polysaccharide vaccine?

Ans: Polysaccharide vaccine is no more in use because of four reasons:
1. *Noneffectiveness < 2 years*: Polysaccharide vaccine antigens include lipopolysaccharides, which is a part of the gram-negative bacterial cell wall. It poorly induces an immunological memory because it is a thymus-independent antigen. Antibodies produced are primarily of the IgM isotype and in lesser quantities IgG2. IgM gives short-duration immunity. Lasting immunity comes by IgG which is T-cell dependent. Therefore, immune responses to these bacteria are relatively insufficient in neonates and infants. (Thymus-dependent antigens consist of soluble proteins or peptides).
2. *It lacks immune memory*: Polysaccharide vaccines elicit a T-cell-independent response, so there is no immune memory. This memory cannot be boosted by additional doses. Lack of immune response to Vi polysaccharide vaccine in <2 years or >65 years is another drawback of the vaccine.
3. *Limited efficacy*: Overall level of protection is not more than 57%. It lasts for not more than 3 years.
4. *Hyporesponsiveness*: Polysaccharide vaccine leads to lower antibody response to revaccination where repeated doses of the vaccine seem to induce a state of immune hyporesponsiveness. When repeat dose of polysaccharide vaccine is given, it leads to apoptosis (cell death and its elimination) of memory B cells in spleen and bone marrow within 12 hours of giving the vaccine. Apoptosis being at least one major mechanism of polysaccharide-induced hyporesponsiveness.

Q4. What is the Indian Academy of Pediatrics (IAP) stand on this situation?

Ans: Conjugation of the Vi antigen with a protein carrier is hence desirable as it would induce a T-cell-dependent immune response which is not only responsible for production of IgG but also for the long-lasting immunity.

Q5. Why conjugate vaccine is a better option?

Ans: There is a T-cell-dependent immune response which lasts long. Immune memory is there. IgM is formed level of which drops rapidly but boosted by repeat immunization. IgG is produced which persists for long time. Efficacy is high and it is effective in <2 years age. Conjugate polysaccharide vaccine induces higher avidity antibodies compared to polysaccharide vaccine. Conjugate vaccine induces multiple IgG subclasses and strong booster response in all ages. Conjugate vaccine is safe and more effective than polysaccharide vaccine in Indian population. Single dose of typhoid conjugate vaccine (TCV) is well-tolerated, induces robust and long-lasting immune response.

Q6. What is conjugation?

Ans: Process where in a poorly immunogenic molecule (polysaccharide) is covalently bound to a carrier protein thereby increasing the immunogenicity of the final product and making it T-cell dependent.

Q7. How the Vi polysaccharide vaccine is conjugated?

Ans: It may be conjugated with *Pseudomonas aeruginosa* exotoxin A, but this is not available in India. The vaccine available in our country is Tetanus toxoid-conjugated vaccine.

Q8. TCV (25 µg) versus TCV (5 µg).

Ans: The IAP considers this 25 µg vaccine to be a promising vaccine, fulfilling the critical gap of providing protection under 2 years of age and recommends its use <1 year of age, preferably between 9 and 12 months (minimum age 6 months). The IAP recommends its single dose and no booster at any age. 5 µg vaccine immunogenicity trial assessed response to only single dose and did not assess duration of immunity; the dosing schedule seemed extremely arbitrary. Booster dose is needed every 10 years. The Advisory Committee on Vaccines and Immunization Practices (ACVIP) does not recommend use of this vaccine as of now.

Q9. What is the dosing schedule for 25 µg TCV?

Ans: TCV 25 µg indicated for active immunization against *Salmonella typhi* infection in adults, children, and infants of age ≥6 months and ≤45 years.

Q10. What are the licensed 25 µg conjugate vaccines available in the Indian market?

Ans: Typbar TCV: Bharat Biotech, Zyvac TCV: Cadila health care, Enteroshield: Abbott.

Q11. Coadministration with other vaccine particularly Measles and MMR (vaccine against measles, mumps, and rubella).

Ans: It is permitted for use together by the IAP as immunogenicity of either is not affected.

Q12. What if one has received typhoid polysaccharide vaccine, can we give TCV now?

Ans: TCV can be given after 4 weeks. TCV booster at 2 years is not recommended as of now.

30 CHAPTER

Hepatitis A Vaccine

KP Sarbhai

Q1. Who is at increased risk for acquiring hepatitis A virus (HAV) infection?

Ans: Travelers to countries with high or intermediate endemicity of HAV infection, men who have sex with men; users of illegal drugs, both injected and noninjected; persons with clotting factor disorders, and persons working with nonhuman primates. Hepatitis A (HA) is contracted 100 times more frequent than typhoid or cholera.

Q2. How long does HAV survive outside the body? How can the virus be killed?

Ans: HAV can live outside the body for months, depending on the environmental conditions. The virus is killed by heating to >185°F (>85°C) for 1 minute. However, the virus can still be spread from cooked food if it is contaminated after cooking. Adequate chlorination of water kills HAV that enters the water supply.

Q3. Can HA become chronic?

Ans: No. HA does not become chronic.

Q4. Can a person become reinfected with HAV after recovering from HA?

Ans: No. IgG antibodies to HAV, which appear early in the course of infection, provide lifelong protection against the disease.

Q5. How is HAV infection prevented?

Ans: There are three ways to get protection against HA: (1) Vaccination, (2) immunoglobulin (Ig), and (3) good hygiene.

Q6. Who is a suitable candidate to get HA vaccine and how many doses?

Ans: Two-dose series of HA vaccine is the best way to prevent HAV infection in children/persons 12 months of age and older. The vaccine is recommended for people:
- Who are more likely to get HAV infection or
- Are more likely to get seriously ill if they get HA
- And for any person wishing to obtain immunity.

Q7. What is the role of Ig in protecting against HA?

Ans: Immunoglobulin is available for short-term protection (approximately 3 months) against HA; it can be used both for pre- and postexposure prophylaxis (PEP). Ig must be administered within 2 weeks after exposure for a maximum protection.

Q8. Who should be vaccinated against hepatitis A?

Ans:
- All children at 1 year of age (i.e., 12–23 months)
- Persons traveling to or working in countries that have high or intermediate rates of HA
- Men who have sex with men
- Users of illegal injectable and noninjectable drugs
- Persons who have occupational risk for infection
- Persons who have chronic liver disease as they have a higher rate of fulminant HA
- Persons who are either awaiting or have received liver transplants also should be vaccinated
- Persons who have clotting factor disorders, who are administered clotting factor concentrates, especially solvent detergent-treated preparations, should be vaccinated
- Household contacts of adopted children newly arriving from countries with hepatitis endemicity.

Q9. How long does protection from HA vaccine last?

Ans: Protective levels of antibody to HAV could be present for at least 25 years in adults and at least 14–20 years in child (A recent review by an expert panel, which evaluated the projected duration of immunity from vaccination.)

Q10. Can HA vaccine be administered concurrently with other vaccines?

Ans: Yes. Hepatitis B, diphtheria, poliovirus (oral and inactivated), tetanus, oral and intramuscular typhoid, cholera, Japanese encephalitis, rabies, and yellow fever vaccines and Ig can be given at the same time that HA vaccine is given, but at a different injection site.

Q11. What HA vaccines are available and what are their peculiarities?

Ans: Two vaccines are available:
1. *Inactivated vaccine*: Havrix (GSK) First vaccine available in Europe in 1991. Approved in the US in 1995. Given IM—two-dose series, 6–18 months apart. Seroconversion is >95%. It cannot replicate. It induces neutralizing antibodies (humoral immunity) antibody titer may diminish with time. Use of second dose after 6 months is mandatory to get a lifelong protective immunity. This is a booster dose. It is relatively expensive.
It contains adjuvant—aluminum hydroxide.
2. *Live attenuated vaccine*: Biovac A (Wockhardt) Earliest attempts to develop a live attenuated vaccine were made in 1980. H-2 strain HAV vaccine has been licensed for use in China since 1992 (Zhejiang Pukang Co) Simulate natural infection produces a complex immune response It produces both humoral and cellular immunity H2 strain—licensed for use above age 1 years. Single dose SC (deltoid) is given.

Observations do not support need for booster in present scenario. Protective antibody persists beyond 10 years in healthy individuals. It is freeze-dried vaccine. (0.5 mL after reconstitution.) Same dose is used for adults and children. It does not contain any adjuvant. It stored at 2–80C. It stimulates cellular immune memory—and gives long-term protection. The Advisory Committee for Vaccines and Immunization Practices (ACVIP) permits use of both the vaccines and considers both, equally efficacious. Inactivated vaccine is used world over but live vaccine use is approved only in China, India, Bangladesh, Thailand, and Guatemala.

Q12. Can a patient receive the first dose of HA vaccine from one manufacturer and the second (last) dose from another manufacturer?

Ans: Yes. Although studies have not been done to examine this issue, there is no reason to believe that using single antigen vaccine from different manufacturers would be a problem. But live vaccine should not be interchanged with killed vaccine and vice versa for subsequent doses.

Q13. Can HA vaccine be given during pregnancy?

Ans: The safety of HA vaccination during pregnancy has not been determined; The risk associated with vaccination, however, should be weighed against the risk for HA in women who might be at high risk for exposure to HAV. With inactivated HAV, risk to the developing fetus is low; therefore, it is the vaccine of choice.

Q14. Can HA vaccine be given to immunocompromised persons (e.g., persons on hemodialysis or persons with AIDS)?

Ans: With inactivated HA vaccine, no special precautions need to be taken when vaccinating immunocompromised persons. Inactivated vaccine is the choice in immunocompromised.

Q15. What are the conditions where inactivated vaccine is the choice over live vaccine?

Ans: It is safe to use killed vaccine in (1) pregnancy, (2) immunocompromised, (3) during an epidemic outbreak, and (4) patients on hemodialysis.

Q16. Is it harmful to administer an extra dose(s) of hepatitis A or hepatitis B vaccine or to repeat the entire vaccine series if documentation of vaccination history is unavailable?

Ans: No. If necessary, administering extra doses of hepatitis A or hepatitis B vaccine is not harmful.

Q17. Should prevaccination testing be performed before administering HA vaccine?

Ans: Prevaccination testing is recommended only in specific circumstances to reduce the costs of vaccinating people who are already immune to HA. Persons who were born in geographic areas with high or intermediate prevalence of HAV infection. Adults in groups that have a high prevalence of infection (e.g., injectable drug users). Prevaccination testing might also be warranted for all older adults. The decision to test should be based on: (1) the expected prevalence of immunity, (2) the cost of vaccination compared with the cost of serologic testing, and (3) the likelihood that testing will not interfere with initiation of vaccination.

Q18. Should postvaccination testing be performed?

Ans: No. Postvaccination testing is not indicated because of:
- The high rate of vaccine response among adults and children
- Not all testing methods approved for routine diagnostic use have the sensitivity to detect low, but protective, anti-HAV concentrations after vaccination. (Concentration of IgG anti-HAV achieved after administration of IM IgG/vaccination are below the level of detection of available diagnostic tests; therefore, it is of no use doing postvaccinaton titer estimation.)

Q19. How soon before travel should the first dose of HA vaccine be given?

Ans: The first dose of HA vaccine should be administered as soon as travel is considered. Previously, vaccination was recommended at least 2–4 weeks before departure. Travelers who were departing in <2 weeks were recommended to receive Ig for short-term protection. However, on the basis of data indicating that Ig and vaccine have equivalent postexposure efficacy among healthy persons aged ≤40 years, the ACIP has amended its guidelines for HA vaccination for travelers. The ACIP now recommends that one dose of single-antigen HA vaccine administered at any time before departure may provide adequate protection for most healthy persons. For optimal protection, older adults, immunocompromised persons, and persons with chronic liver disease or other chronic medical conditions who are planning to depart in ≤2 weeks should receive the initial dose of vaccine and also can simultaneously be administered Ig (0.02 mL/kg) at a separate anatomic injection site.

Q20. What should be done if a traveler cannot receive HA vaccine?

Ans: Travelers who are allergic to a vaccine component, who elect not to receive vaccine, or who are aged <12 months should receive a single dose of Ig (0.02 mL/kg), which provides effective protection against HAV infection for up to 3 months. Travelers whose travel period exceeds 2 months should be administered Ig at 0.06 mL/kg. Administration must be repeated if the travel period exceeds 5 months.

Q21. What should be done for travelers <12 months of age?

Ans: Immunoglobulin is recommended because HA vaccine is currently not approved for use in this age group.

Q22. What are the current Centers for Disease Control and Prevention (CDC) guidelines for postexposure protection against HA?

Ans: Until recently, Ig was the only recommended way to protect people after they have been exposed to HAV. When Ig is administered within 2 weeks of exposure, it is 80–90% effective in preventing HA. Efficacy is greater when administered early in incubation period, when administered later Ig might only attenuate the clinical expression of HAV infection Ig is available in 2-mL and 10-mL vials. It is preservative free. Serious adverse events are rare. Pregnancy, lactation is not a contraindication to use of Ig administration. In June 2007, the US guidelines were revised to allow for HA vaccine to be used after exposure to prevent infection in healthy persons aged 1–40 years. For healthy persons aged 12 months to 40 years, single-antigen HA vaccine at the age-appropriate dose is preferred to Ig because of the vaccine's advantages, including long-term protection and ease of administration as well as the equivalent efficacy of vaccine to Ig. For persons aged 40 years and older, Ig is preferred because of the absence of information regarding vaccine performance in this age group and because of the more severe manifestations of HA in older adults. Vaccine can be used if Ig cannot be obtained. Ig should be used for children aged <12 months, immunocompromised persons, persons with chronic liver disease, and persons who are allergic to the vaccine or a vaccine component.

Q23. If HAV Ig has been used can we use other vaccines without interference?

Ans: Ig does not interfere with oral polio vaccine (OPV), yellow fever, or in general to inactivated vaccines. Ig interferes with response to live attenuated vaccines such as measles, mumps, rubella (MMR) and varicella. Administration of MMR should be delayed by >3 months, and of Varicella by >5 months after administration of HAIg. If these vaccines have been given before hand, the guideline is: Ig should not be administered for <2 weeks after MMR and <3 weeks after Varicella vaccine. If it is mandatory to use HAIg, then in such cases MMR/Varicella have to be given again but with a gap of >3 months in MMR and >5 months in Varicella.

Q24. If a case of HA is found in a school, hospital, or office setting, what should be done?

Ans: If a single case of Hepatitis A is identified in a office, or other work setting, and if the source of infection is outside the school or work setting, PEP (i.e., injection of Ig or HA vaccine) is not routinely recommended. When a person who has HA is admitted to a hospital, staff should not routinely be administered PEP; instead, careful hygienic practices should be emphasized. If HA spreads among students in a school or among patients and staff in a hospital, PEP should be administered to unvaccinated persons who have had close contact with an infected person.

Human Papillomavirus Vaccine

KP Sarbhai

Q1. How is human papillomavirus (HPV) transmitted?

Ans: It can be transmitted through genital skin-to-skin contact during sexual activity, by sharing contaminated sex toys rarely, and during delivery from the infected mother to the baby. HPV cannot be passed by sitting on toilet seats or touching the door knobs.

Q2. A grandmother comes with her granddaughter for her HPV vaccination. Now she asked that she has not received this vaccine because it was not available in her time. Now she wants to know about risk of her getting cervical cancer.

Ans:
- Do not worry if you have not received HPV vaccine because vaccine cannot prevent all cases of HPV (only 4 out of 5).
- Not all HPV infections progress to cervical cancer. Most HPV infection (90% cases) goes away on its own without any treatment.
- Even when it does, it takes up to 20 years to do so.

Q3. Now the grandmother wants to know how safe the vaccine is? Can the vaccine itself produce cervical cancer?

Ans: The vaccine is not a toxic agent. It is not made from an active virus. Rather, it is developed from the outer membrane surrounding the DNA of the HPV virus. By taking the vaccine, a person develops antibody (Ab) against outer shell of virus not the virus itself. But this is enough protection against HPV causing cervical cancer and warts and cannot produce cancer by itself.

Q4. How is HPV related to cervical cancer?

Ans: Some strains of HPV infect the cervix, causing the cells to change. In about 90% of the infection cases, the virus clears by itself and the cells return to normal. In some cases, the infection can persist and causes the cells to grow in an abnormal way. When this goes undetected by a Pap smear at an early stage, some of these abnormal cells may develop into cervical cancer.

Q5. There are 100 strains of HPV virus of which 12 are known to cause cervical cancer. Strains 16 and 18 are responsible for 70% of cervical cancer. What about the remaining 10 strains? Is there any protection against them?

Ans: Yes, there is cross protection for remaining strains by 16 and 18.

Q6. Can HPV be treated?

Ans: The virus itself cannot be treated. Most HPV infection (90% cases) goes away on its own without any treatment. Although HPV virus cannot be treated, regular PAP smear can help to detect changes in the cervical cells caused by HPV infection. With appropriate treatment, the abnormal or precancerous cells can be prevented from developing into cervical cancer.

Q7. Who is at risk of HPV infection?

Ans: Risk factors for HPV infection include:
- *Multiple sexual partners*: Greater the number of sexual partners, the higher is risk of HPV infection.
- Having sexual activity with a partner who has had multiple sex partners can also increase risk.
- People with HIV/AIDS or on immune suppressant are at higher risk of HPV infection, both men and women.
- Gay and bisexual males.

Condoms can help reduce the risk of HPV infection. Condoms however, do not cover whole genital skin and therefore do not guarantee 100% protection.

Q8. Strains 6 and 11 protect 90% of genital warts. Are they important for our country as well?

Ans: There is no Indian data for incidence of genital warts. One lac new cases of genital warts occur in UK every year. If this data is considered as base in our country, approximately 10 lac new cases occur every year (both in males and females).

Every year 9,000 HPV-related cancers occur in males in UK. This can be extrapolated to nearly 1 lac cases in India every year. This makes the male vaccine valid in India as well. Further HPV vaccination of boys is likely to benefit girls by reducing the spread of HPV virus.

Q9. How effective is HPV vaccine?

Ans: Antibody level is much higher after vaccination than after natural infection. Experts predict that protection from vaccine will last for at least 15 years and probably lifelong.

Q10. What is the ideal age HPV vaccination and why?

Ans:
- HPV vaccine works best when a girl is vaccinated before she is sexually active.
- Preteens have a better immune response to a vaccine than older teens. However, vaccine can be given up to 45 years of age keeping in mind that it will not protect against the strains to which one has already been exposed.

Q11. Can HPV vaccine be given during pregnancy?

Ans:
- No, not to be given. If the lady gets pregnant after receiving one or two doses, the remaining doses should be given after delivery in the immediate postpartum period.
- Inadvertently, if vaccine has been given to a pregnant lady, it is not an indication for termination.

Q12. Can it be given to lactating woman?

Ans: Gardasil can be given to lactating females because available data do not indicate any safety concerns.

However, Cervarix safety data for lactating females are not available yet.

Q13. What is latest in immunization schedule of HPV?

Ans: The Strategic Advisory Group of Experts (SAGE) committee on immuni-zation of the World Health Organization (WHO) has recommended two doses for girls <15 years of age with 6-month interval. Three-dose schedule remains necessary after 15th birthday. This 6-month gap between two doses cannot be shortened. 6-month gap gives superior geometric mean concentration (GMC) as compared to shorter interval. However, for immunosuppressed and HIV positives, three-dose schedule is mandatory.

Q14. Is HPV vaccination associated with side effects?

Ans: Both vaccines are safe and well tolerated.

Pain, redness, and swelling around where the shot was given.

Other mild reactions include fever, headache, fatigue, nausea, and vomiting. Some people have experienced fainting as well.

As with any vaccine or medication, there is a possibility of allergic reaction. However, such reactions are rare.

HPV vaccine continues to be monitored for any safety concerns.

Q15. What precaution should be taken for HPV vaccine administration?

Ans: People taking vaccination should be counseled properly and vaccine should be administered in sitting or lying down position and should be observed for 15 minutes postvaccination.

Q16. After receiving HPV vaccine, do one still need to get PAP test done?

Ans: Yes! HPV vaccines will not eliminate all HPV or cervical cancer. The vaccines prevent the HPV types that cause 70% of cervical cancer cases, but there are other types of HPV (not covered in the vaccine) that could cause disease. In addition to regular Pap tests, women 30 and over can also request an HPV test along with their Pap. Unlike a Pap test, which only detects abnormal cell changes, an HPV test can be used to find one or more of the high-risk types of HPV that are most commonly found with cervical cancer. Most women under 30 with HPV will get rid of the virus, so the HPV test for younger women is not helpful.

Q17. How are the two HPV vaccines different?

Ans: Only one of the vaccines (Gardasil) protects against HPV types 6 and 11, the types that cause most genital warts in females and males. Only one of the vaccines (Gardasil) has been tested and licensed for use in males. While both vaccines protect against HPV 16 and 18 responsible for cancers of cervix, vulva, and vagina; only one of the vaccines (Gardasil) has been tested and shown to protect against precancers of penis, anal cancers, anal interepithelial neoplasias, and cancer of oropharynx.

The two vaccines have different adjuvants—(a substance that is added to the vaccine to increase the body's immune response.) Cervarix has ASO4 which is considered as a better adjuvant. Immunogenicity of two vaccines is equivalent with respect to HPV 16, but HPV 18 is more immunogenic in Cervarix.

Q18. How long protection from the HPV vaccine will last?

Ans: Antibody level is much higher after vaccination than after natural infection. This is good as high antibody levels usually mean longer protection. Experts predict that protection from the HPV vaccine will last for at least 15 years and probably lifelong.

Q19. Can the vaccine be given to a young woman who is already sexually active? Is it still advisable to do so?

Ans: The HPV vaccine works best when people are vaccinated before they become sexually active, the vaccine is still recommended for those who are already sexually active.

Most girls and women are infected with HPV, within 2–5 years of becoming sexually active. It is likely that they may not have been infected with HPV during previous sexual activity, and if at all infected, they are unlikely to be infected with all of the types of HPV contained in the vaccine. If her sexual history is fairly limited, seriously consider the vaccine, to protect against the various strains of HPV in the vaccine.

If she has already come into contact with HPV subtype 6, then she will have no protection against that strain responsible for genital warts. But the vaccine will protect her against the other types, if she has not yet been exposed to it. If she has not yet encountered HPV subtypes 16 and 18, vaccination will protect her against dysplasia and possible cervical cancer. There is no way to tell whether exposure has occurred to a particular strains or not, there is no good way to do so at the moment. Thats why the vaccine is recommended for young, presexually active women.

Q20. Should a 41-year-old woman get the vaccine? Is it helpful at such a late age?

Ans: Possibly. Lifestyle is an important variable. Otherwise, a 41-year-old married woman who is not meeting new sexual partners probably would not benefit from vaccination because she is not being exposed to the sexually transmitted HPV viruses that cause a majority of cervical cancers. If a woman has been monogamous for 20 years and her husband has just died, she might want to consider the vaccine before starting to date again. There is a good chance she has not been exposed to at least some of the HPV strains the vaccine protects against.

Q21. Girl at the age of 9–10 years is not sexually active. Why does she need the HPV vaccine?

Ans: Most girls catch HPV infection within 2–5 years of becoming sexually active, so it is important to vaccinate them before they begin sexual activity. Vaccination at this age gives them time to develop an immune response before they begin sexual activity with another person. Additionally, research shows the vaccine actually works best when it is given at a younger age. Thats because preteens have a better immune response to the vaccine than older teens. This means they will be better protected if they are exposed to HPV in the future. Anyone who engages in any kind of sexual activity involving oral or genital contact can get HPV. Sexual intercourse is not necessary to get infected.

Q22. What is DES? DES daughters? DES granddaughters?

Ans: In 1938, DES (diethylstilbestrol) was the first synthetic estrogen to be created. One of the major DES producers was Eli Lilly.

DES was used in the mistaken belief that it prevents miscarriages and premature deliveries.

DES was prescribed primarily between 1938 and 1971 (but not limited to those years). It was considered the standard of care for problem pregnancies.

DES was sometimes even included in prenatal vitamins so there are many individuals who were not actually given a prescription for DES itself, yet were exposed to it anyway.

In the early 1970s cases of a rare vaginal/cervical cancer were being diagnosed in young women.

In November 1971, the Food and Drug Administration (FDA) asked doctors not to use DES for their pregnant patients; however, it was never banned.

DES health issues are extending into the next generation, the so-called DES daughters and grandchildren. This group has been adversely impacted by a drug prescribed to their mothers and grandmothers.

DES daughters are at higher risk for getting HPV than other women.

Many DES daughters have a larger cervical transformation zone than unexposed women, and thats where the HPV virus invades cells. With a bigger area, clearly DES daughters run an increased risk for HPV infection.

This is important for DES daughters to understand—the vaccine works against cervical cancer caused by HPV, and not against *clear cell adenocarcinoma* of the cervix and vagina, linked to DES exposure. This vaccine is safe and effective for DES daughters, granddaughters and otherwise for protection against HPV but does not have any protective effect on clear cell adenocarcinoma which is so specific to DES daughters and granddaughters.

Q23. Who should NOT be vaccinated?

Ans: One should not be vaccinated if: One is sensitive to yeast or to any of the vaccine components, or suffering from moderate or severe acute infectious illness (wait till recovery from the illness) or bleeding disorder, or undergoing anticoagulant therapy.

Q24. Do we need a booster dose?

Ans: No.

Q25. Can this vaccine be given in immunocompromised person?

Ans: There is no evidence to say that it cannot be given in immunosuppressed ones.

Available brands:
- *Gardasil (MSD)*: Quadrivalent; four strains are there—16, 18, 6, and 11. Adjuvant is aluminum-containing substance.
- *Cervarix (GSK)*: Bivalent; two strains are there—16 and 18. Other two strains are not there which protect against genital warts, penile cancers, and anal malignancies. Adjuvant is ASO4.

Both vaccines are manufactured by recombinant DNA technology which produces noninfectious virus-like particles (VLP) which is made up of major capsid protein of HPV (L1).

32 Influenza Vaccine

KP Sarbhai

Q1. When did the first global influenza pandemic occur?

Ans: Pandemic began in May 2009, spread to all over the world, and became global by July 11, 2009. On 10 August, 2010, pandemic was declared. >18,449 deaths reported worldwide by end of the month.

Q2. When did India face the pandemic?

Ans: The first positive case of pandemic H1N1 was reported in May 2009. By end of the 2010, 20,604 cases with 1,763 deaths were reported. Country experienced three waves (2009–2010); first in 2009 September, second wave in December, and third peak in August 2010.

Q3. What is the present status of H1N1 in India?

Ans: After its emergence in 2009, pandemic strain H1N1 virus continues to circulate in India, along with the previously circulating influenza viruses.

Q4. What is the role of environmental temperature?

Ans: Year-round activity is observed in tropical and subtropical regions with annual or biannual peak in different countries. India being a vast country with diverse climate demonstrates three seasonal activities, one during monsoon months which are observed in most part of the country with tropical climate and other in winter period which is observed in the temperate region of extreme northern part of the country.

Q5. How the host immunity develops?

Ans: Pandemic occurs with the emergence of a new virus. Immunity to the new virus is acquired either from exposure to infection or due to vaccination. Decreased rate of infection and severity is expected during the subsequent years due to building up of specific immunity. Waning of host immunity has attributed as the possible cause of resurfacing of the influenza virus. Increased vaccine coverage before the influenza season has been shown to be correlated with decrease influenza activity. Influenza A virus is known for its high rate of mutation. Rate of mutation has been estimated as 6.7 × 10 nucleotides substitution per site/year. Mutations has the capability to prevent the binding of existing antibody resulting in rapid turnover of mutant viral strains. New pandemic virus H1N1 has remained genetically stable since its emergence in 2009.

Q6. What action has been taken by government to control influenza?

Ans: Due to the lack of actual disease burden of influenza, evidence-based vaccination for all high-risk groups was not possible. Vaccination was only recommended for healthcare workers and staff who have the possibility of coming in contact with influenza patients, laboratory personnel who are involved with influenza testing, members of "Rapid response team" who carry out investigation of influenza outbreak.

Q7. What is the burden of influenza in different age groups and different socioeconomic conditions?

Ans: Influenza occurs globally. Annual attack rate estimated at 5–10% in adults and 20–30% in children. Children aged <5 years and particularly those <2 years of age have a high burden of influenza. Burden of influenza is significantly higher in developing countries as compared to developed countries.

Data on the disease burden is less well defined in most of the developing countries including India. Overall risk of influenza complication is much high in high-risk people.

Q8. What are the types of influenza virus?

Ans: This virus belongs to orthomyxoviridae family. Virus is divided into three subtypes: A, B, and C. Influenza A and B cause seasonal epidemics. C causes mild respiratory illness. Influenza A is divided into subtypes based on hemagglutinin (HA) and neuraminidase (NA) proteins. HA and NA genes can be reassorted generating novel subtypes. Different influenza A subtypes result from different combination of HA and NA proteins.

Q9. What are the five protein structure in the virus and their significance?

Ans:
- *Hemagglutinin (H or HA)*: It is responsible for pathogenicity of the virus and allows virus to adhere to epithelial cells in the respiratory tract.
- *Neuraminidase (N or NA)*: It reduces viscosity of the mucus layer in trachea and allows release of newly formed viruses from infected cell.
- *M1 protein*: It is matrix protein which forms the viral capsid.
- *M2 protein channel*: Functioning as anion channel (energy regulators).
- *Ribonucleoprotein*: RNA (genetic code), Nucleoprotein (NP).

These five proteins make the complete structure of virus.

Q10. How does the influenza virus spread?

Ans:
- From person to person primarily through large-particle respiratory droplet transmission. Requires close contact between source and recipient as droplets only travel <1 m.
- By contact with surfaces contaminated with respiratory droplets.
- By airborne transmission of evaporated droplets that may remain in the air for long periods of time (data are limited).
- Virus transmission may be slowed by social distancing.

Q11. What are antigenic drift and shift?

Ans: Influenza strains are constantly mutating. A small change in the in the genetic makeup of strain is called as antigenic drift while a major change is called as antigenic shift.

Antigenic shift is the process by which two or more different strains of virus or two or more different viruses combine to form a new subtype which has a mixture of the surface antigen of the original strains. It occurs when two viruses simultaneously infect the same animal, e.g., Pig carries an endemic strain of influenza and can be infected with both human and avian influenza strain leading to a possibility of antigenic shift. Reassortment of genetic material during shift confers a phenotypic change. Thus a new virus is formed which combines the antigen of both viruses. For example, H3N2 and H5N1 can form H5N2. Human immune system finds it difficult to recognize the new influenza strain, and this may be highly dangerous and result in a new pandemic. Shift is less common, but when it happens, there is no immunity against the new virus and this causes pandemic to take place. It is rare and in past 100 years, only four influenza pandemic have occurred. Influenza A shows antigenic shift as well as drift.

Antigenic drift: Host antibodies recognize virus surface proteins. In drift, the viral genes which code for the surface protein get the mutation. This results in a new strain of virus with new surface protein not recognized and inhibited by existing antibodies. This makes it easy for the changed virus to spread in community which is partially immune. Antigenic drift is responsible for seasonal influenza and needs a new vaccine every year. Influenza B virus shows only antigenic drift.

Influenza C is a stable virus and does not undergo shift or drift.

Q12. What is the advantage of childhood influenza vaccination?

Ans: Vaccine reduces influenza-related hospitalizations. It reduces influenza infection in contacts because it has good herd effect. Reduces circulation of the virus in the community. Immunity following vaccination or natural infection has a very short span. It takes 2 weeks for antibodies to develop and within 8 months, antibody level drops to prevaccination level thus needing annual vaccination. T-cell-mediated immunity persists for a longer time but remains suboptimal. Even the best-matched vaccine provides 60–80% protection.

Q13. What are the types of influenza vaccine?

Ans: Whole-virion vaccines, split-virion vaccines, and subunit virion vaccine, and recombinant flu vaccine.

- *Whole-virion vaccine*: It has surface antigen, internal antigen, and reactogenic lipid (lipopolysaccharides). Immunogenicity of this vaccine is good but reactogenicity is high.
- *Split-virion vaccine*: It has surface antigen, internal antigen but free of reactogenic lipid. It is treated with detergent so as to remove the reactogenic lipid layer which envelops the virus. So it has a good immunogenicity and good tolerance, e.g., vaxigrip. It is also called as detergent-split vaccine.
- *Subunit virion vaccine*: It has surface antigens only. Viral membrane is separated from viral core.
  It lacks internal antigens and is free of reactogenic lipids. So it is highly purified vaccine. Therefore, immunogenicity is moderate and tolerance is good, e.g., influvac.
- *Quadrivalent flu vaccine*: An additional influenza B virus is added to it so that it contributes to additional immune response against added influenza B lineage. Safety and reactogenicity of quadrivalent influenza vaccine (QIV) is consistent with those of trivalent influenza vaccine (TIV). In the US, outbreaks of Influenza B are proving much more risky than H1N1, therefore, QIV is being developed. This will be a fourth-generation vaccine. QIV provides coverage for two influenza B viruses. Present influenza vaccine contains A/California(H1N1)-like virus, A/Switzerland (H3N2)-like virus, and B/Phuket-like virus (Yamagata lineage)

Quadrivalent influenza vaccine has above three viruses and B/Brisbane-like virus (Victoria lineage).

Q14. What is the dosage schedule?

Ans: 0.5 mL at 6 and 7 months of age followed by once every year.

Q15. What is live attenuated influenza vaccine (LAIV)?

Ans: Vaccination with LAIV mimics natural infection; thus induces both cellular and humoral immunities. It was first developed in 1960. LAIV is delivered intranasally and induces longer-lasting antibody titer. LAIV is licensed for use in healthy individuals of 2–49 years age. LAIV should be avoided in children of 2–4 years age who had asthma in preceding 1 year, or adolescents receiving aspirin (because of association of Reye syndrome with wild type of influenza virus infection). Dose schedule: 2–8 years, two doses 4 weeks apart and then one annual dose >8 years, single dose annually.

Q16. What are the contraindications for the use of LAIV?

Ans:
- Contraindicated in persons who have taken influenza antiviral medication within previous 48 hours.
- Contraindicated in persons with history of Guillain-Barré syndrome (GBS) after influenza vaccination.
- Person with any underlying medical condition that serve as an indication for routine influenza vaccination, including asthma, reactive airway disease or other chronic pulmonary or cardiovascular disorder, is a contraindication for LAIV.
- Underlying medical conditions such as metabolic diseases, diabetes, renal dysfunction, and hemoglobinopathies.
- Immunocompromised patient, or in people whose close contact are immunocompromised.
- Not indicated in pregnancy but can be used in lactating mother.

Q17. What precautions should be taken in storage and administration of vaccine?

Ans: Rigorous maintenance of cold chain is required. Vaccine potency once lost cannot be restored. In addition to heat, vaccine is damaged by excessive cold too. All aluminum-adjuvanted vaccine are sensitive to freezing. LAIV is very sensitive to heat. Inactivated vaccine should be stored in middle shelf (2–8°C), if accidentally frozen should be discarded. Inactivated influenza vaccine (IIV) should be given in deltoid with needle length >1 inch. When deltoid mass is sufficient, needle length of 1.25 inch is recommended. Less than this can be insufficient to penetrate muscle mass.

Key points:
- TIV vaccines are safe and well tolerated in infants and young children and reduce the incidence of acute otitis media (AOM), pneumonia, and sinusitis. They reduce influenza-related morbidity among household contacts. Overall efficacy of vaccine is 50–60%. They provides moderate protection against virologically confirmed influenza.
- Herd immunity effect is reasonably good. It reduces mortality from influenza among the elderly. It significantly reduces direct and indirect influenza-related costs in healthy children and their unvaccinated family members.

Q18. What are the benefits of influenza vaccine in preschool children?

Ans: It reduces influenza-related mortality by 83%; AOM by 36%; upper respiratory tract infection (URI) by 33%; and acute bronchitis, wheezing, and pneumonia by 22%.

Q19. What are the benefits in schoolgoing children?

Ans: Missed school days are reduced by 48%. Antibiotic prescriptions are reduced by 32%. Maternal work absenteeism is reduced by 33% and paternal work absenteeism by 43%. It also has a good herd effect so unvaccinated children are also likely to be protected.

Q20. Can influenza vaccine be used in pregnancy and lactating mother?

Ans: Vaccine offers protection both to mother and newborn up to 6 months of infancy. Pregnant woman experiences disproportionately severe sequel of influenza owing to physiological change in pregnancy (reduced lung capacity, increased cardiac output, increased O_2 consumption), and immunosuppression.

Infection in third trimester is most dangerous as there is increased risk of miscarriage, preterm births, and still births. Both LAIV and IIV can be used for lactating mother. Only IIV is indicated for pregnancy. It is recommended that vaccination for pregnant woman is given early in the season regardless of gestation age. India has bimodal seasonal distribution (monsoon and winter) so vaccination of all pregnant woman is recommended. The Centers for Disease Control and Prevention (CDC) and the Food and Drug Administration (FDA) have given safety clearance to vaccination in pregnancy. There is no association of vaccination with adverse obstetric events such as miscarriage, congenital malformation, preterm births, small for gestational age infants. Data regarding first trimester exposure to vaccine is relatively limited.

Q21. Who should be vaccinated?

Ans: The CDC, Indian Academy of Pediatrics (IAP), American Academy of Pediatrics (AAP), and Advisory Committee on Immunization Practices (ACIP) all recommend it to be used in all age groups above the age group of 6 months. The Indian Academy of Pediatrics

Committee on Immunization (IAPCOI) recommends using the influenza vaccine in all children with risk factors, e.g., congenital/acquired immunodeficiency, chronic cardiac, pulmonary, hematologic, liver disease, renal disorders and diabetes mellitus (DM); children on long-term aspirin therapy; any neurologic disease that may cause respiratory compromise or impair ability to handle secretions; and asthma requiring oral steroids.

Q22. How the IAP has suggested prioritization of target group for influenza immunization?

Ans: (1: highest priority, 4: lowest priority)
1. Elderly > 65 years and nursing home residents
2. Individuals with chronic medical conditions including HIV and pregnant women (to protect infants 0–6 months)
3. *Other groups*: Healthcare workers including professionals, individuals with asthma, and children from 6 months to 2 years of age
4. Children aged 2–5 years and 6–18 years, and healthy young adults.

Q23. At which time of the year vaccine should be given?

Ans: Limited influenza activity is usually seen throughout the year in India with a clear peaking during the rainy season. Rainy season in the country lasts from June to August in all the regions, except Tamil Nadu where it occurs from October to December. Flu vaccination should begin soon after vaccine becomes available, if possible by October. As long as flu viruses are circulating vaccination should continue to be offered throughout the flu season, even in January or later.

KEY MESSAGES

Children shed virus for long intervals and are at high risk of flu. Vaccination gives greatest protection between 6 months and 5 years of age and for children suffering from chronic health conditions such as asthma, diabetes, or heart disease. Children < 6 months are not to be vaccinated but can be protected by vaccination during pregnancy. The IAP recommends Influenza vaccine for all high-risk children, HIV patients, and those on long-term salicylate therapy.

CHAPTER 33

Rabies Vaccine

KP Sarbhai

Q1. How does rabies spread?

Ans: Rabies is one of the oldest and most feared zoonotic diseases. All mammals, but mainly carnivores and bats, are susceptible and can transmit rabies virus.

Q2. How is rabies transmitted?

Ans: Rabies is transmitted by infected secretions. Rabies virus can be excreted in saliva, urine, nasal discharge, and respiratory secretions.

Q3. Does kissing a rabies patient calls for antirabies vaccination (ARV)?

Ans: Kissing a rabies patient may transmit the disease because there may be contact with rabies patient's saliva. Full post-exposure immunization must be given either by intramuscular (IM) or intradermal (ID) route. If there are ulcers in the mouth of the exposed person, then rabies immunoglobulin (RIG) must be given by IM route.

Q4. A person has handled or eaten the raw meat of a rabid animal. What should be done?

Ans: If a person has handled or eaten the raw meat of a rabid animal, he should receive full course of ARV. If the person has eaten raw meat of a rabid animal and has oral ulcers/lesions, he may be given RIGs intramuscularly in thigh on day 0 along with the first dose of vaccine.

Q5. Is washing of animal bite wound(s) essential?

Ans: Risk of rabies reduces by about 50% by just washing of wounds and application of antiseptics. The maximum benefit is obtained if cleaned immediately with running tap water for at least 15 minutes. Washing of the wound must be done as long as the wound is raw, irrespective of the time elapsed since the exposure. Care must be taken not to disturb the scab, if formed. After washing with water and soap, disinfectants such as povidone iodine or surgical spirit must be applied. In extraneous circumstances, other alcoholic (>40%) preparations such as rum, whisky, or aftershave lotion may be applied.

Q6. How is RIG lifesaving?

Ans: Protective levels of antibodies (>0.5 IU/mL of serum) are seen 7–14 days after the initial dose of vaccine (window period). When the bites are on the head, neck, face, and hands, the incubation period will be shorter. Thus the patients are during this window period of 7–14 days vulnerable to develop rabies. RIGs are readymade antirabies antibodies and provide passive immunity to rabies.

Q7. How is RIG injected locally? What is the mode of administration of full dose of RIG?

Ans: It is important to infiltrate all wounds with RIG. IM administration of RIG is of very little value. As much of the calculated dose of RIG as is anatomically feasible should be infiltrated into and around all the wounds.

In the event that some volume of RIGs is left after all wounds have been infiltrated, it should be administered deep IM at a site distant from the vaccine injection site. If the calculated dose of RIG is insufficient to infiltrate all wounds, sterile saline can be used to dilute it two or three-fold to permit thorough infiltration.

Q8. Can the wound be deepened for cleaning purpose?

Ans: We should never try to deepen the bite wound. Deepening of wound for cleaning depends on area of injury and extent of injury. The aim should be to preserve as much tissue as possible and to excise only the dead tissue.

Q9. Can RIGs be safely injected into already infected animal bite wounds?

Ans: RIGs can be safely injected following proper wound cleansing and administration of appropriate antibiotics.

Q10. Can RIG be given locally to a healed wound?

Ans: Yes. If ARV has not been started, then RIG can be given locally without disturbing the scab.

Q11. What are the precautions to be taken while administering RIGs?

Ans: Patient should not be on an empty stomach. Warm RIG vial to room/body temperature. Avoid injecting into vessels and nerves. Avoid compartment syndrome (while injecting into finger tips). All emergency drugs must be available. For RIG of equine origin (ERIG), keep the patient under observation for 1 hour. RIGs can be infiltrated even to already sutured wounds without disturbing the sutures.

Q12. Is it essential to perform skin sensitivity test prior to the administration of ERIG?

Ans: Majority of reactions to ERIG result from complement activation and are not IgE mediated and will not be predicted by skin testing.

The recent World Health Organization (WHO) recommendation states that there are no scientific grounds for performing a skin test prior to the administration of ERIG, because testing does not predict reactions and "ERIG should be given whatever the result of the test." However, skin test is mandatory to avoid any possible litigation under the Consumer Protection Act in India.

Q13. What is IM pre-exposure vaccination schedule? What is the importance of pre-exposure vaccination?

Ans: Three IM injections on days 0, 7, and 28 days. Pre-exposure vaccination simplifies postexposure vaccination because after the bite, those who have received full pre-exposure vaccination require only two doses of vaccine at days 0 and 3. RIG is not required (WHO 2007). However, in laboratory-confirmed rabies exposures, irrespective of past rabies immunization, full course of postexposure prophylaxis (PEP) and RIGs is recommended. In rabies, it is safer to overtreat than to undertreat.

Q14. Is there any dietary restriction during PEP?

Ans: Abstain from alcoholic drinks during the course of rabies vaccination as it may affect the immune response.

Q15. Can the vaccine be injected in gluteal region?

Ans: Rabies vaccine must not be administered in gluteal region as the gluteal fat may retard vaccine absorption resulting in delayed and lower seroconversion.

Q16. What is the criterion for "protection" after immunization?

Ans: The rabies virus neutralizing antibody (RVNA) titer of 0.5 IU/mL of serum in the vaccinated person is considered protective. The facility for this test is available at NCDC, Delhi; CRI, Kasauli; Pasteur institute, Coonoor; NIV, Pune; and NIMHANS, Bangalore.

Q17. How to approach a case of irregularities in treatment schedule, e.g., if a patient missed the doses as per the due dates, i.e., dose schedule is broken?

Ans: First three doses of modern rabies vaccine must be very timely. For the fourth and fifth, 1 or 2 days of variation is permissible. If at all there is a break in schedule, vaccine should be given on nearest recommended date. All doses should be completed by 28th day.

Q18. If a person is on antimalarial or steroids or taking immunosuppressant drug, what is the schedule for rabies vaccine?

Ans: The vaccine on day 0 must be doubled and given at two sites. In category II bite, administer RIG + vaccine. Rest of the schedule is same as for any other patient.

Q19. A patient received two doses of modern vaccine (on days 0 and 3) and the dog was well on days 5 and 7 (third injection due, but not given). However, the dog dies on any day between 8 and 15. What should be done?

Ans: In case, day 0 and 3 injections were given and the dose due on day 7 was postponed because the dog was kept under observation but the dog dies between 8 and 15 days, three doses of vaccine must be given as close to the original dates of the schedule. All five injections must be completed by day 28.

Q20. Can a rabies vaccine be given to a pregnant woman?

Ans: Following animal bite, rabies vaccine can be given to a pregnant woman. Medical termination of pregnancy should not be done as a routine clinical practice.

Q21. A pregnant woman develops rabies. What should be done?

Ans: The rabies virus is not known to cross the placental barrier, and so if the mother develops rabies, the fetus is safe. Hence, the pregnant woman with rabies should be clinically managed and if induction of pregnancy or cesarean section is possible, the obstetrician should do it with some "personal precautions" and immune prophylaxis (usually three doses of modern vaccine or if there is any accidental exposure, then full course of post exposure vaccination either by IM or ID route should be given to the obstetrician). Later, the newborn may be given a full course of rabies PEP vaccination.

Q22. Can rabies vaccine be given to a child with chicken pox or measles?

Ans: Since rabies is 100% fatal, there is no contraindication for ARV. ARV can be given to a child with chicken pox or measles and it is effective. If possible administration of measles vaccine should be postponed by a fortnight, after the completion of antirabies immunization.

Q23. Do antibodies from rabies vaccination cross an intact blood–brain barrier?

Ans: No, antibodies from vaccination do not cross an intact blood–brain barrier.

Q24. Can a vaccinated dog transmit rabies? How effective is dog vaccine?

Ans: If a potent veterinary vaccine is given correctly as per pre-exposure schedule, it will mostly prevent rabies in the vaccinated dog, unless the exposure is severe. Ideally, its sera should be tested for protective antibody titer level but this is rarely practicable due to scare facilities in our country. It has been noted that:
- 6% of dogs found rabid have a reliable pre-exposure rabies vaccine history.
- 40% of dogs are vaccinated only one time and loses most of their immunity 4–6 months later.
- PEP vaccination is not very successful in dogs.

Consequently, PEP vaccination is recommended following bites even by vaccinated dogs.

Q25. Can all available antirabies vaccines be used by ID route?

Ans: Not all vaccines produced in India are at present fit for ID usage.

The following vaccines have been approved by the Drugs Controller General of India (DCGI) for use by ID route:
- *PCEC (purified chick embryo cell vaccine)*: Rabipur and Vaxirab-N
- *PVRV (purified verocell rabies vaccine)*: Verorab—vial of 0.5 mL
- *PVRV*: Abhayrab—vial of 0.5 mL (Human Biological Institute)
- *PVRV*: Indirab, vial of 0.5 mL/1.0 mL (Bharat Biotech, Hyderabad)
- *PDEV (purified duck embryo vaccine)*: (Vaxirab)
- *HDCV (human diploid cell vaccine)*: (Rabivax) are approved for IM use only and not for intradermal rabies vaccination (IDRV).
- All CCVs (cell culture vaccines) and PDEV should have antigen content greater than 2.5 IU/IM dose, irrespective of whether it is 0.5 mL or 1.0 mL vaccine by volume.

Rabies vaccines with an adjuvant should not be used as IDRV.

Q26. The IM dose of Verorab (PVRV) and Abhayrab (PVRV) is 0.5 mL that of Rabipur (PCEC) and PVRV (Coonoor) is 1 mL. Is the ID dosage of all vaccines uniformly 0.1 mL?

Ans: The ID dosage of all approved vaccines is uniformly 0.1 mL per ID site, irrespective of their IM dosage.

Q27. How long the immunity persists after a course of PEP?

Ans: Individuals who have taken their vaccination almost 5–20 years earlier show a good an amnestic response after booster vaccination even if antibody level is not detectable.

Q28. What if a person comes several days/months/years after the bite?

Ans: He should be managed in a similar manner as a person who has been bitten recently. Even RIG should be given if indicated. Rabies has a long incubation period; therefore, window of opportunity for prevention remains.

Q29. What is the reduced 4-dose schedule for rabies vaccine?

Ans: 1-1-1-1-0 schedule may be used on 0, 3, 7 and 14 days. This schedule should be used only for healthy, fully immune competent person provided they receive proper wound care plus RIG in category 3 as well as in category 2 bite with the WHO-prequalified vaccine.

Q30. If RIG is not available, what should be done?

Ans: Two doses of vaccine may be given on day 0, one on either hand (though it is not a substitute for RIG).

Q31. What is Zagreb schedule?

Ans: It is 2-1-1 regimen where two doses are given on day 0 and one dose each on day 7 and day 21. This schedule is not approved for use in India.

Q32. How the wound is categorized?

Ans:
- *Category 1*: Touching or feeding animal. Animal licks on intact skin. PEP is not recommended.
- *Category 2*: Minor scratches or abrasions without bleeding. Wound management and ARV are recommended.
- *Category 3*: Single or multiple transdermal bites or scratches, licks on broken skin. Contamination of mucous membrane with saliva. Treatment is done by wound management, RIG, and ARV.

Q33. Comment on ID vaccination.

Ans: Only 0.1 mL is used in one dose; therefore it is cost effective.

Only PVRV and PCEV are approved for ID use. They have to be WHO prequalified. It is in use in Thailand, Sri Lanka, and Philippines. The DCGI has recently approved the use of ID vaccine in certain government antirabies centers. The schedule permitted is 2-2-2-0-1-, i.e., two ID doses in both deltoid on 0, 3, and 7 days and one dose on day 30 and day 90. This is Thai Red Cross Regimen. There is another updated Thai Red Cross Regimen of 2-2-2-0-2-0 where two doses are given on day 0, 3, 7, and 30. ID vaccine is not used for immunocompromised patients and those on chloroquine therapy. ID vaccination is not recommended in individual practice.

Q34. How PEP is done in an immunocompromised patient?

Ans: Patients with low CD4 count (<200) show low antibody response to rabies. In such cases, local infiltration of RIG is of utmost importance followed by ARV. RIG is used even in category 2 bite with full postexposure vaccination. If possible antirabies antibody estimation should be done 10 days after completion of vaccination.

Q35. What is the schedule of vaccination in previously vaccinated child?

Ans: Previously vaccinated by PEP or pre-exposure prophylaxis, two doses are given on day 0 and 3, either by IM/ID route. When ID route is used, 0.1 mL is given at single site only with ID-compliant vaccine.

Q36. What is the significance of pre-exposure prophylaxis?

Ans: It eliminates the need for RIG. (It is important because availability of RIG is a problem and further it is costly also.) It also reduces the PEP to two doses only, i.e., on day 0 and 3. The Advisory Committee on Vaccines and Immunization Practices (ACVIP) recommends pre-exposure prophylaxis to all children at high risk of rabies after discussion with parents. Three doses are used on day 0, 7, and 28. Day 21 may be used if time is limited but day 28 is preferred. ID vaccine may be used in same schedule.

Q37. What RIG are available?

Ans: It is important to provide passive immunity till ARV starts working.

Human monoclonal antibody: Rabishield (Sii) is a recombinant human immunoglobulin. It is superior alternative to Human RIG and ERIG. It avoids adverse reactions of blood borne products. Dose: 3.33 IU/kg. Quantity is less and pain is less. Vial 2.5 mL is available. Each vial contains 100 IU (40 units/mL).

Human RIG (HRIG): Dose—20 IU/kg. Maximum dose is 1,500 units. Equine RIG: Dose—40 IU/kg. Maximum dose is 3,000 IU. HRIG is preferred over ERIG. From 8th day onward, RIG is not indicated because an antibody response to vaccine is presumed to have taken place.

Q38. Can a rabies patient make a valid will?

Ans: A rabies patient can make a valid will. According to the Section 59 in the Indian Succession Act, 1925.

Person capable of making will:
- Every person of sound mind not being a minor may dispose of his property by will.
- A married woman may dispose by will of any property which she could alienate by her own act during her life.
- Persons who are deaf or dumb or blind are not thereby incapacitated for making a will if they are able to know what they do by it.
- A person who is ordinarily insane may make a will during interval in which he is of sound mind.
- No person can make a will while he is in such a state of mind, whether arising from intoxication or from illness or from any other cause that he does not know what he is doing.

Q39. Are there any survivors of human rabies?

Ans: Till date only seven survivors have been recorded. These patients survived not due to any specific antirabies therapy but following intensive life support and excellent nursing care. These patients survived for variable periods with residual neurological deficits. All the survivors had paralytic form of rabies and majority had history of some ARV in the past.

Q40. What does humanizing your dog means?

Ans: Talking to your dog like he/she is a person. Treating your dog like he/she is a person. Allowing dogs to do what they want because it will hurt their " feelings." Dressing them up in little doggie clothes. Remember, humanizing your dog is fulfilling your own human needs, not your dogs. Humanizing dogs does more harm than good.

34 Japanese Encephalitis

KP Sarbhai

Q1. What is Japanese encephalitis (JE)?

Ans: Acute inflammatory disease of brain caused by JE virus. JE comes under the umbrella of acute encephalitis syndrome (AES). JE is clinically similar to encephalitis caused by any other pathogen, and is the most important global cause of arboviral encephalitis. More than 50,000 cases and 15,000 deaths reported each year. 1 in 250 result in symptomatic illness. It affects children between 1 and 15 years of age. Incubation period is 5–14 days. Mortality is up to 30% with half of survivors sustain severe neurological sequel. JE virus is primarily zoonotic in its natural cycle. Natural reservoir hosts are animals and birds. Pigs are amplifier host—which allows virus multiplication without suffering from disease and maintain prolonged viremia. Cattle and buffaloes are mosquito attractants. Man is an accidental "dead-end" host. Man-to-man transmission does not occur. Usual age group is below 15 years with no sex predilection. Adults have serological evidence of previous JE infection.

Q2. What are the features of JE?

Ans: *It is same as AES of any etiology*: Acute onset of fever and change in mental status, confusion, disorientation, coma, inability to talk, etc., with or without new onset to seizure".

Q3. What are the other causes of encephalitis?

Ans: More than 100 different viruses can cause acute encephalitis. Seasonal and geographic distribution can help to narrow differential diagnosis. Examples of common viruses are:
- Arbovirus—dengue, JE, etc., enteroviruses, mumps, varicella, herpes simplex virus, influenza, rabies.
- A large number of reported cases of encephalitis are due to an unspecified cause.

Q4. What one feature differentiates meningitis from encephalitis?

Ans: *Encephalitis*: Altered brain function—altered consciousness, confusion, abnormal behavior, focal neurological signs
- *Meningitis*: Normal brain function, though the person is irritated.

Q5. What are the clinical stages of JE?

Ans: *Incubation period*: 6–16 days.

Course of the disease can be divided into three stages:
1. *Prodromal stage*: Acute-onset fever, chills, headache, and malaise.
2. *Acute encephalitic stage*: High fever (38–40.7°C), neck rigidity, photophobia, nausea, vomiting, seizures, and altered sensorium. Variable neurological signs appear (cranial nerve palsies, tremors, ataxia, abnormal reflexes, paralysis, delirium, and ultimately coma).
3. *Late stage and sequelae*: Active inflammation subsides, neurological signs stable.

Sequelae: Parkinsonism, paralysis, and mental retardation.

Case fatality rate: Exceeds 25%.

Q6. What is the principle of treatment?

Ans: Mainly symptomatic and supportive. Therapeutic norms for the supportive therapy are not established. Fluid and electrolyte balance has to be maintained.

Reduction of intracranial pressure is essential. Control of convulsions, if present and maintenance of airway is crucial. Treatment is mainly supportive, intravenous ceftriaxone is usually used, and empirical acyclovir is used occasionally.

The drug minocycline is a semisynthetic tetracycline. Its neuroprotective properties have since been demonstrated in diverse central nervous system insults. In JE, minocycline's neuroprotective action is associated with marked decrease in neuronal death, microgliosis, and production of cytokine and viral titer.

Treatment with minocycline also improves the behavioral outcome following JE.

Q7. How can we protect from JE?

Ans: Mosquito control and pig control have proved unsuccessful. Since *Culex* has a flight range of 20 km, all local control measures will fail. An effective vaccine is, however, available. Human vaccination is the single most important control measure. Safe and effective vaccines are available.

Q8. What is the efficacy of JE vaccine across the world?

Ans: Vaccination programs showed significant reductions in JE cases.

Japan introduced JE vaccine in 1967. Annual number of JE cases decreased from >1,000 cases to 90 in 1991 and <10 after that.

China introduced vaccine in 1970s; cases decreased from >10,000 in 1996 to 2,541 in 2010.

South Korea: Mass vaccination started in 1983; cases reduced to 10/year (100–1,000 before 1983).

Nepal: JE incidence rate decreased significantly following introduction of JE vaccine.

India: NIP in highly affected areas started in 2006.

Q9. What are the types of vaccines available?

Ans: *Mouse brain-derived inactivated vaccine:*
- Vero cell (culture)-derived live vaccine—government supply only
- Vero cell (culture)-derived inactivated vaccines—private use
- *Newer vaccines:* Chimeric vaccine.

Currently available JE vaccines in India are:
- Vero cell-derived inactivated (SA-14-14-2 strain) vaccine (JEEV)
- Live attenuated (SA-14-14-2 strain) vaccine—only through government agencies
- Vero cell-derived inactivated (821564 XY strain) vaccine (JENVAC Q).

Table 1 compares the two JE vaccine brands available in India.

Points to remember:
- Immunization should be complete at least 1 week prior to potential exposure to JE virus.
- Booster dose is recommended for adults >18 to <49 years of age.
- It should be given 12–14 months after primary immunization.
- It is mandatory prior to potential re-exposure to JE virus, laboratory persons, or persons residing in endemic area. Safety and effectiveness has not been established in pregnant and lactating woman, therefore avoided.
- Excretion in human milk is not established.
- Only symptomatic treatment is available.
- High mortality and morbidity.

TABLE 1: Comparison between JENVAC (BB) and JEEV (BE).

Parameter	JEEV	JENVAC
Year of introduction to market	September 2012	October 2013
Description	Inactivated JE vaccine: Biological E Ltd (BE)	Inactivated JE vaccine: BBIL
Viral strain	SA-14-14-2	821564 XY
Strain isolation	SA 14 wild virus from Culex mosquitoes (China) was developed in PHK cells to obtain SA 14-14-2 virus strain	In early 1980 virus was isolated from blood sample of a clinical case of JE infection from Kolar district of Karnataka
Genotype	• Genotype III • SA-14-14-2 strain provides cross protection against all genotypes (I-IV)	Genotype III
Clinical trials	Multiple international trials done by Intercell in nonendemic and endemic countries, Indian trials done by BE and non-inferiorit with Intercell's vaccine established in human trials	Clinical trial data in India
WHO prequalification	Yes-World's first JE vaccine to get WHO prequalification	No
International approvals	The parent vaccine is approved by USFDA, EMA and many other countries	No
Vaccine usage experience	SA 14-14-2-based vaccines used all over the world. Indian government uses live SA 14-14-2 vaccine for mass vaccination	Vaccine used in Indian private market
Dosage	Two doses of 6 mcg for (3 year and above) 4 weeks apart	Only one dose as per the IAP recommendation
Adjuvant	Adsorbed on aluminium hydroxide	Adsorbed on aluminium hydroxide
Other excipients	No preservatives, no gelatin stabilizers	Thiomrsal used as preservative
Minimum age for primary vaccination	3 years in India (as per PI)	1 year in India (as per PI and the IAP)
Shelf life	3 years for 6 µg vial	2 years

(EMA: European Medicines Agency; JE: Japanese encephalitis; IAP: Indian Academy of Pediatrics; PHK: primary hamster kidney; USFDA: United States of America Food and Drug Administration; WHO: World Health Organization)

Q10. What is chimeric vaccine?

Ans: It is a new genetic approach to develop a live attenuated vaccine. Antigen coding sequence of SA14-14-2 of JEV inserted into genome of 17D yellow fever vaccine strain. Resulting recombinant virus is cultivated on vero-cell. It is safe highly immunogenic and capable of inducing long-lasting immunity. A single dose is sufficient to induce protective immunity similar to that produced in adults by three doses of other vaccine. This vaccine is already licensed in Australia. Clinical development of this vaccine in India is on hold because authorization of phase 3 study is taking too long a time.

Q11. Who are the subjects for use of JE vaccine?

Ans: It is not recommended for routine use but only for individuals living in endemic area. It is a disease of rural area with occasional urban case. Government of India has identified 231 districts as endemic. It is also recommended to travellers going to endemic zone if they are expected to stay for a minimum of 4 weeks.

Q12. At what age the vaccine should be used and in what doses?

Ans: *JEEV*: The immunization committee recommends a primary schedule of two doses of 0.25 mL for children between 1 and 3 years of age, and two doses of 0.5 mL for children >3 years, adolescents and adults given IM on day 0 and 28. How long the immunity will persist and whether booster is needs or not is yet to be established. However, the Advisory Committee on Vaccines and Immunization Practices (ACVIP) has recommended a booster dose in adults.

JENVAC: The company has produced data on Indian trials which are satisfactory.

The ACVIP therefore recommends its clinical use. International trials are however lacking. The committee recommends two doses of vaccine 0.5 mL each given IM at 4 weeks' interval for primary immunization for office practice starting from 1 year of age. Seroconversion and seroprotection both show waning; therefore, booster is needed later. Exact timing of booster needs follow-up study.

Q13. How JE campaign is being run in India?

Ans: JE is primarily a disease of rural India but after epidemic in 2005 cases are being reported from both rural and urban areas. Therefore, all target children in rural and urban areas are now vaccinated to have maximum impact of the program. In endemic states of north east, when childhood vaccine campaign was done; there was an outsurge of adult cases. The ACVIP therefore has recommended that in such districts adult immunization (>15 years) should be taken up. It is not an outbreak-response vaccine. The Indian Academy of Pediatrics (IAP) has urged government to include this vaccine in UIP. Chinese vaccine SA14-14-2 has not been proved to be very effective in high-burden states.

35 CHAPTER

Varicella Vaccine

KP Sarbhai

Q1. What is the structure of varicella zoster virus (VZV)?

Ans: It is a human alpha herpes virus. It is an enveloped DNA virus with double-stranded genome. There is very little antigenic variation and no distinct subtypes of the virus.

Q2. Does infection of varicella gives lifelong immunity?

Ans: After a natural infection, individuals generally acquires lifetime immunity. Virus, however, may reactivates years after to cause herpes zoster (shingles).

Q3. What are the possible complications of varicella?

Ans:
- *Cutaneous*: Bacterial infections, bacteremia, toxic shock syndrome
- *Neurologic*: Acute cellular ataxia, encephalitis, Reye's syndrome
- *Pulmonary*: Pneumonitis, varicella pneumonia.

Q4. How varicella vaccine is developed?

Ans: In 1964, severe chickenpox with high fever and widespread rash lasting 3 days, in a member of Dr Michiaki Takahashi's family stimulated interest in the development of a live varicella vaccine. The Oka strain of VZV was first isolated from vesicles of an otherwise healthy 3-year old boy named Oka, with typical varicella, by Takahashi. The virus was passaged 11 times in human embryonic lung fibroblasts at 34°C and 12 times in guinea pig embryo fibroblasts (GPEFs) at 37°C and 7 times additionally in human diploid cells. The passaged virus was used as a candidate varicella vaccine and proved safe and effective for healthy and immunocompromised children. Varicella vaccines, in use today, are all derived from the original Oka strain but the virus contents may vary from one manufacturer to another.

Q5. What is the minimum concentration of virus in vaccine required to be effective antigenically?

Ans: A serological response was seen in all normal children when a dose of >300 PFU was given and *serological* response to all the strains was similar. The results suggest that the immunogenicity of vaccine virus is stable during at least 15 further passages in human diploid cells.

Q6. The three available brands have to pass through how many passages and how many plaque-forming units are there in different brands?

Ans:
- *Wockhardt (Biovac A)*: 46 passages, 2511.8 PFU
- *GSK (Varicella)*: 35 passages, 1995.3 PFU
- *MSD (Variped)*: 31 passages, >1,350 PFU.

Q7. What happens when vaccine is given intramuscularly (IM)?

Ans: Inadvertent intramuscular injection does not lead to a reduction in immunogenicity and seroconversion to any significant extent. However, efficacy data are based on subcutaneous administration. [Vaccines which contain preservatives and stabilizers may cause local pain and swelling so given IM. Varicella is free of them so given subcutaneously (SC).]

Q8. If there is a doubtful history of chicken pox, whether to vaccinate or not?

Ans: Offer vaccine without performing serology. The vaccine is not dangerous if given to people who are already immune to varicella. Boosting effect of vaccine will be there and it will prevent herpes zoster in older people. Vaccine should not be given to immunocompromised (due to risk of severe reaction) pregnant women, (because of unknown risks to fetus).

Q9. How safe is the vaccine?

Ans: Fever or local reactions at the injection site may occur.

Skin rash occurs in about 7% of healthy vaccinee, either at the injection site or more generalized, and may be vesicular. Rashes caused by the vaccine appear approximately

3 weeks after immunization but may occur up to 6 weeks after vaccination. There is a small potential to transmit the vaccine virus at this time, mainly from direct contact with vesicles at the injection site. Vaccinated individuals do not transmit the vaccine virus by the respiratory route. Papules at the injection site are rarely infectious. Vesicular rash following immunization, can spread the infection. The rash should be covered with clothes if possible. Careful hand washing should be encouraged. The vaccinee should avoid contact with immunocompromised, pregnant women, and should be excluded from school.

Q10. When is the vaccine contraindicated?

Ans: Allergy to vaccine and its constituents:
- *Malignant conditions*:
  - Family history of hereditary immunodeficiency
  - On systemic immunosuppressive therapy
- *Pregnant woman*: If a nonpregnant woman is vaccinated, she should avoid becoming pregnant for 1 month. If a pregnant woman is vaccinated, she should be counseled about potential effects on fetus.

Q11. Can a child with immune thrombocytopenic purpura (ITP) be given varicella vaccine?

Ans: Cases of thrombocytopenia have been reported after measles, mumps, and rubella (MMR) and varicella vaccination. But it is not a contraindication for receiving varicella vaccine.

Q12. Can varicella vaccine be given with other vaccines?

Ans: Varicella zoster virus vaccine can be safely administered at the same time as other vaccines. Although, if it is not given simultaneously, it should be given at least 4 weeks before or after other live vaccines.

Q13. What are primary and secondary vaccine failures?

Ans: Failure to mount protective immune response after a dose of vaccine is primary vaccine failure. (Insufficient number of T memory cells is generated after 1 dose of vaccine.) Gradual loss of immunity after an initial immune response over a period of years after vaccination is secondary vaccine failure or (waning immunity). (Priming has taken place after single dose of vaccine, but initial stimulus was not sufficient for complete protection.)

Q14. Explain whether breakthrough varicella occurs due to primary or secondary vaccine failure.

Ans: Vesicular rash developing 42 days after vaccination is known as breakthrough varicella. Usually it occurs between 2 and 4 years after vaccination. It is controversial. Both primary and secondary failures may lead to breakthrough varicella. Successful primary vaccination gives vaccine effectiveness of 85% which is not enough to prevent breakthrough. More is the time lapsed after vaccination, more are the chances of breakthrough and more is the severity. This suggests that waning immunity with time makes individual susceptible. Second dose of vaccine gives 10-fold boosts to immunity. Give second dose of vaccine after 3 months to cover both *primary/secondary vaccine failure*.

(If second dose is administered 28 days after first dose, second dose is considered valid and does not need repetition.)

Q15. How contagious is breakthrough varicella?

Ans: Breakthrough varicella with <50 lesions are only one third as contagious as unvaccinated person with varicella. Breakthrough varicella with >50 lesions are as contagious as unvaccinated person with varicella.

Q16. Can increasing the virus content of vaccine reduce the risk of breakthrough?

Ans: No, as the quantity of antigen increases, a plateau effect comes about where maximum immune response is achieved and it cannot be made any stronger.

Q17. Can we have breakthrough varicella after two doses of vaccine?

Ans: Quite possible theoretically. Waning immunity is an issue. Immunity may wane over a period of time after second dose as well. Sustained surveillance is mandatory.

Q18. What is the drug interaction of varicella vaccine?

Ans: If a child has undergone blood or plasma transfusion, or immunoglobulin (Ig) or varicella zoster immunoglobulin (VZIG) has been administered, then vaccine should be deferred for at least 5 months. If varicella vaccine has been given, then any Ig/transfusion/VZIG should not be given for 2 months. If either of it has to be given by compulsion, we should repeat the dose of vaccine after a gap of 5 months. Vaccine recipient should avoid the use of salicylates for 6 weeks as Rey syndrome has been reported following salicylates during wild-type varicella infection.

Q19. How effective is the vaccine?

Ans: Overall efficacy of single dose is 85%. Vaccine efficacy against moderate or severe disease is 97%. Immunized children will almost always develop only mild disease. Children immunized >4 years before are at increased risk of breakthrough varicella disease, although they always have mild disease. Despite having mild disease, children with breakthrough disease are contagious and should be subjected to the same school exclusion criteria used for other cases of chickenpox.

Q20. Can the vaccine be used for postexposure prophylaxis?

Ans: The vaccine is preventive if given within 3 days of exposure (90% efficacy). If given up to 5 days after exposure (70% efficacy). Postexposure vaccination is effective in stopping varicella outbreaks. If not effective in preventing the disease, postexposure vaccine may lead to milder disease in vaccine. Postexposure prophylaxis is important.

Q21. How long does vaccine-induced protection last?

Ans: Vaccine is protective for at least 10 years (the proportion of protected people may decline gradually after the first few years). Duration of effectiveness has been studied in an environment where natural boosting of immunity with wild VZV is common. Significant boosting of the varicella immune response has been reported after second injections given 4–6 years after the initial immunization. Recent recommendation is to give booster after 3 months. Booster dose is essential.

Q22. Is there an increased risk of disease in older age groups?

Ans: Proportion of cases in older age is increasing as more children are immunized. Old-age group persons are at greater risk for more severe disease. The overall rates of disease in adults will increase because of waning protection from immunization and reduced boosting from exposure to circulating VZV. The risk increases with old age.

Q23. What is the future risk of herpes zoster after vaccination?

Ans: Immunological boosting from circulating VZV may protect adults from developing shingles. This boosting will not occur as the proportion of children being vaccinated increases, resulting in a short-to-medium-term increase in cases of herpes zoster in adults. Further surveillance will be required. There appears to be a reduced incidence of herpes zoster among immunized people, although the long-term risk is not yet known. Increased immunization coverage has increased the risk of herpes zoster in adults.

Q24. How to protect a newborn who is exposed to a case of varicella?

Ans: Full-term healthy newborn is not at increased risk of complications and thus does not need prophylaxis with VZIG/intravenous (IV) Ig. All premature neonates of <28 weeks gestation/birthweight <1,000 g should be given VZIG. All preterm neonates >28 weeks' gestation should be given VZIG only if mother is –ve for antivaricella IgG.

Q25. What is the risk to newborn of a mother having chicken pox at time of delivery?

Ans: Rash 5 days before or 2 days after delivery is associated with high mortality in newborn. VZIG 125 units/kg IM should be given as soon as possible after delivery. Acyclovir 60 mg/kg in three divided doses is recommended.

Q26. What are the indications for use of VZIG?

Ans: Postexposure prophylaxis in susceptible individuals with significant contact Susceptible:
- All unvaccinated children with no history of Chicken pox.
- All unvaccinated adults who are seronegative for antivaricella IgG.
- Bone marrow transplant (BMT) recipients even if they have received vaccine before BMT.

Significant contact: Any face-to-face contact. Staying in the same room for a period >1 hour with a patient of infectious chicken pox/herpes zoster. (2 days before the rash till all lesions have crusted).

Q27. How late can VZIG be administered to a patient?

Ans: One should be given vaccine as soon as possible but not later than 96 hours following exposure. Protection lasts for 3 weeks and vaccine reduces the risk of disease and complication. VZIG (Varitect) is for intravenous (IV) use at a dose of 0.2–1 mL/kg diluted in normal saline given over 1 hour. Efficacy against death in neonatal exposure case is 100%. VZIG prolongs incubation period, so all exposed should be monitored for 28 weeks for disease manifestation.

Q28. How should the vaccine be stored?

Ans: Vaccines come in lyophilized preparations which require protection from light and should be stored at 2–80°C (or frozen). Varilrix can be stored for up to 2 years, and Varivax refrigerated for up to 18 months from the date of manufacture. The diluents for each vaccine should not be frozen; they can be stored in the refrigerator or at ambient temperatures. Both vaccines should be used promptly after reconstitution: within 90 minutes for Varilrix or within 30 minutes for Varivax. Variped can be stored for 2 years and after reconstitution, it can be used within 30 minutes.

Q29. Who should have the vaccine apart from the children?

Ans:
- Susceptible adults at high risk of exposure, e.g., healthcare workers, women prior to pregnancy, parents of young children, childcare workers, and teachers should be vaccinated.
- All susceptible household contacts of immunosuppressed people should be given priority.
- In general all healthy susceptible people over 12 months of age can be offered the vaccine.

Q30. Can a child on metered dose inhaler (MDI) steroid for asthma since past 6 months receive varicella vaccine?

Ans: Child on inhaled steroid can receive vaccine.

If the child is on systemic steroid and is not otherwise immunocompromised can be vaccinated if they are receiving <2 mg/kg or total of <20 mg/day of prednisolone or its equivalent. If the child is on steroid >2 mg/kg for >2 weeks. Vaccinate, once the steroid has been discontinued for at least 1 month.

Q31. Can a postpartum lactating woman who is seronegative be given varicella vaccine?

Ans: If woman is not immune, vaccination should not be delayed. After vaccination, lady can continue to breastfeed the baby. Virus of live vaccines is not secreted in breast milk. Single-antigen varicella vaccine may be administered to nursing mother.

Q32. Can a child with HIV/AIDS receive the vaccine?

Ans: Screening for HIV infection is not indicated before routine varicella immunization. Vaccine is contraindicated in clinically manifest HIV. The potential risks and benefits should be weighed, only then the vaccination should be considered for HIV-infected children in CDC class 1 with CDC T-lymphocyte percentage of 15%. HIV-infected children should receive two doses of single-antigen vaccine separated by 3 months. They should report to doctor if postvaccination varicella such as rash is seen. Immunogenicity may be lower in HIV-infected adolescents and adults. If inadvertent vaccination of HIV-infected person results in clinical disease, then acyclovir should be used to modify the disease.

Q33. How contagious is the varicella vaccine?

Ans: Transmission of vaccine virus from vaccinee to contacts is rare; therefore, no herd effect is observed with vaccine. Vaccine-related rash is contagious to contacts; therefore, immunocompromised person should avoid contact with vaccine-related rash.

Q34. Should healthy household contacts of immunocompromised be vaccinated?

Ans: The Indian Academy of Pediatrics Committee on Immunization (IAPCOI), Advisory Committee on Immunization Practices (ACIP), and American Academy of Pediatrics (AAP) recommend immunization of healthy contacts. This is most effective way to protect immunocompromised person from exposure to wild-type varicella. Vaccinee should avoid contact with immunocompromised person while the rash is present. If immunocompromised person is inadvertently exposed to vaccine-related rash, then VZIG is not needed because disease associated with this type of transmission is mild.

Q35. What should be the interval between administration of VZIG and varicella vaccine?

Ans: Varicella vaccine should be delayed by 5 months after administration of VZIG if giving vaccine is not contraindicated. Varicella vaccine is not needed if patient has varicella after VZIG administration.

Q36. What is IAPCOI recommendation on varicella vaccine?

Ans:
- Vaccinate all healthy children with no prior history of varicella.
- Children with humoral immunodeficiencies.
- Children with HIV but with CD4 count 15% and above age-related cutoff.
- Leukemia in remission and off chemotherapy for at least 3–6 months.
- Children on long-term salicylates but to be avoided for 6 weeks after vaccination. If on low-dose steroid/alternate-day steroid, vaccinate any time. If on steroid (2 mg/kg) for 2 weeks or more, stop for 4 weeks then vaccinate.
- Household contacts of immunocompromised children.
- Unvaccinated adolescents going to boarding for studies.
- Children with chronic lung or heart disease.
- Adults working as healthcare professionals, school teachers, and military personnel.
- Postexposure prophylaxis within 3 days (90% efficacy), up to 5 days of exposure (70% efficacy). In both cases, efficacy is 100% against severe disease.

36 CHAPTER

Meningococcal Vaccine

KP Sarbhai

Q1. What is the rationale of using meningococcal vaccine?

Ans: Invasive meningococcal disease is potentially fatal. It is rapidly progressive, leaving little time for diagnosis and treatment. Much of invasive meningococcal disease is vaccine-preventable. *Haemophilus influenzae* type b (Hib) and *Streptococcus pneumoniae* are already preventable by conjugate vaccines. Conjugate meningococcal vaccine is available in India and the disease is preventable.

Q2. What are the types of vaccines available?

Ans:

- *Polysaccharide vaccines*:
  - Bivalent (containing A and C serogroups)
  - Quadrivalent [(A/C/W-135/Y), contains 50 µg of each polysaccharide].
- *Conjugated vaccines*: Quadrivalent (A/C/W-135/Y), first licensed in US in 2005 and India in 2012, and now in 27 countries. 4 µg each of polysaccharide is conjugated to 48 µg of diphtheria toxoid. Two doses are recommended in children between 9 and 23 months of age. Apart from minor local side effects, vaccine can occasionally produce Guillain–Barré syndrome (GBS). It is advised not to use this vaccine in those who have already been diagnosed GBS previously unless they are at a very high risk of contracting meningococcal infection. Interference in immune response is noted if it is given with PCV13. Therefore, two vaccines are not given simultaneously on the same day. A gap of 1 month should be there and PCV13 should be given first. In an Indian trial, vaccine has been found to be well tolerated and robust immune response is found in 97–100% subjects.
- *Monovalent serogroup A conjugate vaccine*: It is a lyophilized vaccine which has 10 µg of group A polysaccharide conjugated to tetanus toxoid with alum as adjuvant and thiomerosal as preservative. This vaccine is manufactured by SII and is very cheap. It is licensed in India since 2009 but marketed only in African countries. It is given between 1 and 29 years of age. Need of booster is not established. Vaccine has shown excellent immunogenicity and tolerability in African campaigns. Conjugate vaccines have shown good memory response and herd immunity.

Q3. What is the advantage of conjugate vaccine over polysaccharide?

Ans: Meningococcal conjugate vaccines have several advantages over polysaccharide vaccines. It has ability to induce greater antibody persistence, greater avidity, better immunologic memory and strong herd immunity. Immunity induced by conjugate vaccine provides persistence of immunity and a very good anamnestic response. It also reduces nasopharyngeal carriage of the organism.

Q4. What conjugate vaccine brands are available in India?

Ans: Menactra (Sanofi Pasteur) is indicated for active immunization to prevent invasive meningococcal disease caused by *Neisseria meningitidis* serogroups A, C, Y, and W-135 in 2–55 years of age. Approved for use in individuals 9 months through 55 years of age in US, Argentina, Philippines, and Guatemala.

Menveo (GSK) is also quadrivalent. One dose consists of one vial of Men A which is lyophilized conjugate component to be reconstituted with one vial of Men CWY liquid conjugate component. The two are mixed and product is used immediately.

Q5. What is the Advisory Committee on Immunization Practices (ACIP) recommendation for use of meningococcal vaccine?

Ans: With current burden of disease in India, routine use of vaccine is not recommended. It should be given in high-risk conditions only. Always prefer conjugated meningococcal vaccine if available. High-risk conditions are as follows:

- Persons aged 2 through 55 years with persistent complement component deficiency or asplenia.

- Persons aged 2 through 55 years with prolonged increased risk for exposure.
- Microbiologists routinely working with *N. meningitidis*.
- Travelers to or residents of countries where meningococcal disease is hyperendemic or epidemic.
- Persons with HIV infection where two doses are used at 8 weeks' interval.
- During disease outbreaks, if caused by serogroups included in the vaccine, vaccine should be used to every susceptible.
- Travelers to Saudi Arabia (for Haj) and Africa.
- Students going abroad for higher studies.
- Adjunct to chemotherapy in close contacts.
- Healthcare workers in contact with secretions, household contacts, day care contacts.
- Considering seriousness of invasive meningococcal disease, vaccine should be at least offered to all for individual protection.

The ACIP recommended use of MCV-4 for 9–23 months in 2011.

Q6. Which is the peak season for meningococcal infection?

Ans: It is a dry season from November to March. Cases reduce with monsoon and increase again in November. Outbreak occurs when season is dry and temperature is low. During dry period, there is damage to natural mucosal barrier of nasopharynx, this increases chance of invasion of infecting organism. Most epidemics in India do occur in northern parts of country rather than humid southern part.

SECTION 5: Infectious Diseases

37. Diphtheria
38. Tetanus
39. Pertussis
40. Enteric Fever
41. Measles
42. Mumps
43. Rubella
44. Varicella and Herpes Zoster
45. Leptospirosis
46. TORCH Infections
47. Rickettsial Diseases
48. Malaria
49. Tuberculosis
50. Leprosy
51. Dengue
52. Re-emerging Infections in Pediatrics
53. COVID-19

Diphtheria

SBP Singh

INTRODUCTION

Diphtheria is an acute infectious disease caused by the bacillus *Corynebacterium diphtheriae*, gram-positive bacteria, and is characterized by a primary lesion, usually in the upper respiratory tract, and more generalized symptoms resulting from the spread of the bacterial toxin throughout the body.

Medical reports of a deadly "strangulation" disease first appeared in the early 1600s, emerging as a greater threat with the growth of cities and easier person-to-person spread. The disease was not given its official name diphtérite until 1826; diphtérite was derived from the Greek word for "leather" or "hide," which describes the distinctive coating that appears in the throat of its victims.

The diphtheria bacillus was discovered and identified by German bacteriologists Edwin Klebs and Friedrich Löffler.

ETIOLOGY

Corynebacteria are aerobic, nonencapsulated, nonspore forming, mostly nonmotile, pleomorphic, gram-positive bacilli. *C. diphtheriae* is by far the most frequently isolated agent of diphtheria.

EPIDEMIOLOGY

Corynebacterium diphtheriae is an exclusive inhabitant of human mucous membranes and skin.

Spread is primarily by airborne respiratory droplets, direct contact with respiratory secretions of symptomatic individuals or exudate from infected skin lesions. Asymptomatic respiratory tract carriage is important in transmission. In area where diphtheria is endemic, 3-5% of healthy individuals can carry toxigenic organisms but carriage is exceedingly rare. Skin infection and skin carriage are silent reservoirs of *C. diphtheria* and organisms can remain viable in dust or on fomites for up to 6 months. Transmission through contaminated milk and through in infected food handler has been proved or suspected.

PATHOGENESIS

- Both toxigenic and nontoxigenic *C. diphtheria* cause skin and mucosal infection.
- The organism usually remains in the superficial layers of skin lesions or respiratory tract mucosa, inducing local inflammatory reaction. The major virulence of the organism lies in its ability to produce a potent polypeptide exotoxin, which inhibits protein synthesis and causes local tissue necrosis and resultant local inflammatory response.
- Within the first few days of respiratory tract infection (usually in the pharynx), a dense necrotic coagulum of organisms, epithelial cells, fibrin, leukocytes and erythrocytes forms, initially white and advancing to become a gray brown, leather-like adherent pseudomembrane.
- Removal is difficult and reveals a bleeding edematous submucosa, paralysis of the palate and hypopharynx is an early local effect of diphtheria toxin.
- Toxin absorption can lead to systemic manifestations, kidney tubule necrosis thrombocytopenia, cardiomyopathy, and demyelination of nerves.

CLINICAL FEATURES

- The clinical features of diphtheria depends on immunization status and the site of infection. The incubation period is 1-6 days.
- *Classification* depends on the site of infection nasal, pharyngeal, tonsillar, laryngeal, skin, eye, and genitalia.
- *Nasal diphtheria* presents like common cold, with thin watery secretion becoming serosanguinous and later mucopurulent fowl smelling discharge. Unilateral nasal discharge is pathognomonic. There is minimal systemic symptoms and is considered a mild illness.
- *Tonsillopharyngeal diphtheria* starts with constitutional symptoms of malaise, low-grade fever. A white-gray membrane appears after 1 or 2 days, over tonsils, pharyngeal wall, uvula, and soft palate; the membrane bleeds on removal. The cervical lymph nodes are enlarged may lead to brawny edema around, giving rise to "bull-neck appearance."

- The severity of presentation depends on amount of toxin released in the circulation. In severe case, circulatory and respiratory collapse is there. The heart is affected first, often in the second or third week. Disproportionate tachycardia when compared to body temperature. The patient develops toxic myocarditis which can be fatal.
- *Laryngeal involvement* is usually seen as spread from the surrounding such as from pharynx. It present with progressive stridor, barking cough, and hoarseness.
- *Neurological complication*: Paralysis of the palate and some eye muscles develops in around the third week; this is usually transient and not severe. In severe cases stupor, coma, and death may occur.
- Cutaneous diphtheria is caused by *C. ulcerans* from travel to tropical countries or animal contact has been increasingly reported. Classic cutaneous diphtheria is an indolent, nonprogressive infection characterized by a superficial, ecthyma-like, nonhealing ulcer with a grey-brown membrane.

DIAGNOSIS

Laboratory Criteria
- Isolation of *C. diphtheriae* from a Gram stain or throat culture from a clinicalspecimen.
- Histopathologic diagnosis of diphtheria by Albert's stain.
- Elek test takes 48 hours for the result. Modified Elek test gives result in 16–24 hours.
- Rapid enzyme immunoassay test detects the toxin in 3 hours.
- PCR-specific for portion of diphtheria toxin A and B toxic gene "toxin" is sensitive.

Clinical Criteria
- Upper respiratory tract illness with sore throat.
- Low-grade fever, above 39°C.
- An adherent, dense, gray pseudomembrane covering the posterior aspect of the pharynx.

Case classification:
- *Probable*: A clinically compatible case that is not laboratory-confirmed and is not epidemiologically linked to a laboratory-confirmed case.
- *Confirmed*: A clinically compatible case that is either laboratory-confirmed or epidemiologically linked to a laboratory-confirmed case.

COMPLICATIONS

Cardiac
The first evidence of cardiac toxicity characteristically occurs during the 2nd and 3rd weeks of illness as the pharyngeal disease improves but can appear acutely as early as the 1st week of illness, a poor prognostic sign or insidiously as late as the 6th week. Tachycardia disproportionate to fever is common and may be evidence of cardiac toxicity or autonomic nervous system dysfunction.

Neurological
Neurologic complications parallel the severity of primary infection and are multiphasic in onset. Acutely or 2–3 weeks after onset of oropharyngeal inflammation, hypesthesia, and local paralysis of the soft palate typically occur. Weakness of the posterior pharyngeal, laryngeal, and facial nerves may follow, causing a nasal quality in the voice, difficulty in swallowing and risk for aspiration. Cranial neuropathies characteristically occur in the 5th week leading to oculomotor paralysis. Careful monitoring for diaphragmatic muscle palsy should be done.

TREATMENT

Antidiphtheria Serum (Table 1)
Antidiphtheria serum (ADS) is the mainstay of therapy and should be administered on the basis of clinical diagnosis. Empirical treatment should generally be started in a patient in whom suspicion of diphtheria is high, because it neutralizes only free toxin, antitoxin efficacy diminishes with elapsed time after the onset of mucocutaneous symptoms. Antitoxin is administered as a single dose. Skin testing must be performed before administration of antitoxin. Antitoxin is not recommended for asymptomatic carriers.

TABLE 1: Dose schedule of antidiphtheria serum (ADS) adminstration.

Type of diphtheria	Dose of ADS (units)	Route of administration
Pharyngeal/laryngeal (P/L)	20,000–40,000	Slow IV (can be given IM)
Nasopharyngeal	40,000–60,000	Slow IV (can be given IM)
Severe category of P/L diphtheria	80,000–120,000	Slow IV (can be given IM)
Cutaneous	20,000–40,000	Slow IV (can be given IM)

Sensitivity test: 0.02 mL of a 1:1,000 dilution ADS to be injected intradermally. A wheal of 3 mm after 15–20 minutes is considered sensitive; it should be larger than negative control reaction to isotonic saline. The desensitization of erythema should be done in decreasing dilution order after every 15 minutes.

(IV: intravenous; IM: intramuscular)

TABLE 2: Antibiotics doses, route and duration.

Antibiotic	Dose and frequency	Route	Duration
Aqueous penicillin	100,000–150,000 units/kg/6 hourly	Intravenous	14 days
Procaine penicillin	25,000–50,000 units/kg/d/12 hourly (maximum—1.2 million units)	Intramuscular	To be continued till the patient takes oral penicillin tablets
Erythromycin	40–50 mg/kg/day/6 hourly (maximum 2 g/day)	Orally	14 days

Antibiotics

The antibiotics doses for diphtheria and its route and duration are given in **Table 2**.

Practical Tips

- The drugs amoxicillin, rifampicin, and clindamycin can also be used.
- After 2 weeks of antibiotics, throat culture must be done. If it is positive, give erythromycin for 10 days in same dose.
- Culture test is advised after 2 weeks of antibiotic therapy. If culture is positive a single dose of Benzathine penicillin 600,000 units in children < 30 kg weight, and 12,00,000 units in children > 30 kg weight is given.
- Repeat culture after 2 weeks, at least two to three culture reports should be negative, taken at an interval of 24 hours. If positive, repeat the antibiotic dose again.
- Asymptomatic carrier can be detected by contact surveillance.

PROGNOSIS

- The prognosis for patients with diphtheria depends on the virulence of the organism, patient age, immunization status, site of infection, and speed of administration of the antitoxin.
- The mortality rate is 1% if the treatment has started in first 24 hours, mortality raises to 20% if the treatment has started after 4–5 days.
- The case fatality rate of almost 10% for respiratory tract diphtheria has not changed in 50 years.
- At recovery, administration of diphtheria toxoid is indicated, complete the primary series or booster doses of immunization because not all patients develop antibodies to diphtheria toxin after infection.

PREVENTION

Protection against serious disease caused by imported or indigenously acquired C diphtheria depends on immunization.

Vaccine

Universal immunization with diphtheria toxoid is an ideal way of protection for this infection. (Refer to chapter of DPT vaccine). Remember the ICVAP guidelines.

SUGGESTED READING

1. Textbook of Pediatric Infectious Disease: 2nd Edition; 2019.

PRESCRIPTION ASSISTANCE

Pharmacological salt	Market preparation	Availability	Dosage
Diphtheria antitoxin (enzyme-refined equine globulin solution)	Diphtheria antitoxin	Equine globulin solution 10,000	
Aqueous penicillin	Benzyl penicillin G 500,000 unit	• IU packing: 10 mL vial × 10 • 500,000 units • Injection	100,000–150,000 units/kg/6 hourly IV
Penicillin G Crystalline, Procaine penicillin, Benzyl penicillin	Penicillin G Procaine 600,000	• 600,000 units • 1200,000 units	• IM (AST) • Deep IM (Injection after sensitivity test)
Penicillin + Procaine (a local anesthetic) Benzathine penicillin	1200,000 units Penidure LA	• 600,000 units • 1200,000 units	• <30 kg–6 lac units • >30 kg–12 lac units Deep IM (Injection after sensitivity test)

CHAPTER 38

Tetanus

SBP Singh

INTRODUCTION

Tetanus, also known as lockjaw, is an acute spastic paralytic illness caused by neurotoxin produced by *Clostridium tetani*. Unlike other pathogenic clostridia species, *C. tetani* is not a tissue-invasive organism and instead causes illness through the toxin, tetanospasmin, more commonly referred to as tetanus toxin.

Tetanospasmin is the second most poisonous substance known. *C. tetani* is a motile gram-positive, spore-forming, obligate, anaerobe.

The organism's natural habitat worldwide is soil, dust, and the alimentary tracts of various animals. *C. tetani* forms spores terminally with a classic morphologic appearance resembling a drumstick or tennis racket microscopically. In the most common type, the spasms begin in the jaw and then progress to the rest of the body. Each spasm usually lasts a few minutes. Spasms occur frequently for 3–4 weeks. Some spasms may be severe enough to fracture bones.

Other symptoms of tetanus may include fever, sweating, headache, trouble swallowing, high blood pressure, and a fast heart rate. Onset of symptoms is typically 3–21 days following infection. Recovery may take months. About 10% of cases prove fatal.

Tetanus
- *Other names*: Lockjaw
- Muscle spasms (specifically opisthotonos) in a person with tetanus.
- *Symptoms*: Muscle spasms fever, headache
- *Usual onset*: 3–21 days following exposure
- *Duration*: Months
- *Cause*: C. tetani
- *Risk factors*: Break in the skin
- *Diagnostic method*: Based on symptoms
- *Prevention*: Tetanus vaccine
- *Treatment*: Tetanus immunoglobulin, muscle relaxants, mechanical ventilation
- *Prognosis*: 10% risk of death
- *Frequency*: 209,000 (2015)
- *Deaths*: 56,700 (2015).

Tetanus is caused by an infection with the bacterium *C. tetani*, which is commonly found in soil, saliva, dust, and manure. The bacteria generally enter through a break in the skin such as a cut or puncture wound by a contaminated object. They produce toxins that interfere with normal muscle contractions. Diagnosis is based on the presenting signs and symptoms. The disease does not spread between people.

Tetanus can be prevented by immunization with the tetanus vaccine. In those who have a significant wound and have had fewer than three doses of the vaccine, both vaccination and tetanus immunoglobulin are recommended. The wound should be cleaned and any dead tissue should be removed. In those who are infected, tetanus immunoglobulin, or, if unavailable, intravenous immunoglobulin (IVIg) is used. Muscle relaxants may be used to control spasms. Mechanical ventilation may be required if a person's breathing is affected.

Tetanus occurs in all parts of the world but is most frequent in hot and wet climates where the soil contains a lot of organic matter. In 2015, there were about 209,000 infections and about 59,000 deaths globally. This is down from 356,000 deaths in 1990. In the US, there are about 30 cases per year, almost all of which have not been vaccinated. A nearly description of the disease was made by Hippocrates in the 5th century BC. The cause of the disease was determined in 1884 by Antonio Carle and Giorgio Rattone at the University of Turin, and a vaccine was developed in 1924.

HISTORY

The word tetanus comes from the Ancient Greek: tetavoc, Romanized: tetanus, lit, "taut," which is further from the Ancient Greek: teiveiv, romanized: teinein, lit "to stretch."

Tetanus was well known to ancient people who recognized the relationship between wounds and fatal muscle spasms. In 1884, Arthur Nicolaier isolated the strychnine-like toxin of tetanus from free-living, anaerobic soil bacteria. The etiology of the disease was further elucidated in 1884 by Antonio Carle and Giorgio Rattone, the two pathologists of the University of Turin, who demonstrated the transmissibility of tetanus for the first time. They produced tetanus in rabbits by injecting pus from a person with fatal tetanus into their sciatic nerves. In 1891, *C. tetani* was isolated from a human victim by Kitasato Shibasaburō, who later showed that the organism could produce disease when injected into animals, and that the toxin could be neutralized by specific antibodies.

In 1897, Edmond Nocard showed that tetanus antitoxin induced passive immunity in humans, and could be used for prophylaxis and treatment.

Tetanus toxoid vaccine was developed by P Descombey in 1924, and was widely used to prevent tetanus induced by battle wounds during World War II.

EPIDEMIOLOGY

Tetanus occurs worldwide and is endemic in many developing countries although its incidence varies considerably. Approximately 57,000 deaths were caused by tetanus globally in 2015.

Of these, approximately 20,000 deaths occurred in neonates and 37,000 in older children and adults. It is seen that most of the mortality due to neonatal tetanus occurs in South Asia by maternal tetanus, which results from postpartum or postabortal. In the United States, mortality from neonatal tetanus has declined >95% since 1947. A total of 197 cases and 16 deaths from tetanus were reported in the United States. The majority of US childhood cases of tetanus have occurred in unimmunized children whose parents objected to vaccination.

Most nonneonatal cases of tetanus are associated with a traumatic injury, often a penetrating wound inflicted by a dirty object such as a nail, splinter fragment of glass or unsterile injection. Tetanus may also occur in the setting of illicit drug injection. The disease has been associated with the use of contaminated suture material and after intramuscular injection of medicine most note by quinine for chloroquine-resistant falciparum malaria. The disease may also occur in association with animal bites, abscesses, ear and other body piercing, chronic skin ulceration, burns, compound fractures and frostbite.

Incubation period: The incubation period of tetanus may be up to several months, but is usually about 10 days. In general, the farther the injury site is from the central nervous system, the longer the incubation period. The shorter the incubation period, the more severe are the symptoms. In neonatal tetanus, symptoms usually appear from 4 to 14 days after birth, averaging about 7 days.

CLINICAL MANIFESTATIONS

Tetanus is the most often generalized but may also be localized. In generalized tetanus, the presenting symptom in about half of cases is trismus (masseter muscle spasm or lockjaw).

Headache, restlessness, and irritability are early symptoms, often followed by stiffness, difficulty chewing, dysphagia, and neck muscle spasm. The so-called sardonicus smile of tetanus results from intractable spasm of facial and buccal muscles.

When the paralysis extends to abdominal, lumbar, hip, and thigh muscles, the patient may assume an arched posture of extreme hyperextension of the body or opisthotonos.

Laryngeal and respiratory muscle spasm can lead to airway obstruction and asphyxiation.

Because tetanus toxin does not affect sensory nerves or cortical function, the patient unfortunately remains conscious in extreme pain and in fearful anticipation of the next tetanus seizure. The seizures are characterized by sudden severe tonic contractions of the muscle with fist clenching, flexion and adduction of the arms and hyperextension of the legs. Without treatment, the duration of these seizures may range from a few seconds to a few minutes in length with intervening respire periods. As the illness progresses, the spasms become sustained and exhausting. The smallest disturbance by sight, sound, or touch may trigger a titanic spasm. Dysuria and urinary retention result from bladder sphincter spasm; forced defecation may occur. Fever occasionally as high as 40°C is common and is caused by the substantial metabolic energy consumed by spastic muscles. Notable autonomic effects include tachycardia, dysrhythmias, table hypertension, diaphoresis and cutaneous vasoconstriction. The titanic paralysis usually becomes more severe in the first week after onset, stabilizes in the second week and ameliorates gradually over the ensuing 1-4 weeks.

SIGNS AND SYMPTOMS

Tetanus often begins with mild spasms in the jaw muscles—also known as lockjaw or trismus.

The spasms can also affect the facial muscles resulting in an appearance called risus sardonicus.

Chest, neck, back, abdominal muscles, and buttocks may be affected. Back muscle spasms often cause arching, called opisthotonos. Sometimes the spasms affect muscles that help with breathing, which can lead to breathing problems.

Prolonged muscular action causes sudden, powerful, and painful contractions of muscle groups, which is called "tetany." These episodes can cause fractures and muscle tears.

Other symptoms include fever, headache, restlessness, irritability, feeding difficulties, breathing problems, burning sensation during urination, urinary retention, and loss of stool control. The mortality rate is higher in unvaccinated people and people over 60 years of age.

Generalized Tetanus

Generalized tetanus is the most common type of tetanus, representing about 80% of cases. The generalized form usually presents with a descending pattern. The first sign is trismus, or lockjaw, and the facial spasms called risus sardonicus, followed by stiffness of the neck, difficulty in swallowing, and rigidity of pectoral and calf muscles. Other symptoms include elevated temperature, sweating, elevated blood pressure, and episodic rapid heart rate.

Spasms may occur frequently and last for several minutes with the body shaped into a characteristic form called opisthotonos. Spasms continue for up to 4 weeks, and complete recovery may take months.

Neonatal Tetanus

The infantile form of generalized tetanus, typically manifests within 3-12 days of birth. It presents as progressive difficulty in feeding, associated hunger and crying. Paralysis or diminished movement, stiffness and rigidity to the touch, and spasms with or without opisthotonos are characteristic.

The umbilical stump, which is typically the portal of entry for the microorganism, may retain remnants of dirt during clotted blood or serum, or it may appear relatively benign.

Local Tetanus

Local tetanus is an uncommon form of the disease, in which people have persistent contraction of muscles in the same anatomic area as the injury. The contractions may persist for many weeks before gradually subsiding. Local tetanus is generally milder; only about 1% of cases are fatal, but it may precede the onset of generalized tetanus.

Cephalic Tetanus

Cephalic tetanus is the rarest form of the disease (0.9-3% of cases) and is limited to muscles and nerves in the head. It usually occurs after trauma to the head area, including skull fracture, laceration, eye injury, dental extraction, and otitis media, but it has been observed from injuries to other parts of the body. Paralysis of the facial nerve is most frequently implicated, which may cause lockjaw, facial palsy, or ptosis, but other cranial nerves can also be affected. Cephalic tetanus may progress to a more generalized form of the disease.

DIAGNOSIS

There are currently no blood tests for diagnosing tetanus. The diagnosis is based on the presentation of tetanus symptoms and does not depend upon isolation of the bacterium, which is recovered from the wound in only 30% of cases and can be isolated from people without tetanus.

Laboratory identification of *C. tetani* can be demonstrated only by production of tetanospasmin in mice.

The "spatula test" is a clinical test for tetanus that involves touching the posterior pharyngeal wall with a soft-tipped instrument and observing the effect. A positive test result is the involuntary contraction of the jaw (biting down on the "spatula") and a negative test result would normally be a gag reflex attempting to expel the foreign object. The spatula test had a high specificity (zero false-positive test results) and a high sensitivity (94% of infected people produced a positive test).

PREVENTION

Unlike many infectious diseases, recovery from naturally acquired tetanus does not usually result in immunity to tetanus. This is due to the extreme potency of the tetanospasmin toxin.

Tetanus can be prevented by vaccination with tetanus toxoid. The CDC recommends that adults receive a booster vaccine every 10 years, and standard care practice in many places is to give the booster to any person with a puncture wound who is uncertain of when he or she was last vaccinated, or if he or she has had fewer than three lifetime doses of the vaccine. The booster may not prevent a potentially fatal case of tetanus from the current wound; however, as it can take up to 2 weeks for tetanus antibodies to form.

In children under the age of 7 years, the tetanus vaccine is often administered as a combined vaccine, DPT/DTaP vaccine, which also includes vaccines against diphtheria and pertussis. For adults and children over 7 years, the Td vaccine (tetanus and diphtheria) or Tdap (tetanus, diphtheria, and acellular pertussis) is commonly used.

The World Health Organization certifies countries as having eliminated maternal or neonatal tetanus. Certification requires at least 2 years of rates of less than 1 case per 1,000 live births.

In 1998 in Uganda, 3,433 tetanus cases were recorded in newborn babies; of these, 2,403 died.

After a major public health effort, Uganda in 2011 was certified as having eliminated tetanus.

POSTEXPOSURE PROPHYLAXIS

Tetanus toxoid can be given in case of a suspected exposure to tetanus. In such cases, it can be given with or without tetanus immunoglobulin (also called tetanus antibodies or tetanus antitoxin). It can be given as intravenous therapy or by intramuscular injection.

The guidelines for such events in the United States for nonpregnant people, 11 years and older age are as follows:
- Vaccination status
- Clean, minor wounds, all other wounds
- Unknown or less than three doses of tetanus toxoid-containing vaccine
- Tdap and recommend catch-up vaccination
- *Tetanus immunoglobulin*: Three or more doses of tetanus toxoid-containing vaccine AND less than 5 years since last dose
- *No indication*: Three or more doses of tetanus toxoid-containing vaccine AND 5-10 years since last dose

- Tdap preferred (if not yet received) or Td
- Three or more doses of tetanus toxoid-containing vaccine AND more than 10 years since last dose.

Mild Tetanus

Mild cases of tetanus can be treated with:
- Tetanus immunoglobulin (TIG), also called tetanus antibodies or tetanus antitoxin. It can be given as intravenous therapy or by intramuscular injection.
- Metronidazole IV for 10 days
- Diazepam oral or IV

Severe Tetanus

Severe cases will require admission to intensive care. In addition to the measures listed above for mild tetanus:
- Human tetanus immunoglobulin injected intrathecally (increases clinical improvement from 4 to 35%)
- Tracheotomy and mechanical ventilation for 3-4 weeks. Tracheotomy is recommended for securing the airway because the presence of an endotracheal tube is a stimulus for spasm
- Magnesium sulfate, as an IV infusion, to control spasm and autonomic dysfunction
- Diazepam as a continuous IV infusion
- The autonomic effects of tetanus can be difficult to manage (alternating hyper- and hypotension hyperpyrexia/hypothermia) and may require IV labetalol, magnesium, clonidine, and/or nifedipine.

Drugs such as diazepam or other muscle relaxants can be given to control the muscle spasms. In extreme cases, it may be necessary to paralyze the person with curare-like drugs and use a mechanical ventilator.

In order to survive a tetanus infection, the maintenance of an airway and proper nutrition are required. An intake of 3,500-4,000 calories and atleast 150 g of protein per day is often given in liquid form through a tube directly into the stomach (percutaneous endoscopic gastrostomy), or through a drip into a vein (parenteral nutrition). This high-caloric diet maintenance is required because of the increased metabolic strain brought on by the increased muscle activity. Full recovery takes 4-6 weeks because the body must regenerate destroyed nerve axon terminals.

The antibiotic of choice is metronidazole. It can be given as intravenously, by mouth, or by rectum. Of likewise efficiency is penicillin, but some raise the concern of provoking spasms because it inhibits gamma-aminobutyric acid (GABA) receptor, which is already affected by tetanospasmin.

39 CHAPTER

Pertussis

Raghvendra Singh

INTRODUCTION

- Pertussis is a highly contagious acute respiratory illness caused by *Bordetella pertussis*, occasionally due to *Bordetella parapertussis*. *B. pertussis* is a gram-negative coccobacilli, a strict human pathogen that colonize only ciliated epithelium. Pertussis toxin (PT) is the major virulence protein.
- It is more common and serious in infancy and childhood although all age groups are affected. It is extremely contagious with attack rate of nearly 100% in susceptible individuals exposed to aerosol droplets at close range.
- Neither natural infection nor vaccination provides complete or lifelong immunity against pertussis reinfection or disease.
- Subclinical infection is seen but chronic carriage in humans is not known. The disease is still endemic in India with 25,000 reported cases in 2015.
- Pertussis is now increasingly reported in adolescents and adults because of rapidly waning vaccine-induced immunity and pathogen adaptation.
- Infants are susceptible to infection because maternal antibodies do not appear to give protection against the disease.

CLINICAL MANIFESTATIONS

- Pertussis has incubation period of 3–12 days. The disease spreads mainly by droplet infection and direct contact.
- Infective period begins after 1 week of exposure and is most infective during catarrhal stage; communicability decreases rapidly after this stage. Symptoms are not uniform across ages and symptoms vary with age and immunization status.
- In its classic form, the disease passes through three stages **(Table 1)**.
- *Infants (<3 months old)*: Classic stages are not seen, initial stage goes unnoticed; in paroxysmal stage, well-looking infant will suddenly begin to choke, gasp, gag, and flail extremities with reddening of face. Apnea and cyanosis can follow cough or apnea can occur as only manifestation.
  Paroxysmal stage is prolonged in infants. Cough is not prominent at this time, paradoxically cough/whoop can become louder and more classic in later stages of convalescence.
- *Adolescents and previously immunized children*: Because of a typical presentation and shortening of all stages, pertussis is difficult to recognize in these children. Most commonly they present with sudden feeling of strangulation and suffocation followed by prolonged uninterrupted cough, followed by gasping breath, usually whoop is absent. Post-tussive vomiting and headache can occur. These paroxysmal symptoms followed by hours of well-being can give a clue to the diagnosis. Physical findings are generally uninformative. Conjunctival hemorrhages and petechiae on upper body may be seen.

TABLE 1: Stages of pertussis.

Stage	Duration (weeks)	Symptom
Catarrhal (most infectious)	1–2	Insidious onset with nasal congestion, runny nose, sneezing, mild fever, lacrimation Nose, sneezing, mild fever, lacrimation
Paroxysmal	2–6	Cough which initially is dry and intermittent, soon progresses to relentless episodic paroxysms, which is the hallmark of pertussis, burst of continuous cough, tongue protrusion, bulging and watering eyes, face turns purple until the cough ceases with characteristic whoop as inspired air rushes through the partially closed glottis. Post-tussive vomiting and exhaustion are common. The number and severity of paroxysms increase over days to weeks and remain plateau for weeks
Convalescent	>2	Number, severity, and duration of episodes diminish, general condition improves

TABLE 2: Recommended antimicrobial treatment and postexposure prophylaxis for pertussis.

Age group	Azithromycin	Erythromycin	Clarithromycin
<1 month	10 mg/kg single dose for 5 days	Not preferred	Not recommended
1–5 months	10 mg/kg single dose for 5 days	40–50 mg/kg/day in four divided doses for 14 days	15 mg/kg/day in two divided doses for 7 days
Infants > 6 months	10 mg/kg single dose for 5 days	40–50 mg/kg/ In four divided doses for 14 days	15 mg/kg/day (1 g divided doses for 7 days)
Infants >6 months and children	10 mg/kg single dose day 1 (500 mg maximum) then 5 mg/kg (250 mg maximum) on days 2–5	40–50 mg/kg/day (max 2 g/day) in four divided doses for 14 days	15 mg/kg/day (1 g maximum) in two divided doses for 7 days

DIAGNOSIS

Diagnosis is generally clinical based on symptomatology and suspected in any individual who complains predominantly of cough with normal physical findings. For sporadic cases, clinical case definition of cough >14 days duration of with at least one of the following symptoms of paroxysms, whoop or post-tussive vomiting has high sensitivity of 81% for confirmation of pertussis.

Laboratory Tests

Leukocytosis (15,000–100,000 cells/μL) caused by absolute lymphocytosis is characteristic in early stage. Lymphocytes are normal small cells not the usual large cells as seen in viral infections. More severe course and death are correlated with rapid rise and extreme leukocytosis, especially in infants.

Methods of confirmation are culture, polymerase chain reaction (PCR), and serology. These confirmatory tests are not very practical; they also have limitations of sensitivity and specificity. PCR testing on nasopharyngeal wash specimens is the laboratory test of choice. Results of culture and PCR are expected to be positive in catarrhal and early paroxysmal stages of the disease that too in unimmunized, untreated children. For immunized individuals, serologic tests for detection of change in antibodies to *B. pertussis* antigens between acute and convalescent sample are most sensitive.

Differential Diagnosis

The protracted coughing have to be differentiated from *Mycoplasma*, parainfluenza, influenza, enteroviruses, respiratory syncytial virus (RSV) or adenoviruses, and foreign body.

TREATMENT

- General measures include providing adequate nutrition and hydration and avoiding factors aggravating cough (food, cold air, cold liquids, etc.). Infants <3 months old need to be hospitalized unless witnessed paroxysms are not severe.
- *Antibiotics are used to*: (1) Decrease contagiousness by terminating respiratory tract carriage of *B. pertussis*, (2) afford any possible clinical benefit (generally do not shorten the course of the disease), and (3) early treatment may (within 7 days of symptom onset), antimicrobial therapy may shorten the duration of symptoms and decrease transmission to susceptible contacts.

Recommended antimicrobial treatment and post-exposure prophylaxis for pertussis is given in **Table 2**.

- In rare cases where the patients are allergic to macrolides, Trimethoprim-Sulfamethoxazole can be used as an alternative agent in children above 2 months of age.
- *Isolation*: The patients are placed in isolation with droplet precaution and until 5 days after initiation of azithromycin therapy.
- *Contacts*: Postexposure prophylaxis to all close contacts with same drugs, dose, and duration.

COMPLICATIONS

Infants <6 months have higher morbidity and mortality; complications include apnea, secondary infections (otitis media, pneumonia, etc.), physical sequelae of forceful coughing, seizures, encephalopathy, malnutrition, rarely pulmonary hypertension, and death.

PREVENTION

Universal immunization in children with pertussis containing vaccine beginning in infancy with reinforcing doses through adolescence and adulthood is central to the control of pertussis. DTP (vaccines against diphtheria, pertussis, and tetanus) at 6, 10, and 14 weeks followed by booster doses at 15-18 months and 5 years and dTaP (vaccines against tetanus, diphtheria, and pertussis) at 11-12 years of age. If missed vaccination, then vaccination is completed with age-appropriate immunization.

SUGGESTED READING

1. Parthasarathy A, Kundu R, Yewale VN, Rai A, Shastri DD. Textbook of Pediatric Infectious Disease, 2nd edition. New Delhi: Jaypee Brothers Medical Publishers (P) Ltd.; 2019.

Enteric Fever

Ashwani Agrawal

INTRODUCTION

Typhoid fever is a systemic infection with the bacterium *Salmonella enterica serotype typhi*. Salmonellae are rod-shaped, gram-negative, facultative anaerobic bacteria, most of which are motile by peritrichous flagella [which bear the H antigen(s)].

In addition to the H antigen(s), two polysaccharide surface antigens aid in the further characterization of *S. enterica*, namely the somatic O antigen and the capsular Vi (virulence) antigen.

EPIDEMIOLOGY

- Typhoid is transmitted by contaminated food or water. The incidence in the developing world is ranging from 100 to 1,000 cases/100,000 population.
- The age-specific incidence of typhoid may be highest in children <5 years of age, with comparatively higher rates of complications and hospitalization.
- Estimates of case fatality rates in typhoid fever range from 1 to 4% in patients who receive adequate therapy, but can rise to 10-20% in untreated cases, or treated within appropriate antibiotics.
- The incubation period ranging from 7 to 14 days, depending on the inoculating dose of viable bacteria.

CLINICAL FEATURES

- The classic presentation is fever, malaise, diffuse abdominal pain, and constipation.
- Typhoid fever usually manifests as high-grade fever with a wide variety of associated features such as symptoms of influenza with chills (although rigors are rare), a dull frontal headache, malaise, anorexia, nausea, poorly localized abdominal discomfort, a dry cough, and myalgia, but with few physical signs.
- A coated tongue, tender abdomen, hepatomegaly, and splenomegaly are common.
- A macular or maculopapular rash (rose spots) may be visible around the 7th-10th day of the illness (5-30%). They usually occur on the abdomen and chest and more rarely on the back, arms, and legs.
- If no complications occur, the symptoms and physical findings gradually resolve within 2-4 weeks.
- Vertical intrauterine transmission from an infected mother may lead to neonatal typhoid, a rare but severe and life-threatening illness.

COMPLICATIONS

Complications occur in 10-15% of patients and are particularly likely in patients who have been ill for more than 2 weeks.

Many complications have been:

- *Abdominal*: Gastrointestinal (GI) perforation, GI hemorrhage, hepatitis, cholecystitis (usually subclinical)
- *Cardiovascular*: Asymptomatic electrocardiographic changes, myocarditis, shock
- *Neuropsychiatric*: Encephalopathy, delirium, psychotic states, meningitis, impairment of coordination
- *Respiratory*: Bronchitis, pneumonia
- *Hematologic*: Anemia, disseminated intravascular coagulation (usually subclinical)
- *Other*: Focal abscess, pharyngitis, relapse, chronic carriage.

DIAGNOSIS

The absence of specific symptoms or signs makes the clinical diagnosis of typhoid difficult. In endemic areas such as India, a fever without focus cause that lasts more than 1 week should be considered typhoid until proved otherwise.

- *Complete blood count*: The utility is unremarkable, but it should be the first test to be ordered, apart from other more specific tests. Leukopenia seen in 20-25% cases and eosinopenia in 70-80% cases. A normal eosinophil count in a suspected case of enteric fever makes it less likely. Platelet count may be normal and is reduced in later course of disease.
- *Culture*: Blood culture is the gold standard in the diagnosis of enteric fever. The sensitivity is around 50% in the first week. It should be sent in the early course of disease, before starting antibiotic therapy. The susceptibility

testing for nalidixic acid should be routinely requested from the pathology laboratory. Cultures can be done from the buffy coat of blood, streptokinase-treated blood clots, intestinal secretions (with the use of a duodenal string capsule), and skin snips of rose spots.
- *Widal test*: The test is done from acute serum, after 5–7 days. The titer of both H and O antibodies of 1: 160 dilution (four-fold rise) should be taken as cutoff value for the diagnosis. It is controversial because the sensitivity, specificity, and predictive values of this test vary considerably in endemic areas. It can be negative in 30% of culture-proven case of typhoid fever.
- *Newer diagnostic tests*: The modified widal test, typhidot test, IDL TUBEX test, IgM dipstick test, antigen detection test need evaluation before they are routinely recommended. The polymerase chain reaction (PCR) as a diagnostic modality is still in experimental stage.

Despite these innovations, the mainstay of diagnosis of typhoid remains clinical in most of the developing world, and several diagnostic algorithms have been evaluated in endemic areas.

DIFFERENTIAL DIAGNOSIS

Typhoid must be distinguished from other endemic acute and subacute febrile illnesses. Malaria, deep abscesses, tuberculosis, amoebic liver abscess, encephalitis, influenza, dengue, leptospirosis, infectious mononucleosis, endocarditis, brucellosis, typhus, visceral leishmaniasis, toxoplasmosis, lymphoproliferative disease, and connective-tissue diseases should be considered.

TREATMENT

In areas of endemic disease, more than 60–90% of cases of typhoid fever are managed at home with antibiotics and bed rest. Patients with persistent vomiting, severe diarrhea, and abdominal distention may require hospitalization and parenteral antibiotic therapy.

General Principles of Management

Adequate rest, hydration, and attention are important to correct fluid and electrolyte imbalance and antipyretic therapy (acetaminophen 10–15 mg/kg every 4–6 hours). A soft, easily digestible diet should be continued unless the patient has abdominal distention or ileus.

Principles of Treatment

The treatment of typhoid fever is based on susceptibility.
- As a general principle of antimicrobial treatment, intermediate susceptibility should be regarded as equivalent to resistance. Until susceptibilities are determined, antibiotics should be empiric, for which there are various recommendations. Now it has become necessary to treat all cases presumptively for multidrug resistance (MDR) until sensitivities are obtained.
- The *S. typhi* has developed resistance (MDR) to all the first-line drugs (chloramphenicol, trimethoprim, sulfamethoxazole, and ampicillin). These multidrug-resistant strains also carry the 100,000–120,000-KdIncHI plasmids that encoded the resistance genes.
- Fluoroquinolones are the most effective drug for the treatment of typhoid fever. The organism must be disk tested for sensitivity with nalidixic acid.
- Resistance to nalidixic acid is a surrogate marker for the resistance to fluoroquinolone. The strains of *S. typhi* which are sensitive to nalidixic acid (NASST), a 7-day course is highly effective, and in situation where, nalidixic acid resistance is there 10–14-day course of antibiotics with maximum recommended dose is considered. Fluoroquinolone is not approved by the Drug Controller General of India to be used under 18 years of age. The fluoroquinolones has recently shown the evidence that in children, it neither cause joint toxicity nor impairment of growth.
- *Cephalosporins*: Third-generation cephalosporin like cefixime is now the drug of choice in uncomplicated typhoid fever. In complicated cases, ceftriaxone, cefotaxime, and cefoperazone are considered parenterally.
- *Azithromycin*: Recently it has become an alternative choice in uncomplicated cases.
- Aztreonam and imipenem are used as third line in complicated cases.

Treatment Guidelines

Mild or uncomplicated infections:
- It is appropriate to begin oral therapy with cefixime followed by any of the second-line drugs such as chloramphenicol, amoxicillin, trimethoprim-sulfamethoxazole (TMP-SMX). In uncomplicated typhoid, which is multidrug-resistant cefixime followed by second-line drug azithromycin can be tried **(Table 1)**.

TABLE 1: Treatment of uncomplicated typhoid.

Susceptibility	Antibiotics	Daily dose mg/kg	Days
First line oral drugs fully sensitive	Cefixime	15–20	14
Second line oral drugs fully sensitive	Chloramphenicol	50–75	14–21
	Amoxicillin	75–100	14
	TMP-SMX	8 TMP 40 SMX	14
Multidrug resistant first line drug	Cefixime	15–20	14
Multidrug resistant second line drug	Azithromycin	10–20	14

TABLE 2: Treatment of severe typhoid.

Susceptibility	Antibiotics	Daily dose mg/kg	Days
First line parenteral drugs fully sensitive	Ceftriaxone or Cefotaxime	50–75	14
Second line parenteral drugs fully sensitive	Chloramphenicol	100	14–21
	Amoxicillin	100	14
	TMP-SMX	8 TMP 40 SMX	14
Multidrug resistant parenteral first line drug	Ceftriaxone or Cefotaxime	50–75	14
Multidrug resistant parenteral second line drug	Aztreonam	50–100	14

- Azithromycin offers dual advantages of low risk of resistance and excellent oral absorption. (IAP Task Force Report 2006: Management of Enteric Fever in Children)
- The concept of using dual antibiotic therapy has been revived because of the risk of developing antibiotic resistance; specifically, the combination of cefixime-ofloxacin has been approved by the Indian Regulatory Authority for the treatment of typhoid fever.
- In addition to antibiotics, the importance of supportive treatment and maintenance of appropriate fluid and electrolyte balance is must.
- For severe typhoid, follow the guidelines given in **Table 2**. In rare cases, dexamethasone 3 mg/kg for the initial dose, followed by 1 mg/kg every 6 hours for 48 hours has been recommended for severely ill patients with shock, obtundation, stupor, or coma. Corticosteroids should be use under strict supervision, because it may mask signs of abdominal complications.

Relapses should be treated in the same way as initial infections. The majority of intestinal carriers can be cured by a prolonged course of antibiotics for 5–7 days.

PROGNOSIS

- Prognosis depends on the rapidity of diagnosis and use of appropriate antibiotic therapy. Other factors are age, general state of health, and nutrition of the patient.
- Relapse rate in children are 2–4% even after appropriate treatment.
- The risk to becoming a chronic carrier is low in children (<2%) and increases with age.

IMMUNIZATION

- Three typhoid vaccines are currently recommended by the World Health Organization for control of endemic and epidemic typhoid fever:
  1. Injectable typhoid conjugate vaccine (TCV), consisting of Vi polysaccharide antigen linked to tetanus toxoid protein licensed for children from 6 months of age and adults up to 45 years of age.
  2. Injectable unconjugated polysaccharide vaccine based on the purified Vi antigen (known as Vi-PS vaccine) for persons aged 2 years and above.
  3. Oral live attenuated Ty21, a vaccine in capsule formulation for those over 6 years of age.

Among the available typhoid vaccines, TCV is preferred at all ages for routine programmatic use in view of its improved immunological properties, suitability for use in younger children and expected longer duration of protection.

SUGGESTED READING

1. Parthasarathy A. Textbook of Pediatric Infectious Disease, 2nd edition. New Delhi: Jaypee Brothers Medical Publishers; 2019.

41 CHAPTER

Measles

Ashwani Agrawal

INTRODUCTION

Measles is highly contagious and acute viral disease characterized by generalized maculopapular, erythematous morbilliform rash with catarrhal symptoms. Measles virus is a single-stranded RNA virus belonging to the family Paramyxoviridae and genus *Morbillivirus*. Human being the natural host of the virus, there is no animal reservoir. Mode of transmission is by large and small droplets aerosol which may persist in air for 1 hour. Patients are infectious from 4 days prior to 4–6 days after the appearance of rash.

CLINICAL MANIFESTATIONS

Four phases of measles:
1. Incubation period is 8–12 days.
2. Prodromal phase lasts to 3–5 days and consist of high-grade fever with cough, coryza, and conjunctivitis with photophobia. *Koplik spots* are pathognomonic sign appearing between 1st and 4th days prior to the onset of rash. It is an enanthem (Grayish white or bluish white dots with reddish areola) on inner aspect of cheeks at the level of premolar.
3. *Exanthematous phase*: Rash appears on 4–6 days of fever. Rash generally start from the forehead, and from behind the ears and on the upper neck. Rash spread peripherally over next 3–4 days.
4. *Convalescence phase*: At the onset of the rash, the symptom begins to subside. By the time rashes reach the extremities, they begin to disappear in the same fashion as it evolved. Rash disappears leaving behind the brownish discoloration and desquamation. The cough persists at least for 10 days. In severe cases, cervical and occipital lymphadenopathy may be present.

COMPLICATIONS

Complications from measles have been reported in every organ system. The causes of complications are due to the disruption of epithelial surfaces by measles virus and the causing immune suppression. Measles virus infects CD4+ T cells, resulting in suppression of the Th1 immune response and a multitude of other immunosuppressive effects. Measles virus was the first of the immunodeficiency viruses to be described, and in many respects it resembles AIDS. Uncomplicated measles render lifelong immunity from clinical disease. Complications are more common among <5 years of age (especially <1 years of age) and >20 years of age.

Respiratory Complications
- *Otitis media*: Due to inflammation of the epithelial surface of the Eustachian tube causing obstruction and secondary bacterial infection.
- *Laryngotracheobronchitis*: Due to secondary bacterial infection.
- *Pneumonia*: Most common severe complication of measles and accounts for most measles-associated deaths.
- *Primary interstitial viral pneumonitis.*
- *Measles secondary pneumonia* is due to bacterial infection.
- *Giant cell pneumonia* is due to infected cell fusion and defective cell-mediated immunity.
- *Retropharyngeal abscess.*

Gastrointestinal Complications
Diarrhea (enteritis), mesenteric adenitis, appendicitis, hepatitis, pancreatitis, stomatitis, and noma (cancrum oris).

Neurological Complications
- *Febrile convulsions*
- *Progressive measles inclusion body encephalitis (MIBE)* is due to nuclear inclusions of defective virus and defective cell-mediated immunity
- *Progressive subacute sclerosing panencephalitis (SSPE)* is due to persistent measles virus infection in brain and inclusion bodies in the cytoplasm
- *Postinfectious encephalomyelitis (PIE)* is due to myelin basic protein autoimmunity
- *Guillain–Barre syndrome*
- *Reye syndrome*
- *Transverse myelitis.*

Eye Complications
Keratitis, corneal ulceration, corneal perforation, central vein occlusion, and blindness.

Hematological Complications
Thrombocytopenic purpura and disseminated intravascular coagulation.

Cardiovascular Complications
Myocarditis and pericarditis.

Dermatological Complications
Severe desquamation, cellulitis, hemorrhagic measles or *"black measles"* (hemorrhagic skin eruption) and often fatal.

Others: Hypocalcemia, myositis, nephritis, renal failure, malnutrition, and death.

DIAGNOSIS
- The diagnosis is almost always based on *clinical* and *epidemiological* findings.
- *Serology*: Testing for IgM: antibody in serum, which appears 1–2 days after the onset of the rash and persists for a month. Four-fold rise in serum IgG antibody in acute and convalescent specimens collected 2–4 weeks apart.
- *Viral isolation*: Blood, urine, or respiratory secretions.
- Molecular detection by *polymerase chain reaction (PCR)* is possible.

DIFFERENTIAL DIAGNOSIS
- Measles is to be differentiated from other exanthematous immune-mediated illnesses and infections, e.g., Rubella, Adenoviruses, Enteroviruses, and Epstein–Barr virus
- *Mycoplasma pneumoniae* and Group A *Streptococcus* produce rashes
- Kawasaki syndrome
- Drug eruptions.

TREATMENT
- Management of measles is supportive.
- Maintenance of hydration, oxygenation, and comfort is the goal of the therapy. Antipyretics (Paracetamol) are to be used frequently 6–8 hourly (Avoid aspirin).
- Antiviral therapy is not effective.
- Measles in immunocompromised patient is highly lethal. Ribavirin therapy with or without IV gamma globulin gives some benefit in individual patients but is not approved by the United States Food and Drug Administration (USFDA).
- *Vitamin A supplementation*: Vitamin A deficiency in children has been known to be associated with increased mortality from measles. The World Health Organization (WHO) recommended vitamin A supplements to all children with acute measles. The recommended dosages are:
  - 200,000 IU for children 1 year or older
  - 100,000 IU for children 6–11 months of age
  - 50,000 IU for children less than 6 months of age.

It has to be given once day for 2 days. An additional age-specific third dose is given 4 weeks later to children with ophthalmologic evidence of vitamin A deficiency.

PROGNOSIS
In developing countries, measles case fatality rates are 10- to 100-fold higher than in developed countries. It is due to a young age at infection, crowding, underlying immune deficiency disorders, vitamin A deficiency, and lack of access to medical care. Pneumonia and encephalitis were the common complications in the fatal cases. Immune deficiency conditions were associated in 14–16% of deaths.

PREVENTION
- Isolation of patient is important as measles viruses are shed from 7 days after exposure to 4–6 days after the onset of rash. Immunocompromised patients with measles will shed virus for the duration of the illness, so isolation should be maintained throughout the disease.
- Measles vaccine is available as a monovalent preparation or combined with the rubella (MR) or measles-mumps-rubella (MMR) vaccine. Measles vaccine contains live attenuated measles virus (Edmonston-Zagreb strain).
- Expanded Programme on Immunization (EPI) Policy and National Immunization Program in India recommended measles vaccine at the age of 9 months and 15 months as MMR, and a third dose at 4–6 years.
- The Indian Academy of Pediatrics Advisory Committee on Vaccines and Immunization Practices (IAP-ACVIP) policy also recommends Varicella vaccine along with MMR as MMR-V, at 15 months and second doses of MMR-V at 4–6 years.
- Adverse events from the MMR vaccine include fever (usually 6–12 days following vaccination), rash (5%), and, rarely transient thrombocytopenia.
- Live vaccines should not be administered to pregnant women or to immune-deficient or immune-suppressed patients.

Postexposure Prophylaxis
Susceptible individuals exposed to measles may be protected from infection by either vaccine or immunization with immunoglobulin (Ig).
- The vaccine is effective in prevention or modification of measles if given within 72 hours of exposure.

- Ig may be given up to 6 days after exposure to prevent or modify infection.
- Ig is indicated for susceptible household contacts of measles patients, who are younger than 1 year, pregnant women, and immunocompromised persons.
- Children who have received Ig, measles vaccine is to be deferred for at least 6 months, provided the child age is more than 1 year.
- Immunocompetent should receive 0.25 mL/kg, and immunocompromised children should receive 0.5 mL/kg intramuscularly. Maximum dose in both cases is 15 mL (irrespective of immune status).

SUGGESTED READING

1. Parthasarathy A. Textbook of Pediatric Infectious Disease, 2nd edition. New Delhi: Jaypee Brothers Medical Publishers; 2019.

42 Mumps

Arun Agrawalla

INTRODUCTION

Mumps is an acute self-limiting viral infection of childhood, primarily affecting the salivary glands. Although it is mostly a mild childhood disease, with peak incidence occurring among those aged 5-9 years, the mumps virus may also affect adults, among whom complications such as meningitis and orchitis are relatively more common. Incidence of mumps in the absence of immunization is in the range of 100–1,000 cases/100,000 population, with epidemic peaks every 2-5 years. Natural infection with this virus is thought to confer lifelong protection.

ETIOLOGY

Mumps virus belongs to the genus *Rubulavirus* of the family Paramyxoviridae is a single-stranded RNA genome. There are two surface components: (1) Hemagglutinin-neuraminidase protein and (2) fusion protein. These play a part in virulence. Antibodies against the hemagglutinin-neuraminidase protein are virus-neutralizing.

EPIDEMIOLOGY

Mumps is most often a mild disease of childhood. In hot climates, the disease may occur at any time of year, whereas in temperate climates, the incidence peaks in winter and spring. Many countries experience epidemics at intervals of 2-5 years.

ETIOPATHOGENESIS

Humans are the only known natural host for mumps virus, which is spread via direct contact or by airborne droplets from the upper respiratory tract of infected individuals. The virus appears in saliva from up to 7 days before to 7 days after onset of parotid swelling. The period of maximum infection is from 1-2 days before to 5 days after onset of parotid swelling. The incubation time averages 16-18 days with a range of 2-4 weeks.

The virus proliferates in the upper respiratory tract and then enters the circulation. During viremia, the virus spreads to the meninges, the salivary glands, pancreas, testes, and ovaries. It causes neurosis of infected cell with a lymphocytic inflammatory infiltrate.

CLINICAL FEATURES

Mumps begins with a prodrome of myalgia, headache, malaise, and low-grade fever and within a day, these are followed by the characteristic unilateral or bilateral swelling of the parotid glands which may be unilaterally initially and becomes bilateral in 70% of cases. The parotid gland is tender and is associated with earache on ipsilateral side. Ingestion of sour or acidic food worsens pain. As the swelling increases, there is obliteration of the angle of jaw and the ear lobe is lifted upward and outward. The opening of the Stensen duct may be red and edematous. Other salivary glands are visibly affected in approximately 10% of cases.

After about 1 week, fever and glandular swelling disappear, and unless complications occur, the illness resolves completely.

In approximately 30% of cases, only nonspecific symptoms occur or the infection is asymptomatic. Most infections in children aged <2 years are subclinical.

COMPLICATIONS

Asymptomatic pleocytosis of cerebrospinal fluid is seen in 50-60% of mumps patients. Symptomatic meningitis is seen in around 15%. Mumps encephalitis is reported in 0.02-0.3% of cases.

Although the case-fatality rate of mumps encephalitis is low, permanent sequelae, including paralysis, seizures, cranial nerve palsies, aqueductal stenosis, and hydrocephalus may occur. Acquired sensorineural deafness caused by mumps is one of the leading causes of deafness in childhood, affecting approximately 5/100,000 mumps patients.

Orchitis occurs in 20% of postpubertal males who develop mumps. In 20% of orchitis cases, both testes are affected but mumps orchitis is rarely associated with permanently impaired fertility. Symptomatic oophoritis and mastitis are relatively uncommon and apparently without long-lasting consequences for patients.

Acquisition of mumps during the first 12 weeks of pregnancy is associated with a 25% incidence of spontaneous abortions, but fetal malformations following infection with mumps virus during pregnancy have not been found.

Pancreatitis is reported as a complication in approximately 4% of cases, but the relationship between mumps pancreatitis and diabetes mellitus remains speculative.

DIAGNOSIS

Diagnosis is clinical, based on history of exposure and typical clinical findings. Elevated serum amylase confirms parotitis; there may be leukopenia with relative lymphocytosis. Confirmatory diagnosis can be done with virology or serology. The virus can be isolated in cell culture from upper respiratory secretion, cerebrospinal fluid (CSF), or urine. Viral antigen can be detected by direct immunofluorescence or by identification of nucleic acid by reverse transcriptase polymerase chain reaction (PCR). A sharp increase in serum mumps immunoglobulin G antibody between acute and convalescent phase establishes the diagnosis.

Differential Diagnosis

Parotid swelling may be caused by parainfluenza 1 and 3, influenza A, cytomegalovirus, Epstein-Barr virus, and enterovirus. Purulent parotitis may be caused by *Staphylococcus aureus* but it is usually unilateral and extremely tender. Submandibular or anterior cervical adenitis may be confused with parotitis.

MANAGEMENT

No specific therapy for mumps exists. Treatment is symptomatic and supportive. Adequate hydration and antipyretics for fever are sufficient.

In general, natural infection confers lifelong protection against the disease but recurrent mumps attacks have been reported.

PROGNOSIS

Mumps is a self-limiting disease with excellent prognosis.

PREVENTION

Globally MMR vaccine (vaccine against measles, mumps, and rubella) is used instead of monovalent vaccine. Vaccine strains include Leningrad-Zagreb, Leningrad-3, Jeryl Lynn, RIT 4385 or Urabe AM9 strain and are grown in chick embryo or human diploid cell cultures. The vaccine is available in a lyophilized form. Reconstituted vaccine should be used within 4-6 hours. The dose is 0.5 mL subcutaneously given in a three-dose schedule as MR/MMR vaccine at 9 months, 15 months, and at 4-6 years. Seroconversion rates are >90% but clinical efficacy and long-term protection with single dose is 60-90%. Mumps vaccination is contraindicated in individuals with advanced immune deficiency or immunosuppression, during pregnancy, and allergy to vaccine components, such as neomycin and gelatin.

Routine mumps vaccination is recommended in countries with a well-established, effective childhood, and rubella vaccination (i.e., coverage >80%) and where the reduction of mumps incidence is a public health priority. As with rubella, insufficient childhood vaccination coverage can result in an epidemiological shift in the incidence of mumps to older age groups, potentially leading to more serious disease burden than occurred before immunization was introduced.

SUGGESTED READING

1. Albrecht MA. (2020). Mumps. [online] Available from: https://www.uptodate.com/contents/mumps. [Last accessed June, 2021].
2. Balasubramanian S, Shastri DD, Chatterjee P, Shah AK, Pemde HK, Shivananda S, Guduru VK. 2019 IAP Guidebook on Immunization 2018-19. New Delhi: Jaypee brothers Medical Publishers (P) Ltd; 2019.
3. Vashishtha VM, Yadav S, Dabas A, Bansal CP, Agarwal RC, Yewale VN, et al. IAP Position Paper on burden of mumps in India and vaccination strategies. Indian Pediatr. 2015;52(6):505-14.
4. World Health Organization. (2007). Mumps virus vaccines, WHO position paper. [online] Available from: https://www.who.int/publications/i/item/mumps-virus-vaccines-position-paper. [Last accessed June, 2021].

CHAPTER 43: Rubella

Arun Agrawalla

INTRODUCTION

Rubella is an acute, usually mild, and often exanthematous viral disease of infants and children. Its public health importance is due to its teratologic effects causing fetal death or congenital rubella syndrome (CRS) when infection occurs in early pregnancy.

ETIOLOGY

Rubella is an enveloped single-stranded RNA virus belonging to the family Togaviridae of genus *Rubivirus*. It has three structural proteins: A nucleocapsid associated with nucleus and two glycoproteins E1 and E2 associated with envelope. The virus is sensitive to heat, UV light, and relatively stable at low temperatures. Only one serotype is known.

EPIDEMIOLOGY

Humans are the only known host. It occurs in a seasonal pattern with epidemics every 5-9 years. Secondary attack rate is 50-60% in family contacts. Rubella infection just before conception and during early pregnancy can lead to miscarriage, fetal death, or CRS. The World Health Organization (WHO) estimates that more than 100,000 babies are born with CRS worldwide each year and most of them in developing countries.

ETIOPATHOGENESIS

The virus is transmitted by aerosol droplets from person to person and transplacentally in CRS. The incubation period ranges from 12 to 23 days with a mean of 18 days. After infection, the virus replicates in the respiratory epithelium and then spreads to the regional lymph nodes. Intense viremia occurs 10-17 days after infection. The virus sheds from the nasopharynx 1 week before to up to 2 weeks after onset of rash. Communicability is highest from 5 days prior to appearance of rash and continues till 6 days following its appearance.

Congenital infection occurs during maternal viremia. After infecting the placenta, the virus spreads through the vascular system of the developing fetus and can infect any fetal organ. Maternal infection during the first 8 weeks of gestation results in most severe defects. Risk for congenital defect is 90% for infections occurring before 11 weeks, 33% for infections between 11 and 12 weeks, 11% for infections between 13 and 14 weeks, 24% for infections between 15 and 16 weeks and uncommon for infection after 16 weeks. Infants with CRS may excrete the virus for more than a year.

CLINICAL FEATURES

Postnatal rubella is usually a mild self-limiting disease. Initial prodromal symptoms include malaise, headache, mild catarrh and low-grade fever. Characteristically there is postauricular, occipital, and posterior cervical lymphadenopathy which precedes the rash by 5-10 days. In children, the first manifestation of rubella is usually the erythematous maculopapular rash which is often pruritic. It begins in the face and neck and spreads centrifugally to involve the torso and extremities. Discrete rose-colored spots on the soft palate (Forchheimer spots) are seen in around 20% children. The rash clears rapidly within 3 days without desquamation. Arthritis or arthralgia may occur in 70% of adult women but are less common in men and children.

CONGENITAL RUBELLA SYNDROME

In pregnant women, rubella virus can infect the developing fetus by transplacental infection causing CRS, fetal wastage, or still birth. CRS includes a triad of malformation—cataract, sensorineural hearing loss, and congenital heart disease.

- *Ophthalmic*: Cataracts, microphthalmia, glaucoma, pigmentary retinopathy, and chorioretinitis
- *Auditory*: Sensorineural deafness
- *Cardiac*: Peripheral pulmonary artery stenosis, patent ductus arteriosus, or ventricular septal defects)
- *Craniofacial*: Microcephaly.

Congenital rubella syndrome can also present with neonatal manifestations such as meningoencephalitis, hepatosplenomegaly, hepatitis, interstitial pneumonitis, thrombocytopenia, and radiolucencies in the long bones (a characteristic radiological pattern of CRS).

Neonates who survive suffer from developmental disabilities such as visual and hearing impairments and have an increased risk for developmental delay, including autism.

A progressive encephalopathy resembling subacute sclerosing panencephalitis (SSPE) has been seen in patients with CRS.

COMPLICATIONS

Complications following postnatal is rare and seen more in teenagers and adults. Postinfectious thrombocytopenia can be seen in about 2 weeks after onset of rash as petechiae or epistaxis, gastrointestinal (GI) bleed, and hematuria. It is usually self-limited. Arthralgia is seen commonly in young women. It begins a week after onset of rash involving small joints of the hand. It is usually self-limiting and resolves within weeks without sequelae.

Encephalitis is the most serious complication. It may occur as:
- Postinfectious encephalitis which is rare and appears within 7 days after onset of rash. It may present with headache, confusion, ataxia, seizure, coma, and focal neurological signs may be seen. Cerebrospinal fluid is usually normal or may show pleocytosis with elevated protein. Recovery is usually complete. However, long-term sequelae have been reported.
- Progressive rubella panencephalitis is a rare complication. Its course is similar to SSPE seen in measles. Death occurs 2–3 years after it onset.

DIAGNOSIS

Rubella immunoglobulin M enzyme assay is most commonly utilized for diagnosis. Caution need to be taken as the positive predictive value of this test decreases in population with low prevalence and in immunized individuals. In these situations, the results should be interpreted in context of history of exposure and clinical findings.

The virus can be isolated form the throat and urine from 1 week before to 2 weeks after onset of rash. CRS is most commonly diagnosed by identification of rubella IgG in serum or oral fluids during early month of life. Polymerase chain reaction (PCR) of amniotic fluid in pregnancy can help in diagnosis of CRS. CRS is also associated with thrombocytopenia, deranged liver function test, anemia, and pleocytosis.

DIFFERENTIAL DIAGNOSIS

Rubella can often be confused with mild scarlet fever; rubeola; infection caused by enterovirus, adenovirus, and parvovirus.

TREATMENT

There is no specific treatment for rubella or CRS. Only symptomatic treatment is required.

PROGNOSIS

Prognosis of childhood rubella is excellent whereas that of CRS depends on the gestational age at infection and organs involved.

PREVENTION

Isolation and standard droplet precaution need to be taken in postnatal infection. The goal of rubella vaccination is to prevent CRS. Vaccine contains attenuated Wistar RA 27/3 strain propagated in human diploid cells. One dose of vaccine provides a seroconversion of >95%. It is administered as a subcutaneous injection in a three-dose schedule as MR/MMR (measles-rubella/measles-mumps-rubella) vaccine at 9 months, 15 months, and at 4–6 years.

CATCHUP VACCINATION

All school-aged children and adolescent should have two doses of MMR vaccine with a minimum interval between two doses of 4 weeks. The vaccine is contraindicated in severely immunocompromised individual and in pregnancy. Pregnancy should be avoided for 3 months after vaccination.

Congenital rubella syndrome is a significant public health issue which can be prevented by vaccination of prepubertal girls with rubella-containing vaccine.

SUGGESTED READING

1. Balasubramanian S, Shastri DD, Shah AK, Chatterjee P, Pemde HK, Shivananda S, et al. IAP Guidebook on Immunization 2018-19, 3rd edition. New Delhi: Jaypee Brothers Medical Publishers, 2020.
2. Edwards MS. (2021). Rubella. [online] Available from: https://www.uptodate.com/contents/rubella. [Last accessed August, 2021].
3. Rubella vaccines: WHO position paper. Wkly Epidemiol Rec. 2011;86(29):301-16.

Varicella and Herpes Zoster

Inder Nathani

GENERAL CONSIDERATIONS

Primary infection with varicella-zoster virus results in varicella, which generally confers life-long immunity, but the virus remains latent lifelong in sensory ganglia. Herpes zoster, which represents reactivation of this latent virus, occurs in 30% of individuals at some time in their life. The incidence of herpes zoster is highest in elderly individuals and in immunosuppressed patients, but herpes zoster occurs in immunocompetent children. Spread of varicella from a close contact is by respiratory secretions or fomites from vesicles or pustules, with an 85% infection rate in susceptible persons. Over 95% of young adults with a history of varicella are immune. Many individuals from tropical or subtropical regions fail to develop varicella in their childhood and remain susceptible through early adulthood. Humans are the only reservoir.

CLINICAL PRESENTATION

The incubation period is 14-16 days (range, 10-21 days). Contact may not be recognized, since the index case of varicella is infectious 1-2 days before rash appears. A prodrome of fever, malaise, respiratory symptoms, and headache may occur, especially in older children for 1-3 days. The unilateral, dermatomal vesicular rash, and pain of herpes zoster are very distinctive. The pre-eruptive pain of herpes zoster may last several days and be mistaken for other illnesses.

SYMPTOMS AND SIGNS

- *Varicella*: The usual case consists of mild systemic symptoms followed by crops of red macules that rapidly become small vesicles with surrounding erythema (described as a *"dew drop on a rose petal"*), form pustules, become crusted, and then scab. Scarring occurs, but it is not common. The rash appears predominantly on the trunk and face. Lesions occur in the scalp, and sometimes in the nose, mouth (where they are nonspecific ulcers), conjunctiva, and vagina. The magnitude of systemic symptoms usually parallels skin involvement. Up to five crops of lesions may be seen. New crops stop forming after 5-7 days. Pruritus is often intense. If varicella occurs in the first few months of life (except for the early postpartum period), it is often mild as a result of transplacentally acquired maternal antibody. Once crusting begins, the patient is no longer contagious. A modified form of varicella occurs in about 15% of vaccinated children exposed to varicella, in spite of receiving a single dose of varicella vaccine. This is usually much milder than typical varicella, with fewer lesions that heal rapidly. Cases of modified varicella are contagious.
- *Herpes zoster (Shingles)*: This eruption involves a single dermatome (thus unilateral and does not cross the midline), usually truncal or cranial, occasionally a contiguous dermatome is involved. Especially in older children, this is preceded by neuropathic pain or itching in the same area (designated the "prodrome"). Ophthalmic zoster may be associated with corneal involvement. The closely grouped vesicles, which resemble a localized version of varicella or herpes simplex, often coalesce. Crusting occurs in 7-10 days.

Postherpetic neuralgia is rare in children. Herpes zoster is a common problem in HIV-infected or other immunocompromised children, and is also common in children who had varicella in early infancy (<1-2 years old) or whose mothers had varicella during pregnancy. Herpes zoster can occur infrequently in children who received the varicella vaccine.

LABORATORY FINDINGS

- *Leukocyte counts* are normal or low. Leukocytosis suggests secondary bacterial infection.
- *Fluorescent antibody staining*: The virus can be identified from the smear taken from lesion.
- *Polymerase chain reaction (PCR)* is definitive, when the etiology is critical, as in immunocompromised children and with atypical disease.
- *Serum aminotransferase* levels may be modestly elevated during typical varicella.

- *Imaging* in varicella pneumonia classically produces numerous bilateral nodular densities and hyperinflation. This is very rare in immunocompetent children, but is seen more frequently in adults and immunocompromised children.

DIFFERENTIAL DIAGNOSIS

- *Coxsackievirus infection*: Fewer lesions, lack of crusting.
- *Impetigo*: Fewer lesions, smaller area, no classic vesicles, positive Gram stain, perioral or peripheral lesions.
- *Papular urticaria*: Insect bite history, nonvesicular rash.
- *Scabies*: Burrows, no typical vesicles, failure to resolve.
- *Parapsoriasis*: Rare in children <10 years, chronic or recurrent, often a history of prior varicella.
- *Rickettsial pox*: Eschar where the mite bites, smaller lesions, no crusting.
- *Dermatitis herpetiformis*: Chronic, urticaria, residual pigmentation, and folliculitis. Herpes zoster is sometimes confused with a linear eruption of herpes simplex or a contact dermatitis, e.g., Rhus dermatitis.

COMPLICATIONS AND SEQUELAE

- *Varicella*:
  - *Secondary bacterial infection* with staphylococci or group A streptococci are most common, presenting as impetigo, cellulitis or fasciitis, abscesses, scarlet fever, or sepsis. Bacterial superinfection occurs in 2–3% of children with varicella.
  - *Neurological complication*—Reye syndrome or encephalitis—because Reye syndrome usually occurs in patients who are also receiving salicylates; these should be avoided in patients with varicella. Encephalitis occurs in <0.1% of cases, usually in the first week of illness, and is usually limited to cerebellitis with ataxia, which resolves completely. Diffuse encephalitis can be severe.
  - *Respiratory complication*: Varicella pneumonia usually afflicts immunocompromised children (especially those receiving high doses of corticosteroids or chemotherapy) and adults; pregnant women are at special risk. Cough, dyspnea, tachypnea, rales, and cyanosis occur several days after the onset of rash.
  - *Gastrointestinal tract (GIT) complication*: Unexplained severe abdominal pain and hepatitis.
  - *Varicella exposure in severely varicella-naïve* immunocompromised *children must be evaluated immediately for* postexposure prophylaxis.
  - *Hemorrhagic varicella* lesions may be seen without other complications. This is most often caused by autoimmune thrombocytopenia, but hemorrhagic lesions can occasionally represent idiopathic disseminated intravascular coagulation (Purpura Fulminans).
  - Neonates born to mothers who develop varicella from 5 days before to 2 days after delivery *are at high risk* for severe or fatal (5%) disease and must be given varicella-zoster immunoglobulin and followed closely. Varicella occurring during the first 20 weeks of pregnancy may cause (2% incidence) congenital infection associated with cicatricial skin lesions, associated limb anomalies, and cortical atrophy.
  - *Unusual complications* of varicella include optic neuritis, myocarditis, transverse myelitis, orchitis, and arthritis.
- *Herpes zoster*:
  - Secondary bacterial infection
  - Motor or cranial nerve paralysis, meningitis, encephalitis, keratitis and other ocular complications, and dissemination in immunosuppressed patients. These complications are rare in immunocompetent children.
  - Postherpetic neuralgia occurs in immunocompromised children, but is rare in immunocompetent children.

PREVENTION

- The infectivity of chicken pox starts 2 days before the skin rash. The children suffering from chicken pox are advised not to attend the school so that the infectivity can be minimum.
- *The Advisory Committee on Vaccines and Immunization Practices (ACVIP) recommendation*: The ACVIP recommends two doses of varicella vaccine.
  - *First dose* to be given at 15th month along with MMR (vaccine against measles, mumps, and rubella) separately.
  - *Second dose* to be given at 4–6 years as a separate or in a combination of MMR-V, quadrivalent vaccine.
  - *Catchup vaccine*: For children not vaccinated at recommended age, the catchup schedule to be started.
- The first dose at first visit and second dose after 3 months (Children below 13 years)
- The first dose at first visit and second dose after 4–8 weeks (Children over 13 years of age).
- *Contraindication of varicella vaccine*: Varicella vaccine is contraindicated in patient of immunodeficiency, symptomatic HIV, high dose of steroids (2 g/kg/d or higher), blood dyscrasias, leukemias, lymphoma, and pregnancy.

TREATMENT

- *General measures*:
  - Supportive measures include maintenance of hydration, administration of acetaminophen for discomfort and cool soaks.

- *Antipruritics for itching*: Diphenhydramine 1.25 mg/kg every 6 hours.
- *Hydroxyzine* 0.5 mg/kg every 6 hours.
- General hygiene measures (keep nails trimmed and skin clean).
- Care must be taken to avoid overdosage with antihistaminic agents. Topical or systemic antibiotics may be needed for bacterial superinfection.

■ *Specific measures*:
  - *Oral acyclovir* (80 mg/kg/d, divided in four doses) on varicella in immunocompetent children was modestly beneficial and to be administered within 24 hours after the onset of varicella. Oral acyclovir should be used selectively in immunocompetent children (e.g., when intercurrent illness is present; possibly when the index case is a sibling or when the patient is an adolescent—both of which are associated with more severe disease) and in children with underlying chronic illnesses.
  - *Parenteral acyclovir* is the preferred drug for varicella and herpes zoster infections. Recommended parenteral acyclovir dosage for severe disease is 10 mg/kg (500 mg/m^2) intravenously every 8 hours, each dose infused over 1 hour, for 7–10 days. Parenteral therapy should be started early in immunocompromised patients or high-risk infected neonates. Hyperimmune globulin is of no value for established disease.
  - *Valacyclovir and famciclovir* are superior antiviral agents because of better absorption; only acyclovir is available as a pediatric suspension. Herpes zoster in an immunocompromised child should be treated with intravenous acyclovir when it is severe, but oral valacyclovir or famciclovir can be used in immunocompromised children when the nature of the underlying illness and the immune status support this decision.

PROGNOSIS

Except for secondary bacterial infections, serious complications are rare and recovery is complete in immunocompetent hosts.

SUGGESTED READING

1. Parthasarathy A. Textbook of Pediatric Infectious Disease, 2nd edition. New Delhi: Jaypee Brothers Medical Publishers; 2019.

CHAPTER 45

Leptospirosis

Inder Nathani

GENERAL CONSIDERATIONS

Leptospirosis is caused by a single family of organisms composed of multiple serotypes of many antigenically distinct but morphologically similar spirochetes; it is one of the most widespread zoonoses in the world. Transmission of infection from animal to human can occur by direct contact with the blood, tissue, organs, or urine of infected animals or indirectly by exposure to an environment that has been contaminated by Leptospires. The organism also can be acquired from soil or from fresh water after ingestion. Reports indicate that leptospirosis is not a rare disease, that many infections are not associated with occupational exposure, and that urban and suburban cases are becoming more prevalent.

Clinical manifestations of leptospirosis usually are not specific. More severe disease manifests as icteric leptospirosis, also known as Weil disease.

CLINICAL FINDINGS

Symptoms and Signs

- *Initial phase*: The incubation period is 4–19 days (mean, 10 days). Chills, fever, headache, myalgia (especially lumbar area and calves), conjunctivitis without exudate, photophobia, cervical lymphadenopathy, and pharyngitis commonly occur. The initial leptospiremic phase lasts for 3–7 days.
- *Phase of apparent recovery*: Symptoms typically (but not always) subside for 2–3 days.
- *Systemic phase*: Fever reappears and is associated with headache, muscular pain, and tenderness in the abdomen and back, and nausea and vomiting. Conjunctivitis and uveitis are common. Lung, heart, and joint involvement occasionally occur. These manifestations are due to extensive vasculitis.
  - *Central nervous system (CNS) involvement*: The CNS is involved in 50–90% of cases. Severe headache and mild nuchal rigidity are usual, but delirium, coma, and focal neurologic signs may be seen.
  - *Renal and hepatic involvement*: In about 50% of cases, the kidney or liver is affected. Gross hematuria and oliguria or anuria is sometimes seen. Jaundice may be associated with an enlarged and tender liver.
  - *Gallbladder involvement*: Leptospirosis may cause acalculous cholecystitis in children, demonstrable by abdominal ultrasound as a dilated, nonfunctioning gallbladder. Pancreatitis is unusual.
  - *Hemorrhage*: Petechiae, ecchymoses, and gastrointestinal bleeding may be severe.
  - *Rash*: A rash is seen in 10–30% of cases. It may be maculopapular and generalized or may be petechial or purpuric. Occasionally erythema nodosum is seen. Peripheral desquamation of the rash may occur.

Indian Leptospirosis Society's criteria: These criteria are good clinical indicators of presence of leptospirosis. Any child presenting with high-grade temperature (>39°C), body ache, and headache with any one or more of the following:
- Jaundice
- Oliguria
- Cough and breathlessness
- Hemorrhagic tendency
- Signs of meningeal irritation or altered sensorium or convulsions.

Laboratory Findings

The *WBC count* often is elevated, especially when there is liver involvement. *Serum bilirubin* levels usually remain below 20 mg/dL. Other liver function tests may be abnormal; the *aspartate transaminase* usually is elevated only slightly. An elevated *serum creatine kinase* is frequently found. *Cerebrospinal fluid (CSF)* shows moderate pleocytosis (<500/μL), predominantly mononuclear cells, increased protein (50–100 mg/dL), and normal glucose. *Urine* often shows microscopic pyuria, hematuria, and, less often, moderate proteinuria (or greater). The *erythrocyte sedimentation rate (ESR)* is elevated markedly. *Chest radiograph* may show pneumonitis.

Serological Tests

- Enzyme-linked immunosorbent assay *(ELISA) IgM antibody testing* (positive from 5th day onward), *IgM-specific dot—ELISA test—*is now clinical recommendation; it

TABLE 1: Modified Faine's criteria 2012.

Part A: Clinical data		Part B: Epidemiological factors	
Questions	Score	Questions	Score
Headache	2	Rainfall	5
Fever	2	Contact with contaminated environment	4
Temperature >39°C	2	Animal contact	1
Conjunctival suffusion	4	Total score	10
Meningism	4	**Part C: Bacteriological and laboratory findings**	
Muscle pain	4	*Isolation of leptospirosis in culture*: PCR	25
Conjunctival suffusion		*Positive serology*	Score
+ Meningism	10	ELISA IgM positive	15
+ Muscle pain		SAT: Positive*	15
Jaundice	1	MAT: Single high titer	15
Albuminuria/nitrogen retention	2	Raising titer (paired sera)	15
Hemoptysis/dyspnea	2	Other rapid test†	15
Total score			

*Any one of the tests only should be scored.
†Latex agglutination test/Lepto Dipstick/Leptotel lateral flow/LeptoTek Dri- Dot-Test
Presumptive diagnosis of Leptospirosis is made Part A or Part A + B: 26 or more
Part A B C (Total): 25 or more
A score between 20 and 25: Possible diagnosis of leptospirosis
(ELISA: enzyme-linked immunosorbent assay; IgM: immunoglobulin M; MAT: microscopic agglutination test; PCR: polymerase chain reaction; SAT: standard agglutination test)

has high sensitivity of >80–90%. Two-to four-fold rise is seen in leptospirosis (positive in second to third week of illness).

- The *slide agglutination test*, Dri Dot assay, and others have good sensitivity up to 85%.
- *Microscopic agglutination test (MAT) titer*: It is not for routine clinical purpose. This is test only available for research laboratory.
- *Polymerase chain reaction (PCR)*: It can be used to detect the leptospirosis in the body fluid during the first week of the disease.

Modified Faine's criteria (with amendment) 2012: The World Health Organization (WHO) has introduced *"Faine's criteria"* for diagnosis of leptospirosis. The criteria is very helpful in presumptive diagnosis of leptospirosis diagnosis in older children **(Table 1)**.

DIFFERENTIAL DIAGNOSIS

During the prodrome, malaria, typhoid fever, typhus, rheumatoid arthritis, brucellosis, and influenza may be suspected. Later, depending on the organ systems involved, a variety of other diseases need to be distinguished, including encephalitis, viral or tuberculous meningitis, viral hepatitis, glomerulonephritis, viral or bacterial pneumonia, rheumatic fever, subacute infective endocarditis, acute surgical abdomen, and Kawasaki disease.

TREATMENT
Specific Measures

Response well to *oral antibiotics* if started before the 7th day of illness.

- *Amoxicillin*: 50–100 mg/kg/day × 7 days
- *Cefixime*: 10 mg/kg/day × 7 days
- *Azithromycin*: 10 mg/kg/day × 3 days
- *Doxycycline*: 5–10 mg/kg/day × 7 days, (avoid below 8 years and pregnancy).

In hospitalized patient: Parental aqueous penicillin G (150,000 U/kg/d, given in four to six divided doses intravenously for 7–10 days). Alternative agents include parenteral cefotaxime and ceftriaxone. A Jarisch–Herxheimer reaction may occur.

General Measures

Symptomatic and supportive care, in addition to antibiotics, is indicated. Contact isolation is due to potential transmission from contact with urine.

PREVENTION

Preventive measures include avoidance of contaminated water and soil, rodent control, immunization of dogs and other domestic animals, and good sanitation. Gloves, boots, and other protective clothing can be worn when contact is unavoidable.

PROGNOSIS

Leptospirosis is usually self-limiting and not characterized by jaundice. The disease usually lasts 1-3 weeks but may be more prolonged. Relapse may occur. The mortality rate is 5%, usually from renal failure.

SUGGESTED READING

1. Bandara K, Weerasekera MM, Gunasekara C, Ranasinghe N, Marasinghe C, Fernando N. Utility of modified Faine's criteria in diagnosis of leptospirosis. BMC Infect Dis. 2016;16(1):446.
2. Faine S. Guidelines for the control of leptospirosis. Geneva: World Health Organization; 1982. p. 67.
3. Parthasarathy A. Textbook of Pediatric Infectious Disease, 2nd edition. New Delhi: Jaypee Brothers Medical Publishers; 2019.

CHAPTER 46: TORCH Infections

Sangeetha Balasubramani, Shamsher S Dalal

INTRODUCTION

Congenital and perinatal infections are often referred to by the acronym TORCH that may cause significant morbidity and mortality in neonates. TORCH stands for the following: Toxoplasmosis; other: syphilis, hepatitis B, varicella zoster virus (VZV), human immunodeficiency virus (HIV), parvovirus B19, enteroviruses, lymphocytic choriomeningitis virus; rubella; cytomegalovirus (CMV) and herpes simplex virus (HSV). Even though the TORCH acronym is well recognized in the field of neonatal/perinatal medicine, it is becoming outdated in view of the growing number of infections listed in the "other" category. However, use of the acronym may aid in remembering the causative organisms.

RISK OF TRANSMISSION

The general principles of TORCH infections are:
- Not all infections in mother are transmitted to baby due to placental barrier and not all infected babies are affected.
- Fetal and neonatal infections occur only with primary infection in the mother whereas latent infection or reactivation affects the baby very infrequently.
- The transmissibility and severity of fetal affection depend on the timing of gestation **(Table 1)**.
- Generally, infection during the first trimester has the most devastating consequences.
- Although identification of immunoglobulin M (IgM) antibodies in the newborn is suggestive of congenital

TABLE 1: Risk of transmission of TORCH infections during pregnancy.

Disease	Risk of transmission
Toxoplasmosis	First trimester: 6%, second trimester: 40%, third trimester: 72%
Rubella	First trimester: 80%, second trimester: 25%, third trimester: 100%. However, risk of congenital rubella syndrome after maternal infection is essentially limited to maternal infection in the first 16 weeks of pregnancy
Syphilis	Risk of fetal transmission is 100% during the primary and secondary stages whereas 10–30% during the latent and tertiary syphilis
Cytomegalovirus (CMV)	Primary maternal infection during pregnancy causes fetal transmission rate of 30–40% in contrast to the 1–2% transmission rate in women infected with CMV prior to pregnancy
Herpes simplex virus	Intrapartum transmission is the most common cause of neonatal infection (90%) and the remaining (10%) from postnatal exposure
Hepatitis B virus	Acute maternal infection during late pregnancy results in up to 90% transmission rate in the absence of any prophylaxis
Varicella zoster virus	The congenital varicella syndrome occurs in approximately 0.4% of infants born to women who have varicella during pregnancy before 13 weeks of gestation and in approximately 2% of infants born to women with varicella between 13 and 20 weeks of gestation. Neonatal varicella is seen when maternal varicella occurs in the 5 days before or 2 days after delivery
Human immuno-deficiency virus (HIV)	Infants born to women with HIV acquire infection from their mother, either during pregnancy, labor/delivery (most of the infection is transmitted in late third trimester or at delivery) or through breastfeeding. Rate of transmission depends upon antenatal antiretroviral therapy (ART) of mothers and mode of feeding. Risk of HIV transmission from mother to infant: • No ARV; breastfeeding: 30–45% • No ART; No breastfeeding: 20–25% • *Triple-drug ART with breastfeeding*: 2% • *Triple-drug ART with no breastfeeding*: 1%

(ARV: antiretroviral)

TABLE 2: Specific clinical features of TORCH infections.

Disease	Specific clinical features
Toxoplasmosis	Classic triad of congenital toxoplasmosis consists of chorioretinitis, hydrocephalus, and intracranial calcifications
Syphilis	• Most neonates with congenital syphilis are asymptomatic at birth. Early congenital syphilis presents in <2 years of age as snuffles, pneumonia alba, and osteochondritis • Late congenital syphilis presents after 2 years of age with signs such as Hutchinson teeth, mulberry molars, hard palate perforation, eighth nerve deafness, interstitial keratitis, bony lesions, and saber shins
Rubella	Clinical manifestations of congenital rubella syndrome include sensorineural deafness, cataracts, cardiac malformations and neurologic and endocrinologic sequelae. The "blueberry muffin" lesions that represent extramedullary hematopoiesis is characteristic of rubella infection
Cytomegalovirus (CMV)	Most infants with congenital CMV are asymptomatic, but approximately 10% have symptoms. Clinical manifestations include petechiae, jaundice at birth, hepatosplenomegaly, thrombocytopenia, small size for gestational age, microcephaly, intracranial calcifications, sensorineural hearing loss, chorioretinitis, and seizures
Herpes simplex virus	The manifestations of neonatal herpes can be classified in three ways: primarily skin, eyes, and mucosal involvement (SEM disease); primarily central nervous system (CNS) disease; and disseminated disease with multiple organ involvement
Human immunodeficiency virus (HIV)	Neonates suspected of having perinatally acquired HIV will be asymptomatic and have normal-for-age lymphocyte counts. As the infection evolves, these infants will present with failure to thrive and various opportunistic infections
Hepatitis B virus (HBV)	The majority of neonates who acquire perinatal HBV infection are asymptomatic and become chronic carriers. Rarely, they may demonstrate signs consistent with hepatitis including jaundice, thrombocytopenia, elevated transaminase concentrations, and rash
Varicella zoster virus (VZV)	In pregnancy, VZV may be transmitted across the placenta, resulting in congenital or neonatal chickenpox. Congenital varicella syndrome is characterized by ophthalmologic malformations, cutaneous scarring, limb hypoplasia and damage to the CNS. If maternal infection and subsequent fetal transmission occur later in gestation, the infant may develop the typical signs of varicella after birth

infection (because IgM antibodies do not cross the placenta), indiscriminate screening for TORCH infections with a battery of "TORCH titers" is costly and has a poor diagnostic yield.

CLINICAL FEATURES

The common manifestations of intrauterine infections are abortions (recurrent only with syphilis), intrauterine death, intrauterine growth retardation (IUGR), prematurity, deafness, chorioretinitis, aseptic meningitis, microcephaly, mental retardation, seizures, lymphadenopathy, maculopapular rash, hepatosplenomegaly, neonatal hepatitis, anemia, thrombocytopenia and skeletal abnormalities. The specific clinical features are enumerated in **Table 2**.

DIAGNOSIS

When a congenital infection is suspected, a thorough maternal history should be obtained, including immunization status and past and recent infections and exposures. A careful physical examination of the neonate is vital because different clinical findings may indicate a specific diagnosis. Diagnostic testing **(Table 3)** should be directed only toward those infections that fit the clinical and historical picture. The sometimes employed TORCH titers should *never* be used as a single test to diagnose or to rule out congenital infections. In addition to organism specific tests laboratory evaluation [complete blood count (CBC), liver function test (LFT)], ophthalmic and hearing evaluation, neurologic evaluation including lumbar puncture and neuroimaging, is to be done in all those suspected of having congenital infections.

MANAGEMENT

Congenital Toxoplasmosis

Congenital toxoplasmosis is treated with pyrimethamine, sulfadiazine, and leucovorin for 1 year. Infants who receive treatment have improved hearing loss, although they remain at risk for recurrent chorioretinitis.

Pyrimethamine 2 mg/kg (maximum 50 mg/dose) once daily for 2 days; then 1 mg/kg (maximum 25 mg/dose) once daily for 6 months; then 1 mg/kg (maximum 25 mg/dose) three times per week (i.e., Monday, Wednesday, and Friday) to complete 1 year of therapy,

plus

Sulfadiazine 100 mg/kg per day divided in two doses every day for 1 year,

plus

Folinic acid (leucovorin) 10 mg three times per week during and for one week after pyrimethamine therapy.

Congenital Rubella

There is no specific therapy for either maternal or congenital rubella infection. Congenital rubella syndrome (CRS) can be prevented by effective immunization of all young girls against rubella.

TABLE 3: Organism specific diagnostic investigation for TORCH infections.

Disease	Investigation	Test of choice
Toxoplasmosis	*Peripheral blood serology*: A positive *Toxoplasma* IgM (after 5 days of life) and/or IgA (after 10 days of life) and increase in anti-*Toxoplasma* IgG titers during the first year of life	Isolation of organism from the placenta, serum and cerebrospinal fluid by PCR
Syphilis	Nontreponemal tests such as the VDRL and rapid plasma reagin (RPR) are used for screening and monitoring treatment of the disease	Demonstration of spirochetes under dark-field examination or direct fluorescent antibody (DFA) in fluid from a lesion, CSF, the placenta, or the umbilical cord
Rubella	Detection of rubella specific IgM. Persistently elevated or rising IgG titers	Isolation of rubella virus from certain body fluids, including blood, urine, CSF, and oral and nasal secretions
Cytomegalovirus (CMV)	Antibodies are not useful in diagnosing congenital CMV because assays for IgM have poor sensitivity and specificity	Demonstration of the virus in body fluids such as urine or saliva in the first 3 weeks after birth by PCR or spin enhanced culture (After 3 weeks of age, it is difficult to determine whether the infection was congenital or postnatal)
Herpes simplex virus (HSV)	Serology (HSV IgM) can be done but not all infants seroconvert at the time of presentation	Isolation of HSV from skin lesions, blood or CSF by PCR or culture or detection of viral antigens using rapid direct immunofluorescence assays
Varicella zoster virus (VZV)	Diagnosis of neonatal varicella is usually made clinically. Test for VZV-specific antibodies is confounded by the presence of maternal antibodies. DFA on scrapings from active vesicular skin lesions can provide a rapid diagnosis	PCR is the test of choice for diagnosis of neonatal varicella because it is highly sensitive and specific
Human immunodeficiency virus (HIV)	Nucleic acid amplification tests (NATs) for HIV at birth. If negative, repeat after 4–6 weeks. Infants who are positive for HIV RNA or HIV DNA in the first 3 days of life are considered to have been infected *in utero*; infants who test negative in the first 3 days and positive for HIV thereafter are considered to have peripartum-acquired HIV	
Hepatitis B virus	HBsAg on peripheral venous blood sampling to diagnose intrauterine infection; check infant after age 9 months for anti-HBs and HBsAg	

(anti-HBs: antibodies against hepatitis B surface antigen; CSF: cerebrospinal fluid; HBsAg: hepatitis B surface antigen; Ig: immunoglobulin; PCR: polymerase chain reaction; RNA: ribonucleic acid; VDRL: venereal disease research laboratory)

Congenital CMV

All infants with symptomatic CMV disease should be started on antiviral treatment with valganciclovir as early as possible because efficacy of initiating treatment at more than 1 month of age in symptomatic infants is not known.

Valganciclovir: Dose 16 mg/kg/dose or all twice daily for 6 months. Monitor CBC and LFT during therapy.

Congenital Syphilis

The treatment approach for newborn with congenital syphilis must be made on the basis of (1) identification of syphilis in the mother; (2) adequacy of maternal treatment; (3) presence of clinical, laboratory, or radiographic evidence of syphilis in the neonate; and (4) comparison of maternal (at delivery) and neonatal nontreponemal serologic titers using the same test, preferably conducted by the same laboratory **(Flowchart 1).**

The recommended evaluation for proven and possible congenital syphilis is:
- Cerebrospinal fluid (CSF) analysis for venereal disease research laboratory test (VDRL), cell count, and protein
- Complete blood count (CBC) with differential and platelet count
- Other tests as clinically indicated (e.g., long-bone radiographs, chest radiograph, LFTs, neuroimaging, ophthalmologic examination, and auditory brain stem response).

Perinatally Acquired HSV

The preferred treatment for neonatal herpes infection is intravenous (IV) acyclovir. Treatment with acyclovir improves mortality and neurodevelopmental outcome.
- *Skin, eyes, and mouth (SEM) disease*: IV Acyclovir 20 mg/kg/dose 8 hourly for 14 days
- *Disseminated disease*: IV acyclovir to be given for 21 days
- *Central nervous system infection*: IV acyclovir to be continued till CSF PCR becomes negative

Perinatal HBV

Infants born to HBsAg-positive mothers should receive HBV vaccine and hepatitis B immunoglobulin at birth.

Perinatal HIV

HIV-infected pregnant women should receive antiretroviral therapy (ART), a triple drug regimen as soon as possible to decrease the rate of vertical transmission from 40 to <2%.

Flowchart 1: Treatment approach for newborn with congenital syphilis.

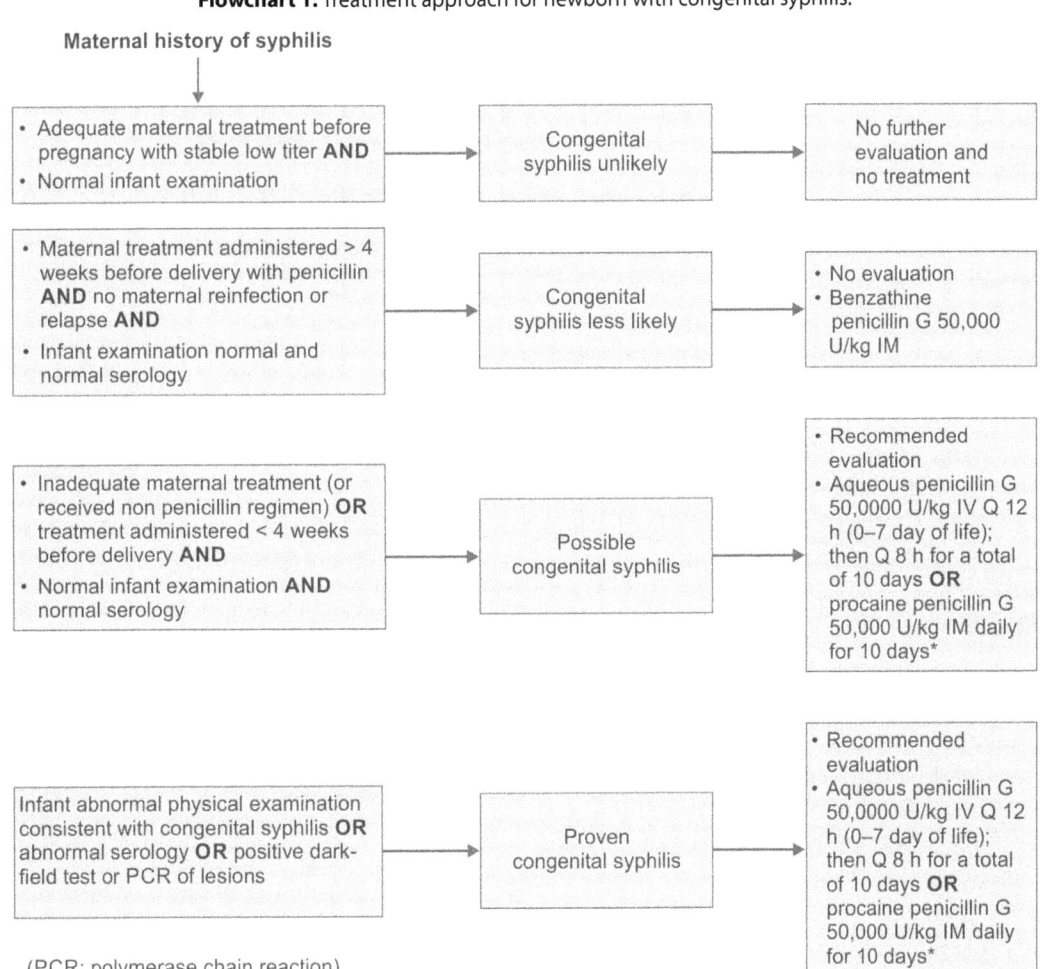

(PCR: polymerase chain reaction)

*Single dose of Penicillin G benzathine can be given if recommended evaluation is normal and follow-up is certain.

TABLE 4: Recommended ARV prophylaxis for HIV-exposed infants.

Infants birth weight	NVP daily dose	AZT daily dose	Duration
Birth weight < 2,000 g	2 mg/kg once daily	5 mg/dose twice daily	• Up to minimum of 6 weeks of age regardless of whether exclusively breastfed or exclusively replacement fed • Extended to 12 weeks, if the duration of ART received by the mother is <4 weeks and she is breastfeeding
Birth weight 2,000–2,500 g	10 mg once daily	10 mg/dose twice daily	
Birth weight > 2500 g	15 mg once daily	15 mg/dose twice daily	

(ARV: antiretroviral; ART: antiretroviral therapy; AZT: azidothymidine; NVP: nevirapine)

Elective LSCS to be planned if the HIV viral load remains >1,000 copies/mL. Mothers should be continued on lifelong ART, regardless of CD4 count and clinical stage. All infants born to HIV-positive mothers should undergo nucleic acid testing (NAT) for HIV infection and should be started on antiretroviral (ARV) prophylaxis with nevirapine (NVP) immediately after birth **(Table 4)**. Syrup azidothymidine (AZT) to be started in place of NVP if mother is infected with HIV-2 as NVP is not effective against HIV-2. At 6 weeks, perform DNA PCR for baby. If DNA PCR is positive, initiate ART (AZT/ABC + 3TC + LPV/r). If DNA PCR is negative, the child has to be followed up at 6 months for rapid antibody test and subsequently DNA PCR (if necessary). Infant to be started on ART if found to be positive. Exclusive breastfeeding for first 6 months of life is recommended; however, choice of breastfeeding should be the decision of woman based on proper information and counseling which should begin during the antenatal period itself. Breastfeeding with concurrent ARV intervention offers HIV-exposed infants the greatest chance of HIV-free survival and is the recommended feeding strategy for them in India.

Cotrimoxazole Preventive Therapy

Cotrimoxazole preventive therapy (CPT) to be initiated for all HIV exposed babies from 6 weeks of age and continued until HIV infection has been reliably excluded by a negative antibody test at 18 months or later if still being breastfed, regardless of ARV initiation. In case the baby is found to be HIV infected at any stage, ART should be initiated and CPT should be continued until 5 years of age.

Congenital/Perinatal Varicella

Pregnant women who are exposed to varicella can be given prophylactic varicella zoster immunoglobulin (VZIg) and those who develop varicella, to be treated with acyclovir. Infants born with congenital varicella are unlikely to have active viral disease, so antiviral therapy is not indicated. Onset of varicella in pregnant women from 5 days before to 2 days after delivery is associated with severe varicella infection in neonates with high risk of mortality. Administration of VZIg to these newborns decreases the rate of complications and fatal outcomes. Neonates who develop active lesions of varicella should be treated with acyclovir.

KEY MESSAGES

- Congenital CMV infection is the most common congenital infection and a leading cause of nonhereditary sensorineural hearing loss.
- Perinatally acquired HSV infection is associated with a high risk of neonatal death and lifelong disabilities, yet the disease can be considerably ameliorated with early use of acyclovir in suspected cases.
- Pediatric HIV-1 infections have been markedly reduced through the use of maternal and/or infant ARV treatment.
- Rubella infection essentially in the first 16 weeks of pregnancy can be catastrophic, resulting in spontaneous abortion, stillbirth, congenital defects and IUGR.

SUGGESTED READING

1. American Academy of Pediatrics, Committee on Infectious Diseases. In: Kimberlin DW, Brady MT, Jackson MA, Long SS. Red Book: 2015 Report of the Committee on Infectious Diseases, 30th edition. Elk Grove Village, IL: American Academy of Pediatrics; 2015.
2. American Academy of Pediatrics. Toxoplasmosis. In: Kimberlin DW, Brady MT, Jackson MA, Long SS. Red Book: 2015 Report of the Committee on Infectious Diseases, 30th edition. Elk Grove Village, IL: American Academy of Pediatrics; 2015:787-95.
3. Kimberlin DW, Baley J; Committee on Infectious Diseases, Committee on Fetus and Newborn. Guidance on management of asymptomatic neonates born to women with active genital herpes lesions. Pediatrics. 2013;131(2):e635-45.
4. Kimberlin DW, Jester PM, Sánchez PJ, Ahmed A, Arav-Boger R, Michaels MG, et al. Valganciclovir for symptomatic congenital cytomegalovirus disease. N Engl J Med. 2015;372(10):933-43.
5. National AIDS Control Organization. (2018). National Technical Guidelines on Antiretroviral Treatment. [online] Available from: https://lms.naco.gov.in/frontend/content/NACO%20-%20National%20Technical%20Guidelines%20on%20ART_October%202018%20(1).pdf. [Last accessed August, 2021].
6. Panel on Antiretroviral Therapy and Medical Management of HIV-Infected Children. (2020). Guidelines for the use of antiretroviral agents in pediatric HIV infection. [online] Available from: https://clinicalinfo.hiv.gov/en/guidelines/pediatric-arv/whats-new-guidelines. [Last accessed August, 2021].

Rickettsial Diseases

Atul Kulkarni, Ashutosh V Yajurvedi

INTRODUCTION

- Rickettsial diseases have gained attention of the clinicians as one of the re-emerging infections. Once thought to be the disease during the wars or the disease of rural population, because of sociodemographic changes, it is not uncommon to see it in urban population as well.
- Rickettsial diseases are group of infections caused by a family of organisms belonging to genus *Rickettsia* within family Rickettsiaceae in order Rickettsiales which are nonmotile, nonspore-forming, highly pleomorphic, obligate intracellular organisms.
- These are arthropod-borne disease transmitted by variety of vectors such as ticks (most common), lice, flea or mites and rodents, dogs, mice, cattle are mammalian reservoirs. Humans are accidental hosts.
- Even though the cases can be seen throughout the year, a surge in number of cases can be seen immediately post rains due to increase in grass.
- The Rickettsial diseases are classified into various groups **(Table 1)**. Out of this extensive list of Rickettsial infections, scrub typhus is most common in India followed by Indian tick typhus and murine typhus.

CLINICAL MANIFESTATIONS

- Symptoms may vary from mild self-limiting illness to life-threatening illness.
- Most common presentation in initial period is non-specific acute febrile illness often associated with anorexia, excruciating headache, myalgia, and arthralgia. Irritability is seen in younger children who cannot speak as a manifestation of headache/myalgia/arthralgia. Fever is usually high grade and is associated with chills.
- The median incubation period is 7 days with range of 2–14 days, rarely up to 28 days.
- Many times, there is a history of travel to the endemic area or contact with domestic animals which carry the vectors.

TABLE 1: Classification of rickettsial infections.

Disease	Rickettsial agent	Insect vector	Mammalian reservoir
Typhus group			
• Epidemic typhus	R. prowazekii	Louse	Humans
• Murine typhus	R. typhi	Flea	Rodent
Scrub typhus	R. tsutsugamushi	Mite	Rodent
Spotted fever group*			
• Indian tick typhus	R. conorii	Tick	Dog/rodents
• Rocky mountain spotted fever	R. rickettsii	Tick	Dogs/rodents
Others			
• Rickettsial pox	R. akari	Mite	Mice
• Q fever	C. burnetii	Nill	Cattle sheep goat
• Trench fever	Rochalimaea quintana	Louse	Humans
• Ehrlichioses	Ehrlichia	Tick	Deer/dog
• Anaplasmosis	Anaplasma phagocytophilum	Tick	Deer/dog

*More than 19 types of spotted fever varieties are described depending upon the geographical area where these are prevelent.
(C.: coxiella; R.: rickettsia)

- Rash which is a part of triad of rickettsial diseases consisting of fever and headache, usually develops 3–5 days after the onset of fever. Rash which is considered to be characteristic finding evolves over the time. To start with, it is a pale rose red blanching discrete macule which becomes petechial or hemorrhagic with advancement in disease. At times, rash can be palpable purpura.
- The frequency of finding rash in different types of rickettsial diseases is different. Almost all cases (90%) of Indian tick typhus have the rash while chances of finding rash in scrub typhus is 40–50%. This is due to transient nature of rash in scrub typhus which is difficult to appreciate in dark skin complexion of Indian population in initial phase of illness. The rarity of the rash in murine typhus is due to the very late appearance almost 10–12 days after the onset of illness by the time usually child is put on treatment and goes into recovery.
- The pathognomonic finding in rickettsial infections is eschar. It is more commonly seen in scrub typhus than spotted fever group. It is single, crusty necrotic, nonpruritic, painless lesion with or without erythematous halo associated with the regional lymphadenopathy. It looks like a cigarette burn and denotes the site of bite of vector. The most common regions are inguinal folds, buttocks, axillae, below the breast and head–neck region. Unless actively search for, there are high chances of missing it.
- Organomegaly, edema of hands and feet, periorbital edema, conjunctival hyperemia are some other manifestations.

COMPLICATIONS

- Generalized vasculitis leading to multiple organ involvement is the cause of complication. Most of the complications are seen after the first week of illness. They occur due to delayed diagnosis and institution of the treatment.
- The complications include meningoencephalitis, pericarditis, myocarditis, nephritis/acute kidney injury (AKI), pneumonitis, acute respiratory distress syndrome (ARDS), liver involvement in a form of elevated transaminases.
- Other complications include sensorineural hearing loss, hemophagocytic lymphohistiocytosis, purpura fulminans and gangrene of digits, ear lobes, buttocks, and scrotum. Gangrene of digits and ear lobe may progress to autoamputation.
- Rickettsial diseases sometimes may progress to disseminated intravascular coagulation (DIC) and shock leading to death.

DIAGNOSIS

- Rickettsial diseases in initial period have nonspecific clinical findings. Also, the available diagnostic tests lack specificity and sensitivity in this period.
- A rapid diagnosis and institution of the right treatment early in course of the illness has lot of bearing on prognosis as delayed diagnosis/treatment is synonymous with sinister complications. A diagnosis of rickettsial infection should be suspected in any acute febrile illness and one or more of the following within 14 days of onset of illness.
- Tick/mite bites or seen on clothes.
- Visit to areas such as high uncut grass or weeds or bushes or rice fields or woodlands (where rodents share habitats with animals) or grassy lawns or river banks or poorly maintained kitchen gardens which are common habitats of vectors.
- Pet animals and cattle at home.
- Residence/visit to endemic area.
- Similar cases in family members/neighborhood.
- Symptoms in the form of fever with rash, edema, headache and myalgia, hepatosplenomegaly and/or lymphadenopathy, cough and pulmonary infiltrates or community-acquired pneumonia, acute kidney injury, acute gastrointestinal or hepatic involvement.

LABORATORY DIAGNOSIS

- No single laboratory test is highly specific or sensitive to rule in or rule out the rickettsial infection in early phases. Laboratory tests such as Weil–Felix or enzyme-linked immunosorbent assay (ELISA) when turns out to be positive in a suspected case increases the probability of infection highly possible. The confirmation of the disease needs detection of rickettsial DNA either by polymerase chain reaction (PCR) or immunofluorescence assay (IFA) which is said to be gold standard. Clinicians must be aware about the inherent advantages and disadvantages of the available serological tests.
- *Weil–Felix test*:
  - It is easily available, simple, and cheap heterophile agglutination test, the results of which are available rapidly but lacks sensitivity and specificity.
  - The principle behind the test is antigenic cross-reactivity between species of *Rickettsia* with certain serotypes of nonmotile *Proteus* species.
  - Test uses OX2 and 19 antigen of *Proteus vulgaris* and OX K of *P. mirabilis*.
  - Type of specific rickettsial disease is suspected depending on agglutination with these antigens of *Proteus* species which is summarized in **Table 2**.
  - Local titer must be defined. Rising titer is more important than single value.
  - Thus, diagnosis is retrospective which is another disadvantage.
  - The result must be considered significant after considering the clinicoepidemiological settings.

TABLE 2: Differentiating rickettsial infections by Weil–Felix test.			
	Weil–Felix test		
Disease	**OX19**	**OX2**	**OX K**
Epidemic typhus	++	+/–	–
Endemic typhus	++	–	–
Scrub typhus	–	–	++
RMSF	+	+	–
Rickettsial pox	–	–	–
Q fever	–	–	–

(RMSF: rocky mountain spotted fever)

- *ELISA*:
  - It has better sensitivity and specificity. Strain-specific IgM ELISA testing is the choice of test.
  - Optical density value of 0.5 is taken as cutoff. Region-specific cutoffs need to be defined.
  - There is a certain time lag before the test becomes positive making it disadvantageous for early diagnosis.
  - Another drawback of the test it being expensive.
- *IFA*:
  - IFA is considered as a gold standard for diagnosis of rickettsial infection.
  - Disadvantage being is unaffordable cost, dearth of availability, and technically challenging nature of the test makes it difficult to integrate in routine clinical practice as a test of the choice. Also, the titer start rising after 5-10 days after the infection reaching peak at 3-4 weeks.
  - Indirect immunoperoxidase assay (IPA): This is similar to IFA in terms of sensitivity, specificity, and disadvantages.
- *PCR*:
  - It is the test of choice during the first week of illness, even before the seroconversion has occurred and even after the treatment.
  - PCR can be done over cerebrospinal fluid (CSF) or eschar apart from the blood thus expanding the possibility of diagnosis.
  - It is highly specific and sensitive.
  - The rapidity, reproducibility, quantitative capability, and low risk of contamination are other advantages.
  - But only handful research centers can perform this making it a major disadvantage.
- *Simple laboratory indicators*: Total leukocyte count can be normal or low with shift to left in initial phases which later with progression in disease becomes leukocytosis. Anemia and thrombocytopenia are also seen. Other nonspecific findings are: Hypoalbuminemia, elevated transaminases and acute phase reactants such as erythrocyte sedimentation rate (ESR) and c-reactive protein (CRP). Pleocytosis in CSF is seen in children with meningoencephalitis, (10-300 cells/μL) with raised albumin (200 mg/dL).

MANAGEMENT

- As delayed initiating of treatment means a significant morbidity and mortality. Thus, early institution of treatment is key to successful management of any child with rickettsial infections.
- Antibiotics are the mainstay of the treatment along with symptomatic care.
  - Doxycycline is the drug of the choice. There are no adverse effects including the tooth staining at the recommended dose and duration, and should not cause any confusion in the pediatricians.
  - The response to doxycycline is dramatic with defervescence of fever occurring in 48 hours. Failure of such response should alert clinician to think about alternate diagnosis though slower response can be expected in children in whom treatment has been started late in course of illness or children with severe illness with multiorgan involvement.
  - Alternately it may suggest resistance to doxycycline where alternate drugs can be started.
  - Chloramphenicol is the alternate drug most commonly used when the child is allergic to doxycycline. On rare occasions, there can be bone marrow depression.
  - Other alternatives are azithromycin and clarithromycin. Fluoroquinolones are not used in pediatric population. The various recommended anti-rickettsial drugs with their dosage, route of administration, and duration have been summarized in **Table 3**.
- Other supportive measures such as paracetamol and adequate hydration should be taken care of. Therapy must be initiated immediately based on high index of suspicion in appropriate clinicoepidemiological setting and consistent laboratory findings. Treatment should never be delayed while pending primary laboratory results.

Treatment of Complications

At the immediate onset of complications, child should be referred to tertiary care center which are skilled and well equipped to take care of these children.

- *Meningoencephalitis*: Apart from routine care, management of airway, breathing circulation, control of seizures with appropriate antiepileptic drugs (AEDs) is required.

Anticerebral edema measures such as hypertonic saline/mannitol needs to be started. Mechanical ventilation may be required in some which can also help in reducing

TABLE 3: Summary of anti-rickettsial drugs.

Drug	Dose, route, and administration	Comments
Doxycycline	2.2 mg/kg/dose BD per oral or IV (maximum 200 mg) 5–7 days or for at least 3 days until the patient is afebrile	• Drug of choice • Rapid defervesce within 48 hours • IV formulation for sick patients
Tetracycline	25–50 mg/kg/dose every 6 hourly per oral (Max 2 gm/day) 5 to 7 days or for at least 3 days until the patient is afebrile 48 hours	• Rapid defervescence within • IV formulation for sick patients
Chloramphenicol	50–100 mg/kg/day every 6 hourly, (Max 3 g/day), 5–7 days or for at least 3 days until the patient is afebrile	• Most common alternative for tetracycline • Most common adverse effect is agranulocytosis
Azithromycin	10 mg/kg/day once daily (maximum 500 mg) 5–7 days or for at least 3 days until the patient is afebrile	• Preferred drug in pregnancy • Recommended when doxycycline resistance is present
Clarithromycin	15 mg/kg/day BD, 5–7 days or for at least 3 days until the patient is afebrile	–
Rifampicin	10 mg/kg, maximum is 300 mg, 5–7 days or for at least 3 days until the patient is afebrile	• Doxycycline resistance cases • Shorter duration of fever with rifampicin in northern Thailand when compared with doxycycline
Fluoroquinolone	–	Not recommended in pediatric age group

cerebral edema. While some authors advocate use of steroids considering the pathology being vasculitis, but the data supporting such practices is lacking.

Pulmonary edema/ARDS can occur due to taxing of already damaged pulmonary vasculature with inadvertent fluid management. Tight input and output balance along with restricted fluids is the strategy. Start with supplemental oxygen. With worsening respiratory status, child may require noninvasive or mechanical ventilation. Lung-protective strategies in a form of smaller tidal volumes and optimum positive end-expiratory pressure (PEEP) should be used. Appropriate antibiotics to cover organisms causing community-acquired pneumonia is warranted.

- Acute kidney injury (AKI) can be treated with fluid restriction or resuscitation depending on the type of AKI. Child may need diuretics as well as peritoneal or hemodialysis.
- Myocarditis does not have any specific management apart from fluid restriction, diuretics, and inotropes. The role of steroids/intravenous immunoglobulin (IVIg) is controversial.
- Multiorgan failure/DIC is one of the dreaded complications. Child is treated like a septic shock with fluids and inotropes/pressors. It is important to note that child should receive a broad-spectrum antibiotic after sending blood culture. Provide other supportive measures such as maintenance of electrolytes, euglycemia, and fluid status. Various blood products such as packed cells, fresh frozen plasma (FFP), and platelet concentrates may be required as per the blood picture and clinical condition. Gangrene of digits, earlobes, digits, buttocks, and scrotum can be managed with low molecular weight heparin.

PREVENTION

- No vaccine is available. No role of postexposure prophylaxis. Mainstay of prevention is control of the vector through controlling the rodents, chopping or burning the vegetations, and spraying of insecticides.
- Prevention of vector bite by avoidance of visit to endemic area, using long-sleeved light-colored cloths sprayed with insecticides, tucking pants inside the shoes and regularly inspecting the cloths for ticks.
- Prompt removal of ticks using tweezers as contact period of minimum 4 hours is needed before ticks can transmit the infection.

PROGNOSIS

The most important determinant of all the prognostic factors is early diagnosis and treatment as delayed diagnosis and treatment invariably leads to complication, death or long-term sequelae.

Other markers of poor prognosis are:

- Younger age
- Male gender
- Shorter incubation period
- Absence of rash
- Comorbidities such as diabetes, cardiovascular disease, glucose-6-phosphate dehydrogenase (G6PD) deficiency
- Treatment with sulfonamides.

KEY MESSAGES

- Rickettsial infections are important re-emerging infections.
- Triad of fever, rash, and headache is the common presenting symptom.
- With high index of suspicion in an ease of nonspecific acute febrile illness with possibility of vector exposure in light or supportive laboratory evidences, rickettsial infections can be diagnosed even in early phases of illness.
- All the serological tests should usually be carried out in second week of illness and interpreted in a light of clinic epidemiological background.
- Drug of choice for rickettsial infections, irrespective of the age, is doxycycline.

SUGGESTED READING

1. Biggs HM, Behravesh CB, Bradley KK, Dahlgren FS, Drexler NA, Dumler JS, et al. Diagnosis and management of tickborne rickettsial diseases. CDC MMWR Recomm Rep. 2016;65:1-44.
2. Dasari V, Kaur P, Murhekar MV. Rickettsial disease outbreaks in India: a review. Ann Trop Med Public Health. 2014;7(6):249-54.
3. Kulkarni A. Childhood rickettsiosis. Indian J Pediatr. 2011;78:81-7.
4. Kulkarni A. Rickettsial infections. IAP textbook of infectious diseases, 1st edition. New Delhi: Jaypee Brothers Medical Publishers; 2013. pp. 376-85.
5. Mahajan SK. Rickettsial diseases. J Assoc Physicians India. 2012: 60:37-43.
6. Martinez JJ, Cossart P. Early signaling events involved in the entry of Rickettsia conorii into mammalian cells. J Cell Sci. 2004;117(Pt 21):5097-106.
7. Paul ML, Ross MJ. Rickettsial and Ehrlichial Diseases. In: Cherry J, Demmler-Harrison GJ, Kaplan SL, Steinbach W, Hotez P. Feigin and Cherry's Textbook of Pediatric infectious Diseases, 7th edition. New York: Saunders Elsevier; 2013. pp. 2647-66.e4.
8. Prakash JA, Sohan LT, Rosemol V, Verghese VP, Pulimood SA, Reller M. Molecular detection and analysis of spotted fever group Rickettsia in patients with fever and rash at a tertiary care centre in Tamil Nadu, India. Pathog Glob Health. 2012;106:40-5.
9. Rahi M, Gupte MD, Bhargava A, Varghese GM, Arora R. Guidelines for diagnosis and management of rickettsial diseases in India. Indian J Med Res. 2015;141(4):417-22.
10. Rathi N, Kulkarni A, Yewale V. IAP guidelines on rickettsial diseases in children. Indian Pediatrics. 2017;54(3):223-9.
11. Rathi N, Maheshwari M, Khandelwal R. Neurological manifestations of rickettsial infections in children. Pediatric infectious Disease. 2016;7:64-6.
12. Rathi N, Rathi A. Rickettsial infections: Indian perspective. Indian Pediatr. 2010;47:157-64.
13. Todd SR, Dahlgren FS, Traeger MS, Beltran-Aguilar ED, Marianos DW, Hamilton C, et al. No visible denial staining in children treated with doxycycline for suspected Rocky Mountain spotted fever. J Pediatr. 2015;166:1246-51.
14. Vaidya S, Kulkarni A, Kulkarni P, Bidri LH, Padwal S. Rickettsial disease-an experience. Pediatr Infect Dis. 2009;1:118-24.

CHAPTER 48: Malaria

AK Rawat

INTRODUCTION

Malaria is an endemic disease in most parts of country with some seasonal variation. It continues to remain an important public health problem with high morbidity and mortality because *Plasmodium falciparum* occurs more commonly. Still malaria is curable with early diagnosis and effective complete treatment. The National plan is to eliminate malaria by 2030. More serious and rapidly deteriorating cases are seen in young age because of their low immunity.

DIAGNOSIS

Clinical diagnosis of malaria has poor accuracy, hence, parasitological confirmation within 1 hour as presumptive treatment is not recommended.

Patency Level of Malaria Parasite Density

Patency level of malaria parasite density for diagnosis by:
- Quality-assured microscopy of peripheral blood film ≥50 parasites/µL
- Quality-assured rapid diagnostic test (RDT) (antigen) ≥200 parasites/µL.

It is possible that malaria parasite density is <50/µL, will be below patency level for microscopy; patients may be suffering from malaria but parasite cannot be detected. To prevent missing such a case, a peripheral smear (PS) for microscopy should be repeated every 12–24 hours for a total of three sets and if all three sets are negative only then diagnosis of malaria can be ruled out.

CLINICAL SUSPICION OF MALARIA

Clinical features of malaria are nonspecific, e.g., fever, chills, rigors, pallor, enlargement of spleen, and gastrointestinal, respiratory or neurological manifestations.

Severe complicated malaria: The World Health Organization (WHO) criteria:
- Impaired consciousness
- Prostration
- Respiratory distress
- Multiple seizures
- Jaundice (serum bilirubin > 3 mg%)
- Hemoglobinuria
- Bleeding
- Severe anemia (Hb < 5 g%)
- Circulatory collapse
- Pulmonary edema.

Additional features of severe malaria:
- Hypoglycemia (blood glucose < 40 mg/dL)
- Parasite density > 5% of RBC
- Parasite count > 10,000/µL
- Serum creatinine > 3 mg/dL.

DIFFERENTIAL DIAGNOSIS

Influenza, hepatitis, sepsis, pneumonia, meningoencephalitis, endocarditis, gastroenteritis, pyelonephritis, brucellosis, leptospirosis, tuberculosis, typhoid, neoplasm, amoebic liver abscess and collagen vascular diseases.

MANAGEMENT

In the first hour of management, stabilize patient, treat complications and arrive at parasitological diagnosis by peripheral blood smear microscopy and/or antigen-based RDT. Next step of treatment depends on species of parasite and complications.

Classifications of malaria for management:
- Uncomplicated malaria:
  - *P. vivax*
  - *P. falciparum*
  - Mixed infection (*P. vivax* and *P. falciparum*)
- Complicated malaria:
  - *P. vivax*
  - *P. falciparum*
  - Mixed infection

Uncomplicated malaria:
- Uncomplicated *P. vivax*: Chloroquine for 3 days and primaquine for 14 days.
- Uncomplicated *P. falciparum*: Artemisinin combination therapy (ACT)—oral for 3 days and primaquine for 1 day.
- Uncomplicated mixed infection: ACT oral for 3 days and primaquine for 14 days.

Complicated malaria: P. vivax, P. falciparum, and mixed infection:
- Injection artesunate followed by oral ACT.
- Primaquine for 1 day in *P. falciparum* and for 14 days in *P. vivax* infection.
- *Quinine*: It remains drug of choice during pregnancy, children weighing < 5 kg, and for treatment of failure.

Confirm recovery: Not only clinical but parasitological recovery by quality-assured microscopy of PS after day 7 and 28 days.

Special precautions: P. malaria and *P. ovale* are rarely seen but still they are seen occasionally in Madhaya Pradesh Chhattisgarh.

SUGGESTED READING

1. Kliegman RM, St. Geme J. Nelsons Textbook of Pediatrics, 21st edition. Canada: Elsevier; 2020.
2. NVBDCP, DGHS, MoHFW, GoI. National strategic plan: Malaria elimination in India: 2017-2022. [online] Available from: http://www.indiaenvironmentportal.org.in/files/file/nsp_2017-2022-updated.pdf. [Last accessed September, 2021].
3. World Health Organization. Guidelines for the treatment of Malaria, 3rd edition. Geneva: World Health Organization; 2015.

CHAPTER 49

Tuberculosis

DY Shrikhande

INTRODUCTION

The disease caused by *Mycobacterium tuberculosis* and its variants has been the scourge of mankind since ancient times and continues to rage in the world population, with deaths several times that of the new entrant COVID-19. The bacterium was identified by Robert Koch on 24 March 1882. Its planned elimination from this world by 2025 for now looks like a distant dream, though the World Health Organization (WHO) and the National Tuberculosis Elimination Programme (NTEP) have this as their objective.

CAUSATIVE ORGANISM

Mycobacterium tuberculosis is weakly gram positive, acid-fast bacillus (AFB), filamentous with a strong lipid-rich wall, resisting penetration by various drugs. Majority of human infections are by *M. tuberculosis hominis*, other subspecies being *M. tuberculosis bovis* and *M. tuberculosis africanus*. Other mycobacteria may also cause disease in immunocompromised individuals and some are commensals.

PATHOGENESIS

Portal of entry is from respiratory tract into lungs in 98% of cases, other being gastrointestinal tract (GIT), skin, or liver (in perinatal period). When the bacterium enters the lungs through droplets, it is engulfed by the alveolar macrophages in the lung parenchyma. The macrophage is unable to neutralize the bacteria which continue to multiply intracellularly and are taken to various organs where seeding occurs. Here granulomas form with macrophages transforming into a boundary wall of epithelioid cells, Langhans giant cells, and lymphocytic infiltration occurs, with the center of the tubercular granuloma showing caseous necrosis. Cellular immune mechanisms come into play and cell-mediated immunity (CMI) develops. If the immunity is good [T-helper (TH) 1 response] the lesions are well contained and majority are destroyed. In case of TH 2 response and poor TH1 response, flare-up of lesions locally or in distant disseminated places takes place. Invasion of the lymphatics and bloodstream with showers of infected emboli may take place leading to miliary tuberculosis (TB). Extrapulmonary TB manifestations may occur as part of the miliary dissemination or flare-up of the distant lesions seeding which had taken place initially.

CLINICAL FEATURES

These are varied and dependent on various factors such as duration and closeness of contact with an open case, the child's own immune status, nutritional state, and any other debilitating conditions which may lower immunity such as measles, pertussis, and HIV.

RISK FACTORS FOR TB INFECTION AND DISEASE IN CHILDREN

Tuberculosis if seen early is likely to be progressive tuberculosis.

Wallgren's Timetable of TB

After the primary infection, dissemination, sensitization, and flare-up or reactivation may occur at any or many foci, especially in low-immunity states, at any time. However, the reactivation in various organs occurs in a certain pattern and timing usually. Hence, Wallgren after observation devised a "timetable" for the appearance of TB in various organs **(Table 1)**. In general, complications occur within 2 years. Tubercular disease >1 year after primary infection is usually due to reactivation.

TABLE 1: Wallgren's timetable of TB.

Event	Conversion time
Mantoux conversion	8–12 weeks
Miliary tuberculosis	2–6 months
Lymph node and endobronchial tuberculosis	3–9 months
Bone and joint disease	1 year
Renal disease	5–15 years
Suprarenal disease	>15 years

No organ is spared by TB but predilection for lungs and some other organs is more; the likely timing of their involvement is what is predicted by Walgreen.

Pulmonary TB

Often mild infection, may go undetected sometimes presents as just a mild fever, dry cough, sometimes just failure to gain weight or loss of weight and failure to thrive, may at times take a turn for the worse and result in rise of fever, productive cough, suggestive of progressive pulmonary TB, or miliary TB, or pleural effusion.

Varied presentations in degree of severity and types:
- Cough, fever, often mild with failure to gain, or loss of weight. Fever may be high and indolent in military TB.
- Breathlessness and pleuritic pain.
- Signs of consolidation, collapse, cavitation, pleural effusion. At times post-tussive increase of crepitations. Often lung signs are more unilateral.
- Extensive signs in progressive pulmonary TB sometimes but a little later in miliary TB.

Central Nervous System TB

"If tuberculosis is not on your mind, it will get into your brain!" A very frequent occurrence in children is sometimes missed or diagnosed late. May present in various forms:
- Central nervous system (CNS) granuloma
- Stroke
- Arachnoiditis
- Spinal tuberculosis with cord compression/invasion as part of military TB
- Hydrocephalus
- Along with miliary TB
- Tubercular meningitis (TBM).

Tubercular Meningitis

The clinical presentation may be divided into three stages:
- *Stage I (lasts for 1–2 weeks):*
  - Fever, malaise
  - No focal neurological signs
  - Infants may show stagnation or loss of developmental milestones.

  Stage I of TBM is often missed. Cerebrospinal fluid (CSF), however, may show evidence of TBM, if done on strong clinical suspicion.
- *Stage II (stage of neurological signs):*
  - Onset abrupt
  - Raised intracranial tension signs with seizures, vomiting, papilledema
  - Signs of meningeal irritation such as Kernig's sign, nuchal rigidity, lethargy
  - Photophobia, hypertonia
  - Cranial nerve palsies and focal neurological deficit may be present.
- *Stage III (stage of sequelae):*
  - Focal neurological deficit
  - Hemiplegia/paraplegia
  - Hypertension
  - Decerebrate posturing
  - Deterioration of vital signs
  - Coma.

Hydrocephalus is often develops as a sequel to TBM, both communicating as well as obstructive type and may require surgical intervention.

Central nervous system granuloma often presents as seizures or features of intracranial space-occupying lesions (ICSOL). Tubercular arteritis may present as a stroke.

Lymph Node TB

Usually of cervical region or axillary, painless, soft-to-firm, nontender, matted lymph nodes (LNs), may be calcified, may have a chronically discharging sinus with scarring.

Abdominal and Gastrointestinal TB

Usual presentation is of anorexia, fever loss of weight, chronic diarrhea. Some signs include abdominal distention, doughy feel of abdomen, and hepatosplenomegaly. Lump, ascites, and peritonitis are not common.

Bone and Spinal TB

It usually comes late as per Wallgren's timetable and presents as signs and symptoms of spondylosis, vertebral pain, kyphosis, and gibbus. It may present later with cold abscess, maybe with features of cord compression. Bone and joints more commonly involved are hip joint and head of femur causing pain, limp, shortening or pseudo lengthening of lower limb.

Other organ involvement include:
- Upper respiratory tract with laryngitis and tracheitis resulting in hoarseness or stridor, and chronic tonsillitis.
- Genitourinary system around puberty with painless hematuria.
- Tubercular pericarditis with effusion or constriction presenting with its symptoms and signs. Cutaneous TB with nonhealing ulcers, middle ear infections.
- No organ is really spared, though above mentioned are the ones more commonly affected.

Some signs of hypersensitivity are often missed or not looked for by clinicians and include phlyctenular conjunctivitis and erythema nodosum, usually seen on shins.

INVESTIGATIONS

Childhood TB is a paucibacillary disease. Hence, history, history of contact, clinical and radiological features are taken into consideration together with the investigations for diagnosing TB.

Visualization of *M. tuberculosis* may not be always be possible. Early morning gastric aspirate, caseous material from lymph node, fine-needle aspiration cytology (FNAC) or excision biopsy, CSF, pleural fluid, ascetic fluid may be taken. Rarely sputum may yield bacilli. From these specimens, evidence of *M. tuberculosis*. It may be seen by Ziehl–Neelsen (ZN) stain as well as other methods such as auramine–rhodamine staining or the newer polymerase chain reaction (PCR)-based tests. Löwenstein–Jensen culture medium is no longer used as the results take about 6 weeks. BACTEC and PCR methods such as CBNAAT (cartridge-based nucleic acid amplification test) yield immediate results within a day.

Radiological: These are very strong indicators of TB when positive.

Three features common to primary infection are:
1. Patient may have nonspecific mild symptoms which can go unrecognized.
2. Primary lung foci are usually quite small relative to large hilar nodes.
3. Primary foci may resemble pneumonia and can be in any lobe. Parenchymal disease in primary TB typically involves areas of greatest ventilation, e.g., middle lobe, superior segments of lower lobes, and anterior segment of upper lobes.

In primary infection, chest radiograph shows paratracheal and/or hilar nodes. There can be associated direct signs (airway narrowing or deviation) or indirect signs of airway compression (collapse and emphysema).

Reactivation TB

Cavitary TB may be a manifestation of recent primary infection or more commonly in endemic settings, of reinfection. From a management point of view, the important distinction between cavitary and noncavitary disease is because of presence of cavities correlates with organism load, treatment outcome, risk of acquiring drug resistance, and infection risk posed to the community.

Skin Tests for TB Hypersensitivity/Sensitization

Mantoux test: The test has low sensitivity but positive result to taken cognizance of along with other findings. Tuberculin protein (2TU PPD RT23) is given intradermally into forearm and induration is measured 48-72 hours. If >10 mm = positive; if <5 mm = negative; 5-10 mm borderline. In immunocompromised cases, after measles, with severe acute malnutrition (SAM), military TB is likely to be negative. Now it is referred to as tuberculin skin test (TST).

Demonstration of Mycobacterium tuberculosis by investigations based on PCR GENE EXPERT, etc., are PCR-based tests and they also show drug sensitivity/resistance to rifampicin and isoniazid (INH) if it is there multidrug resistant (MDR) TB. Drug resistance can also be tested for by similar methods. Result of CBNAAT can be obtained by the patient in a few minutes. CBNAAT has very high specificity, but positivity in children appears low.

Hence, diagnosis of TB in children is not always clear but a conclusion can be obtained by weighing in history of illness, history of close contact, usually from an adult family member, clinical features, radiological, TST and AFB demonstrations. CBNAAT positivity if obtained makes it easier and conclusive.

CBNAAT: The positivity rate is low in children compared to adults. Paucibacillary disease, improper collection of specimen for testing are some of the reasons, however when positive, adds to the confirmation of diagnosis and in addition gives reports of MDR tuberculosis if present.

- Diagnosis of TB should not be made only on clinical features and further investigations are always necessary to establish a diagnosis.
- In case of suspicion of pulmonary TB, sputum examination for *M. tuberculosis* using CBNAAT should be carried out among children who are able to give quality specimens.
- CBNAAT is the preferred investigation of choice over smear examination but its best yield as a test is when it is not ordered based on chest symptoms but on the basis of a positive chest skiagram.
- If CBNAAT is not readily available or testing is not possible even by referral, smear microscopic examination is to be performed.
- For CBNAAT and line probe assay (LPA), only one specimen should be collected.
- If *M. tuberculosis* is detected by either of the methods, child is diagnosed as microbiologically confirmed pulmonary TB.
  - If *M. tuberculosis* is not detected or specimen is not available, diagnosis is inferred from chest X-ray (CXR) and TST by Mantoux technique using 2 TU of PPD RT23.
  - Children with nonspecific radiological shadows with a negative gastric aspirate/induced sputum (GA/IS) by CBNAAT, should be sent for specialist opinion for further evaluation as these children could have a large range of differential diagnoses.
  - All children with TB should be offered HIV testing.

TREATMENT

A combination of drugs has been used for treating TB, considering the bacterium's ability to resist penetration of

TABLE 2: Recommended drug dosages and fixed drug combination pill combination from 0 to 18 years.

Weight band (kg)	Dose
4–7	1 P + 1 E
8–11	2 P + 2E
12–15	3 P + 3E
16–24	4 P + 4E
25–29	3 P + 3E + 1 A
30–39	2 P + 2E +2 A

drugs and its increasing ability to develop resistance to the standard drugs **(Table 2)**. Standard treatment duration is 6 months out of which first 2 months is intensive phase and next 4 months is *continuation phase*. In severe forms of TB, the *continuation phase* is extended to 9–10 months. Thus, principles of treatment include:

- Early diagnosis, early identification of MDR or extensively drug-resistant (XDR) cases
- Combination of drugs, ensuring compliance
- Adequate nutrition, improving living conditions
- Tracing of contacts and their treatment
- Treating intercurrent infections.

Treatment is divided into: (1) *intensive phase* for 2 months and (2) *continuation phase* for next 4 months.

Intensive Phase

- *Isoniazid or isonicotinic acid*: 10–15 mg/kg (standard *10 mg/kg*)
- *Rifampicin*: 7–20 (standard *15 mg/kg*)
- *Pyrazinamide*: 30–40 mg/kg (standard *35 mg/kg*)
- *Ethambutol*: 15–25 mg/kg (standard *20 mg/kg*)
- *Streptomycin*: 15–20 (standard *20 mg/kg*) *not commonly used* because of high incidence of ototoxicity, vestibulotoxicity, and nephrotoxicity.

Pyridoxine 10–15 mg daily given along with antitubercular treatment (ATT) because of increasing the dose of INH.

Continuation Phase

Three drugs are given instead of earlier two.
1. *Isoniazid or isonicotinic acid*: 10–15 mg/kg (standard *10 mg/kg*)
2. *Rifampicin*: 7–20 (standard *15 mg/kg*)
3. *Ethambutol*: 15–25 mg/kg (standard *20 mg/kg*)

In severe TB, the continuation phase is extended for another 3–6 months, e.g., miliary TB, TBM, spinal TB, and extensive cavitary TB.

Pyridoxine 10 mg daily is given in view of the increased dose of INH, to prevent its peripheral neurotoxicity.

In case of hepatotoxicity developing, INH, rifampicin, and pyrazinamide temporary stoppage of these drugs and replacement by ethambutol and streptomycin or amikacin plus levofloxacin can be given and then the original drugs can be reintroduced step by step, one by one.

Corticosteroids (prednisolone): The inflammatory response to the endotoxins from the mycobacteria getting lysed may increase the signs and symptoms temporarily. In certain types of severe cases, it may be prudent to suppress this with corticosteroids.

Indications for prednisolone (as relevant today as before): Neurotuberculosis, miliary TB of serous layers, endobronchial TB, segmental lesions, genitourinary, sinus formation, and other severe forms of TB. 1–2 mg/kg 4 weeks with tapering, up to 8 weeks in neurotuberculosis

Under the NTEP, ease of administration of drugs has been achieved by making fixed drug combinations (FDC). Compliance and follow-up has been further streamlined by proper registry, mobile-based compliance record, and making drugs available free at the periphery.

- Three-drug FDC (H 50, R 75, Z150) (10:15:30) for children, + ethambutol 100
- Four-drug FDC adult (H 75, R 150, Z 400, E 275)

The therapy recommended as per body weight is detailed in **Table 2**.

FOLLOW-UP

It is in two parts: (1) Clinical follow-up and laboratory and (2) investigative follow-up to look for response to the treatment.

1. *Clinical follow-up*: First follow-up may be at 2 weeks to see if there are any side effects of the treatment. After this monthly follow-up is recommended. Signs of improvement may include reduction of cough, fever, absence of appetite, increase and gain in weight besides specific clinical improvement. After completion of treatment, follow-up once in 6 months up to 2 years is recommended. In case, therapy is interrupted <4 weeks, it is resumed again but if noncompliance has been for a longer period, CBNAAT or other methods with a drug sensitivity test (DST) is done and treatment is modified accordingly.
2. *Laboratory and radiological follow-up*: Follow-up radiograph and sputum testing should be done only at the end of therapy unless there is worsening or doubt in diagnosis. Other investigation as and when needed and investigation for hepatotoxicity have to be seen. If there is inadequate healing drugs may be given for another 3–6 months.

NEWER DRUGS

- *Group 1*: First-line oral anti-TB agents—isoniazid (H); rifampicin (R); ethambutol (E); pyrazinamide (Z)
- *Group 2*: Injectable anti-TB agents—streptomycin (S); kanamycin (Km); amikacin (Am); capreomycin (Cm); viomycin (Vm)

- *Group 3*: Fluoroquinolones—ciprofloxacin (Cfx); ofloxacin (Ofx); levofloxacin (Lvx); moxifloxacin (Mfx); gatifloxacin (Gfx)
- *Group 4*: Oral second-line anti-TB agents—ethionamide (Eto); prothionamide (Pto); cycloserine (Cs); Terizidone (Trd); para-aminosalicylic acid (PAS)
- *Group 5*: Agents with unclear efficacy (not recommended by the WHO for routine use in MDR-TB patients)
Clofazimine (Cfz); Linezolid (Lzd); Amoxicillin/Clavulanate (Amx/Clv); thioacetazone (Thz); imipenem/cilastatin (Ipm/Cln); high-dose isoniazid (high-dose H); Clarithromycin (Clr).

Bedaquiline (Sirturo): It holds more promise and can be used alone in MDR and XDR cases; however, it is in use in limited areas under NTEP supervision. It was first described in 2004 and was approved by the Food and Drug Administration (FDA) in December 28, 2012. It is specifically for MDR TB. It affects proton pump for ATP synthetase and should not be coadministered with hepatic enzyme CYP3A inducers: It results in faster metabolism and reduced concentration of drug, and thus avoids use with rifampicin. It should not be used with CYP3A4 enzyme inhibitors to avoid adverse side effects (e.g., ketoconazole).

Adverse effects: Nausea, joint pains, chest pain, headache and cardiac arrhythmias due to long Q-T syndrome. *Delamanid* is another drug which has been approved for such cases and is under trial.

HIV and tuberculosis coinfection: In India, HIV is commonly coassociated with tuberculosis in children and adults. All efforts to isolate mycobacteria must be done. ATT must be started right away along with ART. Treatment regimen is same as in HIV noninfected children. 6-month duration of therapy (with intensive and continuation phases) is optimal. At the end of the continuation phase, give 6 months of INH preventive therapy for 6 months. In case of spinal TB and CNS TB, continuation phase to be prolonged (9–10 months); thus total duration of therapy is 12 months. Pyridoxine supplementation (10 mg/day) should be given till the time INH is prescribed in drug-susceptible TB (DSTB) coinfected children.

Start antiretroviral therapy (ART) regardless of CD4 count. Start ATT first, when well-tolerated, start ART (usually 2 weeks to 2 months).

Neonatal/perinatal TB treatment and prophylaxis: Fortunately, it is rare since TB-affected uteruses, and tubo-ovarian structures result in infertility. If fetus is infected in utero, it may result in hepatic or disseminated form, if in neonatal period, presentation is of miliary or pulmonary form.

The mother should be investigated, if bacteriologically and radiologically positive, and then she should be immediately treated. CXR of child must be done. If negative, she should be put on prophylaxis with INH. If child is positive radiologically, intensive phase of 2 × EHRZ plus continuation phase of 4 × HRE is given. Breastfeeding must continue. If mother is an open case, she can wear a face mask while feeding or handling the child.

PROPHYLAXIS

Bacillus Calmette–Guérin (BCG) vaccine soon after birth, remains to this day a partial protection against TB, particularly disseminated and extrapulmonary TB. About 60% protection to all, significant reduction of extrapulmonary TB or less severity resulting in less morbidity and mortality in in the severe forms such as CNS TB has been shown by various studies. However, improvement of socioeconomic and nutritional status, ensuring strict compliance and regularity of taking medications would ensure better cure and less chances of MDR and XDR TB increasing and spreading.

KEY MESSAGES

- Tuberculosis in children is paucibacillary, hence bacteriological diagnosis, even with newer methods may not be possible; however, all attempts to obtain it must be made.
- High index of suspicion, history of loss of weight, low-grade fever, mild cough, not abating, positive family history of contact would help in establishing diagnosis. Positive radiological features, positive tuberculin test, FNAC of LN or lesion, CSF findings, etc. would establish the diagnosis most of the times. TB, however, is a great mimic and wrong diagnosis is not uncommon.
- Full-treatment compliance would result in a cure and decrease chances of drug-resistant TB. CBNAAT and other tests have come to our aid in this regard. NTEP registration and free drug distribution have contributed toward its control but its elimination by 2025 seems a very difficult objective to achieve.
- Standard treatment is a daily regime, divided into a 2-month intensive phase of 4 drugs (EHRZ) and a 6-month continuation phase of 3 drugs (HRE). Continuation phase maybe extended by another 3–6 months in cases of severe tuberculosis.
- Do DST whenever bacteriological tests, such as CBNAAT, show poor compliance for more than a month, poor response, known drug resistance in that area. There is a possibility of emergence of drug.
- Contact tracing is very important. It is very rare that child-to-child transmission of TB occurs. It is almost always adult-to-child and by a close family contact.
- Nutrition and socioeconomic conditions should also be looked into and improved.

SUGGESTED READING

3. Central TB Division, Ministry of Health and Family Welfare, Government of India, 2019.
2. Kliegman RM, St. Geme J. Nelson's Textbook of Pediatrics, 21st edition. Canada: Elsevier Health Sciences; 2019.
3. Parthasarathy A, Menon PSN, Nair MKC. IAP Textbook of Pediatrics, 7th edition. New Delhi: Jaypee Brothers Medical Publishers; 2019.
4. Seth V, Kabra SK. Essentials of Tuberculosis in Children, 3rd edition. New Delhi: Jaypee Brothers Medical Publishers; 2011.

Leprosy

Vijay P Makhija

GENERAL CONSIDERATION

Leprosy is a chronic granulomatous disease caused by *Mycobacterium leprae*.

It is also called as Hansen's disease.

India contributes to 50% new cases all over the world. India comes in endemic zone for leprosy. It can be easy to diagnose clinically, if our index of suspicion is high. It is easily curable disease with drugs that are easily available free by the government. Early and appropriate treatment and precautions can prevent its many complications and deformities.

CAUSATIVE ORGANISM

Armauer Hansen identified *Mycobacterium leprae* as cause of leprosy in 1873. Previously, humans were thought to be the sole host, but the natural infection was documented in nine-banded armadillos (South American anteaters). Experimental infection is possible in primates, mouse food pad, and armadillos.

MODE OF TRANSMISSION

It is transmitted via droplets from nose and mouth from untreated patient with severe disease.

PATHOGENESIS

Development of disease after being infected greatly depends on host immunity.

Majority (80–90%) of infected patients develop immunity and clear infection without ever development of clinical disease. The pathogenesis is poorly understood. Presently, most infection appears to be transmitted from untreated lepromatous patients. It is transmitted by prolonged contact with infected nasal secretions containing high bacterial load. Nasal droplets of lepromatous leprosy contain thousands of bacilli, from the nasal mucosa *M. leprae* through blood reaches skin and peripheral nerve. It colonizes perineural space and enters interstitium of endoneural space, and macrophages and Schwann cells phagocytose them. The intracellular replication of *M. leprae* in these cells varies according to the host cellular immune response. The varying degrees of skin and peripheral nerve damage occurs depending on host immune response. The vigorous and strong specific cell-mediated immunity leads to *tuberculoid leprosy*; if the cell-mediated response is poor it may lead to *lepromatous leprosy*. Bacilli are found in enormous numbers in skin, nasal mucosa, and peripheral nerves.

CLINICAL TYPES OF LEPROSY (TABLE 1)

- Indeterminate leprosy (IL)
- Tuberculoid leprosy (TL)
- Borderline leprosy
- Lepromatous leprosy (LL)
- Polyneuritic leprosy.

The borderline group is further subdivided into following:
- Borderline tuberculoid (BT)
- Mid borderline (BB)
- Borderline lepromatous (BL).

INVESTIGATIONS IN LEPROSY (ACID-FAST BACILLI DETECTION)

- *Skin smears*: Smear is taken from the most affected skin by "slit and scrap" method, and stained by Ziehl–Neelsen staining. The site of smear is thickened skin, ear lobule, and buttocks. Smear is positive in LL, BL, and BB.
- *Bacillary index*: Semi-quantity estimation of bacilli is done from skin smear and biopsies.
- *Lepromin test*: This is not used for diagnosis of the disease, but for the classification of the disease. This test indicates the cell-mediated immunity to the antigen. It is positive in TT and BT and negative in LL, BL, weakly positive in BB leprosy.
- *Serological assays*:
  - Fluorescent leprosy antibody absorption test (FLA-ABS)
  - Radioimmunoassay
  - Enzyme-linked immunosorbent assay (ELISA)—[PGL (phenolic glycolipid)-ELISA, dot-ELISA, dipstick-ELISA].
- *Molecular diagnosis*: Polymerase chain reaction (PCR) is used to amplify the *M. leprae*-specific gene sequence.

TABLE 1: Clinical type of leprosy.

Indeterminate leprosy (IL)
- Earliest clinical detectable form of leprosy
- There is a single hypopigmented macule 2–4 cm in diameter with poorly defined border but having no erythema or induration
- Anesthesia is minimal or absent, especially if lesion is present on face
- In 50–75% of patients with IL lesions heal spontaneously. In remaining they progress to one of other classic forms

Tuberculoid leprosy (TL) (Paucibacillary leprosy)
- Often single macule with well-demarcated erythematous rim
- Interior of lesion is flat, atrophic, hypopigmented, occasionally scally and anesthetic
- Associated with loss of hair follicles and sweating
- Closest supplying nerve thickened significantly
- Ulnar, post-tibial, and great auricular nerves are most commonly affected

Borderline tuberculoid (BT)
- Lesions are greater in number but size smaller
- Small satellite lesions present around older lesions
- Margins of BT lesions are less distinct
- Usually associated with thickening of two or more superior nerves

Mid borderline (BB)
- Inverted saucer pattern seen
- Lesions more numerous but more heterogeneous
- May become confluent and plaques may be present
- Borders poorly defined and erythematous rim fades into surrounding skin
- Anesthesia may be present but hyperesthesia is more common
- Mild-to-moderate nerve thickening common

Borderline lepromatous (BL)
- Many asymmetrically distributed heterogeneous lesions
- Macules, papules, plaques, and nodules may all coexist
- Individual lesions small unless confluent
- Anesthesia is mild and superior nerve trunks are spared
- Response to therapy dramatic. It flattens nodules/plaques within 2–3 months
- With continued therapy, lesions become macular and almost invisible

Lepromatous leprosy (LL) (Multibacillary disease)
- Lesions innumerable often confluent and symmetric
- As disease progresses, lesions become increasing papular and nodular
- Diffuse thickening and infiltration of skin/ear lobes
- Characteristic leonine facies may be seen with loss of eyebrows
- Anesthesia less severe than tuberculoid but a symmetrical peripheral sensory neuropathy develops in late disease
- Testicular infiltration azoospermia/infertility
- Gynecomastia common in adults tuberculoid but a symmetrical peripheral sensory neuropathy develops in late disease
- Testicular infiltration azoospermia/infertility
- Gynecomastia common in adults
- Bacilli are demonstrable in most internal organs other than central nervous system

Pure neural tuberculoid leprosy
- It presents as either pure sensory or combined sensory and motor dysfunction
- Prominent nerve thickenings are seen, but no cutaneous lesions
- Histopathology is mandatory to establish this diagnosis
- Nodular or fusiform nerve thickening
- This thickening has greater diagnostic value than a smooth and symmetrically enlarged palpable nerve

MANAGEMENT OF LEPROSY: MULTIDRUG THERAPY

- Multidrug therapy (MDT) is used for its cure.
- Resistance to drugs and duration of therapy has decreased with use of MDT.
- Drugs are efficacious, economical, and widely available.

Mainly three drugs are used: Dapsone, rifampicin, and clofazimine **(Table 2)**.

Lepra Reaction

Sudden exacerbations of clinical activity of disease process in leprosy are termed lepra reactions.

They represent hypersensitivity reactions. Mainly of two types—type I and II **(Table 3)**.

Management of Type II Lepra Reaction
- High-dose systemic steroids are given promptly and tapered gradually to avoid nerve/tissue damage.
- Oral nonsteroidal anti-inflammatory drugs (NSAIDs)
- *Clofazimine*: 200–300 mg/d for many weeks
- Chloroquine/colichine/zinc supplement steroid action and allow smooth tapering
- In unresponsive/relapsing reactions, thalidomide 100 mg tid/qid daily is the drug of choice. Absolutely contraindicated in women of child-bearing age.

New Drugs in Leprosy
- Ofloxacin/minocycline/clarithromycin
- Treatment duration may be reduced to 1 month in multibacillary and 1 day in paucibacillary leprosy
- Unfortunately, resolution of lesions is not hastened by them.

What is ROM single dose MDT for single lesion leprosy?
- Rifampicin 600 mg
- Ofloxacin 400 mg
- Minocycline 100 mg

TABLE 2: Multidrug therapy in leprosy.

Dapsone	Rifampicin
• Cornerstone of therapy because of its low cost, minimal toxicity and wide availability • Its adult dose is 100 mg given once daily orally. Pediatric dose is 1 mg/kg • Contraindicated in G6PD deficiency • Always test for G6PD deficiency before starting it in any patient *Side effects of dapsone:* • Dermatitis, hepatitis, and methemoglobinemia • Granulocytopenia rare but potentially fatal *Dose-related hemolytic anemia in G6PD deficiency patient:* • The WHO-recommended MDT regimen (Paucibacillary leprosy) IL/TT/BT leprosy • Dapsone 100 mg once daily for 6 months • Rifampicin 600 mg once monthly for 6 months supervised (DOT) • Duration of therapy is 6 months	• Most rapidly mycobactericidal drug for *Mycobacterium leprae* • It achieves excellent levels inside cells where most leprosy bacilli live. • Hepatitis/thrombocytopenia/flu-like symptom/OCP failure/red discoloration urine, sweat, tears, and contact lenses are its some side effects • 600 mg monthly dose in adults • 10 mg/kg monthly dose in children *Clofazimine:* • It is a phenazine dye • It is used in treatment of Hansen's as well as in decreasing the incidence of reactional states • It is avidly taken up by epithelial cells, results in *cutaneous hyperpigmentation* • Multibacillary disease BL/LL • Dapsone 100 mg once daily (self-administration) × 1 year • Clofazimine 50 mg once daily (self-administration) × 1 year • Rifampicin 600 mg once monthly DOT • Clofazimine 300 mg once monthly DOT • Duration of therapy is for 1 year

(BL: borderline lepromatous; BT: borderline tuberculoid; DOT: directly observed therapy; G6PD: glucose-6-phosphate-dehydrogenase; IL: intermediate leprosy; LL: lepromatous leprosy; MDT: multidrug therapy; OCP: oral contraceptive pill; TL: tuberculoid leprosy)

TABLE 3: Types of lepra reaction.

Type I lepra reaction	Type II lepra reaction
• Occur in first 6 months of beginning of therapy • Existing skin lesions change by developing erythema, tenderness, edema, and hyperesthesia • New lesions are uncommon. No/mild constitutional features • Nerve trunk neuritis in vicinity is common • Neuritis is an indication for systemic steroids, it prevents nerve damage • Oral chloroquine (CQ) 250 mg tid or ibuprofen 400 mg tid helpful, if neuritis absent • Occurs in borderline leprosy • Type IV hypersensitivity	• Common after 6 months of therapy • New lesions called erythema nodosum leprosum (ENL) appear as crops of transient (7-10 days) red, tender, dermal or subcutaneous nodules over face and extremities • New lesions seen called as ENL • Existing lesions are unaffected • Associated with severe constitutional features • Systemic affection common as iritis, arthritis, periostitis, orchitis, GN and lymphadenitis • Occurs in lepromatous or borderline leprosy • Type III hypersensitivity (immune complex disease)

(GN: glomerulonephritis)

HANSEN'S DISEASE SUMMARY

- India accounts for >50% new cases in past 20 years
- Chronic infection is caused by *M. leprae*
- More common in low-socioeconomic status people
- It is not very contagious
- Believed to be transmitted by droplet infection
- May remain asymptomatic for 5–20 years
- Mainly two types—pauci- and multibacillary
- Paucibacillary have poorly pigmented numb patches (Hypopigmented maculoanesthetic) five or fewer lesions. Multibacillary have more than five lesions
- Diagnosis is confirmed by finding acid-fast bacilli skin biopsy or by detecting DNA in PCR
- Leprosy is curable with treatment
- Treatment for paucibacillary leprosy is dapsone and rifampicin for 6 months
- Treatment of multibacillary is dapsone, rifampicin, and clofazimine for 12 months. A number of other antibiotics may also be used.

SUGGESTED READING

1. Parthasarathy A. Textbook of Pediatric Infectious Disease, 2nd edition. New Delhi: Jaypee Brothers Medical Publishers; 2019.
2. World Health Organization. (2011). Leprosy: Global burden at the end of 2010. Weekly Epidemiological Report. [online] Available from: https://www.who.int/publications/i/item/who-wer8535. [Last accessed September, 2021].

Dengue

Neelam Verma

INTRODUCTION

Dengue is an acute febrile illness, characterized by biphasic fever, myalgia, arthralgia, rash, leukopenia, and lymphadenopathy. It is caused by dengue virus, a Flavivirus transmitted by *Aedes aegypti*. Each virus elicits lifetime immunity against the same serotype as well as short-term cross immunity against the other three serotypes. Dengue virus infection can present with different manifestations ranging from a mild illness to a very serious life-threatening illness.

CLASSIFICATION

Dengue is classified into three categories (**Flowchart 1**):
- *Group A*: Dengue
- *Group B*: Dengue with warning signs
- *Group C*: Severe dengue

The clinical course can be divided into three phases: (1) Febrile, (2) critical, and (3) recovery phase.

ETIOLOGY

There are four distinct dengue viruses 1, 2, 3, and 4 of Flaviviridae family. Dengue virus is an RNA virus transmitted by mosquito. *A. aegypti* is a mosquito, which bites during daytime and has a highly domesticated breeding in stagnant water stored for drinking or bathing. It also breeds in rainwater collected in old tyres or other small containers discarded by people. The mosquito has a limited flight range and the spread of virus is mainly by mobile viremic human beings.

Humans are the primary reservoir.

In the tropics, outbreaks of dengue coincide with the onset of the monsoon season. Biting rates increase with increasing temperature and humidity.

PATHOPHYSIOLOGY

The major pathophysiological abnormalities that occur in dengue hemorrhagic fever (DHF) and dengue shock syndrome (DSS) are plasma leakage and bleeding. Plasma leakage is caused by increased capillary permeability and it may be manifested by hemoconcentration leading to pleural effusion and ascites. Bleeding is caused by capillary fragility and thrombocytopenia, which may range from simple petechial skin hemorrhage to life-threatening gastrointestinal or central nervous system (CNS) bleeding. Focal hemorrhage may occur in liver, lungs, adrenal and subarachnoid spaces. Yellow, watery, and blood-tinged effusions are present in serous cavities. Liver enlarges with fatty changes.

CLINICAL FEATURES

The clinical features of dengue virus infection vary from asymptomatic to severe life-threatening illness in the form of DHF or DSS. In young children, the manifestation is generally asymptomatic or mild febrile illness undistinguishable from other febrile illnesses.
- *Group A*: Dengue fever:
  - *Febrile phase*: After an incubation period of 2–7 days, patients experience a sudden onset of fever, which rapidly rises to 103–106°F, accompanied by frontal headache and retro-orbital pain. Oliguria and hepatomegaly may be seen during this phase. Sometimes back pain may precede fever and a generalized macular rash may appear for a short period that blanches under pressure within 22–24 hours of fever. Generalized lymphadenopathy, aberration in taste and anorexia may be there. Rashes disappear in 1–5 days. Edema of palm and sole may be seen. Some patients may present with biphasic fever.
  - *Critical phase*: Defervescence occurs between 3 and 7 days of illness. After this, the patient may either improve or deteriorate. Those who improve have dengue without warning signs and those who deteriorate have dengue with warning signs. Children typically have temperature lower than 38°F in this stage. There is an increase in capillary permeability during this stage, which may lead to third spacing and some children may develop complications such as respiratory distress, shock, bleeding or organ dysfunction.

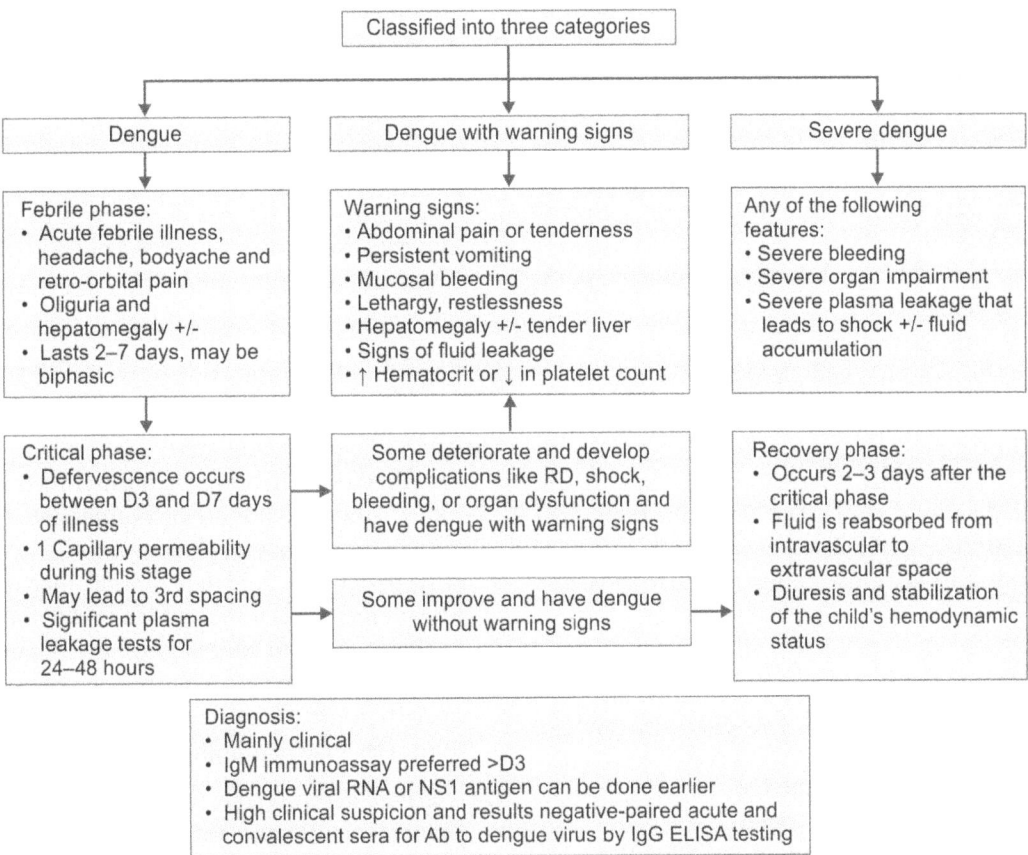

Flowchart 1: Algorithm for classification of dengue.

(IgM: immunoglobin M; NS1: nonstructural protein 1; ELISA: enzyme-linked immunosorbent assay; RD: retinal detachment)

Significant plasma leakage generally lasts for 24–45 hours. An increasing hematocrit, progressive leukopenia, and thrombocytopenia are seen at this stage. The degree of hemoconcentration reflects the severity of plasma leakage.

- *Recovery phase*: Recovery phase occurs 2–3 days after the critical phase. Now the fluid is reabsorbed from the intravascular to extravascular space. It manifests as diuresis and stabilization of the child's hemodynamic status. Some patients may manifest a rash during this phase.
- *Group B*: Dengue with warning signs: The following are the warning signs, which must alert the physician during the critical phase:
    – Abdominal pain or tenderness
    – Persistent vomiting
    – Mucosal bleeding
    – Lethargy, restlessness
    – Hepatomegaly +/– tender liver
    – Sign of fluid leakage
    – Increase in hematocrit or fall in platelet count
- *Group C*: Severe dengue: A patient is considered a case of severe dengue, when a suspected case presents with the following features:
    – Severe bleeding
    – Severe organ impairment
    – Severe plasma leakage that leads to shock +/– fluid accumulation.

INVESTIGATIONS

- *Enzyme-linked immunosorbent assay (ELISA)-based NS1 antigen test*: A highly conserved glycoprotein is abundant in the serum of patients during the early stages of dengue infection and has been found to be useful in diagnosis of acute dengue infection. NS1 is very specific and shows high sensitivity.
- *IgM capture enzyme linked immunosorbent assay (MAC-ELISA)*: MAC ELISA test is based on detecting the dengue-specific IgM antibodies in the test serum by capturing them using anti-human IgM. It is detectable on day 5 of the illness. It is especially useful for hospitalized patients, who are admitted at a later stage of the illness when detectable IgM is already present in the blood.
- *Isolation of dengue virus*: Isolation of most strains of dengue virus from specimen can be done if the sample is taken in the first 5 days of illness and processed without delay or used in autopsy.
- *Polymerase chain reaction (PCR)*: Real-time reverse transcriptase (RT)-PCR has gradually replaced the virus isolation method as the new standard for the detection of dengue virus in acute phase serum sample.
- *IgG ELISA*: This test is used to differentiate primary and secondary dengue infections. It indicates past infections only.

- *Serological tests*: There are few like H1 (hemagglutination inhibitor), CF (compliment fixation) and NT (neutralization test), which are not commonly used due to technical problems.
- *Rapid diagnostic test (RDT)*: It is a commercial test, which gives result within 15-25 minutes. Accuracy is neither proven, nor is it properly validated. Specificity and sensitivity vary from batch to batch, hence it is not recommended.
- Complete blood count (CBC) shows thrombocytopenia and increased hematocrit.
- X-ray chest reveals pleural effusion.
- USG of chest shows ascites and pleural effusion.
- Urine input and output.

DIFFERENTIAL DIAGNOSIS

The differential diagnosis of dengue fever includes viral respiratory and influenza-like diseases, the early stages of malaria, mild yellow fever, scrub typhus, viral hepatitis, and leptospirosis.

TREATMENT

Treatment of dengue is according to the classification of the disease **(Flowcharts 2 and 3)**:
- *Group A cases*: Outpatient management
- *Group B cases*: Inpatient management
- *Group C cases*: Emergency treatment and referral

Group A: Outpatient management—
- Patients who can tolerate oral liquids, have an adequate urine output and do not have warning signs are fit for outpatient management.
- Adequate rest and fluid intake must be ensured in these children.
- Paracetamol is the antipyretic of choice. Nonsteroidal anti-inflammatory drugs (NSAIDs) and steroids should be avoided.
- The parents must be informed about the warning signs such as vomiting, abdominal pain, petechiae, black tarry stool, blood in vomitus or bleeding through nose, pale and cold extremities, lethargy, failure to pass urine for >6 hours and breathing difficulty.

Group B: Inpatient management—Indoor management should be done for patient with warning signs, or in a comorbid condition.

Dengue without warning signs:
- Oral fluids should be given. If the child is not able to take orally, isotonic fluids are recommended. IV 0.9% NaCl or ringers lactate may be given.
- If the patient has mild dehydration, then the fluid needed for volume correction is added to the maintenance fluid to decide the total fluid requirement. One half of the fluid is given over the first 8 hours and the rest half over the next 16 hours. Periodic assessment is needed, and the fluid is given accordingly.

Dengue with warning signs:
- Before starting the therapy, a reference hematocrit should be obtained.
- Only isotonic fluid is to be recommended. Start with 5-7 mL/kg/h for 1-2 hours, followed by 3-4 mL/kg/h for 2-4 hours, and then 2-3 mL/kg/h depending on the clinical response.

Algorithms for Dengue Management

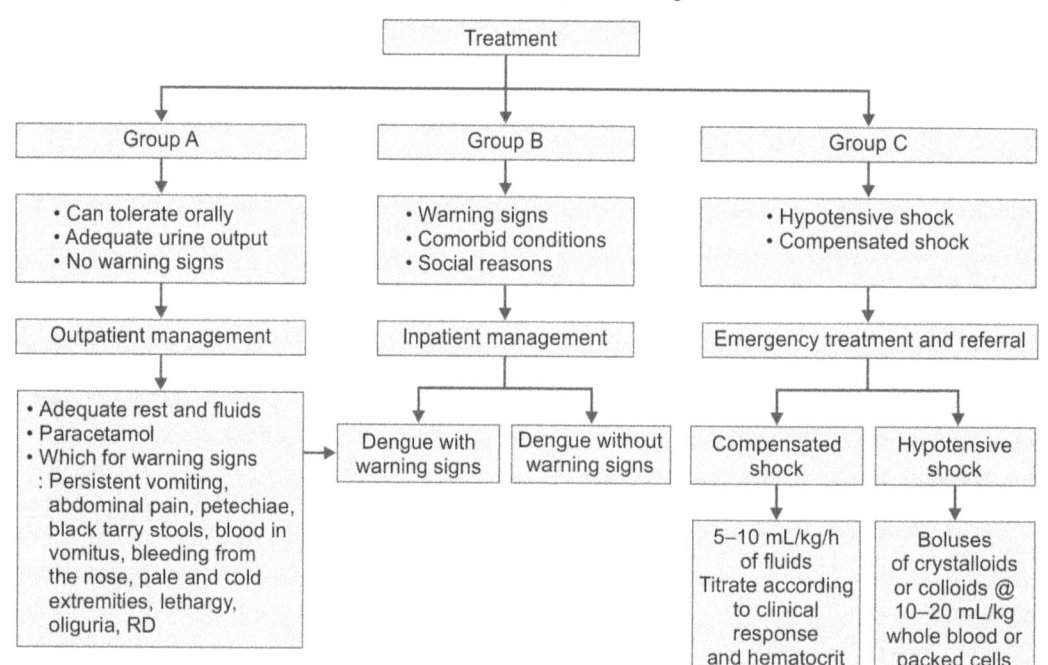

Flowchart 2: Treatment plan for dengue.

(RD: retinal detachment)

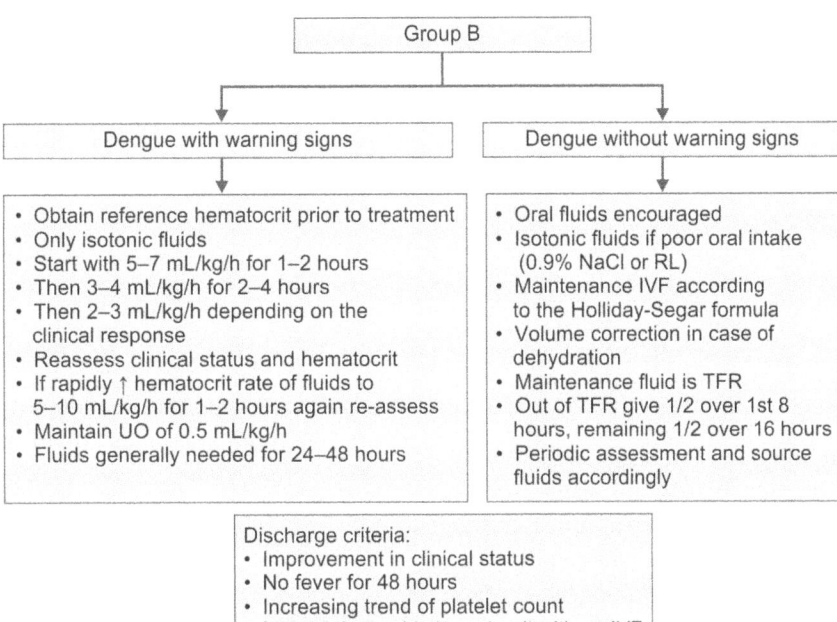

Flowchart 3: Algorithm for treatment of dengue.

(IVF: in vitro fertilization; TFR: total fertility rate)

- The clinical status and the hematocrit should be monitored, if the hematocrit rises rapidly, the rate of fluids should be increased to 5-10 mL/kg/h for 1-2 hours, again reassessment must be done. Fluids should be titrated to maintain adequate perfusion and urine output of 0.5 mL/kg/h.
- Fluid is generally needed for 24-48 hours, then it should be gradually reduced if the plasma leakage decreases, as indicated by adequate intake of fluid and urine out put and fall in hematocrit to below the baseline level.

Group C: Emergency treatment and referral: It consists of patients who need urgent fluid resuscitation. They generally present with hypotensive or compensated shock.

Dengue with compensated shock: These patients should be started on fluid at the rate of 5-10 mL/kg/h and further requirement should be titrated based on the clinical response and serial hematocrits.

Dengue with hypotensive shock: These patients should be started on bolus of IV crystalloids or colloids at a rate of 10-20 mL/kg over 15 minutes. Periodic reassessment should be done to ascertain further course of action. Blood transfusion may be needed in case of hemorrhage. Severe bleeding may manifest as a rapid fall in hematocrit, or shock that does not respond to fluids. Fresh whole blood or packed cells are recommended for the transfusion. Platelets, cryoprecipitate, and fresh frozen plasma (FFP) are not routinely advised for hemorrhage and must be given judiciously as they can cause fluid overload.

DISCHARGE CRITERIA

- Appetite and urine output improve
- There is no respiratory distress
- Hemodynamic stability is achieved without intravenous fluids
- No fever for 48 hours
- Increasing trend of platelet count is seen.

PREVENTION

Prophylaxis, in the absence of vaccine, consists of avoiding daytime household mosquito bites by:
- Using insecticides or repellents
- Covering the body with clothes
- Screening of houses and destruction of *A. aegypti* breeding sites

SUGGESTED READING

1. Gupte S. Dengue Fever. Recent Advances in Pediatrics. New Delhi: Jaypee Brothers Medical Publishers; 2014. pp. 1-10.
2. Kliegman RM, St. Geme J. Nelson Textbook of Pediatrics, 21st edition. Canada: Elsevier; 2019. pp. 1760-4.
3. Parthasarathy A. Dengue & chart. Dengue and chart. IAP Management and Algorithm for Common Pediatrics illnesses. New Delhi: Jaypee Brothers Medical Publishers; 2016. pp. 71-4.
4. World Health Organization. (2012). Global strategy for dengue prevention and treatment. [online] Available from: https://www.who.int/immunization/sage/meetings/2013/april/5_Dengue_SAGE_Apr2013_Global_Strategy.pdf. [Last accessed September, 2021].

Re-emerging Infections in Pediatrics

Ashok Bhandari

INTRODUCTION

Human infection emerges and re-emerges due to interaction of multiple complex factors and leads to major epidemics. During 1950-60, many developing countries were undergoing mass vaccination campaigns against polio, small pox, measles, and few other common diseases. These campaigns decreased the incidence of vaccine-preventable diseases and strengthened the belief of disappearance of major infections from the world. In last few years, there is emergence of old diseases and new diseases are coming up. There is a difference between emerging and re-emerging infectious disease.

Emerging disease is one which has not been described or identified before. Re-emerging infectious diseases are one which were under control or eradicated in specific geographic area, but have later resurfaced and became health problem again.

This chapter highlights re-emergence of infectious diseases in children such as diphtheria, congenital rubella syndrome (CRS), cholera, plague, Nipah, and corona and specific preventive measures.

DIPHTHERIA

The World Health Organization (WHO) report indicates primary immunization coverage for diphtheria remained between 56 and 72% in past two decades. Persistence or re-emergence of diphtheria in India and other countries is because of low coverage of primary immunization and booster.

Etiology

Diphtheria is caused by *Corynebacterium* species, typically *Corynebacterium diphtheriae* and, less often, toxigenic strains of *C. ulcerans*.

Clinical Manifestation

Major virulence is due to potent polypeptide exotoxin, causing pseudomembrane formation. Its removal is difficult and reveals a bleeding edematous submucosa. Paralysis of the palate and hypopharynx is an early local effect of diphtheria toxin. Toxin absorption can lead to systemic manifestations such as renal tubular necrosis, thrombocytopenia, cardiomyopathy, and demyelination of nerves.

Diagnosis

Nose and throat swabs and portion of membrane along with exudate are used for culture. Selective culture media used for primary isolation of organism are tellurite agar or specially enriched Loeffler, Mueller, or Tinsdale media.

Treatment

Equine diphtheria antitoxin is administered as a single empirical dose of 20,000–100,000 units based on the degree of toxicity, site and size of the membrane, and duration of illness. The role of antimicrobial therapy is to halt toxin production, treat localized infection, and prevent transmission of the organism to contacts. Erythromycin or penicillin are main drugs used as antimicrobial.

Prevention

The WHO advises primary series of three doses of diphtheria toxoid-containing vaccine with the first dose as early as 6 weeks of age and third dose completed by 6 months of age with minimum of 4 weeks interval between two doses. The WHO also recommends three booster doses during childhood and adolescence with at 12–23 months of age, 4–7 years of age, and 9–15 years of age. To further promote immunity against diphtheria, the use of Td/Tdap (tetanus and diphtheria/tetanus, diphtheria, and pertussis) rather than tetanus toxoid is recommended during pregnancy to protect against maternal and neonatal tetanus, diphtheria and pertussis.

CONGENITAL RUBELLA SYNDROME

According to the WHO, every year there are 1 lac babies born with CRS all over the world. As there is no specific treatment available for CRS, it can only be prevented. There is recent re-emergence of rubella in form of large outbreaks in Japan and other countries due to incomplete rubella vaccination programs. Studies in Indian population revealed that 10–30% of adolescent girls and 12–30% of women in the reproductive age group are susceptible to rubella infection.

Etiology

Rubella virus is the sole member of the genus *Rubivirus* in the family Togaviridae. It is transmitted via primary maternal infection (85% chance of transmission if maternal infection occurs before 12 weeks of gestation).

Clinical Presentation

Intrauterine growth restriction (IUGR), cataracts, glaucoma, cardiac anomalies (patent ductus arteriosus and peripheral pulmonic stenosis), deafness, and "blueberry muffin rash."

Diagnosis

IgM at birth. Level typically would increase within in first 6 months of life. Diagnosis can be confirmed by stable or increasing IgG level over first 7–11 months.

Treatment

Supportive care, with evaluation by ophthalmologist and cardiologist.

Prevention

India introduced a rubella initiative as a part of the nationwide measles-rubella (MR) campaign in two stages—the first stage targeted to cover a wide age range of children and adolescents aged 9 months to 15 years with the MR vaccine. This was followed by the second stage and included MR vaccine in the routine immunization programs in a two-dose schedule at 9–12 months and at 16–24 months of age.

CHOLERA

Cholera is one of the infections which also re-emerged as outbreak.

Etiology

Cholera results from infection by *Vibrio cholerae*, a gram-negative, facultative anaerobic rod in the family Vibrionaceae. Two serogroups, 01 and 0139 ("Bengal"), can cause disease.

Clinical Features

Transmission is by the fecal–oral route. Infections are particularly common after ingesting contaminated water or food. Cholera appears abruptly with painless, watery diarrhea, sometimes accompanied by vomiting. Infections may be subclinical, mild and self-limiting, or fulminant and severe. Severe fluid loss can be seen in more serious cases; thirst, oliguria, severe dehydration, acidosis, muscle cramps, and shock may result.

Diagnosis

Cholera can be diagnosed by observing the organism's characteristic motility during direct, bright-field or dark-field microscopic examination of the feces; the addition of specific antibodies to *V. cholerae* stops the movement. Bacteria can also be identified in the feces by immunofluorescence.

Treatment

Fluid replacement and the restoration of electrolyte balance. Antibiotics reduce the stool volume, decrease shedding of organism, and shorten the course of the disease.

Prevention

Development of oral cholera vaccine (OCV) when given in two-dose schedule is found to be efficacious. Providing clean water and proper sanitation to population is important in prevention of re-emergence of this disease. Currently there are three WHO prequalified OCV: Dukoral®, Shanchol™, and Euvichol®. All three vaccines require two doses for full protection.

PLAGUE

Etiology

It is an acute communicable disease caused by a bacterium called *Yersinia pestis* and transmitted to man by the bite of infected rat fleas. It is primarily a zoonosis, being a disease of rodents, and humans are affected incidentally. This caused three major pandemics in human history, changing the path of our civilization.

Recent outbreaks of disease: In India, focal outbreaks of plague observed in 1994, 2002, and 2004. In 1994, there was plague outbreak in Surat in Gujarat, resulted in considerable negative social, political and economic impact. The outbreak of plague in Himachal Pradesh during 2002 came after a gap of 8 years. Plague infection continues to exist in sylvatic foci in many parts of India which is transmitted to humans occasionally. Since 2001, a total of 14 major outbreaks have been reported to the WHO from all over the world. This re-emergence is attributed to spill over from an epizootic cycle of plague in wild rodents to commensal rodent.

Clinical Features

There are three forms of plague:
1. *Bubonic plague* causes the tonsils, adenoids, spleen, and thymus to become inflamed. Symptoms include fever, aches, chills, and tender lymph glands.
2. *Septicemic plague*: Bacteria multiply in the blood. It causes fever, chills, shock, and bleeding under the skin or other organs.

3. *Pneumonic plague*: It is the most serious form. Bacteria enter the lungs and cause pneumonia. People with the infection can spread this form to others.

Diagnostic Tests

F1 rapid diagnostic test, paired serology, polymerase chain reaction (PCR), culture.

Treatment

Injection streptomycin is the drug of choice, alternative is injection gentamicin; other drugs which are effective are ciprofloxacin, doxycycline, and chloramphenicol.

Prevention

Plague vaccines, live attenuated and formalin killed at one time, were widely used but have not proven to be an approach that could prevent plague effectively. The vaccine does not protect against primary pneumonic plague. During outbreak, preventive measures are handwashing, social distancing, mask and disinfective measures as used for other diseases such as influenza and corona.

NIPAH VIRUS

Nipah virus was first recognized in year 1999 to cause disease outbreak in pig farmers in Malaysia. After this, there are multiple outbreaks of this viral infection in south Asia. The Nipah outbreak reported in Kozhikode and Malappuram districts of Kerala in May 2018 was the third of Nipah virus Outbreaks in India, the earlier being in 2001 and 2007, both in West Bengal.

Etiology

This virus belongs to the family Paramyxoviridae and genus *Henipavirus*. The name, Nipah virus, was proposed because the first isolate was made from clinical material from a fatal human case from Kampung Sungai Nipah, a village in Negeri Sembilan, Malaysia.

Clinical Features

These range from asymptomatic infection (subclinical) to acute respiratory infection and fatal encephalitis. The case fatality rate is estimated at 40–75%. Nipah virus can be transmitted to humans from animals (such as bats or pigs), or contaminated foods and can also be transmitted directly from human to human. Fruit bats of the Pteropodidae family are the natural host of Nipah virus.

Treatment

Measures were largely supportive and consisted of anticonvulsants, treatment of secondary infection, mechanical ventilation, and rehabilitation.

Prevention

Currently there is no effective vaccine, interventions to prevent farm animals from acquiring Nipah virus by eating fruit contaminated by bats. Farms should be designed to reduce overcrowding to avoid rapid spread of disease between animals and should not be near fruit trees that attract bats.

Consumption of contaminated sap should be avoided.

CORONAVIRUS

First coronavirus infections were reported in 1960 as a cause for the common cold. Since then, until 2002, four subtypes of coronaviruses were reported to infect humans, two alpha (α) coronaviruses—229 E and NL6 3 and 2 beta (β) coronaviruses—OC4 3 and HKU1, which routinely produce noncomplicated infections of the upper and/or lower respiratory tract. Similarly to SARS-CoV-2, the original SARS-CoV emerged in Guangdong Province in China in 2002, spreading through human transmission chains to infect at least 8,096 individuals in 29 countries and succumb 774 patients in 2002–2003. In 2012, a novel β-coronavirus that had not previously been observed in humans was detected for the first time in a patient in Saudi Arabia. Since then, the new coronavirus, which causes Middle Eastern Respiratory Syndrome and is now known as MERS-CoV, has infected >2,494 individuals across 27 countries and led to the death of at least 858 individuals through a series of emergence and re-emergence from camelid hosts. On December 8, 2019, in Wuhan, Hubei Province, China, the first case was reported of a new coronavirus that produces pneumonia. Since then, the new virus first named 2019-nCoV and subsequently renamed SARS-CoV-2.

Etiology

Coronaviruses are positive-stranded RNA viruses with a crown-like appearance under an electron microscope (coronam is the Latin term for crown) due to the presence of spike glycoproteins on the envelope. Thus, SARS-CoV-2 belongs to the β-CoVs category.

Clinical Features

- From asymptomatic to influenza-like illness, respiratory distress with respiratory failure.
- Children are also presenting with Kawasaki disease and toxic shock syndrome-like feature.

Diagnosis

Definitive diagnosis is by RT-PCR of nasal and throat swabs. Serological tests are being developed to look for evidence of infection in general population.

Prevention

Vaccine is in a developing state and not yet available. Main steps of prevention is isolation and quarantine of cases, wearing mask, social distancing, handwashing, and cough etiquette.

This pandemic of COVID-19 resulted into unprecedented situation with enormous impact on economy, daily lifestyle, and policy decisions. Tremendous efforts are on to develop vaccine against this ongoing pandemic which can be seen as ray of hope in preventing this deadly infection.

CONCLUSION

Re-emerging infectious diseases will continue to challenge health facilities, health infrastructure. They continually pose threat to communities and countries due to devastating effect of these infections on economy, lifestyle and health. To overcome these deleterious effects, health system of countries should strengthen surveillance and rapid response mechanism, should comply with international health regulations, strengthening of laboratory and network, more emphasis on research and development and must share correct information about disease extent and spread.

SUGGESTED READING

1. Dikid T, Jain SK, Sharma A, Kumar A, Narain JP. Emerging & re-emerging infections in India: an overview. Indian J Medical Res. 2013;138(1):19-31.

COVID-19

Rama Krishnan Sanjeev

INTRODUCTION

Coronaviruses (Covs) are enveloped single-stranded zoonotic RNA viruses of the family Coronaviridae, order Nidovirales. They are classified into alpha-, beta-, gamma- and delta-coronaviruses. The causative virus, 2019 novel coronavirus, SARS-Cov-2 (severe acute respiratory syndrome coronavirus 2), is a beta coronavirus with a crown-like appearance on electron microscopy. It was first noted in Wuhan city, China where cases of a pneumonia of unknown etiology among adults were identified to be caused by the virus. Many of them were epidemiologically linked to a local seafood and animal market. Disease caused by the virus has been named the 2019 coronavirus disease (COVID19) by the World Health Organization (WHO). Host response is important in the pathogenesis. Children account for 1–5% of diagnosed COVID-19 cases.

EPIDEMIOLOGY AND TRANSMISSION

The incubation period for the disease is 2–7 days, up to 14 days. It has a basic reproductive number of 2.2–3.58. The basic reproductive number is the number of infections arising from one case in a susceptible population. No evidence of intrauterine transmission has been documented as of now. Transmission through breastfeeding is unclear, as breast milk has not been found to have the virus. Majority of children are infected by a close household contact. The mode of transmission is droplets or fomites, with the virus being found in respiratory secretions or saliva. The virus can be transferred from the hands to eyes, nose, and mouth. Shedding of the virus is greater during the early stages of infection and may precede the symptoms by 1–2 days.

Since being declared a global pandemic by the WHO on 11th March 2020, the virus has affected countries all over the world disrupting everyday life and commerce, with considerable mortality and sickness, particularly among the elderly. Children are affected to a much lesser extent, though, they constitute an important means of community transmission.

PATHOGENESIS

The virus utilizes the angiotensin-converting enzyme-2 (ACE-2) receptor for cell entry. The ACE 2 receptors are present in the ciliated epithelial cells of respiratory and gastrointestinal tract, thereby contributing to the initial symptoms. Mechanisms underlying pathogenesis are ill understood. In autopsy studies, extensive lung damage is linked to high initial virus titers, increased infiltration in the lungs by mononuclear phagocytes and neutrophils with elevated levels of proinflammatory cytokines are seen. This suggests a disease induced by a cytokine storm secondary to a heavy viral load in severe disease. The profile of the cytokine storm appears to be similar to secondary hemophagocytic lymphohistiocytosis (HLH) secondary to viral infections. The cytokine storm leads to peripheral lymphopenia, higher interleukin levels, higher d-Dimer and fibrin degradation products leading to increased thrombosis and multi-organ injury. Lesser susceptibility in children is hypothesized to be due to lesser viral loads, fewer comorbidities, differences in ACE-2 receptor expression, bacillus Calmette–Guérin (BCG) vaccination and other viral coinfections leading to decreased replication of SARS-CoV-2.

CLINICAL FEATURES

Children have less severe disease in comparison to adults. Some children may require hospitalization and intensive care. Children < 1 year old, with serious comorbidities, are more at risk of severe disease. There are reports of clusters of children with multisystem inflammatory disease syndrome with features of Kawasaki disease and toxic shock syndrome requiring intensive care (**Fig. 1**).

Symptoms seen in children are:
- Fever
- Cough
- Malaise
- Anorexia
- Shortness of breath
- Sore throat
- Rhinorrhea

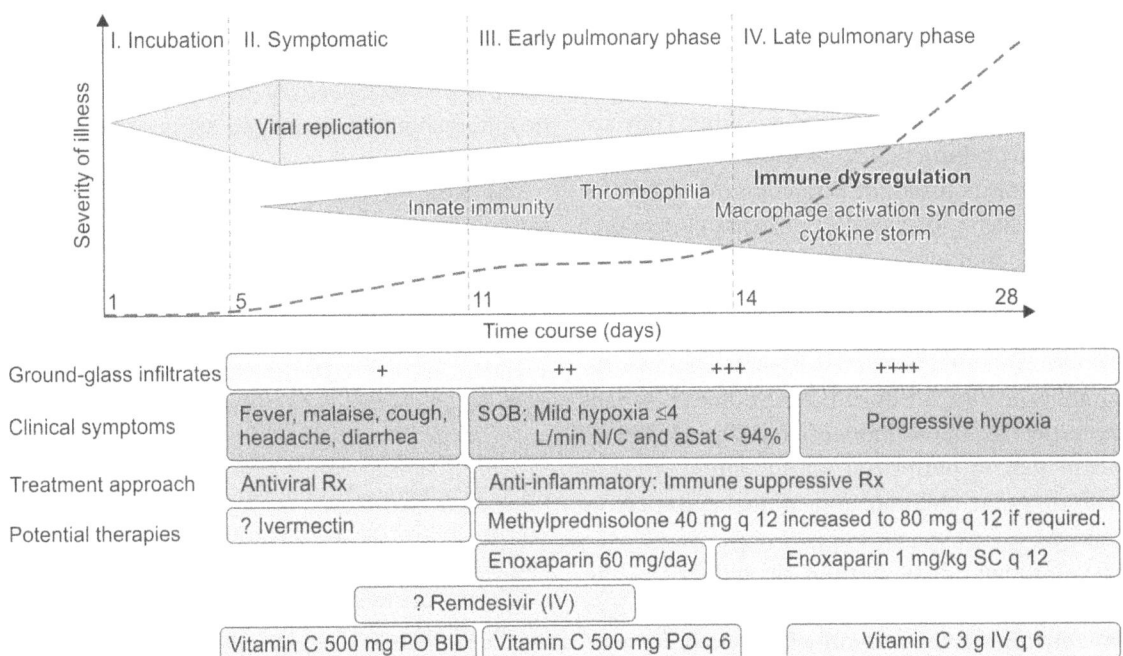

Fig. 1: Typical course and stages of COVID-19 disease integrated with clinicoradiologic features and management.
(COVID19: 2019 coronavirus disease; IV: intravenous; N/C: nasal cannula; PO: per oral; SC: subcutaneous; SOB: shortness of breath)
Source: Marik P. EVMS Critical care COVID 19 management protocol: Updated guidelines. [online] Available from https://www.evms.edu/covid-19/. [Last accessed September, 2021].

- Myalgia
- Fatigue
- Headache
- Nausea
- Vomiting
- Diarrhea
- Seizures—febrile and nonfebrile.

The disease is divided into four types among a population ranging from neonates to adolescents. There is no age and sex preponderance.

1. *Mild*: Asymptomatic or some upper respiratory infection signs only.
2. *Moderate*: The above manifestations with pneumonia on clinical grounds or imaging study.
3. *Severe*: Disease progression with danger signs:
   - Cyanosis or oxygen saturation (SpO_2) < 90%
   - *Fast breathing (in breaths/min)*: <2 months: ≥60; 2–11 months ≥ 50; 1–5 years ≥ 40
   - General danger signs such as inability to breastfeed or drink, lethargy, unconsciousness, or convulsions.
4. *Critical*: Shock or organ failure needing intensive care.

In severe cases, multiorgan dysfunction (MODS) with acute respiratory distress syndrome (ARDS), acute kidney injury, cardiac dysfunction, and liver injury is possible.

CRITICAL DISEASE

Sepsis: Suspected or proven infection and ≥2 age-based systemic inflammatory response syndrome (SIRS) criteria of which one must be abnormal temperature or white blood count.

Septic shock: Any hypotension or two/three of the following—altered mental status/bradycardia/tachycardia/prolonged capillary refill time/tachypnea/mottled or cool skin/high lactate/reduced urine output/hyperthermia/hypothermia.

Acute respiratory distress syndrome: Onset is within 1 week of known pneumonia or new or worsening respiratory symptoms. Chest imaging (and/or echocardiography) will show bilateral lung opacities not fully explained by volume overload, lobar or lung collapse, or nodules.

Kawasaki disease-like manifestations in COVID-19-positive patients usually presents in the older age group on day 6 of fever (on average) with both classic and incomplete form of Kawasaki disease. The classic form in about half the patients presents with nonexudative conjunctivitis, polymorphous rash, hand or feet or lip/face abnormalities and laterocervical lymphadenitis. Respiratory and gastrointestinal involvement, meningeal signs and signs of cardiovascular involvement with shock-like features may be there. The disease is now described as *multisystem inflammatory syndrome temporally associated with COVID-19 in children and adolescents.*

Various cutaneous rashes have been observed in some pediatric patients.

WORKUP

Workup is to be guided by local epidemiology and clinical features so as to exclude malaria, enteric fever, dengue, etc.

Confirmatory diagnosis is by nucleic acid amplification methods such as reverse transcriptase polymerase reaction

(RT-PCR) or TrueNAT of nasopharyngeal, respiratory, and other tissue specimens such as urine and stool.

Antigen tests detect presence of viral protein in a sample, utilizing antibodies on a paper strip and read out. They are shorter and easier to perform than PCR-based tests.

Antibody tests can be used for screening using IgG- or IgM-specific antibodies to look for past or current infection.

Chest X-ray and computed tomography (CT) scanning show patchy or segmental consolidation with ground-glass opacities in some of the moderate-to-severe cases. CT scanning in children should be used with discretion in view of high radiation exposure. Advanced disease shows evident consolidation especially in posterobasal regions with ARDS-like widespread patchy peripheral consolidation. Overall radiological findings in children appear to be similar to adults but milder.

Laboratory findings show normal or reduced white blood cell count. Frequently there may be leukocytosis and neutrophilia. Leukopenia is common with a small fraction demonstrating lymphopenia. Raised C-reactive protein (CRP), procalcitonin, with raised d-Dimer levels, elevated hepatic and muscle enzymes are variably seen. Lymphocyte count and CRP can be used to monitor severe infections while procalcitonin can be used for detecting bacterial coinfection.

MANAGEMENT

General principles: The four main principles of good management are early identification, isolation, diagnosis, and treatment. Isolation of all suspected cases, as per the current WHO guidelines, is preferable. Supportive care with adequate nutrition, caloric intake, and oxygen administration, as needed, should be practiced. Fluid and electrolyte management should be appropriate. Cautious hydration should be practiced in well-perfused patients. Application of timely, effective, and safe supportive therapies is the cornerstone of management of patients with severe symptoms. Home-based care and telemedicine should be used whenever possible, particularly for asymptomatic patients and those with mild disease. *As per the WHO, infants should not be separated from suspected or confirmed COVID-19 mothers and breastfeeding should be continued.*

Regular monitoring of vital signs, including pulse oximetry and medical early warning scores, as applicable, to look for signs of deterioration. Supplementary oxygen therapy to any patient with SpO_2 < 90% or with emergency signs (obstructed or absent breathing, severe respiratory distress, central cyanosis, shock, coma, or convulsions). Nasal prongs or nasal cannula in children are preferred as they are better tolerated. Case notification of patients being tested is a must. Coinfections must be sought and treated. Parental and patient anxiety should be alleviated. Children with suspected or confirmed COVID-19 should be kept with caregivers in child-friendly places with an aim to ensure medical and nursing care while attending to the nutritional and psychosocial needs of the child. Transportation between hospitals should be managed with necessary precautions by medical transport teams.

In mild cases, pending diagnosis, Oseltamivir for influenza, may be given. Mild cases can be treated with symptomatic relief medication such as paracetamol. Ibuprofen should be avoided. Aerosol bronchodilators should be avoided in favor of metered-dose inhalers with spacers. Children < 5 years of age can be given oral antibiotics such as amoxycillin/clavulanic acid.

Respiratory care: Consider tachypnea on the basis of the IMNCI (Integrated Management of Neonatal and Childhood Illness) guidelines with respiratory rates ≥ 60 in <2 months, ≥50 in 2–11 months, ≥40 in 1–5 years.

Severe acute respiratory illness (SARI) is defined by the presence of cough and fast breathing plus at least one of the following: (1) SpO_2 < 90%, (2) severe chest indrawing and grunting, and (3) altered mental status. SARI is the most common reason for ICU transfer.

The norm is to use nasal prong oxygen and shift to ventilation (NIV or invasive with adequate filters for inspiratory and expiratory circuits) as needed. High-flow nasal cannula (HFNO), bubble continuous positive airway pressure (CPAP) or noninvasive ventilation (NIV) should be used with airborne precautions in view of potential for aerosolization. Bag-valve masks too have potential for aerosolization.

Standard procedures such as preoxygenation, sedation with fentanyl or ketamine, and rapid sequence intubation should be utilized, as needed. Protective mechanical ventilation can be done using pressure-controlled or volume-cycled modes, with a low tidal volume of 6 mL/kg and plateau pressure of ≤30 mm Hg. Positive end-expiratory pressure (PEEP) of 5–6 mm Hg can be used to begin with and titrated as per requirement. Prone positioning has been utilized with benefit in critical cases.

Shock management: Septic shock management is on common lines with fluid therapy and use of vasoactive/inotrope agents. Dobutamine and milrinone can be used for normal arterial pressure with pulmonary hypertension and a low cardiac index. Epinephrine can be used for patients with hypotension. Conservative fluid strategy avoiding colloids is advocated with fluid restriction of up to 50%, in hemodynamically stable cases. Fluid therapy is however, dictated by clinical conditions. D-dimer levels, if available, can be used for detecting thrombotic events such as strokes. Vigilance should be exercised against coagulopathy. Use of low-molecular-weight heparin or intermittent pneumatic compression devices should be considered in adolescents, as appropriate.

Coinfections are treated with broad-spectrum antibiotics. Side effects of medication or drug interactions should be carefully monitored.

Acute kidney injury should be managed with renal replacement therapy as required.

Kawasaki disease-like presentation may be treated with adjunctive steroids in addition to intravenous immunoglobulin (IVIg) in view of the more severe clinical course seen in these children.

For management of delivery to mothers with confirmed COVID-19, the healthcare personnel [with full personal protective equipment (PPE)] should use adequate distancing from mother while handling neonate, while following standard neonatal protocols for resuscitation using self-inflating bag mask while avoiding T-piece resuscitator. They should be isolated, baby should be breastfed with mother wearing a mask. If neonatal care is required, a separate room with adequate ventilation can be utilized. Two consecutive negative tests 48–72 hours apart would be required before declaring baby negative.

Investigational Therapies (Recommendations as per the WHO and Center for Disease Control, USA)

Remdesivir, which was developed for Ebola, has shown promising results. It has been approved by the Center for Disease Control (CDC) for the management of severe disease.

Plasma from convalescent patients is being used in the settings of clinical trials.

Ritonavir/lopinavir has been recommended against use by the CDC in view of unfavorable pharmacodynamic and negative clinical trial data.

Hydroxychloroquine/chloroquine/azithromycin: Present status is to avoid use in view of high side effects.

Corticosteroids can be used to combat inflammation as per protocol used.

For interleukin (IL)-6 inhibitors, studies are ongoing for IL-6 inhibitors such as Tocilizumab.

For IL-1 inhibitors, such as emapalumab and anakinra, trials are ongoing, in view of biomarkers in disease progression [high ferritin, high alanine aminotransferase (ALT) and low platelets] resembling markers of macrophage activation syndrome.

For convalescent sera of patients with SARS-CoV-2, there are no recommendations for or against use.

Recommendations are against non-SARS-Cov-2 IVIg being used for the treatment of COVID-19.

For cytokine storm syndromes or suspected hemophagocytic syndrome, IL-1, IL-6 inhibitors and Janus kinase inhibitors (JKI) are being considered.

The MATH+ protocol uses a combination of methylprednisolone, ascorbic acid (IV), thiamine, and heparin early in disease course when oxygen requirements are there. The + indicates drugs such as magnesium, melatonin, famotidine, and zinc. The + indicates that the management of COVID 19 is a work in progress with new treatments being added as they prove beneficial.

Prevention

Community level measures such as contact tracing, social distancing, avoidance of crowded areas as well as public transportation with early detection of clusters of infection, and quarantine measures form the core of disease containment strategy. Rationale of the 2-week quarantine being the fact that 95% of patients develop symptoms within 12.5 days of infection. Shedding by asymptomatic people may represent 25–50% of total infections and hence, the emphasis on universal mask use to prevent spread of the disease.

Prevention of contact from infected subjects in hospital by healthcare providers is by means of:
- Frequent handwashing between examining patients
- Use of alcohol-based hand sanitizers between handling patients
- Universal use of PPE such as N95 masks, exchange surgical face masks, caps, and goggles, particularly while doing high-risk procedures such as suction, intubation, and surgery.
- Safe waste management and disinfection practices as per the guidance issued by the Ministry of Health and Family Welfare (MOHFW) should be followed.

Lastly, delayed or neglected presentation of other childhood illnesses and the severe economic impact of the pandemic on those from the lower socioeconomic strata is seen as a major contributor to childhood morbidity and mortality in India currently.

KEY MESSAGES

COVID-19 disease, caused by the novel Coronavirus SARS CoV-2, is a pandemic, affecting all age groups, particularly the elderly. Pediatric subjects have relatively mild disease with few having multi-organ dysfunction including ARDS. Kawasaki-like disease is increasingly being recorded in large outbreak clusters. Transmission is by droplets or fomites with children being vehicles for community spread. Diagnosis is by use of PCR-based tests, antibody tests, and radiology (CT scanning and chest X-ray). Prevention is by frequent handwashing, use of PPE, universal use of masks, social distancing norms and early case detection by contact tracing coupled with quarantine measures. Treatment is essentially supportive utilizing current pediatric intensive care management guidelines. Use of anti-inflammatory drugs such as steroids is key to managing complications of the disease which are mostly due to an exaggerated immune response to the viremia. Other life-threatening illnesses should not be neglected in the process of managing this pandemic.

SUGGESTED READING

1. Balasubramanian S, Rao NM, Goenka A, Roderick M, Ramanan AV. Coronavirus Disease (COVID-19) in Children – What We Know So Far and What We Do Not? Indian Pediatr. 2020;57(5):435-42.
2. Carlotti APCP, Carvalho WB, Johnston C, Rodriguez IS, Delgado AF. COVID-19 diagnostic and management protocol for pediatric patients. Clinics (Sao Paulo). 2020;75:e1894.
3. COVID-19 Treatment Guidelines Panel; National Institutes of Health. Coronavirus Disease 2019 (COVID-19) Treatment Guidelines. [online] Available from: https://www.covid19treatmentguidelines.nih.gov/. [Last accessed September, 2021].
4. Dong Y, Mo X, Hu Y, Qi X, Jiang F, Jiang Z, et al. Epidemiology of COVID-19 among children in China. Pediatrics. 2020;145(6):e20200702.
5. Marik P. EVMS Critical care COVID 19 management protocol: Updated guidelines. [online] Available from: https://www.evms.edu/covid-19/. [Last accessed September, 2021].
6. Ministry of Health and Family Welfare. [online] Available from https://www.mohfw.gov.in.
7. Ravikumar N, Nallasamy K, Bansal A, Angurana SA, Basavaraja GV, Sundaram M, et al. Novel coronavirus 2019 (2019-nCoV) infection: Part I – Preparedness and management in the pediatric intensive care unit in resource-limited settings. Indian Pediatr. 2020;57:324-34.
8. Verdoni L, Mazza A, Gervasoni A, Martelli L, Ruggeri M, Ciuffreda M, et al. An outbreak of severe Kawasaki-like disease at the Italian epicentre of the SARS-CoV-2 epidemic: An observational cohort study. Lancet. 2020;395(10239):1771-8.
9. World Health Organization. (2020). Clinical management of COVID-19: Interim guidance. [online] Available from: https://apps.who.int/iris/handle/10665/332196. [Last accessed September, 2021].

SECTION 6: Gastroenterology

54. Chronic Pain Abdomen in Children
55. Chronic Constipation
56. Recurrent Vomiting in Infants and Children
57. Celiac Disease in Children
58. Gallstones in Children
59. Upper Gastrointestinal Bleeding in Children
60. Lower Gastrointestinal Bleed
61. Acute Pancreatitis in Children
62. Ascites
63. Cholestasis in Newborns and Infants
64. Abnormal Liver Function Tests
65. Asymptomatic Hepatomegaly
66. Acute Viral Hepatitis
67. Acute Liver Failure
68. Chronic Hepatitis B
69. Metabolic Liver Disease in Children
70. Liver Mass on Imaging in Children
71. Liver Transplantation
72. Foreign Body Ingestion in Children

CHAPTER 54: Chronic Pain Abdomen in Children

Smita Malhotra

INTRODUCTION

Abdominal pain is one of the most common problems encountered in pediatric office practice. As many as 18–38% of these children may have weekly symptoms and up to 24% of these pain may last for >8 weeks. Only about 5–10% of children with abdominal pain have an organic cause.

DEFINITIONS

- *Recurrent abdominal pain*: At least three episodes of pain over at least 3 months that are severe enough to affect the child's ability to perform normal activities.
- *Chronic abdominal pain*: Long lasting, at least 1 month but commonly >3 months, intermittent or constant abdominal pain that is functional or organic.
- *Functional abdominal pain*: Recurrent abdominal pain with specified clinical criteria where after appropriate medical evaluation, the symptoms cannot be attributed to another medical condition.

Functional abdominal pain disorders (FAPDs) represent a subgroup of functional gastrointestinal disorders (FGIDs) that include four defined diagnoses **(Table 1)**:
1. Functional dyspepsia (FD)
2. Irritable bowel syndrome (IBS)
3. Abdominal migraine (AM)
4. Functional abdominal pain—not otherwise specified (FAP-NOS).

Although chronic abdominal wall pain (CAWP) is not included in the FGIDs group, but is another kind of long-term, intermittent, abdominal pain in which the pain arises from the abdominal wall rather than from visceral organs, with minimal or no relationship to food intake or defecation **(Table 2)**.

MANAGEMENT

Where the Rome IV criteria are met, extensive investigations are not required and are strongly discouraged. A thorough

TABLE 1: Rome IV criteria for functional abdominal pain disorders.	
H2 a. Functional dyspepsia (FD)	Postprandial fullness, early satiation, epigastric pain, or pain not associated with defecation on at least 4 days per month for at least 2 months
H2 b. Irritable bowel syndrome (IBS)	Abdominal pain at least 4 days per month for at least 2 months that is associated with defecation or with a change in frequency or form of stools, and in children with constipation, pain does not resolve with resolution of constipation
H2 c. Abdominal migraine (AM)	At least two paroxysmal episodes over 6 months of intense periumbilical, midline, or diffuse abdominal pain lasting for more than 1 hour and affecting normal activities, and pain associated with two or more additional symptoms (anorexia, nausea, vomiting, headache, photophobia, or pallor)
H2 d. Functional abdominal pain-not otherwise specified (FAM-NOS)	Occurs at least four times per month for at least 2 months and includes episodic or continuous abdominal pain not associated with eating or menses; does not meet criteria for pain with dyspepsia, irritable bowel syndrome, or abdominal migraine
The phrase "no evidence of an inflammatory, anatomic, metabolic, or neoplastic process that explain the subject's symptoms" has been removed from diagnostic criteria, thus taking away the emphasis from detailed investigations and shifted the focus to clinical criteria	

TABLE 2: Differential diagnosis: Organic etiologies of chronic/recurrent abdominal pain.

Gastrointestinal	Genitourinary	Metabolic	Others
• Esophagitis • Gastritis (peptic, *Helicobacter pylori*) • Peptic ulcer • Gastroenteritis • Colitis • GERD • Hiatal hernia • Parasitic infestations • Inflammatory bowel disease • Irritable bowel syndrome • Pancreatitis • Cholelithiasis • Food allergies	• Recurrent UTI • PUJ obstruction • Uro/Nephrolithiasis • Testicular pain • Menstrual cramps • Mittelschmerz • Ovarian cyst • Pelvic inflammatory disease • Endometriosis	• Adrenal crisis • Diabetic ketoacidosis • Porphyria • Musculoskeletal • Anterior cutaneous nerve entrapment • Neurologic • Spinal tumor • Transverse myelitis	• Pneumonia • Lead poisoning • Lymphoma • Peritoneal abscess/tumor • Polyarteritis nodosa/vasculitis • Sickle cell disease • Familial • Mediterranean fever

(GERD: gastroesophageal disease; PUJ: pelviureteric junction; UTI: urinary tract infection)

BOX 1: Alarm symptoms/red flag signs that point to an organic etiology.

- Family history of inflammatory bowel disease, celiac disease, or peptic ulcer disease
- Persistent right upper or right lower quadrant pain
- Dysphagia, odynophagia
- Persistent vomiting
- Gastrointestinal blood loss
- Chronic, severe or nocturnal diarrhea
- Arthritis
- Perirectal disease
- Involuntary weight loss, deceleration of linear growth
- Delayed puberty
- Unexplained fever
- Genitourinary tract symptoms
- Pain that awakes the child from sleep
- Jaundice, pallor
- Organomegaly
- Localized tenderness
- Abdominal mass
- Ascites
- Costovertebral angle tenderness/back pain with lower extremity neurologic findings

history about the abdominal pain and any other associated symptoms, including onset, duration, frequency, site, characteristics, and triggering or relieving factors and meticulous clinical examination (including pelvic and scrotal examination in adolescence) to pick up red flags **(Box 1)** is mandatory and targeted investigations is then planned as per suspected etiology.

INVESTIGATIONS

- Hemogram, CRP, ESR
- Urine examination, stool examination
- Fecal calprotectin. LFT, electrolytes
- *Radiologic imaging*: USG, CT, barium studies, MR enterography
- *Endoscopy with biopsies*: Gastroscopy/colonoscopy/enteroscopy/capsule endoscopy
- *Serology*: EMA, anti-tTG, ASCA, ANCA
- *Others*: D-xylose, ELISA breath tests, endocrine evaluation, pancreatic function tests

(ANCA: antineutrophil cytoplasmic antibody; ASCA: anti-*Saccharomyces cerevisiae* antibody; CT: computed tomography; CRP: C-reactive protein; ELISA: enzyme-linked immunosorbent assay; EMA: endomysial antibody; ESR: erythrocyte sedimentation rate; LFT: liver function test; MR: magnetic resonance; tTG: tissue-transglutaminase; USG: ultrasonography)

- X-ray abdomen is not mandatory to diagnose functional constipation but may be ordered when fecal impaction is suspected.
- Stool examinations for ova and parasites should be repeated on three samples to increase the diagnostic yield.
- Stool for occult blood is a good screen for lower gastrointestinal (GI) inflammation.
- Stool calprotectin is a noninvasive screen for inflammatory bowel disease (IBD) and a negative value can help to rule out Crohn's disease.
- *Upper GI endoscopy (UGIE)*:
  - Not routinely required for the diagnosis of FD.
  - Indicated if there is family history of peptic ulcer disease, *Helicobacter pylori* infection, child >10 years with symptoms >6 months or severe symptoms that affect activities of daily living including sleep are present.
  - Along with serology (antitissue transglutaminase and antiendomysial antibodies) UGIE is indicated to rule out celiac disease.

- Mandated along with colonoscopy in the work up of IBD.
- Esophagitis, gastritis, and hiatus hernia are other etiologies picked up by UGIE.
- The American Academy of Pediatrics recommends that CT abdomen is not required in the routine evaluation of abdominal pain.

TREATMENT

- Establishing a rapport and winning over the confidence of the child and family is the cornerstone of effective therapy. Though the underlying problem is benign in the majority, the child and family are considerably distressed and anxious which vitiate the symptoms.
- Every attempt should be made to restore routine and school attendance at the earliest.
- The most important step is to arrive at a correct and precise diagnosis. If specific causes for the pain are discovered, then the management is etiology specific.
- When there are no alarming signs with a normal physical examination, organic cause is unlikely and the pain is labeled functional.
- However, this does not imply that the child does not require therapy as the physical and psychological distress are genuine and commonly perceived by families and treating practitioners as difficult to manage due to lack of specific cure.
- A biopsychological approach with aim to improve the quality of life by pharmacological and non-pharmacological interventions based on different aspects of behavioral habits of affected children, such as specific diet, gut microbiota, defecation pattern, stress, and psychosocial aspects of the illness, may represent targets of treatment on a case-by-case basis.

Nonpharmacological Treatment Strategies

- *Dietary interventions*:
  - High fiber and/or lactose-free diets have not been found helpful but reducing the fructose load reduces abdominal pain intensity and frequency.
  - Diet low in fermentable oligosaccharides, disaccharides, monosaccharides, and polyols (FODMAPs) has been found to be efficacious as these food products are poorly absorbed in the gut and increase the osmotic load.
  - A low-gluten diet may relieve symptoms in children with nonceliac gluten sensitivity.
  - Chocolate, caffeine, spicy, and fatty foods, nitrite- and amine-containing foods; and nonsteroidal anti-inflammatory drugs need to be avoided in children with gastritis and reflux disease.
- *Probiotics*:
  - Probiotics are a safe and a possible therapy for FAPD, especially in children with suspected IBS or when symptoms have been triggered following an episode of gastroenteritis or after an antibiotic course.
  - *Lactobacillus rhamnosus* GG (LGG) and VSL#3 have shown treatment response. *L. reuteri* DSM 17938 supplementation for 4 weeks has been shown to significantly reduce intensity of abdominal pain.
- *Biopsychosocial modifying therapies*:
  - *Hypnotherapy*: Proven beneficial effect which persists for up to 5 years after the completion of therapy and may even be regarded as first-line therapy.
  - *Cognitive behavior therapy*: Potential tool but needs multiple sessions
  - Yoga and acupuncture may be helpful.
  - Physiotherapy is helpful for CAWP.

Pharmacological Therapies

- *Antispasmodics*:
  - Peppermint oil has a proven role in adults with IBS, few studies in children have shown benefit after 2 weeks of therapy.
  - Drotaverine and mebeverine have shown some treatment response after 4 and 8 weeks of therapy.
  - Trimebutine is underevaluation for use in children.
- *Antidepressants*:
  - Amitriptyline has proven efficacy in adults with IBS and FD but these effects are not confirmed in children though improvement in quality of life has been observed.
  - Citalopram is being evaluated but it has a higher rate of side effects.
- *Antihistaminic agents*:
  - Cyproheptadine that has calcium channel and antiserotonin effects has been found efficacious as 5-hydroxytryptamine (HT) alterations in the gut may be responsible for dysmotility and visceral hypersensitivity.
  - Side effects are sleepiness and weight gain, more so in nonresponders.
- *Calcium channel blockers*: Flunarizine in AM improves both abdominal pain and headache
- *Serotonin antagonists*: Pizotifen in AM is promising.
- *Laxatives*: Polyethylene glycol (PEG) 3350 useful in IBS constipation
- *Antibiotics*: Rifaximin and cotrimoxazole not found beneficial
- *Placebo*: A meta-analysis of 21 trials has shown that the placebo effect can have a therapeutic role in children with FAPD.

MANAGEMENT OF FUNCTIONAL ABDOMINAL PAIN

- *General measures*:
  - Reassurance

- Cognitive behavior therapy, hypnotherapy, probiotics/synbiotics
- Subspecialist referral as indicated
■ *Acid reflux/FD*:
  - Trial of antacids, proton pump inhibitors or anti-H2 histamine antagonists
  - Omeprazole is superior to ranitidine, famotidine, and cimetidine
  - Low-dose amitriptyline and imipramine in difficult cases
  - Prokinetics: Domperidone reduces early satiety and bloating
  - Cyproheptadine is helpful for dyspeptic symptoms
  - Gastric electrical stimulation in refractory cases
■ *Chronic constipation or constipation-predominant irritable bowel syndrome*:
  - Dietary modification: Increased intake of fluids, fiber, fruit juices (i.e., papaya, mango, pear, and apple)
  - Behavioral intervention: Scheduled toilet times, stool diary, reward system
  - Polyethylene glycol (PEG 3350)
  - Severe constipation: Manual disimpaction, enemas, suppositories, nonpolyethylene glycol laxatives
■ *Diarrhea-predominant irritable bowel syndrome*:
  - Partially hydrolyzed guar gum, peppermint oil; consider loperamide or rifaximin
  - Low FODMAP diet
■ *Abdominal migraines*:
  - *First line*: Simple analgesics (e.g., acetaminophen, ibuprofen), antiemetics (e.g., ondansetron)
  - *Second line*: Triptans (rizatriptan, almotriptan), sumatriptan/naproxen, nasal zolmitriptan, nasal sumatriptan, injectable sumatriptan
  - *Prophylaxis*: Cyproheptadine, propranolol, pizotifen, and amitriptyline
■ *FAP-NOS*:
  - Amitriptyline, citalopram
  - Hypnotherapy and cognitive behavior therapy
  - Partially hydrolyzed guar gum, peppermint oil; consider loperamide or rifaximin
  - Low FODMAP diet.

KEY MESSAGES

- Chronic abdominal pain has an organic cause in only 5–10% cases.
- The term recurrent abdominal pain is obsolete and FAPD is the new terminology.
- Red flags on history and physical examination should not be missed.
- A normal physical examination with absence of red flags rules out need for additional diagnostic interventions.
- Functional abdominal pain disorders are treated on a biopsychosocial model of care.
- Family dynamics and behavior patterns of child and parents need to be addressed.
- Treatment strategies include pharmacological, non-pharmacological, and placebo interventions.

SUGGESTED READING

1. Berger MY, Gieteling MJ, Benninga MA. Chronic abdominal pain in children. BMJ. 2007;334:997-1002.
2. Brusaferro A, Farinelli E, Zenzeri L, Cozzali R, Esposito S. The management of paediatric functional abdominal pain disorders: latest evidence. Paediatr Drugs. 2018;20(3):235-47.
3. Hyams JS, Di Lorenzo C, Saps M, Shulman RJ, Staiano A, van Tilburg M. Childhood functional gastrointestinal disorders: child/adolescent. Gastroenterology. 2016;150(6):1456-68.
4. Reust CE, Williams A. Recurrent abdominal pain in children. Am Fam Physician. 2018;97(12):785-93.
5. Santucci NR, Saps M, van Tilburg MA. New advances in the treatment of paediatric functional abdominal pain disorders. Lancet Gastroenterol Hepatol. 2020;5(3):316-28.

CHAPTER 55: Chronic Constipation

Bhaswati C Acharyya

INTRODUCTION

Chronic constipation accounts for 3–5% of all visits to pediatricians and up to 30% of visits to gastroenterologists. The common perception in South Asia is that functional constipation is uncommon as diet here is rich in fiber. However, in Asia too functional constipation is the most common type of constipation encountered. The Rome IV criteria for functional constipation are given in **Boxes 1 and 2**.

THE TRIGGERING FACTORS

These factors precipitate or exaggerate the bowel habit:
- *Toilet training*: Rigorous training, punishments and scolding during toilet training can precipitate problem in smooth defecation. Change of house, change of school, and frequently neglecting the call for passing stool may produce excessive hard stool which is difficult to pass and eventually results in constipation.
- *Painful defecation*: The most common cause of avoidance to pass stool is pain on passing the fecal matter. Passing one hard stool often creates anal fissure to cause pain while passing it again. If pain is not relieved, bowel movement becomes a horrifying experience to avoid as much as possible. Though not very common in our country but sexual abuse may be a cause of painful defecation which needs to be elicited by careful history-taking.
- *Dietary changes*: Sometimes excessive refined foods and lack of fiber can precipitate hard fecal matter.

Secondary Causes

Sometimes secondary etiologies exist which may or may not be exacerbated by the behavioral problem.
- Cow's milk (or other dietary protein) intolerance
- Celiac disease
- Cystic fibrosis
- Lead poisoning
- Intestinal obstruction
- Severe mental retardation
- Depression.

MANAGEMENT

Diagnosis should be established with proper history-taking and physical examination. In history, the following points should be noted: (1) Meconium passage, (2) frequency of bowel movement, (3) diet, (4) school/travel, (5) painful defecation, (6) soiling, (7) family history, (8) failure to thrive, (9) clogging of the commode, and (10) drug history.
- *Physical examination* should find out growth, abdominal distention, fecal mass felt on abdominal examination, fecal soiling, anogenital index (to know anteriorly situated anus), anal fissure, signs of trauma (abuse), signs of spinal defects (spina bifida) and neurological defects if any.
- *Investigations*: Needed only in 15% of children. Abdominal X-ray is not routinely indicated. If intestinal obstruction is suspected X-ray may be done.

BOX 1: Diagnostic criteria for functional constipation in child at or above 4 years.

Must include two or more of the following occurring at least once per week for a minimum of 1 month with insufficient criteria for a diagnosis of irritable bowel syndrome:
- Two or fewer defecations in the toilet per week in a child of a developmental age of at least 4 years
- At least 1 episode of fecal incontinence per week
- History of retentive posturing or excessive volitional stool retention
- History of painful or hard bowel movements Presence of a large fecal mass in the rectum
- History of large-diameter stools that can obstruct the toilet

---

BOX 2: Diagnostic criteria for functional constipation in infants and toddlers.

Must include 1 month of at least two of the following in infants up to 4 years of age:
- 2 or fewer defecation per week
- History of excessive fewer defecations stool retention
- History of painful or hard bowel movements
- History of large-diameter stools
- Presence of a large fecal mass in the rectum; in toilet-trained children, the following additional criteria may be used:
  – At least 1 episode/week of incontinence after the acquisition of toileting skills
  – History of large-diameter stools that may obstruct that may obstruct the toilet

Other tests include urine analysis and culture, celiac screening, thyroid.

Function test, electrolytes, creatinine and calcium, lead level. These can be undertaken when long-standing constipation seems difficult to treat. Other investigations, such as anorectal manometry, are done when Hirschsprung's disease is suspected. Colonic transit time or colonic manometry is indicated in cases of refractory constipation.

- *Treatment*: The goal of therapy is the passage of soft stools, ideally once per day, and no less than every other day. The four principles of treatment include:
  - *Education*: In the education aspect, reassure that avoiding bowel movement is not a willful or defiant behavior, parents should maintain consistent, positive, supportive attitude; avoid punishment and establish a reward system.
  - *Disimpaction*: This is the second important aspect of management. It comprises removing all the hard fecal mass in colon and rectum being deposited for prolonged period. Different methods are in vogue. It can be done being hospitalized or at home.
    - *In hospital*: Polyethylene glycol (PEG) solution as lavage at 25 mL/kg/h orally or via nasogastric tube is used.
    - *At home*: PEG at 1.5–2 g/kg in 10r2 doses given over 3–6 days until the rectal effluent is clear. At home, varying combination of osmotic and stimulant laxatives are used.

    Many prefer using enemas for disimpaction but the National Institute for Health and Care Excellence (NICE) guidelines recommend not to use enemas until oral medications fail to elicit response.
  - *Maintenance*: This is the phase where regular laxatives are maintained and patient is monitored at regular interval. This phase should last long period (at least 6 months to 1 year). The most preferred laxative is the osmotic laxatives.

    Osmotic laxatives
    - *PEG*: Usually PEG 3,350/4,000 is given at a dose of 0.4–0.8 mg/kg/day in a noncarbonated beverage.
    - Lactulose/Lactitol is the second most common osmotic laxative used in a dose of 1–3 mL/kg/day in single or divided doses.

    Stimulant laxatives
- *Sodium picosulfate*
  - Elixir (5 mg/5 mL)
  - *Child 1 month to 4 years*: 2.5–10 mg once a day
    Child/young person: 4–18 years: 2.5–20 mg once a day
  - *Senna syrup (7.5 mg/5 mL)*:
    - *Child 1 month to 4 years*: 2.5–10 mL once a daily
    - *Child/young person 4–18 years*: 2.5–20 mL once a daily.
- *Docusate not available in India*:
  - *Child 6 months–2 years*: 12.5 mg three times daily (use pediatric oral solution)
  - *Child 2–12 years*: 12.5–25 mg three times daily
  - *Child/young person 12–18 years*: Up to 500 mg daily in divided doses.

Dietary intervention: It is controversial whether dietary modification can treat constipation in children. In mild constipation, increased fluid intake and dietary fiber intake (Goal: age + 5 g fiber) can help. But in severe constipation, diet alone is unlikely to produce any result.

- *Behavioral modification includes*: (1) Routine toilet sitting, (2) 5 minutes after meals (two or three times/day), (3) Developing a regular habit, (4) Maintaining stool diary, and (5) supporting the leg in western type toilet. Positive reinforcement, avoidance of punishment and addressing psychological issues if any go a long way in management of constipation.

Surgery:
- Surgery and other procedures are indicated in case of refractory constipation after appropriate investigations:
- Anal sphincter release
- Antegrade continence enema (ACE)—appendix is used as conduit to insert cecostomy button (Chait trapdoor button) to give enema
- Primary intestinal diversion (ileostomy or colostomy)
- Colonic resection
- Percutaneous nerve stimulation.

The NICE recommendations:
- Relieve anal pain use Sitz Bath and local cream/ointment.
- Add another laxative such as docusate if stools are hard.
- Continue medication at maintenance dose for several weeks after regular bowel habit is established–this may take several months.
- Do not stop medication abruptly: Gradually reduce the dose over a period of months.

KEY MESSAGES

- Chronic constipation requires a comprehensive approach.
- After disimpaction, a long-term maintenance treatment is the mainstay to manage constipation.
- Refractory cases need investigations and specific individualized intervention.

SUGGESTED READING

1. Tabbers MM, DiLorenzo C, Berger MY, Faure C, Langendam MW, Nurko S, et al. Evaluation and treatment of functional constipation in infants and children. J Pediatr Gastroenterol Nutr. 2014;58(2):258-74.
2. Yachha SK, Srivastava A, Mohan N, Bharadia L, Sarma MS. Management of Childhood Functional Constipation: Consensus Practice Guidelines of Indian Society of Pediatric Gastroenterology, Hepatology and Nutrition and Pediatric Gastroenterology Chapter of Indian Academy of Pediatrics Indian Pediatr. 2018;55(10):885-92.

Recurrent Vomiting in Infants and Children

Vibhor Borkar

INTRODUCTION

Vomiting encompasses all retrograde ejection of gastro-intestinal (oroesophageal) contents from the mouth. Some commonly confused terms are given in **Table 1**. The three temporal patterns of vomiting and their causes are given in **Tables 2 and 3**.

EVALUATION AND APPROACH

Once the child with vomiting reports in the office or emergency room, do the basic screening evaluation and then do the specific tests **(Table 4)**.

In few children, metabolic work up is required if certain red flags are identified **(Table 5)**. If there are no red flags and no organic etiology is found, then suspect a functional cause.

Table 6 gives elaborative definitions of the episodic functional causes associated with vomiting.

TREATMENT

1. *Acute phase*:
    a. Hydration correction. Ensure good hydration and normal glycemia. One can give one and half times maintenance for 1-2 days

TABLE 1: Definitions.

Terms	Clinical features
Nausea	Unpleasant, vaguely epigastric or abdominal sensation accompanied by a variety of autonomic changes: decreases in gastric tone, contractions, secretion, and mucosal blood flow; increases in salivation, sweating, pupil diameter, and heart rate; and changes in respiratory rhythm
Retching	Strong, involuntary efforts to vomit, which may be seen as preparatory maneuvers to vomiting
Vomiting (emesis)	Differs from retching in that material is expelled from the mouth
Regurgitation	Form of gastroesophageal reflux and, as such, is caused predominantly by lower esophageal sphincter dysfunction
Rumination	Similar to regurgitation in its effort less appearance and its probable propulsion by somatic muscle contraction

TABLE 2: Features distinguishing different types of vomiting.

Clinical features	Acute	Recurrent chronic	Recurrent cyclic
Epidemiology	Most common	Two third of recurrent vomiting	One third of recurrent vomiting
Vomiting pace	Moderate to severe	Mild, 1–2 emeses/hour at peak	Severe, >4 emeses/hour at peak
Acuity	Moderate to severe, ± dehydration	Not acutely ill or dehydrated	Severe, dehydrated
	Severe	Hour at peak	Emeses/hour at peak
Acuity	Moderate to severe, ± dehydration	Not acutely ill or dehydrated	Severe, dehydrated
Stereotype	NA	None	Yes
Recurrence rate	No	Yes, >2 episodes/week	Yes, <2 episodes/week
Onset	Variable	Daytime	Early morning
Symptoms	Fever, diarrhea	Abdominal pain, diarrhea	Pallor, lethargy, abdominal pain
Household contacts	Affected	Uncommon	No
Family history of migraine	No	14% positive	80% positive

TABLE 3: Causes of vomiting by temporal pattern.

Category	Acute	Chronic recurrent	Recurrent cyclic
Infections	Gastroenteritis, hepatitis, pharyngitis, UTI, meningitis, otitis media, sinusitis	*Helicobacter pylori* gastritis, giardiasis, chronic sinusitis	Chronic sinusitis
Gastrointestinal	Hernia, intussusception, appendicitis, cholecystitis, pancreatitis, intestinal obstruction	Anatomical obstruction, GERD, gastritis, achalasia, SMA syndrome, food allergies	Malrotation with volvulus
Genitourinary	Pyelonephritis	Pyelonephritis, pregnancy, uremia	Hydronephrosis secondary to PUJ
Endocrine-metabolic	Diabetic ketoacidosis	Adrenal hyperplasia	Diabetic ketoacidosis Addison disease MCAD deficiency Partial OTC deficiency MELAS syndrome Acute intermittent porphyria
Neurological	Concussion Subdural hematoma Encephalitis Migraine	Arnold–Chiari malformation, Subtentorial neoplasm	Abdominal migraine, migraine headaches, Arnold–Chiari malformation, subtentorial neoplasm, metabolic encephalopathy
Other	Toxic ingestion Chronic marijuana use Food poisoning	Rumination Functional Bulimia Pregnancy	Cyclic vomiting syndrome, factitious disorder by proxy (e.g., ipecac poisoning)

(GERD: gastroesophageal reflux disease; MCAD: Medium-chain acyl-coenzyme A dehydrogenase; MELAS: mitochondrial myopathy, encephalopathy, lactic acidosis, and stroke; PUJ: pelviureteric junction; OTC: ornithine transcarbamylase; SMA: superior mesenteric artery; UTI: urinary tract infection)

TABLE 4: Initial test for evaluation for different temporal patterns of vomiting.

Tests	Acute	Chronic	Episodic
Screening tests	Electrolytes BUN Creatinine	CBC, ESR, LFT, amylase, lipase, urine analysis Stool for giardiasis	CBC LFT, glucose Amylase, lipase, ammonia Lactate, carnitine, amino acids, organic acids—plasma and urine Urine analysis Porphobilinogen, cortisol levels
Definitive tests	Abdominal radiographs Sonography Surgical consults	Endoscopies with biopsy Sinus CT, UGI/small bowel series Abdominal USG	Endoscopies with biopsy, sinus CT, UGI/small bowel series Abdominal USG Head MRI Metabolic testing

(BUN: blood urea nitrogen; CBC: complete blood count; CT: computed tomography; ESR: erythrocyte sedimentation rate; LFT: liver function test; MRI: magnetic resonance imaging; UGI: upper gastrointestinal; USG: ultrasonography)

TABLE 5: Red flags to consider metabolic workup.

Nutritional abnormalities	Failure to thrive, anorexia
Dietary provocation	Fructose, galactose, fasting, protein
Neurologic abnormalities	Lethargy, coma, developmental delay, change in muscle tone, seizures
Liver abnormality	Hepatosplenomegaly, jaundice, coagulopathy
Respiratory abnormality	Apnea, hyperapnea
Odd odors (breath, urine, eat wax)	*Cabbage*: Tyrosinemiaa *Sweaty feet*: Isovaleric acidemia *Musty*: Phenylketonuria, hepatic coma (fetor hepaticus) *Fruity*: Ketones (many, nonspecific) *Maple syrup*: Maple syrup urine disease *Other*: 3- methylcrotonyl-CoA carboxylase deficiency Multiple carboxylase deficiency Acyl-CoA dehydrogenase deficiency *Putrid*: Sinusitis *Alcohol*: Alcohol ingestion

Contd...

Contd...

Miscellaneous abnormalities	Eye abnormalities (cataracts) Hair abnormalities (fragile) Pigmentation of skin ("tan") and mucosa Adrenal calcifications Ambiguous genitalia Cardiomyopathy Family history of fetal or neonatal deaths; Consanguinity
Screening study abnormalities	Metabolic acidosis Hypoglycemia (hyperketonuric or hypoketonuric) Hyperkalemia (with hyponatremia) Hyperammonemia Hypertransaminasemia anemia, leukocytopenia, thrombocytopenia Urinary non-glucose-reducing substance Urinary Fanconi syndrome

TABLE 6: Diagnostic criteria for episodic diseases (As per ROME IV criteria).

Diagnosis/disorder	Diagnostic criteria
Infant regurgitation	Must include both of the following in otherwise healthy infants 3 weeks to 12 months of age: 1. Regurgitation 2 or more times per day for 3 or more weeks 2. No retching, hematemesis, aspiration, apnea, failure to thrive, feeding or swallowing difficulties, or abnormal posturing

Infantile rumination syndrome	Must include all of the following for at least 2 months:
	1. Repetitive contractions of the abdominal muscles, diaphragm, and tongue
	2. Effort less regurgitation of gastric contents, which are either expelled from the mouth or rechewed and reswallowed
	3. Three or more of the following:
	  a. Onset between 3 and 8 months
	  b. Does not respond to management for gastroesophageal reflux disease and regurgitation
	  c. Unaccompanied by signs of distress
	  d. Does not occur during sleep and when the infant is interacting with individuals in the environment

Adolescent rumination syndrome	Must include all of the following:
	1. Repeated painless regurgitation and rechewing or expulsion of food that
	  a. Begin soon after ingestion of a meal
	  b. Do not occur during sleep
	  c. Do not respond to standard treatment for gastroesophageal reflux
	2. No retching
	3. No evidence of an inflammatory, anatomic, metabolic, or neoplastic process that explains the subject's symptoms

Cyclic vomiting syndrome	Must include all of the following: 1. Two or more periods of unremitting paroxysmal vomiting with or without retching, lasting hours to days within Process that explains the subject's symptoms Must include all of the following: 1. Two or more periods of unremitting paroxysmal vomiting with or without retching, lasting hours to days within a 6-month period 2. Episodes are Stereotypical in each patient 3. Episodes are separated by weeks to months with return to baseline Health between episodes of vomiting

Abdominal migraine	Must include all of the following:
	1. Paroxysmal episodes of intense, acute periumbilical pain that lasts for 1 hour or more
	2. Intervening periods of usual health lasting weeks to months
	3. The pain interferes with normal activities
	4. The pain is associated with two or more of the following:
	  a. Anorexia
	  b. Nausea
	  c. Vomiting
	  d. Headache
	  e. Photophobia
	  f. Pallor
	5. No evidence of an inflammatory, anatomic, metabolic, or neoplastic Process considered that explains the subject's symptoms

TABLE 7: Symptomatic treatment for vomiting.

Drug	Mechanism of action	Dose	Indications	Side effects
Anti-histaminics				
Diphenhydramine	Vestibular suppression, anti ACH effect, and H1 antagonist	12.5–30 mg PO 4–6 hourly	Motion sickness	Sedation, anti-ACH effects
Meclizine		12.5–50 mg 1 hour before travel (>12 years old)		
Substituted Benzamide				
Metoclopramide	D2 antagonist, at CTZ, 5HT4 agonist in gut	0.1 mg/kg IV/IM/PO q 6–8 hourly	GERD, gastroparesis	Irritability and extrapyramidal reaction
Benzimidazole derivatives				
Domperidone	D2 antagonist on gut	0.1–0.2 mg/kg 8 hourly PO	Gastroparesis	Headache
5HT-3 receptor antagonist				
Ondansetron	5HT3 Antagonist at CTZ, and depresses vagal afferents from gut	0.1 mg/kg q8 hourly		

b. *Electrolyte imbalance*: Watch for disturbances in serum electrolytes and bicarbonate and correct adequately.

c. Keep empty stomach if any obstruction or pancreatitis is suspected.

2. Symptomatic treatment for vomiting **(Table 7)**.

Celiac Disease in Children

Vibhor Borkar

INTRODUCTION

Celiac disease (CeD) is an immune-mediated systemic disorder elicited by gluten in genetically susceptible individuals. Gluten is a major protein component of wheat, rye, and barley. The major predisposing genes are *HLA-DQ 2* and *HLA-DQ 8* genotype found in at least 95% of patients. CeD is a common disorder with about 1% prevalence of biopsy-proven disease. The pathogenesis of CeD is not yet completely understood. CeD is considered a T-cell mediated chronic inflammatory disorder with an autoimmune component.

CLINICAL PRESENTATION

Clinical features of CeD vary considerably. They can remain asymptomatic or have varied manifestations. It can complicate at times if severe and untreated as celiac crisis, or can lead to refractory CeD, jejunoileitis, enteropathy-associated T-cell lymphoma, etc.

- *First 2 years of life*: Intestinal symptoms are more common as a result of malabsorption. Child can have failure to thrive, chronic diarrhea, vomiting, abdominal distention, muscle wasting, anorexia, irritability, recurrent intussusception, and even constipation occasionally.
- *Older age group children*: Extra intestinal manifestations such as iron-deficiency anemia, which is usually unresponsive to iron therapy, osteoporosis, short stature, delayed puberty, arthritis, arthralgia, epilepsy with bilateral occipital calcifications, peripheral neuropathies, isolated hypertransaminasemia, dental enamel hypoplasia, and aphthous stomatitis.
- *Classical CeD*: Signs and symptoms of malabsorption are present.
- *Nonclassical CeD*: Without signs and symptoms of malabsorption.
- *Silent CeD (subclinical)*: No apparent symptoms or signs in spite of histological evidence of mucosal damage and positive serology
- *Latent CeD*: Confusing term; better to avoid
- *Potential CeD*: Normal mucosa, asymptomatic patient and positive serology
- *Association*: Some diseases with autoimmune pathogenesis are found with a higher than normal incidence in CeD patients. Among these are type 1 diabetes, autoimmune thyroid disease, Addison disease, Sjögren syndrome, rheumatoid arthritis, autoimmune cholangitis, autoimmune hepatitis, and primary biliary cholangitis. Other associated conditions include selective IgA deficiency and Down, Turner, and Williams syndromes.

DIAGNOSIS

The diagnosis of CeD is based on a combination of symptoms, antibodies, HLA status, and duodenal histology.

- *Serologies of CeD*: The initial approach to symptomatic patients is to test for anti-tissue transglutaminase immunoglobulin A (anti-TG2IgA) antibodies and for total IgA in serum to exclude IgA deficiency. IgA anti-TG2 decline if the patient is on a gluten-free diet. In patients with selective IgA deficiency, testing is recommended with IgG antibodies to TG2. **Table 1** gives the various serological tests and their utility.

TABLE 1: Various serological tests and their utility.

Serology	Sensitivity	Specificity	Comment
IgA TTG-2	74–94%	99–97%	Reliable, affordable and easily available—Preferred serology
IgA EMA	83–95%	95–100%	Operator dependant, and expensive
IgG DGP	90–99%	92–95%	May be used in children with IgA deficiency
IgA DGP	92–99%	93–98%	Comparable to TTG
IgA AGA	61–88%	89%	Not to be used

(AGA: anti-gliadin antibody; DGP: deamidated gliadin peptide; EMA: endomysial antibodies; IgA: immunoglobulin A; IgG: immunoglobulin G; TTG-2: anti-tissue transglutaminase)

TABLE 2: Modified Marsh-Oberhuber grading.

Grade	Description	Comment
Marsh 0	Normal mucosa and villous architecture	
Marsh 1	Infiltrative increased IEL > 25/100 enterocytes	
Marsh 2	1+ hyperplastic crypts	
Marsh 3	2+destructive–villousatrophy 3a-partialvillousatrophy • 3b: Subtotal villous atrophy • 3c: Total villous atrophy	More consistent with celiac disease
Marsh 4	Hypoplastic flat atrophic mucosa –total villous atrophy with crypt hypoplasia	More consistent with celiac disease

(IEL: intraepithelial lymphocytes)

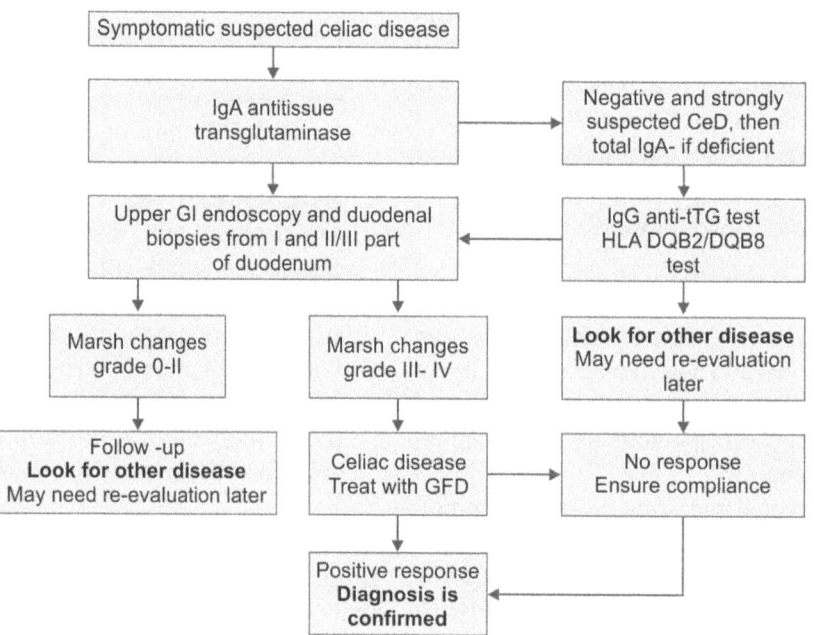

Flowchart 1: Diagnostic algorithm for celiac disease.

- *Intestinal biopsy*: It is very important part in diagnostic workup. At least two biopsies from first part of duodenum and 4 biopsies from second part of duodenum are required. Histopathological changes of CeD are given as modified Marsh grading **(Table 2)**.

Role of intestinal biopsy in diagnosis of CeD: Need of intestinal biopsy for confirmation of CeD is currently matter of debate. The American college of Gastroenterology recommends intestinal biopsy as an integral part of diagnostic workup. However, the European Society for Paediatric Gastroenterology, Hepatology and Nutrition (ESPGHAN) 2012 introduced concept that small intestinal biopsies can be omitted in children with CeD symptoms, high TTG-2 (10 times upper limit of normal) and predisposing *HLA* genotype. However, this new guideline needs validation in respective countries to be followed. In India, the Indian Council of Medical Research (ICMR) guidelines (2016) advise that diagnosis of CeD should not be based on only very high TTG.

Gallstones in Children

Aabha Nagral

INTRODUCTION

Gallstone (GS) or cholelithiasis has been described in 0.1–2% of children in worldwide studies although the incidence is increasing. GS can present in all age groups and the proportion varies: 50% in adolescents >12 years of age, 40% in 2–12 years of age, and 10% in infants <2 years. GS are more common in girls compared to boys in the adolescent age group (as in adults) but girls and boys have similar prevalence in childhood.

TYPES OF GALLSTONES

In the past, hemolytic disease was thought to be a cause of majority of GSs in children. Recent studies suggest a lower prevalence to 20–25% as other causes such as childhood obesity have become more common. Determining the type of GS may help in planning the management.

The types of GS seen in children are different from those seen in adults:

- *Pigment stones* constitutes more than half of GS in children. Black pigment stones are secondary to hemolysis and brown pigment stones are usually secondary to parasitic infection.
- *Cholesterol stones* are related to obesity and genetic factors.
- *Calcium carbonate stones* are seen in sick neonates and patients with Down syndrome.

CAUSES/ASSOCIATIONS WITH GALLSTONES

In adults, GS disease does not have a single identified cause. On the other hand, in children a cause can be identified in a significant number, which are as follows:

- *Hemolysis*: Excessive breakdown of RBCs usually secondary to sickle cell disease or hereditary spherocytosis. These are pigment stones
- Children with a family history of GSs are more predisposed
- Childhood obesity
- Prolonged fasting usually due to an illness
- Long-term total parenteral nutrition, especially post ileal bypass or resection (e.g., infants with necrotizing enterocolitis)
- Use of drugs such as ceftriaxone and diuretics
- Use of hormonal pills
- Cardiopulmonary bypass operations (through hemolysis)
- Prematurity
- Down syndrome.

Ceftriaxone-related gallbladder sludge:

- Treatment with ceftriaxone can cause calcium ceftriaxone precipitates or pseudolithiasis or ceftriaxone sludge to develop in 25–40% of patients on ceftriaxone and was first described in 1961.
- The liver secretes an abnormal bile with high concentration of ceftriaxone, far exceeding the calculated solubility product.
- The gallbladder provides an environment for precipitation of calcium ceftriaxone for sludge to develop.
- The ceftriaxone sludge can rapidly form and disappear and is often asymptomatic.
- It can occasionally become a calcium ceftriaxone GS.

SYMPTOMS/COMPLICATIONS

- *Incidental*: GSs are often incidentally detected when the child undergoes an ultrasound for an unrelated problem or recurrent abdominal pain not suggestive of biliary disease. The GSs lying in the gallbladder per se are asymptomatic (**Flowchart 1**).
- *Biliary colic*: This is the pain which occurs in the epigastrium or right upper quadrant and lasts for 15 minutes to few hours to a day and may radiate to the right shoulder or back. It is often associated with vomiting. It is manifested when the gallbladder contracts and causes a GS to temporarily block the cystic duct which drains the gallbladder. The pain usually settles when the GS usually drops back into the gallbladder. The classic biliary colic and associated complications are seen in children and adolescents.

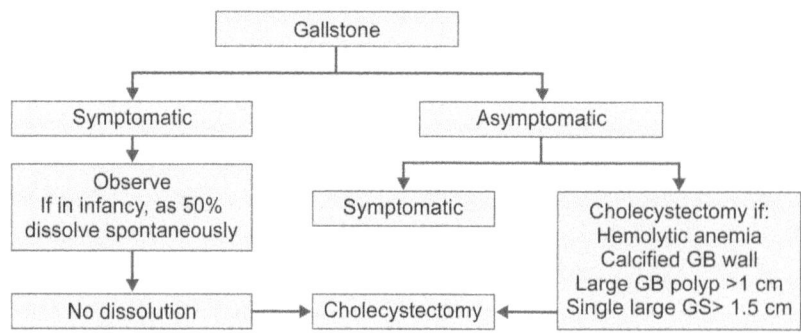

Flowchart 1: Algorithm for approach to gallstone treatment in children.

- *Infants*: GSs are often asymptomatic in infants and can manifest as sepsis, vomiting, jaundice, and colics.
- *Acute cholecystitis*: If the gallstone remains in the cystic duct, it may cause distension of the gallbladder and inflammation and thickening of the walls. There is tenderness over the gallbladder on deep inspiration (Murphy's sign) and fever. The pain here lasts much longer.
- *Chronic cholecystitis*: The acute attacks of cholecystitis may settle or keep recurring to cause a chronically inflamed and thickened gallbladder—chronic cholecystitis.
- *Choledocholithiasis (bile duct stones)*: When the gallstone (small stones are more likely) slips into the bile duct there is pain usually in the epigastrium with or without vomiting. It may pass off through the papilla into the duodenum or get stuck in the bile duct causing jaundice, fever, and pain—the Charcot's triad of cholangitis.
- *Acute pancreatitis*: Gallstones may get stuck at the papilla causing obstruction to flow of pancreatic juice and ensuing inflammation of the pancreas—acute pancreatitis.

INVESTIGATIONS

- *Biochemical tests* show a rise in liver enzymes during passage of GSs in the bile duct and may even go above 1,000 IU/L. If the GS gets impacted in the bile duct, there is direct hyperbilirubinemia with more than three-fold rise in alkaline phosphatase and gamma-glutamyl transferase (GGT). There is leukocytosis in acute cholecystitis or cholangitis or pancreatitis. Acute pancreatitis will also have a more than three-fold rise in amylase or lipase enzymes.
- *Ultrasound (USG)*:
  - GSs are best and easily diagnosed on ultrasound of the abdomen in a fasting state. If the USG is performed after eating, the gallbladder is often collapsed and the GSs may be missed. GSs are seen as mobile hyperechoic are as in the dependent part of the gallbladder with posterior acoustic shadowing.
  - *Biliary sludge*: Bile is a transparent aqueous solution. When precipitates occur, the sediments are referred to as biliary sludge. Sludge most commonly consists of cholesterol monohydrate and calcium bilirubinate. There is no posterior acoustic shadowing in sludge. However, calcium ceftriaxone sludge produces posterior acoustic shadowing as the sludge can be very dense and can be mistaken for a GS.
  - *Cholecystitis* is recognized by thickened gallbladder wall > 3 mm and presence of pericholecystic fluid with USG demonstration of probe tenderness over the gallbladder. Chronic cholecystitis is diagnosed by a thickened gallbladder wall with a contracted gallbladder.
- *Computed tomography (CT) scan*: Complications of acute cholecystitis include empyema, emphysematous/gangrenous cholecystitis, gallbladder perforation and need a CT scan for diagnosis.
- *Magnetic resonance cholangiopancreatography (MRCP)*: When common bile duct stones are found, with a hugely dilated bile duct a choledocalcyst with anomalous pancreatobiliary duct junction needs to be excluded. MRCP should be performed in this situation.

TREATMENT

- Most asymptomatic GSs do not merit any treatment. Smaller stones often pass off on their own.
- *Prophylactic cholecystectomy*: The indications for prophylactic cholecystectomy in the asymptomatic group are not well defined. However, for practical purposes, the accepted indications are hemolytic disease; large stones >1.5 cm; situations which predispose to development of carcinoma of the gallbladder—porcelain or calcified GB; gallbladder polyps >1 cm in size; anomalous pancreatobiliary duct union.
- The GS colic may be temporarily managed by NSAID injections or suppositories (Ketorolac, diclofenac) or antispasmodics such as drotaverine.
- *Cholecystectomy*: Symptomatic GSs need definitive treatment in the form of a cholecystectomy usually laparoscopic. Open cholecystectomy may be needed

PRESCRIPTION ASSISTANCE

Biliary colic.

Pharmacological agent	Market preparation	Availability	Dosages
Ketorolac (>6 months of age)	Cadolac, Ketorol	IM/IV injection—1 mL, 30 mg/mL	0.5–1 mg/kg IM/IV
Diclofenac sodium	Diclonac, Jonac	Tablets 50 mg Suppository 12.5 mg and 100 mg Injection 3 mL 25 mg/mL	1–3 mg/kg
Drotaverine	Drotin	Tablet 40 mg Syrup 10 mg/5 mL Injection 40 mg/2 mL	20 mg per dose for 4–6 years of age 40 mg for >6 years of age

(IM: intramuscular; IV: intravenous)

when laparoscopic route is technically not feasible. It does not help by just removing stones as they are very likely to recur as the gallbladder wall itself is diseased which predisposes to formation of stones. In acute cholecystitis, the patient is started on antibiotics and cholecystectomy is advocated in the same admission.
- In infants, even in symptomatic stones, one may have a case for waiting at least up to a year as 50% may dissolve, especially if there are no complications.
- *Endoscopic retrograde cholangiopancreatography (ERCP):* Bile duct stones merit removal endoscopically through ERCP (through sphincterotomy and extraction) when feasible in an older child or through the percutaneous biliary route when endoscopic removal is not feasible.

Role of UDCA

- There is no role of ursodeoxycholic acid (UDCA) in treatment of GS since these are usually pigment stones.
- Studies in children, both in asymptomatic and symptomatic groups, have shown a very low incidence of dissolution with UDCA and high recurrence ranging from a third of patients to 100%.
- In a study from Toronto comprising 382 children with GS diagnosed over a 6.5 years period, in the 194 who were asymptomatic, the complication rate, indication for cholecystectomy was much lower than seen in the symptomatic group and was statistically significant.
- Of the 58 (15.1%) diagnosed in infancy, 81% were asymptomatic. The infant group also had low rates of complications (8.6%) and cholecystectomy (1.7%). In cases with sonographic follow-up, resolution of GSs was demonstrated in 16.5% of asymptomatic patients and in 34.1% of infants.

Do GSs disappear in children?

- Natural dissolution of asymptomatic GS has also been reported in children.
- It is as high as 50% in neonates, 34% in infants and is <16% in children.
- The dissolution usually occurs in 14–24 months.
- Diagnosis of GS at age <2 years, small-sized stone (<5 mm) and a solitary stone are more likely to undergo spontaneous dissolution.
- Dissolution may be related to change in the bile composition or removal of the factor responsible for stone formation.
- Asymptomatic passage of the stone into the duodenum is also a possibility.

KEY MESSAGES

- Gallstones are uncommon in children although the incidence is increasing.
- Asymptomatic/incidental gallstones do not require any intervention as risk of complications is low.
- Prophylactic cholecystectomy may be warranted in a specific subgroup of patients with asymptomatic GSs.
- In infants, natural dissolution rate of GS is high and observation may be warranted even in symptomatic stones up to 1–2 years of age.
- There is no role for UDCA in management of gallstones.
- Cholecystectomy is the definitive treatment for gallstones-preferably laparoscopic whenever feasible.

SUGGESTED READING

1. Bogue CO, Murphy AJ, Gerstle JT, Moineddin R, Daneman A. Risk factors, complications, and outcomes of gallstones in children: a single-center review. J Pediatr Gastroenterol Nutr. 2010;50:303-8.
2. Debray D, Pariente D, Gauthier F, Myara A, Bernard O. Cholelithiasis in infancy: a study of 40 cases. J Pediatr. 1993; 122:385-91.
3. Deepak J, Agarwal P, Bagdi RK, Balagopal S, Madhu R, Balamourougane P. Pediatric cholelithiasis and laparoscopic management: a review of twenty two cases. J Minim Access Surg. 2009;5:93-6.
4. Kim YS, Kestell MF, Lee SP. Gall-bladder sludge: lessons from ceftriaxone. J Gastroenterol Hepatol. 1992;7:618-21.
5. Serdaroglu F, Koca YS, Saltik F, Koca T, Dereci S, Akcam M, et al. Gallstones in child-hood: etiology, clinical features, and prognosis. Eur J Gastroenterol Hepatol. 2016;28:1468-72.
6. St-Vil D, Yazbeck S, Luks FI, Hancock BJ, Filiatrault D, Youssef S. Cholelithiasis in newborns and infants. J Pediatr Surg. 1992;27: 1305-7.

Chapter 59: Upper Gastrointestinal Bleeding in Children

Shrish Bhatnagar, Saman Beg

INTRODUCTION

Upper gastrointestinal bleeding (UGIB) refers to the intraluminal hemorrhage proximal to the ligament of Treitz. The incidence is approximately 100 per 100,000 cases per year. UGIB is more common and massive than lower gastrointestinal bleeding (LGIB).

ETIOLOGY

In western countries, the most common causes are gastric and duodenal ulcers, esophagitis, gastritis, and varices whereas in India and some other parts of the world, variceal bleeding predominates **(Table 1)**.

DIFFERENTIAL DIAGNOSIS

It includes vomited blood originating from structures or organs other than the GI tract and ingested blood or blood-like substances:

- *Swallowed maternal blood*: Neonates and infants may swallow maternal blood during delivery or while nursing, and this can mimic UGIB. One method with which to distinguish maternal blood is the Apt-Downey test. The principal is that fetal hemoglobin is resistant to denaturation in an alkaline solution and remains red or pink and adult hemoglobin discolors to a brownish yellow.
- *Epistaxis*: Swallowed blood from the patient's nasopharynx or respiratory tract may be very difficult to distinguish from UGIB. To evaluate this possibility, the physical examination should include inspection of the nares for evidence of venous injury of the anterior medial septum. Some patients may require endoscopic evaluation to adequately assess for lesions in the nasopharynx, larynx, or respiratory tract.
- *Substances that resemble blood*: Red food colorings and dyes (e.g., red-colored drinks or liquid medications) also may be confused with blood, particularly after vomiting. While this can frequently be suspected from this history, bedside tests for occult blood also can be helpful. It is preferable to use a kit designed specifically to detect blood in gastric secretions (e.g., Gastroccult), which incorporates additional alkali to neutralize the gastric acid present in emesis.
- *Medical child abuse*: Factitious illness (Munchausen syndrome by proxy), caused by surreptitious administration of blood or blood-like substance to simulate UGIB, should be considered in patients with unexplained GI bleeding.

CLINICAL PRESENTATIONS

- *Hematemesis*: It refers to the passage of blood in vomiting. Depending upon the severity of hemorrhage and the duration, it stayed in contact with gastric juices, vomitus may be bright red or coffee ground in color.
- *Melena*: It is the production of dark sticky feces commonly referred as black tarry stool.

TABLE 1: Etiologies of UGIB.

Neonates	Infants and children
Swallowed maternal blood	Mallory-Weiss tear
Hemorrhagic disease of newborn	Esophageal/GI foreign body
Stress gastritis	Esophagitis
Congenital anomalies: Intestinal duplication/vascular anomaly	Peptic ulcer and gastritis
Coagulopathy/sepsis	Bleeding from esophageal varices
Milk protein allergy	*Arterial bleeding*: Dieulafoy's lesion, peptic ulcer

(UGIB: upper gastrointestinal bleeding)

- *Hematochezia*: It refers to passage bright red color blood in stool. Due to short intestinal transit time, neonates and infants with UGI bleeding are more likely to present with hematochezia.
- *Clinical features suggesting a severe UGIB*:
  - Melena or hematochezia
  - Heart rate >20 bpm above the mean heart rate for age
  - Prolonged capillary refill time
  - Decrease in hemoglobin of >2 g/dL
  - Need for fluid bolus
  - Need for blood transfusion (given if hemoglobin <8 g/dL)

MANAGEMENT

Initial Assessment and Resuscitation

- Monitor important parameters of patient such as heart rate, blood pressure, pulse volume, poor peripheral perfusion, peripheral cyanosis, and urine output.
- Oliguria can develop secondary to reduced renal perfusion.
- Increase in heart rate by 20 bpm and drop in systolic blood pressure by 10 mm Hg from baseline are reliable markers of significant blood loss in children.
- Patients with hemodynamic instability (shock and orthostatic hypotension) should be admitted to an intensive care unit for resuscitation and close observation.

History

The clinical history should include information concerning the time course of the bleeding episode, estimated blood loss, and any associated symptoms.
- The presence of hematemesis, melena, or hematochezia should be documented; these characteristics provide clues about the source and rate of bleeding.
- History of (H/o) dyspepsia, heart burn, abdominal pain, dysphagia, and weight loss in children whereas poor feeding and irritability in infants.
- Recent onset of jaundice, easy bruising, or change in stool color (underlying liver disease).
- Recent or recurrent epistaxis (nasopharyngeal source of bleeding).
- H/o easy bruising or bleeding (coagulation disorder, platelet dysfunction, or thrombocytopenia).
- Personal or family history of liver, kidney, or heart disease, or coagulation disorders.
- Drug history related to nonsteroidal anti-inflammatory drugs (NSAIDs), corticosteroids, ibuprofen, tetracycline intake.

Physical Examination

The rapid assessment of hemodynamic status is described above. Rule out possible sources for the bleeding **(Flowchart 1)**:
- Examination of the skin and mucus membranes for bruising, petechiae, or mucosal bleeding is done. Depending on the presentation and pattern, these findings may suggest a bleeding disorder [e.g., immune thrombocytopenia (ITP)], trauma, or liver disease.
- Abdominal examination for evidence of portal hypertension, such as splenomegaly or a prominent cutaneous abdominal and hemorrhoidal vessels and ascites.
- Inspection of the nasopharynx for evidence of disrupted mucosa and inspection of the anterior nares for evidence of venous injury of the anterior medial septum.

Laboratory Evaluation

- Hematocrit and hemoglobin should be monitored frequently to assess severity of blood loss.
- Coagulation studies, liver function tests, blood urea nitrogen (BUN), and serum creatinine.
- For patients with epigastric abdominal pain, pancreatitis also should be ruled out with screening amylase and lipase; pancreatitis occasionally is associated with gastritis, duodenitis, and peptic ulcer disease.
- Elevation of BUN secondary to absorption of intestinal blood also points to an UGI cause.

Imaging

- *Plain radiographs* to identify a foreign body if this is suspected by the clinical history.
- *Abdominal ultrasound* can be used to evaluate splenomegaly and portal hypertension and should be performed in patients with severe acute UGIB suggestive of variceal bleeding, known or suspected liver disease, or those with signs of portal hypertension on examination (e.g., splenomegaly, prominent abdominal wall vessels).
- *UGI barium studies* should NOT be performed in the setting of UGIB, because the contrast will interfere with subsequent endoscopy or angiography.

Upper Gastrointestinal Endoscopy

- The indications for upper GI endoscopy are both diagnostic and therapeutic purposes in a hemodynamically stable patient.
- It is useful for evaluating the cause and site of bleeding and also for treating the lesion.

Other diagnostic tests include angiography and radionucleotide studies but not widely used.

Treatment

- *In hemodynamically stable patients*: Supportive care with observation generally is sufficient, usually with acid suppression to treat any peptic component and reduce the risk for rebleeding.
- *In hemodynamically unstable patients*:
  - Good venous assess, intake output monitoring, oxygen inhalation, and charting of vitals are mandatory.

Flowchart 1: Algorithm of management of UGIB.

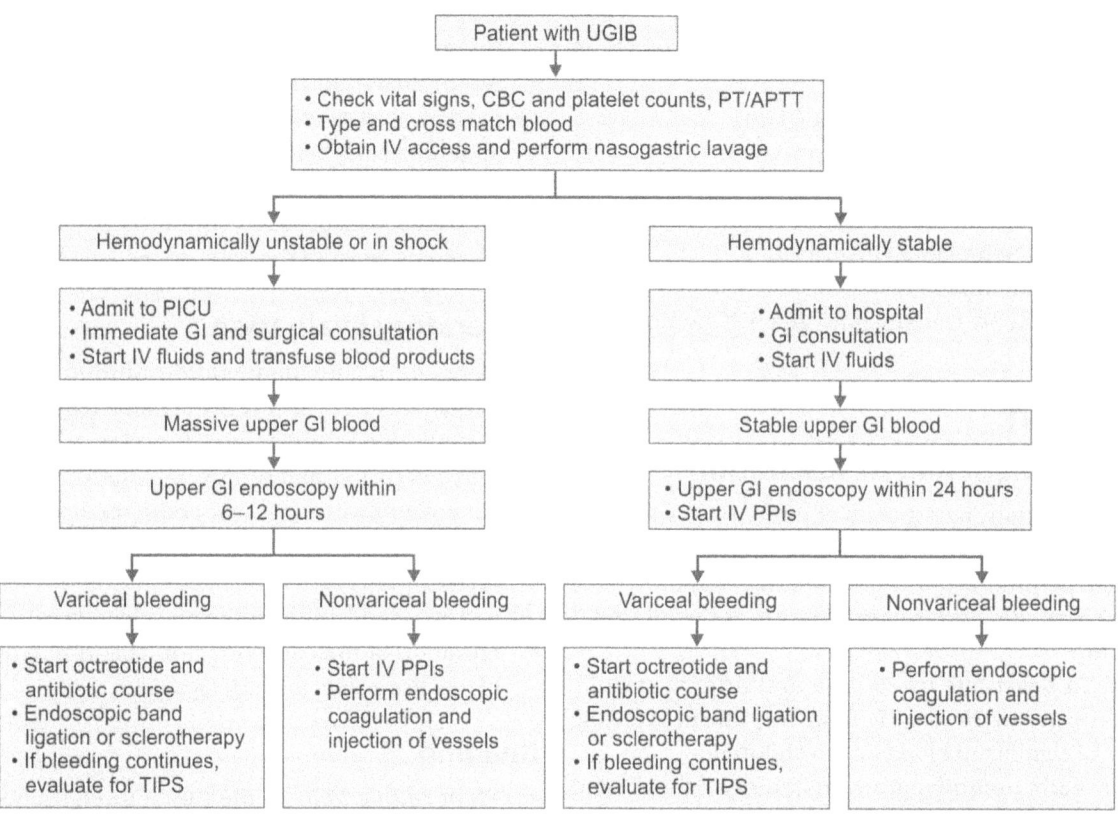

(APTT: activated partial thromboplastin time; CBC: complete blood count; IV: intravenous; PICU: pediatric intensive care unit; PPIs: proton-pump inhibitors; PT: prothrombin time; TIPS: transjugular intrahepatic portosystemic shunt; UGIB: upper gastrointestinal bleeding)

- Hemodynamic resuscitation with blood transfusion and crystalloid/colloid infusion for maintenance and to replace the ongoing losses.
- Nasogastric (NG) tube should be left in situ for gravity drainage to detect any recurrence of bleeding for 24 hours and vigorous NG suction should be avoided to prevent mucosal trauma. The lavage may be performed with either water or normal saline at room temperature. Ice water lavage is not recommended as it may induce iatrogenic hypothermia, particularly in infants and small children.
- Correction of coagulopathy and thrombocytopenia by fresh frozen plasma (FFP) and/or platelet transfusion.
- Correction of electrolytes and acid–base abnormality.
- *Pharmacological agents include acid suppression and vasoactive agents*:
  - *Acid suppression*: Intravenous proton-pump inhibitors (PPIs) should be initiated. Intravenous pantoprazole dose for ulcer bleed is 2 mg/kg (maximum 80 mg) loading followed by 0.2 mg/kg/h infusion (maximum 8 mg/h). High-dose infusion PPI is thought to promote clot stability and facilitate hemostasis by raising the intragastric pH.
- *Vasoactive agents*, somatostatin and octreotide, decrease the splanchnic and azygous blood flow thus reducing the pressure in the varices and they also reduce the gastric secretions. Overall this therapy is well tolerated, with mild side effects such as hyperglycemia, abdominal discomfort, nausea, and diarrhea. Dose of octreotide is 1 µg/kg bolus and then 1 µg/kg/h infusion (maximum 5 µg/kg/h).

  Infusion should be given for at least 24–48 hours after the bleeding has stopped to prevent recurrence and care should be taken not to stop the infusion abruptly.
- Short-term antibiotic prophylaxis (third-generation cephalosporin for 7 days) reduces bacterial infection.
- *Endoscopy* should be performed within 24–48 hours for infants and children presenting with UGIB that is acute and severe.

  Hemodynamically unstable patients should be stabilized prior to endoscopy, including transfusion and correction of coagulopathy if present.
- *Endoscopic sclerotherapy of varices (EST)*:
  - The varices are inspected and their location, size, and extent are documented with a fiberoptic endoscope.

PRESCRIPTION ASSISTANCE

Drug	Market preparation	Availability	Dosages
Ranitidine	Rantac, Zantac, Rantid	• Drops 150 mg/10 mL • Syrup 75 mg/5 mL • Tablet 75, 150, 300 mg • Injection 50 mg/2 mL amp	2–4 mg/kg/day PO q 8–12 hours, (maximum 10 mg/kg/day)
Sucralfate	Sucral, Ucracid, Sucralwell	• Syrup 1 g/10 mL • Tablet 1 g	0.5–1.0 g PO q 6 hour
Lansoprazole	Lanzol Jr	Tablet 15 mg, 30 mg	• <30 kg: 15 mg/day • >30 kg: 30 mg/day
Pantoprazole	Pantop, Pantocid	• Tablet 20 mg, 40 mg • Injection 40 mg/vial	2 mg/kg (maximum 80 mg) loading f/b 0.2 mg/kg/h infusion (maximum 8 mg/h)
Octreotide	Sandostatin	• Injection (amp): 0.05, 0.1, 0.5 mg/mL • Injection (MDV): 0.2, 1 mg/mL (5 mL)	1 µg/kg bolus f/b 1 µg/kg/h infusion (maximum 5 µg/kg/h)

- A flexible needle is inserted through the endoscope to inject 2–3 mL of sclerosant into engorged vessel.
- Following emergency EST, the varices are then sclerosed at interval of 2–3 weeks until all varices are obliterated.
- Emergency EST is very effective (>90%) in controlling esophageal variceal bleeding. Major complications include esophageal ulceration, perforation, and stricture of esophagus.
- *Endoscopic variceal ligation (EVL)*:
  - EVL is done with a device called multiple band ligator. First a diagnostic UGI endoscopy is done to note the details of the varices and there after the space is removed, banding apparatus is loaded on the scope and the scope is reintroduced.
  - EVL can easily be performed in children >2 years of age and it is desirable to give sedation in order to minimize the risk and increase the ease of performing the procedure.

KEY MESSAGES

- Early resuscitation
- NG lavage and look for ongoing bleeding
- High-dose PPIs therapy for at least 72 hours
- Urgent endoscopy for severe UGIB
- Combination therapy preferred over only medical management.

SUGGESTED READING

1. Kleinman K, McDaniel L, Molloy M. The Harriet Lane Handbook, 20th edition. Philadelphia, PA: Saunders; 2015.
2. Singh M. Medical Emergencies in Children, 5th edition. New Delhi: CBS Publishers & Distributors Pvt Ltd; 2016.
3. Villa X. (2021). Approach to upper gastrointestinal bleeding in children. [Online] Available from: https://www.uptodate.com/contents/approach-to-upper-gastrointestinal-bleeding-in-children. [Last accessed June, 2021].

Lower Gastrointestinal Bleed

Gautam Ray

INTRODUCTION

Gastrointestinal bleeding may be upper gastrointestinal (UGI) or lower gastrointestinal (LGI) depending on the site of bleeding. When the source of bleeding is distal to the ligament of Treitz, which is situated at duodenojejunal junction, it is called LGI bleeding (LGIB). Though UGI bleeding is more common than LGIB, LGIB is a fairly common clinical problem in pediatric office practice.

Blood in stool/bleeding per rectum (PR) may occur in three forms:
1. *Hematochezia*: Bright red blood or dark red color of the blood; the sources are usually colonic; maroon-color stools indicate small bowel bleeding.
2. *Melena*: Black tarry stools with a distinct offensive odor; source of bleed is proximal to the ligament of Treitz.
3. *Occult GI bleed*: Blood is not visible but can be detected by the stool occult blood test.

ETIOLOGY AND DIFFERENTIAL DIAGNOSIS (TABLE 1)

- Appropriate initial management (choosing the proper diagnostic and therapeutic modality) of LGIB would require a pragmatic clinical approach to the possible differential/provisional diagnosis. To achieve this, the importance of a proper history and physical examination cannot be overemphasized.
- *The approach is based on*:
  - *Age*: Infancy, toddlers (2–5 years), and older children
  - *Appearance of the child*: Well/ill appearing
  - Character of the blood/bleeding rate
  - Stool characteristics
  - *Associated symptoms*: Painless/painful, constipation, diarrhea, abdominal distention, rash/purpura, etc.
- When infants present with LGIB, commonly think of a fissure or an allergic proctocolitis, e.g., cow milk protein allergy (CMPA).
- In sick babies, necrotizing enterocolitis (NEC), Hirschsprung-associated enterocolitis, mid-gut volvulus need to be kept in mind, among others.
- For young children, the most common condition presenting with painful bleeding PR is an anal fissure, and acute self-limiting colitis/infectious diarrhea when there is associated pain abdomen (other causes such as intussusception may present similarly, but are rarer).
- The common causes of painless bleeding are colonic polyps (small-volume bleed), Meckel's diverticulum or enteric duplication cyst (large-volume bleed).
- For older children, anal fissures and polyps remain the most common causes.
- Inflammatory bowel diseases (IBD), though less common in young children, can present with LGI bleeding, especially when there is associated diarrhea and failure to thrive.
- Henoch–Schönlein purpura (HSP) (pain abdomen, buttock rash, bleed PR), Hemolytic uremic syndrome (HUS) [(history of (h/o) preceding bacterial infection], pseudomembranous colitis (h/o preceding antibiotic usage), CMV colitis (immunocompromised children) and other less commonly seen causes are suggested by the appropriate clinical presentation/associated symptoms.
- Location of the lesion can also be judged based on the character of bleeding; red blood coating the stool indicates an anorectal pathology, altered colored blood indicates colonic bleeding and maroon color indicates small bowel bleeding; while bloody diarrhea (blood and mucus mixed with stools) signifies colonic pathology; melena indicates UGI bleeding.
- *Digital rectal examination (DRE)*: A per-rectal examination is a MUST in all cases of LGIB. It consists of inspection of anal canal/perianal region, followed by a DRE.
- DRE should not be done if a fissure is found on external anal examination. In a sick child, gross blood on finger stalk is a predictor of severe bleeding.

INVESTIGATIONS

Before ordering fancy investigations, it should be remembered that there are some mimickers of rectal bleeding.

TABLE 1: Causes of lower gastrointestinal bleeding in children based on age, appearance, and bleed rate.

	Ill-looking child	Otherwise well-looking child	
		High bleeding rate	Low bleeding rate
Infants	Infectious colitis	Meckel's diverticulum	Anal fissure
	Necrotizing enterocolitis	Enteric duplication cyst	Eosinophilic proctocolitis/cow milk protein allergy
	Hirschsprung's enterocolitis	Vascular malformation	Infectious colitis
	Volvulus		Nodular lymphoid hyperplasia
Age: 2–5 years	Intussusception	Meckel's diverticulum	Infectious colitis
	Volvulus	Sloughed juvenile polyp	Juvenile polyp
	Henoch–Schönlein purpura (HSP)	Inflammatory bowel disease	Nodular lymphoid hyperplasia
	Hemolytic uremic syndrome	Enteric	*Inflammatory bowel disease*: Ulcerative
	HSP	Inflammatory bowel disease	Hyperplasia
	Hemolytic uremic syndrome	Enteric duplication cyst	*Inflammatory bowel disease*: Ulcerative colitis/Crohn's disease
Older child	Infectious colitis	Ulcerative colitis	Infectious colitis
	Inflammatory bowel disease (Ulcerative colitis/Crohn's disease)	Enteric duplication cyst	Ulcerative colitis/Crohn's disease
	HSP	Vascular malformations	Juvenile polyp
	Intestinal ischemia		Hemorrhoids

Dark-colored stools may be seen in children receiving oral iron therapy for anemia, or sometimes with intake of foods such as spinach. Red color of stools may be seen in those consuming beetroot, some fruit punches, or those on rifampicin therapy. A proper history can delineate the same.

First-line Investigations

- *Complete blood count (CBC):* In a large volume acute bleeding, the initial hematocrit may be misleading (it takes a few hours to decrease). It needs to be repeated 6 hourly to assess the impact of ongoing bleeding. Increased eosinophil counts may point toward an allergic etiology such as CMPA. The platelet counts may be low in sepsis, hypersplenism, or in HUS. Schistocytes in peripheral smear are seen in HUS.
- *Coagulation profile:* For suspected disorders of coagulation, prothrombin time/partial thromboplastin time is needed.
- Azotemia may be seen in HUS, HSP, or massive bleeding of any etiology.
- Urine testing is of significance in HUS and HSP.
- Stool needs to be tested for occult blood in anemia due to suspected GI blood loss.

Endoscopy

- The next step in evaluation is to find out the site and cause of LGI bleeding and endoscopy plays an important role.
- Elective full-length colonoscopy after proper bowel cleansing (best done with polyethylene glycol taken orally or through nasogastric tube) has the highest yield.
- Though polyps are commonly seen in the left colon, a third of children have lesions proximal to the rectosigmoid too.
- A short colonoscopy/sigmoidoscopy in an unprepared colon (with biopsies) is done in cases of acute severe colitis, where time is at a premium, and full colonoscopy carries a higher risk of perforation.
- Uncommonly massive UGI bleeding may manifest as LGI bleeding and in such cases upper GI endoscopy also indicated.
- Diagnoses classically made on colonoscopy (and histology) are polyps, IBD, other causes of colitis (CMPA enterocolitis, CMV colitis, pseudomembranous colitis, etc.), among others.
- Contraindications to the performance of endoscopy should be remembered; they are significant cardiopulmonary compromise, peritonitis, and bowel perforation.
- *It would be a good practice for the primary pediatrician to seek pediatric gastroenterology opinion for the following patients with LGIB—children with persistent (>1 week)/recurrent/severe bleeding. Endoscopy would* be needed in such situations.

Scintigraphy

- Technetium-99m pertechnetate disodium scintigraphy (Meckel's scan) should be requested before colonoscopy in patients with suspected Meckel diverticulum (young children with large-volume painless bleeding).

- Of note, a negative Meckel's scan does not rule out the diagnosis of a heterotrophic gastric mucosa, as this may happen in about a quarter to a third of all such children.
- Meckel's scan also detects the heterotopic gastric mucosa present in a duplication cyst.
- Nuclear bleeding scan (Technetium-99-labeled red blood cell scan) is not much used these days.

Angiography

- Whenever there is a suspicion of small bowel bleeding and when bidirectional endoscopy (both UGI and LGI) has remained inconclusive, angiography is the investigation of choice.
- Magnetic resonance angiography (MRA)/computed tomography angiography (CTA) are the modalities utilized, and though MRA has the advantage of lack of radiation, CTA remains the workhorse for such situations.

Enteroscopy (Video Capsule Endoscopy and Deep Enteroscopy)

For nonemergency patients [mostly for obscure GI bleed, (OGIB)], small bowel enteroscopy (double-balloon/single-balloon enteroscopy) has been shown to be the most cost-effective modality in adults, though for children double-balloon enteroscopy (DBE) is generally done after video capsule enteroscopy. The diagnostic utility of these modalities for OGIB is >50%.

TREATMENT

- The first question that needs to be answered is whether the child is hemodynamically stable, and those requiring stabilization should be managed emergently as per protocol [ABC: airway, breathing (oxygen supplementation) and circulation (crystalloid infusion and blood transfusion)].
- Of equal priority is identification of those children whose LGIB is due to intestinal obstruction or due to a surgical cause (volvulus, intussusception, NEC, etc.). A pediatric surgery consultation should be urgently arranged in such cases.
- Treatment basically involves treatment of the underlying etiology. Since treatment of all individual diseases is beyond the scope of this chapter, a few salient features are highlighted.
  - *Endoscopic therapy*: Common lesions which can be tackled by endoscopy are polyps (polypectomy), ulcer or vascular lesions (injection/hemoclip/local ablation therapy). For a bleeding ulcer or a vascular lesions, there are three modalities are used for arrest of bleeding. These are injection therapy (adrenaline, sclerosants, glue, etc.), mechanical therapy (e.g., hemoclips, bands), and ablation therapy. Ablation therapy may be through contact devices (commonly using bipolar electric probes; heater probes are used rarely) or noncontact devices (e.g., argon plasma coagulation, which is being increasingly used, and remains a modality of choice for vascular malformations).
  - Polypectomy during colonoscopy is common practice among gastroenterologists.
  - *Conventional angiography [Digital subtracting angiography (DSA) and coil embolization]*: DSA has therapeutic potential for arterial sources of bleeding, with the radiologist performing coiling or embolization of the culprit artery documented by CT angiography or MR angiography.
  - Among enteroscopy devices, DBE is superior as it can be used to obtain tissue for histology, and has therapeutic applications as well.

PROGNOSIS

Most LGIB is due to benign or self-limiting causes. The overall reported mortality has varied from <1 to <5%. Recurrence of LGIB is seen in 10–20% of children. Prognosis depends on the underlying cause.

KEY MESSAGES

- *Classification is useful*: Painful/painless; colitic/noncolitic; age of onset; severity of bleeding.
- A proper history and physical examination are essential for arriving at a provisional diagnosis.
- Per-rectal examination is a MUST.
- In <2 years age group, anal fissure/CMPA is a common cause.
- Infant/toddler presenting with pain abdomen/tenderness associated with LGIB think of intussusception.
- *Large amount of bright/maroon-colored blood in a well-child*: Meckel's diverticulum.
- *Toddlers/older children*: Polyps and fissures are the common causes.
- Obtain pediatric gastroenterology opinion for persistent/recurrent/severe diverticulum.
- Involve a pediatric surgeon for suspected intestinal obstruction/surgical causes.

SUGGESTED READING

1. Lawrence Jr WW, Wright JL. Causes of rectal bleeding in children. Pediatrics in Review. 2001;22:94.
2. Romano C, Oliva S, Martellossi S, Miele E, Arrigo S, Giovanna M, et al. Pediatric gastrointestinal bleeding: perspectives from the Italian Society of Pediatric Gastroenterology. World J Gastroenterol. 2017;23(8):1328-37.
3. Sahn B, Bitton S. Lower gastrointestinal bleeding in children. Gastrointest Endoscopy Clin N Am. 2016;26:75-98.
4. Teach SJ, Fleisher GR. Rectal bleeding in the pediatric emergency department. Ann Emerg Med. 1994;23:1252-8.

CHAPTER 61: Acute Pancreatitis in Children

Rimjhim Shrivastava

INTRODUCTION

Acute pancreatitis (AP) is an inflammatory condition of pancreas and its surroundings due to the release of the enzymatic cascade initiated by the conversion of trypsinogen to trypsin, leading to autolysis. The most common etiology of AP in pediatric population is idiopathic followed by trauma, systemic illness, structural abnormalities of biliary tree or pancreas, drugs, and infections.

DIAGNOSIS

A detailed history, complete physical examination, and biochemical markers are sufficient for the diagnosis of AP. Imaging in the early phase of AP usually is not required.

Diagnosis of AP requires at least two of the following:
1. Abdominal pain compatible with AP
2. Serum amylase and/or lipase values ≥3 times upper limits of normal
3. Imaging findings consistent with AP.

CLINICAL FEATURES

Abdominal pain or irritability is the most common finding of AP, followed by epigastric tenderness, nausea, and vomiting. Abdominal pain can be localized to epigastrium or diffuse and is persistent or minimally easing. Only 1.6–5.6% patients present with the classic epigastric pain radiating to the back.

CLASSIFICATION

Acute recurrent pancreatitis: Two or more than two episodes of AP with normal intervening period are termed acute recurrent pancreatitis. The intervening period should be of at least 4 weeks and pain-free or there should be a pain-free interval of any duration with complete normalization of serum pancreatic enzyme levels.

Chronic pancreatitis: It is diagnosed if there is typical abdominal pain or exocrine pancreatic insufficiency or diabetes, along with characteristic imaging findings.

INVESTIGATIONS

- *Complete blood count*: A complete blood count demonstrating leukocytosis can point toward infective pancreatitis. Hemoconcentration at admission has been proposed as a negative predictor. Low hemoglobin can be seen in traumatic pancreatitis.
- *Serum amylase*: Rise in levels is seen in the early phase of the disease and can normalize by 24 hours after onset of symptoms.
- *Serum lipase*: Elevation in serum lipase concentration is detected within 6 hours of symptoms, the peak serum level is attained at 24–30 hours, and it remains elevated for >1 week. Levels over seven times the upper limit of normal within 24 hours of presentation may indicate severe disease.
- *Liver function test (LFT)*: Biliary pancreatitis can be suspected with abnormal LFTs. All patients undergoing evaluation for the first episode of AP should have LFTs done.
- *Genetic mutation analysis*: It is reserved for recurrent or chronic pancreatitis. They have mutations in the *cationic trypsinogen (PRSS1), cystic fibrosis transmembrane generator (CFTR), serine protease inhibitor Kazal type 1 (SPINK1), carboxypeptidase1 (CPA1) genes.*
- *Imaging*: In AP, it is required to document complications as fluid collection, necrosis, or anatomical abnormalities.
- *USG*: Ultrasound is noninvasive and safe but has lower sensitivity in visualizing the pancreas compared to contrast-enhanced computed tomography (CECT). Nevertheless, it is recommended as the first choice for imaging. In AP, it shows characteristic pancreatic parenchymal edema, changes in echogenicity, or peripancreatic fluid collections. Severe necrosis can also be picked up.
- *CECT*: *It is the gold standard*. It is usually utilized in ambiguous situations when there is delayed presentation and serum enzymes are low. If required, it should be done after 96 hours of presentation as the evolution of several complications may not be seen in early phase.

- *Magnetic resonance imaging (MRI)*: It is generally reserved for the detection of late complications.
- *Magnetic resonance cholangiopancreatography (MRCP)* in AP is used if there is suspicion of biliary or pancreatic ductular causes of AP.

MANAGEMENT

- *Fluid management*: Fluid resuscitation is the mainstay of AP management.
  Early fluid replacement with the correction of hypovolemia increases the perfusion of the pancreas and reduces necrosis and other complications.
  Though there is lack of consensus but Ringer lactate, normal saline, or dextrose-containing crystalloids are the choices of fluids. Fluid therapy should be aggressive with a rate of 1.5–2 times the maintenance rate in the first 24 hours.
- *Pain management*: Management of pain in AP is very crucial but should be given only when indicated. For mild pain, paracetamol or ibuprofen is the drug of choice. Opioids as meperidine can be used in severe pain.
- *Nutrition*: Early nutrition therapy is considered another important modality for AP management. Oral, enteral, or parentral nutrition should be initiated within 72 hours for a better outcome. Nutrition maintains gut barrier function, prevents bacterial translocation thus lowering the risk for infection.
- *Antibiotics*: Prophylactic antibiotics are not recommended in AP. It is indicated only if there is infected necrosis of pancreas or noninfected necrosis without clinical improvement. The choice of antibiotics is third-generation cephalosporins, metronidazole, or carbapenem.
- *Endoscopic retrograde cholangiopancreatography (ERCP)*: It can be considered as a therapeutic modality if there is biliary pancreatitis secondary to choledocholithiasis or sludge, pancreatic ductal stones, strictures, pseudocyst, and pancreatic duct leak or laceration. It should be done within 24–72 hours for better outcome.
- *Surgery*: Surgical intervention is required for severe abdominal trauma, cholecystectomy for biliary pancreatitis, open pseudocyst drainage or necrosectomy. In mild disease, cholecystectomy can be done within 48 hours and after 2 weeks for severe AP.

COMPLICATIONS

Acute pancreatitis in pediatric age group is mild in most cases and resolves without serious complications. Most commonly seen complication is *pseudocyst of pancreas* which rarely requires any intervention. Symptomatic pseudocyst can be managed by endoscopic or surgical drainage. Others might develop severe pancreatic inflammation and necrosis, systemic inflammatory response syndrome or multi-organ failure.

PROGNOSIS

Overall there is a favorable outcome in pediatric population with hospital stay ranging from 3–8 days and mortality <5%. Recurrence is seen in 15–35% of patients and is associated with anatomical abnormalities and metabolic and hereditary etiologies.

PHARMACOLOGICAL ASSISTANCE

Pharmacological salt	Market preparation	Availability (drops/syrup/tablet/injection)	Dosages
Acetaminophen	Crocin, Pyrigesic, p. 250, Calpol	• *Tablet*: 500 mg • *Syrup*: 125 mg/5 mL; 250 mg/5 mL • *Drops*: 100 mg/mL; 150 mg/mL • *Injection*: 150 mg/mL	• *Oral*: 15 mg/kg/dose 4–6 hourly • *Injection*: 5 mg/kg IM
Ibuprofen	Ibugesic, Brufen	• *Tablet*: 200 mg, 400 mg • *Suspension*: 100 mg/5 mL • *Injection*: 100 mg/mL	*Oral*: 10–15 mg/kg/dose 4–6 hourly
Meperidine	Pethidine	*Injection*: 50 mg/mL	*Dose*: 1–2 mg/kg/dose IV/IM
Ceftriaxone	Monocef, Oframax	250 mg, 500 mg. 1A Wg Vials	50–75 mg/kg/day IV 12 hourly
Metronidazole	Metrogyl, Aristogyl	• *Tablet*: 200mg, 400mg • *Suspension*: 200 mg/5 mL • *Injection*: 500 mg/100 mL	• *Oral*: 15–20 mg/kg/day 8 hourly • *IV*: 20 mg/kg/day 6 hourly
Imipenem	Iminem	• *Injection*: 500 mg, 100 mg, 1,500 mg • Powder for solution	• *Injection*: 60–100 mg/kg/day • 6 hourly IV/IM

CONCLUSION

- Acute pancreatitis is quite often seen in pediatric population and is a medical emergency.
- Most of the cases are mild.
- Serum biomarkers (Serum amylase and lipase) and USG are the recommended choice of initial evaluation.
- Further investigations and interventions are kept reserved for specific cases.
- Hydration, pain management, and nutrition are the main pillars of treatment.
- The prognosis of AP is very good in pediatric population but follow-up is required to identify any complication.

SUGGESTED READING

1. Abu-El-Haija M, Kumar S, Quiros JA, Balakrishnan K, Barth B, Bitton S, et al. The management of acute pancreatitis in the pediatric population: a clinical report from the NASPGHAN Pancreas Committee. J Pediatr Gastroenterol Nutr. 2018;66(1): 159-76.
2. Grzybowska-Chlebowczyk U, Jasielska M, Flak-Wancerz A, Więcek S, Gruszczyńska K, Chlebowczyk W, et al. Acute pancreatitis in children. Gastroenterology Rev. 2018;13(1):69-75.
3. Párniczky A, Abu-El-Haija M, Husain S, Lowe M, Oracz G, Sahin-Tóth M. EPC/HPSG evidence-based guidelines for the management of pediatric pancreatitis. Pancreatology. 2018;18(2):146-60.

CHAPTER 62: Ascites

Yogesh Waikar

INTRODUCTION

Ascites has been derived from the Greek word "askos," which means a bag or sack. Presence of fluid in abdomen or peritoneal cavity is termed ascites. Peritoneal fluid generally gravitates to flanks and intestine and generally floats in periumbilical region. It is a consequence of hepatic, cardiac, and renal diseases; infections; or malignancy. Development of ascites in cirrhotic patients is associated with poor mortality.

CLINICAL FEATURES

- Gradual distension of abdomen noted by mother or parent
- Tightening of clothes and weight gain with or without reduced urine output
- Associated symptoms such as yellow eyes, yellow urine, ecchymotic patches, and edema elsewhere.

SIGNS

Distended abdomen is noted with flank fullness or everted umbilicus.

Abdominal veins may or may not be distended. Hernial orifices and genital examination to rule out scrotal edema is must. Liver or spleen palpability should be checked along with abdominal tenderness or pain. Positive fluid wave and associated edema increases the possibility of ascites. In flanks tympanic note or absence of edema reduces the possibility of ascites. Flank dull note on percussion or bulging flanks suggests ascites. Shifting dullness or fluid thrill or wave is another sign well elicited in ascites.

PARACENTESIS AND ASCITIC FLUID ANALYSIS

Indications

- A diagnostic paracentesis should be performed in all patients with new-onset grade 2 or 3 ascites **(Table 1)**.
- In hospitalized patient for worsening of ascites or any complication of cirrhosis as per the European Association for the Study of the Liver (EASL) guidelines.

TABLE 1: Grading of ascites.

Grade 1 ascites	Mild detected by ultrasound only
Grade 2 ascites	*Moderate ascites evident on examination*: Moderate distension of abdomen
Grade 3 ascites	Large or gross ascites

- Ascitic fluid examination is used to determine cause, presence or absence of infection, or other pathologies.

Paracentesis is the procedure to collect fluid from peritoneal cavity for examination. It is either *diagnostic* or *therapeutic*.

Paracentesis should be done with proper aseptic preparations.

Diagnostic Clues in Ascitic Fluid

- Chylous ascites is due to raised triglycerides seen in congenital lymphatic abnormalities. By definition, chylous ascites have ascitic fluid triglyceride >200 mg/dL and greater than corresponding serum triglyceride level. Usually it is >1,000 mg/dL.
- Pseudochylous ascites is associated with bacterial infection, peritonitis, pancreatitis, or perforated bowel. Both chylomicrons and high concentration of triglycerides are there in true chylous ascites.
- Hemoperitoneum is a sign of the benign or malignant tumors, hemorrhagic pancreatitis, or perforated ulcer. High ascitic fluid lactic dehydrogenase (LDH) values had high sensitivity but low specificity to diagnose malignancy.
- Ascitic fluid bilirubin >6 mg/dL and correspondingly greater than serum level is diagnostic of biliary ascites.
- *Serum ascitic albumin gradient (SAAG)*:
  - SAAG correlates with portal pressure.
  - SAAG is calculated by subtracting the ascites albumin concentration from the serum albumin concentration.
  - SAAG ≥ 1.1 g/dL suggests portal hypertension, cirrhosis, fulminant hepatic failure, Budd–Chiari syndrome, and portal vein thrombosis.

- SAAG < 1.1 g/dL suggests peritoneal carcinomatosis, pancreatic or biliary ascites, peritonitis, ischemic or obstructed bowel.
- Ascitic adenosine deaminase (ADA) analysis is valuable in differentiating tubercular peritonitis and malignancy. ADA > 40 IU/L suggests diagnosis of tuberculous ascites. GeneXpert MTB is the newer test available for diagnosing peritoneal tuberculosis.
- *Tumor marker levels*: Alpha fetoprotein (AFP), carcinoembryonic antigen (CEA), cancer antigen (CA) 19-9, and CA125 in ascitic fluid must be interpreted with caution when differentiating malignant ascites from other types of ascites. Presence of malignant cells in cytology is more diagnostic.
- Pancreatic ascites is due to leakage of pancreatic secretions into the peritoneum. Pancreatic ascites is suggested by an amylase level over 1,000 IU/L. The calculated SAAG is <1.1 g/dL. Raised ascitic fluid amylase can also be seen in small bowel ischemia or mesenteric vein thrombosis. Concurrent raised ascitic fluid lipase supports diagnosis of pancreatic ascites.
- Spontaneous bacterial peritonitis (SBP) is defined by the presence of neutrophils ≥ 250/μL or a positive bacterial culture in the ascitic fluid without evidence of an abdominal source.
- Monomicrobial non-neutrocystic ascites is defined as positive ascitic fluid culture with ascitic fluid neutrophil count < 250/μL without evidence of surgical intra-abdominal pathology. While culture-negative neutrocytic ascites (CNNA) is defined by negative culture but neutrophil count is >250 cell/μL. Recent recommendations do not differentiate between SBP and CNNA for treatment purpose.
- Ascitic fluid inoculation (10 mL) in blood culture bottles should be performed at the bedside in all patients for ascitic fluid culture.
- Granulocyte elastase (GE) latex immunoassay and leukocyte esterase (LE) reagent strips can be used for the diagnosis of SBP in hepatic children with ascites with 86% accuracy. Predominance of ascitic fluid eosinophils suggests possibility of serosal eosinophilic ascites secondary to eosinophilic gastroenteritis.
- In uncertain case, *laparoscopic peritoneal examination* and biopsy are useful.
- *Relative contraindication* to ascitis tapping is severe thrombocytopenia or severe coagulopathy.

TREATMENT

- Treatment of underlying cause is essential. In grade 1 ascites low-sodium diet (1-2 mEq/kg/day) is recommended. The EASL guideline suggests that there is no data to support the use of fluid restriction in patients with ascites with normal serum sodium concentration. Moderate restriction of salt intake is an important component of the management of ascites.
- Spironolactone is started in 2 mg/kg/day maximum 100 mg, given as single dose in morning, if no response loop diuretic can be added in dose of 1 mg/kg/day or in cases of recurrent ascites. Weight loss should be monitored. 300-500 g/day of weight loss is acceptable. If serum albumin is <2.5 g/dL, one may consider albumin transfusion. Maximum dose of albumin should not exceed 1.5 g/kg or 100 g.
- Large-volume paracentesis (LVP) is defined as removal of 50 mL/kg of ascitic fluid. It should be supported with 8 g/L of ascitic fluid drained.
LVP should be completed in a single session. The goal of long-term treatment is to maintain one free of ascites with the minimum dose of diuretics. Diuretics should be discontinued in patients with refractory ascites who do not excrete >30 mmol/day of sodium under diuretic treatment. Transjugular intrahepatic portosystemic shunt (TIPS) should be considered in patients with very frequent requirement of LVP, or in those in whom paracentesis is ineffective. TIPS cannot be recommended in patients with severe liver failure, current hepatic encephalopathy grade 2 or chronic hepatic encephalopathy, concomitant active infection, progressive renal failure, or severe cardiopulmonary diseases. Once goal is achieved, diuretics should be reduced and discontinued later, whenever possible. Electrolyte monitoring is essential.
- Diuretics are generally contraindicated in patients with overt hepatic encephalopathy. Diuretics should be discontinued if there is severe hyponatremia (serum sodium concentration <120 mmol/L), progressive renal failure, worsening hepatic encephalopathy and incapacitating muscle cramps. Furosemide should be stopped if there is severe hypokalemia (<3 mmol/L). Aldosterone antagonists should be stopped if patients develop severe hyperkalemia (serum potassium > 6 mmol/L). Nonsteroidal anti-inflammatory drugs are contraindicated in patients with ascites because of the high risk of developing further sodium retention, hyponatremia, and renal failure. Angiotensin-converting enzyme (ACE) inhibitors, angiotensin II antagonists, or alpha 1-adrenergic receptor blockers should be avoided in patients with ascites because of increased risk of renal impairment. One should be careful while using aminoglycoside with diuretics. Contrast media should also be used with caution while performing radiological procedure.
- Blood cultures and ascitic fluid culture should be performed in all patients with suspected SBP before starting antibiotic treatment. Empirical antibiotics should be started immediately following the diagnosis of SBP. Third-generation cephalosporins are preferred. Resolution of SBP should be proven by demonstrating

- a decrease of ascitic neutrophil count to <250/mm³ and sterile cultures of ascitic fluid, if positive at diagnosis.
- Ascites that cannot be treated or the early recurrence cannot be prevented because of a lack of response to sodium restriction and diuretic treatment is defined diuretic-resist ant ascites. While ascites that cannot be reduced or the early recurrence cannot be prevented because of the development of diuretic-induced complications that preclude the use of an effective diuretic dosage is diuretic intractable ascites. Maximum dose of spironolactone is 400 mg/day and of furosemide 40 mg/day. But these doses should be used with extreme caution and monitoring.
- Hepatorenal syndrome (HRS) is diagnosed by demonstrating a significant increase in serum creatinine and excluding other known causes of renal failure. For therapeutic purposes, HRS is usually diagnosed only when serum creatinine increases to >133 µmol/L (1.5 mg/dL). HRS is classified into two types: Type 1 HRS, characterized by a rapid and progressive impairment in renal function (increase in serum creatinine of ≥100% compared to baseline to a level higher than 2.5 mg/dL in <2 weeks), and type 2 HRS characterized by a stable or less progressive impairment in renal function gradual rise in serum creatine to >1.5 mg/dL.
- Urinary biomarkers of tubular damage can be used to differentiate between HRS, prerenal acute kidney injury (AKI), and renal AKI are *neutrophil gelatinase-associated lipocalin (NGAL), kidney injury molecule-1 (KIM-1) interleukin-18 (IL-18) and liver fatty acid-binding protein (L-FABP)*. These are significantly raised in patients with AKI secondary to acute tubular necrosis (ATN)/ischemic AKI. More studies are needed in pediatric populations before wide use. Urinary neutrophil gelatinase-associated lipocalin > 110 ng/mL is studied to be predictive of inpatient mortality and suggests tubular injury. In HRS, values may not be high as compared to AKI-induced tubular damage. Similarly cystatin C level of >1.23 mg/L is thought to be better at predicting AKI than serum creatinine.
- HRS-1 is acute and is commonly associated with multi-organ failure. HRS-2 is the true form of AKI in patients with cirrhosis. LVP with albumin may be needed in type 1 HRS. All diuretics should be stopped in patients at the initial evaluation and diagnosis of HRS. Furosemide may be useful to maintain urine output and treat central volume overload if present. Spironolactone is contraindicated. Terlipressin (1 mg/4-6 h intravenous bolus) in combination with albumin can be considered the first-line therapeutic agent for type 1 HRS. In few studies, terlipressin is used as an infusion as compared to a bolus with a better response in reducing serum creatinine. Infusion dose: 10-20 µg/kg/day. More studies are needed. Noradrenaline at a dose of 0.5-1 µg/kg/min can be used if terlipressin is not available. If there is no response to terlipressin in the form of decreasing serum creatinine or sustained blood pressure increment, the dose of terlipressin can be doubled at 48 hours. Patients should be monitored for development of cardiac arrhythmias or signs of splanchnic or digital ischemia, and fluid overload. Renal replacement therapy may be useful in patients who do not respond to vasoconstrictor therapy after approximately 1 week. Terlipressin and albumin are effective in 60-70% of patients with type 2 HRS. Liver transplant may be needed. Prolonged renal support (>12 weeks) with HRS may need both liver and kidney transplant.
- Administration of album in 1.5 g/kg at diagnosis and 1 g/kg on day 3, decreases the frequency of HRS and improves survival in patients with SBP. In patients with gastrointestinal bleeding and severe liver disease ceftriaxone is the prophylactic antibiotic of choice to prevent SBP. For less severe liver involvement, oral norfloxacin 5 mg/kg once a day following first episode of SBP in cirrhotic is recommended.

Without prior SBP, norfloxacin prophylaxis may be used but needs further validation.
- Fluid restriction is effective in increasing serum sodium concentration in only a minority of patients with hypervolemic hyponatremia. Vaptans may be considered in patients with severe hypervolemic hyponatremia (<125 mmol/L). Rapid increases in serum sodium concentration (>8-10 mmol/day) should be avoided. Neither fluid restriction nor administration of saline should be used in combination with vaptans to avoid a too rapid increase in serum sodium concentration.
- Involvement of pediatric gastroenterologist who manages these patients routinely is essential. Management of these patients with cirrhosis, need for endoscopy to rule out gastroesophageal varices and treatment of underlying cause where possible is must.

PROGNOSIS

Development of grade 2 or 3 ascites in patients with cirrhosis is associated with reduced survival, liver transplantation should be considered in appropriate cases. Clinically detectable ascites is associated with decreased 1-year survival of children with biliary atresia, one of the most common cause of chronic liver disease in children.

KEY MESSAGES

- Diagnostic paracentesis should be performed in all patients with new-onset grade-2 or 3 ascites.
- SAAG is must in analyzing ascitic fluid.
- Spironolactone with or without furosemide can be used with judicious monitoring.
- Blood cultures and ascitic fluid culture should be performed in all patients with suspected SBP.

- Early suspicion and diagnosis of HRS and other complications of portal hypertension is recommended.

SUGGESTED READING

1. Bes DF, Fernández MC, Malla I, Repetto HA, Buamscha D, Lopez S, et al. Management of cirrhotic ascites in children. Review and recommendations. Part 1: Pathophysiology, diagnostic evaluation, hospitalization criteria, treatment, nutritional management. Arch Argent Pediatr. 2017;115(4):385-90.
2. Bes DF, Fernández MC, Malla I, Repetto HA, Buamscha D, Lopez S, et al. Management of cirrhotic ascites in children. Review and recommendations. Part 2: Electrolyte disturbances, nonelectrolyte disturbances, therapeutic options. Arch Argent Pediatr. 2017;115(5):505-11.
3. Deep A, Saxena R, Jose B. Acute kidney injury in children with chronic liver disease. Pediatr Nephrol. 2019;34 (1):45-59.
4. El-Hakim Allam AA, Eltaras SM, Hussin MH, Salama E-SI, Hendy OM, Allam MM, et al. Diagnosis of spontaneous bacterial peritonitis in children using leukocyte esterase reagent strips and granulocyte elastase immunoassay. Clin Exp Hepatol. 2018;4(4):247-52.
5. European Association for the Study of the Liver. EASL clinical practice guidelines on the management of ascites spontaneous bacterial peritonitis, and hepatorenal syndrome in cirrhosis. J Hepatol. 2010;53:397-417.
6. Huang LL, Xia HH, Zhu SL. Ascitic fluid analysis in the differential diagnosis of ascites: focus on cirrhotic ascites. J Clin Transl Hepatol. 2014;2(1):58-64.

Cholestasis in Newborns and Infants

Rimjhim Shrivastava

INTRODUCTION

Cholestasis in newborns or infants refers to the stasis of biliary substances within the liver due to mechanical or functional obstruction to the bile flow. It implies hepatobiliary dysfunction. Early evaluation and management are imperative for a favorable outcome. Though there are many markers of cholestasis but direct hyperbilirubinemia is considered most informative.

DEFINITION

Direct hyperbilirubinemia is defined as serum direct bilirubin level >1 mg/dL if the total bilirubin is ≤5 mg/dL, or direct bilirubin level >20% of the total bilirubin level if the total bilirubin is >5 mg/dL.

ETIOLOGY

Biliary atresia (BA) is the most frequent cause of cholestasis in the first 3 months of life followed by genetic disorders and infections. **Flowchart 1** depicts the important causes of cholestasis in newborns and infants.

CLINICAL FEATURES

- Newborns or infants may present with jaundice, bleeding manifestations, pruritic, or acute liver failure.
- Babies who have sepsis or metabolic disorder may appear sick whereas babies with BA appear playful.
- Dysmorphic features may be seen in Alagille syndrome but rarely before 6 months of age.
- They may have hearing defects or cataract associated with congenital infections or storage disorders.
- Congenital heart disease may be seen along with Alagille syndrome or BA with splenic malformation.
- Hepatomegaly is a consistent feature except in some newborns with sepsis-induced cholestasis.
- Splenomegaly with or without ascites is seen in later stages of decompensated disease.
- *Stool color*: Persistently pale stools **(Fig. 1)** are seen in 95% of infants with BA. The sensitivity and specificity of stool color to pick BA is 72–97% and 99.9%, respectively. Stool color should be examined for at least three occasions.
- Mean age of presentation of BA to a tertiary care center is 2.8–3.9 months compared to the desired age of evaluation, that is 4–6 weeks.
- Timely diagnosis of BA is important for optimal response to Kasai's hepatic portoenterostomy (HPE), which is the palliative surgery for BA. If HPE is done before 60 days of life, the bile flow is re-established in almost 70% of the

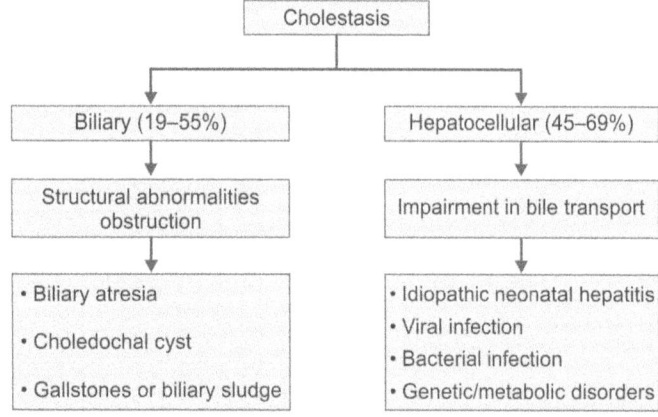

Flowchart 1: Etiologies of cholestasis.

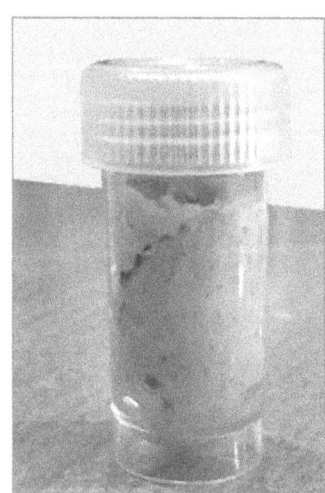

Fig. 1: Pale stool in a cholestatic newborn management.

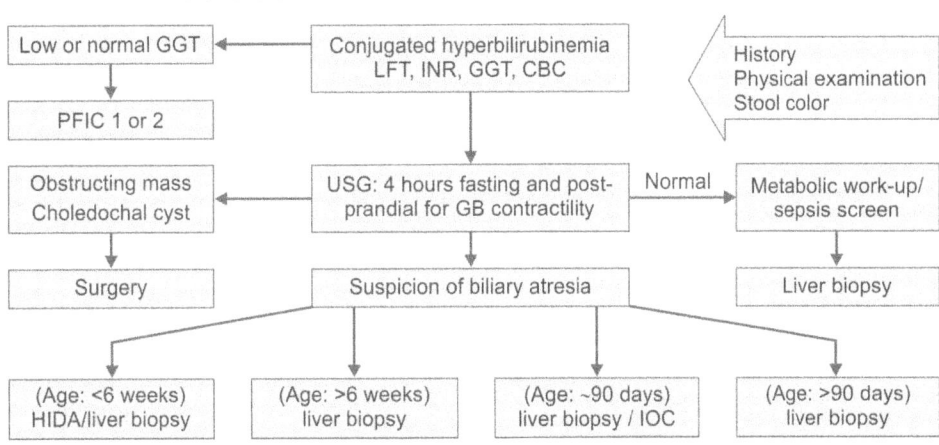

Flowchart 2: Evaluation of cholestasis in newborns and infants.

(CBC: complete blood count; GB: gall bladder; GGT: gamma-glutamyl transferase; HIDA: hepatobiliary iminodiacetic acid; INR: international normalized ratio; IOC: intraoperative cholangiography; LFT: liver function test; PFIC: progressive familial intrahepatic cholestasis; USG: ultrasonography)

children whereas this percentage goes down to 25% if HPE is performed after 90 days of life.
- The ideal goal should be to complete the diagnostic evaluation or at least rule out BA before 45–60 days of life. The management algorithm is outlined in **Flowchart 2**.

INVESTIGATIONS (TABLE 1)

Liver function test: It confirms the diagnosis. In tyrosinemia and neonatal hemochromatosis, liver enzymes are normal or marginally raised.

Gamma-glutamyl transferase (GGT): In progressive familial intrahepatic cholestasis (PFIC) 1 and 2, GGT is low or normal; in rest of the cholestatic conditions, it is high.

International normalized ratio (INR) gives a clue regarding the extent of liver's functioning. INR of a normal newborn can extend up to 2. So, acute liver failure might best be defined as INR > 3 in newborns. As it is very difficult to detect, encephalopathy in newborns has been removed from essential diagnostic criteria by the pediatric acute liver failure (PALF) study group.

Ultrasonography (USG) is a very good imaging modality for initial evaluation.
- A 4-hour fasting USG followed by a postprandial scan to look for gall bladder (GB) contractility is must for all cholestatic baby.
- Pointers toward BA are absent, small, or atretic GB; triangular chord sign; poor or noncontractility of GB; abnormal common bile duct. A normal USG does not rule out BA.
- USG can also give clues regarding other obstructing conditions as choledochal cyst, sludge or very rarely gall stones.

Hepatobiliary scintigraphy (HBS): The principle of scan is that the radioactive material injected is excreted in the intestine within 24–48 hours. The sensitivity and specificity for obstruction is 83–100% and 33–100%, respectively. With an excretory scan, obstruction is highly improbable; however,

TABLE 1: Specific investigations for cholestatic disease.

Disease	Investigations
Biliary atresia	Intraoperative cholangiogram
Galactosemia	• Nonglucose-reducing substances in urine • Serum galactose-1-phosphate uridyl transferase level
Tyrosinemia	• Serum tyrosine and methionine levels • Serum α-fetoprotein levels • Succinylacetone detection in urine
Hemochromatosis	Ferritin, TIBC, liver biopsy/buccal mucosal biopsy MRI
Hereditary fructosemia	Fructose-1-phosphate aldolase B

(MRI: magnetic resonance imaging; TIBC: total iron binding capacity)

we must keep in mind the entity incompletely evaluated BA in the initial days of life where the scan can be excretory. Nonexcretory scan can also be seen in severe cholestasis due to other reasons as well. Scan requires priming with phenobarbitone or ursodeoxycholic acid (UDCA) for 5 days. Because of the time delay and low specificity, scan is not widely used.

Liver biopsy: Liver biopsy has high sensitivity (99%) and specificity (92%) for diagnosing BA. In 90–95% of patients, biopsy can help in taking decision regarding surgery. With the advent of various immunohistochemistry modalities, it can also diagnose other conditions as paucity of intrahepatic bile ducts, giant cell transformation, metabolic and storage diseases, PFIC, neonatal sclerosing cholangitis, etc., with high accuracy.

TREATMENT

- The goal of the treatment is to provide adequate nutrition and micronutrients.
- The calorie requirement is approximately 125% of the recommended dietary allowances (RDA) based on ideal body weight.

PHARMACOLOGICAL ASSISTANCE

Pharmacological salt	Market preparation	Availability (drops/syrup/tablet/injection)	Dosages
UDCA	Udcament, Udiliv	• Tablet: 150 mg, 300 mg • Syrup: 125 mg/5 mL	20 mg/kg/day
Vitamin A	Aquasol	Capsule: 50,000 IU	5,000–25,000 IU/day
Vitamin D	Vitanova D3, D3 must	Oral: 400 IU/mL, 800 IU/mL	400–1,200 IU/day
Vitamin E	Evion, Evit	• Drops: 500 mg/mL • Pearls: 30 mg, 100 mg	50–400 IU/day
Vitamin K	Menadione	Injection: 100 mg/mL	• IV/IM • 2.5–5 mg twice/week
Calcium	Coralium D3, Gemical-P	Syrup: 200 mg/5 mL	Syrup: 200 mg/5 mL

(IM: intramuscular; IV: intravenous; UDCA: ursodeoxycholic acid)

- In breastfed babies, breastfeeding should be continued along with medium-chain triglycerides (MCT) oil 1–2 mL/kg/day. In older children, energy-dense food should be given.
- They also require oral supplementation of fat-soluble vitamins.
- UDCA is a choleretic agent and is helpful in establishing the bile flow and decreasing the stasis. Details are given in Prescription Assistance.

Specific Treatments

- Galactosemia, fructosemia, and tyrosinemia require special infant formula along with dietary restrictions.
- Nitisinone (1 mg/kg/day) is an important drug for tyrosinemia.
- Antiviral agents such as ganciclovir are given in CMV infection with central nervous system (CNS) manifestations.
- Kasai's portoenterostomy (PE) is the palliative surgery for BA and consists of removal of the atretic extrahepatic tissue and a Roux-en-Y jejunal loop anastomosis to the hepatic hilum.
- Liver transplantation is the standard therapy for decompensated cirrhosis for all types of cholestatic diseases.

CONCLUSION

- Conjugated hyperbilirubinemia at any age in a newborn is pathological and requires evaluation.
- Newborns with physiological jaundice should be followed up after 2 weeks of life to confirm the resolution of jaundice.
- The evaluation of a cholestatic newborn should be completed or at least BA should be ruled out, before 45–60 days of life.
- There is no particular test which would differentiate biliary obstruction from other causes of cholestasis.
- Malnutrition adversely affects the outcome in infants with cholestasis, so nutritional support is very crucial.

SUGGESTED READING

1. Bhatia V, Bavdekar A, Matthai J, Waikar Y, Sibal A. Management of neonatal cholestasis: consensus statement of the Pediatric Gastroenterology Chapter of Indian Academy of Pediatrics. Indian Pediatr. 2014;51(3):203-10.
2. Fawaz R, Baumann U, Ekong U, Fischler B, Hadzic N, Mack CL, et al. Guideline for the evaluation of cholestatic jaundice in infants: Joint Recommendations of the North American Society for Pediatric Gastroenterology, Hepatology, and Nutrition and the European Society for Pediatric Gastroenterology, Hepatology, and Nutrition. J Pediatr Gastroenterol Nutr. 2017J;64(1):154-68.
3. Pandita A, Gupta V, Gupta G. Neonatal Cholestasis: A Pandora's Box. Clin Med Insights Pediatr. 2018;12:1179556518805412.

CHAPTER 64

Abnormal Liver Function Tests

Malathi Sathiyasekaran, Suresh Natarajan

INTRODUCTION

The term "liver function test" (LFT) is a misnomer as this test also helps to assess liver cell injury, cholestasis, and fibrosis, apart from excretory, synthetic, and clearance functions by the liver. Hence, it is preferable to call them as "laboratory investigations or biochemical tests of the liver." There are some limitations as they lack sensitivity (the tests are normal in presinusoidal portal hypertension and compensated cirrhosis), specificity [e.g., aspartate aminotransferase (AST) is raised not only in liver injury, but also in muscle and cardiac diseases, and serum albumin may be low not only in liver disease but also in intestinal, nutritional, and renal diseases]. Therefore, these tests should be always correlated with history and clinical examination. We can divide these tests into two levels (I and II).

Level I

Essential investigations which should be done in all children with liver disease are as follows:

Serum Bilirubin

- Jaundice or yellowish color of sclera parallels increase in level of serum bilirubin.
- Serum bilirubin is an important test to assess the metabolic and excretory functions of liver.
- Increase in bilirubin can occur due to increased production (hemolysis), defective conjugation (decreased UDP-glucuronosyltransferase), and decreased excretion (biliary atresia and obstructive jaundice).
- It is essential that both total and fractionated bilirubin (direct) are estimated.
- When indirect bilirubin is persistently elevated, one should consider hemolytic jaundice. A dual rise of both direct and indirect bilirubin may be seen in hepatocellular jaundice, whereas in obstructive jaundice, the direct component is predominant.
- In congenital hyperbilirubinemia such as in Crigler–Najjar and Gilbert syndrome, the indirect bilirubin is persistently high at variable levels.
- An increasing or persistently elevated bilirubin in a sick child is not a good prognostic index and may indicate progression to acute liver failure (ALF) or acute-on-chronic liver failure.
- Hyper hyperbilirubinemia is a term used when the total bilirubin is >25 mg/dL and indicates combination of both hepatocellular and hemolytic jaundice.
- *Limitations*: Serum bilirubin alone can be elevated in hemolytic jaundice and congenital hyperbilirubinemia. Bilirubin may be normal in a child with hepatitis or chronic liver disease.

Serum Transaminases

- Transaminases or aminotransferases are catalyst enzymes which are detected in low levels.
- The two enzymes AST or serum glutamic oxaloacetic transaminase (SGOT) and alanine aminotransferase (ALT) or serum glutamic pyruvic transaminase (SGPT) are sensitive indicators of hepatocyte injury.
- SGPT is primarily from liver cytosol, whereas SGOT is distributed in a wide variety of tissues such as liver (cytosol 20% and mitochondria 80%), cardiac muscle, kidneys, brain, pancreas, lung, and WBC and RBC.
- *Elevated transaminases* is the term used when the level is more than 2 times the upper limit of normal (ULN) and is characteristic of various acute or chronic hepatitis. It may be present without elevation of bilirubin (anicteric hepatitis). The normal range is 1–40 U/L but this may vary. Studies have shown that the 95th centile for SGPT (ALT) is 25.8 U/L and 22.1 U/L in adolescent boys and girls, respectively. However, for practical purposes, the laboratory values can be used.
- Abnormal serum transaminases may suggest possible etiology and also guide therapy:
  - *Acute hepatitis*: The levels are classified as mild >2–3 ULN (sepsis, cholestasis and steatohepatitis), moderate >3–20 ULN (bacterial, spirochetal, metabolic hepatitis) and marked or severe 20 ULN (acute hepatitis due to hepatotrophic viruses, hypoxic and toxic hepatitis). There is no direct correlation

between the transaminase level and the severity of liver disease and therefore they are not used as prognostic indices in ALF. Falling levels may indicate recovery, but a rapid fall may indicate poor prognosis and suggest impending ALF.
- *Chronic hepatitis*: Level of transaminases is useful for categorizing the phase of chronic hepatitis B, initiating therapy and monitoring response. During therapy, an abrupt increase may indicate flare of disease. Similarly, the transaminases are useful in autoimmune hepatitis.
- *Cirrhosis*: The levels may be variable. An elevated SGOT/AST is seen in cirrhosis; however; they can also be normal in cirrhosis and end-stage liver disease.
- *Ratio of SGOT/SGPT*: The normal SGOT/SGPT ratio is 1. Ratio >2 indicates mitochondrial injury and may be seen in drug-induced liver injury (DILI), Wilson disease, dengue Shock syndrome, ethanol-induced liver disease and Reye-like syndrome.
- *Limitations*: 6% of healthy asymptomatic individuals have elevated liver enzymes. Transaminases may increase due to nonhepatic causes, e.g., muscular dystrophy and celiac disease.

Serum Alkaline Phosphatase

- *Normal value*: 250–700 U/L.
- Alkaline phosphatase (ALP) is a family of zinc metalloenzymes and detects cholestasis.
- BLIP is a simple mnemonic to recap the sources of ALP (bone, liver, intestine, and placenta).
- Low levels may be seen in hypophosphatasia, zinc deficiency, hypothyroidism, and pernicious anemia. Approach to elevated ALP is shown in **Flowchart 1**.
- *Limitation*: ALP values vary with age and are relatively high in growing children.

Serum Albumin

- This is an important plasma protein, synthesized exclusively by the liver and helps to assess synthetic function.
- Normal values range from 3.5 to 4.5 g/dL.
- Albumin has a half-life of 21 days.
- Decreased albumin <3 g should raise the suspicion of chronic liver disease (CLD).
- Persistently low albumin is not a good prognostic index in CLD and is an important parameter used in Child–Pugh–Turcotte, PELD (pediatric end-stage liver disease) and PELD Na scoring systems. Approach to hypoalbuminemia is shown in **Flowchart 2**.

Gamma Glutamyl Transpeptidase

- This cholestatic enzyme is secreted by the biliary epithelium and is dependent on the bile salt transport.
- The enzyme may be induced by medications such as rifampicin, griseofulvin, and alcohol.

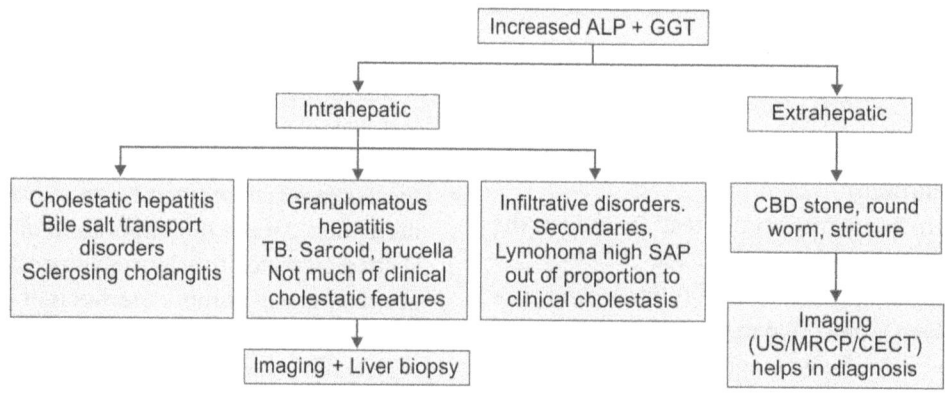

Flowchart 1: Approach to elevated ALP.

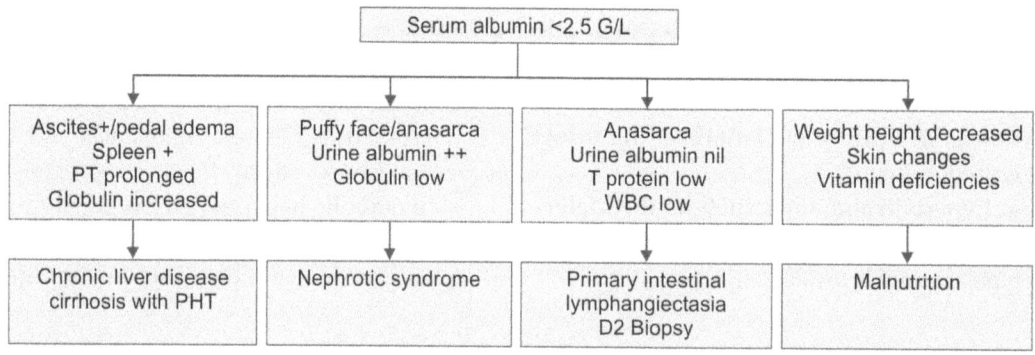

Flowchart 2: Approach to hypoalbuminemia.

- Normally, gamma glutamyl transpeptidase (GGT) increases in parallel with ALP in cholestatic disorders, except in progressive familial intrahepatic cholestasis (PFIC) 1, 2, 4, 5, 6 and bile acid synthesis defect. Hence, this test should be included in all infants presenting with cholestatic features.
- *Limitations*: The levels of GGT may be very high in normal neonates and infants.

Prothrombin Time

- Normal prothrombin time (PT) is 9–11 seconds and is prolonged when test is 3 seconds more than control.
- PT is a sensitive test for synthetic function.
- International normalized ratio (INR) is the ratio between patient's PT and mean normal PT and the normal value is 1.
- If PT normalizes or improves by 30% with a single dose of vitamin K, it indicates good parenchymal function.
- PT/INR is useful to identify risk of bleeding in planned therapeutic procedure, e.g., liver biopsy, monitoring progression of CLD.
- Elevated INR > 2 is diagnostic of ALF and for assessing progress of disease and prioritizing liver transplant.
- *Limitations*: PT may be prolonged in disseminated intravascular coagulation (DIC) and in children on anticoagulants.

Level II

Specific tests which may help in confirming diagnosis are given in the following text.

Bile Acids

- Bile acids (BAs) are synthesized from cholesterol in the liver and are the only liver specific tests.
- They are disproportionately increased in inherited bile salt transport defects PFIC 1–6.
- BAs are decreased in bile acid synthesis defect (BASD) and this helps us to differentiate PFIC and BASD since GGT is low or normal in both these conditions.
- *Limitations*: BAs are elevated in healthy neonates and decrease within the first year of life.

Serum Ammonia

- The ammonia produced by the large intestine is cleared by the liver mainly by the urea synthesis.
- The serum ammonia is elevated in hepatic encephalopathy and is useful in monitoring these patients.
- The levels increase at the onset of coma, and return to normal 48–72 hours before neurological improvement.
- High concentrations are seen in urea cycle disorders, organic acidemias, fatty acid oxidation defects, congenital or acquired portosystemic shunts and Reye syndrome.
- *Limitations*: Sodium valproate can cause increase of ammonia independent of hepatotoxicity.

Serum Ceruloplasmin

- This α2 globulin is synthesized by the liver and is a simple screening test for Wilson disease (WD).
- The normal value is 20–40 mg/dL. A value <10 mg/dL is more or less diagnostic of WD in any child with liver disease.
- *Limitations*: Ceruloplasmin (Cp) may be high in a child with WD in the presence of infections or low in protein-losing enteropathy and nephrotic syndrome without WD.

Lactate Dehydrogenase

- This cytoplasmic enzyme has wide distribution and elevation is seen in acute and chronic liver disease.
- In ischemic hepatitis, it is high but transient.
- A persistent elevation with high ALP indicates malignant infiltration.
- ALT/LDH (lactate dehydrogenase) ratio >1.5 helps to differentiate viral hepatitis from ischemic hepatitis. This ratio is also used to differentiate viral from typhoid hepatitis which is >4 in the former and <4 in the latter.
- *Limitations*: Not liver specific since elevated LDH is seen in skeletal and myocardial injury, hemolysis, and renal infarction.

Alpha Fetoprotein

- This is a protein produced by the fetal hepatocytes and the levels fall rapidly minutes after birth to <10 mg/dL.
- It is an important oncofetal antigen used for screening hepatic malignancy.
- High values are seen in hepatoblastoma and hepatocellular carcinoma and tyrosinemia.

Fibroscan (Transient Elastography)

- It is a good noninvasive test to detect and grade liver fibrosis.
- *The advantages of fibroscan are*: It is painless; quick (<5 minutes); highly reproducible and easy to perform in the outpatient clinic or bedside and may replace liver biopsy in some select situations.
- *Limitations*: The cost of the machine and the inability to identify characteristic changes seen on liver biopsy.

KEY MESSAGES

- Abnormal liver tests help in screening and documenting liver injury and dysfunction, assess pattern of hepatitis, determine a broad etiology, assess severity and prognosis in ALF and monitor response to treatment.
- A single abnormal liver function test should not be interpreted categorically.

- Some of these tests are abnormal even in nonhepatic conditions.
- Investigations may be repeated if there is a discrepancy between clinical diagnosis and the values.
- Level I investigations should be done in all children with liver disease. This can be followed with selective tests from level II.

SUGGESTED READING

1. Hall P, Cash J. What is the real function of the liver 'function' tests? Ulster Med J. 2012;81(1):30-6.
2. Kang KS. Abnormality on liver function test. Pediatr Gastroenterol Hepatol Nutr. 2013;16(4):225-32.
3. Limdi JK, Hyde GM. Evaluation of abnormal liver function tests. Postgraduate Medical Journal. 2003;79:307-12.

Asymptomatic Hepatomegaly

Sakshi Karkra, Rohan Karkra

INTRODUCTION

Hepatomegaly is defined as a liver edge 3.5 cm and 2 cm below the right costal margin in newborns and older children, respectively. The average liver span (distance between the upper edge, determined by percussion, and lower edge by palpation, in the midclavicular line) is 4–5 cm in newborns at 1 week of age, 7–8 cm for boys and 6–6.5 cm for girls at 12 years of age. Hepatomegaly with no other symptoms can be a normal variant of right lobe (Riedel lobe), may represent intrinsic liver disease or may be the presenting physical finding of a generalized disorder. Early diagnosis and treatment of children with hepatomegaly is important because specific treatments are available for some diseases that can prevent disease progression or hepatic failure.

CAUSES OF HEPATOMEGALY

The causes have been tabulated **(Table 1)** based on the mechanism of hepatomegaly and age of the patient. Most of the acute illnesses such as infection, sepsis, trauma, and abscess would have signs and symptoms to suggest the etiology.

MANAGEMENT (FLOWCHART 1)

This is based on age, history, examination, and laboratory and possible radiographic studies.

History

- *Age of onset*: Early age suggest congenital infection or metabolic disorder.
- History of jaundice suggests hemolysis, bile duct abnormalities, liver inflammation while additional itching, acholic stools and dark urine suggest biliary obstruction.
- Failure to thrive, diarrhea, vomiting, aversion to feeds, developmental delay, neurological deterioration, seizures may indicate metabolic cause.
- Melena, hematemesis suggests portal hypertension and have associated splenomegaly.
- *Family history*: Liver disease, metabolic disease, neurodegenerative disease.
- Maternal infections during pregnancy [TORCH (Toxoplasmosis, Other (syphilis, varicella-zoster, parvovirus B19), Rubella, Cytomegalovirus (CMV), and Herpes infections)], risk factors for hepatitis A, B, C, D, and E, drug exposure, recurrent abortions, eclampsia might suggest metabolic cause.
- Difficulty in breathing and feeding suggest cardiac cause.

Examination

Incidentally detected hepatomegaly on examination should always be confirmed with liver span and a complete systemic examination.

- Vitals should include temperature, which if high suggests a systemic infection, viral hepatitis, liver abscess, or infiltration.
- *Anthropometry*: Weight, height, head circumference (HC) should be taken to detect failure to thrive [glycogen storage diseases (GSD), hereditary fructose intolerance (HFI), organic acidemia, Wolman disease], obesity [nonalcoholic fatty liver disease (NAFLD)] or neurological involvement.
- *Facies*: Dysmorphic features suggest mucopolysaccharidoses (MPS) (coarse features), GSD (doll-like), Alagille syndrome, Zellweger syndrome (mongoloid).
- *Eye*: Cataracts [galactosemia, Wilson's disease (WD)], Kayser-Fleischer (KF) ring (WD), chorioretinitis (TORCH), posterior embryotoxon (Alagille syndrome), cherry-red spots (sphingomyelinosis), icterus, and pallor.
- Hemangiomas and bruits anywhere on body might suggest one on liver.
- Generalized lymphadenopathy suggests infection, leukemia or neoplasia.
- Splenomegaly suggests portal hypertension, infiltration, storage or hemolytic disease.
- Ascites and edema suggest portal hypertension and hypoalbuminemia.
- Developmental delay and neurologic deterioration (peroxisomal disorders, Zellweger syndrome, Lysosomal

TABLE 1: Causes of hepatomegaly.

Mechanism	Neonate	Children
Inflammation/infection*	• TORCH • Neonatal hepatitis • Drug induced	• Chronic HBV, HCV, EBV, CMV • Autoimmune hepatitis • Drug induced • Parasitic cyst
Storage/metabolic	• Total parenteral nutrition • Wolman disease • FAOD • Tyrosinemia • Galactosemia • Hemochromatosis	• Glycogen storage diseases • Disorders of lipid storage • FAOD, NAFLD • Hereditary fructose intolerance • *Metals*: Wilson's disease (copper), hemochromatosis (iron) • Tyrosinemia • Gaucher disease, Niemann–Pick • Mucopolysaccharidosis • Alpha1 antitrypsin deficiency
Infiltration†	• Hemangioendothelioma • Hepatoblastoma (rare)	• *Primary neoplastic tumors*: Hepatoblastoma/hepatocellular carcinoma • Primary non-neoplastic • *Tumors*: Hemangioma, hemangioendothelioma, teratoma, focal nodular hyperplasia, simple hepatic cyst • *Metastatic*: Leukemia, lymphoma, neuroblastoma, histiocytosis • Extramedullary hematopoiesis • ‡HLH
Congestion†	Congenital heart disease with congestive heart failure (CHF)	• CHF • Restrictive pericarditis • Budd–Chiari
Obstruction of biliary system	Biliary atresia progressive familial intrahepatic cholestasis (PFIC)	• PFIC • Alagille syndrome
Pseudohepatomegaly system	Pectus excavatum, pneumothorax, retroperitoneal mass, choledochal cyst PFIC	• Pectus excavatum, pneumothorax, retroperitoneal mass, choledochal cyst, or intrahepatic cholestasis (PFIC) • Alagille syndrome
Pseudohepatomegaly	Pectus excavatum, pneumothorax, retroperitoneal mass, choledochal cyst	Pectus excavatum, pneumothorax, retroperitoneal mass, choledochal cyst, or perihepatic abscess
Normal variant	Riedel lobe	Riedel lobe

*Acute viral infections such as Hepatitis A, E, B and liver abscess will have hepatomegaly with pain, fever, vomiting, etc.
†Most of the patients with CHF and infiltrative disorders, especially metastatic group might have other symptoms and on examination have hepatomegaly+/- splenomegaly, lymphadenopathy.
‡HLH patients are very sick.
[EBV: Epstein–Barr virus; FAOD: fatty acid oxidation disorder; HBV: hepatitis B virus; HCV: hepatitis C virus; HLH: hemophagocytic lymphohistiocytosis; TORCH: toxoplasmosis, other (syphilis, varicella-zoster, parvovirus B19), rubella, cytomegalovirus (CMV), and Herpes infections; NAFLD: nonalcoholic fatty liver disease]

storage disease, Niemann–Pick disease, Gaucher disease, GM1 gangliosidosis, MPS, WD)
- Presence of any cardiac murmur or prominent neck veins points toward cardiac cause
- Chest deformity (pectus excavatum), unusual odor (organic acidemia, tyrosinemia)

Laboratory Evaluation

Results of the history and physical examination should tailor the laboratory evaluation and suggest the need for further diagnostic testing. Stepwise investigations are planned and tabulated in **Table 2**.

Imaging

Computed tomography (CT) or magnetic resonance imaging (MRI) may be superior to ultrasonography in detecting small focal lesions, such as tumors, cysts, or abscesses **(Table 3)**.

Biopsy

- Liver biopsy may demonstrate parenchymal changes, presence of storage materials, and tissue for enzyme identification.
- Bone marrow biopsy may help to rule out infiltrative and storage disorders.

CHAPTER 65 | Asymptomatic Hepatomegaly

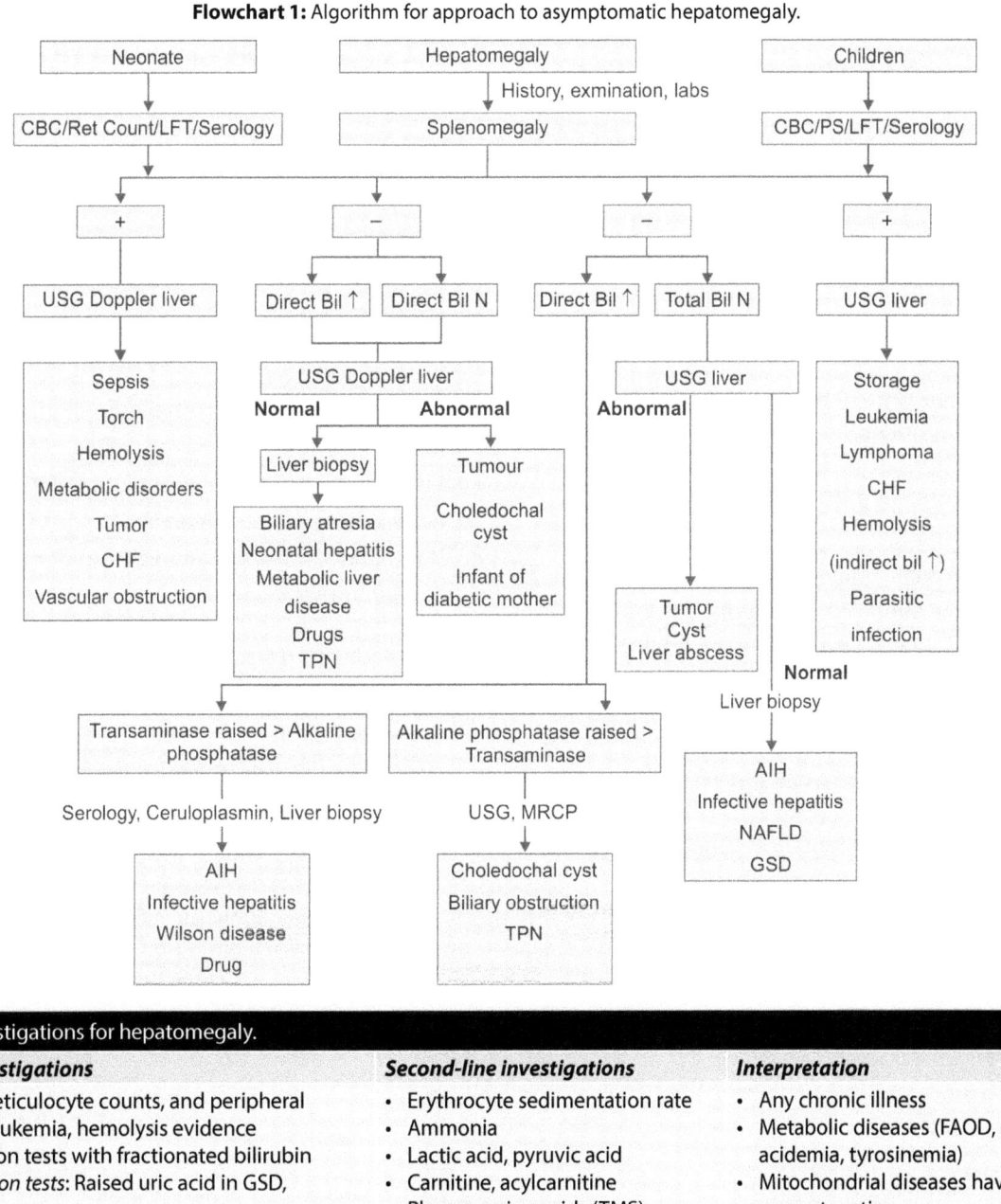

Flowchart 1: Algorithm for approach to asymptomatic hepatomegaly.

TABLE 2: Investigations for hepatomegaly.		
First-line investigations	**Second-line investigations**	**Interpretation**
• CBC, DLC, reticulocyte counts, and peripheral smear for leukemia, hemolysis evidence • Liver function tests with fractionated bilirubin • *Renal function tests*: Raised uric acid in GSD, electrolytes • *Venous blood gas*: Acidosis in organic academia, normal anion gap in RTA PT, APTT, INR: Liver disease • Fasting glucose with urinary ketones for GSD, FAOD • *Serology*: Hepatitis A, B, and C • Urine analysis and culture	• Erythrocyte sedimentation rate • Ammonia • Lactic acid, pyruvic acid • Carnitine, acylcarnitine • Plasma amino acids (TMS) • Urine organic acids (GCMS) • Hepatitis serologies • Alpha-fetoprotein • Serum ceruloplasmin • 24-hour urinary copper excretion • Antinuclear antibodies • Anti-smooth muscle antibodies • Anti-liver/kidney microsomal Ab • Serum alpha-1-antitrypsin • Sweat chloride • TORCH titers • *Fibrinogen, D-dimers, • Ferritin, triglycerides	• Any chronic illness • Metabolic diseases (FAOD, organic acidemia, tyrosinemia) • Mitochondrial diseases have lactate/pyruvate ratio • Chronic Hepatitis B, C in hepatoblastoma, hemachromatosis, tyrosinemia • Low and raised in Wilson's disease • Autoimmune hepatitis • Alpha-1-antitrypsin deficiency • Cystic fibrosis • TORCH infection • HLH, hemochromatosis • Hypertriglyceridemia with raised uric acid and hypoglycemia suggest • GSD

Note: In suspected metabolic diseases or syndromes diagnosis can be confirmed by clinical exome or whole genome to confirm the mutation and for genetic counseling.
*Patients are usually very sick in HLH and neonatal hemochromatosis
[CBC: complete blood count; DLC: differential leukocyte count; FAOD: fatty acid oxidation disorder; GSD: glycogen storage diseases; GCMS: gas chromatography–mass spectrometry; HLH: hemophagocytic lymphohistiocytosis; PT: prothrombin time; TMS: Tandem Mass Spectrometer; TORCH: toxoplasmosis, other (syphilis, varicella-zoster, parvovirus B19), rubella, cytomegalovirus (CMV), and Herpes infections; INR: international normalized ratio; RTA: renal tubular acidosis; APTT: activated partial thromboplastin time]

TABLE 3: Stepwise imaging for hepatomegaly.

First line	Second line
Abdominal ultrasonography with Doppler flow	• Abdominal computed tomography (CECT) • Magnetic resonance cholangiopancreatography (MRCP) • Radionuclide biliary scan • Cholangiography • Echocardiography

(CECT: contrast-enhanced computed tomography)

TREATMENT

Usually these patients need detailed investigations to rule out any underlying disease and treatment planned as per diagnosis.

FOLLOW-UP

Child should be kept under follow-up and should be examined in OPD and with laboratory parameters [liver function test (LFT)] every 3 months even if major illnesses are ruled out.

KEY MESSAGES

- Hepatomegaly on palpation should always be confirmed by liver span.
- Pseudohepatomegaly should be ruled out by detailed physical examination.
- Asymptomatic hepatomegaly can suggest intrinsic liver disease or generalized systemic illness.
- The cause of hepatomegaly varies with age.
- Detailed history and physical examination are very important.
- Baseline blood tests include complete blood count (CBC), peripheral smear (PS), LFT, international normalized ratio (INR), electrolytes, blood sugar and urine routine.
- Second-line tests are based on history and baseline reports.
- Metabolic tests are advised if history, examination and liver biopsy suggests.
- Ultrasonography (USG) abdomen should be done as first radiological test.
- Liver biopsy is done once structural defects, cyst, tumor, or abscess are ruled out on USG.
- Bone marrow examination is done to rule out storage and infiltrative disorders.

SUGGESTED READING

1. Fishbein M, Mogren J, Mogren C, Cox S, Jennings R. Undetected hepatomegaly in obese children by primary care physicians: a pitfall in the diagnosis of pediatric nonalcoholic fatty liver disease. Clinical Pediatrics. 2005;44(2):135-41.
2. Pietro Vajro, Sergio Maddaluno, Claudio Veropalumbo. Persistent hypertransaminasemia in asymptomatic children: a stepwise approach. World J Gastroenterol. 2013;19(18):2740-51.
3. Wolf AD, Lavine JE. Hepatomegaly in neonates and children. Pediatr Rev. 2000;21(9):303-10.

Acute Viral Hepatitis

Gautam Ray

INTRODUCTION

Acute viral hepatitis (AVH) is an important public health problem in India. The common causes are: Hepatitis A virus infection (HAV) (almost two thirds of all cases), hepatitis E virus infection (HEV) and hepatitis B virus infection (HBV). A proportion of cases (10–25% cases) is due to combinations of these (commonly HAV along with HEV). Hepatitis C virus (HCV) rarely causes AVH.

CLINICAL FEATURES

Hepatotropic viral infections may present in four different ways: (1) Asymptomatic, (2) anicteric hepatitis, (3) icteric hepatitis or AVH, and (4) acute liver failure (ALF). The classic AVH presentation is more common in older children. This classic form of AVH starts with a prodromal phase (anorexia—most specific feature, weakness, fever, malaise, vomiting, diarrhea, pain abdomen in varying combinations) for a few days, followed by the icteric phase when the clinical jaundice appears. In this classic form, the prodromal features start improving with the onset of the jaundice, including a return of the appetite and most children improve in 2–3-week time. If fever, loss of appetite, etc., continue after the onset of jaundice, causes other than those due to hepatotropic viral infection such as malaria, enteric fever, leptospirosis, scrub typhus, etc., should be looked into. A proportion of children (10–25%) with HAV-related AVH develop atypical features such as prolonged cholestasis (jaundice for ≥3 months, pruritus and serum bilirubin >10 mg/dL), ascites, relapsing hepatitis (recurrence of acute hepatitis symptoms after a period of remission for 1–4 months), intravascular hemolysis, etc. ALF occurs in <1–2% of cases, though recent hospital-based studies report a higher incidence.

MANAGEMENT

The diagnosis of AVH is made on basis of history, supported by liver function tests (LFTs), and the etiology is confirmed by viral serology.

Investigations

- *LFT*: It shows conjugated hyperbilirubinemia with high transaminases [alanine aminotransferase/aspartate aminotransferase (ALT/AST)] in hundreds to thousands, with normal serum albumin, and a variable elevation of alkaline phosphatase. A decline in serum albumin is seen in the ascitic form of AVH and in the rare patient with underlying chronic liver disease. This characteristic picture (especially ALT/AST in thousands, with ALT > AST) is generally present in the initial stages only, hence, it is important to order a complete LFT when seeing patients with jaundice first time.
- *Prothrombin time (PT)/international normalized ratio (INR)* should always be requested without fail, as it is the single most important laboratory marker which reliably indicates prognosis individually. In uncomplicated cases of AVH, prolongation of PT is <5 seconds from the control value or INR is <1.5. In those being managed on an outpatient basis, PT should be repeated to see the trend in the event of the slightest doubt about the clinical status/progress of the child.
- *Serology*: Etiological diagnosis is established by doing IgM anti-HAV, IgM anti-HEV and HBsAg with IgM anti-HBc. They are already positive by the time icterus appears, and remain so for months. If HBsAg is positive, then IgM anti-HBc needs to be done, to differentiate HBV-related AVH (positive anti-HBc IgM, in high titers) from HBsAg carrier with some other cause of AVH (such as HAV).
Rarely, a flare of chronic HBV infection (CHB) (negative/low titer of IgM anti-HBc) infection may mimic AVH, and the confusion regarding the same warrants a referral to hepatologist (HBV DNA is >10⁴ copies/mL in chronic HBV flare, and less than that in HBV-related AVH).
- *Imaging*: In classical AVH, there is no role of ultrasound abdomen. Its role lies in looking for complications, or for the confirmation of clinically suspected underlying comorbidities (irregular margin of the liver in cirrhosis, choledochal cyst or gallstones, Doppler of hepatic veins—IVC in suspected Budd–Chiari syndrome).
- *Follow-up investigations*: As mentioned, the single most important test that needs to be done for prognostication is PT. A normal value reassures the treating pediatrician, as well as the parents (who often remain anxious due to the high values of bilirubin/ALT/AST, often in spite of explaining that such high values are expected in a child with AVH).

- *Other investigations*: If there is ascites (except for those patients with a "chink of fluid" reported on ultrasound only), a characterization of the fluid (total protein, albumin, concomitant serum albumin) and cytology (TLC/DLC) to rule out infection must always be done without fail. Testing for Wilson, autoimmune hepatitis, etc., becomes important only if viral serology is negative, or the clinical picture is one of acute-on-chronic liver failure (ACLF), not AVH.

TREATMENT

- *Diet*: There is no role of restriction of fat, spices, turmeric, nonvegetarian items in a patient with AVH. The best advice is to allow home-based tasty food based on the child's preferences. Similarly, there is no need for extra glucose, sugarcane juice, etc. In fact, these cause bloating and further compromise appetite.
- *Rest*: Bed rest is not mandatory, and the child may perform activities which he voluntarily wishes to do.
- *Drugs*: The role of drugs in AVH is limited to paracetamol for fever, antiemetics for nausea/vomiting, and ursodeoxycholic acid (UDCA) for those with pruritus only. The practice of prescribing UDCA for every patient of jaundice is strongly discouraged. There is no role of liver tonics in the management of AVH too. Prescribing B-complex vitamins interferes with the assessment of urine color, which is a reliable clinical marker of the decreasing trend of cholestasis (scleral icterus takes a longer time to clear). Ascites is easily managed with salt restriction and a short course of diuretics.
- *Indications for admission*: Patients with red flag signs should be managed on an inpatient basis. These include persistent vomiting, features of hepatic encephalopathy (altered sensorium), nonimproving clinical status including continued fever/increasing jaundice/worsening of appetite, cola-colored urine, coagulopathy. ALF should be managed aggressively with adequate supportive measures as per protocol in an intensive care setting, as the child with hepatotropic virus-related ALF starts improving as soon as the progression of the liver necrosis stops spontaneously. The presence of spontaneous bacterial peritonitis (SBP) on ascitic fluid examination warrants treatment with parenteral antibiotics on an inpatient basis.

PROGNOSIS AND FOLLOW-UP

Acute viral hepatitis has an excellent prognosis, with complete recovery in almost all cases. It becomes guarded in those developing ALF. HBV-related AVH results in clearance of the virus in approximately 95% of the cases, the remaining going on to develop CHB. HAV and HEV do not cause chronic infection. An infection with HAV provides life-long immunity to the same. Repeated LFTs need not be done for follow-up of a typical AVH child who is being managed on out patient basis. Since it may takes months for the parameters to improve, an LFT at the 6-month follow-up is a pragmatic approach to document normalization (and HBsAg/anti-HBs antibody for HBV-related AVH).

IMMUNIZATION

Epidemiological studies have suggested that India is possibly transitioning from a high-endemicity region for HAV to one with intermediate endemicity. Based on this premise, it would need large-scale seroprevalence data (IgG anti-HAV) and cost-effective analysis of mass HAV vaccination, before considering inclusion of HAV vaccination in the national schedule. Introduction of vaccination with sparse coverage in a high-endemicity zone would shift the epidemiology to an intermediate-endemicity pattern. This is an undesirable outcome, as symptomatic AVH, ALF, etc., would paradoxically increase with this.

KEY MESSAGES

- AVH in children is commonly caused by hepatitis A virus, and less commonly by hepatitis E and hepatitis B.
- It has an excellent prognosis, with complete recovery being the rule in the overwhelming majority.
- Atypical features (prolonged cholestasis, relapsing hepatitis, etc.) may be present, and do not necessarily indicate a poor prognosis.
- A complete LFT and PT must be done initially.
- PT is the most important prognostic marker, and repeated LFTs are not necessary for the common garden variety.
- There is no role of UDCA (except in pruritus) or liver tonics in the management. There is no role of dietary restrictions in any form (except salt restriction in ascites). A bland diet, excess glucose/sugarcane juice may be deleterious.
- Acute HBV infection clears in 95% cases.
- Alarm features such as encephalopathy, protracted vomiting, clinical nonimprovement/worsening, coagulopathy, and spontaneous bacterial peritonitis should be kept in mind.
- ALF requires management in a pediatric intensive care setup.

SUGGESTED READING

1. Aggarwal R, Goel A. Hepatitis A. Epidemiology in resource-poor countries. Curr Opin Infect Dis. 2015;28:488-96.
2. Poddar U, Ravindranath A. Is time ripe for hepatitis a mass vaccination? Indian Pediatr. 2019;56:731-32.
3. Poddar U, Thapa BR, Prasad A, Singh K. Changing spectrum of sporadic acute viral hepatitis in Indian children. J Trop Pediatr. 2002;48:210-13.
4. Rosenthal P. Hepatitis A and hepatitis E virus infection. In: Suchy FJ, Sokol RJ, Balistreri WF (eds). Liver Disease in Children, 4th edition. New York: Cambridge University Press; pp. 265-75.
5. Singh SK, Borkar V, Srivastava A, Mathias A, Yachha SK, Poddar U. Need for recognizing atypical manifestations of childhood sporadic acute viral hepatitis warranting differences in management. Eur J Pediatr. 2019;178:61-7.
6. Yachha SK. Sporadic acute viral hepatitis in children. Pediatric Infectious Disease. 2011;3:1-6.

Acute Liver Failure

Sakshi Karkra, Rohan Karkra

INTRODUCTION

Pediatric acute liver failure (ALF) is rare but life-threatening illness that occurs in children without preexisting liver disease. Over the last few decades the outcome of ALF has transformed from near fatal, to one with overall improving prognosis since emergency liver transplantation (LT) has been established as a treatment option.

DEFINITION

The Pediatric Acute Liver Failure (PALF) study group used the following criteria:
- No evidence of a known chronic liver disease
- Biochemical evidence of acute liver injury
- Hepatic-based coagulopathy uncorrectable by parenteral vitamin K [international normalized ratio (INR) > 1.5 with encephalopathy and INR > 2 without encephalopathy]

It is subclassified (International Association for the Study of the Liver) on the basis of duration between encephalopathy and onset of symptoms as this provides clinicians clues about probable etiology and outcome **(Table 1)**:
- Hyperacute (<10 days)
- Fulminant (10–30 days)
- Subacute (5–24 weeks).

EVALUATION

It should determine the status of major organs and establish the etiology **(Table 2)**.
- *History*:
  - Jaundice preceded by fever, myalgia, and nausea suggests a viral etiology.

TABLE 1: Causes of acute liver failure.

Etiology	Neonate	Children
Infections	• Herpes simplex • Parvovirus B19 • Adenovirus, echovirus • Hepatitis B, measles, HHV6, VZV	• Hepatitis A, B, C, D, E • Leptospirosis • EBV • Dengue fever and dengue shock syndrome (DSS)
Metabolic liver disease (MLD)/other	• Galactosemia • Tyrosinemia • Fatty acid oxidation defects (FAOD) • Mitochondrial defects • Hereditary fructose intolerance (HFI)	• Wilson's disease (WD) mitochondrial defects • Niemann-Pick type C
Drugs/toxins	• Valproate • TMP/SMX • Paracetamol overdose	• Rifampicin • TMP/SMX • Valproate, Halothane • Paracetamol overdose • MAO inhibitor • Mushroom poisoning • Herbal medication
Immune/Infiltrative	• Neonatal hemochromatosis • Hemophagocytic lymphohistocytosis (HLH)	• Leukemia • HLH • Autoimmune hepatitis (AIH)
Cardiac	• Birth asphyxia • Myocarditis • Congenital heart disease and cardiac surgery	• Cardiomyopathy, myocarditis • Budd-Chiari syndrome, congestive heart failure • Heat stroke, shock
Genetic	NBAS mutation	• NBAS mutation • SCYL1 mutation

(EBV: Epstein-Barr virus; VZV: varicella zoster virus; TMP/SMX: trimethoprim/sulfamethoxazole; INH: isoniazid; MAO: monoamine oxidase; HHV6: human herpesvirus 6)

- In an infant, symptoms can be nonspecific (vomiting, irritability) with jaundice developing subsequently.
- Symptoms worsening after feeds [aversion to sweets in hereditary fructose intolerance (HFI) or lactose in galactosemia with recurrent sepsis].
- History of altered sleep pattern with irrelevant speech, incoherent thought process or seizures suggest neurological involvement and hepatic encephalopathy.
- Passing dark cola colored urine, decreased urine output suggest hemolysis and points Wilson's disease (WD), leptospirosis.
- Fever with rash [leptospirosis, human herpesvirus 6 (HHV6), herpes, dengue, Epstein-Barr virus (EBV), measles], exposure to rats (leptospirosis), drugs, toxins especially herbal medications.
- Failure to thrive, diarrhea, vomiting suggest HFI, tyrosinemia.
- Past and family history of jaundice usually suggests autoimmune hepatitis (AIH) or WD while recurrent ALF preceded by fever suggest genetic cause.
- A sibling or a relative dying of similar illness suggests metabolic cause.
- History of abortion in mother or sibling death in neonatal age with similar complain suggest alloimmune hemochromatosis.
- *Physical examination*:
  - *Anthropometry*: Failure to thrive
  - *Vitals*: A febrile child in shock suggest dengue or other infective causes
  - Petechiae suggest dengue, WD; maculopapular rash (viral, leptospira) rash
  - Extreme pallor suggest parvovirus B19 (suppression) or WD (hemolysis)
  - Skeletal deformity suggest genetic cause, rickets suggest (renal tubular acidosis)
  - *Eyes*: Cataract (galactosemia, WD), Kayser–Fleischer (KF) ring (WD)
  - A rapidly shrinking liver suggests massive hepatocellular necrosis (poor *prognosis*)
  - Ascites is mostly seen in ACLF, rather than ALF, except acute Budd-Chiari syndrome
  - A complete central nervous system examination
- *Investigations*: Laboratory, radiological, and other investigations are tabulated in **Tables 3 and 4**.

TABLE 2: Classification of hepatic encephalopathy (HE) in infants/children.

Grade	Clinical findings	Reflexes
Grade 0	Normal	Normal
Grade 1	Confused, mood changes, inconsolable crying	Normal or hyper-reflexic
Grade 2	Drowsy, inappropriate behavior, inconsolable crying	Normal or hyper-reflexic
Grade 3	Stupor, somnolence, combativeness but may obey simple commands	Hyper-reflexic, Babinski
Grade 4	Comatose, +/- response with pain	Normal

TABLE 3: Diagnostic tests to evaluate child of ALF.

First line (assess severity)	Second line (assess etiology)	Interpretation
• Complete blood cell count (CBC) with platelets • *Liver function tests*: Very low serum alkaline phosphatase • Ratio of alkaline phosphatase to total bilirubin < 4 and AST to ALT>2.2 suggest WD • *Renal function tests*: Creatinine, sodium, potassium, uric acid, calcium, Mg • PT, INR, aPTT • *Blood gas*: glucose pH, lactate, bicarbonate • Arterial ammonia • Serum osmolarity • *Septic profile*: Procalcitonin, CRP, blood cultures, urine cultures, tracheal cultures • *For DIC*: Fibrinogen, D – dimer, FDP • Blood group, cross match • Urine routine	• Anti-HAV antibody (IgM) • HbsAg, anti-core antibody (HbcAb IgM) • Anti-HEV IgM • Anti-HCV • Other serologies for infection • ANA, ASMA, anti-LKM1 in dilution, immunoglobulin (IgG) • Bone marrow aspiration (typical cells), raised ferritin, raised triglycerides, low/absent NK cell activity • Buccal mucosal biopsy, raised ferritin, high transferrin saturation, high AFP • Toxicology screen • Galactose-1-phosphate uridyl transferase assay (No transfusion in last 3 months) • High urinary succinylacetone, TMS, high AFP, gene study • 24 hr urinary copper, KF ring, Coombs negative hemolytic anemia, low serum ceruloplasmin, gene study • TMS • Carnitine - acyl carnitine profile • Muscle, liver biopsy for quantitative assay of respiratory chain enzymes	• Hepatitis A infection • Hepatitis B infection • Hepatitis E Infection • Hepatitis C infection • CMV; EBV; VZV; echovirus; parvovirus B19; malaria; dengue; leptospirosis • AIH • HLH • NH /Congenital alloimmune hepatitis • Acetaminophen, opiates, barbiturates • Galactosemia • Tyrosinemia • WD • Urea cycle defect (UCD) • FAOD • Mitochondrial hepatopathies

(ANA: antinuclear antibody; ASMA: antismooth muscle antibody; anti-LKM: antiliver, kidney microsome; NK: natural killer; OTC: ornithine transcarbamylase; TMS: tandem mass spectrometry; AFP: alpha fetoprotein)

MANAGEMENT

Due to potentially devastating course, the patient is managed in an pediatric intensive care unit with a facility of mechanical ventilation, renal replacement therapy (RRT), intracranial pressure monitoring, blood bank, with facility of emergency LT if needed. Management is divided into general and specific management for the etiology. Emphasis is to maintain hemodynamics and functions of other organs while avoiding and treating any complications during the process **(Table 5)**.

TABLE 4: Other tests for acute liver failure (ALF) evaluation.

	First line	*Second line*
Imaging	Chest radiograph, abdominal ultrasound (USG) with Doppler study of the liver	• Doppler USG computed tomography/magnetic resonance imaging (CT/MRI): Rule out veno-occlusive disease/malignancies • CT brain: Intracranial bleed/edema
Cardiac	Electrocardiogram	Echocardiography
Central nervous system (CNS)	EEG, bispectral index (BIS)	? Intracranial pressure (ICP)

TABLE 5: Management of acute liver failure (ALF).

	General management
Electrolytes and sugar	• Blood sugar monitoring (every 2 hours) • IV glucose (6–8 mg/kg/min) is recommended in patients who develop hypoglycemia • For Dextrose concentration > 12.5% - Use Central line • Correct hypokalemia, hypophosphatemia, hypomagnesemia
Fluid therapy and hemodynamics	• Maintain hydration/renal function, avoid cerebral edema and fluid overload • Restrict fluids to 2/3rd maintenance except in hypovolemia and dehydration • Shock (Warm d/t to hyperdynamic circulation and low SVR secondary to intense arterial vasodilatation because of released endogenous nitric oxide): They need fluids with inotrope (Nor-epinephrine preferred) • Bedside echocardiography can guide fluid therapy, by assessing pre-load, contractility, ejection fraction • Refractory hypotension: Injection hydrocortisone

Respiratory system with ventilation	*Indications of intubation*:
	• > Grade 2 encephalopathy
	• Raised intracranial pressure (ICP)
	• Respiratory failure
	• Hypotension and shock
	   – Propofol and fentanyl suggested for sedation
	   – Avoid propofol > 24 hours (infusion syndrome)
	   – Aim SpO_2 >90 % and $PaCO_2$ 35–45 mm Hg
	   – Excessive hyperventilation should be avoided except to reduce ICP in impending herniation
	   – High PEEP, low TV can increase cerebral edema
	   – Sedation before tracheal suction to avoid ICP surges

Cerebral edema and intracranial hypertension	*Avoid hyperammonemia:* • Reduce endogenous (control bleeding and infection) or exogenous (avoid unjustified FFP) nitrogen intake • Insufficient evidence to support Lactulose/Lactitol • Neomycin is not recommended • Ornithine aspartate and sodium benzoate have been proposed to decrease serum ammonia, in Reye syndrome and urea cycle defects • Hemofiltration *Osmotic therapy:* • 20% Mannitol as first line therapy (2 mL/kg/dose) and repeated, till serum osmolality is < 320 mOsm/L (avoided in significant kidney injury or shock.) • Hypertonic saline (target sodium 145–155 mEq/L) till serum osmolality <360 mOsm/L. Raise the head end of bed to 20–30 degree (if no shock). Avoid neck rotation *Refractory raised ICP:* • Moderate hypothermia (32°C–33°C) with paralysis • Barbiturate coma—reduce brain metabolism • Hepatectomy—rarely considered when all measures to neuroprotect exhausted (potential donor identified) No consensus exists on the use of invasive ICP monitoring non invasive methods of neuromonitoring • Transcranial Doppler examination, near-infra red spectroscopy, tympanic membrane displacement, optic nerve sheath diameter (evidence insufficient) Treat seizure with phenytoin or levetiracetam (prophylactic anti-epileptics not recommended)

Contd...

Contd...

Infections	*Empirical broad spectrum antibiotics (cephalosporins) with antifungals are recommended in following:* • Cultures positive • Advanced stage (III/IV) hepatic encephalopathy • Persistent hypotension • Systemic inflammatory response syndrome • Patients listed for liver transplant (LT)
Coagulopathy	• Prophylactic correction should not be done without overt bleeding except procedures (target INR ~1.5, platelet count 50,000/mm^3) • TEG should be used for finer management. • Cryoprecipitate (40 mg/kg) is recommended for significant hypofibrinogenemia (<100 mg/dL) • Recombinant factor 7a (rF7) can be considered for bleeders not responding to FFP and Cryo
N-acetylcysteine (NAC)	• *The optimal duration (not clear)*: 3 to 7 days protocol. • *Dose for non acetaminophen ALF*: -100–150 mg/kg/day; diluted in 5–10% dextrose IV infusion
Complications: GI Bleed	• Coagulopathy and thrombocytopenia corrected • IV Vitamin K 5–10 mg (except G6PD deficiency) • Injection Octreotide (0.5–1 µg/kg/min) to reduce portal pressure • H2 blockers (ranitidine 1–3 mg/kg TDS) • PPIs (pantoprazole 0.5 to 1.0 mg/kg/day up to 20 mg for children <40 kg) or sucralfate
Acute Kidney Injury	• Ensure urine output >1 mL/kg/hr • *Oliguria*: Early fluid challenge followed by a trial of diuretic (if child is hemodynamically stable) • Low dose dopamine is no longer advisable. • Early CRRT (AKI, reduce NH_3 in grade III/IV HE if NH_3 > 200 µmol/L, lactate and fluid overload
Nutrition	• Higher caloric density feeds to avoid excessive free water and hypo-osmolality • TPN (35–40 kcal/kg per day) reserved for patients with contraindications to enteral nutrition • Normal protein intake till stage I and II HE and thereafter restriction (0.5–1 g/kg/day) recommended • MLD presenting as ALF need special diet plan
Specific treatment	
Acetaminophen poisoning	• Activated charcoal 1 g/kg orally • NAC 150 mg/kg IV in 15 min, then maintenance dose 50 mg/kg over 4 hrs, then 100 mg/kg over 16 hrs
HSV	Acyclovir 10 mg/kg 8 hourly or 150 mg/m^2/day IV
Neonatal hemochromatosis	• IVIG • Deferoxamine 30 mg/kg/day IV in 3 doses • Selenium 2–3 µg/kg/day IV • NAC 140 mg/kg, then 70 mg/kg orally or IV • Tocopherol glycolsuccinate 20 IU/kg/day orally
Mushroom poisoning	• Penicillin G 300,000–1 million units/kg/day IV • Silymarin 30–40 mg/kg/day IV or orally
Autoimmune hepatitis	• Methyl prednisolone 1–2 mg/kg IV (max 60 mg) • Azathioprine may be added to steroids
Tyrosinemia	NTBC
Galactosemia	Galactose-free formula

(TEG: thromboelastography; SVR: systemic vascular resistance; NTBC: 2-(2-nitro-4-trifluoro-methylbenzoyl)-1,3-cyclohexandion)

EMERGENCY LIVER TRANSPLANTATION

In children, fulminant WD and undetermined ALF carry grim prognosis and require emergency liver transplantation (ELT), whereas hepatitis A and acetaminophen-induced ALF have good recovery without transplantation. Commonly used criteria are Kings College criteria though they are not very accurate for children. Recently, in nonacetaminophen-induced ALF in children it is recommended that an INR > 4 or factor V concentration of <25% is best available criteria for listing for LT **(Table 6)**.

Contraindications for LT

- Metastatic malignant disease
- Lymphohistiocytosis
- Systemic metabolic
- Systemic mitochondrial respiratory chain disorders
- Uncontrolled sepsis
- Fixed dilated pupils
- Severe respiratory failure.

TABLE 6: King's College Hospital criteria for acute liver failure (ALF).

ALF secondary to acetaminophen overdose	ALF with other causes
pH < 7.30 (irrespective of encephalopathy grade), following volume resuscitation >24 hours post overdose Or Hepatic encephalopathy (HE) III–IV, prothrombin time (PT) > 100 seconds [international normalized ratio (INR) > 6.5], and Serum creatinine over 300 µmol/L (3.4 mg/dL) Or *The extended King's College Hospital Criteria (KCH) criteria*: Serum lactate > 3.5 mmol/L after early resuscitation Serum lactate > 3.0 mmol/L 24 hours post overdose and adequate volume resuscitation	Prothrombin time >100 seconds (INR > 6.5) (irrespective of encephalopathy grade) Or Any three of the following (irrespective of HE grade) 1. Age under 10 or over 40 years – Non-A, non-B or drug-induced hepatitis 2. Duration of jaundice before encephalopathy over 7 days 3. Serum bilirubin > 300 µmol/L (17.6 mg/dL) 4. PT > 50 seconds (INR > 3.5)

Prognosis

Mortality is mainly attributed to cerebral edema, multiorgan dysfunction syndrome and sepsis.

KEY MESSAGES

- Presence of encephalopathy is not an essential criterion for diagnosing ALF in children.
- An infant or child with recurrent ALF may have mutation in SCYL1/NBAS.
- Early referral must be made to a liver transplant center as they deteriorate rapidly.
- FFP should be avoided as long as no active bleeding is present.
- An excellent ICU care is needed for good outcome.
- Specific treatment for some causes can prevent LT.
- Fulminant WD has poor outcome without LT and emergency LT has drastically changed prognosis of pediatric ALF.

SUGGESTED READING

1. Agarwal B, Wright G, Gatt A, et al. Evaluation of coagulation abnormalities in acute liver failure. J Hepatol. 2012;57:780-6.
2. Dhaliwal M, Raghunathan V, Mohan N, Deep A. Acute liver failure in children – a constant challenge for the treating intensivist. J Pediatr Crit Care. 2016;3(4):37-51.
3. Jia-Qi Li, Jing-Yu Gong, Knisely AS, et al. Recurrent acute liver failure associated with novel SCYL1 mutation: a case report. World J Clin Cases. 2019;7(4):494-9.
4. Shanmugam NP, Dhawan A. Selection criteria for liver transplantation in paediatric acute liver failure: the saga continues. Pediatr Transplant. 2011;15:5-6.
5. Squires Jr RH, Shneider BL, Bucuvalas J, et al. Acute liver failure in children: the first 348 patients in the pediatric acute liver failure study group. J Pediatr. 2006;148:652-8.

Chapter 68: Chronic Hepatitis B

Shrish Bhatnagar, Alok Kumar

INTRODUCTION

India is a region of intermediate endemicity for hepatitis B virus (HBV) infection, as its prevalence is about 3% in general population. Chronic hepatitis B (CH-B) disease is defined as hepatic necroinflammation resulting from the persistent presence of HBV infection. World Health Organization (WHO) case definition of CH-B requires the detection in serum of hepatitis B surface antigen (HBsAg) on two occasions over a 6-month period. Liver biopsy is an important component in defining the severity of liver disease in these patients. Abnormal liver enzyme levels are defined as an alanine aminotransferase (ALT) of >17–20 IU/mL in women and >25–30 IU/mL in men.

World Health Organization places CH-B in the top 10 causes of death worldwide. CH-B in children is mostly due to mother-to-child transmission (60%) and risk of chronicity is highest when exposed in early infancy. The risk of chronicity after exposure to hepatitis B is 90% in the newborn, 30% in children <5 years, and 5% in adolescents. Though CH-B is seemingly innocuous during childhood, risk of cirrhosis is 3–5% and risk of hepatocellular carcinoma (HCC) is 0.01–0.03% even before reaching adult hood.

NATURAL HISTORY OF CHRONIC HEPATITIS B

Clinical course of CH-B is divided in various phases **(Table 1)** which are described using:

- Hepatitis B e-antigen (HBeAg) status (a secreted protein represent active replication of wild-type HBV)
- HBV-DNA (HBV-deoxyribonucleic acid)
- ULN (upper limit of normal) of ALT/AST (aspartate aminotransferase) as marker of liver inflammation

1. *HBeAg (+), chronic HBV infection/immune tolerant phase*:
   a. Characterized by dormancy of immune system against the virus, thus allowing uncontrolled replication of HBV.
   For example: Perinatally acquired HBV or transmission of HBV in the first 2 years of life. Transplacental transmission of HBeAg induces immune tolerance thus explaining establishment of infection without any inflammation.
   b. There is minimal/no parenchymal inflammation.
   c. There is continuous integration of HBV-DNA into the hepatocytes and formation of covalently closed circular (ccc) DNA which forms the transcription template for rapid viral replication. This phase form a fertile background for development of HCC because of the random insertion of viral DNA into the host genome.

2. *HBeAg-positive chronic hepatitis B/immune active phase*:
   a. There is activation of the immune system against the virus.
   b. Liver histopathology will show varying degree of necroinflammation.
   c. Activated immune system can cause HBeAg sero conversion in 65–90% in the long run. However, repeated flares of inflammation lead to progression of fibrosis.
   d. In children, early seroconversion is a risk factor for developing HCC as the severe necroinflammation forms an ideal background for carcinogenesis.

TABLE 1: Summarizing various phases of chronic hepatitis B (CH-B).

	HBeAg positive chronic infection (Immune tolerant)	HBeAg positive chronic hepatitis (Immune active)	HBeAg negative chronic infection (Inactive carrier)	HBeAg negative chronic hepatitis
HBeAg	Positive	Positive	Negative	Negative
HBV-DNA (Copies/ml)	>20,000	2,000–20,000	<2,000	>20,000
ALT	Normal	>ULN	Normal	>ULN
Liver Histopathology	Normal	Moderate to severe Necroinflammation/fibrosis	Minimal activity	Moderate to severe Necroinflammation/fibrosis
Treatment	No	Yes	No	Yes

(ALT: alanine aminotransferase; DNA: deoxyribonucleic acid; HBeAg: hepatitis B e-antigen; HBV: hepatitis B virus; ULN: upper limit of normal)

3. *HBeAg-negative chronic HBV infection/inactive carrier phase/nonreplicative phase*:
   a. Necroinflammatory activity is low and risk of progression to cirrhosis is low.
   b. These patients are at risk for relapse to active liver disease and replication of virus as well as HBV-DNA integration into the hepatocyte nuclear DNA with the attendant risk of developing HCC later in life.
4. *HBeAg-negative chronic hepatitis B*:
   a. Virus at this phase has mutations in the core and precore regions that prevent HBeAg expression but still allow replication.
   b. There is a risk of rapid disease progression and risk of HCC.
   c. Reactivation can occur naturally or with the use of immunosuppressive therapy.
   d. Individuals in this phase tend to be older and to have more advanced liver disease with a higher likelihood of adverse clinical outcomes.
5. *HBsAg-negative phase/occult HBV/resolved infection*:
   a. If this phase occurs before development of cirrhosis there is hardly any risk of disease progression or HCC.
   b. There is persistence of cccDNA in the hepatocytes would lead to reactivation when exposed to immunosuppression.
   c. The standard is to treat these patients during chemotherapy with a nucleoside or nucleotide analog.

TREATMENT

Goal of treatment is eradication of HBV which in turn will stall disease progression HCC development. HBsAg loss signifies intense suppression of viral replication and is a desirable goal. HBeAg seroconversion is a less desirable end point as there still remains the risk of seroreversion. Relative levels of HBV-DNA often correlate inversely with the degree of necroinflammatory activity in the liver, reflecting attempts by the host's immune response to control and eliminate the virus. The serum level of HBV DNA can be used for prognosis **(Flowchart 1)**.

Indications for Treatment

Patients with HBeAg positive or negative chronic HBV infection are not offered treatment unless they have extrahepatic manifestations, history of HCC/cirrhosis or age >30 years. In children, a decision to treat should take into account the slow progression of the disease in children, risk of complications and side effects of prolonged treatment **(Table 2)**.

Drugs for Treatment

The two classes of drugs approved for treatment of CH-B in children are:
1. Pegylated interferon (Peg IFN)
2. Nucleos(t)ide analogs (NA)

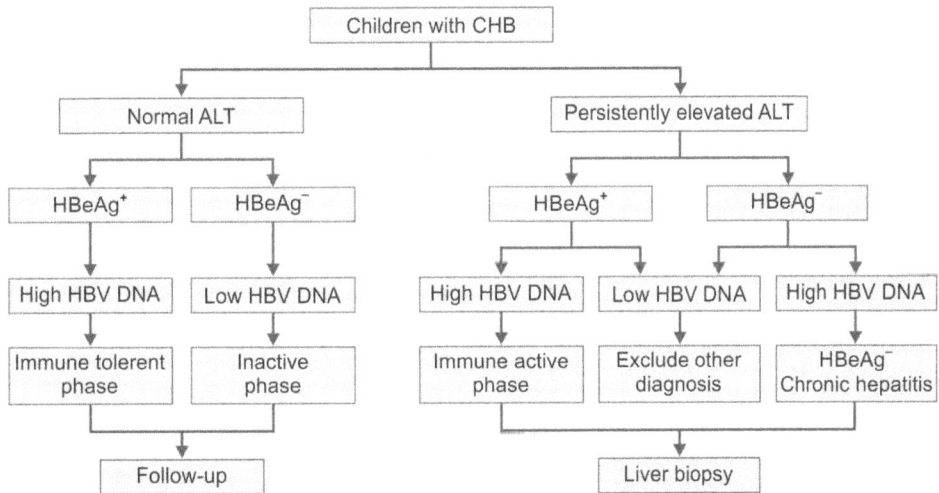

Flowchart 1: Algorithm for management for chronic hepatitis B.

TABLE 2: Suggested intervals of monitoring children with chronic HBV.

Phase of disease	Parameter monitored	Frequency of monitoring
At diagnosis	LFTs, AFP, HBV-DNA, HBV serology	Baseline
Immune tolerance	LFTs, HBeAg, HBeAb, HBV-DNA, AFP	Every 6–12 months
Immune clearance	LFTs, HBeAg, HBeAb, HBV-DNA, AFP	Every 3 months
Inactive carrier	LFTs, HBV-DNA	Every 6–12 months

(AFP: alpha-fetoprotein; DNA: deoxyribonucleic acid; HBV: hepatitis B virus; HBeAg: hepatitis B e-antigen; LFTs: liver function tests)

1. *Peg IFN*: Interferon-α: It is the first drug to be approved for treating children with CH-B, in which the addition of a polyethylene glycol (PEG) moiety increases its half-life and reduces the frequency of injection to once weekly rather than 3 times/week.
   - Immunomodulatory role
   - Antiviral effect

   Advantages of Peg IFN therapy:
   - Finite duration of therapy
   - High barrier against resistance
   - Low risk of relapse

   Adverse effects:
   - Subcutaneous injections
   - Contraindication in decompensated cirrhosis
2. *Nucleos(t)ide analogs*:
   - Lamivudine
   - Adefovir
   - Telbivudine
   - Entecavir
   - Tenofovir DF

Duration of treatment: After achieving HBeAg seroconversion and undetectable HBV-DNA, NAs should be continued for at least 12 months more to consolidate the treatment.

In those who do not seroconvert or in those with HBeAg negative chronic hepatitis B therapy with NAs should be continued indefinitely.

LIVER TRANSPLANTATION

- Liver transplantation (LT) for decompensated liver disease due to CH-B should receive NA and hepatitis B immunoglobulin (HBIG) after transplantation which reduces the chances of graft infection to <5%.
- HBV-DNA (-) at the time of LT HBIG can be discontinued but NA's to be continued.
- HBV-DNA (+) at the time of LT prolonged therapy with NA and HBIG would be required.
- Liver transplantation from a donor who is anti-HBc IgG (+), lifelong NA should be continued to prevent reactivation with immunosuppression.

Prevention

For children born to HBV-infected mothers, prevention of perinatal and early horizontal transmission with injection of HBIG [0.5 mL, intramuscular (IM)] combined with HBV vaccine within 48 hours of birth has higher efficacy than vaccine alone, protecting >98% of infants. Understanding of risk factors and intervention aimed at each of the major routes of transmission [e.g., homo/heterosexual contact, intravenous (IV) drugs, mother to child transmission, renal dialysis, etc.] is the key for preventing HBV transmission. The combination of education, prevent ion strategies, and vaccination could lead to eradication of the disease.

- Persistence in serum of HBsAg on two occasions over a 6-month period is CH-B.
- Chronic hepatitis B is among leading cause of death worldwide and India is a zone of intermediate endemicity.
- Treatment depends upon the phases of CH-B and should be individualized.
- Children born to HBV positive mothers should be vaccinated as recommended.

SUGGESTED READING

1. Kelly DA (Ed). "Diseases of the Liver and Biliary System in Children", 4th edition. Wiley Blackwell; 2017.
2. "Pediatric Gut and Liver Journal" Official E-Journal of Indian Society of Pediatric Gastroenterology Hepatology and Nutrition.
3. Ronald KE, Sanderson IR (Eds). "Walker's Pediatric Gastrointestinal Diseases" 6th edition. People's Medical Publishing House-USA; 2018.

PRESCRIPTION ASSISTANCE

Pharmacological salt	Market preparation	Availability (drops/syrup/tablet/injection)	Route of administration	Dosage
Peg INF	Pegasys	Injection	Subcutaneous	180 µg/1.73 m²/week for 6 months
Lamivudine	Epivir-HBV/Epivir/Zeffix/Heptodin	Tablet 100, 150, 300 mg Syrup 5 mg/mL	Oral	3 mg/kg/OD; Max 100 mg/day (<2 years of age) Renal dose modification
Entecavir	Baraclude	Tablet 0.5, 1 mg Syrup 0.5 mg/mL	Oral	0.5 mg/PO/q Day (>2 years of age) For CH-B with e/o active viral replication
Adefovir	Adefovir-dipivoxil/Hepsera	Tablet 10 mg	Oral	10 mg/PO/q Day (>12 years of age) Renal dose modification
Tenofovir DF	Viread	Tablet 150, 200, 250 mg 40 mg/g of powder (i.e., 1 scoopful)	Oral	8 mg/kg/PO/q Day (>2 years of age and weight >10 kg)

(CH-B: chronic hepatitis B; HBV: hepatitis B virus; INF: interferon)

Metabolic Liver Disease in Children

Malathi Sathiyasekaran, Ganesh Ramaswamy

INTRODUCTION

Metabolic liver diseases (MLDs) are inherited inborn errors of metabolism (IEM) which include liver disease as a clinical entity. Hepatomegaly, hepatosplenomegaly, and/or disturbed liver function or structure form an integral part of this disorder. IEM accounts for 2% of hospital admissions and metabolic liver disease accounts for 13-43% of acute liver failure in young children and 5-20% in older children. Since liver plays a pivot al role in several anabolic and catabolic biochemical reactions involving carbohydrates, protein, lipid, and minerals, it is the target in several IEM. Many inherited metabolic disorders are treatable and therefore performing appropriate investigations, making a definitive diagnosis and initiating prompt treatment are essential to ensure a good outcome.

PATHOPHYSIOLOGY

The manifestation of liver disease depends on the substrate involved, duration of disease, and degree of injury. The majority of MLDs are inherited as autosomal recessive inheritance though inheritance from autosomal dominant, X linked or from maternal mitochondrial DNA may also occur.

The pathophysiology of MLD is very complex and is diagrammatically represented in **Figure 1**.

The disorders can be classified into three main groups **(Fig. 1)**:
1. *Disorders of synthesis or catabolism of complex molecules*: For example, lysosomal and peroxisomal disorders. The partly degraded molecules accumulate in the affected organs, including the liver and disrupts the organ function.
2. *Energy metabolism disorders*: These are caused by a deficiency in energy production and its consequences, e.g., glycogen storage disorders (GSDs), fat oxidation, and mitochondrial disorders.
3. *Disorders caused by the accumulation of toxic compounds*: Arising as a consequence of the enzyme defect, as occurs in galactosemia and tyrosinemia type I.

APPROACH TO MLD

- *History*: Since MLD is a genetic disorder, the history **(Table 1)** should extend to include gestation and also extended family members. Galactosemia should be suspected in a neonate with recurrent vomiting. Children born to mothers with acute fatty liver pregnancy or HELLP (hemolysis elevated liver enzymes low platelet) during pregnancy should be followed up for fatty acid oxidation (FAO). Similarly, if there is a history of intrahepatic cholestasis of pregnancy, there is a possibility of progressive familial intrahepatic cholestasis (PFIC) in the child. Poor scholastic performance in a child may be a clue for Wilson disease (WD). Dietary history includes symptoms which occur after ingestion of fructose-rich foods such as honey, fruit juices, syrups as in fructose intolerance. Aversion to protein-rich foods points toward urea cycle disorders.
  Craving for protein-rich foods and aversion to carbohydrates points toward citrin deficiency.
- *Physical examination*: Assessment of growth and development is essential in all MLDs and a thorough examination is an important step in evaluation **(Table 2)**.
- *Clinical presentation and common causes of MLDs*: Many MLDs present in the neonatal period and early infancy but some may manifest later in childhood.
1. *MLD in neonatal period and infancy*:
    a. *Hydrops fetalis*: Neonatal ascites and nonimmune hydrops fetalis can be due to IEMs such as Gaucher disease, Niemann-Pick disease, Barth syndrome, GM 1 gangliosidoses, congenital disorders of

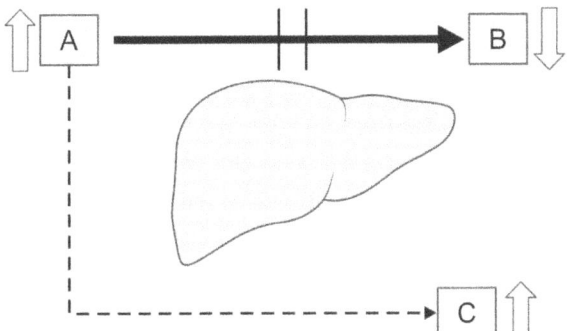

Fig. 1: Schematic representation of pathogenesis of metabolic liver disease.

TABLE 1: Clues in history and examination to suspect MLD.

Positive family history of liver disease	Recurrent episodes of similar illness at times of catabolic stress
Unexplained sibling deaths	Episodes of unexplained metabolic derangement or hypoglycemia
Recurrent fetal loss, AFLP, and HELLP during pregnancy	History of (H/o) change or avoidance of specific diet or amount of intake before
H/o parental consanguinity	H/o abnormal growth or development
Unusual body odors	Microcephaly, macrocephaly, coarse features, mental retardation
Acute neonatal illness	FTT, rickets, dysmorphic features
Presence of unexplained coma	Cataracts, impaired vision
Developmental delay, unexplained convulsions, hypotonia, hypertonia	Unexplained hepatomegaly, hepatosplenomegaly, elevated serum transaminases, recurrent jaundice

(AFLP: acute fatty liver of pregnancy; FTT: failure to thrive; HELLP: hemolysis elevated liver enzymes low platelet; MLD: metabolic liver disease)

TABLE 2: Clues in general physical examination to suspect MLD.

Facial dysmorphism	Mucopolysaccharidoses and peroxisomal disorders
Doll-like facies, Chubby cheeks (**Fig. 2**)	Glycogen storage disorder I and citrin deficiency
Inverted nipples, abnormal fat pads	Congenital disorder of glycosylation Ia, b
Extensive mongolian spots	GM1 gangliosidosis
Hypopigmented, thin, brittle, kinky hair	Menkes kinky hair disease
Cataract	Galactosemia, Wilson disease (WD)
Cherry red spots	Niemann-Pick disease, Tay Sachs disease
Supranuclear vertical gaze palsy	Gaucher disease type 3, Niemann-Pick C disease
Scratch marks	Chronic cholestatic disorders, PFIC, BASD
Fractures	Chronic cholestasis, Gaucher disease
Rickets	WD, HFI, Fanconi Bickel syndrome, tyrosinemia
Skeletal dysplasia (dysostosis multiplex), large skull, spinal deformities, and short, thick tubular bones	Mucolipidosis, Mucopolysaccharidosis
Reye-like illness	LCHAD, FAO
Neurodevelopmental regression	Mucolipid disorder
Multisystem disease	Mitochondrial hepatopathy

(BASD: bile acid synthesis defect; FAO: fatty acid oxidation; HFI: hereditary fructose intolerance; LCHAD: long chain 3 hydroxyacyl coenzyme a dehydrogenase; PFIC: progressive familial intrahepatic cholestasis)

glycosylation (CDG), and glycogen storage disease type IV. Although the prognosis is poor, it is important to establish the diagnosis for genetic counseling.

b. *Neonatal cholestasis syndrome (NCS)*: In India, 4–12% of NCS is due to metabolic liver disease. The common metabolic disorders are tyrosinemia, galactosemia, bile salt transport disorders (PFIC 1-6), and bile acid (BA) synthesis defects.

c. *Acute liver failure (ALF)/sick infant with FTT*: The important metabolic causes in this group are tyrosinemia, galactosemia, mitochondrial hepatopathy, and congenital disorders of glycosylation.

d. *Hyperbilirubinemia*: In the new born period, the two important causes are Crigler–Najjar (CN) I and II.

e. *Organomegaly*: The important causes of isolated hepatomegaly or hepatosplenomegaly are Wolman disease, GSD, FAO defect, and citrin deficiency.

f. *Others*: Some neonates and infants with MLD may appear normal on clinical examination, e.g., organic acidemia and FAO. These manifest during an intercurrent infection or at the times of catabolic stress.

2. *MLD in older children*:
   a. *Isolated hepatomegaly*: There are some metabolic disorders like GSD I, hereditary fructose intolerance, and FAO which present with isolated hepatomegaly.
   b. *Hepatosplenomegaly/splenohepatomegaly*: Glycogen storage disease, WD, Gaucher disease, Niemann-Pick disease, and mucopolysaccharidosis may present with hepatosplenomegaly.
   c. *Chronic liver disease*: Some metabolic disorders present with cirrhosis with portal hypertension (PHT). The common ones are WD, Gaucher disease, GSD IV, hereditary fructose intolerance, cystic fibrosis, and tyrosinemia.

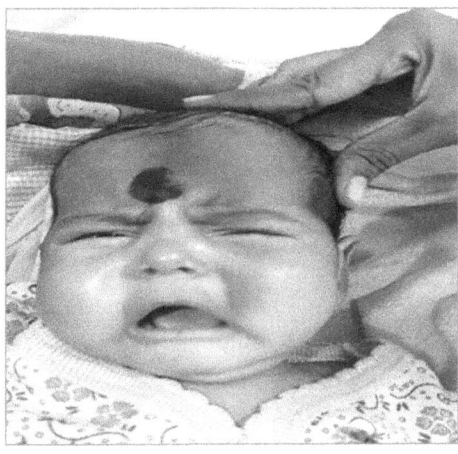

Fig. 2: Chubby Cheeks in infant /Citrin deficiency/GSD.

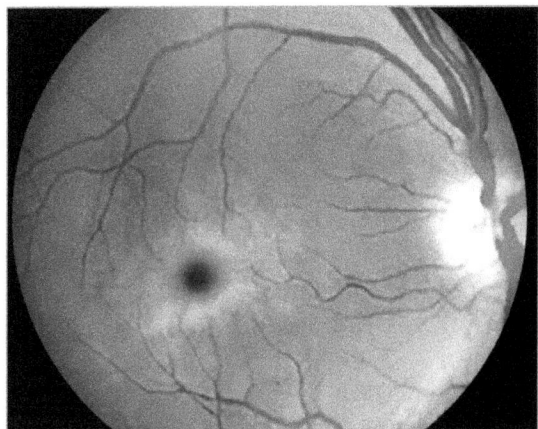

Fig. 3: Fundus showing cherry red spot.

d. *Acute liver failure and acute on chronic liver failure (ACLF)*: In India WD and Bile salt transport defects PFIC 3 are important MLDs presenting as ALF or ACLF.
e. *Recurrent jaundice*: Crigler–Najjar syndrome II, Gilbert's syndrome, Dubin Johnson syndrome, and Rotor Syndrome are common metabolic disorders presenting as recurrent jaundice in older children.
f. *Chronic cholestasis*: The two MLDs which present with chronic cholestasis in older children are PFIC and inborn error of BA synthesis.
g. *Others*: Apart from the abdominal examination a meticulous assessment of the neurological, cardiac, and respiratory systems is essential. Ophthalmological examination should be included in the protocol and performed by an experienced ophthalmologist for cataract, Kayser-Fleischer (KF) ring, cherry red spot **(Fig. 3)**, and retinal pigmentary changes.

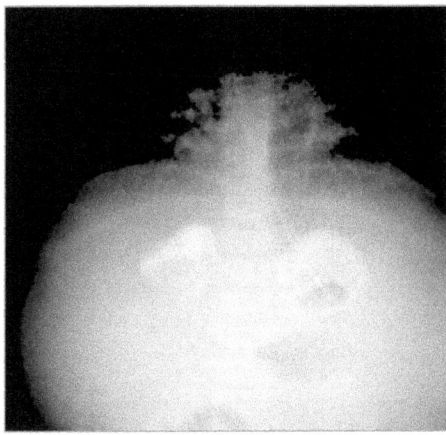

Fig. 4: X-ray abdomen adrenal calcification in wolman disease.

Investigations:
A. *Basic investigations*:
 1. *Blood*:
    a. *Complete blood count and peripheral smear*: Anemia may be a feature of Wolman and Gaucher disease. Acanthocytosis on smear is suggestive of abetalipoproteinemia. vacuolated lymphocytes in Wolman disease or Lysosomal disorders.
    b. *Liver function tests*: Though these tests may be abnormal in several non-MLDs, it may help in diagnosis of some MLD. Normal or low gamma-glutamyl transpeptidase (GGT) levels are seen in PFIC 1–6 (except PFIC 3) and in bile acid synthesis defects (BASDs) and thus low GGT is an excellent marker to diagnose a subset of metabolic cholestatic disorders.
    c. *Serum BAs*: BAs are disproportionately increased in inherited bile salt transport defects PFIC 1–6 but decreased in BASD. This helps us to differentiate PFIC and BASD since GTP is low or normal in both these conditions.
    d. *Serum uric acid*: High levels of serum uric acid points toward Lesch Nyhan syndrome and low levels point toward xanthine/hypoxanthine disorders and molybdenum cofactor deficiency.
    e. *Serum ceruloplasmin (Cp)* is useful as a screening test for WD. The normal value is 20–40 mg/dL. A value < 10 mg/dL is more or less diagnostic of WD.
    f. *Serum iron/ferritin*: Levels are increased in hemochromatosis.
    g. *Lipid profile*: Abnormal lipid profile points toward GSDs, lipid storage disorders, Wolman disease, and Niemann-Pick disease.
    h. *Creatinine phosphokinase*: Levels are increased in GSDs III with muscle involvement and mitochondrial disorders.
    i. *Serum alphafetoprotein*: A high AFP in the absence of hepatic malignancy is a sensitive marker for tyrosinemia.
 2. *Urine*: Reducing substance for glucose may indicate diabetes but nonglucose-reducing substance is more important and is seen in galactosemia and fructosemia.
 3. *Imaging*:
    a. *X-ray*: Adrenal calcification is seen in Wolman disease **(Fig. 4)**; epiphyseal stippling is seen in Zellweger syndrome.

b. Ultrasonography (USG) of abdomen may show the changes seen in chronic liver disease such as coarse echotexture of liver, ascites, and dilated portal vein, or collaterals.
4. *Bone marrow examination*: Presence of large macrophages with crinkled paper cytoplasm is seen in Gaucher disease and foamy cells in Niemann-Pick disease.
5. *Liver biopsy*:
   a. *GSD I and III*: Swollen hepatocytes filled with glycogen, periodic acid–Schiff (PAS) positive and diastase sensitive.
   b. *Hereditary fructose intolerance*: Characteristic "fructose holes"
   c. *Wilson disease*: Nuclear vacuolation and steatosis with positivity for copper
   d. *PFIC I*: Bland cholestasis and Byler's bile on electron microscopy
   e. *Steatosis*: Cystic fibrosis, Fatty Acid Oxidation defect and citrin deficiency.
B. *Basic metabolic investigations*: (Mnemonic: GALAK)
   a. *Glucose*: Hypoglycemia [(blood glucose levels 1 < 40 mg/dL) (plasma glucose levels < 45 mg/dL)] is seen in GSDs, gluconeogenesis defects, galactosemia, FAO disorders, and congenital disorders of glycosylation.
   b. *Ammonia*: Ammonia estimation should be done from a free flowing blood sample obtained from either arterial or venous puncture and the normal values are <100 µmol/L (neonates), <80 µmol/L (infants), and <50 µmol/L (older children). Hyperammonemia is seen in urea cycle disorders, organic acidemias, and liver failure.
   c. *Lactate*: Lactate estimation should also be done from a free flowing blood sample and the normal values are 0.2–2.5 mmol/L. Increased lactate levels are seen in poor perfusion states, organic acidemias, FAO disorders, defects in pyruvate metabolism, and electron chain defects.
   d. *Acid–base status*: Acidosis is defined as pH < 7.3. Metabolic acidosis is seen in organic acidemias, defects in pyruvate metabolism, and mitochondrial disorders. Alkalosis is seen in urea cycle disorders.
   e. *Ketones*: Ketonuria, an increase in the urinary excretion of ketones, points to organic acidemia. Ketonuria in fed and fasting states can occur in ketone body handling disorders such as succinyl-CoA transferase (SCOT) deficiency or beta-ketothiolase (BKT) deficiency.
C. *Advanced investigations*: Advanced metabolic tests are tabulated in **Table 3**.

TABLE 3: Advanced metabolic tests for confirming diagnosis in MLD and treatment.

Probable MLD diagnosis	Common hepatic presentation	Confirmatory tests for diagnosis	Treatment
Galactosemia	NCS, ALF in neonate	• GAL-I-PUT galactose1phosphate uridyltransferase activity in RBC decreased • DNA mutation analysis	• Elimination of lactose from the diet. • Galactose free special formulas available
GSD	• Massive hepatomegaly GSDI • Hepatosplenomegaly GSD III	Mutation analysis or by enzyme analysis on a liver biopsy specimen	• Uncooked corn starch for children > 6 months of age • Avoid fructose, sucrose, lactose and sorbitol
HFI	Hepatomegaly cirrhosis	Mutation analysis	Elimination of fructose, sucrose and sorbitol from the diet
Tyrosinemia	NCS, ALF in NB CLD in older child	Urine succinyl acetone elevated	NTBC oral tablets Liver transplant
Niemann-Pick disease	Hepatosplenomegaly NCS: transient CLD/Cirrhosis	• Sphingomyelinase assay (leukocytes, lymphocytes, or skin fibroblasts) • Mutation analysis • Plasma chitotriosidase levels may be modestly elevated (20–30-fold), • Intracytoplasmic unesterified cholesterol in skin fibroblasts (by filipin staining)	Supportive therapy
Gaucher disease	Splenomgaly/Splenohepatomegaly	• Glucocerebrosidase assay (leukocytes or cultured fibroblasts). • Mutation analysis	• Enzyme replacement therapy[Imiglucerase] • Substrate reduction therapy with miglustat, eliglustat

Contd...

Contd...

Probable MLD diagnosis	Common hepatic presentation	Confirmatory tests for diagnosis	Treatment
FattyAcid Oxidation	Hepatomegaly	Plasma acyl carnitine assay	Avoiding fasting, Carnitine
Wolman disease	Hepatomegaly /ALF-Fatal	Acid lipase assay (leukocytes or cultured fibroblasts) and/or DNA sequencing	Enzyme replacement therapy [sebelipase alfa]
Mitochondrial disorders	Multisystem disease	• Mutation analysis for known mitochondrial and nuclear • DNA defects	Supportive therapy
Organic acidemia	Sick infant with hepatomegaly	• Urine organic acids. Plasma Acylcarnitine • Gene testing	Special formulas
Urea cycle disorders	Hepatomegaly with vomiting/hyperammonemia/encephalopathy	• Plasma amino acids assay • Urine orotic acid • Gene testing	Special formulas
Zelleweger	NCS	Mutational analysis	Supportive treatment
PFIC	NCS, Chronic cholestasis, progressive liver disease	Mutational analysis	Supportive therapy[choloretics, Vitamin supplements, antipruritic agents, Biliary diversion procedures, Liver transplant
BASD	Progressive cholestasis	Mutational analysis	Supportive therapy[choloretics, Vitamin supplements, antipruritic agents, Biliary diversion procedures, Liver transplant
Wilson disease	Asmptomatic to a range of symptomatic ALF to ESLD	Mutational Analysis	D-Penicillamine, Zinc, Liver transplant
Crigler Najjar	Hyperbilirubinemia	Mutational Analysis	Phenobarbitone, phototherapy, liver/hepatocyte transplant
Cystic fibrosis	NCS, Hepatomegaly, FTT	Mutational analysis	Supportive treatment

(ALF: acute liver failure; CLD: chronic liver disease; GSD: glycogen storage disorder; HFI: hereditary fructose intolerance; MLD: metabolic liver disease; NCS: neonatal cholestasis syndrome; RBC: red blood cell)

Molecular gene testing: Genetic testing by next generation sequencing in MLDs is important for accuracy of diagnosis to provide information on prognosis for cascade carrier testing and for prenatal or pretransplantation diagnosis. Both biochemical tests and NGS are complimentary to each other.

TREATMENT

The treatment of MLD ranges from modification of diet in certain conditions like galactosemia, hereditary fructose intolerance and GSDs, special formulas in aminoacidopathies, organic acidemia and urea cycle disorders, drugs in Crigler-Najjar syndrome type II, tyrosinemia and WD, enzyme replacement, and substrate reduction therapies in lysosomal storage disorders to liver transplant and gene therapy. The treatment also includes supportive therapy such as choloretics in cholestatic disorders, Vitamin supplementation, apt management of hepatic encephalopathy, blood products, and vitamin K in coagulopathies and appropriate recognition and treatment of complications.

PREVENTION

Prevention is better than cure goes the saying. Though definitive treatment is available for select MLDs, for many only symptomatic/supportive treatment. The preventive components in MLDs include genetic counseling, sibling screening, and antenatal diagnosis. Immunization with hepatitis B and A vaccines is essential to prevent worsening of underlying disease.

KEY MESSAGES

- Metabolic liver diseases are an important cause of acute and chronic liver disease in children of all age groups.
- However, presentation is varied there are some clues which point to the etiology.
- Complete clinical and biochemical evaluation baseline and metabolic investigations are essential.
- Molecular gene testing is nowadays a big boon to the diagnosis of MLDs.
- Therapy is now available either as special diet, medication, enzyme replacement, or liver transplant.

SUGGESTED READING

1. Alam S, Sood V. Metabolic liver disease: when to suspect and how to diagnose? Indian J Pediatr. 2016;83(11):1321-33.
2. Demirbas D, Brucker WJ, Berry GT. Inborn errors of metabolism with hepatopathy: metabolism defects of galactose, fructose, and tyrosine. Pediatr Clin North Am. 2018;65(2):337-52.

CHAPTER 70: Liver Mass on Imaging in Children

Bhaswati C Acharyya

INTRODUCTION

Liver tumors in children are rare. It accounts for 0.5–2% of all neoplasms in the pediatric age group. Common tumors occurring in different age group are given in **Table 1**. When a mass or tumor is suspected in imaging then the history, examination, and investigations should be according to the age and primary suspicion.

INFANTILE HEMANGIOMATA

- Benign vascular tumor
- Occurs almost exclusively in the first year of life
- Relatively common in the skin and mucous membranes but can affect any organ system
- In the liver, two histological types of lesions have been described:
  - Capillary hemangioendothelioma
  - Cavernous hemangioma
- Presenting features are hepatomegaly and abdominal distension
- Involvement can be as a single tumor or multifocal
- Complications include high-output cardiac failure, often life-threatening due to the presence of significant shunting Kasabach–Merritt syndrome (anemia, consumptive coagulopathy, cholestasis); vascular malformation involving other organs, and rarely intraperitoneal hemorrhage secondary to rupture. Hypothyroidism can occur associated with increased activity of type 3 iodothyronine within the tumor
- Diagnosis is made on imaging including ultrasound scan (USS) with Doppler, computed tomography (CT), and magnetic resonance imaging (MRI).

Needle liver biopsy is contraindicated because of the high-risk bleeding. Liver tissue can be obtained at laparotomy in selected cases, when malignancy cannot be excluded on imaging.

Management

- Asymptomatic—does not warrant treatment because of the spontaneous resolution of the lesion over time
- Symptomatic—depends on its severity
- Medical treatment consists of symptomatic treatment of high-output cardiac failure with digoxin, diuretics, and angiotensin-converting enzyme (ACE) inhibitors. Propranolol is the treatment of choice for all uncomplicated

TABLE 1: Common tumor occurring in different age group.

Age	Benign	Malignant primary	Metastatic
Infancy (0–1 year)	• Hemangioendothelioma • Mesenchymal hamartoma • Teratoma	• Hepatoblastoma (HB) • Rhabdoid tumor • Yolk sac tumor	• Langerhans cell • Histiocytosis • Leukemia • Neuroblastoma
Early childhood 1–3 years	• Hemangioendothelioma • Mesenchymal hamartoma • Inflammatory myofibroblastic tumor	• HB • Rhabdomyosarcoma	• Leukemia • Neuroblastoma
Later childhood (3–10 years)	Angiomyolipoma	• HCC, embryonal sarcoma • Angiosarcoma	–
Adolescent (10–16 years)	Adenoma, focal nodular hyperplasia, biliary cyst adenoma	• HCC, fibrolamellar carcinoma • Nested stromal-epithelial tumor, leiomyosarcoma	Hodgkin's and non-Hodgkin's lymphoma

(HCC: hepatocellular carcinoma)

large hemangiomas or hemangioendotheliomas. Surgical management includes resection of the lesion by hepatic lobectomy or hepatic artery ligation, depending on the size and localization of the lesion.
- Liver transplantation should be reserved for cases that do not respond to any of the above treatment options.

Mesenchymal Hamartoma
- Rare benign tumor
- *Multicystic appearance*: Typically affects children during the first 2 years of life
- Presentation can be with symptoms of abdominal distension but is often an incidental finding on clinical examination or imaging and is rarely symptomatic
- Biochemically, alpha fetoprotein (AFP) can be mildly raised, liver function tests are usually normal
- Imaging with USS, CT, and MRI
- Final diagnosis is made on the basis of histology usually obtained at the time of resection. Spontaneous regression has been described.

Focal Nodular Hyperplasia (FNH)

Benign Epithelial Tumors
- The lesion, typically well circumscribed and lobulated, can vary in size and be single or multiple.
- Seen in all age groups, more common in females, has been reported in older patients with glycogen storage disorder (GSD) type 1.
- Presentation with abdominal pain is common.
- Imaging with USS, CT, and are usually diagnostic.
- Three treatment strategies are employed:
  1. Conservative management with regular clinical and radiological follow up.
  2. Surgical incision of the mass
  3. Interventional treatment with embolization or ligation of the hepatic artery
- No reports of malignant transformation.

Nodular Regenerative Hyperplasia (NRH)
- Rare in pediatric population
- Usually asymptomatic; hepatosplenomegaly is detected fortuitously
- CT and MRI usually went the diagnosis
- Can involve the whole liver and lead to portal hypertension and its complications
- Treatment is management of the complications.

Hepatoblastoma
- Embryonal tumors derived from the epithelial cells of the fetal liver and characterized by a rapid growth.
- Most frequent malignant liver tumor in children, most common diagnosed in the first 3 years of life.
- Male preponderance.
- Spreads by vascular invasion, typically in the lungs.
- Presentation usually with abdominal distension, abdominal pain, and failure to thrive.
- Anemia and thrombocytosis are common, very high AFP levels are characteristic and are a marker of response to therapy.
- CT or MRI is necessary for an accurate differentiation between tumor and normal liver tissue.
- Diagnosis is by liver biopsy.
- Treatment consists of chemotherapy and complete tumor resection by partial hepatectomy or, if the tumor is unresectable, by liver transplantation.
- Adverse prognostic factors are low serum AFP (<100 ng/mL), lack of response to chemotherapy and presence of metastases at diagnosis.

Hepatocellular Carcinoma (HCC)
- Rare in pediatric age group, but when present, is typically seen in older children/teenagers.
- Most commonly, HCC develops in the presence of an underlying liver disease such as chronic viral hepatitis (e.g., hepatitis B) or a metabolic disorder (e.g., tyrosinemia or progressive familial intrahepatic cholestasis syndromes).
- Typical presentation is with abdominal pain and an abdominal mass.
- AFP is often elevated, though not as much as in hepatoblastoma.
- CT and MRI can help to determine whether tumor resection is an option.
- Liver biopsy under USS guidance is indicated if no underlying liver pathology is present.
- Treatment consists of resection, chemotherapy or combined chemotherapy and resection, but the prognosis is very poor, with a reported 10–20% long-term survival.

Inflammatory Pseudotumor
- Rare benign lesion that can arise in different organs and tissues with the liver being a relatively common site of origin.
- Histology consists of proliferation of spindle-shaped cells, myofibroblasts, mixed with inflammatory cells consisting of plasma cells, lymphocytes, and occasional histiocytes.
- Since 1971, 15 pediatric cases have been reported in the literature ranging in age from 10 months to 15 years.
- The lesion can be solitary or multiple.
- Presentation is commonly with nonspecific symptoms such as fever, jaundice, and paired growth with raised inflammatory markers on biochemistry.

- There are no specific laboratory or radiological findings and differential diagnosis with FNH can be difficult on imaging.
- A final diagnosis is made at the time of surgical resection, which is the most common form of treatment; prognosis in generally good.

Fibropolycystic Liver Disease

- Heterogeneous group of disorders
- Often associated with fibrocystic anomalies in the kidneys and share the same genetic defect
- Gene was localized to chromosome region 6p21 in 1994 and described as PKHD1 in 2002: 119 different mutations have been reported so far. Four types have been described:
  1. *Congenital hepatic fibrosis*:
     - It is associated with autosomal recessive polycystic kidney disease
     - Presentation during childhood or adolescence with isolated hepatomegaly or variceal bleeding secondary to portal hypertension.
     - It can be associated with carbohydrate-deficient glycoprotein syndrome type Ib (CDGS Ib), characterized by congenital hepatic fibrosis associated with cyclical vomiting, protein-losing enteropathy and prothrombotic tendency, as well as neurological impairment screening with transferrin isoelectrofocusing for a glycosylation defect.
     - Management is symptomatic treatment of portal hypertension.
  2. *Caroli disease*:
     - It is caused by malformation of the larger bile ducts: hepatic fibrosis is absent.
     - Clinical presentation is often with recurrent episodes of cholangitis.
     - Management involves aggressive antibiotic therapy.
  3. *Caroli syndrome*:
     - Ductal plate malformation of larger bile ducts associated with hepatic fibrosis
     - Complications of portal hypertension and recurrent cholangitis are common
  4. *Von Meyenburg complexes*: It is known as biliary hamartomas, discrete foci of ductal plate malformation affecting the smallest bile ducts, commonly present as an incidental finding on liver histology.

Management

With this basic knowledge in mind a good history and physical examination should be undertaken. Age and physical findings should decide further blood tests. Liver function, prothrombin time, complete blood count, and an AFP should be the initial investigation. CT and MRI followed by image-guided biopsy (except in hemangiomas) will decide character and stage of the lesion. Further treatment will be decided according to the nature of the lesion.

SUGGESTED READING

1. Di Bisceglie AM, Befeler AS. in Feldman M, Friedman LS, Brandt LJ (eds). Sleisenger and Fordtran's Gastrointestinal and Liver Disease, 11th edition. Elsevier, Philadelphia. 2021:1509-32.
2. López-Terrada D, Finegold MJ. In Kleinman RE, Goulet OJ, Vergani G (eds). Walker's Pediatric Gastrointestinal Disease; Pathophysiology, Diagnosis, Management. 6th edition. People's Medical Publishing House—USA; 2018:3576-649.

Liver Transplantation

Prasanth KS

INTRODUCTION

Liver transplantation (LT) is a state-of-the-art treatment for children with acute liver failure (ALF), end-stage liver disease (ESLD), hepatic tumors, and some genetic/metabolic diseases. Improvement in pretransplant management, patient selection, surgical techniques using split liver grafts and living donors, organ preservation, immunosuppression and post-transplant follow-up has led to outstanding results in patient and graft survival and quality-of-life (QOL). LT has been well established in India for more than two decades now.

Common indications for pediatric LT are listed in **Box 1**.

BOX 1: Indications for pediatric liver transplantation.

- Cholestatic conditions
- Biliary atresia
- Primary sclerosing cholangitis (PSC)
- Parenteral nutrition-associated cholestasis
- Alagille syndrome
- Progressive familial intrahepatic cholestasis (PFIC)
- Metabolic disease
- Alpha 1 antitrypsin deficiency
- Cystic fibrosis
- Crigler–Najjar type 1
- Urea cycle defects
- Tyrosinemia
- Wilson disease
- Organic acidemia
- Primary hyperoxaluria
- Glycogen storages disorders
- Immune mediated
- Autoimmune hepatitis
- Tumors
- Hepatoblastoma
- Hemangioendothelioma
- Hepatocellular carcinoma (HCC)
- Miscellaneous
- Acute liver failure
- Gestational alloimmune liver disease
- Caroli disease
- Cryptogenic cirrhosis
- Budd–Chiari syndrome

Contraindications to LT in children are the following: nonresectable extrahepatic malignant tumor; multisystem organ failure with concomitant end-stage organ failure that cannot be corrected by a combined transplant; uncontrolled sepsis; irreversible serious neurologic damage and uncorrectable life-limiting defects in critical organs such as heart, lungs, and kidneys.

When to refer for transplant?

Referral to LT depends on the child's clinical circumstances: Emergent in ALF or acute on chronic liver failure (ACLF). Those patients with chronic liver disease (CLD) who start demonstrating deteriorating liver function should also be referred in anticipation for enhanced medical support and listing for transplantation. In some metabolic diseases, early referral may offer the benefit of avoiding multisystem complications and irreversible organ damage.

The criteria for listing for LT in children with CLD are pediatric end-stage liver disease (PELD) score >10 for age <12 years and model for end-stage liver disease (MELD) score >15 in children >12 years. PELD takes into account the total serum bilirubin, international normalized ratio (INR), albumin, and growth failure and MELD is calculated using the total serum bilirubin, INR, and serum creatinine.

Complications of liver disease that suggest consideration for LT are given in **Box 2**.

BOX 2: Complications of liver disease.

- Failed portoenterostomy for extrahepatic biliary atresia
- Refractory ascites
- Spontaneous bacterial peritonitis
- Persistent hyponatremia
- *Portal hypertensive complications*:
  - Severe hypersplenism
  - Variceal bleeding
- Hepatorenal syndrome
- Hepatopulmonary syndrome
- *Hepatic osteodystrophy*:
  - Recurrent fractures
- Growth failure
- *Poor quality of life*:
  - Severe debilitating pruritus
  - Fatigue

ROLE OF PEDIATRICIAN IN PRETRANSPLANT CARE

Optimization of a patient's health prior to transplantation is essential to improve transplant outcomes. Special attention should be paid to immunization status, nutritional support, and neurodevelopment.

Immunization

Children with CLD cannot be transplanted for 3–4 weeks after a live vaccine is administered, it is important that early vaccination against varicella, measles, mumps and rubella, is ensured for all children who are listed for LT. Vaccination against pneumococcal disease, influenza, typhoid, and hepatitis A and B should similarly be advanced to complete the vaccination schedule. While every effort should be made to vaccinate prior to transplantation, inactivated vaccines are safe after transplantation. Live attenuated vaccines are generally contraindicated after transplantation. It is preferred that close contacts be vaccinated against measles, mumps, rubella, and varicella, weeks before the transplant so as to prevent the transplanted patient from having contact with wild type viruses.

Nutrition

Growth failure is common in children with CLD as they require 20–80% more calories to achieve adequate growth. Increased nutritional support pre-transplant is associated with improved patient and graft survival as well as neurodevelopment outcomes post-transplant. Special attention should be paid to fat soluble vitamin deficiencies (A, D, E, K) and should be supplemented accordingly.

Neurodevelopment

Reduced global cognitive functioning with specific weakness in gross motor and receptive language skills is seen in children post-LT. Children with CLD should undergo neurocognitive and developmental assessment early on with referral to appropriate early intervention therapy when indicated pretransplant to minimize long-term cognitive delays.

SURVIVAL OUTCOME IN PEDIATRIC LIVER TRANSPLANT RECIPIENTS

According to recent US Organ Procurement and Transplantation Network and Studies in Pediatric Liver Transplantation (SPLIT), patient survival rates at 1 and 5 years after a pediatric LT are now 91–91.4% and 84–86.5%. Based on the experience of 200 pediatric living donor liver transplantation (LDLT) from India over a period of 12 years the overall 1 year survival rate stood at 94% and 5 years actuarial survival was 87% with no statistically significant difference between children weight <10 kg vs. >10 kg. Outcome in acute liver failure did not differ significantly between those with acute on chronic liver failure vs. those with chronic liver disease.

ROLE OF PEDIATRICIAN IN POST-TRANSPLANT CARE

- *Ensure optimum adherence to immune suppression*: Most immunosuppression protocols from pediatric LT programs include calcineurin inhibitors (CNIs) (tacrolimus or cyclosporine), corticosteroids, and mycophenolate mofetil (MMF). Typically, patients are placed on 2 or more immunosuppressants postoperatively as induction. Most of these children then continue on tacrolimus monotherapy lifelong. Tacrolimus has become the preferred CNI due to reduction in steroid-resistant acute rejection, improved graft survival, and reduced rates of nephrotoxicity compared with cyclosporine.

  In order to ensure their immunomodulating effect while minimizing toxicity, drug levels and dosing have to be monitored closely. Dosages and target therapeutic drug levels vary depending on the time since transplantation and should be personalized to the individual patient. Care must be taken in balancing risk of overimmunosuppression [side effects, infection, post-transplant lymphoproliferative disease (PTLD), etc.] and under immunosuppression (rejection).

- *Infections*: Infectious issues that one should be aware of include the avoidance of live virus vaccinations post-transplant, and an escalated response to exposures such as varicella, cytomegalovirus (CMV), and Epstein-Barr virus (EBV). Varicella and CMV infections can cause debilitating consequences for LT recipients and should be treated aggressively.

  Epstein-Barr virus disease can present insidiously with fever, lymphadenopathy, and tonsillitis, but if ignored consequences can be serious, including PTLD, which in its extreme form manifests as lymphoma and needs to be treated as such with the help of an oncologist.

- *Growth*: Patients often fully recover and gain weight after successful LT; however, linear growth may lag behind by 2 years. Obesity post-transplant is also a growing issue among pediatric LT recipients. Height, weight, and BMI should be monitored at each office visit to screen for both growth failure and obesity.

- *Psychosocial development and neurocognitive function*: Studies suggest that pediatric LT patients have lower physical and psychosocial function.

  The follow-up of school-aged LT recipients should include an assessment of school functioning and school absence. Be aware of post-traumatic stress disorder or other mental health issues and refer a patient for a formal psychiatric evaluation if significant symptoms are present. The onset of liver disease in infancy impairs neurodevelopment. Provide rehabilitation immediately after transplantation: physical therapy for infants with delayed motor development and speech and occupational therapy for older children with deficits.

Screen neurocognitive function before transplantation for LT candidates older than 5 years and at key junctures afterward to determine special education needs. Assess recipients for hearing loss in the first postoperative year and periodically thereafter as indicated.

- *Endocrine issues*: Due to their ESLD and subsequent corticosteroid use post-transplant, children undergoing LT are at risk for several endocrine problems including hepatic osteodystrophy, growth failure, and pubertal delay.

  Hepatic osteodystrophy includes all of the metabolic bone disease associated with ESLD such as low bone mass, growth delay, fractures, spinal problems, and vitamin D deficient rickets. Many of these issues resolve post-transplant; however, osteopenia may persist for up to 1 year.

  Patients, especially those with cholestatic liver disease, often have low vitamin D levels that should be monitored at least biannually and supplemented until levels normalize. Tacrolimus can cause renal phosphate and calcium loss, so it is important that patients have adequate intake of these minerals. Children who have osteopenia prior to LT should be monitored for scoliosis, and those children age ≥5 years should be monitored for fractures with a dual-energy X-ray absorptiometry (DEXA) scan and lateral thoracic spine X-ray.

- *Dermatologic care*: Patients who have had a LT are at increased risk of skin cancer due to decreased tumor immunosurveillance on immunosuppression, DNA damage from antimetabolite medications and chronic inflammation. Use of protective clothing, sunscreen, and regular screening for skin lesions is recommended. A yearly screen by a dermatologist is encouraged.

- *Chronic rejection*: Chronic rejection occurs in 5–10% of transplanted patients and leads to long-term graft dysfunction and fibrosis. Patients may present with jaundice, pruritus, elevated bilirubin and GGT, or elevated transaminases. Diagnosis is confirmed by liver biopsy. Patients with a history of steroid-resistant acute rejection or more than one episode of acute rejection are at increased risk of late graft loss.

- *Monitor adverse effects of immunosuppression*: Long-term use of CNIs is associated with an increased risk of hypertension, hyperlipidemia, diabetes mellitus, renal insufficiency, obesity, and metabolic syndrome. Corticosteroids are used for the first 3–6 months post-transplant and they carry an added known side-effect profile.

  Renal insufficiency is a common long-term complication post-transplant. Therefore, serum creatinine should be monitored regularly as an estimate of glomerular filtration rate (GFR).

  Hypertension that arises either as an adverse effect of the immunosuppressant therapy or due to renal insufficiency should be managed with angiotensin-converting enzyme inhibitors or angiotensin receptor blockers for renal protection.

  Post-transplant patients are at increased risk for the development of premature cardiovascular disease given their increased risk of diabetes mellitus, obesity, hyperlipidemia, hypertension, and metabolic syndrome; therefore, all patients should be monitored for body mass index (BMI), blood pressure, and fasting lipids, and any abnormalities found on this screening should be treated with age-appropriate recommendations.

- *Dealing with the adolescent patient*: Adolescent patients present a distinct population with unique issues.

  Medication nonadherence (NA) and inadequate follow-up checks pose serious problems and are associated with increased rates of rejection and poor outcomes.

  Adolescents should be discouraged from using drugs or alcohol due to the toxic effects on the liver as well as potential medication interactions.

  Adolescents should also be counseled on safe sexual practices as they are at increased risk of sexually transmitted diseases. Although healthy pregnancies are possible post-transplant, contraception is recommended in the adolescent girl as pregnancies should be avoided for at least 12-months post-transplant and are associated with increased risk of pregnancy-induced hypertension and preeclampsia.

- *Facilitate transition to adult care*: As patients mature into young adulthood, a process of transition has to take place to allow safe and effective transfer of care from a pediatric facility to the care of adult providers. In the absence of a transfer process, patients may experience anxiety, confusion, distress, inability to manage the requirements of the new setting, increased risk of NA, rejection, and even mortality.

KEY MESSAGES

- Liver transplantation has come of age in India as a life-saving intervention for children with ESLD.
- These patients need extra attention pre- and post-transplant.
- Special attention should be given to vaccination and growth of the children.

PRESCRIPTION ASSISTANCE

Pharmacologic salt	Market preparation	Availability	Dosages
Corticosteroids Methyl prednisolone	Solu-medrol	*Injection*: 125 mg/250 mg/500 mg/1 g/4 g	Induction with high-dose methylprednisolone IV
Prednisolone	Omnacortil	• *Tablet*: 2.5 mg/5 mg/10 mg/20 mg/30 mg/40 mg • *Syrup*: (5 and 15 mg/5 mL)	• 20 mg/kg/dose (maximum 1 g) • Taper over 5 days to maintenance • Prednisolone (approximately 0.2–0.3 mg/kg/dose po daily)
Tacrolimus	• Tacrocord • Tacsant	• *Tablet*: 0.25 mg/0.5 mg/1 mg/2 mg • *Tablet*: 0.5 mg/1 mg/2 mg	0.15–0.2 mg/kg/day po divided q12 h
Cyclosporine	• Panimun • Bioral • Conimune ME • Neoral	• *Tablet*: 25 mg/50 mg/100 mg • *Tablet*: 25 mg/50 mg • *Suspension*: 100 mg/mL)	15 mg/kg/day po divided q12 h for 2 weeks post-transplant, then 4–12 mg/kg/d po divided BID
Mycophenolate mofetil	• Cellcept • Tacsant	*Tablet*: 250 mg/500 mg 1 mg/2 mg *Tablet*: 0.5 mg/1 mg/2 mg	10–15 mg/kg/dose po BID divided q12 h

SUGGESTED READING

1. Cuenca AG, Kim HB, Vakili K. Pediatric liver transplantation. Semin Pediatr Surg. 2017;26(4):217-23.
2. European Association for the Study of the Liver. EASL Clinical Practice Guidelines: Liver transplantation. J Hepatol. 2016; 64(2):433-85.
3. Spada M, Riva S, Maggiore G, Cintorino D, Gridelli B. Pediatric liver transplantation. World J Gastroenterol. 2009;15(6): 648-74.
4. Yazigi NA. Long term outcomes after pediatric liver transplantation. Pediatr Gastroenterol Hepatol Nutr. 2013;16(4): 207-18.

72. Foreign Body Ingestion in Children

Vishnu Biradar

INTRODUCTION

Foreign body (FB) ingestion in children usually occurs inadvertently. In some children with behavioural disorders, ingestion of inedible material could be a part of their illness. Presentation is obvious if seen by parents or caretakers, but majority of times the ingestion may not have been witnessed. Hence, many a times the child himself or a friend will report about the ingestion. In case of suspected ingestion first question to them is to verify and search if anything is missing from the area where the child was playing. Unfortunately, in majority, symptoms do not occur immediately and complications can set in.

CLINICAL FEATURES

Child may have pain while swallowing, drooling of saliva, bleeding, coughing, persistent vomiting, abdominal distension, abdominal pain, fever or even in shock from either intestinal perforation or toxin ingestion.

Common sites of impaction of FBs in gastrointestinal tract (GIT):

- Narrowest part of GIT is upper esophageal stricture (UES). FB can get impacted at cricopharynx above UES, at level of aortic arch, gastroesophageal GE junction, pylorus, duodenal cap, ileocaecal (IC) junction or rectoanal area.
- On occasion, children with eosinophilic esophagitis (EoE) present with food bolus impaction. In fact, this is a known presentation of EoE in children.

CHARACTERISTICS OF SOME FOREIGN BODIES

- *Button battery*:
  - Button batteries impacted in lumen can have electrical discharge because of leakage and pressure necrosis. Leaked sodium hydroxide accumulates and allows continued injury in spite of removal.
  - Mucosal damage can start within 2 hours of ingestion of button battery and unfortunately does not depend upon whether it is old and used or non-used button battery.
  - So careful observation is needed for 24 hours after removal of the button battery.
  - Button battery ingestions can lead to perforation, fistula formation, mediastinitis or peritonitis, massive bleeding from esophageal-aortic fistula, empyema, abscesses, spondylodiscitis or late sequaele such as dysphagia or stricture formation.
- *Magnet*: In case of more than one magnet being ingested, the magnets get attracted to each other and leads to pressure necrosis of intestine and perforation or bleeding.
- *Glass*:
  - Careful evaluation by endoscopy is needed and if glass particles are seen, they need to be removed.
  - While introducing endoscope, please use basket or cap at insertion end so as to avoid mucosal injury while taking out sharp objects.

MANAGMENT INVESTIGATIONS

- *X-ray*:
  - Always ask for X-ray chest and abdomen including neck immediately after knowing child has ingested FB.
  - Sometimes, to differentiate coin from button battery, lateral X-ray of neck is required to see difference in thickness of FB if parents were not sure of what type of ingestion.
  - A battery may show a double rim. Occasionally two coins stuck together can give a similar impression.
  - Nonmetallic FBs are difficult to assess on the X-ray, but it is still worthwhile doing one film. In case of nonopaque FB, contrast study may be helpful such as Barium swallow
- Ultrasonography (USG) has very limited ability to localize the foreign body.
- *Magnetic resonance imaging (MRI) or computed tomography (CT) scan*: In case of a sharp FB that seems to have perforated a viscus or presence of significant bleeding, or there is a history of ingestion of a button battery more than 24–48 hours earlier that is lodged in the esophagus then child should undergo CT scan/MRI to see extent of involvement.

Referral to Pediatric Gastroenterologist

- Inform and discuss with pediatric gastroenterologist before sending the child home.
- If not available then discuss with adult gastroenterologist or pediatric surgeon.
- ENT surgeon's role will be if FB is in nose, ear and above or in cricopharynx.
- A simple way to determine this would be if the FB is above the clavicles or below (**Fig. 1A**). The ENT surgeons often tackle the former FB.

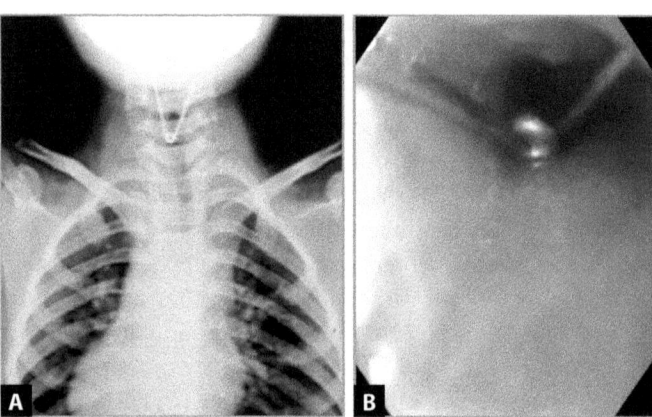

Figs. 1A and B: Impacted safety pin in esophagus: (A) X-ray; (B) Endoscopy.

- Parents often are advised to give bananas or something to eat, as perception is that it will facilitate movement of the FB.
- Practically, we should ask to keep the child empty stomach till we decide next plan of action for two reasons:
  1. If anesthesia is needed the child should be fasting to avoid risk of aspiration.
  2. It becomes difficult to locate the FB within the food material.

Endoscopic Removal

It is important to ask about the type of FB, number ingested, time since it was swallowed, what has child eaten before or after the FB ingestion and history of any surgery performed on the GIT or comorbidities (**Table 1**).

- *Indication for removal*: Button batteries, more than one magnet ingestion, sharp objects, any large diameter FB >2.5 cm or long FB >6 cm length, toxic FB (lead balls, mercury containing FB, etc.) as they can lead to perforation, obstruction, or poisoning.
- *Time of removal*: It is recommended to remove blunt foreign bodies and coins or impacted food from the esophagus urgently (<24 hours), even in asymptomatic children.

If the child is symptomatic, an emergent (<2 hours) removal is indicated.

TABLE 1: Guidelines to manage FB ingestions.

Sr. No.	Type of FB	Site	Symptomatic	Action endoscopy/surgery/wait and watch	Time period	Endoscopy accessory needed
1.	Coin or blunt object	Esophagus	NA	Removal	<24 hours	Rat tooth forceps
		Stomach/duodenum	Yes	Remove		
			No	Wait and watch	Up to 4 weeks*	
		Intestine	Yes	Surgery		
			No	Wait and watch	Up to 4 weeks*	
2.	Sharp objects	Esophagus	NA	Emergent removal	<2 hours	Rat tooth forceps
		Stomach/duodenum		Emergent removal	<2 hours	
		Intestine		Wait and watch with serial X-ray 12 hours apart*		
3.	Button/disk batteries	Esophagus	NA	Emergent removal	<2 hours	Roth net
		Stomach/duodenum		Emergent removal	<2 hours if disk battery or within 48 hours if button battery	
		Intestine	Yes	Surgery		
			No	Wait and watch*		
4.	Magnets single	Any site	Yes	Removal	24 hours	Roth net/magnet forceps
			No	Wait and watch*		

*Surgery is indicated in case of symptomatic or signs of obstruction present. But we can wait and watch up to 4 weeks.

- If blunt FB is in stomach or duodenum then removal of objects more than 2.5 cm wide in diameter or >6 cm in length.
- Otherwise, blunt FB in stomach can be followed and retrieved if symptomatic or does not pass spontaneously after 4 weeks.
- Sharp pointed object or if more than one magnet is ingested, it should be removed emergently in less than 2 hours regardless of where it is lodged **(Fig. 1B)**.
- Any button batteries if in esophagus should be removed immediately. But if in in stomach or duodenum can be observed and removed if symptomatic or stays in stomach for more than 48 hours.

CONCLUSION

- Foreign body ingestion in children is common.
- What we should know is type of FB, number ingested, time since ingestion, food taken by child before and after the FB ingestion.
- We should ask for appropriate X-ray of the chest and abdomen which should include the neck and pelvis.
- Button battery, magnet (more than one) or sharp objects needs to be removed emergently even though child is asymptomatic because of high rates of complication that may prove to be fatal.

SUGGESTED READING

1. He S, Zuo Z-L. Different anatomical sites of the foreign body injury with 2999 children during 2012-2916. Chinese J Traumatol. 2018;21(6):333-7.
2. Krom H, Visser M, Hulst JM, Wolters VM, Vanden Neucker AM, de Meij T, et al. Serious complications after button battery ingestion in children. Eur J Pediatr. 2018;177(7):1063-70.
3. Lin A, Chan LCN, Hon KLE, Tsui SYB, Pang K, Cheung HM. Magnetic foreign body ingestion in children: the attractive hazards. Case Reports in Pediatrics. Case Rep Pediatr. 2019; 2019:3549242.
4. Tringali A, Thomson M, Dumonceau J-M, Tavares M, Tabbers MM, Furlano R, et al. Pediatric gastrointestinal endoscopy: European Society of Gastrointestinal Endoscopy (ESGE) and European Society for paediatric Gastroenterology Hepatology and Nutrition (ESPGHAN) guideline executive summary. Endoscopy. 2017;49:83-91.

SECTION 7: Hematology–Oncology

73. ABC of CBC
74. Approach to Normocytic Anemia
75. Iron Deficiency Anemia
76. Megaloblastic Anemia
77. Sickle Cell Disorders
78. Thalassemia
79. Aplastic Anemia in Children
80. Leukemias in Children
81. Lymphoma in Children
82. Immune Thrombocytopenia in Children
83. Hemophilia
84. Hematopoietic Stem Cell Transplantation
85. Blood Component Therapy

CHAPTER 73: ABC of CBC

Prachi Chaudhary

INTRODUCTION

- Complete blood count (CBC) is the first-line investigation in any sort of illness but it is of utmost value for diagnosis of blood and immune system disorders. There is a lot that can be inferred from this basic and simple investigation. Some additional parameters such as retic count, cell morphology have to be analyzed manually.
- A CBC is performed by running a blood sample on an automated analyzer. The automated CBC analyzer calculates few basic parameters namely, hemoglobin, hematocrit, red blood cell (RBC) count, white blood cell (WBC) count with differential, and platelet count. The analyzer counts red and white blood cells and platelets by flow cytometry, isolating single cells and measuring characteristics such as light scattering and electrical impedance to distinguish between different types of cells and collect information about their size and structure.
- Hemoglobin is measured by spectrophotometry. Others are derived parameters, namely mean corpuscular volume (MCV), mean corpuscular hemoglobin (MCH), mean corpuscular hemoglobin concentration (MCHC), red cell distribution width (RDW), men platelet volume (MPV), platelet distribution width (PDW), histograms, and scattergrams.
- Manual techniques are used to confirm the results of automated testing. Approximately 10–25% of CBC samples are flagged for manual blood smear review, which requires the blood to be stained and viewed under a microscope by a medical laboratory technologist to verify that the analyzer results are correct and look for abnormal changes in the appearance of blood cells.
- Causes of faulty results are hemolyzed specimens, lipemic specimens, clotted specimens, diluted specimens, presence of cold agglutinins, platelet clumps, or platelet satellitosis.
- CBC broadly analyzes RBC, WBC and platelets. For the health of RBCs, RBC count, hemoglobin, hematocrit, MCV, MCH, MCHC, RDW, and reticulocyte count are assessed. For WBC, total count, neutrophils, lymphocytes, monocytes, basophils and eosinophils are assessed; and for platelets, platelet count and MPV are assessed on CBC.

RED BLOOD CELLS

The normal values of RBC count and conditions causing their number to increase or decrease are described in **Table 1**.

Hemoglobin

Hemoglobin lower than normal is anemia while higher than normal is polycythemia. Age wise normal hemoglobin level is given in **Table 2**. Clues to the cause of anemia come from MCV, RBC count, reticulocyte count, MCH, and other findings on the smear. History and other relevant investigations also play a major part but here discussion will be limited to CBC parameters.

Hematocrit (Table 3)

It measures the portion of your blood made up of RBCs. Hematocrit = MCV (fL) × RBC count (millions/microliters)/1,000.

TABLE 1: Red blood cells (RBC).		
Normal values	**Conditions with increased RBC count**	**Conditions with decreased RBC count**
• Newborn: 4.1–6.1 million/mm³ • Children: 3.6–5.5 million/mm³ • Adult male: 4.6–6 million/mm³ • Adult female: 4.2–5.0 million/mm³	• Polycythemia vera • High altitude • Pulmonary hypertension • Congestive cardiac failure • Sleep apnea • Poor blood flow to kidneys	• Blood loss • Decreased production due to marrow dysfunction • Increased destruction

TABLE 2: Age-wise normal hemoglobin values.

Age	Hemoglobin values (g/dL)
Newborn	15.5–24.5
0.5–1.9 years	11–12.5
2–4 years	11–12.5
5–7 years	11.5–13
8–11 years	12–13.5
12–14 years	• 12–13 (females) • 12.5–14 (male)
15–17 years	• 12–14 (females) • 13–15 (male)
Adult: • Male • Female	 • 13.5–16.5 • 12–15.5

TABLE 3: Hematocrit (Hct).

Normal values	Conditions with increase Hct	Conditions with decreased Hct
• Newborn: 14–68 • Up to 1 year: 29–41 • Adult male: 39–47 • Adult female: 36–44	• Dengue shock syndrome • Polycythemia vera • COPD • Erythropoietin use • Dehydration • Capillary leak syndrome • Anabolic steroid use	• Anemia • Blood loss • Hemolysis • Bone marrow aplasia • Malnutrition

(COPD: chronic obstructive pulmonary disease)

TABLE 4: Normal mean corpuscular volume (MCV) values.

Age	Range (fL)
Neonate	88–123
1–3 months	91–112
3–6 months	74–108
6 months to 1 year	70–85
Child/adult	80–95

TABLE 5: Causes of anemia based on MCV.

Causes of low MCV	Causes of anemia with normal MCV	Causes of high MCV
• Iron deficiency anemia • Thalassemia • Chronic disease/infiltration • Lead poisoning • Sideroblastic anemia • Copper deficiency anemia • Iron refractory iron deficiency anemia	• RBC aplasia • Anemia of chronic disease • Endocrinopathies • Acute bleeding • Hypersplenism • Dyserythropoietic anemia II • Renal failure • Malignancy • Hypersplenism • Antibody-mediated hemolysis • Microangiopathies • Membranopathies • Enzymopathies • Hemoglobinopathies	• Folate deficiency • Vitamin B_{12} deficiency • Acquired aplastic anemia • Congenital aplastic anemia • Drug induced • Trisomy 21 • Hypothyroidism • Orotic aciduria • Dyserythropoietic anemia I and III

(MCV: mean corpuscular volume; RBC: red blood cell)

TABLE 6: Causes of anemia based on RDW.

Causes of low RDW	Causes of anemia with normal RDW	Causes of high RDW
Thalassemia minor	• Thalassemia minor • Anemia of chronic disease • Hereditary spherocytosis • Aplastic anemia • Myelodysplastic anemia	• Iron deficiency anemia • Sickle cell anemia • Vitamin B_{12} and folate deficiency

(RDW: red cell distribution width)

Mean Corpuscular Volume

It measures the size of the RBCs. MCV = Hematocrit/RBC count × 100 fL; this is a very important clue for etiology of anemia. Values change during childhood. The normal values are given in **Table 4**. The causes of anemia based on MCV values are described in **Table 5**.

Red Cell Distribution Width

Red cell distribution width is a quantitative measure or numerical expression of anisocytosis. It is a coefficient of variation of the distribution of individual RBC volume.

- *RDW-SD (red cell distribution width-standard deviation):* It is the actual measurement of the width of the RBC distribution curve in femtoliters (fL) at the point that is 20% above the baseline values 35–45 fL.
- *RDW-CV (red cell distribution width-coefficient of variation):* It is the measure of the width of RDW curve. RDW-CV = standard deviation of MCV/mean MCV × 100. The normal value is 11.5–14.5%.

Low value indicates uniformity in size of RBCs. High value indicates mixed population of small and large RBCs. Immature RBCs tend to be larger. False high RDW value can be found if ethylenediaminetetraacetic acid (EDTA) is used as an anticoagulant instead of citrate. **Table 6** enumerates the causes of anemia based on RDW values.

MCH and MCHC

Mean corpuscular hemoglobin is the average mass of hemoglobin per RBC in a sample of blood. The result is reported by a very small weight called a picogram (pg). MCH is hemoglobin/red cell count × 100 pg. Normal range for newborn is 36–38 pg, up to 1 year age: 23–27 pg, and in adults: 26.7–31.9 pg. Low MCH is seen in microcytic as well as normocytic anemia, whereas high MCH is seen in macrocytic anemia.

Mean corpuscular hemoglobin concentration is the measure of hemoglobin in a given volume of packed RBC. It is calculated as hemoglobin/hematocrit × 100. Normal range for newborn: 34–36%, up to 1 year age: 31–33%, and for adults: 32–36%. MCHC is decreased in hypochromic microcytic anemia. MCHC is increased in hereditary spherocytosis, in presence of auto agglutinins and cold agglutinins, marked leukocytosis, hemolysis and in rouleaux formation.

Reticulocyte Count

Absolute reticulocyte count (ARC) is the actual number of reticulocyte in 1 microliter of blood.

ARC = % reticulocyte × RBC count/100

Corrected reticulocyte count = % reticulocyte × (Patient's Hct/normal Hct)

In the setting of anemia, a low reticulocyte count indicates a condition is affecting the production of RBCs such as bone marrow disorder or damage, or a nutritional deficiency (iron, B12 or folate) where as a high reticulocyte count generally indicates peripheral cause, such as bleeding or hemolysis, or response to treatment (e.g., iron supplementation for iron deficiency anemia).

WHITE BLOOD CELLS

White blood cells consist of neutrophils, lymphocytes, monocytes, basophils, and eosinophils. The normal range of WBCs for different ages: 0–3 days: 9,000–35,000/mm^3; up to 1 month: 5,000–19,000; 1 month to 2 years: 6,000–17,000; 2–5 years: 5.5–15,000; 5–12 years: 4,500–13,000; adults: 4,500–11,000. The differential count also varies with age **Table 7**.

Neutrophils

- Neutrophil series matures in an orderly fashion, from myeloblast to promyelocyte to myelocyte to metamyelocyte to band form to mature neutrophil. Only the last of these stages are normally present in the peripheral smear.
- Metamyelocytes can sometimes be seen in infection, pregnancy, leukemoid reaction, and recovery from myelosuppression but forms less mature than a myelocyte if present in the peripheral smear exclusively suggests hematologic malignancy.
- Increase in the number of immature forms or band cells, presence of toxic granulations, Dohle bodies, and cytoplasmic vacuoles are suggestive of acute bacterial infections.
- Presence of more than five lobes in a nucleus of a neutrophil is called hypersegmentation and suggests either a megaloblastic process or rarely iron deficiency anemia.
- Absolute neutrophil count (ANC) is (% of neutrophils + % of bands) × WBC/100.
- Neutrophilia is defined as at least 2 SD above the mean.
- Neutropenia means ANCs more than 2 SD below the normal mean.
- Generally, this term is used when neutrophils counts is <1,500/μL. It can be classified as mild; ANC between 1,000 and 1,500/μL, moderate 500–1,000/μL, severe <500/μL and very severe <200 /μL.
- Pseudoleukopenia can be seen at the onset of infection. In early infection, leukocytes (predominantly neutrophils) may be low in circulation as they migrate to the site of infection. **Table 8** enumerates the conditions of neutrophilia and neutropenia.

Lymphocytes

Lymphocytosis is increase in absolute lymphocyte count (age specific) or >45% lymphocytes of total peripheral WBC count, in children >5 years of age. Causes of lymphocytosis as well as lymphocytopenia are described in **Table 9**.

TABLE 7: White cell diffential according to age.

Age	Lymphocytes (%)	Neutrophils (%)
6 months to 1 year	61	32
2 years	59	33
4 years	50	42
6 years	42	51
8 years	39	53
10–16 years	35–38	54–57
Adults	34	59

TABLE 8: Causes of neutrophilia and neutropenia.

Causes of neutrophilia	Causes of neutropenia
- Acute inflammation, e.g., tissue necrosis (myocardial infarctions and burns) - Sterile inflammation, e.g., tissue necrosis (myocardial infarctions and burns) - Myeloproliferative disorders such as CML, JMML - Sweet syndrome - Asplenia - Leukocyte adhesion deficiency - Drugs such as steroids, ATRA - Acute stress	- Infections (typhoid fever, pertussis, brucellosis, gram-negative sepsis) - Post infectious especially viral - Nutritional (B$_{12}$/folate/copper deficiency) - Aplastic anemia or bone marrow failure syndromes - Arsenic poisoning - Hereditary disorders (e.g., congenital neutropenia, cyclic neutropenia) - Radiation - Chemotherapy - Hemodialysis - Hypersplenism - Immune neutropenia - Medications such as clozapine, sulfasalazine

(ATRA: all-trans retinoic acid; CML: chronic myeloid leukemia; JMML: juvenile myelomonocytic leukemia)

TABLE 9: Causes of lymphocytosis and lymphocytopenia.

Causes of lymphocytosis	Causes of lymphocytopenia
• *Reactive lymphocytosis*: Acute viral infections (e.g., chicken pox, CMV, EBV, herpes, rubella, hepatitis A); bacterial infections such as pertussis. Drug-induced, post splenectomy and autoimmune conditions such as RA and thyroiditis • Clonal lymphocytosis or malignant lymphocytosis	• Infections (e.g., HIV, viral hepatitis, typhoid fever, influenza, histoplasmosis) • Autoimmune disorders [e.g., lupus, rheumatic arthritis (RA)] • Bone marrow damage (e.g., chemotherapy, radiation therapy) • Congenital immunodeficiency disorders

(CMV: cytomegalovirus; EBV: Ebstein–Barr virus; HIV: human immunodeficiency virus)

BOX 1: Causes of monocytosis.

- Chronic infections (Tuberculosis, fungal infections)
- Rickettsiosis
- Malaria
- Infection within the heat (bacterial endocarditis)
- Collagen vascular diseases (systemic lupus erythematosus, vasculitis)
- Monocytic or myelomonocytic leukemia (acute or chronic)
- Inflammatory bowel disease (ulcerative colitis)

BOX 2: Causes of eosinophilia.

- Allergies
- Asthma
- Urticaria
- Addison's disease
- Skin infections (eczema, psoriasis, pemphigus, dermatitis herpetiformis)
- Drug reactions
- Parasitic infestations (round worms, hookworms, filiariasis, trichinosis)
- Neoplasms
- Collagen vascular disorders
- Atheroembolic diseases (transient)

TABLE 10: Causes of increased and decreased platelets.

Causes of thrombocytosis	Causes of thrombocytopenia

• Chronic infection
• Chronic inflammation
• Malignancy
• Hyposplenism (post splenectomy)
• Iron deficiency
• Acute blood loss in myeloproferative disorders—platelets are both elevated and activated
• Essential thrombocytosis
• Polycythemia vera associated with other myeloid neoplasms
• "Congenital" cancer (lung, gastrointestinal, breast, ovarian, lymphoma)
• Kawasaki disease
• *Soft-tissue sarcoma*: Osteosarcoma dermatitis (rarely)
• Bacterial diseases, including pneumonia, sepsis, meningitis, urinary tract infections, and septic
	• *Decreased production*: Selective impairment of platelets production: Drug induced, alcohol, thiazide, cytotoxic drugs
	  – *Infections*: Measles, HIV
	  – Nutritional deficiency. Vitamin B_{12}, folate
	• *Deficiency*: Inherited bone marrow failure syndromes
	  – Acquired aplastic anemia
	  – *Bone marrow replacement*: Leukemia, ineffective hematopoiesis
	  – Myelodysplastic syndromes
	• *Decreased platelets survival*: Immunological destruction
	  – Primary autoimmune (CITP, AITP)
	  – Secondary autoimmune (SLE)
	  – Alloimmune (post-transfusion)

(AITP: autoimmune thrombocytopenia; CITP: chronic immune thrombocytopenia; HIV: human immunodeficiency virus; SLE: systemic lupus erythematosus)

Monocytes

Monocytes develop in the bone marrow and circulate before entering the tissues where they differentiate into either macrophages or dendritic cells. These are the largest normal cells encountered in a peripheral smear.

Repeated low monocyte counts can indicate bone marrow damage or failure or hairy cell leukemia. Conditions with increased monocytes in peripheral blood are enlisted in **Box 1**.

Eosinophils

They are predominantly tissue dwelling cells whose function in health are not entirely understood. They are most likely involved in host response to infection, tissue remodeling, tumor surveillance, and maintenance of other immune cells. The normal value is 0–500 cells/µL. **Box 2** enlists causes of Eosinophilia. Alcohol abuse and Cushing's disease are associated with persistently low eosinophil counts.

Basophils

These are the least common of all circulating blood cells, comprise <1% of total WBCs. **Box 3** enumerates causes of basophilia.

PLATELETS

Platelets are cytoplasmic fragments of bone marrow megakaryocytes. They circulate in blood for 7–10 days. Their primary function along with the coagulation factors is hemostasis or prevention of bleeding. They also contribute

> **BOX 3:** Causes of basophilia.
> - Myeloproliferative disorders such as CML, primary myelofibrosis
> - Hypersensitivity or inflammatory reactions
> - Hypothyroidism
> - Infections such as chicken pox, TB
>
> (CML: chronic myeloid leukemia; TB: tuberculosis)

to the inflammatory process, microbial host defense, wound healing, angiogenesis, and remodeling.

The number and size of platelets give us important information about the disease state.

Platelet Count (Table 10)

Normal platelet counts are in the range of 150,000–400,000/µL. Spurious thrombocytopenia can be caused by improper collection, delayed processing, or inadequate anticoagulation of blood sample. EDTA-dependent antibodies which are present on some individuals also may cause falsely low platelet counts.

Mean Platelet Volume

Mean Platelet Volume (MPV) is a measure of the size of Platelets. It varies from 9 tp 12 femtolites. High MPV indicates a larger number of young platelets in circulation, seen in recent blood loss, or platelet destruction with a normal functioning marrow, eg ITP. Low MPV suggests higher number of old platelets in circulation, seen in contions like bone marrow failure, Wiscott Aldrich Syndrome, Lupus.

SUGGESTED READING

1. Pediatric Heamatology and Hemato Oncology by Dr M R Lokeshwar.
2. Practical Hematology by Dacie and Lewis.

CHAPTER 74: Approach to Normocytic Anemia

Atish N Bakane, Gaurav Kharya

INTRODUCTION

- Anemia in children is responsible for poor growth, developmental delays, and increased susceptibility to infection and in adults it is accountable for lost productivity, premature deaths, and perinatal complications.
- Overall, 47% of children <5 years of age and about 42% of pregnant women in developing countries are anemic. According to the study carried by the National Nutrition Monitoring Bureau, iron deficiency anemia (IDA) prevalence among children under 5 years of age was 66% in India. Anemia incidence is more in rural areas.
- Timely screening coupled with appropriate diagnostic testing will offer the most optimal identification and management of childhood anemia.

DEFINITION

- The Greek word *"Anemia"* means "without blood." Anemia refers to red blood cell (RBC) mass or amount of hemoglobin (Hb) in blood, and/or volume of packed RBCs less than normal, determined either as a hematocrit (Hct) or Hb concentration > 2 standard deviations below the normal mean for age **(Table 1)**.
- Normal ranges for Hb and Hct vary substantially with age, race, and sex.

TABLE 1: The WHO Hb thresholds used to define anemia.

Age or gender group	Hb threshold (g/dL)	Hb threshold (mmol/L)
Children (0.5–5.0 years)	11.0	6.8
Children (5–12 years)	11.5	7.1
Teens (12–15 years)	12.0	7.4
Women, nonpregnant (>15 years)	12.0	7.4
Women, pregnant	11.0	6.8
Men (>15 years)	13.0	8.1

(Hb: hemoglobin; WHO: World Health Organization)

CLASSIFICATION OF ANEMIA

Anemia can occur as a result of decreased production which in turn can be due to ineffective erythropoiesis, bone marrow suppression due to any cause, increased blood loss as a result of hemorrhage or increased destruction. Anemia can be classified in many ways:
- *Etiological classification*
- *Morphological classification* **(Box 1)**

BOX 1: Classification based on RBC size.

Microcytic anemias:
- Iron deficiency (nutritional, chronic blood loss)
- Chronic lead poisoning
- Thalassemia syndromes
- Sideroblastic anemias
- Chronic inflammation
- Some congenital hemolytic anemias with unstable hemoglobin

Macrocytic anemias:
- With megaloblastic bone marrow:
  - Vitamin B_{12} deficiency
  - Folic acid deficiency
  - Hereditary orotic aciduria
  - Thiamine-responsive anemia
- Without megaloblastic bone marrow:
  - Aplastic anemia
  - Diamond–Blackfan syndrome
  - Hypothyroidism
  - Liver disease
  - Bone marrow infiltration
  - Dyserythropoietic anemias

Normocytic anemias:
- Congenital hemolytic anemias:
  - Hemoglobin mutants
  - Red cell enzyme defects
  - Disorders of the red cell membrane
- Acquired hemolytic anemias:
  - Antibody mediated
  - Microangiopathic hemolytic anemias
  - Secondary to acute infections
- Acute blood loss
- Splenic pooling
- Chronic renal disease (usually)

(RBC: red blood cell)

- *Pathophysiological classification*
- *Based on severity.*

RELEVANT CLINICAL DETAILS WHILE EVALUATING A CHILD WITH ANEMIA

Age

The normal values of Hct and Hb vary greatly with age, and because different causes of anemia are present at different ages.

Birth to 3 Months

- The most common cause of anemia in young infants is "physiologic anemia", which occurs at approximately 6-9 weeks of age.
- Common causes of pathologic anemia in newborns include blood loss, immune hemolytic disease, congenital infection, twin-twin transfusion, and congenital hemolytic anemia.
- Hyperbilirubinemia in the newborn period suggests a hemolytic etiology; microcytosis at birth suggests chronic intrauterine blood losts or thalassemia.
- Compared with term infants, preterm infants are born with lower Hct and Hb, have shorter RBC life span, and have impaired erythropoietin production due to immature liver function. Hence, the decline in RBC production occurs earlier after birth and is more severe than the anemia seen in term infants. This is referred to as "anemia of prematurity."

Infants 3–6 Months

Hemoglobinopathy is the likely cause for anemia in this age group. Nutritional iron deficiency is an unlikely cause of anemia before the age of 6 months in term infants.

Toddlers, Children and Adolescents

In toddlers, older children, and adolescents, acquired causes of anemia are more likely, particularly iron deficiency anemia.

Gender

X-linked disorders in male, glucose-6-phosphate dehydrogenase (G6PD) deficiency and pyruvate kinase (PK) deficiency can cause hemolysis at any age.

Race

Sindhi, Punjabi, and Gujarati communities from our country tend to have thalassemia syndromes more commonly.

Ethnicity

Thalassemia syndromes are more common in patients of Mediterranean origin. G6PD deficiency is more common in north Indians and Sephardic, Greeks, Sardinians around the world.

Diet

- Document sources of iron, vitamin B_{12}, folic acid, or vitamin E in the diet.
- Commonly observed practices in India like giving too much (>500 mL/day) of cow milk or delay in initiation of supplementary diet can be responsible for IDA.
- Likewise, practicing vegan diet (vegetarian diet not even including milk can be responsible for megaloblastic anemia).
- Pica suggests the presence of iron deficiency.

Drugs

Oxidant-induced hemolytic anemia, drug-induced megaloblastic anemia, or aplastic anemia.

Infection

Hepatitis-induced aplastic anemia infection-induced red cell aplasia, and hemolytic anemia are also considered.

Inheritance

Family history of anemia, jaundice, gall stones, blood transfusion, and splenomegaly, cholecystectomy shall be asked for.

Persistent Diarrhea

Suspect small bowel disease with malabsorption of folate or vitamin B_{12}; inflammatory bowel disease with blood loss; protein-losing enteropathy with blood loss.

Past Medical History

- Focus on characterizing past episodes of anemia and identifying underlying medical conditions.
- *Birth history*: Gestational age, duration of birth hospitalization, and history of jaundice and/or anemia in the newborn period. Results of newborn screening if done.
- *History of anemia*: Previous complete blood counts (CBCs) should be reviewed, and if prior anemic episodes occurred, they should be characterized (including duration, etiology, therapy, and resolution). Prior recurrent episodes of anemia might suggest an inherited etiology, whereas anemia in a patient with previously documented normal CBC may be suggestive of an acquired etiology.
- *Underlying medical conditions*: Past medical history/recent illnesses and review of symptoms. Travel to/from areas of endemic infection (e.g., malaria, hepatitis, tuberculosis) should be noted.

Developmental History

Developmental delay can be associated with iron deficiency, vitamin B_{12}/folic acid deficiency, and Fanconi anemia.

SIGNS TO LOOK FOR WHILE EVALUATING A CHILD WITH ANEMIA

Skin

- Skin can act as mirror for diagnosis for many diseases including anemia in childhood. Hyperpigmentation and caféau-lait-spots can be suggestive of Fanconi anemia.
- Petechiae, purpura can be seen with autoimmune hemolytic anemia (AIHA) with thrombocytopenia, hemolytic uremic syndrome, bone marrow aplasia or bone marrow infiltration.
- Presence of jaundice can suggest hemolytic anemia, hepatitis, or aplastic anemia.
- Hemangioma can give clue toward microangiopathic hemolytic anemia (MAHA) or vice versa. Ulcers on lower extremities can be seen commonly with S and C hemoglobinopathies or thalassemia syndromes.

Facies

Frontal bossing, prominence of the malar and maxillary bones can be seen in congenital hemolytic anemias, transfusion-dependent thalassemia or even severe IDA.

Eyes

- Microcornea is a feature of Fanconi anemia.
- Tortuosity of the conjunctival and retinal vessels and microaneurysms of the retinal vessels are seen in S and C hemoglobinopathies.
- Presence of cataract can suggest galactosemia with hemolytic anemia.

Mouth

- Glossitis is a feature of vitamin B_{12} deficiency and iron deficiency. Angular stomatitis can be seen along with glossitis.

Digital Anomalies

- Triphalangeal thumbs are seen in pure red cell aplasia.
- Hypoplasia of the thenar eminence is a characteristic feature of Fanconi anemia.
- Spoon-shaped nails can be a feature of IDA.

Spleen

Splenomegaly can be seen in congenital hemolytic anemia, leukemia, lymphoma, acute infection or portal hypertension.

DIAGNOSTIC SIGNIFICANCE OF RBC INCLUSION BODIES

- *Basophilic stippling (Wright stain)*: **Figure 1** represents aggregated ribosomes.
  Causes: Thalassemia, IDA, Pyrimidine 5′-nucleotidase deficiency; unstable hemoglobino-pathies and lead poisoning.
- *Howell–Jolly bodies (Wright stain)*: **Figure 2** represents nuclear remnants; solitary round mass, relatively large.
  Causes: Asplenic and hyposplenic states, pernicious anemia, congenital dyserythropoietic anemia (CDA), severe IDA, erythroblastosis, myelodysplasia, megaloblastic anemia, or post chemotherapy.
- *Cabot's rings (Wright stain)* **(Fig. 3)**.
- *Heinz bodies (Brilliant cresyl blue, methyl violet)*: **Figure 4** represents denatured or aggregated Hb.
  Causes: Thalassemia syndromes or unstable Hb, after oxidant stress in patients with enzyme deficiencies of the pentose phosphate pathway, and asplenia or chronic liver disease.
- *Siderocytes (Prussian blue counter stained with safranin O)*: **Figure 5** represents nonhemoglobin iron within erythrocytes.

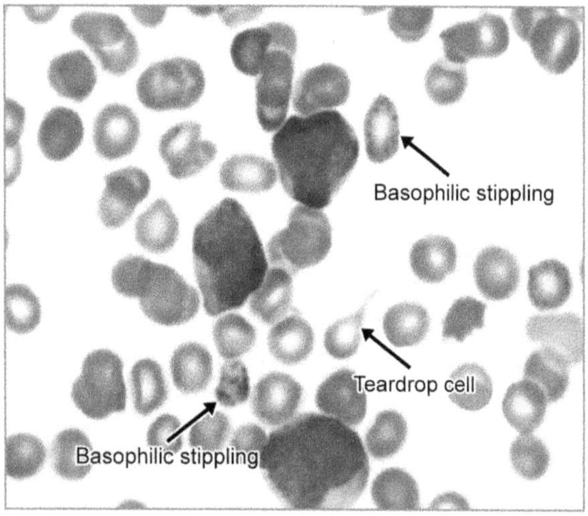

Fig. 1: Basophilic stippling (Wright stain).

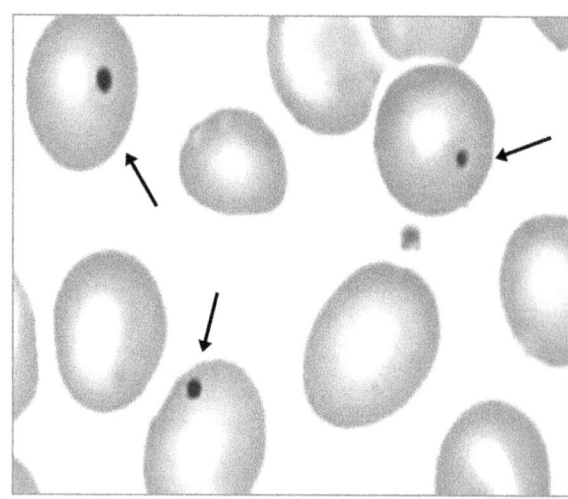

Fig. 2: Howell–Jolly bodies (Wright stain).

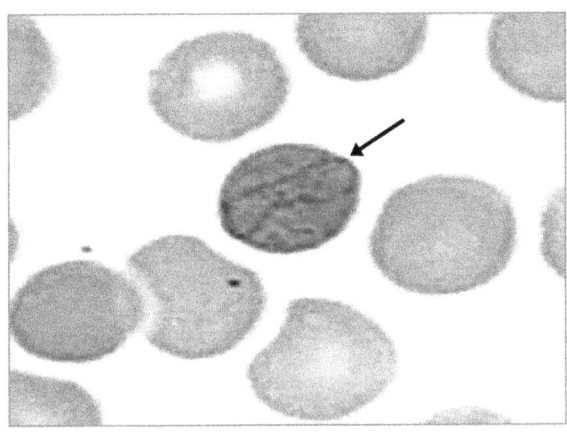

Fig. 3: Cabot's rings (Wright stain).

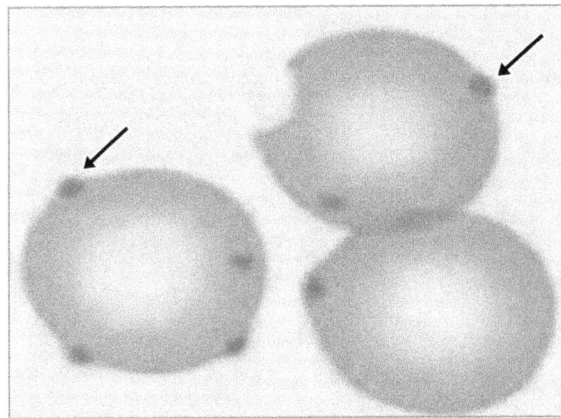

Fig. 4: Heinz bodies.

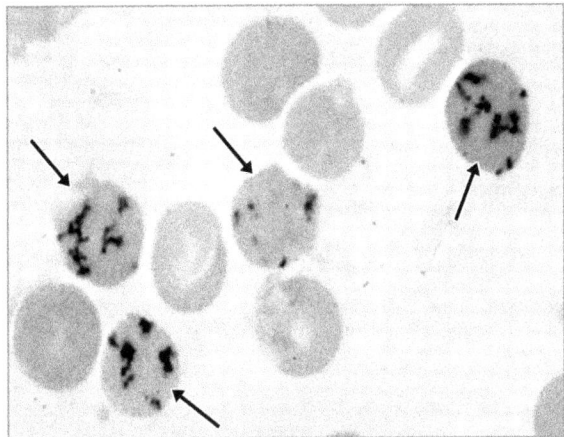

Fig. 5: Siderocytes (Prussian blue counterstained with safranin O).

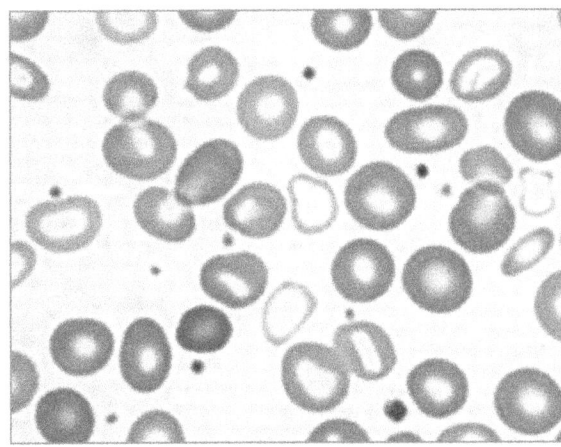

Fig. 6: Anisochromia.

Causes: After splenectomy, observed in increased numbers in patients with chronic infection, aplastic anemias, or hemolytic anemias.

COMMON RED BLOOD CELL MORPHOLOGIC FINDINGS AND POSSIBLE CAUSES

- *Anisochromia*: **Figure 6** shows variation in the amount of central pallor among a population of RBCs.
  Causes: IDA, myelodysplastic syndrome (MDS), hypochromic anemia posttransfusion.
- *Anisocytosis*: **Figure 7** shows variation in size among a population of RBCs. Common nonspecific finding.
  Causes: IDA, moderate or severe thalassemia, megaloblastic anemia, partially treated anemia of several causes, posttransfusion.
- *Echinocyte (Burr cell)*: RBC has regularly distributed, equally sized, rounded projections of fits surface **(Fig. 8)**.
  Causes: Artifact, renal failure, post-transfusion, phosphate deficiency, burns.
- *Acanthocyte (Spur cell)*: RBCs have irregularly distributed, variably sized, pointy projections off its surface **(Fig. 9)**.
  Causes: Advanced liver disease, hyposplenism, dyslipidemias, PK deficiency, McLeod phenotype.

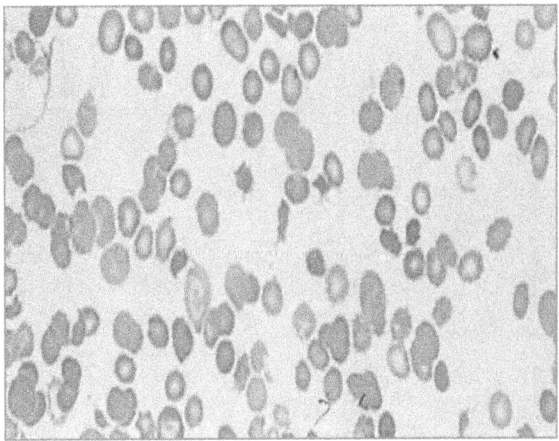

Fig. 7: Anisocytosis.

- *Elliptocyte*: RBC is oval shaped **(Fig. 10)**.
  Causes: Iron deficiency, megaloblastic anemia, hereditary elliptocytosis, and postchemotherapy.
- *Hypochromia*: The zone of central pallor is >one third the diameter of the RBC.
  Possible etiologies: IDA, thalassemia or anemia of chronic diseases.

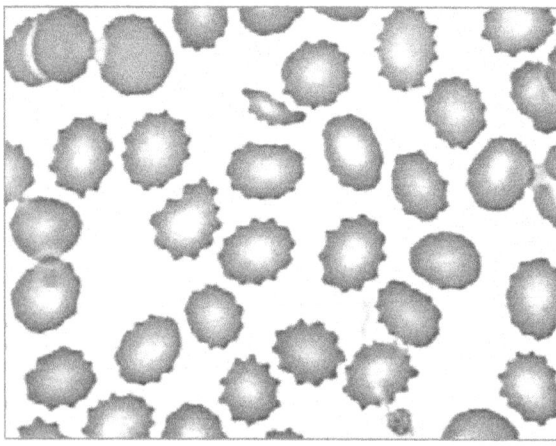

Fig. 8: Echinocyte (Burr cell).

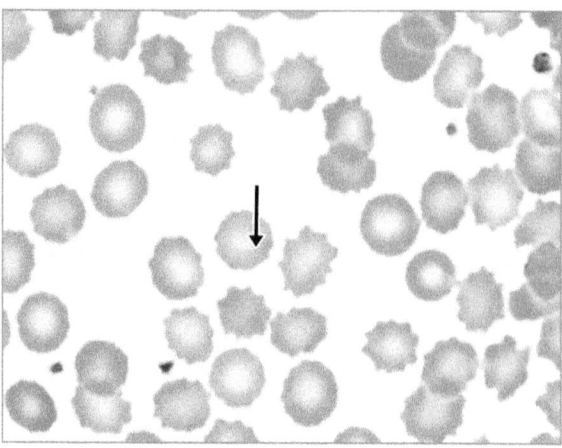

Fig. 9: Acanthocyte (Spur cell).

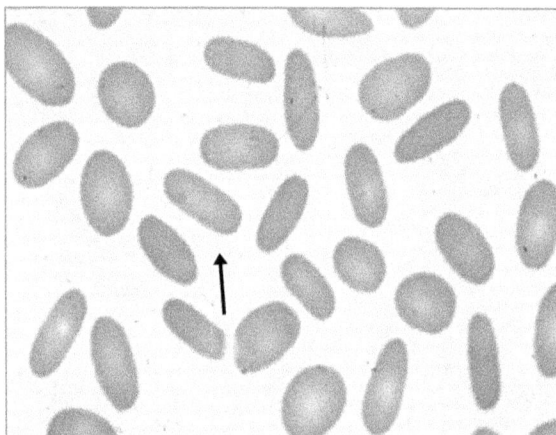

Fig. 10: Elliptocyte.

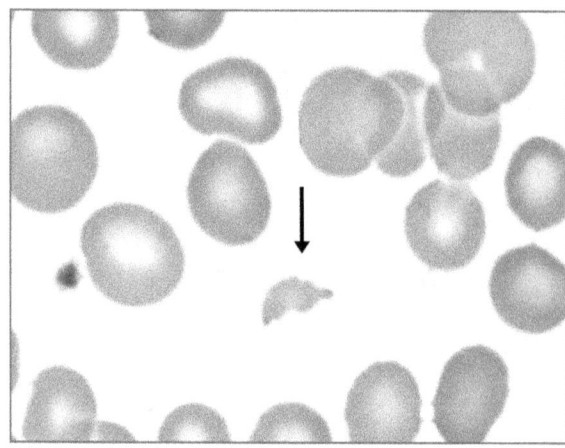

Fig. 11: Schistocyte.

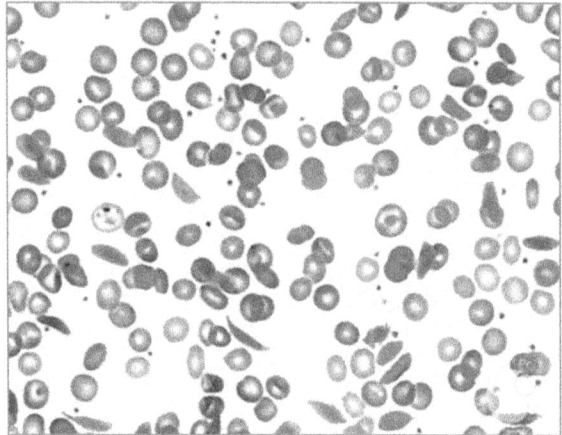

Fig. 12: Sickle cell.

- *Schistocyte*: Fragmented RBC, the zone of central pallor is often missing **(Fig. 11)**.
  Causes: MAHA and hemolysis secondary to cardiac valve.
- *Sickle cell*: Sickle RBC morphologies **(Fig. 12)**:
  - Crescentic
  - Boats

  Causes: Severe sickling syndrome, e.g., Homozygous Hb S disease, Hb SC disease, Hb SD disease.

- *Spherocyte*: The RBC is smaller and darker than normal, there is no zone of central pallor, the outer edge must be almost perfectly round **(Fig. 13)**.
  Causes: AIHA (hemolytic disease of the newborn), hereditary spherocytosis.
- *Target cell*: The RBC has a central red area within the zone of central pallor **(Fig. 14)**.
  Causes: Thalassemia, liver disease, hyposplenism, Hb C disease or SC disease, hereditary xerocytosis, may be seen in iron deficiency.

DIAGNOSTIC EVALUATION (FLOWCHART 1)

Initial Evaluation

- CBC/DLC/PS/reticulocyte count
- Hemoglobin variants identification [high-performance liquid chromatography (HPLC) or isoelectric focusing preferred]
- *Iron studies*: Serum iron, serum transferrin, serum ferritin, total iron binding capacity (TIBC)
- *Hemolysis indicators*: Bilirubin (total and direct), lactate dehydrogenase (LDH) (for intravascular hemolysis)
- G6PD screening test

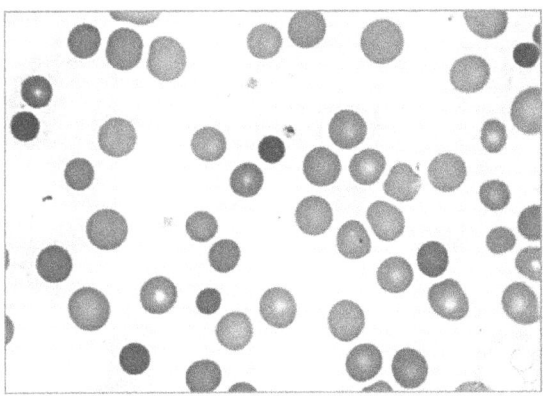

Fig. 13: Spherocyte.

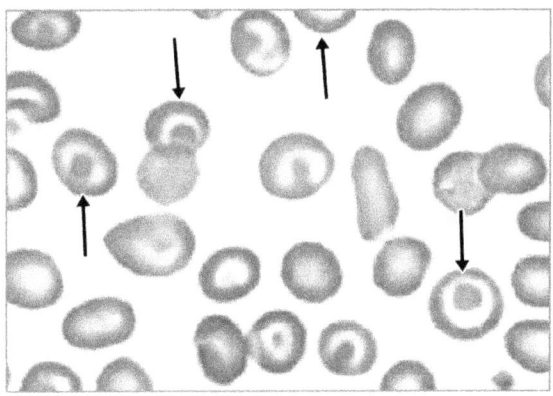

Fig. 14: Target cell.

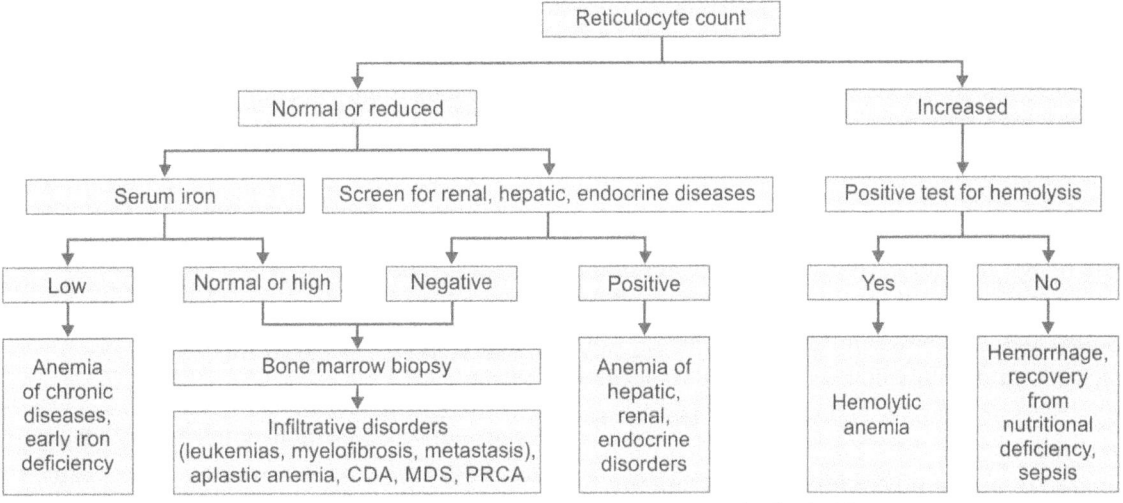

Flowchart 1: Approach to normocytic anemia.

(CDA: congenital dyserythropoietic anemia; MDS: myelodysplastic syndromes PRCA: pure red cell aplasia)

Further Evaluation

- Serum B_{12}, folate, red cell folate, and serum/urine methyl malonic acid
- Osmotic fragility
- Serum haptoglobin, serum/plasma Hb, urine hemosiderin
- Direct antiglobulin test and indirect antiglobulin test. Unstable Hb screen (isopropanol or thermal stability), Heinz bodies preparation
- Paroxysmal nocturnal hemoglobinuria (PNH) testing by flow cytometry: (red blood cell and white blood cell)
- Erythrocyte adenosine deaminase (ADA) activity
- *Human parvovirus B19*: IgM and G titers, viral DNA detection tests
- Serum erythropoietin, serum α-fetoprotein, mitomycin, or diepoxybutane test
- Acid serum lysis test with ABO-compatible serum.

Advanced Evaluation

- Bone marrow aspirate/biopsy
- Electron microscopy
- Complementation test (Fanconi anemia subtyping)
- Molecular genetic studies (CDA types I and II, Blackfan-Diamond syndrome and other inherited anemias).

SUGGESTED READING

1. Beutler E, Waalen J. The definition of anemia: what is the lower limit of normal of the blood hemoglobin concentration? Blood. 2006;107(5):1747-50.
2. Brugnara C, Mohandas N: Red cell indices in classifcation and treatment of anemias: from M.M. Wintrobes's original 1934 classifcation to the third millennium. Curr Opin Hematol. 2013;20(3):222-30.
3. Diagnostic approach to the anemic patient. Nathan and Oski's hematology and oncology of infancy and childhood, Vol. 1, 8th edition. pp 423-36.
4. Ford J. Red blood cell morphology. Int J Lab Haematol. 2013; 35:351-7.
5. Holland BM, Jones JG, Wardrop CA. Lessons from the anemia of prematurity. Hematol Oncol Clin North Am. 1987;1:355.
6. Kling PJ, Schmidt RL, Roberts RA, Widness JA. Serum erythropoietin levels during infancy: associations with erythropoiesis. J Pediatr. 1996;128:791.
7. Matoth Y, Zaizov R, Varsano I. Postnatal changes in some red cell parameters. Acta Paediatr Scand. 1971;60:317.
8. Means RT, Glader B. Anemia: General Considerations. In: Greer JP, Foerster J, Rodgers GM, et al. (eds). Wintrobe's Clinical Hematology, Vol. 1, 12th edition, Philadelphia: Lippincott Williams and Wilkins; 2009. p. 784.
9. Rapaport SI. Diagnosis of Anemia. Introduction to Hematology. Philadelphia: JB Lippincott; 1987. p. 15.
10. Sandoval C. Thrombocytosis in children with iron deficiency anemia: series of 42 children. J Pediatr Hematol Oncol. 2002;24:593.
11. Wintrobe MM. Classification of the anemias on the basis of differences in the size and hemoglobin content of the red corpuscles. Proc Soc Exp Biol Med. 1930;27(9):1071-3.

Iron Deficiency Anemia

Tripty Naik

INTRODUCTION

The World Health Organization (WHO) estimates that 42% of children <5 years are anemic. In India 59% children have some degree of anemia [National Family Health Survey (NFHS-4), 2015-16]. Nutritional deficiencies, particularly iron deficiency, are the most common cause of anemia.

Iron deficiency anemia (IDA) most commonly affects young children and adolescent females.

Iron deficiency even without anemia in children under 2 years of age can cause irreversible effects on brain development and learning (role of iron in myelin production, synaptogenesis, and neurotransmitter metabolism). Iron is important for immune function. IDA is also associated with febrile seizures and various behavioral and psychiatric disorders in children.

In children, IDA occurs due to intake of less amount of iron in diet and/or its impaired absorption of from proximal small intestine: Delayed introduction of complementary feeding, increased phytates and/or decreased vitamin C in diet, drinking tea or coffee with or soon after meals, celiac disease, and probably *Helicobacter pylori* infection.
- *Increased loss of iron (blood)*: During menstruation, hookworm or schistosomiasis infestation, cow's milk protein allergy.
- *Increased demand or impaired utilization of iron*: During inflammation and active periods of growth like babies born prematurely, preschool years, and adolescence.

CLINICAL FEATURES

- *Hematological consequences*: Pallor [starts at hemoglobin (Hb) 7-8 g/dL], fatigue, irritability, and exercise intolerance.
- *Nonhematological consequences*: Cognitive impairment in infancy. It produces geophagia (eating mud), amylophagia (eating raw rice), pagophagia (eating ice cube). Epithelial abnormalities such as glossitis and koilonychias, behavioral manifestation, growth retardation, impaired collagen synthesis (blue sclera).

LABORATORY DIAGNOSIS

Iron deficiency anemia is a laboratory diagnosis. Careful history and examination is needed to identify etiology of iron deficiency, and to rule out other causes of anemia. Symptomatic iron deficiency is infrequent; hence, routine screening will be useful at 9-12 months of age and again at 18-24 months of age (if on cow milk), adolescent females should be screened after 1-2 years of menarche. IDA causes microcytic hypochromic anemia; refer to **Table 1** for various causes of microcytic anemia and their laboratory account. IDA is diagnosed by following tests:
- *Complete blood count (CBC)*: Low Hb and hematocrit (Hct), reduced total number of red cells, increased platelet count, normal leukocyte count, low mean cellular volume (MCV), and low mean cell hemoglobin concentration (MCHC). Red cell distribution width

TABLE 1: Comparative account of laboratory findings in various causes of microcytic anemia.

	FEP	Serum iron	TIBC	Ferritin
IDA	Increase	Decrease	Increase	Decrease
Alpha-thalassemia	Normal	Normal	Normal	Normal
Beta-thalassemia	Normal	Normal	Normal	Normal
Lead poisoning	Increase	Normal	Normal	Normal
Anemia of chronic disease	Increase	Decrease	Normal	Normal to increase

(IDA: iron deficiency anemia; FEP: free erythrocyte protoporphyrin; TIBC: total iron binding capacity)

(RDW) is variability in red cell volume, less the 14.5% is highly sensitive to IDA.
- *Reticulocyte count*: Baseline *reticulocyte count* to monitor the response.
- *Peripheral blood smear*: Microcytic hypochromic red cells, anisopoikilocytosis, thrombocytosis or thrombocytopenia, tear drop cells, and target cells.
- Serum ferritin will be low; the level of <12 ng/mL is almost diagnostic.
- *Serum iron studies*: *Serum iron* will be low and total iron binding capacity (TIBC) will be increased. Transferrin saturation <14% is sensitive enough to diagnose the deficiency.
- *C-reactive protein (CRP)*: To rule out falsely elevated serum ferritin in the presence of infection and/or inflammation.
- *High-performance liquid chromatography (HPLC)*: To rule out thalassemia trait (total red cells are increased in thalassemia, with a normal RDW).
- Stool tests for routine microscopy and presence of hemoglobin tests.
- *Other tests*: Serum or tissue lead levels, and bone marrow aspirate for stainable iron, reticulocyte hemoglobin content (CHr).

TREATMENT

Diet

- Iron-rich foods include meat, especially liver, poultry, fish, green leafy green vegetables, broccoli, legumes, "*munga*," and iron-fortified foods.
- Acid, vitamin C, and meat increase iron absorption, whereas presence of food, phytates and phosphates decrease its absorption.

Oral Iron Therapy

- Recommended treatment dose of oral iron is 3–6 mg/kg/day of elemental iron taken on an empty stomach.
- Ferrous salts have higher iron content and are better absorbed than ferric salts.
- Ferrous sulfate (20–32% iron) is the cheapest and preferred form.

All oral iron preparations cause some gastric intolerance and staining of teeth **(Table 2)**.

Parenteral Iron Therapy

- Reserved for use in chronic kidney disease (along with erythropoietin), malabsorption like inflammatory bowel disease, and nonresponse or nontolerance of oral iron.
- Intravenous route is preferred to intramuscular route.
- Different formulations available are iron–dextran, ferrous sucrose, and ferric carboxymaltose, and iron isomaltoside 1000.
- Ferrous sucrose is better tolerated, newer formulations such as iron isomaltoside 1000 have better safety profile.

Transfusion of Packed Red Blood Cells

- In severe anemia with congestive cardiac failure and in severe ongoing blood losses.
- *Follow-up*: Response to oral iron is the best available conformation for the diagnosis.

Increase in reticulocyte count after 5–7 days gives you the earliest clue, followed by achievement of normal hemoglobin level in 2 months. Total duration of 3 months is sufficient to replete stores after which maintenance nutritional need must be met.

PREVENTION

- The World Health Organization recommends daily 30–60 mg of elemental iron supplementation in menstruating adult women and adolescent girls, living in settings where anemia is highly prevalent (≥40% anemia prevalence), for the prevention of anemia and iron deficiency.

TABLE 2: Properties of various iron preparations.

Iron salt	Elemental Fe	Role of dietary inhibitor	Staining of teeth	Side effect	Availability
Ferrous sulfate	20%	Yes	Yes	GIT	Syrup
Ferrous fumarate	33%	Yes	Yes	Less	Syrup
Ferrous ascorbate	16.6%	Less	Yes	Less	Syrup
Ferrous bisglycinate	20%	Less	Yes	Less	Syrup
Na-Feredetate	14.3%	No	No	Less	Syrup
IPC	25–40%	No	No	No	Syrup
Colloidal	50%	Yes	Yes	GIT	Syrup
Carbonyl	100%	Yes	No	GIT	Syrup

(GIT: gastrointestinal tract; IPC: iron(III)-hydroxide polymaltose complex)

PRESCRIPTION ASSISTANCE

Pharmacological salt	Market preparation	Availability	Dosage
Ferrous calcium Citrate + Folic acid	Raricap L	Syrup–Ferrous Calcium citrate 25 mg + Folic acid 0.3 mg	
Ferrous Ascorbate + Folic acid + Methylcobalamin	Feronia-Max	Syrup–Ferrous ascorbate 30 mg + Folic acid 500 µg + Methylcobalamin 500 µg	
Ferrous ascorbate + Folic acid	Imax XT	Ferrous ascorbate 30 mg + Folic acid 550 µg	

- Encourage exclusive breastfeeding with timely introduction of complementary feeding and hand hygiene to prevent infections.
- Good antenatal care and delayed cord clamping.

PROGNOSIS

Iron deficiency anemia is easily treatable with good outcome, but prolonged untreated iron deficiency can slow growth in children and cause irreversible brain damage, so early diagnosis and treatment are important.

KEY MESSAGES

- Iron deficiency ± anemia in children impairs growth, development, and immunity; well child visits include enquiry into risk factors for the same for early detection and treatment of IDA.
- Regular follow-up during therapy with iron is important to ensure compliance and completion of therapy.
- Compliance, associated micronutrient deficiencies, blood loss or lead poisoning and review diagnosis are common causes of nonresponse to iron therapy.

SUGGESTED READING

1. Cusick SE, Georgieff MK, Rao R. Approaches for reducing the risk of early-life iron deficiency-induced brain dysfunction in children. Nutrients. 2018 Feb 17;10(2):227.
2. Pivina L, Semenova Y, Doşa MD, Dauletyarova M, Bjørklund G. Iron deficiency, cognitive functions, and neurobehavioral disorders in children. J Mol Neurosci. 2019;68(1):1-10. doi: 10.1007/s12031-019-01276-1.
3. WHO guideline on use of ferritin concentrations to assess iron status in individuals and populations. Geneva: World Health Organization; 2020. Licence: CC BY-NC-SA 3.0 IGO.

Megaloblastic Anemia

Nilay Mozarkar

INTRODUCTION

Megaloblastic anemia (MA) is characterized by macrocytic RBC with nuclear dysmaturity. It can occur due to nutritional and congenital etiologies more common being B_{12} and folate deficiency. Nutritional MA is commonly seen in India in nutritionally challenged pediatric populations in which B_{12} deficiency is more prevalent.

ETIOLOGY

B_{12} Deficiency

- *Nutritional inadequacy*: Breast milk infant of B_{12}-deficient mothers, strict vegetarian diet for long as older children have sufficient stores of B_{12} in liver.
  - *Inherited disorders*: Imerslund–Gräsbeck syndrome, transcobalamin deficiency, transcobalamin receptor defects, methylmalonic aciduria, homocystinuria.
- *Pernicious anemia*: Intrinsic factor deficiency.
- *Drug induced*: Para-aminosalicylic acid, colchicine, and zidovudine therapy.

Folate Deficiency

- *Nutritional inadequacy*: Exclusive goat milk ingestion, boiling vegetables for long, concurrent vitamin C deficiency.
- *Inherited disorders*: Difolate reductase deficiency and congenital folate malabsorption.
- *Increased requirements*: In hemolytic anemia and leukemia
- *Drug induced*: Anticonvulsants, antifolate/antimetabolite drugs such as methotrexate, sulfonamides, azathioprine, hydroxyurea, and sulfasalazine

CLINICAL FEATURES

- Anemia, anorexia, mental apathy, fatigability, glossitis, and diarrhea.
- Knuckle and terminal phalanges hyperpigmentation are seen in Asian communities.
- Hepatosplenomegaly seen in 30–40% cases.
- Skin bleed and hemorrhagic manifestation are seen in 25% cases. The anemia with bleeding tendency has to be differentiated from aplastic anemia.
- The severe anemia with hepatosplenomegaly has to be differentiated from acute leukemia.
- *Infantile tremor syndrome*: Abnormal body movement with coarse tremors, hypotonia, psychomotor retardation, apathy, and failure to thrive.
- *Microcephaly with developmental delay* has been seen even before the appearance of anemia. Magnetic resonance imaging (MRI) brain reveals diffuse Frontotemporal parietal cortical atrophy.
- MA also manifests with pancytopenia. It has been seen in Indian studies that MA is more common cause of pancytopenia than aplastic anemia and leukemia.

APPROACH TO DIAGNOSIS (FLOWCHART 1)

- *Cellular characteristics of MA*:
  - A characteristic finding in bone marrow smears for MA would be the appearance of nuclear-cytoplasmic (N:C) asynchrony in all cell lines. N:C asynchrony describes the inability of the cell's chromatin to mature normally giving the nucleus a more immature, more fine, looser, and larger appearance than expected compared to that of the cytoplasm. Cytoplasm maturation is not affected and matures normally. Due to these characteristics, the cells are described as megaloblastic. In peripheral blood, RBC becomes large and displays a great deal in variation in their shapes; these macrocytes are generally normochromic but can become hypochromic in mixed deficiencies.
  - The second most likely cells to display morphologic finding are neutrophils showing hypersegmentation in peripheral blood smear. Hypersegmentation is described when either observation is present—5% or more neutrophils have 5 lobes or one neutrophil with ≥6 lobes. This is the most sensitive and specific sign of MA.

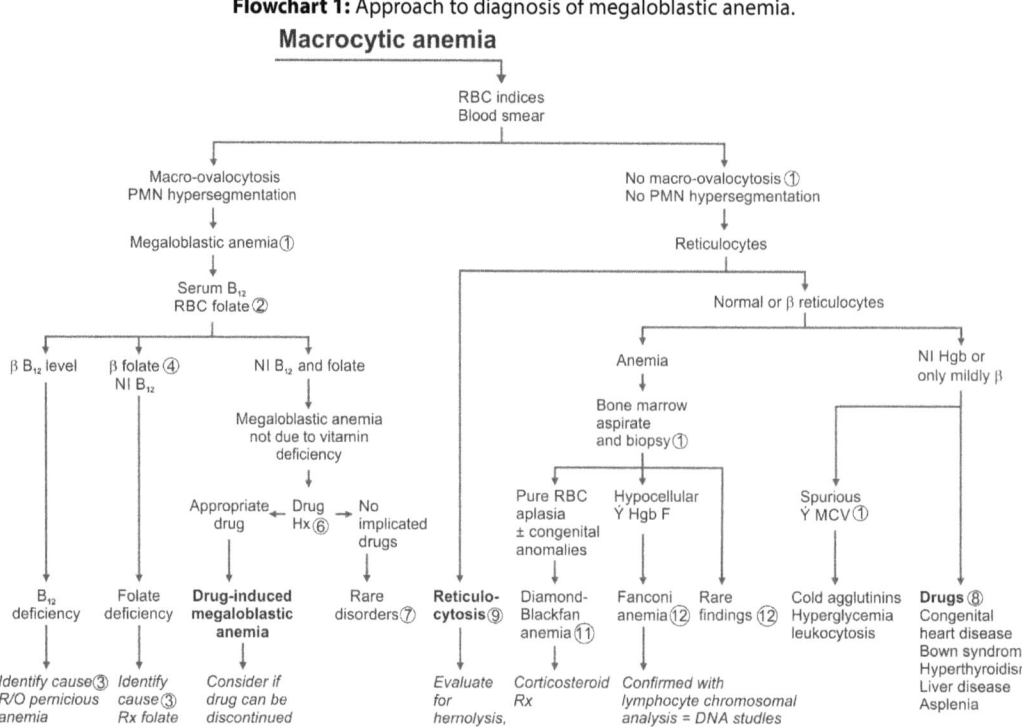

Flowchart 1: Approach to diagnosis of megaloblastic anemia.

TABLE 1: Hematologic laboratory features of megaloblastic anemia.

CBC	PBS	BM
RBC, WBC, PLT, Hb, Hct, decreased	Macroovalocytes, anisocytosis	M:E ratio: decreased (Ineffective erythropoiesis)
MCV: Usually > 110 fL	Hypersegmented neutrophils	Hypercellular
MCH: Increased	Howell–Jolly bodies	N:C asynchrony
MCHC: Normal	Teardrop cells, schistocytes	Enlarged precursors
Reticulocyte count: Normal to decreased		Giant metamyelocytes and bands

(BM: bone marrow; CBC: complete blood count; Hb: hemoglobin; Hct: hematocrit; M:E ratio: the ratio of myeloid to erythroid precursors in bone marrow; MCH: mean corpuscular hemoglobin; MCHC: mean corpuscular hemoglobin concentration; MCV: mean corpuscular volume; N:C: nuclear-cytoplasmic; PLT: platelets; PBS: peripheral blood smear; RBC: red blood cell; WBC: white blood cell)

- The most severe and prolonged MA ultimately may lead to moderate thrombocytopenia with large bizarre platelets in peripheral blood smear.
- Hematologic laboratory features of MA is given in **Table 1**.
- Biochemical abnormalities to differentiate between B_{12} and folic acid deficiency:
- *Serum levels of B_{12} and folate levels* are subjected to fallacies of false positivity and negativity. RBC folate levels are more accurate to reflect negative folate balance. A cutoff level of *100-150 pg/mL* of vitamin B_{12}, and *3-5 ng/mL* of folate have been used to define the deficiency of respective vitamins.
- *Serum lactate dehydrogenase (LDH)* level which are elevated in the range of 2,000-5,000 μg/dL with appropriate clinical and hematological situation is a useful surrogate marker. Reverse isozyme pattern (LDH1 > LDH2) was found to have good adjunct to differentiate MA from hemolytic anemia.
- *Serum homocystine level is increased in vitamin B_{12} and FA deficiency.*
- *Serum methylmalonic acid (MMA) is increased in only vitamin B_{12}.*
- *Holotranscobalamine (HoloTC) level or transcobalamine-bound vitamin B_{12}, which is biologically active form of B_{12} is said to be sensitive marker of vitamin B_{12} deficiency. Normal range of HoloTC is ≥42.48 pmol/L. HoloTC performs better than total vitamin B_{12} level.*

It is recommended that the diagnosis of vitamin B_{12} deficiency must be based on two sets of investigations (**Table 2**):
1. *One functional marker, i.e., MMA or homocystine level*
2. *One marker of level of vitamin, i.e., either HoloTC or serum vitamin B_{12} level*

TABLE 2: Biochemical diagnosis of vitamin B_{12} deficiency.

	B_{12}	Folic acid	Homocystine	Methylmalonic acid
B_{12} deficiency	↓	Normal	↑	↑
Folic acid deficiency	Normal	↓	↑	Normal

PRESCRIPTION ASSISTANCE

Pharmacological salt	Market preparation	Availability (drop/syrup/tablet/injection)	Dosages
Folic acid	Tablet Folvite, Tab FH12, Tablet fol5	Tablet 5 mg	1–5 mg/day
Cyanocobalamin (synthetic, inactive, less recommended)	• Neurobion tablet • Folired tablet • Optineuron • Injection Vitocofol capsule • Eldervit capsule • Vitcofol injection	• Neurobion tablet cyanocobalamin 15 mg plus iron folic acid OPTINEURON injection cyanocobalamin 1,000 meg, plus other B complex/mL • VITCOFOL capsule: B_{12} 7.5 µg. µg plus iron folic acid, B_6 and zinc • ELDERVIT capsule vitamin B_{12} 15 µg folic acid 1.5 mg vitamin C 150 mg • Vitcofol injection folic acid 15 mg, vitamin B_{12} 0.5 mg nictoinamide/1 mL	1,000 µg/day I/M or oral 100–250 µg/day or weekly or monthly oral or IM
Hydroxocobalamin (inactive, can be used)	• Injection hydrox • Only injectable preparations	• Mydrox-12 injection 1,000 µg x 1 mL • TRINEUROSOL HP injection 5 mg x 1 mL	
Methylcobalamin (natural, active, best choice)	• Nervijen capsule • Nervijen injection • Neurobion forte-RF injection • Methycobal injection • Methycobal tablet • Neuromet capsule	• *Nervijen capsule*: Benfodiamine, methylcobalamin 750 µg, calcium pantotherate, alpha lipoic acid, B_6, nicodnamide, folic acid • Nervijen injection methylcobalamin 1,500 µg plus B_1, B_6, niacinamide D panthenol folic acid/2 mL • Neurobion forte-RF • Injection mecobalamin 1,000 µg pyostacine, niacinamide/2 mL • Methycobal injection 500 µg, mL • Methycobal tablet 500 µg • Neuromet capsule mecobalamin 1,500 µg, folic acid, alpha lipoic acid, pyridoxine	
Adenosylco-balamin (natural, active, storage from, 2nd best choice)	Adenosyl capsule AHB 15 capsule only oral preparations	Adenosyl capsule 500 and 1,000 µg AHB 15 capsule 500 µg, iron 50 mg, folic acid 5 mg	

MANAGEMENT

Folate 100–200 µg daily is needed for treatment; however, it is given in a dose 1–5 mg daily for 3 weeks for therapeutic response then continued for 2 months for replenishment of body stores.

B_{12}: 500–1,000 µg given IM per irrespective of age and weight on alternate day for 2–3 weeks. This should be followed by 100–250 µg/dose IM every month till complete correction. Vitamin B_{12} orally is not universally effective due to poor patient compliance and erratic absorption.

Treatment alone with folate can produce hematologic response but does not correct neurological impairment.

Response to Therapy

Symptomatic response in the form of alert-ness and improved appetite usually occurs in few days. Brisk reticulocytosis in a week along with normalization of LDH, homocysteine, and MMA occurs in 1 week. Normalization of hemoglobin takes at least 2 months.

SUGGESTED READING

1. Brandow Amanda M. Pallor and anemia. In: Kliegman RM, Lyepatricia S, Bordinibret J, Toth H, Basel D (eds). Nelson pediatric symptom based diagnosis, volume 3. USA: Elsevier; 2018. pp. 661-7.
2. Choudhary P. Iron deficiency anemia. In: Lokeshwar MR, Shah N, Agrawal B, Sachdeva A (eds). IAP Speciality Series on Hematology

and Oncology. Mumbai: Indian Academy of Pediatrics; 2006. pp. 28-35.
3. Cooper JD, Tersakjean M. Hematology and oncology. In: Zitellibasil J, Mcintire SC, Nowalk AJ (eds). Atlas of Pediatric Physical Diagnosis, volume 2. USA: Elsevier; 2018. pp. 419-21.
4. Schendurnikar N. Nutritional anemia in infancy and childhood. Parthsarathy A, Menon PSN, Nair MKC (eds). IAP Textbook of Pediatrics. Mumbai: Indian Academy of Pediatrics; 2019. pp. 869-73.
5. Sills RH, Deters A. Macrocytic anemia: Red cell disorders. In: Silla RH, Albany NY (eds). Practical Algorithms in Pediatric Hematology and Oncology. Basel: Karger; 2003. pp. 10.
6. Sills R. Iron deficiency anemia In: Kliegman RM, St. Geme J. (eds). Nelson Textbook of Pediatrics, Volume 2. USA: Elsevier; 201. pp. 2323-6.

Sickle Cell Disorders

Jyotish Patel

INTRODUCTION

Sickle cell anemia is a common and complex inherited blood disorder affecting Hb structure. After first case report of sickle cell in the year 1910, sickle cell anemia is documented as a common most genetically inherited blood disorder. With high prevalence in Africa, America, Europe, Asia and less in other parts of the World, even today every child born has variable lifespan due to many reasons. The mutations Benin, Bantu, Senegal, and Asian haplotypes were reported years before. Every country affected, reports variable prevalence rates from 0 to 35%. Sickle cell anemia is autosomal recessive disorder. Sickle cell trait (SCT) is a heterozygous and *sickle cell disease* (SCD) is a homozygous state. In SCT, one of parents inherit *Sickle* gene while in SCD both inherit *Sickle* gene to child. There is a chance to have double heterozygous state in sickle cell hemoglobinopathy such as S Bet a0/+ thalassemia, SHbD Punjab, and SHbE thalassemia. The sickle cell anemia has been coded as "ICD-10-CM code", by International classification of diseases, under which various sickle cell disorders and combinations are classified and allotted codes **(Box 1)**.

BOX 1: ICD classification.

ICD-10-CM code:
- D57 Sickle cell disorders
- D57.00 Hb-SS disease with crisis, unspecified
- D57.01 Hb-SS disease with acute chest syndrome
- D57.02 Hb-SS disease with splenic sequestration
- D57.1 Sickle-cell disease without crisis
- D57.2 Sickle-cell/Hb-C disease
- D57.20 Sickle-cell/Hb-C disease without crisis
- D57.21 Sickle-cell/Hb-C disease with crisis
- D57.3 Sickle-cell trait
- D57.4 Sickle-cell thalassemia
- D57.40 Sickle-cell thalassemia without crisis
- D57.41 Sickle-cell thalassemia with crisis
- D57.8 Other sickle-cell disorders
- D57.80 Other sickle-cell disorders without crisis
- D57.81 Other sickle

(ICD: International Classification of Diseases)

CLINICAL FEATURES

Sickle Cell Trait (Heterozygous)

Sickle cell trait individuals represent a carrier state and do not require any treatment. Usually they are diagnosed as a population screening for sickle cell or as a parental study of affected case of SCD. If they become symptomatic, the clinician must try and search for other causes than to attribute it to SCT. SCT cases have urinary tract infection as a common morbidity for which necessary investigations and management should be done. Rarely, in a severe hypoxic state, SCT individual can have manifestations of painful crisis. The clinical signs such as pallor, jaundice, and splenomegaly are not found in SCT. The Hb level is normal but if found low than it is to be investigated for nutritional deficiency or other causes. SCT individuals are to be considered as a healthy person of society and must not have any social stigma attached. On the contrary, they have added advantage of relative resistance to *Plasmodium falciparum* malaria than normal and SCD individual. They can marry to a person who is not a carrier for sickle cell, i.e., HbS or other hemoglobinopathy such as beta-thalassemia trait, HbD Trait, HbE Trait. SCT individuals can be given medicine as per need and no drug is contraindicated.

Sickle Cell Disease (Homozygous or Double Heterozygous)

Sickle cell disease case demands treatment on daily basis as well as during symptomatic period. Such cases can manifest early before 1-year age to late at age 20s/30s/40s or even beyond 50s. Pain is the most common symptom located in upper or lower limbs (one side or both sides). This pain is constant in nature and increases in intensity during night disturbing sleep. If untreated, pain intensity increases and spread to areas such as chest, abdomen, back, hip, and head. A sudden change in a stable case of SCD is termed as *sickle cell crisis*.

The reason for such episode could be sudden change in weather, physical or mental stress, and bacterial-viral-malarial infection. Every symptom needs thorough evaluation and treatment. On examination, pallor and jaundice are common in majority. Such cases have increased size of spleen except case with autosplenectomy and

TABLE 1: Types of sickle cell crisis.

Crisis	Symptom	Sign	Investigation
Painful crisis	• Pain • Fever+/−	• *Pain score*: 3 to 10/10 • Tachycardia or bradycardia • Spleen same or decreased in size	• CBC • CRP • Reticulocyte count • Chest PA view • Blood C/S to judge precipitating factor
Sequestration crisis	• Pain in abdomen • Vomiting • Nausea • Cold skin	• Tachycardia • Low BP • Low temperature • SpO_2: Low • Pallor++++ • Jaundice ++ • *Spleen size*: Increased • *Liver size*: Increased	• Fall in Hb >1.5 g% • *Reticulocyte count*: Raised • *USG abdomen*: Markedly increased spleen size and liver size
Acute chest syndrome	• Chest pain • Difficulty in breathing • Coughing • Increased pain intensity	• Fall in SpO_2 • Increased respiratory rate • RS: Crepitation and rhonchi	• Chest X-ray s/o • Pulmonary edema and/or Pneumonia—Echo s/o • Pulmonary HT and tricuspid regurgitation • Blood gas s/o hypoxia with acidosis
Hemolytic crisis	• Fatigue • Pallor • Deep jaundice • Red-color or dark urine	• Pallor++++ • Jaundice++ • Spleen+++/− • Liver++	• Declining Hb • High normoblast count • Peripheral smear shows sickle cells, fragmented RBCs • High reticulocyte count • High indirect serum bilirubin
Aplastic crisis	• Fatigue • Pallor • Fever+/−	• Pallor+++ • Jaundice++ • Spleen+/−	• Repeated fall in Hb even after blood transfusion • High indirect serum bilirubin • Low reticulocyte count • *Test for Parvovirus*: Positive

(BP: blood pressure; CBC: complete blood count; CRP: C-reactive protein; C/S: culture and sensitivity; Echo: echocardiography; Hb: hemoglobin; HT: hypertension; PA: posteroanterior; RBC: red blood cells; RS: respiratory sounds; USG: ultrasonography)

occasionally increased size of liver. The examination finding depends on type of sickle cell crisis patient has. Fever, abdomen tightness, distension of abdomen, swelling in left side of abdomen, chest pain, difficulty in breathing, deep yellow eyes, pallor, fatigue, nausea, vomiting, difficulty in walking, perioral altered sensation, loose teeth with painful jaw, swelling of bone and joints anywhere in body, sudden cough, cold extremities, and red urine are various symptoms with which sickle cell crisis patient presents.

Along with different clinical features and investigation, types of sickle cell crisis are described; **Table 1** lists clinical features and relevant investigation.

APPROACH TO A CASE OF SICKLE CELL CRISIS

Any stable case of SCD, which suddenly becomes symptomatic, demands an urgent attention and action. This should be considered a case of sickle cell crisis. Such situation arises due to precipitating factors such as sudden change in weather, physical or mental stress and bacterial-viral-malarial infection. During sickle cell crisis, patient is in discomfort with altered vital signs and change in stable laboratory parameters. With clinical evidence and laboratory parameters, type of sickle cell crisis can be defined **(Table 1)**. The internal process of sickle cell crisis is too complex and just not sickling of red blood cells (RBCs). There is interplay of precipitating factor, ongoing RBCs sickling and its interaction with WBCs-platelet-endothelium of vessel. A patient presented as one type of sickle cell crisis can progress or change to other type or combination type of sickle cell crisis, e.g., painful crisis case progress and start manifestations of acute chest syndrome. Such a change could be sudden and critical in few minutes demanding high-end intensive care unit (ICU) care equipped with well-experienced sickle cell ICU care team. Such ICU should be equipped with ventilators, central medical gas pipeline, portable X-ray, in-house CT scan and echocardiography, blood gas analyzer, central monitoring system. Such patients occasionally demand surgical, neurosurgical or obstetric management for splenectomy-cholecystectomy-laparotomy, intracranial hemorrhage and difficult delivery of baby, respectively.

As suggested shown in **Table 1**, type of sickle cell crisis can be differentiated as below:
- *Painful crisis* has pain as a major symptom.
- *Sequestration crisis* has signs of shock with sudden fall in Hb, which could be 1.5 g% or more. Splenic sequestration is common with increase in size of spleen, but hepatic sequestration is not uncommon.
- *Acute chest syndrome* case predominates with fall in oxygen saturation, increasing respiratory rate, crepitation plus rhonchi; X-ray chest suggests evidence of pneumonia or pulmonary edema; echocardiography suggests tricuspid regurgitation with pulmonary arterial hypertension.
- *Hemolytic crisis* has pallor and jaundice with fall in Hb and rise in indirect serum bilirubin and reticulocyte count.
- *Aplastic crisis* has evidence of recurrent fall in Hb level with low reticulocyte count suggestive of bone marrow suppression. Such cases have evidence of parvovirus infection with raised IgM level.

Appropriate laboratory test should be carried out on emergency basis. The report of complete blood count (CBC) should be available in *less than 30-minute time* to decide on urgent need of blood transfusion (BT). A treating doctor must insist on availability of CBC report within 30 minutes. If there is a limitation, then patient should be sent to a place where such facility is available.

After admission, patient may show constant and steady improvement or may not. At times, the patient becomes more critical. Repeated clinical examination with repeat investigations would help in early detection of most dreadful complication, namely acute chest syndrome, intracranial hemorrhage, and sequestration. There should be a faster communication about clinical data and investigation data with repeated re-evaluation of critical case to decide on ongoing treatment plan, required change in treatment and seeing response.

Sickle cell crisis requires more monitoring than a critical cardiac case because it is a multivessel systematic disease affecting every organ of body.

TREATMENT APPROACH

The principle of management is mentioned which can be used as per clinical status and type of sickle cell crisis. Majority patients would become stable in 72-96 hours. In case patient is not showing desired response to treatment, then rethink about factors responsible and revise treatment plan.

Pain Management

The most common symptom demands recurrent medicine throughout life. Pain is a subjective feeling. Pain score evaluation is a supportive guide to actual pain experienced but believes in patient complain and chooses medicine which are beneficial, less harmful, and nonaddictive.

Analgesic
For Mild Pain
- Paracetamol is safe and effective.
- *Dose*: 5 mg/kg/dose can be given every 4-6 hours for 3-5 days.
- *Adult dose*: 500 mg qid.
- Oral preparations are preferred than injection because they are equally effective.

For Moderate Pain
- *Codeine dose*: 0.5-1.0 mg/kg/dose can be repeated at 4-6-hour interval.
- *Adult dose*: 15-60 mg PO q4-6 h PRN; not to exceed 360 mg/day in naïve patients to be given alone or with paracetamol.
- Both drugs can be given alternatively at 3-hour interval for best analgesic effect.
- *Nonsteroidal anti-inflammatory drugs (NSAID)*: Ibuprofen (Dose: 5-10 mg/kg orally every 6-8 hours as needed; Maximum dose: 40 mg/kg/day or 4 doses per day Adult dose: 200-400 mg 6-8 hours) can be an alternative as a single or as combination with paracetamol. Another NSAID Ketorolac (Dose: 0.5 mg/kg 6 hourly oral, IM or IV maximum dose in adult: 60 mg/day) can be given. It is a well-tolerated safe analgesic agent which be given for 5 days maximum.

For Severe Pain
This is a real challenge. Patient is restless with constant pain and needs relief earliest. Such pain needs expertise and frequent assessment to judge efficacy of selected regimen. Such pain needs multiple drugs round the clock to achieve adequate analgesic effect covering 24 hours.
- *Regimen 1*: Ketorolac plus paracetamol
- *Regimen 2*: Ketorolac plus paracetamol plus buvalor patch (5 mg or 10 mg)
- *Regimen 3*: Ketorolac plus buvalor patch (5 mg or 10 mg)
- *Regimen 4*: Tramadol plus paracetamol
- *Regimen 5*: Tramadol plus paracetamol plus carbamazepine/eptoin

The response to regimen differs from case to case. *A pain intensity of sickle cell crisis is most severe human* can experience. After patient is controlled with a selected regimen, it must be given for 5 days. Such cases may need other analgesic for next 5 days, which is given orally.

Apart from drug mentioned, to achieve optimum analgesia, the patient needs adjuvants from antihistaminic, antiepileptic, antidepressant group of drugs. Such combinations are used more frequently now.

Withdrawal of drug must not be sudden. It should be one by one depending on clinical response and need of a case.

Fluid and Electrolyte

Oral intake of fluids must be encouraged to maintain proper hydration. In case of dehydration intravenous fluid is given. The precision in judgment of hydration is mandatory. One of serious complications of inadvertent use of intravenous fluid is precipitation of acute chest syndrome. It is desired that every case of sickle cell crisis be monitored with inferior vena cava (IVC) collapse study by echocardiography to judge on fluid requirement. On the contrary, diuretics are indicated if s/o volume overload like <50% IVC collapse or tricuspid regurgitation or pulmonary hypertension. Isotonic fluid is to be selected whenever needed. 5% dextrose and 0.45% dextrose saline are preferred isotonic solution. Use of other intravenous fluids to be decided on electrolyte studies. Sodium bicarbonate is to be given only if there is deficit. The routine use of oral or intravenous sodium bicarbonate is no more recommended.

Oxygen

Use of pulse oximeter is routine now, oxygen saturation > 95% is normal. 3% decline in oxygen saturation is to be considered as significant fall and needs oxygen therapy. It is important to maintain patients' baseline oxygen saturation level by giving adequate oxygen. Allowing hypoxia to manifest in form of respiratory distress is late and allow patient to become more critical.

Antibiotics-Antivirals-Antimalarials

Sickle cell disease cases are prone to infection including malaria. Based on clinical features and investigation, antibiotics-antivirals-antimalarial drugs are given orally or parenterally.

Antibiotics: In India, community-acquired bacterial infection is common.

Antibiotics indicated, if total leucocyte count and C-reactive protein are raised with neutrophilia >80%.

Choice of antibiotics:
- Amoxycillin-clavulanic combination, cefixime, azithromycin can be first-line oral antibiotics.
- Ceftriaxone and amoxycillin-clavulanic combination with amikacin can be first-line parental antibiotics.

Depending on clinical response and blood culture report, change in antibiotics can be done.

Antiviral drug: Chicken pox and herpes zoster are common viral infection encountered. Oral or parenteral acyclovir is to be given.
- *Antimalarial drug:* Malaria is a vital cause of fever and sickle cell crisis. As mentioned earlier, only SCT individuals are partially protected against *Plasmodium falciparum* and not SCD. Due to *P. vivax* or *P. falciparum* malaria, SCD cases have significant fall in Hb level. All cases of fever and SCD give full course of oral chloroquine or lumefantrine. Depending on clinical status, early choice of injection artesunate must be done. Please do not wait for positive rapid diagnostic test (RDT) or positive slides (PS) for malarial parasite (MP), such tests have many limitations. In case of *P. vivax*, radical cure with primaquine must be done. Get test for G6PD before starting primaquine.

Blood Transfusion

Like beta-thalassemia major, SCD case does not require regular BT. There are specific indications of BT, especially during sickle cell crisis. Decision of BT often depends on stable-state Hb of patient. *Stable-state Hb differs in every case of SCD. It may vary low as 4 g% to high as 11 g%. At this level of Hb, patient is stable and asymptomatic.*

If fall in Hb is >1.5 g% then BT is considered. If fall in Hb is <1.5 g% and patient have tachycardia without fever and oxygen saturation is falling then also BT is to be given. In acute chest syndrome and intracranial hemorrhage, consider partial exchange BT.

IMMUNIZATION

As per the National Immunization Program of India, additional typhoid, pneumococcal, and meningococcal vaccines are be given.

MONITORING DURING SICKLE CELL CRISIS

Such cases need careful monitoring for early detection of serious complication such as intracranial hemorrhage, acute chest syndrome, and multiorgan failure.

Clinical monitoring supported by laboratory and radiology investigation is most important. Every symptom, sign, or investigations have significance. Why there is sudden fall in Hb? Why there is sudden breathlessness? Why there is sudden change in sensorium? Why fall in SpO_2 occurs? Why there is persistence of fever? Why there is tachycardia? The key is constant monitoring and answering question one by one. Frequent assessment will help to define the cause, which inturn demands redefining of treatment.

MORTALITY

With better understanding and facility of specialized center of excellence for sickle cell treatment, survival is increasing, and mortality is decreasing. Multiorgan dysfunction syndrome, acute chest syndrome, and intracranial hemorrhage are the leading causes of mortality.

DISCLAIMER

The views expressed are based on scientific data and work experience of managing sickle cell cases over 35 years. These are guidelines, which need to be utilized and modified as per clinical status of every case the doctor manages.

SUGGESTED READING

1. Brandow AM, DeBaun MR. Key components of pain management for children and adults with sickle cell disease. Hematol Oncol Clin North Am. 2018;32(3):535-50.

Thalassemia

Sunil Bhat

INTRODUCTION

Definition and Type

Thalassemia is group of blood disorders characterized by absent or decreased synthesis of normal globin chains. They are called α-, β-, γ-, δ-, δβ-, or εγδβ-thalassemias based on which globin chain synthesis is abnormal. Most thalassemias are inherited as recessive disorders. Phenotypically thalassemia syndromes are classified into *nontransfusion-dependent thalassemia (NTDT)* and *trans-fusion-dependent thalassemia (TDT)* based on transfusion requirement and clinical severity **(Fig. 1)**. TDT is also called *Thalassemia Major*.

From the clinical point of view, α- and β-thalassemias are the most relevant types which result from the impaired production of one or two types of polypeptide chains that form the normal adult human hemoglobin molecule (HbA, α2β2). In this chapter, the focus will mainly be on β-thalassemia.

PATHOPHYSIOLOGY

β-thalassemia refers to decreased or absent production of β-globin chains with relative excess of α-chains. This leads to decrease of hemoglobin production and an imbalance in the globin chain synthesis which leads to ineffective erythropoiesis.

DIAGNOSIS

Clinical Diagnosis

- β-thalassemia major should be suspected in any child <2 years of age with clinical findings of anemia, jaundice, hepatosplenomegaly, failure to thrive, and hemolytic facies.
- β-thalassemia intermedia should be suspected in individuals who present at a later age, mostly after 2 years of age.
- β-thalassemia minor/trait/carrier is clinically asymptomatic.

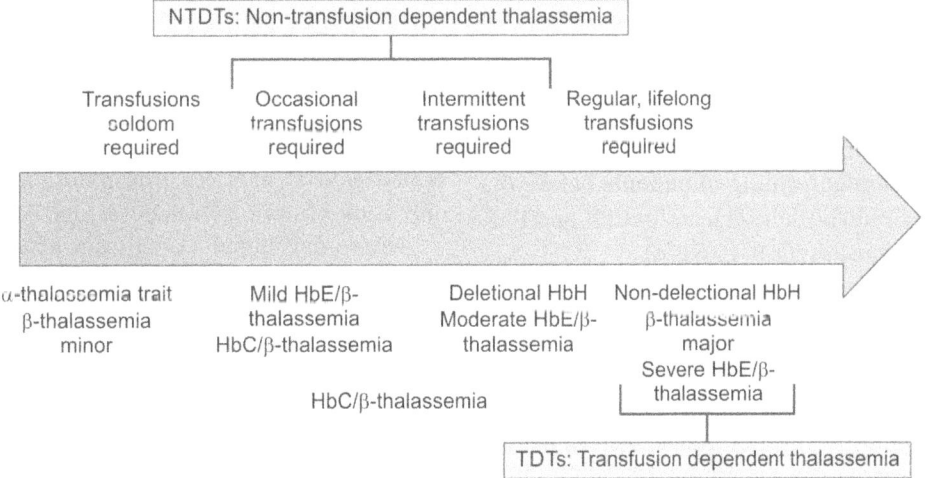

Fig. 1: Spectrum of thalassemia syndromes.

(Hb: hemoglobin)
Source: Cappellini MD, Cohen A, Porter J, Taher A, Viprakasit V. Guidelines for the management of transfusion dependent thalassemia (TDT), 3rd edition. Nicosia (CY): Thalassaemia International Federation; 2014.

Laboratory Investigations (Table 1)

TABLE 1: Laboratory investigations to diagnose thalassemia.

Complete blood count	Hemoglobin (Hb) low, low MCV (mean corpuscular volume) and MCH (mean corpuscular hemoglobin) red blood cell count is increased
Peripheral smear examination	Microcytic hypochromic anemia with polychromasia, target cells and anisopoikilocytosis, inclusion bodies/HbH: α-thalassemia
Reticulocyte count	Increased
Liver function test	Indirect hyperbilirubinemia
Qualitative and quantitative hemoglobin analysis	To identify the amount and type of hemoglobin present
High-pressure liquid chromatography (HPLC) or cellulose acetate electrophoresis or capillary Electrophoresis (CE) and DE-52 microchromatography	Hb A2 ≥4%, normal HbA, HBF: β-thalassemia trait • *High HbF, low HbA*: β-thalassemia disease Hb A2 ≥4%, HbF <1%: Possible α-thalassemia trait Hb A2 ≥4%, HbF <5–25% ± Hb • *CS/PS*: HbH disease + other Hb variants: Hb E, Hb C, Hb S disorders and others
Molecular/genetic analysis	DNA analysis of α and β globin mutations by PCR-based techniques
Antenatal diagnosis	• Chorionic villus sampling amniocentesis • Fetal blood sampling • Preimplantation genetic diagnosis

MANAGEMENT

Main goals in management are:
- Correction of anemia with blood transfusion
- *Removal of excess iron*: Chelation therapy
- Management of complications
- Pharmacological methods to increase gamma-chain synthesis.

Blood transfusion: To correct anemia and suppress erythropoiesis, basic principles of transfusion are as follows:
- Packed red blood cell (RBC) transfusion.
- Leukodepleted and nucleic acid testing (NAT)-tested blood transfusion.
- ABO, Rh (D)-compatible blood. Matching for C, E, and Kell antigen is highly recommended.
- Extended red cell antigen typing of patients before the first transfusion should be done at least for C, E, and Kell.
- *To keep the pretransfusion Hb*: 9–10.5 g/dL.

Iron chelation: Iron overload occurs as a result of RBC transfusions or increased absorption of iron through the gastrointestinal tract. Iron accumulation is toxic to many tissues in the body causing hepatic, cardiac, growth retardation, and multiple endocrinopathies. Chelation therapy balances the rate of iron accumulation from blood transfusion by increasing iron excretion in urine and or faeces with chelator. Most of the times chelation drugs are used in combination **(Table 2)**.

Fetal hemoglobin inducers:
- Decreases the α- and β-imbalance
- *DNA methylation inhibitors*: 5-Azacitidine and decitabine
- Hydroxyurea
- Erythropoietin-stimulating and other agents, e.g., thalidomide
- *Others*: Short-chain fatty acids.

Splenectomy:
- *Indications in thalassemia major*:
  - Hypersplenism
  - Increased blood requirement that prevents adequate control with iron chelation therapy
  - Symptomatic splenomegaly.

Treatment of complications: Based on the complications-associated treatment, e.g., hypothyroidism can be treated with thyroxine supplement.

Hematopoietic stem cell transplantation: This remains the only curative option for thalassemia.

Pesaro developed a prognostic scheme to predict transplant outcomes in patients younger than 17 years of age (Lucarelli 1993, Lucarelli 1990). These prognostic adverse risk factors were as follows:
1. Lifetime quality of chelation received prior to transplantation (regular vs nonregular).
2. Hepatomegaly (defined as more than 2 cm below the costal margin).
3. Presence of liver fibrosis pretransplant, by hepatic biopsy examination.

- Class 1: No adverse risk factors.
- Class 2: 1 to 2 adverse risk factors.
- Class 3: Exhibits all 3 adverse factors.

TABLE 2: The pharmacological properties of the three chelators.

Compound	Desferrioxamine (DFO)	Deferasirox (DFX)	Deferiprone (DFP)
Stoichiometry	Hexadentate (1:1)	Tridentate (2:1)	Bidentate (3:1)
Route of administration	Subcutaneous/intravenous	Oral	Oral
Dosage	30–60 mg/kg/day (over 8–12 hours) × 5–7 days, every week	20–40 mg/kg/day once a day	75–100 mg/kg/day in three divided doses
Half-life of iron-free drug	2–3 minutes	12–16 hours	3–4 hours
Excretion	Urinary and fecal	Fecal	Urinary
Adverse effect	Auditory, ocular, bone growth retardation, reactions at infusion site, *Yersinia* infection	Gastrointestinal (GI) disturbances, increase in creatinine and liver enzymes	GI disturbances, arthralgia, agranulocytosis/neutropenia

TABLE 3: Monitoring a child with thalassemia.

Timeline	Clinical and laboratory evaluation
At each transfusion	CBC, fasting blood sugar
Every 3 months	*Growth assessment*: Height and weight serum ferritin, AST, ALT, GGT, bilirubin level, albumin serum creatinine, urea calcium, ionized calcium, fasting blood sugar
Every 6 months	Growth velocity, Tanners staging, urine analysis, zinc level, vitamin D level
Every 12 months	• Bone age assessment • Audiology, ophthalmology, and dental examination • Hepatitis A, B, C serology testing • Liver iron • T2 MRI of liver and heart (from age of 8 years) USG liver • Glucose tolerance test (perform annually after the age of 10 years) • Free T4, TSH • ECG, 2D ECHO
Delay in puberty: 12 years for girl, and 14 years for boys	• Estradiol FSH • LH • IGF 1, IGF BP 3

(AST: aspartate aminotransferase; ALT: alanine transaminase; 2D ECHO: two-dimensional echocardiography; ECG: electrocardiography; GGT: gamma-glutamyl transferase; T2 MRI: T2-weighted magnetic resonance imaging; T4: thyroxine; TSH: thyroid-stimulating hormone; USG: ultrasonography)

Gene therapy by autologous transplantation of genetically modified stem cells represents a novel therapeutic approach. The goal of gene therapy is to achieve introduction of functional globin genes into the patient's own stem cells in order to correct hemolytic anemia and ineffective erythropoiesis, thus obviating the need for transfusion.

- Genetic counseling
- Long-term follow-up is essential in a patient of thalassemia and the timeline for monitoring is shown in **Table 3**.

New Approaches

Luspatercept-aamt is an erythroid maturation agent. The Food and Drug Administration (FDA) has approved this drug in 2019. This is indicated for the treatment of anemia in adult patients with β-thalassemia who require regular RBC transfusions. This drug seems to reduce the RBC transfusion burden in these patients.

KEY MESSAGES

- Thalassemia is genetic disorder and hence genetic counseling plays an important part of management.
- Complete blood count, Hb analysis, and mutational studies are important tests to diagnose thalassemia.
- RBC transfusion and iron chelation are the basis for treatment of thalassemia.
- Pretransfusion Hb should be 9–10.5 g/dL.
- Packed RBC should be leukodepleted, NAT tested and ABO, Rh, and other minor blood group compatible.
- Most of the chelating agents are used in combination.
- Hematopoietic stem cell transplant is the only curative option at present.

SUGGESTED READING

1. Cappellini MD, Cohen A, Porter J, Taher A, Viprakasit V. Guidelines for the management of transfusion dependent thalassemia (TDT), 3rd edition. Nicosia (CY): Thalassaemia International Federation; 2014.
2. Taher A, Musallam K, Cappellini MD. Guidelines for the management for the non-transfusion dependent thalassemia (NTDT), 2nd edition. Nicosia (CY): Thalassaemia International Federation; 2017.

Aplastic Anemia in Children

Sunil Jondhale

INTRODUCTION

- Hemoglobin is important blood component which carries oxygen and nutrients to tissues. Hemoglobin level in children varies with age. Anemia is defined as a hemoglobin level of less than the 5th percentile for age. Anemia may result from blood loss, a destructive process (ie, hemolysis), nutritional deficiency, or poor production (eg, ineffective erythropoiesis or hypoplastic or aplastic marrow).
- Anemia caused by suppression of bone marrow, either due to congenital bone marrow failure syndrome or acquired causes, is called aplastic anemia (AA).
- Acquired AA has to be distinguished from inherited bone marrow failure syndromes (IBMFS) and from hypoplastic myelodysplastic syndrome (MDS). Distinguishing between acquired AA and IBMFS can be difficult in patients with inherited conditions lacking classical congenital anomalies or in patients without a supporting family history.
- Aplastic anemia is characterized by low reticulocyte count and increased mean corpuscular volume (MCV).
- It encompasses peripheral blood single cytopenias as well as pancytopenia, due to inability of the bone marrow to effectively produce blood cells.
- Aplastic and hypoplastic anemias are characterized by impaired erythropoiesis due to decreased hematopoietic cells in the bone marrow.
- Acquired AA is a rare disorder with an incidence of about 2 per 1,000,000 children per year in North America and Europe and two- to threefold higher in Asia. The majority of these cases are categorized as idiopathic because their primary etiology is unknown.
- In 15–20% of patients, the disease is constitutional/inherited where it can present with one or more somatic abnormalities.
- At least 25% of childhood AA is on a background of known marrow failure genes; these patients must be identified since the inherited and acquired disorders differ significantly in treatment and prognoses.
- The earliest and most frequent life-threatening complication in Fanconi anemia (FA) (reported in approximately 90%) is AA, with usual onset in childhood, manifest by thrombocytopenia, neutropenia, and macrocytic anemia, and associated with a hypocellular fatty bone marrow with decreased myeloid and erythroid precursors and megakaryocytes.

PATHOGENESIS

- Aplastic anemias are characterized by impaired erythropoiesis due to decreased hematopoietic cells in the bone marrow.
- An immune-mediated pathogenesis has been postulated for AA because immunosuppressive therapy (IST) is often successful in the treatment of AA and bone marrow lymphocytes from AA patients can suppress normal bone marrow *in vitro*.
- Acquired conditions may include parvovirus infection of erythrocyte precursors or T-cell-mediated destruction of hematopoietic cells in acquired AA.
- Inherited defects in marrow function can present at any point throughout the life span with progressive anemia.
- The diagnosis of acquired AA also requires the exclusion of other conditions associated with pancytopenia.

ETIOLOGY

In large number of cases of AA, no cause could be identified and it is assumed to be immune mediated. Only in few cases, specific underlying cause could be demonstrated. AA causes include congenital or acquired.

Causes of predominant red cell aplasia are:
- Inherited conditions
- Diamond–Blackfan anemia (pure red cell aplasia)
  - Congenital dyserythropoietic anemia
  - Pearson syndrome
  - Congenital sideroblastic anemias
- *Acquired*:
  - Idiopathic
  - Transient erythroblastopenia of childhood (TEC)

- Infection—parvovirus B19 infection in immunodeficiency patients (chronic bone marrow failure).

Aplastic anemia associated with physical or other hematologic anomalies of the other cell lines are called complex AA) include following conditions:
- *Inherited AA syndromes*:
  - Fanconi anemia
  - Shwachman-Diamond syndrome (SDS)
  - Diamond-Blackfan syndrome
  - Dyskeratosis congenita
  - Other rare genetic disorders
- *Acquired*:
  - Unknown etiology (?Immune mediated)
  - *Infections*: Hepatitis B surface antigen (HBsAg), human immunodeficiency virus (HIV), cytomegalovirus (CMV), Epstein-Barr virus (EBV), varicella, *Mycoplasma*, etc.
  - *Drugs*: Azathioprine, zidovudine, etc.
  - Autoimmune disorders
  - Paroxysmal nocturnal hemoglobinuria
- *Secondary*:
  - Drugs
  - Autoimmune neutropenia of infancy
  - Other autoimmune associated [systemic lupus erythematosus (ELE), etc.]
  - Exposure to radiations.

In majority of cases, causative agents/factors could not be demonstrated but if identified could help in prognosis and for management in some cases.

CLINICAL PRESENTATION

The clinical symptoms of acquired AA depend on the degree of cytopenia and on the time required for it to develop.
- Severe cytopenia may cause fever, bleeding, and life-threatening infections.
- Often these are young patients, otherwise healthy, sometimes with a preceding history of a recent febrile illness, and occasionally following an episode of elevated serum transaminases with or without cholestasis.
- Most children with AA present with signs and symptoms resulting from advanced pancytopenia, while others are diagnosed by incidental laboratory findings.
- Thrombocytopenia may manifest as easy bruising or petechiae. Epistaxis and menorrhagia in postmenarchal girls are other common complaints at presentation.
- Anemia may manifest as pallor, fatigue, or exercise intolerance.
- Neutropenia may predispose to infections and thus fever or focal signs of infection can occur as initial complaints.
- Hepatosplenomegaly and lymphadenopathy are typically absent.
- A history of jaundice often occurring 2-3 months prior to discovery of pancytopenia is consistent with hepatitis-associated AA.
- Infants and children with anemia may display irritability, poor feeding, or growth failure.

DIAGNOSIS AND INVESTIGATIONS

Aplastic anemia should be considered in a patient with two or more persistent cytopenias. The diagnostic criteria of acquired AA have been defined, and require an empty or hypoplastic marrow, with peripheral blood cytopenia.

Severity of AA is graded as given in **Table 1**.

Following investigations are required to establish diagnosis, identify etiology and management:
- *Complete blood count (CBC)*: Reveal anemia along with thrombocytopenia and/or neutropenia.
- *Reticulocyte %*: A normal or decreased reticulocyte count in the setting of anemia generally represents an inappropriate compensatory response and may be an indication of impaired erythropoiesis.
- *Peripheral blood smear*: Anemia is usually normocytic or macrocytic with decreased variable cell lines.
- Liver function tests, serum bilirubin, and lactate dehydrogenase (LDH)
- Vitamin B_{12} and folate level
- *Bone marrow examinations*: Bone marrow aspirate and biopsy are needed to establish the diagnosis marrow hypoplasia. Cellularity in the bone marrow biopsy need to be <25%. Absence of marrow dysplasia and reticulin increase rule out MDS.
- HIV, CMV, EBV, HBsAg, parvovirus serology, or polymerase chain reaction (PCR)
- Copper, ceruloplasmin, and zinc
- Cytogenetic studies including a karyotype and fluorescence In situ hybridization (FISH), and bone marrow cytogenetics.

TABLE 1: Severity of AA.

Nonsevere/moderate AA	• Hemoglobin level < 10 g/dL • ANC < 1,500/mL • Platelet count <50 × 10³/mL • ARC < 4 0 × 10³/mL • Bone marrow cellularity: 25–50%
Severe AA (SAA)	Bone marrow cellularity <25% and at least tw • Neutrophil count < 500 × 10⁶/L • Platelet count < 20,000 × 10⁶/L • Reticulocyte count < 60,000 × 10⁶/L
Very SAA	Fulfilling criteria for SAA plus: Neutrophil cou

(AA: aplastic anemia; ANC: absolute neutrophil count; ARC: absolute reticulocyte count)

- Human leukocyte antigen (HLA) typing for the patient and any full siblings to facilitate timely hematopoietic stem cell transplantation (HSCT) if the sibling is a match.
- Consider additional diagnostic and genetic testing for IBMFS if suspected.

Exclusion of inherited bone marrow failure syndromes (IBMFs):
- Clinical history, family history, and physical examination
- Chromosomal breakage studies in peripheral blood
- Telomere length measurement in peripheral blood
- Increased fetal hemoglobin (Hb) (several IBMFS)

DIFFERENTIAL DIAGNOSIS

There are wide variety of potential causes of bicytopenia or pancytopenia in children, hence, following differential diagnosis needs to be consider before labeling diagnosis of AA:
- Vitamin B_{12} deficiency
- Severe sepsis leading to transient myelosuppression
- *Viral infection with transient bone marrow suppression*: Viral and other infections may account for as many as 10–20% of children presenting with pancytopenia
- SLE
- Systemic-onset juvenile idiopathic arthritis (JIA)
- Hemophagocytic lymphohistiocytosis (HLH) secondary to infections or drug
- Paroxysmal nocturnal hemoglobinuria (PNH)
- Leukemia
- Myelodysplastic syndrome (MDS).

MANAGEMENT OF ACQUIRED APLASTIC ANEMIA

In the absence of significant bleeding or severe infection, nonsevere/moderate AA (NSAA) does not require treatment but need to be followed regularly for increase in severity and complications. For NSAA patients who show signs of progression, or who are transfusion dependent, IST is suggested as the first choice of treatment. Only severe or very severe AA need to be treated aggressively.

Supportive Care

- Blood transfusion required to maintain Hb > 8. Leukodepleted and irradiated blood products should be given to reduce the risk of transfusion associated graft-versus-host disease (GVHD) and HLA sensitization.
- Iron chelation is initiated for patients who remain transfusion dependent over a prolonged time period. Iron chelation is performed with deferoxamine or deferasirox.
- Platelet transfusions given for bleeding or when < 20,000 platelet. Transfusions should be considered to prevent bleeding in asymptomatic patients with platelet counts < 10,000/μL. Higher thresholds for platelet transfusions are reserved for patients with either active bleeding or a history of significant bleeding complications or in patients at risk for worsening thrombocytopenia.
- Treatment of febrile neutropenia and infections with appropriate antibiotics and antifungals as per prevalent microbial in region
- Granulocyte colony stimulating factor (G-CSF) use for patients with AA is controversial and should not be given routinely for treatment of AA. G-CSF is given when neutrophil counts < 500/μL in combination with IST. Prolonged use of high doses of G-CSF may increase the risk of clonal hematopoiesis and malignant transformation to MDS/acute myeloid leukemia (AML).
- *Prevention of infection by chemoprophylaxis, vaccinations, and maintaining good hygiene*: Use prophylactic antifungals for AA patients with prolonged (>7 days) neutrophil counts < 500/μL or for AA patients on IST. In AA patients with lymphopenia < 500/μL or those receiving IST also need *Pneumocystis jiroveci* pneumonia (PJP) prophylaxis. Three times weekly Trimethoprim/sulfamethoxazole (TMP/SMX) (cotrimoxazole) has been shown quite beneficial. Vaccination with use of inactivated vaccines can be done but until 1 year after the cessation of IST.
- Patients with AA needs to be monitored for bleeding, infections, malignancy, and drug side effects.

Once a diagnosis is firmly established, bone marrow transplantation (BMT) and IST are currently the primary treatment options for AA patients in children. Primary AA is treated with immunosuppression, with cyclosporine with or without corticosteroids achieving the most durable responses. Treatment of secondary AA is usually directed at the underlying etiology. IST with horse antithymocyte globulin and cyclosporine is the recommended first-line therapy for patients without an HLA-matched sibling donor. Survival rates are similar to BMT with a matched-sibling donor but relapse, clonal hematopoiesis, leukemia, autoimmunity, and cancer remain concerns that require long-term follow-up.

Immunosuppressive Therapy for Severe AA

Immunosuppressive therapy for AA is associated with response rate of 50–70% at 6 months, relapse rate about 20%, and survival up to 80% after 5–10 years **(Table 2)**.

Follow-up After IST

- CBC, reticulocyte counts, CRP, initially at least weekly
- CSA level, creatinine, liver enzymes, serum bilirubin, magnesium monitoring
- Transfusion support if hemoglobin < 8g/dl, platelets <10,000/mcl
- Close monitoring for infections, Autoimmune diseases and malignancy.
- Repeat bone marrow aspirate, biopsy and cytogenetics at 3 months and 12 months or at sustained worsening of cytopenia.

TABLE 2: IST protocol for AA.

Drug	Dose	Route	Schedule
Antithymocyte globulin (ATG)	40 mg/kg/day	IV	Day 1–4: Initial dose over 8–10 hours, subsequent doses over 6–8 hours
Cyclosporine	5–15 mg/kg/day divided in two doses	PO	• Starting on day 5: Target trough blood level 200–400 ng/mL • For 12 months after stable CR or PR: Then taper over 12 months
Methylprednisolone	1 or 2 mg/kg/day	IV/PO	• Day 1–5 before ATG infusion • Change to 1 mg/kg/day prednisone PO day 6–10, then individualize taper over 14 days
Granulocyte colony stimulating factor	Starting dose 3–5 µg/kg/daily		

(AA: aplastic anemia; CR: complete response; IST: immunosuppressive therapy; IV: intravenous; PO: per oral; PR: partial response)

Hematopoietic Stem Cell Transplantation

Various studies showed excellent survival after matched sibling-donor (MSD) HSCT with pediatric series showing disease-free survival rates ranging from 64% to 97%. Bone marrow transplantation (BMT) is the recommended first-line therapy for patients with an HLA-matched sibling donor, with 5-year survival rates exceeding 90%. BMT with an HLA-matched unrelated donor should be offered to all IST non responders early in the course of disease and may be considered as a first-line treatment in selected cases of Severe and very severe AA as the first-line therapy transfusion-dependent non-severe AA after failure of first-line IST (IST-1). Factors associated with favorable outcomes in children with AA undergone HSCT include young age, less transfusion history, no intervening therapy and a short interval from diagnosis to transplantation. But non availability of HSCT facility at most centre, cost and affordability remain limiting factors for same.

Response to IST or HSCT in AA is assessed by response complete, partial or no response defined as Complete Response (CR)
- Red blood cell and platelet transfusion independence
- Absolute neutrophil count >1,500 × 10^6/L
- Platelet count > 150,000 × 10^6/L.

Partial Response (PR)
- Improvement of cytopenia with absolute neutrophil count ≥500 × 10^6/L
- Platelets ≥20,000 × 10^6/L
- +/– Transfusion dependent

No response or relapse defined by same criteria as of original criteria of aplastic criteria.

Complications of Aplastic anemia
- Recurrent infections-in fact this is the commonest cause of mortality in AA
- Iron overload due to frequent blood transfusion
- Recurrent bleeding and occasionally severe bleed leading to death
- Malignancy like Myeloid leukemia
- Growth failure due to recurrent infection and severe anemia
- Endocrine disorder
- Auto immune disease
- Complications associated with IST
- Compilations related to HSCT like graft vs Host disease (GVHD) and secondary malignancy.

PROGNOSIS

- Advancement management of AA have been made in the care of children with AA, which is now associated with excellent overall survival upto 90%.
- Allogenic BMT offers the opportunity for cure in children if a suitable histo-compatible donor is available.
- Comparable long-term survival in SAA is achieved with IST.
- However, 25% of AA children will likely do not respond to primary IST and will require second-line therapy, 10–30% of responders will relapse, and there is an increased risk of leukemia, autoimmunity, and cancer that requires a long-term follow-up.
- With an increased understating of the pathogenesis of AA and its specific late manifestations targeted preventative strategies and more personalized treatment options are likely to further improve outcomes and decrease late complications in children with acquired AA.

SUGGESTED READING

1. Bacigalupo A, Passweg J. Diagnosis and treatment of acquired aplastic anemia. Hematol Oncol Clin N Am. 2009;23:159-70.
2. Blanche P. Alter. Bone marrow failure syndromes in children Pediatr Clin N Am. 2002;49:973-88.
3. ET Korthof et al. Management of acquired aplastic anemia in children. Bone Marrow Transplantation. 2013;48:191-5.
4. Hartung HD, Olson TS, Bessler M. Acquired aplastic anemia in children. Pediatr Clin North Am. 2013;60(6):1311-36.
5. Kurre P, Johnson FL, Deeg HJ. Diagnosis and treatment of children with aplastic anemia. Pediatr Blood Cancer. 2005;45(6):770-80.
6. Niemeyer C, Baumann I. Classification of childhood aplastic anemia and myelodysplastic syndrome. Hematol Am Soc Hematol Educ Program. 2011;2011:84-9.
7. Noronha SA. Aplastic and hypoplastic anemias. Pediatrics in Review. 2018;39;601.

CHAPTER 80

Leukemias in Children

Suman Mittal

INTRODUCTION

Leukemia is the most common malignancy of childhood, accounting for 30% of cases of childhood cancer. Although there are some associations between environmental or host factors, most leukemia diagnoses in children are sporadic. There are three main subtypes of leukemia: (1) Acute lymphoblastic leukemia (ALL), (2) acute myelogenous leukemia (AML), and (3) chronic myelogenous leukemia (CML). ALL is the most common subtype, accounting for approximately 80% of cases. CML is the least common, and this review touches on this subtype only briefly. There are many subgroups within ALL and AML.

SIGNS AND SYMPTOMS

Children with ALL often present with signs and symptoms that reflect bone marrow infiltration and/or extramedullary disease. When leukemic blasts replace the bone marrow, patients present with signs of bone marrow failure, including anemia, thrombocytopenia, and neutropenia.

Other presenting signs and symptoms of pediatric ALL include the following:

- *Patients with B-precursor ALL*: Bone pain, arthritis, and limping; fevers (low or high); neutropenia; fatigue, pallor, petechiae, and bleeding; lymphadenopathy; and hepatosplenomegaly.
- *Patients with mature-B ALL*: Extramedullary masses in the abdomen or head/neck; CNS involvement (e.g., headache, vomiting, lethargy, nuchal rigidity).
- *Patients with T-lineage ALL*: Respiratory distress/stridor due to a mediastinal mass.

Symptoms of central nervous system (CNS) involvement are rarely noted at initial diagnosis but are more common in T-lineage and mature B-cell ALL. Testicular involvement at diagnosis is also rare; if present, it appears as unilateral painless testicular enlargement.

DIAGNOSIS

Testing

Complete morphologic, immunologic, and genetic examination of the leukemic cells is necessary to establish the diagnosis of ALL.

- Routine laboratory studies in pediatric ALL include the following:
  - Complete blood count (CBC)
  - Peripheral blood smear
  - Serum chemistries (e.g., potassium, phosphorus, calcium)
  - Uric acid level
  - Lactate dehydrogenase (LDH) level
  - Coagulation studies such as prothrombin time (PT), activated partial thromboplastin time (aPTT), levels of fibrinogen and D-dimer.

Laboratory tests that help classify the type of ALL include the following:

- *Immunophenotyping*: To detect surface immunoglobulin on leukemic blasts (diagnosis of mature B-cell leukemia) or the expression of T-cell—associated surface antigens (diagnosis of T-lineage ALL).
- *Cytogenetic studies*: To identify specific genetic alterations in leukemic blasts.
- *Molecular studies [e.g., fluorescence in situ hybridization (FISH), reverse transcriptase-polymerase chain reaction (RT-PCR), Southern blot analysis]*: To identify translocations more rapidly and those not detected on routine karyotype analysis; to distinguish lesions that appear cytogenetically identical but are molecularly different.
- *Minimal residual disease studies*: To detect chimeric transcripts generated by fusion genes, detect clonal T-cell receptor (TCR) or immunoglobulin heavy-chain (*IgH*) gene rearrangements, or identify a phenotype specific to the leukemic blasts.
- *Genome-wide association studies*: To detect the presence of genetic changes where routine techniques are unhelpful (e.g., activated tyrosine kinase pathways in Ph-like ALL), not in clinical use yet.
- *Imaging studies*:
  - *Chest X-ray*: No other imaging studies other than chest radiography to evaluate for a mediastinal mass are routinely required in pediatric ALL. However, the following radiologic studies can be helpful:

- *Ultrasonography*: To evaluate for testicular infiltration in boys with enlarged testes; to evaluate for leukemic kidney involvement as a risk assessment for tumor lysis syndrome.
- *Echocardiogram (ECG)*: To identify any preexisting cardiac dysfunction before administration of anthracycline (baseline studies); to monitor heart function during treatment with anthracyclines.
■ *Procedures*:
  - *Lumbar puncture with cytospin morphologic analysis*: To assess for CNS involvement before administration of systemic chemotherapy and to administer intrathecal chemotherapy.
  - *Bone marrow aspiration and biopsy*: To confirm the diagnosis of ALL.

Central nervous system disease is divided into the following groups:
■ *CNS 1*: Absence of blasts on cere fluid (CSF) cytospin preparation, regardless of the WBC count.
■ *CNS 2*: WBC count of <5/mL and blasts on cytospin findings, or WBC count of >5/mL but negative by Steinherz-Bleyer algorithm findings (if traumatic tap).
■ *CNS 3*: WBC count of 5/mL or more and blasts on cytospin findings and/or clinical signs of CNS leukemia (e.g., facial nerve palsy, brain/eye involvement, hypothalamic syndrome).

MANAGEMENT

Leukemia is a systemic disease, and treatment is primarily based on chemotherapy. However, the different forms of ALL require different approaches for optimal results. Treatment of subclinical CNS leukemia is an essential component of ALL therapy.

Treatment for ALL typically consists of the following phases:
■ *Remission*: Induction phase (e.g., dexamethasone or prednisone, vincristine, asparaginase, daunorubicin).
■ *Intensification/consolidation phase*: The importance of this phase is undisputed, but consensus is scarce on the best regimens and duration of treatment. Current Children's Oncology Group (COG) ALL protocols use a therapeutic backbone that was originally introduced in Berlin-Frankfurt-Muenster (BFM) clinical trials in the 1980s. This includes administration of cytarabine, cyclophosphamide, dexamethasone, asparaginase, doxorubicin, methotrexate (MTX), 6-mercaptopurine (6-MP), 6-thioguanine, and vincristine.
■ The CNS-directed therapy consists of systemic chemotherapy that enters the CSF, as well as intrathecal chemotherapy administered throughout the entire course of treatment, which is primarily MTX but sometimes includes hydrocortisone and cytarabine ("triple-intrathecal therapy").
■ Continuation therapy targeted at eliminating residual disease (e.g., MTX, 6-MP, vincristine, and glucocorticoid pulses).

Pharmacotherapy

Medications used in the treatment of pediatric ALL include the following:
■ Antineoplastics (e.g., vincristine, asparaginase *Escherichia coli*, asparaginase *Erwinia chrysanthemi*, calaspargase pegol, daunorubicin, doxorubicin, MTX, 6-MP, cytarabine, cyclophosphamide, dasatinib, imatinib).
■ Corticosteroids (e.g., prednisone, dexamethasone).
■ Antimicrobials [e.g., Trimethoprim/sulfamethoxazole (TMX/SMP), pentamidine].
■ Antifungals (e.g., fluconazole).

Blood transfusions or antibiotics may be required to deal with complications of ALL therapy. Do not administer folate supplementation owing to interactions with MTX.

Other treatments involved in managing pediatric ALL may include the following:
■ *Initial administration of IV fluids*: Without potassium, with or without sodium bicarbonate.
■ *Cranial irradiation*: Effectively prevents overt CNS relapse but potentially causes neurotoxicity and brain tumors; largely replaced by intensive intrathecal and systemic chemotherapy.
■ *Allogeneic hematopoietic stem cell transplant (HSCT)*: Usually following second complete remission after relapse (if early) or first remission in high risk patients; potentially prevents relapse and/or mortality versus chemotherapy alone.

Acute Myeloid Leukemia

■ In general, treatment for AML uses higher doses of chemotherapy over a shorter period of time (usually less than a year).
■ Treatment of children with AML is divided into two main phases of chemotherapy: (1) Induction and (2) consolidation (intensification).
■ *Induction*: The chemotherapy drugs most often used to treat AML are daunorubicin (daunomycin) and cytarabine (ara-C), which are each given for several days in a row.
■ Consolidation (intensification) begins after the induction phase.
■ Maintenance chemo is not needed for children with AML.

Chronic Myeloid Leukemia

■ Chronic myeloid leukemia is typically a slower-growing cancer of early (immature) myeloid bone marrow cells.
■ CML is not common in children, but it can occur.

- CML does not have subtypes. Instead, the course of CML has three phases, based mainly on the number of immature white blood cells—myeloblasts (or blasts)—that are seen in the blood or bone marrow.
- CML can sometimes progress to more advanced phases over time.
- *Chronic phase of CML*: In this earliest phase, children usually have fairly mild symptoms (if any), and the leukemia usually responds well to standard treatments. Most children are in the chronic phase when they are diagnosed.
- Accelerated phase of CML children whose CML is in accelerated phase may have symptoms such as fever, night sweats, poor appetite, and weight loss. CML in the accelerated phase might not respond as well to treatment as CML in the chronic phase.
- *Blast phase (also called acute phase or blast crisis) of CML*: In this phase, the leukemia cells often spread to tissues and organs outside the bone marrow. Children with CML in this phase often have fever, poor appetite, and weight loss. At this point the CML acts much like an aggressive acute leukemia (AML or, less often, ALL).

SURVIVAL RATES FOR CHILDHOOD LEUKEMIAS

- *Acute lymphocytic leukemia*: The 5-year survival rate for children with ALL has greatly increased over time and is now about 90% overall. In general, children in lower-risk groups have a better outlook than those in higher risk groups.
- *Acute myelogenous leukemia*: The overall 5-year survival rate for children with AML has also increased over time, and is now in the range of 65–70%. However, survival rates vary depending on the subtype of AML and other factors.

CHAPTER 81: Lymphoma in Children

Vikas Goel

INTRODUCTION

Lymphoma consists of a diverse group of malignant neoplasms of the lymphoid tissues variously derived from B-cell progenitors, T-cell progenitors, mature B cells, or mature T cells. Broadly, they are classified as non-Hodgkin's and Hodgkin's. Of these two types, non-Hodgkin's lymphoma (NHL) is the more common lymphoma in children, and it occurs more frequently between the ages of 10 and 20 years than under 10 years. Hodgkin's lymphoma (HL) is rare in children under 5 years of age. In children under age 10 years, it is more common in boys than in girls.

PRESENTING SYMPTOMS AND SIGNS

- Common presenting symptoms and signs of lymphoma in children include lymphadenopathy, systemic complaints, and mediastinal mass. Results of cooperative group studies show that 80–85% of pediatric lymphoma patients present with only lymph node and/or splenic involvement (stage I to III). The remaining have liver, lung, or bone marrow involvement and are stage IV.
- *Lymphadenopathy*: Most children with lymphoma present with painless lymphadenopathy, usually cervical, supraclavicular, axillary, or, less often, inguinal. The affected lymph nodes typically feel rubbery and more firm than inflammatory adenopathy.
- *Mediastinal mass*: Up to 75% of children with lymphoma have a mediastinal mass on chest radiograph at the time of presentation. Bulky mediastinal disease may cause dysphagia, dyspnea, orthopnea, cough, stridor, or the superior vena cava syndrome.
- *Systemic symptoms*: Patients with lymphoma may present with nonspecific systemic symptoms including fatigue, anorexia, and weight loss. Fever (>38.0°C), drenching night sweats, and weight loss (≥10% loss within 6 months before diagnosis), classified as "B" symptoms, have important implications for staging and prognosis.
- *Other*: Hepatic and/or splenic enlargement may be present in patients with advanced-stage lymphoma. Rarely, patients present with autoimmune disorders such as autoimmune hemolytic anemia, thrombocytopenia, or neutropenia. Cases presenting with nephropathy have also been described.

DIAGNOSTIC EVALUATION

- A complete evaluation of patients with suspected lymphoma is mandatory before beginning treatment. The goal is to evaluate the extent of disease, which, in turn, determines the clinical and pathologic stage, treatment, and prognosis.
- *History*: The routine evaluation of a patient with suspected HL should include a complete history, with emphasis on constitutional symptoms such as fever, night sweats, weight loss as well as evidence of underlying immune deficiencies and familial cancer, including HL.
- *Physical examination*: A complete physical examination includes assessment of general health, measurement of height and weight, and documentation of the size and location of lymphadenopathy, and liver and spleen size. The tonsils, base of the tongue, and nasopharynx (i.e., Waldeyer's ring) must be included in this evaluation.
- *Imaging*: The goal of imaging is to define the extent of disease and guide tissue biopsy.

The following studies should be obtained:

- Chest radiograph (anteroposterior and lateral)
- 18-fluoro-2-deoxyglucose (FDG)-positron emission tomography (PET) scan

  PET scan is more sensitive for detecting both nodular and diffuse disease, and may be more sensitive than bone marrow biopsy in detecting bone marrow involvement.

- *Tissue biopsy*: The diagnosis of lymphoma is established by histologic examination, usually by excisional biopsy of an enlarged lymph node. Fine-needle aspirates do not provide adequate amounts of material for proper histologic classification. Bone marrow aspirate and biopsy are recommended to know the bone marrow involvement. Advances in diagnostic imaging and the use of systemic chemotherapy in all pediatric lymphoma treatment protocols have made routine staging laparotomy unnecessary.

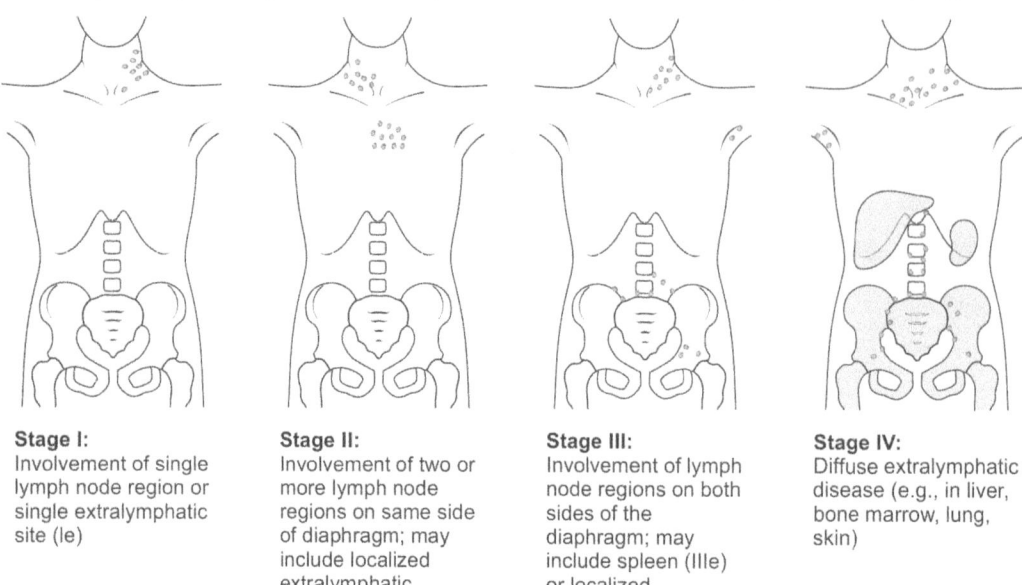

Stage I: Involvement of single lymph node region or single extralymphatic site (Ie)

Stage II: Involvement of two or more lymph node regions on same side of diaphragm; may include localized extralymphatic

Stage III: Involvement of lymph node regions on both sides of the diaphragm; may include spleen (IIIe) or localized

Stage IV: Diffuse extralymphatic disease (e.g., in liver, bone marrow, lung, skin)

Fig. 1: Ann Arbor staging.

LABORATORY EVALUATION

- Routine laboratory tests, including complete blood count with white blood cell differential and platelet count, erythrocyte sedimentation rate, renal and liver function tests, lactate dehydrogenase (LDH), and urinalysis, should be obtained.
- Although not routinely studied, patients who have a past medical history of recurrent infections, autoimmune and inflammatory disorders, disease occurrence in children younger than 5 years of age, or a family history of immune deficiency undergo a detailed immunologic evaluation.

STAGING

Therapy and prognosis are based upon the stage of the disease, as currently defined by the Ann Arbor staging system with Cotswolds modifications used both in children and adults (**Fig. 1**).

Ann Arbor Staging System with Cotswolds Modification

Additional substaging variables:
- A: Asymptomatic
- B: Presence of B symptoms (including fever, night sweats and weight loss of over 10% of body weight over 6 months)
- X: Bulky nodal disease: nodal mass >one third of intrathoracic diameter or 10 cm in dimension.

TREATMENT

Whenever possible, children with lymphoma should be treated in a comprehensive pedia-tric oncology center by a multidisciplinary team experienced in the diagnosis and care of children with cancer. Management of lymphoma depends on type and stage of the disease and it consist of combination chemotherapy and/or radiotherapy. Type of lymphoma and preferred chemotherapy regimens are as follows:

- *Hodgkin's lymphoma*: ABVD (adriamycin, bleomycin, vincristine, dacarbazine); ICE (ifosfamide, carboplatin, etoposide).
- *Non-Hodgkin's lymphoma*: CHOP [cyclophosphamide, adriamycin, oncovin (vincristine), Prednisolone] BR (bendamustine, rituximab).

PROGNOSIS

With latest therapy, prognosis has significantly improved for pediatric lymphoma such as children with HL have a 5-year survival of 94% since 2002 compared with an 81% survival in the early 1970s.

SUGGESTED READING

1. Adolescent non-Hodgkin lymphoma and Hodgkin lymphoma: state of the science. Br J Haematol. 2009;144(1):24-40.
2. Non-Hodgkin Lymphoma in Children. Curr Hematol Malig Rep 2015;10(3):237-43.

Immune Thrombocytopenia in Children

AK Ganju

INTRODUCTION

Immune thrombocytopenia (ITP), which was earlier called idiopathic thrombocytopenic purpura, is one of the most common hematologic disorders encountered by pediatricians. Its prevalence is approximately 8 per 1 lac children. It usually presents in an otherwise well child whose blood count is normal except for isolated but sometimes quite severe thrombocytopenia. ITP is an immune-mediated condition attributable to antibodies directed against platelet membrane antigens.

CLINICAL PRESENTATION

It commonly affects children between 1 and 7 years of age. Mean age was 5-7 years with peak incidence at 2-4 years of age in one study done by Kuhne. Most children with ITP develop sudden onset petechiae, bruises, and sometimes mucous membrane bleeding often preceded by history of infection or vaccination. Intracranial hemorrhage (ICH) is the most serious consequence of thrombocytopenia; but is fortunately a rare complication of ITP in children, with reported rates ranging from 0.1 to 0.8%. In majority of the patients it runs a benign, self-limiting course, with or without treatment. Complete remission occurs within 6 months from diagnosis and commonly within 6-12 weeks.

However, 20-30% of children will continue to have persistent low platelets count with bleeding symptoms beyond 6 months from diagnosis.

PATHOPHYSIOLOGY

Studies on pathogenesis of ITP are largely done in adult patients; there is less information available specifically on ITP in children.

In ITP, usually immunoglobulin G (IgG) autoantibodies are directed against platelet membrane antigens, such as the glycoprotein (GP) IIb/IIIa complex, GP Ib/IX, GP Ia/IIa, and GP VI. The antibody-coated platelets are cleared by tissue macrophages, predominantly those in the spleen. These antibodies may inhibit platelet production too. The net effect is shortened platelet survival and decreased platelet count.

Only 60% of children have detectable antiplatelet antibodies and hence measurement of antiplatelet antibodies is not helpful and moreover the test is not sensitive nor specific.

In some patients, there may be alternative immunologic mechanism of T-cell-mediated cytotoxicity. Mechanisms rupturing self-tolerance also appear to be active.

TERMINOLOGY

Immune thrombocytopenia can be:
- *Primary ITP*: ITP in the absence of other causes or disorders.
- *Secondary ITP*: It is immune-mediated thrombocytopenia with an underlying cause, including connective tissue disorders, drugs or associated with systemic illness {e.g., infection [hepatitis C virus (HCV), HBV, *Helicobacter pylori*, and human immunodeficiency virus (HIV)], and other causes} such as vaccination [measles, mumps, and rubella (MMR)].

Primary ITP is categorized into three phases, depending on the duration of the disease course:
1. Newly diagnosed ITP—<3 months of diagnosis
2. Persistent ITP—3-12 months from the initial diagnosis
3. Chronic ITP—>12 months from diagnosis.

EVALUATION

The diagnosis is by exclusion. We need to exclude all the secondary causes of thrombocytopenia as discussed above.

In primary ITP, mostly the presenting platelet count is <30,000/uL. Clinically the child presents with acute onset bleeding (petechiae, purpura, and ecchymosis) and no significant systemic signs. Complete blood count (CBC) and peripheral smear examination show only thrombocytopenia.

Initial evaluation: It includes the following—complete blood counts, peripheral smear with reticulocytes, blood group, and direct antiglobulin test (DAT).

Some experts recommend Ig levels to investigate the possibility of underlying common variable immuno-deficiency (CVID).

Further evaluation is needed if there are systemic signs and symptoms, chronic thrombocytopenia or any abnormality in CBC/peripheral smear. Following are some of the indicators.

If thrombocytopenia is associated with neutropenia and/or anemia one needs to investigate further. Hemolytic uremic syndrome (HUS), thrombotic thrombocytopenic purpura (TTP), and DIC need to be diagnosed earlier as that needs an urgent management. Leukemia, aplastic anemia, connective tissue disorders have distinct clinical manifestations and CBC findings. Thrombocytopenia in childhood needs special considerations. The childhood inherited genetic syndromes have variable platelet size. Wiskott–Aldrich syndrome is X-linked disorder associated with small size platelets. Large platelets are seen in Bernard-Soulier syndrome and MYH9-related disorders.

Normal size platelets are seen in congenital amegakaryocytic thrombocytopenia, TAR (thrombocytopenia with absent radius) syndrome, etc. Children with familial inherited thrombocytopenia's are often misdiagnosed as having ITP. Inherited disorders should be suspected if thrombocytopenia has been present since early life with a positive family history for a similar disorder. The characteristic features are present, or there is failure to respond to first-line treatment. Occasionally von Willebrand disease (vWD) type 2B is associated with excessive bleeding manifestations which is disproportionate to the number of platelets. The children with CVID or autoimmune lymphoproliferative disorder also need evaluation for the thrombocytopenia.

INDICATION FOR BONE MARROW EXAMINATION

When the platelets are extremely low and clinical examination and initial CBC is suggestive of some other cause for thrombocytopenia and moreover if the low platelet counts warrants an early diagnosis to initiate the treatment, an urgent bone marrow examination is needed.

We need to look for the adequacy of Megakaryocytes and normal erythropoiesis, and granulopoiesis.

MANAGEMENT

Less than 4% of children with newly diagnosed ITP have severe (grade 4) bleeding requiring immediate intervention **(Table 1)**. About 30-56% of patients may require treatment. The incidence of ICH in children with ITP is <1%. Before starting therapy, multiple factors need to be considered including grade of bleeding symptoms, the platelet count, recent trauma, existence of headache, recent medication use, and psychosocial and lifestyle issues, such as activity profiles and economic impacts.

Wait and Watch Policy

At diagnosis, mild or moderate bleeding on a pediatric bleeding assessment tool (grade 1-2) may be managed with supportive advice.

All patients need regular follow up to monitor for worsening, HRQoL (health related quality-of-life) and evolution to a serious bone marrow disorder or a secondary form of ITP (Grade C recommendation).

Most children with newly diagnosed ITP do not have significant bleeding symptoms or other risk factors and may be managed conservatively. Reasons to institute therapy are associated with increased bleeding severity and with risk factor for ICH.

Children with ITP and their parents need to understand the risks of serious or life-threatening hemorrhage with or without treatment.

They should also be aware that drug therapy is often effective but may have side effects and, thus, is usually reserved for children at higher risk for serious hemorrhage.

Recommendations for when to start initial treatment in children newly diagnosed with ITP: (international on Acute ITP 2019).

- Most children can be managed with watchful waiting.
- Any severe (grade 4) bleeding requires immediate hospital admission and treatment to increase platelet levels until bleeding has decreased.
- Any moderate (grade 3) bleeding requires hospital review and consideration for admission and therapy.
- Treatment should be administered, and hospitalization should be strongly considered in the following cases:
  - Worsening bleeding or significant comorbidities
  - Risk of ICH (e.g., head trauma or unexplained headaches): The patients at higher risk for ICH include those with a history of moderate or severe bleed in the preceding 28 days, recent administration

TABLE 1: Management of immune thrombocytopenia.

Grade	Bleeding		Management approach
Grade 1	Minor	Few petechiae (<100) and or <5 small bruises and no mucosal bleeding	Consent for observation
Grade 2	Mild	Many petechiae (>100) and >5 Bruises and no mucosal bleeding	Consent for observation
Grade 3	Moderate	Bleeding, overt mucosal bleeding, troublesome lifestyle	Intervention to reduce to grade 1 or 2
Grade 4	Severe	Bleeding Reducing Hb by 2 g/dL/suspension of internal bleeding	Intervention

(within 8 hours) of nonsteroidal anti-inflammatory drugs (NSAIDs), and another clinically significant coagulopathy (e.g., vWD). In the case of head trauma, treatment should precede a head CT scan.
- A change in behavior or mood consistent with significant depression or irritability.
- Parents are anxious about bleeding and do not believe that they can control (young child) or restrict (older child) their child's activity.
- Parents cannot be relied upon to bring the child back readily if there is an emergency (e.g., they live too far away, they cannot afford to return, there are additional social concerns).
- Child has not spontaneously improved and must be overly restricted in activities.
- Child needs to take an anticoagulant or antiplatelet agent.
- Higher risk of bleeding due to another medical or psychological issue.

Recommendations for initial treatment of children with ITP when required:
- If there is moderate/severe bleeding, intravenous immunoglobulin (IVIg) or anti-D can increase the platelet count to hemostatic levels (50,000/uL) within 24–48 hours. Dose of IVIg is 0.8–1.0 g/kg. (Grade A recommendation, evidence level Ib). Anti-D has similar efficacy to IVIg when given as a single dose of 75 mg/kg.
- In general, corticosteroids are used for grade 1 or 2 bleeding or for patients not responsive to IVIg.
- Prednisolone should be given at 4 mg/kg per day in 3 or 4 divided doses for 4 days with no taper, with a maximum daily dose of 200 mg or at 1–2 mg/kg, with an 80-mg maximum daily dose, even in patients weighing 80 kg, for 1 to 2 weeks. Steroids should be tapered and stopped in 3 weeks.
- IV anti-D can be used if the patient is Rh positive, not splenectomized, does not have a positive direct Coombs test (DAT), and has hemoglobin (Hb) 9 g/dL.

Recommendations for emergency treatment in children at any stage of their ITP:
- Platelet transfusion, IV corticosteroids, and IVIg, with or without anti-D, are recommended. A second dose of IVIg and IV steroids may be required if a platelet response is not seen within 24 hours of the initial dose.
- If there is an ICH, emergency splenectomy and/or neurosurgical control of bleeding should be considered in conjunction with emergency.
- *Thrombopoietin receptor agonists (TPO-RAs)* should be considered; they may aid the acute response in patients and prevent a decrease in platelet count if initial response to emergency therapy is lost.

Recommendations for treatment of persistent or chronic ITP in children:
- Multiple pediatric studies support the use of TPO-RAs demonstrating good response and reduction in bleeding frequency with an absence of side effects in most patients.
- If there is no response to TPO-RA or there is a response that is lost switch to an alternative TPO-RA and/or consider combining with MMF or another immunosuppressant. (Grade C recommendation).
- In those who fail TPO-RAs, especially adolescent females, rituximab and dexamethasone should be considered (evidence level III; Grade C recommendation).

Recommendations for splenectomy in children with chronic ITP:
- Splenectomy is very rarely indicated in childhood ITP (Grade C recommendation) and should be undertaken in consultation with a hematologist experienced in the management of children with ITP. It should only be considered in children who have failed all available medical therapies, are having thrombocytopenia-related bleeding, and whose life is at risk or whose HRQoL is substantially impaired.
- Splenectomy should be avoided if possible before 5 years of age and within 1 year of disease onset.
- Before considering splenectomy, reassess the diagnosis of ITP by excluding alternative diagnoses, including inherited thrombocytopenia, bone marrow failure, drug-induced thrombocytopenia, subclinical viral infections, immunodeficiency syndromes (e.g., CVID, autoimmune lymphoproliferative syndrome), and myelodysplastic syndrome (Grade C recommendation).
- Prior to splenectomy, vaccinations should be up to date according to national policy. Vaccination, as a minimum, should include pneumococcal 13-valconjugate vaccine, followed by pneumococcal 23-valent vaccine 4 weeks later; *Haemophilus influenzae* type B; and both meningococcal vaccines to cover all 5 species subtypes.
- If there is any concern for an immunodeficiency-related ITP, even if undocumented, reducing the risk for postsplenectomy sepsis by assessing response to pneumococcal vaccines preprocedural is advisable.

CONCLUSION

Immune thrombocytopenia affects young children between 1 and 7 years of age who present with acute onset bleeding symptoms often preceded by infection. Majority of them do not require treatment. Mainstay of treatment is IVIg, anti-D, and steroid in acute onset ITP. Few of them have chronic course needing long-term treatment. In such cases we need to rule out secondary causes. For chronic cases TPO-RA and rituximab can be used. Splenectomy is avoided as far as possible and if required should be delayed beyond 5 years of age. It affects quality of life of the child substantially. The risk of bleeding and information about ITP should be provided to the school in a way that facilitates inclusion, not isolation (Grade C recommendation). Active participation in low-risk activities should be maintained, irrespective of platelet count and treatment. Participation in high-risk activities should be discouraged.

SUGGESTED READING

1. Grainger JD, Rees JL, Reeves M, Bolton-Maggs PH. Changing trends in the UK management of childhood ITP. Arch Dis Child. 2012;97(1):8-11.
2. Grimaldi-Bensouda L, Nordon C, Leblanc T, Abenhaim L, Allali S, Armari-Alla C, et al. Childhood immune thrombocytopenia: a nationwide cohort study on condition management and outcomes. Pediatr Blood Cancer. 2017;64(7):e26389.
3. Guidelines for the investigation and management of idiopathic thrombocytopenic purpura in adults, children and in pregnancy. British Committee for Standards in Hematology General Hematology Task Force. Br J Haematol. 2003;120(4):574.
4. Kühne T, Buchanan GR, Zimmerman S, Michaels LA. A prospective comparative study of 2540 infants and children with newly diagnosed idiopathic thrombocytopenic purpura (ITP) from the Intercontinental Childhood ITP Study Group. J Pediatr. 2003;143(5):605.
5. Kuhne T, Imbach P, Bolton-Maggs PHB, Berchtold W, Blanchette V, Buchananm GR, et al. Newly diagnosed idiopathic thrombocytopenic purpura in childhood: an observational study. Lancet. 2001;358:2122-55.
6. Provan D, Stasi R, Newland AC, Blanchette VS, Bolton-Maggs P, Bussel JB, et al. International consensus report on the investigation and management of primary immune thrombocytopenia. Blood. 2010;115(2):168-86.
7. Rosthøj S, Hedlund-Treutiger I, Rajantie J, Zeller B, Jonsson OG, Elinder G, et al., NOPHO ITP Working Group. Duration and morbidity of newly diagnosed idiopathic thrombocytopenic purpura in children: A prospective Nordic study of an unselected cohort. J Pediatr. 2003;143(3):302.
8. Terrell DR, Beebe LA, Neas BR, Vesely, SK, Segal JB, George JN. Prevalence of primary immune thrombocytopenia in Oklahoma. (Research Support, N.I.H., Extramural Research Support, Non-U.S. Govt). Am J Hematol. 2012;87:848-52.
9. Zeller B, Rajantie J, Hedlund-Treutiger I, Tedgård U, Wesenberg F. Childhood idiopathic thrombocytopenic purpura in the Nordic countries: epidemiology and predictors of chronic disease. Acta Paediatr. 2005;94(2):178.
10. Zufferey A, Kapur R, Semple JW. Pathogenesis and therapeutic mechanisms in immune thrombocytopenia (ITP). J Clin Med. 2017;6(2).

Hemophilia

Aradhana Mishra

BASIC CONSIDERATION

- Hemophilia is a rare and inherited (X-linked recessive condition) bleeding disorder that affects males in which the affected individual may present with spontaneous hemorrhage or persistent bleeding even after minor trauma. Females are carriers.
- It is estimated that about 1 in 10,000 people have hemophilia A or B.
- Many people with hemophilia are still undiagnosed or inadequately treated. Even when treated, people may suffer from chronic pain and limited mobility mainly due to bleeds in the joints, and if undertreated or not treated at all, risk of dying at a young age.
- Patients with hemophilia A have either no, decreased, or defective production of the blood clotting protein, factor VIII (FVIII). Those with hemophilia B have similar impairments with factor IX (FIX).
- Hemophilia A is four times more common than hemophilia B. Hemophilia C is a rare genetic bleeding disorder with deficiency of factor XI. About one third of babies who are diagnosed with hemophilia have a new mutation not present in other family members.

SUSPECT HEMOPHILIA

- Whenever a patient presents with excessive bleeding to trivial trauma or overt bruising or with a history of repeated bleeding (**Flowchart 1**).
- Bleeding within joints, swelling and pain, or tightness in the joints.
- Bleeding in to the skin, muscle, and soft tissue (hematoma).
- Bleeding of mouth and gums and bleeding that is hard to stop after losing a tooth.
- Bleeding after circumcision.
- Bleeding or hematoma at vaccination site.

PRESENTATION

- Severe hemophilia usually becomes apparent in the first years of life—often when the child starts to move about independently.

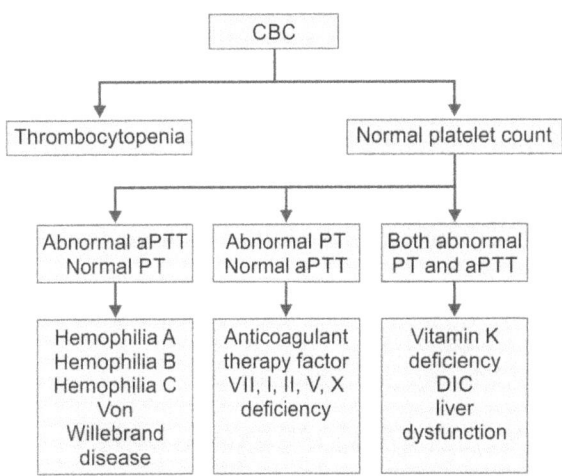

Flowchart 1: Diagnostic algorithm to identify the cause.

Note: In Hemophilia: Abnormal aPTT and normal PT, normal platelet count (CBC: complete blood count; aPTT: activated partial thromboplastin time; DIC: disseminated intravascular coagulation; PT: prothrombin time)

- Hemorrhages often occur in the joints (particularly the weight-bearing joints such as knees and ankles). These joint bleeds can cause severe pain and often permanent damage and disability if not treated properly.
- Mild-to-moderate or even life- or limb-threatening bleeds can occur in the muscles, soft tissues, gastrointestinal tract, or even the brain. In addition, trauma, major surgery, tooth extractions, or other minor surgical interventions require medical treatment to manage the associated bleeding.
- Severe hemophilia is often associated with spontaneous bleeding (i.e., bleeding not caused by trauma or injury).
- Hemophilia is referred to as "moderate" when clotting factor activity is between 1 and 5% of normal, and "mild" when the relevant clotting factor activity is greater than 5%, but less than normal.
- Approximately 30–50% of hemophilia patients (depending on the type of hemophilia) have severe disease and can require treatment for bleeding several times per month.

APPROACH TO HEMOPHILIA

Factor assays are done to confirm the disease and severity.

The severity of hemophilia that person has is determined by the amount of the factor in the blood **(Table 1)**. The lower the amount of the factor, the more likely it is that bleeding will occur which can lead to serious health problem.

TREATMENT

- The initial treatment of early and moderate bleeds should aim for a peak factor VIII of 50–60 IU.
- Early bleeds often do not require a second infusion, and moderate bleeds often respond to a single infusion but may require up to two infusions.
- Children may require more frequent or higher doses as they have a shorter factor half-life than adults.
- For joint immobilizing bleeds, higher initial doses are recommended which aim to raise the peak factor VIII level to 60–80 IU, doses should be administered every 24 hours until complete resolution of pain.
- Dose calculation of factor VIII = % desired (rise in f8) × body weight (kg) × 0.56
- Dose calculation of factor IX = % desired (rise in f9) × body weight × 1.4
  Table 2 lists the hemostatic agents.

PROGNOSIS AND LIFE EXPECTANCY

- Life expectancy in hemophilia varies, depending on whether patients receive appropriate treatment. Many patients still die before adulthood due to inadequate treatment. Overall, the death rate for people with hemophilia is about twice that of the rate for healthy men. For severe hemophilia, the rate is four to six times higher.
- The most important life-threatening complications of the disease are intracranial bleed responsible for a third of hemophilia deaths (10% patients may have bleed and 30% of those die, lifetime risk of bleed is 8%). Other hemorrhages in soft tissue around airways or other internal organs can also be fatal.
- These patients can develop chronic debilitating joint disease. About 25% of children with severe hemophilia have below-normal motor skills, academic performance, and emotional and behavioral problems.
- Preventive measures and early treatment have significantly improved the long-term outlook. Clotting factor concentrates prevent serious bleeding.
  The comprehensive care to keep the disease from worsening in many patients increases their life expectancy and improves their quality of life.
- With proper treatment and education, life expectancy is only about 10 years less than healthy men and people with hemophilia can have fulfilling and productive lives.

KEY MESSAGES

- Hemophilia A is about four times as common as hemophilia B, and about half of those affected have the severe form.
- Lifestyle modification to prevent bleeding by avoiding trauma. Start clotting factor concentrates as indicated.
- Avoid nonsteroidal anti-inflammatory drugs drugs.
- Early treatment of joint hemorrhage with higher doses factor concentrate.
- Newer drugs such as *hemlibra* also known as *ACE910* or *emicizumab* and the use of *amicar* (epsilon amino caproic acid) may hold promise for better management.

TABLE 1: Level of factor VIII and factor IX in the blood.

Level of factor VIII and factor IX in the blood	Diagnosis and severity of hemophilia
50–100%	Normal (person who do not have hemophilia)
Between 5 and 50%	Mild hemophilia
1–5%	Moderate hemophilia
<1%	Severe hemophilia

TABLE 2: Hemostatic agents.

Component	Contents	Dose	Disadvantage
Fresh frozen plasma	1 unit/mL of each	10–15 mL/kg	Large volume
Cryoprecipitate (bag)	100 units factor VIII/bag 150 mg fibrinogen/bag	0.2 bag/kg	Infectious risk
Platelet (units)	$5-7 \times 10^{10}$ platelets in 30–60 mL of plasma	0.2 U/kg	Infectious risk
Factor concentrate (unit)	Unit as labeled	Factor VIII: 20–50 U/kg Factor IX: 30–130 U/kg	Recombinant
1-deamino-8-D-arginine vasopressin	4 µg/mL	0.3 µg/kg/dose	Increase factor VII and von Willebrand factor three to four fold

SUGGESTED READING

1. Peyvandi F, Garagiola I, Young G. The past and future of haemophilia: diagnosis, treatments, and its complications. Lancet. 2016;388(10040):187-97.
2. Bhatnagar N, Hall GW. Major bleeding disorders: diagnosis, classification, management and recent developments in haemophilia. Arch Dis Child. 2018;103(5):509-13.
3. Marijke van den Berg H. Preventing bleeds by treatment: new era for haemophilia changing the paradigm. Haemophilia. 2016;22 (Suppl 5):9-13.
4. Croteau SE; Evolving complexity in hemophilia management. Pediatr Clin North Am. 2018;65(3):407-25.
5. Ling G, Nathwani AC, Tuddenham EGD. Recent advances in developing specific therapies for haemophilia. Br J Haematol. 2018;181(2):161-72.
6. Kizilocak H, Young G. Diagnosis and treatment of hemophilia. Clin Adv Hematol Oncol. 2019;17(6):344-51.
7. Mannucci PM. Hemophilia therapy: the future has begun. Haematologica. 2020;105(3):545-53.

Hematopoietic Stem Cell Transplantation

Dinesh Bhurani

INTRODUCTION

- Hematopoietic stem cell transplantation (HSCT) has become a well-established therapy for many severe congenital or acquired disorders of the hematopoietic system and for chemosensitive, malignancies in children.
- Aim of HSCT is to re-establish hematopoietic function in patients whose bone marrow or immune system is damaged or defective.
- Autologous SCT is used to allow patients with cancer to receive higher doses of chemotherapy than bone marrow can usually tolerate.

INDICATIONS FOR HSCT

- Autologous transplants (*Using patient's own stem cells for infusion*):
  - Non-Hodgkin lymphoma
  - Hodgkin lymphoma
  - Acute myeloid leukemia
  - Neuroblastoma
  - Germ cell tumors
  - Autoimmune disorders
- Allogenic transplants (Stem cells from other normal donors):
  - *Malignant indications*:
    - Acute myeloid leukemia
    - Acute lymphoblastic leukemia
    - Chronic myeloid leukemia
  - *Nonmalignant indications*:
    - Aplastic anemia
    - Fanconi anemia
    - Diamond–Blackfan anemia
    - Thalassemia major
    - Sickle cell anemia
    - Severe combined immunodeficiency (SCID)
    - Wiskott–Aldrich syndrome
    - Hemophagocytic lymphohistiocytosis
    - Inborn errors of metabolism
    - Severe congenital neutropenia
    - Shwachman–Diamond syndrome
    - Leukocyte adhesion deficiency.

Human leukocyte antigen (HLA) matching for allogenic HSCT:

- HLAs are expressed on the surface of various cells, in particular white blood cells.
- These antigens are also known as the major histocompatibility complex (MHC) and occupy the short arm of chromosome 6.
- Traditionally, the loci critical for matching are HLA-A, HLA-B, and HLA-DR.
- HLA-C and HLA-DQ are also now considered when determining the appropriateness of a donor.

Sources of stem cells are as follows:

- Bone marrow (traditional source)
- Peripheral blood (now preferred for many transplantations)
- Umbilical cord blood

Donor selection for HSCT: Preference for selection of donor as given in **Flowchart 1**.

- Donors for HSCT must be in generally good health.
- There should be no comorbid conditions, and should in general have the same qualifications as a blood donor.
- The donor must have a performance status that permits safe collection of cells and have adequate cardiac, pulmonary, hepatic, and renal function.

Procurement of stem cells:

- The traditional source of hematopoietic stem cells has been bone marrow.

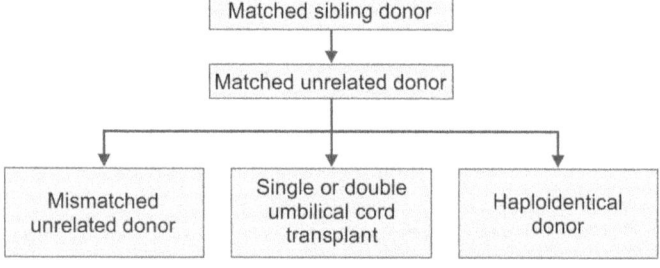

Flowchart 1: Types of allogenic hematopoietic stem cell transplantation.

- The use of peripheral blood as a source of these cells has replaced bone marrow for most autologous transplantations and a significant proportion of allogeneic transplantations.

Procedural considerations:
- The purpose of the preparative regimen is to provide immunosuppression sufficient to prevent rejection of the transplanted graft and to eradicate the disease for which the transplantation is being performed.
- Preparative or conditioning regimens involve delivery of maximally tolerated doses of multiple chemotherapeutic agents with nonoverlapping toxicities.

INFUSION OF STEM CELLS AND ENGRAFTMENT

Infusion of either bone marrow or peripheral blood progenitor cells is a relatively a simple process like any blood transfusion that is performed at the bedside.

Infection prophylaxis may include the following:
- Care in high-efficiency particulate air (HEPA)–filtered, positive air pressure-sealed rooms, with strict hand hygiene.
- Antifungal prophylaxis with fluconazole or amphotericin B or voriconazole.
- Acyclovir prophylaxis (herpes simplex-positive patients).
- Pneumocystis prophylaxis with trimethoprim-sulfamethoxazole or pentamidine.

COMPLICATIONS ASSOCIATED WITH HSCT

Early-onset problems:
- Mucositis
- Hemorrhagic cystitis
- Prolonged, severe pancytopenia
- Infection
- Graft-versus-host disease (GVHD)
- Graft failure
- Pulmonary complications
- Hepatic veno-occlusive disease

Late-onset problems:
- Infection
- Chronic GVHD
- Ocular effects
- Endocrine effects
- Pulmonary effects
- Musculoskeletal effects
- Neurologic effects
- Immune effects
- Congestive heart failure
- Subsequent malignancy.

Infections

Many factors predispose to the development of infections in a transplant patient.

- *Early after transplantation (0–30 days)*: Mucosal and skin injury, as well as neutropenia, contribute to infections with aerobic bacteria (particularly gram-negative bacilli), *Candida* species, and herpes simplex.
- *About 1–3 months after transplantation*: T-cell dysfunction, hypogammaglobulinemia, and acute GVHD predispose to infections with gram-negative bacilli, encapsulated bacteria (e.g., *Pneumococcus*, *Haemophilus influenzae*), Viruses [e.g., cytomegalovirus (CMV)], *Pneumocystis jiroveci*, molds (e.g., *Aspergillus*, Zygomycetes) and *Candida* species.
- *Between 3 and 12 months after transplantation*: Slow T-cell reconstitution and chronic GVHD predispose patients to infections with encapsulated bacteria, CMV, *P. jiroveci*, and herpes zoster virus.

Graft-versus-Host Disease

- GVHD occurs when immunocompetent T cells and natural killer cells in the donor graft recognize host antigens as foreign targets and mediate a reaction.
- *Acute* GVHD is a common complication of allogeneic transplantation within the first 100 days after the procedure. Acute GVHD involves skin, mucosal, surfaces, gut, and liver.
- Chronic GVHD develops 2–12 months after HSCT and involves the skin, eyes, mouth, liver, fascia, and almost any organ in the body.

PROGNOSIS

Currently, overall and event-free survival rates are based on the individual's disease pathology and on the stage of disease. Patients undergoing HLA-matched sibling allogeneic transplantation have the best 5-year survival rate of all treated patients.

THALASSEMIA

The ideal candidate is a child who has undergone rigorous therapy with transfusions and iron chelation and who has an HLA-identical sibling donor or unrelated donor; such a patient has a more than 90% likelihood of cure and <5% risk of transplant-related mortality.

APLASTIC ANEMIA

Bone marrow transplantation (BMT) is the recommended first-line therapy for patients with an HLA-matched sibling donor, with 5-year survival rates exceeding 90%.

REVACCINATION

- Many studies suggest that most vaccine-acquired immunity wanes after HSCT.
- Most killed vaccines are considered safe, but the use of live virus vaccines is generally contraindicated until at least 18 months post-transplantation.

- The appropriate timing for revaccination is 12–18 months after transplantation, although this period may need to be individualized based on the patient's immune function, especially in the presence of GVHD.

MY ROLE AS PRIMARY PEDIATRICIAN

- Confirmation of primary diagnosis.
- Initial discussion with family regarding available treatment options including transplant.
- Counseling of family about pros and cons of transplant, prognosis, and cost.
- Coordinate HLA typing
- Informing about possible transplant center
- Coordinating donor physical examination and testing
- Involvement in post-transplant care.
- Monitoring growth
- Treatment of infections in post-transplant period in coordination with transplant center.
- Post-transplant vaccination
- Monitoring for transplant-related long-term complications.

SUGGESTED READING

1. Carreras E, et al. (eds.), The EBMT Handbook, https://doi.org/10.1007/978-3-030-02278-5.
2. Lucarelli G, Isgro A, Sodani P, Gaziev J. Hematopoietic stem cell transplantation in thalassemia and sickle cell anemia. Cold Spring Harbor Perspectives in Medicine. 2012;2(5):a011825.
3. Yesilipek M, Karasu G. Hematopoetic stem cell transplantation in children. Journal of Pediatric Sciences. 2010;2(3).

CHAPTER 85: Blood Component Therapy

Kiran Makhija

INTRODUCTION

The transfusion therapy is to correct any deficiency by replacing with one or more component of blood which is not possible by other means.

The available components in the blood center for clinical use are:
- *Oxygen-carrying components*: Whole blood, red cell components, leuko-poor red cells and irradiated red cells
- *Platelet products*: Single or random donor platelet concentrate
- *Plasma product*: Fresh frozen plasma, cryoprecipitate, and cryo poor plasma.

WHOLE BLOOD

- *Prepared/stored*: Unit volume is 450 mL (63 mL anticoagulant), stored at 2–6°C and shelf life of blood in CPDA (citrate-phosphate-dextrose solution with adenine) is 35 days.
- *Advantage*: Hemoglobin will be raised approximately 1.2 g% in children and 3 g% hemoglobin (Hb) in infants with no functional platelets and factor V (FV), FVIII.
- *Administration*: Blood must be ABO and RhD compatible with recipient. For transfusion 1 unit of 10–20 mL/kg body weight is required. Transfusion should be started within 30 minutes given by standard 150–180 microfilter BT set.
- Rate of transfusion depends on clinical circumstances generally 3–5 mL/kg/h and increased in hypovolemic shock. The transfusion should be completed within 4 hours of beginning.

Precautions

- Examine blood bag for any damage and clots, abnormal dark color. If anything seems abnormal, check with blood center. Red blood cells (RBCs) will usually be dark red in color.
- Invert the bag several times to ensure resuspension of red cells.
- Never add medication in blood unit.
- Antihistamines, steroids prior to transfusion given to patient may mask features of acute tricuspid regurgitation (TR).
- Change the transfusion set after 2 units of blood.

Indications

Acute blood loss if >20–30% total blood volume (TBV), i.e., hypovolemia.

Contraindications

- Chronic anemia
- Risk of volume overload in cardiac or renal disease
- Should not be used in coagulopathies bleeding as it does not contain sufficient viable platelets or coagulation factors.

PACKED RED CELLS

- Obtained after centrifugation of whole blood and with removal of most of plasma.
- 1 unit bag gives 150–200 mL of packed cells. Fresh blood (<7 days) is used to avoid biochemical overload.
- Indicated to increase the oxygen capacity of blood and to correct anemia.
- Not to be given for general well-being, asymptomatic and nutritional anemia even when Hb is <7 g%.

Leuko-reduced red cells
- Advantage being almost 99.9% of WBCs are removed by freezing-thawing-wash technique (removal of buffy coat) or filtration by readymade leuko-filters
- There is reduced human leukocyte antigen (HLA) alloimmunizations, effective in reducing cytomegalovirus (CMV) and other infections but reduces incidences of graft-vs-host disease (GVHD)
- Useful in multiple transfused patients who had previous febrile reactions (hemato-oncology, thalassemia major, aplasia, hemodialysis patients).

Irradiated red cells
- Gama radiation given to bag to kill lymphocytes which prevents GVHD
- Blood is given to immune compromised patients like BMT patients
- Congenital immunodeficiency syndrome
- Hodgkin's lymphoma.

PLATELETS CONCENTRATES

Random donor: Platelet concentrate (60 mL) is separated by centrifugation from freshly drawn blood units.

Single donor: PC (150-300 mL) platelet pheresis/apheresis technique is used to get 6-8 times more platelet and which result in higher increase in counts, i.e., 30-60 thousands/cc³.

Platelets concentrates stored at 20-24°C under gentle and constant agitation and kept not >5 days as bacterial contamination is a problem.

Administration

ABO match is used (Rh negative is given to Rh negative patient).

1 unit PC per 10 kg body weight is required and transfusion is to be completed in 20-30 minutes due to the risk of bacterial contamination. At last entrapped platelets should be rinsed from BT set by isotonic saline through it.

Indications
Bone marrow failure:
- Rx of bleeding and thrombocytopenia
- Prophylactic use in thrombocytopenia

Massive blood transfusion: Dilution thrombocytopenia
- *DIC*: For procedures such as LP, insertion of lines, biopsies.

Maintain platelet count
- >20 × 10⁹/L in infections
- >10 × 10⁹/L in other patients
- >50 × 10⁹/L
- >20 × 10⁹/L
- >50 × 10⁹/L

Contraindications

Idiopathic thrombocytopenic purpura, thrombotic purpura (TTP), untreated DIC, thrombocytopenia associated with septicemia, and hypersplenism.

FRESH FROZEN PLASMA

Volume of 200-300 mL is prepared from blood within 8 hours of collection and rapidly frozen to −25°C and can be kept for 1 year.

Advantage: Rich in clotting FV and FVIII, protein C and S, complements, and immunoglobulin.

Administration is done by normal BT set, measured dose of 15 mL/kg and to be used within 6 hours of thawing as labile coagulation factors rapidly degraded. It should be transfused quickly like platelets.

Indications
- DIC with microvascular bleeds and when prothrombin time (PT) and/or partial thromboplastin time (PTT) is >1.5 times normal (sepsis, liver, and renal disease)
- C1 esterase inhibitor deficiency (specific concentrate is not available)
- TTP
- Contraindications
- As volume expander
- As prophylaxis for massive whole blood transfusion
- Inherited coagulation inhibitor deficiencies where specific concentrate is unavailable, e.g., von Willebrand disease, hemophilia A.
- Urgent warfarin effect reversal (5-8 mL/kg)
- Massive blood transfusion
- As nutrition support.

CRYOPRECIPITATE

- Prepared from fresh frozen plasma, contain plasma concentrate, rich in factors like VIII, vWF, fibrinogen and XIII, volume of pack is 15 mL which gives 100 clotting units of FVIII and 250 mg of fibrinogen, stored life is 1 year if frozen at −18°C to −25°C.
- Other plasma derivative is prepared like albumin, coagulation factor concentrates and immunoglobulin.
- Administered—aspirate all cryoprecipitate in a syringe from bag with connected needle and infused within 6 hours of thawing as quickly as possible.

GRANULOCYTE CONCENTRATE

- Produced by apheresis from family members for administration to a cancer patient. Gives 1.0 × 10.10 granulocytes, pretreatment with recombinant G-CSF, and dexamethasone can yield 4-8 times.
- Stored at 24°C and transfused within 24 hours of collection.

Criteria

- Absolute neutrophil count (ANC) < 500
- Documented infection of bacteria/fungus
- Unresponsive to appropriate antibiotics
- Reasonable hope of BM recovery.

TRANSFUSION REACTIONS

Acute Blood Transfusion Reaction

Reactions type	Characteristics
Febrile nonhemolytic	- Most frequent type - In multiple transfused patients, caused by cytokines developed in stored component and antileukocytes antibodies in recipient - Rx–PCM, should use blood filter
Allergic urticarial (hives or rash)	Due to plasma having traces of IgA. Cytokines occasionally cause broncho-/vasoconstriction and rarely, IgA deficiency in recipient causes very severe anaphylaxis Rx—diphenhydramine

Acute Hemolytic TR

- Worst reaction
- Due to ABO group mismatch, clerical errors—misidentified patient, collect ion vials, mismatch bag label, and blood group on patient's file.
- C/F—fever, chills, anxiety, chest pain, pain at site, shock, dyspnea and dark urine (hemoglobinuria) soon after transfusion.
- Rx—intravenous (IV) fluids, diuretics can be given

Other reactions	Characteristics
Sepsis	- In 1–2% of platelet concentrates - Donor's skin bacteria (staphylococci grows at +20°C to +24°C), during collection (Yersinia), gram-negative pseudomonas +2°C to +6°C - C/F—high fever, vomiting, diarrhea, and shock - M/M: Proper check on processing and handling of bag and antibiotics given
Transfusion-related acute lung injury (TRALI)	- Caused by donor antibodies against patient's WBC - C/F—fever, dyspnea, hypoxia, bilateral chest infiltrate (d/d with ARDS) - M/M—intensive, respiratory, and general support - Most common cause of death, better prognosis than ARDS
Transfusion-associated circulatory overload	- Associated with excess and rapid transfusion, chronic severe anemia or any underlying cardiovascular or renal disease - C/F—heart failure and pulmonary edema - M/M—given blood slowly and diuretics

Diagnosis and Management of Acute Blood Transfusion Reaction

Category 2: Moderate reactions

Features	Immediate management
- Headache - Flushing - Restlessness - Palpitations - Mild dyspnea - Possible cause—hypersensitivity	- Stop transfusion and keep IV line open with normal saline - Notify senior doctor attending the patient and blood center immediately - Return blood unit with transfusion set, freshly collected urine and new blood samples (1 clotted and 1 anticoagulated), drawn from a vein opposite to transfusion site, sent to center for laboratory - Give IM antihistamine, oral or rectal antipyretic - IV corticosteroids and bronchodilators if anaphylactoid features seen - If patient is stable, restart transfusion slowly with new WBC filter unit and watch carefully - If patient is not well, treat as category 3

Category 3: Life-threatening reactions

Features	Possible causes
- Chest pain, dyspnea/SOB, Loin/back pain - Hypotension (fall in systolic BP by 20%) - Tachycardia (rise in heart rate by 20%)	- Acute intravascular hemolysis, sepsis and shock - Fluid overload, anaphylaxis - Transfusion related acute lung injury (TRALI)

Hemoglobinuria: Unexplained Bleeding

Disseminated intravascular coagulation (DIC)

Immediate management—1
- Maintain airway and give high-flow oxygen by mask.
- Infuse normal saline (2 times normal maintenance) to flush hemoglobin from kidney and to support systolic BP.
- Give adrenaline (as 1:1,000 solution) 0.01 mg/kg body weight by slow IM injection.
- Give IV corticosteroids and bronchodilators if there are anaphylactoid features.
- Give diuretic, e.g., furosemide 1 mg/kg IV or equivalent.
- Check a fresh urine specimen visually for signs of hemoglobinuria.

Immediate management—2
- Start a 24-hour urine collection.
- Assess if bleeding from puncture sites or wounds.

- If DIC-treat with platelets and cryoprecipitate/FFP.
- *If fall in BP*: Give further normal saline and inotrope if required.
- *If urine output falls and acute renal failure (high potassium, urea, creatinine)*:
  - Maintain fluid balance accurately.
  - Diuretic, e.g., frusemide 1 mg/kg IV.
  - Dopamine infusion.
  - Renal dialysis if required.
- If infection/sepsis: IV broad-spectrum antibiotic.

Transfusion Notes Detail

Patient ID	Diagnosis	Source of blood	Amount of blood
• Date • Patient Name • Age/Sex	• Ward/Bed • Blood group • Pretransfusion • Hb g/dL	• Bag number • Collection date • Type of component	• Cross match and screening laboratory ID • Transfusion start time

- Transfusion was successful without any adverse reaction
- Transfusion was deferred due to adverse reaction of severe category
- Transfusion was completed with management of febrile/allergic reaction
- *Time transfusion completed*: Signature of doctor.

Transfusion Monitoring Chart

Parameter	Start	15 min	30 min	1 h	2 h	3 h	4 h
• Pulse • BP • Temp • RR • Urine • Color • Dp • Rate							

Delayed Transfusion Reactions

Hemolytic TR
- 5-10 days after transfusion.
- C/F: Fever, anemia, jaundice occasionally hemoglobinuria.
- Severe shock, renal failure, and DIC are rare.

Post-transfusion purpura
- 5-10 days after transfusion.
- Transfused antibodies against platelet-specific antigens in recipient.
- C/F: Bleeding, severe thrombocytopenia (<1 L) rare but potentially fatal.
- *Rx*: Corticosteroids, IV immunoglobulin, 2 g/kg or 0.4 g/kg for 5 days, plasma exchange. Recovery usually after 2-4 weeks.

Transfusion-associated graft-vs-host disease (TA-GVHD)
- 10-12 D after transfusion. Fatal condition unlike transplant-associated
- GVHD occurs in:
  - Immunodeficient recipients of BMT
  - Immunocompetent transfused with blood with a compatible HLA tissue type, usually relative's blood particularly first degree
  - C/F: Fever, skin rash, desquamation, diarrhea, hepatitis, and pancytopenia.

Transfusion transmitted infections
- Easily be overlooked as it occur days, weeks, or months after the transfusion
- Infects like HIV, hepatitis B and C, syphilis, and malaria
- Others are—CMV, human parvovirus B19, brucellosis, EB virus, toxoplasmosis, Chagas disease, infectious mononucleosis and Lyme's disease.

SECTION 8: Respiratory System

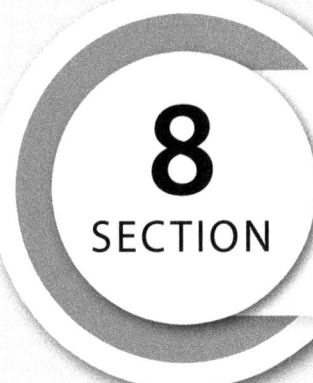

86. Common Cold
87. Allergic Rhinitis
88. Rhinosinusitis in Children
89. Croup and Epiglottitis
90. Acute Bronchiolitis
91. Wheezing in Children
92. Community-acquired Pneumonia
93. Pleural Effusion
94. Empyema Thoracis
95. Lung Abscess
96. Pneumothorax
97. Hydrocarbon Aspiration
98. Foreign Body in Lungs

86 Common Cold

Subroto Chakrabartty

INTRODUCTION

The common cold is the most common respiratory tract illness in children, essentially of viral origin. It may be called a benign illness but understanding it properly will certainly add to improving the quality of life and also prevent unnecessary use of antibiotics.

Its commonness can be understood by the fact that it occurs in young children at an average of six to eight colds per year, but 10–15% of children have at least 12 infections per year.

The incidence of illness decreases with increasing age, with two to three illnesses per year by adulthood.

ETIOLOGY

The most common pathogens causing common cold are types of human rhinoviruses (HRV). Other viruses are also involved in causing the syndrome such as respiratory syncytial virus (RSV), human metapneumovirus, parainfluenza virus and adenovirus but HRV causes >50% of the colds.

PATHOGENESIS

Common cold being a viral illness presents so frequently can be explained by the fact that the viruses have evolved different strategies to overcome the host defenses. HRV has 200 different serotypes and the immunity developed is serotype specific. The influenza viruses change the antigens on the surface by genetic drift, thus they behave as though they are multiple viral serotypes. The symptoms of the disease are generated by host immune system in response to viral infection rather than damage to respiratory tract. Infected cells of the respiratory epithelium release cytokines and attract polymorphonuclear cells.

Human rhinoviruses also increases the vascular permeability of the nasal submucosa contributing to the symptoms.

Modes of spread of the viruses can be by three mechanisms. It can be by self-inoculation by one's own nasal mucosa after touching contaminated person or object. It can also be by aerosol or droplet infection expelled during coughing and sneezing or normal talking.

LABORATORY FINDINGS

Routine laboratory studies do not help in the management of cold. A nasal smear for eosinophils (Hansel strain) may help if allergic rhinitis is suspected.

TREATMENT

Treatment consists of supportive care.

For nasal obstruction, adrenergic agents such as xylometazoline, oxymetazoline, or phenylephrine are often used as intranasal drops or nasal sprays. Diluted formulations of these drugs are available for use in younger children but they are not recommended for use in children younger than 6 years.

Rhinorrhea can be treated by first-generation antihistamines; second-generation antihistamines are ineffective for common cold symptoms because the symptoms are relieved by anticholinergic effect and not by antihistaminic effect. It can also be treated with ipratropium bromide a topical anticholinergic drug. The most common side effect of ipratropium are nasal irritation and bleeding.

Sore throat associated with cold is not severe and is relieved by acetaminophen. Cough suppression is generally not necessary. Cough due to postnasal drip may be helpful. Cough lozenges may be helpful but should be avoided in children younger than 6 years because of potential risk of aspiration. Honey 5–10 mL may have a modest effect in relieving nocturnal cough in children older than 1 year. Codeine and dextromethorphan are ineffective.

It has to be remembered always that cough could be because of virus-induced reactive airways disease and will be relieved by bronchodilators.

SUGGESTED READING

1. Nelson's Textbook of Pediatrics, 21st edition.

87. Allergic Rhinitis

Subroto Chakrabartty

INTRODUCTION

Allergic rhinitis (AR) is probably the most common respiratory tract disease which is underdiagnosed and undertreated by the pediatricians. The timely diagnosis and treatment will reduce the long-term morbidity and definitely will improve the quality of life.

Allergic rhinitis affects 20–30% of children according to western figures but in our country, the figures would be higher because of the greater exposure to allergens. The unique presentation of the disease is that it may appear as early as infancy and should be diagnosed by the time the child reaches the age of 6 years. The prevalence peaks late in childhood.

The most important point to remember is that the childhood AR is associated with three-fold increase in risk of asthma at an older age. There is an important clinical correlation between occurrence of three or more episodes of rhinorrhea in the first year of life and development of AR at 7 years of age.

CLINICAL TYPES

Allergic rhinitis is expressed as a sensitivity to allergen in the environment. It may be seasonal or perineal.

Both the types can be intermittent (mild intermittent and moderate-to-severe intermittent) and persistent (mild persistent and moderate-to-severe persistent). Intermittent AR occurs in response to air-borne pollens, weeds and mold sporulation, etc. Persistent AR is most often associated with indoor allergens (house dust mites, animal danders, mice, and cockroaches).

Intermittent symptoms are said when it lasts <4 days/week or <4 weeks at a time and persistent if it is equal to >4 days/week or ≥4 weeks at a time.

The symptoms are considered as mild if they are not troublesome, the sleep is normal, there is no impairment in daily activities and school performance.

Otherwise it is called severe.

CLINICAL FEATURES

The most common error done is ignoring AR as temporary infection. It has to be remembered that AR is often associated with conjunctivitis, sinusitis, serous otitis media, hypertrophic tonsils and adenoids, and eczema.

Classical complaints include intermittent nasal congestion, clear rhinorrhea, and conjunctival irritation.

Nasal congestion is often more severe at night interfering with sleep and waking up episodes. Mouth breathing and snoring can also be present.

The signs often encountered in AR is "Allergic Salute" (upward rubbing of the nose with open palm), "Nasal Crease" (horizontal skin fold over the bridge of the nose), "Allergic Gape" (mouth breathing) and "Allergic Shiners" (dark circles under the eyes).

DIFFERENTIAL DIAGNOSIS

Allergic rhinitis is basically a clinical diagnosis which necessitates considering the allergen exposure to the child, i.e., environment, diet, and family history of allergic conditions.

- Nonallergic inflammatory rhinitis with eosinophils imitates AR but without raised IgE antibodies.
- Vasomotor rhinitis is characterized by excessive responsiveness of nasal mucosa to physical stimuli.
- Rhinitis medicamentosa is caused by overuse of topical vasoconstrictors.
- Other nonallergic conditions such as infectious rhinitis, structural problems (nasal polyp, septal deviation) have to be considered.

COMPLICATIONS

- *Affects the quality of life*: The most common and often overlooked complication of AR is that it lowers the quality of life. More than 70% of children experience allergic conjunctivitis, especially in older children and adults. Overall experience of the child is frustrating.

- Rhinitis that coexists with asthma is often overlooked. Aggravation of AR coincides with exacerbation of asthma.
- Chronic sinusitis is a common complication of AR.
- Postnasal drip associated with AR causes chronic or recurrent cough.
- Eustachian tube blockade and middle ear effusion are frequent complications.
- AR can cause sleep disturbances and daytime fatigue which can seriously affect child's learning process.

LABORATORY DIAGNOSIS

Presence of eosinophils in nasal smear supports the diagnosis of AR whereas neutrophils will suggest infection. Epicutaneous skin tests can be the best method of diagnosis of AR.

Eosinophilia and measurement of total serum IgE concentration have relatively low sensitivity.

TREATMENT

Allergic Rhinitis and its Impact on Asthma (ARIA) guidelines provide the appropriate treatment options for the treatment of AR.

Antihistamines help reduce the sneezing, rhinorrhea, and ocular symptoms. Both first- and second-generation antihistamines can be used but second generation is preferable because they cause less sedation.

Pseudoephedrine-containing preparations have been used for relief of nasal and sinus congestion, but better to avoid them because they cause irritability and insomnia in children. It has also been suggested that it increases infant mortality.

The anticholinergic nasal spray ipratropium bromide can be used for the treatment of serous rhinorrhea. The intranasal decongestants (oxymetazoline and phenylephrine) relieve nasal congestion but should be used for <5 days at a time and should not be repeated for more than once a month to avoid rebound congestion.

Sodium cromoglycate is effective but requires frequent administration, every 4 hours.

Leukotriene-modifying agents are very frequently used in AR but it has only a modest effect.

Nasal saline is not a placebo but does have a adjunctive action with other modes of therapy.

Intranasal corticosteroids remain the most effective therapy for AR but preferably should be reserved for more persistent and severe symptoms. Budesonide, fluticasone mometasone and ciclesonide have been used.

Mometasone is safer option for children below 4 years.

SUGGESTED READING

1. Nelson's Textbook of Pediatrics, 21st edition.

CHAPTER 88: Rhinosinusitis in Children

Anindya Kundu

INTRODUCTION

Rhinosinusitis is an inflammation and infection of the paranasal and nasal sinus mucosae. It is a more accurate term than "Sinusitis" since it is almost always preceded by or associated with symptoms of rhinitis. It is classified according to the duration of signs:

- Acute (up to 1 month)
- Subacute (1–3 months)
- Chronic (>3 months)

Acute bacterial rhinosinusitis (ABRS) is diagnosed in a child based on several criteria. Persistent upper respiratory tract symptoms >10 days (cough or nasal discharge or both); or recurrence of symptoms after initial improvement: Fever, worsening cough, or severe onset of symptoms such as fever or purulent nasal discharge lasting >3 consecutive days associated with facial tenderness or headache. Common pathogens involved in rhinosinusitis in children are *Streptococcus pneumoniae, Haemophilus influenzae,* and *Moraxella catarrhalis*. Up to 5–10% of viral upper respiratory tract infec-tions (URIs) in children progress to rhinosinusitis, with a number of them developing into chronic rhinosinusitis (CRS). The presentation of viral rhinosinusitis is similar to ABRS and it is difficult to differentiate between them since they both have the same clinical and radiological findings. ABRS complicates between 5 and 10% of viral URIs in children. A recent cohort published in Pediatric Infectious Disease Journal found that viruses were found in 63% during the initial URI infection visit and rhinovirus detection was highly associated with ABRS risk (p = 0.01).

Compared to ABRS, CRS typically has a complex pathophysiology resulting from multiple environmental and genetic factors. If left untreated, it can significantly affect the quality of life, more than any chronic respiratory or arthritic disease.

The diagnosis of acute bacterial sinusitis is made when a child with an acute URI presents with: (1) Persistent illness [nasal discharge (of any quality) or daytime cough or both lasting >10 days without improvement], (2) a worsening course (worsening or new-onset of nasal discharge, daytime cough, or fever after initial improvement), or (3) severe onset [concurrent fever (temperature ≥ 39°C/102.2°F) and purulent nasal discharge for at least 3 consecutive days].

Predisposing factors for rhinosinusitis are given in **Table 1**.

TABLE 1: Predisposing factors for rhinosinusitis.

Local predisposing factors	Systemic predisposing factors
Allergic rhinitis	Immune deficiency
URI	IgA deficiency
Anatomic abnormality	Panhypogamma-globulinemia
Deviated septum	IgG subclass deficiency
Concha bullosa	HIV
Enlarged adenoids	Cystic fibrosis
Nasal polyps	Ciliary disorder
Tumor	Wegener's granulomatosis
Foreign body	
Trauma	
Barotrauma	
Diving, swimming	
Smoke, topical decongestant abuse	
Nasal intubation, nasogastric tube	

(Ig: immunoglobulin; HIV: human immunodeficiency virus; URI: upper respiratory tract infection)

DIAGNOSIS

The Infectious Disease Society of America (IDSA) guidelines suggest that ABRS can be diagnosed with each of the following clinical scenarios:

- URI symptoms lasting >10 days without any improvement
- Severe onset of signs and symptoms lasting >3–4 consecutive days, such as high-grade fever (>39°C), facial pain, or purulent nasal discharge
- Worsening of signs and symptoms following atypical viral URI that lasted 5–6 days and were initially improving,

such as new onset of fever, headache, or increase in nasal discharge "double-sickening".

Confirmation is by nasal examination and by documenting purulent discharge beyond the nasal vestibule by rhinoscopy or endoscopy; or posterior pharyngeal drainage. CT scan is not recommended for routine management, but may be helpful in complex cases or if complications are suspected. Other clinical symptoms associated with ABRS include tenderness overlying the sinuses, nasal erythema, increased posterior pharyngeal secretions, periorbital edema, halitosis, eustachian tube dysfunction on ear examination. The clinical presentation of pain in ABRS may provide the clinician with clues as to which sinus is infected.

Imaging

Plain radiographic studies are not sufficiently sensitive or specific to detect sinusitis and are essentially not recommended for either diagnosis or follow-up of acute or chronic rhinosinusitis.

Computerized tomography (CT) is the imaging of choice and both coronal and axial images are obtained. Use of contrast with the CT scan is usually reserved for cases where abscess formation is suspected in either the orbit or the brain. Rim enhancement allows the improved detection of possible abscesses and facilitates the decision for surgical intervention if necessary.

Three radiographic findings indicate sinusitis:
1. Air-fluid level
2. Opacification (partial or complete)
3. 4-6-mm thickening of the mucus membrane.

Although imaging is not routinely recommended in the diagnosis of sinusitis, a negative CT effectively eliminates the diagnosis. Addition of magnetic resonance imaging may be useful when complications of sinusitis are suspected. In this situation, fluid collections that require surgical drainage may be identified.

Flexible or rigid nasal endoscopy is adequate in visualization of purulent discharge, adenoid hyperplasia or infection, nasal polyps, mucosal edema, and septal deviation.

Sinus Aspiration

Indications for sinus aspiration include sinusitis unresponsive to multiple courses of antibiotics, severe facial pain, and suspected sinusitis in an immunocompromised child in whom unusual pathogens such as fungi may be present. It can be performed on an outpatient basis but is usually poorly tolerated in children without anesthesia.

Additional testing to complete the workup for refractory CRS may include:
- Testing for a primary immunodeficiency, i.e., quantitative immunoglobulins, immune profile, vaccine titers. There is a high prevalence of CRS in individuals with common variable immune deficiency (CVID) and selective IgG3 subclass deficiency weakens host defense against *M. catarrhalis* and the M component of *S. pyogenic*.
- *Testing for allergies*: Skin prick testing or specific allergens IgE levels.
- Sweat chloride test and genetic testing for cystic fibrosis.
- Nasal and preferably bronchial biopsy and genetic testing for primary ciliary dyskinesia.

COMPLICATIONS

Complications of sinusitis may be divided into those involving the orbit (optic neuritis, orbital and periorbital cellulitis, orbital, and subperiosteal abscesses), the central nervous system (meningitis, subdural and epidural empyema, brain abscess and venous sinus thrombosis), or the bone [maxillary osteitis, frontal osteitis (Pott puffy tumor)].

TREATMENT

Acute Rhinosinusitis

High-dose amoxicillin (90 mg/kg/day) should be considered as a first-line agent for the treatment of sinusitis because of its activity against sinus pathogens. Because the proportion of cases caused by *Haemophilus influenzae* is likely increasing and the rate of β-lactamase production by this organism is also increasing, the addition of clavulanic acid to amoxicillin provides an advantage over amoxicillin alone. Using (90 mg/kg/day) of the amoxicillin component provides better coverage for penicillin nonsusceptible *S. pneumoniae*. Cephalosporins are alter-native antibiotics, although they are less active against *S. pneumoniae* than amoxicillin-clavulanate. For those children in whom amoxicillin-clavulanate or second-or third-generation cephalosporins fail, a combination of cefixime (or cefdinir) and linezolid may be used as an alternative to the use of parenteral antimicrobial agents.

For patients in whom beta-lactam antibiotics are contraindicated, respiratory fluoroquinolones (levofloxacin or moxifloxacin) or doxycycline may be used. Reference to local antibiotic susceptibility patterns may aid in choosing appropriate therapy.

Response to therapy is rapid in children who have sinusitis and are adherent to therapy with an appropriate antimicrobial agent. Symptoms typically improve within 48 hours (i.e., fever, cough, discharge). If symptoms worsen within 72 hours or are not improved within 3–5 days, then clinical reassessment is warranted (If the diagnosis remains unchanged, a second-line antimicrobial should be prescribed). Alternatively, sinus aspiration may be considered for precise identification of the causative organism.

The appropriate duration of antimicrobial therapy has not been studied thoroughly. For children who have a rapid response to the initiation of antimicrobial, 10 days of therapy usually is appropriate. For those who respond at a slower rate, treating until the patient has no more symptoms plus an additional 7 days is reasonable.

Chronic Rhinosinusitis

In pediatric CRS associated with allergic rhinitis, allergen avoidance, antihistamines, and nasal steroids will help in ameliorating the symptoms.

Moreover, allergen immunotherapy may be an underused option that could benefit patients with persistent allergic rhinitis and can change the natural course of the disease by reducing the symptoms and medications use.

Whereas data supports the efficacy of immunotherapy for the treatment of allergic rhinitis, there is no evidence for this treatment modality in patients with CRS.

The role of empiric antireflux medication, topical antibiotics, and antral irrigation are not supported for the treatment of pediatric CRS.

Surgery

Surgical intervention is not the mainstay of treatment of CRS and is only used in the presence of complications, in failure of medical treatment and in patients with suspected anatomic abnormalities.

Adenoidal tissue acts as a bacterial reservoir in children with CRS, regardless of their size and removing them improves outcomes. Adenoidectomy is highly effective as an initial surgical therapy in children aged up to 6 years; it has been found that the efficiency of this treatment decreases between the age of 6 and 12 years.

Surgeries such as adenoidectomy, balloon sinuplasty, sinus puncture and lavage, endoscopic sinus surgery, turbinectomy, and open surgical approaches are reserved for patients who fail medical management.

Endoscopic sinus surgery in pediatric chronic rhinosinusitis (PCRS) is performed in case of failure of medical management and/or adenoidectomy in controlling the symptoms of PCRS.

SUGGESTED READING

1. Nelson's Textbook of Pediatrics, 21st edition.

Chapter 89: Croup and Epiglottitis

Raghvendra Singh

CROUP

INTRODUCTION

- The term "croup" includes heterogeneous group of conditions, which are generally caused by viruses, are acute processes that are characterized by bark-like or brassy cough and may also have hoarseness of voice, inspiratory stridor and respiratory distress, all these resulting from inflammation of larynx and subglottic airway.
- It is the most common cause of upper airway obstruction in children. The hallmark of croup in infants and young children is barking cough, whereas hoarseness is more common in older children.
- Inflammation of vocal cord and structures below it are termed laryngitis, laryngotracheitis, or laryngotracheobronchitis depending upon the extent of involvement of larynx, trachea, and bronchi.
- Croup typically affects larynx, trachea, and bronchi. It occurs commonly in age groups 3 months to 5 years, although other age groups are also affected.
- Croup is usually a mild, self-limited illness but rarely, it can be fatal.
  Recurrent croup can occur and is defined as two or more croup-like episodes. Patients with recurrent croup have higher incidence of asthma and allergies. Some patients have family history of croup.

ETIOLOGY

Parainfluenza viruses (types 1, 2, and 3) account for majority of cases; other viruses include influenza A and B, adenovirus, respiratory syncytial virus (RSV), and measles, adenovirus, enterovirus, etc.

CLINICAL FEATURES

- After initial symptoms of upper respiratory tract infection for 1–3 days, signs and symptoms of upper airway obstruction become apparent, with characteristic barking cough, hoarseness, and inspiratory stridor.
- In occasional patients, respiratory difficulty may ensue due to increasing airway obstruction. Fever may or may not be present.
- Children generally prefer upright position; symptoms tend to worsen at night, and also with agitation. In usual scenario, symptoms resolve within a week.
- History of affected family members with upper respiratory tract infection might be there.
- On examination, hoarse voice, coryza, inflamed pharynx may be present. Degree of respiratory distress is variable and is proportional to the degree of airway obstruction. Hypoxia is rare and occurs when there is nearly complete airway obstruction.

CLASSIFICATION OF CROUP

- *Mild*: No stridor at rest (stridor on crying may be present), barking cough, no or minimal chest retractions.
- *Moderate*: Stridor at rest, mild respiratory distress.
- *Severe*: Stridor at rest, severe retractions, anxious, agitated, fatigued child.

LABORATORY INVESTIGATIONS

- Croup is a clinical diagnosis; laboratory investigations are not required.
- X-ray neck, although not required, for diagnosis shows typical subglottic narrowing or steeple sign on posteroanterior view though it may be absent in some patients.

COMPLICATIONS

- Otitis media and pneumonia can occur.
- Bacterial tracheitis may occur as a complication and should be suspected if, after croup-like illness, high-grade fever persists with worsening of respiratory distress at the time when usually recovery is expected.

TREATMENT

- Airway management is the mainstay of therapy in croup. Fortunately majority is mild and can be managed at home.

- *Mild croup*:
  - Humidity, antipyretics, hydration.
  - Oral dexamethasone (as effective as IM route) in single dose 0.6 mg/kg (maximum dose 16 mg) decreases duration of symptoms, complications, need for epinephrine nebulization and hospitalization.
  - Alternatively prednisolone single oral dose 1 mg/kg can also be given.
- *Moderate-to-severe croup*:
  - Humidification, fluids, antipyretics, and oxygen.
  - *Corticosteroids*: Decrease edema in airways by their anti-inflammatory action.
  - Oral/IM/IV dexamethasone in the dose of 0.6 mg/kg (maximum 16 mg) single dose.
  - Alternatively single dose of nebulized budesonide (2 mg/2 mL solution via nebulizer) can also be used.
    - *Nebulized epinephrine/racemic epinephrine*: Racemic epinephrine is a 1:1 mixture of D- and L-isomers of epinephrine (not available easily). The duration of action of racemic epinephrine is 2 hours, consequently, observation is mandated. L-epinephrine is administered as 0.5 mL/kg per dose (maximum of 5 mL) using the 1 mg/mL strength (also referred as 1:1,000 dilution); it is given via nebulizer over 15 minutes. Current evidence does not support the use of racemic epinephrine over L-epinephrine in terms of efficacy or safety.
  - Helium-oxygen mixture (heliox) may be used in children with severe croup where intubation is being considered, although evidence is inconclusive.
  - *Not useful*: Antibiotics and over-the-counter cough–cold medicines.

DIFFERENTIAL DIAGNOSIS

Spasmodic croup is usually a benign recurring disease affecting children aged 6 months to 3 years.
- It always occurs at night; symptom duration is short with abrupt onset and cessation.
- Similar episodes can occur for few successive nights.
- Fever is absent but upper respiratory tract symptoms (e.g., coryza) may be present.
- The disease is more common in children with family history of allergies.
- Treatment is comforting the anxious child and administering humidified air.

EPIGLOTTITIS

INTRODUCTION

- Inflammation of epiglottis and adjacent supraglottic structures.
- Rare nowadays due to universal immunization, this condition is characterized by acutely onset of high fever, sore throat, dyspnea, and rapidly progressing respiratory obstruction and is lethal if not treated on time.
- Median age of children involved is 6–12 years age.

ETIOLOGY

In the past, *Haemophilus influenzae b* was most common cause but its incidence declined after immunization; *Streptococcus pyogenes*, *S. pneumoniae*, nontypeable *H. influenzae*, and *Staphylococcus aureus* are more common in immunized children now.

CLINICAL FEATURES

- In children, the most common presentation is of an otherwise healthy child who acutely develops sore throat, anterior neck pain, and fever. Within hours, the child becomes sick, anxious, swallowing becomes difficult, and breathing is labored, drooling is usually present, and voice may be muffled.
- The child may assume tripod position, to open the airway which is the child prefers sitting upright, with hyperextended neck and trunk leaning forward with the chin up and mouth open. The child refuses to lie down.
- Stridor, if present, is a late finding and suggests near-complete airway obstruction.
- Untreated, air hunger with restlessness may be followed by rapidly increasing respiratory obstruction leading to cyanosis, coma, and death can ensue unless treatment measures are instituted promptly.
- Cough typical of croup is rare. Usually no other family members are sick.

COMPLICATIONS

Pneumonia, cervical lymphadenitis, otitis media, meningitis or septic arthritis can occur.

DIAGNOSIS

- It is suspected based on rapidly developing clinical features.
- *Laryngoscopy*: Under controlled circumstances (operating room or ICU and never in outpatient settings), a large, cherry red, swollen epiglottis is visualized by laryngoscopy.
- Lateral X-ray of upper airway can be done in doubtful cases. In classic cases, "*thumb sign*" (swollen epiglottis) is seen, for which proper positioning of the patient in form of adequate hyperextension of the head and neck is necessary while doing X-ray.

TREATMENT

- It is a medical emergency requiring immediate treatment with an artificial airway placed under closed conditions.
- Until the airway is secured, anxiety-provoking measures such as IV line insertion, phlebotomy, or trying to place the child supine should be avoided.

- Cultures of blood, epiglottic surface should be collected after the airway is stabilized.
- Ceftriaxone/cefepime/meropenem should be given parenterally; pending culture reports, antistaph, vancomycin can also be added.
- After the insertion of the airway patient should improve immediately, and respiratory distress and cyanosis should disappear. Duration of intubation is variable and is determined by frequent direct laryngoscopy or flexible fiber optic laryngoscopy. Most patients have concomitant bacteremia.
- Antibiotics should be continued for 7–10 days.

Chemoprophylaxis

Ii is not routinely recommended for close contacts but close careful observation is necessary.

Indication for chemoprophylaxis:
- For all household members if there is a child younger than 4 years of age and incompletely unimmunized.
- Child 12 months and younger and not completed the primary vaccination series.
- Immunocompromised.

DOC: Rifampicin 20 mg/kg (maximum 600 mg) orally OD for 4 days.

PROGNOSIS

With prompt diagnosis and management, prognosis is excellent.

SUGGESTED READING

1. Nelson's Textbook of Pediatrics, 21st edition.

CHAPTER 90: Acute Bronchiolitis

Kripasindhu Chatterjee

INTRODUCTION

- Acute bronchiolitis is commonly caused by viral lower respiratory tract infection (LRTI) in infants.
- It is most common cause of hospitalization due to LRTI in infants and children.
- It is defined as acute inflammation, edema, and necrosis of epithelial cell lining of small airways, and increased mucus production.
- Oski's Pediatrics Principles and Practice defines as first episode of wheezing in a child <24 months with physical findings of viral respiratory infection and no other explanation for wheezing-like atopy, etc.

ETIOLOGY

Causative agents are respiratory syncytial virus (RSV)—50–80% of cases, rhinovirus— 30–40%. Parainfluenza, influenza, adenovirus, and Coronaviruses are found in lesser number of patients.

Newer respiratory viruses also cause bronchiolitis such as human metapneumovirus (hMPV) and human bocavirus (HboV).

EPIDEMIOLOGY

In India, outbreaks occur between September and March. Acute bronchiolitis occurs in small children. 76% of cases occur in <1 year of age and 94% in <2 years. The peak incidence is between 2 and 6 months. Preterm infants (<37 weeks) had similar rates as compared to term infants of 5.2 per 1,000 but highest hospitalization rate is higher 18.7 children per 1,000.

DIAGNOSIS

Diagnosis is basically clinical. It presents with upper respiratory features of rhinitis and cough and fever for 1–2 days followed by worsening of cough, tachypnea, respiratory distress and wheezing. Majority improve with mild course in 3–5 days but some may continue to worsen and may develop respiratory failure with irritability or drowsiness, decreased intake, cyanosis with decreased SaO_2, grunt, marked retractions, and hyperexpanded chest.

Course is usually self-limiting up to around 4 weeks.

Radiology: Radiographic changes associated are atelectasis or hyperinflation.

Chest radiography do not correlate with disease severity and routine chest radiography in children with bronchiolitis is not recommended and should be reserved for severe disease needing intensive care unit (ICU) admission or suspicion of complication (such as pneumothorax).

Laboratory investigations: Common laboratory tests are not useful and routinely not indicated. Higher values of nasal fluid lactate dehydrogenase (LDH) indicate good antiviral response and decreased need of hospitalization in some studies.

Virology:

- Viral antigen may be detected from respiratory secretions by immunofluorescence or polymerase chain reaction (PCR).
- Positivity rate of PCR varies in studies from 60% to 75% for RSV, and coinfections in up to one third of infants.
- PCR should be done for infants on monthly prophylaxis, if testing for RSV is positive suggesting breakthrough infection, monthly palivizumab prophylaxis should be discontinued because of the very low likelihood of a second RSV infection in the same year.

Different parameters in *scoring systems to predict severity* are used in different studies but none are universally acceptable. Tal et al. proposed a similar scoring system **(Table 1)**.

Prediction of severity: There are several risk factors that are associated with severe disease **(Box 1)**.

Environmental factors include family history of older sibling, inutero smoke exposure, overcrowding, etc.

Host factors associated more with progression to severe disease or mortality include prematurity, low birth weight, age <6–12 weeks, preexisting pulmonary disease hemodynamically significant congenital heart disease,

TABLE 1: Scoring system to predict severity.

Score: RR min	Wheeze	Cyanosis	Accessory use
0: <30	None	None	None: No chest indrawing
1: 30–45	Terminal expiration only	Perioral on crying only	Lost visible intercostal indrawing, no head bobbing/tricheal tag
2: 46–60	Entire expiration and inspiration with stethoscopy only	Perioral at rest	Moderate intercostal indrawing. No head bobbing/tracheal tag
3: >60	Entire explanation and inspiration without stethoscope	Generalized at rest	Intercostal indrawing with head bobbing/incheal tag

(RR: respiratory rate)

BOX 1: Prediction of severity.

- *Host factors:*
  - Prematurity
  - Low birth weight
  - Age < 6–12 weeks
  - Pre-existing pulmonary disease
  - Hemodynamically significant CHD—CHF requiring medication
  - Moderate-to-severe pulmonary hypertension
  - Immunodeficiency
- *Environmental factors:*
  - Family history in older sibling
  - Passive smoking
  - Overcrowding
- *Clinical predictors:*
  - Toxic or ill appearance
  - SaO_2 < 95% in room air
  - RR ≥ 70/min
  - Moderate-to-severe retractions
  - Atelectasis on CXR

Repeated observation over a period is more informative.

(CHD: congenital heart disease; CHF: congestive heart failure; CXR: chest X-ray; RR: respiratory rate)

BOX 2: Treatment options.

- *Clearly effective:* Supportive care including oxygen, IV fluids
- *Possibly effective:*
  - Nebulized bronchodilators—SABA/epinephrine
  - Nebulized hypertonic saline dexamethazone + Inhaled epipnephrine
- *Possibly effective severe cases:*
  - CPAP
  - Surfactant
  - Heliox
  - Aerosolized ribavirin
- *Possibly ineffective:*
  - Oral bronchodilators
  - Leukotriene antagonists
  - Corticosteroid inhaled/Systemic
  - Chest physiotherapy
  - Steam inhalations
  - RSV polyclonal immunoglobulin
  - Inhaled furosemide
  - Inhaled interferon alfa

(CPAP: continuous positive airway pressure; IV: intravenous; RSV: respiratory syncytial virus; SABA: short-acting beta-agonist)

chronic lung disease (bronchopulmonary dysplasia), and congenital anomalies. Clinical predictors include toxic or ill appearance; SaO_2 < 95% in room air; respiratory rate (RR) ≥ 70/min, moderate-to-severe retract ions, atelectasis on chest X-ray (CXR). Repeated observation over a period is more informative than a single assess mention anytime.

Risk of mortality increases in some conditions such as age < 6 months, prematurity, underlying lung disease, cyanotic congenital heart disease, and immunodeficiency.

TREATMENT (BOX 2)

- Acute bronchiolitis is a mild-to-moderate disease with chance progressive disease in some cases.
- Best treatment options are still not clear and there exist a lot of controversies about best possible evidence based management in moderate-to-severe cases.

Nutrition and Hydration

- The essential part of treatment is nutrition, hydration, and electrolyte balance.
- Oral feeding may be given frequently to those who can feed.
- Parenteral fluids should be given if RR is more than 60–70 breaths per minute or the child refuses to take orally. Parenteral fluid should be isotonic fluids to reduce chance of hyponatremia.

Oxygen

- Oxygen saturation is a poor predictor of respiratory distress but is a primary determinant for need for hospitalization in infants with bronchiolitis.
- Supplemental oxygen is indicated if SaO_2 falls persistently below 90% in previously healthy infants and may be

discontinued when SaO$_2$ is persistently at or above 90% and infant is feeding well and has minimal respiratory distress.
- There are several new approaches to oxygen delivery in bronchiolitis, two of which are home oxygen and high-frequency nasal cannula. There is emerging evidence for the role of home oxygen in reducing hospitalization stay or admission rate for infants with bronchiolitis, including two randomized trials.
- Use of humidified, heated, high-flow nasal cannula to deliver air-oxygen mixtures provides assistance to infants with bronchiolitis through multiple mechanisms such as improving respiratory effort, generation of continuous positive airway pressure reducing work of breathing, and may decreasing need for intubation.
- One very large retrospective study from Australia showed a decline in intubation rate in the subgroup of infant with bronchiolitis (n = 330) from 37 to 7% after the introduction of high-flow nasal cannula.

Continuous Positive Airway Pressure
- In severe bronchiolitis, continuous positive airway pressure (CPAP) is used to reduce mechanical ventilation. CPAP helps by recruiting collapsed alveoli, and reducing airway pressure thus reducing air trapping.
- A systematic review in 2011 showed no conclusive evidence that CPAP reduces intubation in severe bronchiolitis. Another randomized trial in 2013 comparing nasal CPAP (NCPAP) and oxygen-inhalation concluded that NCPAP resulted in rapid improvement in 6 hours.
- Current evidence is inconclusive on routine use of CPAP in severe cases of acute bronchiolitis.

Mechanical Ventilation
Major indication of intubation and mechanical ventilation are clinical deterioration on conventional management or respiratory failure from beginning and usually needed in around 10% of cases and median duration is about 5 days.

Heliox (mixture of helium and oxygen) reduces airway resistance and respiratory distress as it flows more linearly. Current evidence on benefits of heliox in moderate-to-severe bronchiolitis is inadequate.

Bronchodilators
- Most RCTs have failed to demonstrate a consistent benefit from α- or β-adrenergic agents.
- In a recently updated Cochrane systematic review involving 1,992 infants from 12 countries, Godamsky A Min 2014, indicated no benefit in the clinical course.
- *Epinephrine*: Most studies have compared L-epinephrine to placebo or albuterol. A Cochrane meta-analysis by Hartling et al. found no evidence for utility in the inpatient setting.
- Another multicenter trial by Skierven HO et al. found even longer hospital stay when epinephrine was used on a fixed schedule compared with an as-needed schedule and suggests epinephrine should be used only as a rescue agent in severe disease.

Hypertonic Saline
- Nebulized hypertonic saline is an increasingly studied therapy for acute viral bronchiolitis because it involves airway inflammation and resultant mucus plugging and physiologic evidence suggests that hypertonic saline increases mucociliary clearance in both normal and diseased lungs.
- A Cochrane review by Zhang et al. on infants with mild-to-moderate disease suggests that 3% saline is safe and effective at improving symptoms of mild-to-moderate bronchiolitis after 24 hours of use and reducing hospital stay when average stay exceeds 3 days.

Corticosteroids

Systemic Steroids
- Corticosteroids are effective in respiratory diseases, such as asthma and croup. Initial studies suggested that steroid may favorably influence treatment of bronchiolitis.
- Fernandes RM et al. in Cochrane Systemic Review showed that corticosteroids by any route (IM, IV, Oral, ICS) do not reduce outpatient admissions and do not reduce hospital stay.
- Another meta-analysis by Davison C et al. stated no role of systemic steroid in critically ill infants with bronchiolitis but may lead to prolonged virus shedding.

Inhaled Corticosteroid
- A systematic review by Blom DJM failed to show that use of inhalation method (ICS) during acute bronchiolitis prevents postbronchiolitis wheeze.
- Hence, there is no evidence use of ICS during acute bronchiolitis prevents postbronchiolitis wheeze.

Antibiotics
Antibiotics showed no benefit from routine antibacterial therapy for children with bronchiolitis and should be given when there is a definite evidence of infection.

PREVENTION
Acute bronchiolitis is a common infection without any effective therapy, so preventive measures are very useful.

General measures: Measures include among others tobacco smoke avoidance and promotion of breastfeeding.

Tobacco smoke: Tobacco smoke exposure increases the risk and severity of bronchiolitis evidenced in different meta-analysis studies.

Breastfeeding: The American Academy of Pediatrics in 2012 stated that respiratory infections were shown to be significantly less common in breastfed children. Meta-analysis from the Agency for Healthcare Research and Quality that showed that hospitalization risk secondary to respiratory diseases was reduced by 72% in infants who were exclusively breastfed for 4 or more months.

Immunoprophylaxis:
- Passive immunoprophylaxis using monoclonal or polyclonal antibodies in high-risk infants have shown to reduce risk of RSV transmission.
- *Polyclonal antibodies*: Studies did not support its usefulness.
- *Monoclonal antibodies*:
  - These include palivizumab (humanized mouse IgG1 directed against RSV) and its variants such as Motavizumab and Numax-YTE, second-and third-generation monoclonal antibodies, respectively.
  - Monthly palivizumab prophylaxis should be restricted to infants < 29 weeks, except chronic lung disease of infancy and continue to require treatment may receive till 2 years.
  - Data show that infants born at or after 29 weeks 0 days' gestation have an RSV hospitalization rate similar to the rate of full-term infants.

CONCLUSION

- Acute bronchiolitis is the most common cause of hospitalization due to LRTI in infants and children.
- Current evidence do not support a routine bronchodilators or corticosteroid.
- Acute bronchiolitis is the most common cause of hospitalization due to LRTI in infants and children.
- Current evidence do not support a routine broncho dilators or corticosteroid.
- Hypertonic saline reduces hospital stay when average duration of stay exceeds 3 days. High-flow nasal cannula oxygen (HFNCO) leads to decline in intubation rate in bronchiolitis.
- Tobacco smoke exposure increases both severity of illness and risk of hospitalization for bronchiolitis.
- Exclusive breastfeeding for 4 months reduces risk of hospitalization secondary to respiratory diseases by 72%.

SUGGESTED READING

1. AAP Subcommittee on Diagnosis and Management of Bronchiolitis. Diagnosis and management of bronchiolitis. Pediatrics. 2014;134:e1474-502.
2. American Academy of Pediatrics; Committee on Infectious Diseases and Bronchiolitis Guidelines Committee. Technical report: updated guidance for palivizumab prophylaxis among infants and young children at increased risk of hospitalization for respiratory syncytial virus infection. Pediatrics. 2014; 134(2):e620-38.
3. Arora B, Mahajan P, Zidan MA, Sethuraman U. Nasopharyngeal airway pressures in bronchiolitis patients treated with high-flow nasal cannula oxygen therapy. Pediatr Emerg Care. 2012;28(11):1179-84.
4. Bajaj L, Turner CG, Bothner J. A randomized trial of homeoxygen therapy from the emergency department for acute bronchiolitis. Pediatrics. 2006;117(3):633-40.
5. Blom DJM, Ermers M, Bont L. Inhaled corticosteroid during acute bronchiolitis in the prevention of postbronchiolitis wheezing. Cochrane Database Syst Rev. 2007;1:CD004881.
6. Cherian T, Simoes EA, Steinhoff MC, Chitra K, John M, Raghupathy P, et al. Bronchiolitis in tropical South India. Am J Dis Child. 1990;144(9):1026-30.
7. Corneli HM, Zorc JJ, Holubkov R, Bregstein JS, Brown KM, Mahajan P, et al; Bronchiolitis Study Group for the Pediatric Emergency Care Applied Research Network. Bronchiolitis: clinical characteristics associated with hospitalization and length of stay. Pediatr Emerg Care. 2012;28(2):99-103.
8. Davison C, Ventre KM, Luchetti M. Efficacy of interventions for bronchoilitis in critically ill infants: a systemetic review and metaanalysis. Pediatr Crit Care Med. 2004;5:482-9.
9. Donlan M, Fontela PS, Puligandla PS. Use of CPAP in acute viral bronchiolitis: a systematic review. Pediatr Pulmonol. 2011;46:736-46.
10. Fernandes RM, Bialy LM, Vandermeer B, Tjosvold L, Plint AC, Patel H, et al. Glucocorticoids for acute viral bronchiolitis in infants and young children. Cochrane Database Syst Rev. 2013;(6):CD004878.
11. Friis B, Andersen P, Brenøe E, et al. Antibiotic treatment of pneumonia and bronchiolitis. A prospective randomised study. Arch Dis Child. 1984;59(11):1038-45.
12. Gadomski AM, Scribani MB. Bronchodilators for bronchiolitis. Cochrane Database Syst Rev. 2014;(6):CD001266.
13. Hall CB. Nosocomial respiratory syncytial virus infections: The" Cold War " has not ended. Clin Infect Dis. 2000;31(2):590-6.
14. Hanson IC, Shearer WT. Bronchiolitis. Oski's Pediatrics: Principles and Practice, 4th edition. USA: Lippincott Williams and Wilkins; 2006. pp. 1391
15. Hartling L, Fernandes RM, Bialy L, Milne A, Johnson D, Plint A, et al. Steroids and bronchodilators for acute bronchiolitis in the first two years of life: systematic review and meta-analysis. BMJ. 2011;342:d1714.
16. Kallappa C, Hufton M, Millen G, Ninan TK. Use of high flow nasal cannula oxygen (HFNCO) in infants with bronchiolitis on a paediatric ward: a 3-year experience. Arch Dis Child. 2014;99(8):790-91.
17. Laham FR, Trott AT, Bennett BL, Kozinetz CA, Jewell AM, Garofalo RP, et al. LDH concentration in nasal wash fluid as a biochemical predictor of bronchiolitis severity. Pediatrics. 2010;125(2):e225-33.
18. Meissner HC. Selected population at increased risk from RSV infection. Pediatr Infect Dis J. 2003;22:S40-44.
19. Milder E, Arnold JC. Human metapneumovirus and human bocavirus in children. Pediatr Res. 2009;65:78R-83R
20. Milesi C, Matecki S, Jaber S, Mura T, Jacquot A, Pidoux O, et al. 6 cm of H_2O CPAP versus conventional oxygen therapy in severe viral bronchiolitis: a randomised trial. Pediatr Pulmonol. 2013;48(1):45-51.
21. Pham TM, O'Malley L, Mayfield S, Martin S, Schibler A. The effect of high flow nasal cannula therapy on the work of breathing in infants with bronchiolitis. Pediatr Pulmonol. 2015;50(7):713-20.

22. Roghman KJ. Parental smoking and family history of asthma increases risk of bronchiolitis. Am J Dis Child. 1986;140:806-12.
23. Russell KF, Liang Y, O'Gorman K, Johnson DW, Klassen TP. Glucocorticoids for croup. Cochrane Database Syst Rev. 2011;(1):CD001955.
24. Section on Breastfeeding. Breastfeeding and the use of human milk. Pediatrics. 2012;129(3):e827-41.
25. Skjerven HO, Hunderi JO, Brugmann-Pieper SK, Brun AC, Engen H, Eskedal L, et al. Racemic adrenaline and inhalation strategies in acute bronchiolitis. N Engl J Med. 2013;368(24):2286-93.
26. Strachan DP, Cook DG. Health effects of passive smoking. 1. Parental smoking and lower respiratory illness in infancy and early childhood. Thorax. 1997;52(10):905-14.
27. Swingler Gh, Hussey GD. Duration of illness in ambulatory children diagnosed as acute bronchiolitis. Arch Pediatr Adolesc Med. 2000;154:997-1000.
28. Tal A, Bavilski C, Yohai D, Bearman JE, Gorodischer R, Moses SW. Dexamethasone and salbutamol in the treatment of acute wheezing in infants. Pediatrics. 1983;71:13-18.
29. Voets S, van Berlaer G. Clinical predictors of severity of bronchiolitis. Eur J Emerg Med. 2006;13:134-8.
30. Wang EE, Law BJ. Pediatric Investigators Collaboration Network on Infections in Canada (PICNIC) Prospective study of risk factors and outcome in patients with RSVLRTI. J Pediatr. 1995;126:212-9.
31. Wang J, Xu E, Xiao Y. Isotonic versus hypotonic maintenance IV fluids in hospitalized children: a meta-analysis. Pediatrics. 2014;133(1):10513.
32. Zhang L, Mendoza-Sassi RA, Wainwright C, Klassen TP. Nebulized hypertonic saline solu-tion for acute bronchiolitis in infants. Cochrane Database Syst Rev. 2008;(4):CD006458.

Wheezing in Children

Atanu Bhadra

INTRODUCTION

Wheezing is associated with or contributory to a large proportion of childhood acute respiratory infection (ARI). For logistic reasons, World Health Organization (WHO) strategy for control of ARI has focused only on case management of pneumonia. In last two decades researchers from developing countries have raised serious concerns over the applicability of these guidelines in children having wheeze. The diagnosis and management of "Wheeze" has largely been ignored resulting in over use of bronchodilator medications at the community level.

To rationalize the prescriptions at community level, accurate diagnosis of wheeze is to be made using simple clinical tools.

1. **How common is wheeze?**
Ans: Almost 50% of children have at least 1 episode of wheeze by the time the child reaches 5 years.

2. **What is wheeze?**
Ans: Wheezing is a musical sound produced when the air flow from the lungs is obstructed, due to contraction of the smooth muscles surrounding the airways or swelling of the lining of bronchioles.

3. Mechanism of wheeze production:
   - Toy trumpet whose sound is produced by vibrating reed.
   - Pitch of wheeze depends on the elasticity of airway walls.
   - Modern model: Mathematical analysis of the stability of airflow through a collapsible tube.
   - Wheezes are produced by fluttering of the airway walls and fluid together with a critical airway velocity. The oscillations began when the airflow velocity reaches a critical value called "Flutter Velocity." The flutter velocity is dependent on the mechanical and physical characteristics of the tube and gas.
   - Grotberg model predicts the critical flow velocity inducing oscillations, as well as frequency of these oscillations.

4. Inspiratory wheezing/squawking inspiratory sound—hypersensitivity pneumonitis.

5. Wheeze and severity of airway obstruction.
   - Intensity has no correlation with degree of obstruction.
   - Tw/Total and FEV1 and forced expiratory volume in 1 second (FEV1) has (the total proportion of respiratory cycle occupied by wheeze) significant relationship.

6. Wheezes for diagnosis of bronchial hyper-responsiveness.
   - PCzo concentration of methacholine inducing 20% fall in FEV1. (Audible without stethoscope)
   - *Stridor*: Audible wheeze extremely high pitched, both inspiration/expiration (significant upper airway obstruction).
   - *Wheeze*: Expiratory sound usually high pitched, continues (>250 ms). (Inspiratory also in case of severe obstruction) ≥ 400 Hz especially upper airway.
   - *Polyphonic*: Differ pitches originating from different caliber airway.
   - *Rhonci*: 200 Hz/low-pitched continuous sound.

7. Wheezes for monitoring nocturnal asthma.
   Asthma is the most common chronic disease of childhood and leading cause of childhood morbidity in terms of school absence, emergency hospital visit, and admission.
   It consists of different phenotypes. Recurrent wheezing occurs in a large proportion of children 5 years and younger. It is typically associated with upper respiratory tract infection (URTI) which occurs 6–8 times/years. Rhinovirus and respiratory syncytial virus (RSV) are the most common causative organism. Wheezing <5 years of age is a heterogeneous group and not all wheezing is asthma.

8. Wheezing phenotypes symptom based:
   - *Episodic wheeze*: Symptoms are absent between episodes.
   - *Multitrigger wheeze*: Symptoms are present in-between episodes and trigger such as activity, laughing crying.

- Children with (+)ve loose index 2.6/5.5 times more likely to have asthma between 6 and 13 years.
- 59% of (+)ve loose index active asthma.
- Children with (+)ve stringent index 4.3-9.8 time more likely to have asthma.
- 76% had active asthma.
- Over 95% of children with (-)ve stringent index never had asthma between 6 and 19 years.
- Time trend based.
- Transient wheeze (symptoms began and ended before 3 year).
- Persistent wheeze symptoms began before 3 year and continued beyond 6 years.
- Late-onset wheeze symptoms began 3 years with the present state of knowledge; we now know the above phenotypes are not watertight compartments.

ASTHMA

Will my child have asthma?

Probability-based Approach

Keeping in mind that not all wheezes are asthmatic and it is not routinely possible to assess airflow limitation or bronchodilator responsiveness in this age group, parents/caregivers are now directed to have the probability approach.

Symptoms (cough, wheeze heavy breathing for <10 days during URTI 2-3 episodes/year).

No symptom between episodes.

Few have asthma: Symptoms >10 days during URTI > 3 episodes/year/night working/severe. In between, occasional cough and wheeze.

Some have asthma: Symptoms >10 days during URTI > 3 episodes/years/severe/night working/cough/wheeze during play and laughing. Allergic sensitive, atopic dermatitis (AD), and food allergy.

Tucson's Children Respiratory Study

Arizona: 1,246 newborns born between 1980 and 1984 were enrolled for a longitudinal study Stringent index:
Frequent wheeze first year of life +

1. Major criteria
   a. Asthma
   b. Eczema
   Parents (diagnosed by physician)

1. or 2.

2. Minor criteria
   a. AR
   b. Wheezing without cold
   c. Eosinophilia > 4%

Caveat: Use of "eosinophilia" certain is not studied in areas of helminthic infection.

Loose index: Any wheezing <3 years and the same combination of major and minor criterion.

Key Indications for Alternative Diagnosis
- Failure to thrive
- Neonatal or early onset of symptoms
- Wheezing not responsive to [inhaled corticosteroid (ICS)/short-acting β2-agonist (SABA)]
- No triggers identified
- Hypoxemia out of proportion to clinical assessment.

Alternative Diagnosis
- Gastroesophageal reflux disease (GERD)
- Foreign body (FB) aspiration
- Tracheomalacia
- Tuberculosis
- Coronary heart disease (CHD)
- Cystic fibrosis (CF)
- Primary ciliary dyskinesia
- Vascular ring
- Bronchopulmonary dysplasia (BPD)
- Immune deficiency.

Goals of Management
- To achieve good control
- To minimize risk of flare ups.

Asthma Control

In last 4 weeks:
- Daytime asthma symptoms > few minutes > once/week
- Activity limitation
- Reliever medication > once/week
- Night waking
  Well controlled—none (of the above)
  Partly controlled—1 and 2 (of the above)
  Uncontrolled—3 and 4 (of the above).

Steps of Treatment (Children under 5 Years)

Step 1: Reliever—as needed SABA (use of SABA > 2 time/week/over 1 month → trial of ICS)

Step 2: Controller—regular daily low-dose ICS + As needed SABA (Reliever)

Alternative: Daily leukotriene receptor antagonist (LTRA/intermittent ICS)

Step 3: Before stepping up consider:
- Alternative diagnosis
- Check inhaler skills
- Compliance
- Double daily low-dose 1CS (or, low-dose 1CS + LTRA)

Step 4: Referred to "Specialist"

Preferred device:
- 0-3: Pressurize metered-dose inhaler plus spacer with face mask

- 4-5: Pressurized metered dose inhaler with space ± mask
- Nebulizers with face mask is the only other alternative for the minority of children who cannot be thought the use of spacer device.

Asthma Self-management Education for Caregivers

- Training about inhalation technique
- Information of the importance of child's adherence to medication
- Written asthma action plan
- Recognizing worsening symptoms

Re-Flag Signs of Acute Exacerbation

- Onset of symptoms of RTI
- Acute increase in wheeze and shortness of breath
- Increase in cough (sleep)
- Lethargy/reduced exercise tolerance
- Impairment of daily activities, including feeding
- A poor response to reliever medication.

Mild/Moderate Attack

- Pulse ≤ 180 beats/min (0-3 year), ≤150 beats/min (4-5 years)
- $SPO_2 ≥ 92\%$
- Breathless

↓

Treatment
- (SABA)/Salbutamol 2 puffs (100 mg) + every 20 minute to 1 hour
- O_2—Target SPO_2 94-98%

↓

- No response/? response/compromise SPO_2

↓

- Transfer to critical care

Severe Attack/Life-threatening Attack

- Unable to speak
- Central cyanosis
- Respiratory rate (RR) > 40
- $SPO_2 < 92\%$
- Silent chest
- Pulse rate >180 beats/min (0-3 years), >150 beats/min (4-5 year) (while waiting give salbutamol 100 mg 6 puff/20)

↓

Transfer to critical care

Asthma—6 to 11 Years

Asthma is described as symptoms of wheeze, breathlessness, and cough. Time has come to revise this. The proper response of a family whose child has been given a diagnosis of asthma is "What sort of asthma does my child have?" The airway disease (asthma) should be deconstructed into identifiable aspect such as:

- Airflow limitation
- Eosinophilic airway inflammation
- Airway infect ion
- Impaired airway defenses
- Attend cough reflex sensitivity.

Wheeze and Asthma—6 to 11 Years

Asthma as discussed is a heterogeneous disease, characterized by chronic airway inflammation and hyper-responsiveness.

History: Respiratory symptoms wheeze, short ness of breath, and chest tightness.

Pattern typical of asthma:
- More than one symptoms
- Vary in intensity and overtime
- Triggers, example—smoke, viral RTI, allergen exposure
- Symptoms worse at night/early morning

Diagnosis: Evidence of variable airflow limitation.

Confirmed variable expiratory airflow limitation:
- Positive bronchodilator reversibility test (bronchodilator not to be used SABA ≥ 44, long-acting β2-agonist (LABA) ≥ 15, and FEV1 > 12% predicted [FEV1/FVC (forced vital capacity) < 0.90].
- Increase variability in twice daily peak expiratory flow (PEF) over 2 weeks. PEF variability >13%.
- Significant increase in lung function after 4 weeks of treatment.
- Excessive variation in lung function in between visit: FEV1 > 12%, PEF > 15%.

Management

- Assess asthma control (over last 4 weeks)
- Assess treatment issues (including inhales techniques)
- *Assess comorbidities*: Rhinitis, rhinosinusitis, GER, obstructive sleep apnea (OSA), depression, and food allergy.

Steps of Treatment

Customized management of wheeze in children < 5 years (Diagnosed Asthma)

Step 4: Asthma not well-controlled on double ICS
- Eferred to specialist or ICS frequently
- Reliever: As needed SABA

Step 3: Asthma diagnosed not well controlled
- Controller: Double low dose ICS or, low dose ICS + LTRA
- Reliever: As needed SABA

Step 2: Wheezing ≥ 3/year Diagnostic trail for 3 month
- Controller: Daily low dose ICS or, Daily LTRA or, Intermittent ICS
- Reliever: As needed SABA

Step 1: Infrequent viral wheezing
- Reliever: As needed SABA

Initial in children aged 6–11 years (Diagnosis as Asthma)

Step 5: Phenotypic assessment
- Low dose OCS
- Reliever: As needed SABA

Step 4: Low lung function
- Reliever: Medium dose ICS –LABA
- Refer: High dose ICS – LABA or add on TRITROPIUM
- Reliever: As needed SABA

Step 3: Symptom most days/waking once per week
- Controller: Low dose ICS/LABA or, medium dose ICS or, low dose ICS + LTRA
- Reliever: As needed SABA

Step 2: (Symptom > 2 time/month)
- Controller: Daily low dose ICS or, daily LTRA or, low dose ICS whenever SABA taken
- Reliever: As needed SABA

Step 1: (Symptom < 2 time/month)
- Controller: daily low dose ICS or, low dose ICS alongside SABA (whenever needed)
- Reliever: As needed SABA

Difficult to Treat Asthma

Uncontrolled asthma even after step 4/5 treatment:
- Confirm diagnosis
- Check adherence
- Refer to specialist

Type 2 Inflammation

Asthma phenotype:
- Blood eosinophil ≥ 150/µL
- FeNO ≥ 20 ppb
- Sputum eosinophil ≥ 2%
- Clinically allergen driven.

ALLERGEN IMMUNOTHERAPY

Asthma where the allergy component plays a prominent role (asthma with rhinoconjunctivitis) allergen-specific immunotherapy can be given.

Subcutaneous Immunotherapy

Sublingual immunotherapy (especially house dust mites allergic rhinitis).

VACCINATIONS

Yearly influenza vaccinations are recommended.

CAUSES OF WHEEZING IN UNDER-5 YEARS

- Bronchiolitis
- FB aspiration
- Bronchial asthma
- Compression of airways (tumor or lymph node)
- Pulmonary edema
- Audible wheeze and auscultatory wheeze.

RISK FACTORS

- *Nonmodifiable*: Preterm, low-birthweight (LBW)
- *Modifiable*: Triggers, viral infection, and smoking noncompliance.

CHAPTER 92: Community-acquired Pneumonia

Indranil Halder

INTRODUCTION

Community-acquired pneumonia (CAP) is a common and a serious disease which is defined as signs and symptoms of an acute infection of the pulmonary parenchyma in an individual who acquired the infection in the community, as distinguished from hospital-acquired (nosocomial) pneumonia.

EPIDEMIOLOGY

Incidence and hospitalization: The incidence of childhood pneumonia varies geographically.

- *Resource-rich countries*: In resource-rich countries, the annual incidence of pneumonia is estimated to be 3.3 per 1,000 in children younger than 5 years and 1.45 per 1,000 in children 0–16 years and half of the children younger than 5 years require hospitalization.
- *Resource-limited countries*: The annual incidence of pneumonia in children younger than 5 years from resource-limited countries in 2015 was estimated to be 231 per 1,000; about 50–80% of children with severe pneumonia required hospitalization.
- *Mortality*: In 2015, lower respiratory tract infections (LRTIs) accounted for nearly 800,000 deaths among children ≤ 19 years worldwide (31.1 per 100,000 population), second only to neonatal/preterm birth complications.
- *Seasonality*: Although both viral and bacterial pneumonia occur throughout the year, they are more prevalent during the colder months, presumably because direct transmission of infected droplets is enhanced by indoor crowding.
- *Risk factors*: Lower socioeconomic groups have a higher prevalence of LRTIs, which correlates best with family size, a reflection of environmental crowding. School-age children often introduce respiratory viral agents into households, resulting in secondary infections in their parents and siblings.
- Underlying cardiopulmonary disorders and other medical conditions predispose to pneumonia and contribute to increasing severity. These include:
  - Congenital heart disease
  - Bronchopulmonary dysplasia
  - Cystic fibrosis
  - Asthma
  - Sickle cell disease
  - Neuromuscular disorders, especially those associated with a depressed consciousness
  - Some gastrointestinal disorders (e.g., gastroesophageal reflux, tracheoesophageal fistula)
  - Congenital and acquired immunodeficiency disorders.
- Cigarette smoke compromises natural pulmonary defense mechanisms by disrupting both mucociliary function and macrophage activity. Exposure to cigarette smoke, especially if the mother smokes, increases the risk for pneumonia in infants younger than one year of age.
- *Effect of vaccines*: Immunization with the *Haemophilus influenzae* type b (Hib) and pneumococcal conjugate vaccines protects children from invasive disease caused by these organisms. Pneumococcal vaccination also reduces the risk of viral pneumonia.

ETIOLOGY

The etiology of community-acquired pneumonia is age related as given in **Table 1**.

CLINICAL PRESENTATION

The clinical presentation of childhood pneumonia varies depending upon the responsible pathogen, the particular host, and the severity. The presenting signs and symptoms are nonspecific; no single symptom or sign is pathognomonic for pneumonia in children.

Symptoms and signs of pneumonia may be subtle, particularly in infants and young children. The combination of fever and cough is suggestive of pneumonia; other respiratory findings (e.g., tachypnea, increased work of breathing) may precede the cough. Cough may not be a feature initially since the alveoli have few cough receptors. Cough begins when the products of infection irritate cough receptors in the airways. The longer fever, cough, and respiratory findings are present, the greater the likelihood of pneumonia.

TABLE 1: Age-based etiologies of childhood community-acquired pneumonia.

Age	Common etiologies	Less common etiologies
2–24 months	• Respiratory syncytial virus • Human metapneumovirus • Parainfluenza viruses • Influenza A and B • Rhinovirus • Adenovirus • Enterovirus • Streptococcus pneumoniae • Chlamydia trachomatis	• Mycoplasma pneumoniae • Haemophilus influenzae (type B and nontypable) • Chlamydophila pneumoniae
2–5 years	• Respiratory syncytial virus • Chlamydia trachomatis • Human metapneumovirus • Parainfluenza viruses • Influenza A and B • Rhinovirus • Adenovirus • Enterovirus • S. pneumoniae • M. pneumoniae • H. influenzae (B and nontypable) • C. pneumoniae	• Staphylococcus aureus (including methicillin-resistant S. aureus) • Group A Streptococcus pneumoniae
Older than 5 years	• M. pneumoniae • C. pneumoniae • S. pneumoniae • Rhinovirus • Adenovirus • Influenza A and B	• H. influenzae (B and nontypable) • S. aureus (including methicillin-resistant S. aureus) • Group A Streptococcus • Respiratory syncytial virus • Parainfluenza viruses • Human metapneumovirus

Neonates and young infants may present with difficulty feeding, restlessness, or fussiness rather than with cough and/or abnormal breath sounds. Neonates, young infants, and young children (i.e., <5–10 years of age) may present only with fever and leukocytosis.

Older children and adolescents may complain of pleuritic chest pain (pain with respiration), but this is an inconsistent finding. Occasionally, the predominant manifestation may be abdominal pain (because of referred pain from the lower lobes) or even neck rigidity (because of referred pain from the upper lobes).

The agents commonly responsible vary according to the age of the child and the setting in which the infection is acquired.

Immunocompromised: The causes of pneumonia in immunocompromised hosts include all of the pathogens mentioned above as well as a variety of other organisms, such as gram-negative bacilli, and *S. aureus* are common etiologies in neutropenic patients or in those with white blood cell defects.

Clinically significant legionellosis usually is seen only in immunocompromised hosts with an exposure to an aquatic reservoir of *Legionella pneumophila*, such as a river, lake, air conditioning cooling tower, or water distribution systems

Viral causes of pneumonia, which may be life-threatening in the immunocompromised host, including the post-solid organ and stem cell transplant populations, include:

Common community-acquired viral agents are:
- Respiratory syncytial virus (RSV)
- Adenovirus
- Influenza
- Parainfluenza
- Rhinovirus
- Human metapneumovirus
- SARS-CoV-2
- Rubeola (Hecht giant-cell pneumonia)
- Varicella zoster virus (VZV)
- Cytomegalovirus.

- In children younger than 5 years, viruses are most common. However, bacterial pathogens, including *Streptococcus pneumoniae, Staphylococcus aureus*, and *S. pyogenes*, also are important.
- In otherwise healthy children older than 5 years, *S. pneumoniae, Mycoplasma pneumoniae*, and *Chlamydia pneumoniae* are most common.
- Community-associated methicillin-resistant *S. aureus* is an increasingly important pathogen in children of all

ages, particularly in those with necrotizing pneumonia. *S. pneumoniae* is another frequent cause of necrotizing pneumonia.

RADIOLOGICAL EVALUATION

Radiographs

Chest radiography is often used to diagnose CAP. Routine chest radiographs are not necessary to confirm the diagnosis of suspected CAP in children with mild, uncomplicated LRTI who are well enough to be treated as outpatients. Chest imaging is most useful when the diagnosis is uncertain or when the findings from the history and physical examination are inconsistent.

Indications for radiographs in children with clinical evidence of pneumonia include:
- Severe disease
- Confirmation/exclusion of the diagnosis when clinical findings are inconclusive
- Hospitalization
- History of recurrent pneumonia
- Exclusion of alternate explanations for respiratory distress (e.g., foreign body aspiration, heart failure)
- Assessment of complications, particularly in children whose pneumonia is prolonged and unresponsive to antimicrobial therapy
- In children older than 4 years, the frontal posteroanterior (PA) upright chest view is usually obtained to minimize the cardiac shadow. In younger children, position does not affect the size of the cardiothoracic shadow, and the anteroposterior (AP) supine view is preferred because immobilization is easier and the likelihood of a better inspiration is improved.

Other imaging techniques: High-resolution computed tomography and ultrasonography are required for patients who require more extensive imaging or clarification of radiographic findings.

Etiologic clues: Certain radiographic features that are more often associated with bacterial, atypical bacterial, or viral etiologies. However, none can reliably differentiate between them.

Segmental consolidation is reasonably specific for bacterial pneumonia but lacks sensitivity, again pneumatoceles, cavitations, large pleural effusion, and necrotizing processes are supportive of bacterial etiology.

Significant mediastinal/hilar adenopathy suggests a mycobacterial or fungal etiology.

LABORATORY EVALUATION

The laboratory evaluation of the child with CAP depends on the clinical scenario, including the age of the child, severity of illness, complications, and whether the child requires hospitalization.

Young infants in whom pneumonia is suspected, particularly those who are febrile and toxic appearing, require a full evaluation for sepsis and other serious bacterial infections.

- Complete blood count (CBC) usually is not necessary for children with mild LRTI who will be treated as outpatients, unless the CBC will help determine the need for antibiotic therapy. CBC should be obtained in infants and children who require hospital admission.
- WBC count > 15,000/µL is suggestive of pyogenic bacterial disease. However, children with *M. pneumoniae*, influenza, or adenovirus pneumonia may also have WBC count > 15,000/µL.
- Peripheral eosinophilia may be present in infants with afebrile pneumonia of infancy, typically caused by *C. trachomatis*.
- *Acute phase reactants*: Acute phase reactants, such as the erythrocyte sedimentation rate, C-reactive protein (CRP), and serum procalcitonin (PCT), need not be routinely measured in fully immunized children with CAP managed as outpatients. However, for those with more serious disease requiring hospitalization, measurement of acute phase reactants may provide useful information to assist clinical management.
- *Serum electrolytes*: Measurement of serum electrolytes may be helpful in assessing the degree of dehydration in children with limited fluid intake and whether hyponatremia is present (as hyponatremia often accompanies CAP).

DIAGNOSIS

Clinical

The diagnosis of pneumonia should be considered in infants and children with respiratory complaints, particularly cough, tachypnea, retractions, and abnormal lung examination.

Common physical findings include fever, tachypnea, increasingly labored breathing, rhonchi, crackles, and wheezing. Hydration status, activity level, and oxygen saturation are important and may indicate the need for hospitalization. Tachypnea seems to be the most significant clinical sign. To be measured accurately, the respiratory rate must be counted over a full minute when the child is quiet. In febrile children, the absence of tachypnea has a high negative predictive value (97.4%) for pneumonia. Conversely, the presence of tachypnea in febrile children has a low positive predictive value (20.1%).

Fever alone can increase the respiratory rate by 10 breaths per minute per degree Celsius. In febrile children with tachypnea, findings of chest retractions, grunting, nasal flaring, and crepitation increase the likelihood of pneumonia. The World Health Organization uses tachypnea in the presence of cough as the diagnostic criterion of pneumonia

TABLE 2: World Health Organization tachypnea thresholds for diagnosing pneumonia in the presence of cough.

Age	Normal respiratory rate (breaths per minute)	Tachypnea threshold (breaths per minute)
2–12 months	25–40	50
1–5 years	20–30	40

Source: World Health Organization. The Management of Acute Respiratory Infections in Children: Practical Guidelines for Outpatient Care. Geneva, Switzerland: World Health Organization; 1995.

in developing countries where chest radiography is not readily available **(Table 2)**.

Radiographic confirmation: An infiltrate on chest radiograph confirms the diagnosis of pneumonia in children with compatible clinical findings, although chest radiographs must be interpreted with caution in children with asthma and comorbid viral infection.

Etiologic

Children with mild disease who are treated as outpatients usually can be treated empirically, based on age and other epidemiologic features, without establishing a microbiologic etiology.

Although the etiologic agent is suggested by host characteristics, clinical presentation, epidemiologic considerations, and the results of nonspecific laboratory tests and chest radiographic patterns neither clinical nor radiologic features reliably distinguish between bacterial, atypical bacterial, and viral pneumonia.

Accurate and rapid diagnosis of the responsible pathogen can be helpful in making treatment or cohorting decisions for infants and children who are admitted to the hospital with CAP.

If possible, a microbiologic diagnosis should be established in children:
- With severe disease
- With potential complications
- Who require hospitalization
- In whom an unusual pathogen is suspected, particularly if it requires treatment that differs from standard empiric regimens (e.g., *S. aureus* including methicillin-resistant strains, *Mycobacterium tuberculosis*)
- Who fail to respond to initial therapy.

Microbiologic diagnosis should also be established if there appears to be a community outbreak.

Microbiologic diagnosis can be established with culture or rapid diagnostic testing [enzyme immunoassay (EIA), immunofluorescence, or polymerase chain reaction (PCR)].

Among children who are hospitalized with CAP, the investigations that may be sent are:
- Blood cultures, particularly in children with complications
- Sputum gram stain and culture in children who are able to produce sputum
- Pleural fluid gram stain and culture in children with more than minimal pleural effusion
- *Rapid diagnostic tests (e.g., PCR-based assays):* Rapid diagnostic tests include molecular tests that use PCR techniques (including multiplex PCR panels) and immunofluorescence. They can be performed on samples from the NP, pleural fluid or throat (for *M. pneumoniae*)
- *Serology:* Routine serologic testing for specific pathogens (e.g., *S. pneumoniae*, *M. pneumoniae*, *C. pneumoniae*) is not required because the results usually do not influence the treatment but the other tests include:
  - Urine antigen testing for legionellosis
  - Serum and urine antigen and antibody (complement fixation, immunodiffusion, and EIA IgM/IgG) testing for histoplasmosis.

Invasive studies: Invasive procedures may be necessary to obtain lower respiratory tract specimens for culture and other studies in children in whom an etiologic diagnosis is necessary and has not been established by other means:
- Bronchoscopy with bronchoalveolar lavage (BAL)
- Percutaneous needle aspiration of the affected lung tissue guided by ultrasonography or computed tomography.

DIFFERENTIAL DIAGNOSIS

Although pneumonia is highly probable in a child with fever, tachypnea, cough, and infiltrate(s) on chest radiograph, alternate diagnoses and coincident conditions must be considered in children who fail to respond to therapy or have an unusual presentation/course.

Noninfectious mimics of pneumonia may include foreign body aspiration which must be considered in young children. The aspiration event may not have been witnessed.

Other causes of tachypnea, with or without fever and cough, in infants and young children include:
- Bronchiolitis
- Heart failure
- Sepsis
- Metabolic acidosis.

These conditions usually can be distinguished from pneumonia by history, examination, and appropriate laboratory tests.

TABLE 3: Choice of antibiotics.

6 months to 5 years	
Typical bacterial	*Amoxicillin*: 90 mg/kg per day in two or three divided doses (maximum: 4 g/day)
	Amoxicillin-clavulanate: 90 mg/kg per day of the amoxicillin component in two or three divided doses (maximum 4 g/day amoxicillin component)
	For patients with non-type 1 hypersensitivity to penicillins: Cefdinir 14 mg/kg per day in two divided doses (maximum 600 mg/day)
	For patients with type 1 hypersensitivity to penicillins: • Levofloxacin 16–20 mg/kg per day in two divided doses (maximum 750 mg/day) • Clindamycin 30–40 mg/kg per day in three or four divided doses (maximum 1.8 g/day) • Erythromycin 40–50 mg/kg per day in four divided doses (maximum 2 g/day as base, 3.2 g/day as ethylsuccinate), • *Azithromycin*: 10 mg/kg on day 1 followed by 5 mg/kg daily for 4 more days (maximum 500 mg on day 1 and 250 mg thereafter) • Clarithromycin 15 mg/kg per day in two divided doses (maximum 1 g/day)
	In communities with a high rate of pneumococcal resistance to penicillin: • Levofloxacin 16–20 mg/kg per day in two divided doses (max 750 mg/day) • Linezolid 30 mg/kg per day in 3 divided doses (maximum 1,800 mg/day)
≥5 years *Mycoplasma pneumoniae* or *Chlamydia pneumoniae*	• *Azithromycin*: 10 mg/kg on day 1 followed by 5 mg/kg daily for 4 more days (maximum 500 mg on day 1 and 250 mg thereafter) • *Clarithromycin*: 15 mg/kg per day in two divided doses (maximum 1 g/day) • *Erythromycin*: 4,050 mg/kg per day in four divided doses (maximum 2 g/day as base, 3.2 g/day as ethylsuccinate) • Doxycycline 4 mg/kg per day in two divided doses (maximum 200 mg/day) • Levofloxacin 8–10 mg/kg once daily for children 5–16 years (maximum 500 mg/day); 500 mg once per day for children for children ≥16 years • Moxifloxacin, 400 mg once per day

COMPLICATIONS

Bacterial pneumonias are more likely than atypical bacterial or viral pneumonias to be associated with complications involving the respiratory tract:
- Pleural effusion and empyema
- Necrotizing pneumonia
- Lung abscess
- Pneumatocele
- Hyponatremia.

TREATMENT

Amoxicillin is recommended as first choice for oral antibiotic therapy in all children because it is effective against the majority of pathogens which cause CAP in this group, well tolerated, and cheap. Alternatives are coamoxiclav, cefaclor, erythromycin, azithromycin, and clarithromycin. Macrolide antibiotics may be added at any age if there is no response to first-line empirical therapy. Macrolide antibiotics should be used if either *Mycoplasma* or *Chlamydia pneumonia* is suspected or in very severe disease.

Antibiotics administered orally are safe and effective for children presenting with even severe CAP. Intravenous antibiotics should be used in the treatment of pneumonia in children when the child is unable to tolerate oral fluids or absorb oral antibiotics (e.g., because of vomiting) or presents with signs of septicemia or complicated pneumonia. Recommended intravenous antibiotics for severe pneumonia include amoxicillin, coamoxiclav, cefuroxime, and cefotaxime or ceftriaxone. These can be rationalized if a microbiological diagnosis is made.

The choice of antibiotics may be summarized in **Table 3**.

93 CHAPTER

Pleural Effusion

Swapan Kumar Ray

INTRODUCTION

Pleural effusion is an accumulation of fluid within pleural cavity. However, pleurisy means inflammation of pleura.

Pleurisy is of three types: (1) Dry pleurisy, (2) serosanguineous or serofibrinous, and (3) purulent pleurisy or empyema.

CAUSES

Pleurisy may precede pleural effusion. The most common cause of pleural effusion is bacterial pneumonia. Other causes are heart failure, rheumatological disorder, metastatic intrathoracic malignancy, tuberculosis, Lupus erythematosus, aspiration pneumonitis, uremia, pancreatitis, subdiaphragmatic abscess, and rheumatoid arthritis.

In tuberculosis, pleurisy can be caused by a severe delayed-type hypersensitivity reaction to *Mycobacterium tuberculosis*.

PATHOGENESIS

- Pleural fluid originates from the capillaries of the parietal pleura and is absorbed from the pleural space via pleural stomas and the lymphatics of the parietal pleura.
- Fluid movement is determined by the balance of hydrostatic and osmotic pressures in the pleural space and pulmonary capillary bed, and the permeability of the pleural membrane.
- Normally, approximately 10–15 mL of fluid is present in the pleural space. But if formation exceeds clearance, fluid accumulates within pleural cavity.

CLINICAL MANIFESTATIONS

- Initially the child presents with chest pain which may be dull aching in nature.
- But as more fluid accumulates within the pleural cavity, the pain subsides.
- Large fluid causes respiratory distress, cough, tachypnea, orthopnea, and dyspnea. There may be fever. In case of tuberculosis, there may be evening rise of temperature.

CLINICAL EXAMINATION

- The child may be symptomatic or asymptomatic, depending upon the amount of fluid within pleural space.
- If a large amount of fluid accumulates, the child is usually dyspneic and orthopneic. The child prefers to lie down on lateral decubitus on the affected side, to restrict movement on that side.
- Inspection revels bulge in huge effusion. Movement of the chest is also diminished on the affected side.
- Palpation reveals decreased mediastinal shift (tracheal shift as well) and decreased tactile vocal fremitus.
- On percussion, we find dull note (Stony Dull).
- There may be decreased breath sound, egophony and whispering pectoriloquy.

INVESTIGATIONS

- *Complete blood count* is usually non-contributory except leukocytosis at times.
- *Chest X-ray* is very helpful as it is easily available tool of investigation. PA and lateral decubitus films, both are required to exclude free fluid in pleural cavity. With change of position of patient, fluid shift can be appreciated, if it is not loculated one. Moreover, therapeutic interference is also dependent on the thickness of fluid along the inner thoracic wall, and for prognostication as well as treatment response.
- *Ultrasonography (USG) chest* is nowadays a better tool for diagnosis, and therapeutic maneuver as it guides to diagnostic thoracocentesis. Yield of USG is very good. It can pick up as small as 20 mL of pleural fluid, where chest X-ray requires minimum 150–200 mL of fluid to detect.
- *Computed tomography (CT) chest* is also a sensitive too and septations are better visualized in CT. But it incurs lot of radiation to the child.
- *Pleural fluid testing*: Pleural fluid is tested after diagnostic thoracocentesis. Pleural fluid should be tested for cytology, biochemical analysis and culture sensitivity. Pleural fluid adenosine deaminase (ADA) is important to exclude tuberculosis. *Exudates usually have at least one of the following features*: protein level >3.0 g/dL,

Pleural fluid:serum protein ratio > 0.5; pleural fluid lactic dehydrogenase values >200 IU/L; or fluid:serum lactic dehydrogenase ratio >0.6.

COMPLICATIONS
- It persists somewhat longer in tuberculosis or a connective tissue disease. May recur or remain for a long time if caused by a neoplasm.
- Pleural thickening may develop and is occasionally mistaken for small quantities of fluid or for persistent pulmonary infiltrates. Pleural thickening may persist for months, but the process usually disappears, leaving no residue.

TREATMENT
- Therapy should address the underlying disease. If the effusion is <10 mm in size on a chest X-ray, then there is no need for drainage.
- With a large effusion, draining the fluid makes the patient more comfortable. When a diagnostic thoracentesis is performed, as much fluid as possible should be removed for therapeutic purposes. Rapid removal of ≥1 L of pleural fluid may because of pulmonary edema.
- In older children with suspected parapneumonic effusion, tube thoracostomy is considered necessary if the pleural fluid pH is <7.20 or the pleural fluid glucose level is <50 mg/dL.
- If the fluid is thick, loculated, or clearly purulent, tube drainage with fibrinolytic therapy or less often video-assisted thoracoscopic surgery (VATS) is indicated.

SUGGESTED READING
1. Kliegman RM, St Geme J. Nelson's Textbook of Pediatrics, 21st edition. Philadelphia: Elsevier; 2019.

Empyema Thoracis

Swapan Kumar Ray

INTRODUCTION

Empyema is accumulation of pus in the pleural space. It is most often associated with pneumonia caused by *Staphylococcus aureus*. Empyema is most frequently encountered in infants and preschool children. Although rates of bacterial pneumonia have decreased, the incidence of parapneumonic effusions has increased because more virulent organisms are emerging.

CAUSATIVE AGENTS

- *Streptococcus pneumoniae*
- *Staphylococcus aureus*
- *Haemophilus influenzae type B*
- Gram-negative bacilli
- *Mycobacterium tuberculosis*
- Fungi
- Malignancy.

PATHOLOGY

- *Exudative stage*: Increased permeability of inflamed pleura
- *Fibrinopurulent phase*: Accelerated fibrin deposition→loculation→pus formation
- *Organization phase*:
  - Begins 2 weeks after infection
  - Multiloculated cavities containing pus
  - Pleural peeling.

CLINICAL FEATURES

- Persistent high fever
- Malaise
- *Decreased appetite*: Cough, chest pain, and dyspnea: Patient lie on the affected side for splinting (provide temporary analgesia)
- Weight loss if occurs >2 weeks
- Tachypnea
- *Shallow breaths*: Tracheal deviation and mediastinal shift to opposite side: Asymmetrical chest expansion (decreased movement over the affected part of the chest and fullness on the affected side)
- Stony dull on percussion
- Tenderness on percussion
- Decreased breath sounds on auscultation
- Pulse oximetry < 92% indicates severe disease.

Children with severe pneumonia who do not show sign of recovery 48 hours after initiation of the antibiotic therapy should raise the suspicion of empyema.

INVESTIGATIONS

- *X-ray*: Frontal view/lateral decubitus view:
  - Obliteration of the costophrenic angle
  - White homogeneous opacity of the affected hemothorax
  - Shifting of trachea and mediastinum to the opposite side.
- *Ultrasonography (USG)*: Anechoic to echoic fluid in empyema. No shift of fluid with position change in case of loculated empyema. It is used to find out loculi for therapeutic thoracentesis as well as diagnostic thoracentesis.
- *Computed tomography (CT) scan*: Split pleura sign (parietal and visceral layers are separated by interposed empyema pus).

Other Investigations

- Fluid aspirated before starting antibiotic
- *Gross*: Pus (turbulent with putrid odor)
- Protein > 30 g/L
- Pleural fluid protein: serum protein > 0.5
- *Pleura fluid lactate dehydrogenase (LDH)*: serum LDH > 0.6a } Modified Light's criteria
- Pleural fluid LDH >2/3 times upper normal limit of serum LDH
- Pleural fluid pH < 7.2
- Cartridge-based nucleic acid amplification test (CBNAAT) to diagnose TB

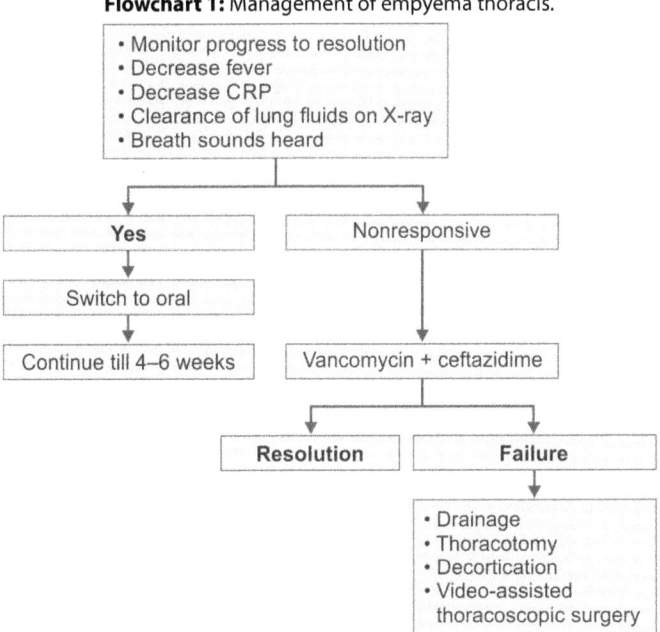

Flowchart 1: Management of empyema thoracis.

(CRP: C-reactive protein)

- Gram staining for detecting bacteria
- Bacterial culture
- Acid-fast bacilli (AFB) staining to detect tuberculosis
- Latex agglutination
- Counter immunoelectrophoresis
- *Complete blood count (CBC)*: Leukocytes, secondary thrombocytosis may be there
- C-reactive protein (CRP) to monitor progress
- Serum electrolytes to detect syndrome of inappropriate antidiuretic hormone secretion (SIADH).

Modified Light's Criteria

- *Pleural fluid protein*: serum protein > 0.5
- *Pleura fluid LDH*: serum LDH > 0.6
- Pleural fluid LDH > 2/3 times upper normal limit of serum LDH
- Pleural fluid pH < 7.2.

MANAGEMENT (FLOWCHART 1)

Supportive:
- When PaO_2 < 92%, give oxygen by nasal hood/mask
- Intravenous (IV) fluids (counter poor intake and increased loss)
- *Paracetamol*: 15–20 mg/kg body weight

- *Antibiotics*: For 4–6 weeks, IV then oral after the child become afebrile or chest tube drain removed.

    Ampicillin + cloxacillin (IV) or cloxacillin + third-generation cephalosporin (IV) (ceftriaxone).

Dose:
- *Ampicillin*: 50–100 mg/kg/day
- *Cloxacillin*: 50–100 mg/kg/day
- *Ceftriaxone*: 50–75 mg/kg/day
- Intercostal water-sealed drainage to be done as soon as child arrives
- Left in place until fluid drainage is minimal (<15 mL/day)
- Open decortication
- Video-assisted thoracoscopic surgery (VATS)
- Rib resection (thoracoplasty/lobectomy)
- Antitubercular therapy
- If there is poor response even after 3 days of IV antibiotics and chest tube drainage, VATS, or thoracostomy surgery to be undertaken. If pus is obtained by thoracentesis or pleural fluid septation is detected on radiographic studies, then closed-chest tube drainage with fibrinolytics is the initial procedure, followed by VATS when there is no improvement
- The optimal fibrinolytic drug and dosages have not been determined. Streptokinase 15,000 units/kg in 50 mL of 0.9% saline, urokinase 40,000 units in 40 mL saline, and alteplase (tPA) 4 mg in 40 mL of saline have been used in the pediatric population.

Management of Complications

Complication that may arise:
- *Bronchopleural fistula* (air leaks persists, pus through bronchus coughed out)
- *Empyema necessitates*: When pus escapes from pleural cavity and dissects through the intercostal muscles, causing a bulge underneath the skin.

The long-term clinical prognosis for adequately treated empyema is excellent, and follow-up pulmonary function studies suggest that residual restrictive disease is uncommon, with or without surgical intervention.

SUGGESTED READING

1. Kliegman RM, St Geme J. Nelson's Textbook of Pediatrics, 21st edition. Philadelphia: Elsevier; 2019.

CHAPTER 95

Lung Abscess

Swapan Kumar Ray

INTRODUCTION

Lung abscess is a thick-walled cavitary lesion of lung parenchyma containing purulent necrotic material, formed as a result of lung infection.

Types:
- *Primary lung abscess*: In previously healthy patients with no underlying disease.
- *Secondary lung abscess*: Occurs in patients with underlying or predisposing conditions and may be multiple.
  Primary abscess usually develops on right side, where as secondary abscess, if immunocompromised, occurs on left side.

RISK FACTORS

- Aspiration pneumonia (aspiration is one of the predominant causes of lung abscess)
- Gastroesophageal reflux disease (GERD)
- Tracheoesophageal fistula
- Cystic fibrosis.

ORGANISMS

- *Bacteroides* spp. anaerobic
- *Fusobacterium* spp.
- *Peptostreptococcus*
- *Streptococcus*
- *Staphylococcus* aerobic
- *Escherichia coli*
- Fungus in immunocompromised children.

CLINICAL FEATURES

- Cough with purulent expectoration
- Fever
- Tachypnea
- Dyspnea
- Chest pain
- Reversible clubbing
- Vomiting
- Retraction with accessory muscle
- Dull note on affected site on percussion
- Crackles
- Cavernous breath sounds over deep cavity communicating with a bronchus.

INVESTIGATIONS

- *Chest X-ray*:
  - Parenchymal inflammation
  - Cavity containing air fluid level
- *Computed tomography (CT) scan*: Abscess is usually a thick-walled lesion with low-density center progressing to an air fluid level.

SPECIMEN COLLECTION

To avoid contamination from oral flora include:
- Direct lung puncture
- Bronchoalveolar lavage
- Percutaneous (CT guided)
- Transtracheal aspiration.

The secretions obtained are subjected to following:
- Gram staining
- Sputum culture.

DIAGNOSIS

Lung abscess should be suspected when there is:
- Persistent consolidation
- Volume of involved lobe increased
- Bulging fissure sign.

MANAGEMENT

- The organism needed to be isolated by lung aspiration under USG- or CT-guided technique or bronchoalveolar lavage.
- Treatment regimen should include a penicillinase-resistant agent against *Staphylococcus aureus* and anaerobic coverage typically *clindamycin/ticarcillin + clavulanic*

acid. Gram-negative infection → aminoglycoside is added.
- *Duration*: 4–6 weeks. Systemic antibiotic should be administered for initial 2–3 weeks, then oral antibiotics to be given for another 2–3 weeks.
- *Failure of resolution (after 72 hours)*: Needle aspiration/catheter drainage (diagnostic and therapeutic).
- At least 3 weeks of IV antibiotic therapy before lobectomy is considered. Minimally invasive percutaneous aspiration techniques, often with CT guidance, are the initial and, often, only intervention required.

COMPLICATIONS
- Intracavitary hemorrhage which can cause spillage of abscess contents with spread of infection to other areas
- Bronchopleural fistula
- Empyema
- Septicemia
- Cellular abscess.

SUGGESTED READING
1. Janahi IA, Fakhoury K. (2020). Epidemiology, clinical presentation, and evaluation of parapneumonic effusion and empyema in children. [online] Available from: https://www.uptodate.com/contents/epidemiology-clinical-presentation-and-evaluation-of-parapneumonic-effusion-and-empyema-in-children?search=epidemiolgy-clinical-presentation-and-evaluation-of-parapneumonic-effusion-and-empyema-in-children&source=search_result&selectedTitle=1~150&usage_type=default&display_rank=1. [Last accessed August, 2021].
2. Kliegman RM, St Geme J. Nelson's Textbook of Pediatrics, 21st edition. Philadelphia: Elsevier; 2019.

Pneumothorax

Kinshuk Sarbhai, Saurabh Gupta

DEFINITION

The abnormal presence of air in the pleural cavity leads to separation of visceral pleura from parietal pleura.

CLASSIFICATION

Spontaneous Pneumothorax

Pneumothorax occurring without any antecedent trauma or obvious cause comes under spontaneous pneumothorax. It is further classified into **(Flowchart 1)**:

- *Primary spontaneous pneumothorax*:
  - Pathogenesis of this type of pneumothorax is not clearly understood. It usually occurs suddenly with no identifiable underlying lesion.
  - One of the probable causes is rupture of small air sacs in lungs which leads to air leak from apical subpleural blebs and bullae.
  - It usually occurs in men aged 20–40 years who are tall and thin.
- *Secondary spontaneous pneumothorax*:
  - It occurs as a complication of underlying lung disease, most commonly chronic obstructive pulmonary disease (COPD).
  - Pneumothorax can be the first and foremost presenting symptom of these any underlying disease.
- Other causes can be tuberculosis (TB), cystic fibrosis, asthma, interstitial lung disease (ILD), necrotizing pneumonia, *Pneumocystis carinii* pneumonia (PCP), Langerhans cell histiocytosis, lymphangioleiomyomatosis, Marfan's syndrome, esophageal rupture, lung cancer, catamenial pneumothorax, and pulmonary infarction.

Traumatic Pneumothorax

- *Noniatrogenic pneumothorax*: It occurs due to direct or indirect trauma to the chest. Any blunt trauma which may or may not lead to fracture of ribs or any penetrating injury such as stab wound or gunshot wound that disrupts parietal or visceral pleura can cause pneumothorax.
- *Iatrogenic pneumothorax*: It includes pneumothorax occurring secondary to diagnostic or therapeutic maneuver such as thoracentesis, central venous pressure line, tracheostomy, lung biopsy, etc. Pneumothorax and pneumomediastinum may occur in up to 1% of cases and it is most often occurs during subclavian catheter placement. Risk factors for pneumothorax are larger catheter size and number of attempted insertions.

RISK FACTORS

- *Age*: 20–40 years
- *Built*: Usually taller and thinner people

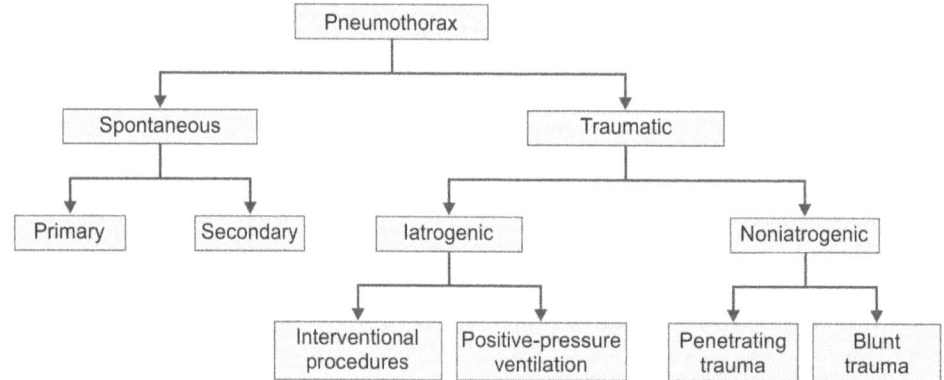

Flowchart 1: Classification of pneumothorax.

- *Genetics*: Birt-Hogg-Dube syndrome
- *Familial pneumothorax*: Association with HLA haplotypes: Marfan's syndrome homocystinuria, Ehlers-Danlos syndrome, alpha-1-antitrypsin deficiency
- *The bronchial abnormalities*:
  - Disproportionate bronchial anatomy (smaller than normal dimensions and deviating anatomic arrangements of airways at various locations)
  - An accessory bronchus or a missing bronchus
- Underlying lung lesions such as cavitary lung lesions, emphysematous bullae, pneumatocele, etc.

CLINICAL FEATURES

Pneumothorax usually manifests as acute onset of pleuritic chest pain and/or breathlessness. Breathlessness is often minimal in young patients and is more severe in secondary spontaneous pneumothorax.

Uncommon manifestations: Cough, hemoptysis, orthopnea, and cyanosis.

CLASSIFICATION BASED ON TYPE OF PLEURAL TEAR

Open Pneumothorax

In this type, pleural tear remains open so that there is constant connection between atmosphere and the thoracic cavity. As a result, the pleural cavity pressure becomes equal to atmospheric pressure. It occurs mostly in traumatic injury or fall.

Closed Pneumothorax

In this type, there is no connection between atmosphere and thoracic cavity. Hence, the atmospheric pressure and plural pressure would be same in this condition. It is mostly due to underlying lung parenchymal dysfunction which leads to air leak due to any bullous or alveolar rupture.

Tension Pneumothorax

In this type, there is progressive accumulation of intrapleural air so that it exerts a positive pressure on mediastinal and intrathoracic structures.

It is a life-threatening occurrence requiring rapid recognition and treatment is required if a cardiorespiratory arrest is to be avoided.

INVESTIGATIONS

Chest X-ray

Standard erect chest X-rays in inspiration are recommended for the initial diagnosis of pneumothorax. We need to notice the outer margin of the visceral pleura (and lung) is separated from parietal pleura (and chest wall) by a lucent space which is devoid of pulmonary vessels on chest radiograph.

Some signs seen in chest X-ray are:
- *Visceral pleural line*: Presence in this line demarcates the boundary between lung parenchyma and the pneumothorax. Presence of this line is mostly a confirmatory marker of presence of pneumothorax in chest X-ray. This line should not be confused with skin fold of patient which mimics visceral pleural line. A way to differentiate between two is that skin fold line might extend beyond the chest wall and secondly the lung markings can be seen beyond the skin-fold line. Another confusing line is scapular line. One must trace the scapular medial boundary to get rid of confusion.
- *Deep sulcus sign*: Extension of costophrenic angle deeper than normal.
- Lucent cardiophrenic sulcus.
- Double diaphragm sign.

Computed Tomography Scanning

- "Gold standard" in the detection of small pneumothoraces and in size estimation.
- Useful in presence of surgical emphysema and bullous lung disease.

Light Index

Differentiation of a "large" from a "small" pneumothorax: There are two guidelines to differentiate small and large pneumothorax, which are as follows:
1. *The British Thoracic Society (BTS) guidelines*: Large pneumothorax: Visible rim of air > 2 cm between the lung margin and the chest wall (at the level of hilum).
2. The American College of Chest Physicians (ACCP) guidelines:
   - *Large pneumothorax*: Apex-to-cupola distance > 3 cm
   - Accurate pneumothorax size calculations are best by CT scanning.

Ultrasonography

Ultrasonography (USG) is not a very good investigation method for diagnosing pneu-mothorax. Since it is hard to decode the signs of pneumothorax and signs may not be always apparent in some cases, especially minimal pneumothorax.

Signs

- *Loss of lung sliding*
- Loss of comet tails
- Loss of sea shore sign (M mode)
- *Stratosphere sign* or *Bar code sign* (in pneumothorax, the granular pattern of lung parenchyma is lost and horizontal, linear lines are seen throughout the display).

TREATMENT

- There are no specific guidelines for pneumothorax in pediatric age group.
- To begin with, the *distinction between primary and secondary spontaneous pneumothorax* should be made at the time of diagnosis to guide appropriate management. Primary spontaneous pneumothorax has better prognosis compared to secondary.
- *Breathlessness* in the patient indicates the need for *active intervention* and supportive treatment.

During management we want to achieve two goals:
1. To rid the pleural space of its air
2. To decrease the likelihood of a recurrence:
   - Observation and supplemental oxygen
   - Simple needle aspiration
   - Tube thoracostomy with or without the instillation of a sclerosing agent
   - Medical thoracoscopy with insufflation of talc
   - Video-assisted thoracoscopic surgery (VATS) with stapling of blebs
   - VATS with instillation of a sclerosing agent or pleural abrasion
   - Open thoracotomy.

Observation and Supplemental Oxygen

It is treatment of choice for small PSP without significant breathlessness. Selected asymptomatic patients with a large PSP may be managed by observation alone. Mean rate of absorption of pneumothorax is approximately 2.2% per day. So we can say that pneumothorax occupying <15% of hemithorax takes approximately 12 days for complete reabsorption.

Giving supplemental oxygen accelerates the rate of pleural air absorption by a factor of six times.

Simple Aspiration

We will consider undergoing therapeutic thoracocenteses in a patient if the pneumothorax is occupying more than 15% of volume of hemithorax. Patient should be kept in continuous high flow oxygen to augment absorption in the meantime.

Location: Second anterior intercostal space at midclavicular line after local anesthesia is considered ideal position. But alternative site should be considered if there are adhesions present or pneumothorax is loculated in nature.

Procedure: Under all aseptic conditions, 14–16-G needle is inserted in the pleural space after giving local anesthesia. As per the BTS guidelines, needle (14–16 G) aspiration is as effective as large-bore (>20 F) chest drains and associated with reduced hospitalization and length of stay. Needle aspiration should not be repeated many times as per the guidelines since it is associated with risks such as life-threatening hemorrhage. If needle aspiration was unsuccessful, instead of repeating the procedure, it is advised to undergo tube thoracostomy or VATS.

Administration of oxygen creates a partial pressure gradient between the pleural cavity and the pulmonary capillary web; diminished nitrogen partial pressure in the blood produces an increase in the pressure gradient of the gases between the pleura and the venous blood which will favor the absorption of air.

Tube Thoracostomy

Indications:
- Following failed needle aspiration
- Large pneumothorax
- Recurrent pneumothorax
- Hydropneumothorax
- *Location:* In upper most part of the pleural space, where residual air accumulates
- Large-bore chest drains are not needed for pneumothorax. Small tubes of 7–14 F are recommended as small tubes are less painful.

Tube Thoracostomy with Instillation of Sclerosing Agent

Different methods have been used to treat persistent air leaks, including prolonged use of pleural drainage, chemical pleurodesis by via injection of sclerosing agents, such as tetracycline, pleurodesis with autologs blood patch or surgical repair.

- If intercostal tubes (ICTs) are removed too soon after the lung re-expands and the air leak ceases, there is a high likelihood of a nearly recurrence.
- Injecting various agents into pleural space creates an intense inflammatory reaction and obliterating the space.
- *Best sclerosing agents:* Talc slurry, tetracycline derivatives.
- Pleurodesis is usually painful and injection 4 mg/kg of xylocaine maximal dose of 250 mg to be preceded by administration of sclerosing agent.

Medical Thoracoscopy

Indications:
- Treatment of PSP
- Persistent or recurrent spontaneous pneumothorax
- Less role in pneumothorax than in pleural effusion.

Referral to Thoracic Surgeons

In cases of persistent air leak or failure of the lung to re-expand, an early (3–5 days) thoracic surgical opinion should be sought:

Accepted indications for surgical advice:
- Lung remains unexpanded after 5 days
- Persistent air leak > 7 days

- Recurrent pneumothorax
- First contralateral pneumothorax
- Bilateral pneumothorax
- Spontaneous hemothorax
- High-risk operation (pilot/diver)
- In AIDS patients, lymphangioleiomyomatosis patients as there are high chances of pneumothorax.

Surgical Strategies

- Open thoracotomy and pleurectomy
- VATS with pleurectomy and pleural abrasion

Two primary objectives:
1. To treat the bullous disease responsible for pneumothorax
2. To create a pleurodesis

The primary alternatives are:
- Mechanical abrasion of the pleura partial parietal pleurectomy
- Talc insufflation
- Argon beam coagulation.

If there is no resolution and the air leak persists (3–5 days), or if there is recurrence, the use of VATS should be considered. VATS with stapling of bullae is very effective at managing spontaneous pneumothorax with an overall recurrence rate of approximately 3%.

Treatment Options for Recurrent Pneumothorax

- *Medical treatment*: Chemical pleurodesis should be considered in patient with recurrent pneumothorax.
- *Surgical treatment*: VATS with partial pleurectomy or talc poudrage, thoracotomy with partial or complete pleurectomy.

COMPLICATIONS

- Recurrence of spontaneous pneumothorax
- Tension pneumothorax
- Encysted pneumothorax
- Hydropneumothorax
- Failure of expansion of collapsed lung
- Re-expansion pulmonary edema
- Bronchopleural fistula
- Pneumomediastinum.

SUGGESTED READING

1. Benbow MK, Nanagas MT. Pneumothorax beyond the newborn period. Pediatr Rev. 2014; 35:356.
2. Bhutta ST, Culp WC. Evaluation and management of central venous access complications. Tech Vasc Interv Radiol. 2011;14:217-24.
3. Dotson K, Johnson LH. Pediatric spontaneous pneumothorax. Pediatr Emerg Care. 2012;28: 715-20.
4. Light RW. Pleural controversy: optimal chest tube size for drainage. Respirology. 2011;16: 244-8.
5. MacDuff A, Arnold A, Harvey J. BTS Pleural Disease Guideline Group. Management of spontaneous pneumothorax: British Thoracic Society Pleural Disease Guideline 2010. Thorax. 2010;65(Suppl 2):ii18-31.
6. Manley K, Coonar A, Wells F, Scarci M. Blood patch for persistent air leak: a review of the current literature. Curr Opin Pulm Med. 2012; 18:333-8.
7. McGee DC, Gould MK. Preventing complications of central venous catheterization. N Engl J Med. 2003;348:1123-33.
8. Robinson PD, Cooper P, Ranganathan SC. Evidence-based management of paediatric primary spontaneous pneumothorax. Paediatr Respir Rev. 2009;10:110-7.
9. Vats HS. Complications of catheters: tunneled and nontunneled. Adv Chronic Kidney Dis. 2012;19:188–94.

Hydrocarbon Aspiration

Taraknath Ghosh

INTRODUCTION

With advancement of modern society use of hydrocarbon is gradually increasing. Hydrocarbon constitutes 1-4% of total poisoning cases and case fatality rates vary from 1 to 12%. Accidental ingestion of hydrocarbon (commonly kerosene oil, incidence 33-60%) is the most common orally consumed poison among Indian children because hydrocarbon-based products are easily available in most households of our poverty-stricken country. Moreover, storage of kerosene oil in a transparent container looks like drinking water. As the toddlers (children of 1-3 years) have the innate curiosity for exploring things by taking anything into mouth, they are generally the most susceptible for poisoning. So they are easily attracted to this kind of materials.

On the other hand, careless, overburden parents contribute to it. Aspiration and resulting chemical pneumonitis are the most dangerous consequences of acute hydrocarbon ingestion.

CLASSIFICATION

Hydrocarbon includes wide varieties of chemical substances found in different commercial preparations. Specific nature and amount of each product will determine the range and severity of toxicity. It may be classified in following ways on the basis of chemical and clinical characteristics:

- Aliphatic hydrocarbon, e.g., kerosene, mineral spirits, gasoline, naphtha, mineral seal oil easily aspirated following ingestion, poorly absorbed from gastrointestinal (GI) tract with minimal systemic effect.
- Aromatic hydrocarbon (commonly used for inhalation), e.g., benzene, toluene, xylene.
- Halogenated hydrocarbons, e.g., chlordane, lindane, trichloroethane (minimal aspiration, more systemic effect).

PATHOPHYSIOLOGY

The most import ant pathogenetic mechanism of hydrocarbon toxicity is chemical pneumonitis through inactivation of type II pneumocytes resulting in surfactant deficiency and its consequences.

The physical properties (lower viscosity, low surface tension and high volatility) are the prime factors for aspiration potentiality and its consequence.

Hydrocarbon having above properties can easily be aspirated into the lung during coughing and gagging at the time of ingestion and aspiration also may occur during vomiting following ingestion. Aliphatic hydrocarbon such as kerosene oil, gasoline, and naphtha have high aspiration potential as they have lower viscosity and surface tension with high volatility and these properties help in spreading of the liquid in lung tissue. Moreover hydrophobic nature of hydrocarbon enhances penetration into tracheobronchial tree, producing inflammation. Volatile nature of the hydrocarbon helps displacing alveolar oxygen resulting in hypoxia. Direct contact to alveolar membrane may lead to hyperemia, leukocytic infiltration, edema, surfactant inactivation resulting in chemical pneumonitis and atelectasis. Sometimes, pneumatoceles may occur in areas of lung where densest infiltrates are seen in X-ray.

CLINICAL FEATURES

Clinical features depends upon the nature, amount of intake of hydrocarbon, and also on the amount aspirated in lung.

- Immediately after ingestion, there is irritation in the throat and sensation of choking with cough followed by nausea, vomiting, abdominal pain. Transient mild central nervous system (CNS) depression may occur.
- Chemical findings including cough, tachypnea, chest pain, refraction, grunting, wheeze, cyanosis suggests pulmonary aspiration which may occur as soon as 30 minutes after aspiration may be delayed for several hours. Respiratory distress may remain mild or may progress rapidly to acute respiratory distress syndrome (ARDS) and respiratory failure.
- Fever may follow after few hours or days, the presence of which does not necessarily indicate bacterial infection. This usually subsides after 24-48 hours but may last as long as 7 days.

Other symptoms may be related to systemic involvement:
- *Cardiovascular*: Cardiac arrhythmia, congestive heart failure.
- *Neurological*: Euphoria, CNS depression, headache, vertigo, etc.
- *Miscellaneous*: Renal and hepatic damage.

INVESTIGATIONS

Chest radiography is the investigation of choice which is usually done after 6-8 hours of ingestion. Characteristic radiographic changes—perihilar opacities, atelectasis, and bibasilar infiltrates—usually occur within 2-8 hours, peaking at 48-72 hours. These findings may remain long after clinical recovery. Other radiographic findings—pneumatoceles, pleural effusion, and pneumothorax—are related to complications. Pneumatocele may appear on the chest radiograph after 2-3 weeks of exposure. Repeat X-ray is recommended in those cases where clinical deterioration occurs. However, chest X-ray (CXR) should be done after 6 hours in asymptomatic patient planning for discharge.

Blood pictures show leukocytosis which does not necessarily indicate superadded infection.

Pulse oximetry should be done in every patient with respiratory distress. Arterial blood gases monitoring is useful in severely affected patients with mechanical ventilation. Electrocardiogram should be done if cardiac arrhythmia is suspected.

MANAGEMENT

Initial Assessment
- All asymptomatic patient should be admitted.
- In asymptomatic patient, observe for at least 6 hours, discharge if the patient remains asymptomatic and CXR is normal after 6 hours.
- Determine accurately the product ingested and duration of ingestion from meticulous history-taking.
- Assess vital signs, chest findings, mental status, gastrointestinal and cardiovascular system (CVS) findings.
- Nothing should be allowed orally.
- Induction of emesis, gastric lavage, and activated charcoal is contraindicated.

Treatment of Symptomatic Patient

Treatment is mainly supportive as there is no specific antidote.
- In every respiratory distressed patient, SPO_2 monitoring should be done.
- O_2 should give to maintain saturation >95%.
- IV fluid (maintenance fluid) should be given in every patient.
- Use of corticosteroids have no proven benefit.
- Prophylactic antibiotics have no role, start antibiotics if evidence of bacterial infection present.
- If O_2 requirement and respiratory distress gradually increases, consider mechanical ventilation after shifting the patient in intensive care unit. Mechanical ventilators with standard mode or high-frequency oscillatory ventilators are very effective in ARDS and respiratory failure. In refractory cases, extracorporeal membrane oxygenation may be used where facilities are available.
- Cardiac arrythmia if occurs, should be treated with β-blocker (usually esmolol).

PREVENTION

Patient and parent education is the key factor for preventing hydrocarbon or any kind of poisoning. Parents should know how to keep materials out of reach from the children. Parents should teach young children about the danger aspect of these materials.

SUGGESTED READING

1. Nelson's Textbook of Pediatrics, 21st edition.

Foreign Body in Lungs

Saurabh Gupta, Kinshuk Sarbhai

INTRODUCTION

Foreign body in a child is a common presentation usually brought immediately but often present late as a complicated pneumonia due to unnoticed inhalation and due to inability to communicate. There are reported incidences of late presentation up to 12 years. Objects have been variety in nature from a simple seed to metallic pin. Most common object which recovered later is peanuts. Threat and complication depend not only size of foreign body as well as nature of it, e.g., a button battery is more dangerous than a simple coin despite its small size due to its tendency to react and initiate an early reaction to surrounding.

Foreign body are mostly seen between 2 and 6 years of life (due to curiosity of child to keep everything in mouth). However, accidental aspiration cases can present at any age.

CLASSIFICATION

- *Reactive*: Organic objects such as seeds, peanuts. nonorganic such as button battery or other reactive metals.
- *Nonreactive* such as plastic-made objects, metals.

Classification of foreign bodies by its cause:
- *Foreign body as a result of accident/injury*: Bullet injuries, blast injuries in thorax, etc.
- *Accidental aspiration*: Accidental aspiration of seeds, pin, coins, small toys, etc.
- *Iatrogenic*: Gauze granuloma, thoracic plombage.

CLINICAL PRESENTATION

Presenting complains depends upon site of obstruction:
- *Above larynx*: Patient will have a choking effect. If object is large enough to occlude the larynx, death may happen (Heimlich maneuver to be done). If object is very small, will present as a throat irritation. Biphasic rhonchi can be heard if sufficient obstruction occurs.
- *In trachea*: Intractable cough, wheeze, or whistling sound can be heard.
- *In bronchus*: Late presentation, nonresolving pneumonia, intractable cough may present as pyrexia of unknown origin.

Types of obstruction in bronchus:
- Partial obstruction.
- *One-way obstruction (ball valve mechanism)*: Toward lungs, air can go in inspiration only, will develop emphysema and pneumothorax subsequently. Toward larynx, air can pass in expiration only; will develop atelectasis in due course.
- Total obstruction will develop resorption atelectasis in due course.

CASE HISTORY

A 3-year-old male presented with complains of shortness of breath, cough, vomiting since 2 days. At evaluation, patient had temperature of 101°F, tachypnea, tachycardia, and cough. On auscultation, patient had biphasic rhonchi in left infraclavicular and mammary area and posteriorly in UISA and LISA. There was no history of any foreign body ingestion. Chest X-ray (CXR) on day 1 was suggestive of whiteout lung on left side with slight lower mediastinal shifting toward left side suggestive of collapse consolidation of left side. Patient was admitted as a case of left-side pneumonia and started with antibiotics and oxygen support. Repeat X-ray on day 4 showed a shifting of lower mediastinum toward left side suggestive of resorptive atelectasis. High-resolution computed tomography (HRCT) done on day 4 showed bronchus cutoff sign at T-5 with a intraluminal obstruction or growth. Bronchoscopy done on day 5 showed a foreign body (broken tooth in left main bronchus). Post bronchoscopy X-ray done on day 7 showed a normal CXR. This is almost what happens in most of the scenarios of foreign body in children.

APPROACH TO A CASE OF FOREIGN BODY

Luckily most of the foreign body aspiration events gets noticed by caregivers due to a severe acute cough and choking phenomenon in kids. An evident history of accidental aspiration of objects is a first clue toward diagnosis. Presence of stridor, hoarseness, and respiratory difficulty may or may not present in all cases. However, biphasic rhonchi can be heard in most of the cases.

Chest X-ray

A careful examination of CXR posteroanterior view and lateral view are basic investigation to start with. However, a normal X-ray does not rule out possibility of foreign body. X-ray can be repeated in inspiration and expiration view can show atelectasis and emphysema as secondary sign of obstruction with emphysema.

Findings: Metallic objects can be localized easily. Coin will look like a radiopaque round shadow in trachea or bronchus or it may look like a ring.

Organic substances will have edema in surrounding area looking like a radiopaque shadow. A collapse of segment or lobe due to complete obstruction causing resorption atelectasis may be seen. In late cases of partial obstruction, consolidation can be seen.

It is wise to repeat X-ray in 24–48 to hours to identify a reactionary edema surrounding foreign body if CT scan is not available.

Fluoroscopy/Video Fluoroscopy

A small pneumomediastinum or shallow pneumothorax can be identified which develops as a complication to foreign body inhalation.

High-resolution Computed Tomography Thorax

With recent advances and increased resolution of scanning, HRCT has become an investigation of choice as it not only provides a confirmation it also provides an overview about the location of object facilitating bronchoscopic intervention to remove the object.

Fiberoptic Bronchoscopy

It helps in direct visualization of foreign body till lower divisions. By using baskets, one can attempt removal also at same time.

Rigid Bronchoscopy

It allows visualization of small or very thin foreign bodies such as fish bone, which may get missed in HRCT thorax. It also allows simultaneous removal of object thus having its own advantages. However, it cannot negotiate beyond primary carina.

SUGGESTED READING

1. Dhingra PL, Dhingra S. Diseases of Ear, Nose and Throat. India: Elsevier; 2017.
2. Leitch AG. In: Leitch AG, Seaton A, Seaton D. Crofton and Douglas's Respiratory Diseases. India: Wiley India Pvt. Limited; 2008.
3. Mason RJ, Broaddus VC, Martin TR, King TE, Murray JF, Schraufnagel D, et al. Murray & Nadel's Textbook of Respiratory Medicine, 5th edition. Philadelphia: Elsevier Health Sciences; 2010.
4. Patel MS, Knipe H. Airway foreign bodies in children. [online] Available from: https://radiopaedia.org/articles/airway-foreign-bodies-in-children. [Last accessed September, 2021].
5. Rovin JD, Rodgers BM. Pediatric foreign body aspiration. Pediatr Rev. 2000;21(3):86-90.
6. The Royal Children's Hospital Melbourne. [online] Available from: https://www.rch.org.au/clinicalguide/guideline_index/Foreign_bodies_inhaled/. [Last accessed September, 2021].

SECTION 9: Neurology

99. Cerebral Palsy
100. Autism Spectrum Disorder
101. Febrile Seizure
102. Childhood Absence Epilepsy
103. Childhood Epilepsy with Centrotemporal Spikes
104. Juvenile Myoclonic Epilepsy
105. West Syndrome
106. Breath-holding Spells
107. Neurotuberculosis
108. Neurocysticercosis
109. Headache in Children
110. Acute Rheumatic Chorea
111. Neuro-Wilson's Disease
112. Ataxia
113. Duchene Muscular Dystrophy
114. Spinal Muscular Dystrophy
115. Benign Acute Childhood Myositis
116. Bell's Palsy
117. Traumatic Brain Injury

Cerebral Palsy

Sheffali Gulati, Rahul Sinha, Sonali Singh

INTRODUCTION

Cerebral palsy (CP) is a chronic neurodevelopmental disorder characterized by disturbances in posture, tone, and motor skills resulting from a nonprogressive (static) insult to the developing brain. It was first described in 1862 by an orthopedic surgeon named William James Little. As per the International Consensus definition 2005, it is defined as group of permanent disorders of the development of movement and posture, causing activity limitation, that are attributed to nonprogressive disturbances that occurred in the developing fetal or infant brain.

EPIDEMIOLOGY

The worldwide incidence of CP is approximately 2–2.5/1000 live births. The prevalence and most common cause of CP has varied overtime in different geographical locations based on the development of perinatal pediatric care. Mostly in the developed countries, it is prematurity and extremely low birth weight (ELBW)-related morbidities. In the developing countries, it is mostly related to perinatal asphyxia, TORCH [(T)oxoplasmosis, (O)ther agents, (R)ubella, (C)ytomegalovirus, and (H)erpes simplex], infections, and neonatal hyperbilirubinemia. In India, the estimated incidence is around 3/1,000 live births. In an analysis of 1,000 cases of CP, it was found that spastic quadriplegia constituted 61% of cases followed by diplegia 22%.

ETIOLOGICAL RISK FACTORS/CLASSIFICATION/PATTERN OF INVOLVEMENT

In about 50% cases of CP, the underlying etiology is not established. The common etiology depends on the timing of insult which can be prenatal (most common), intranatal, or postnatal. The etiology can be acquired (traumatic, infectious, hypoxic, ischemic, TORCH infections) or congenital (developmental, malformations, syndromic) **(Table 1)**. Perinatal asphyxia is a cause in only 8–15% of all cases. Chorioamnionitis and maternal infections have been shown to be risk factors for hypoxic-ischemic encephalopathy (HIE) and CP. Periventricular leukomalacia is considered strongest and most independent risk factor for the development of CP.

CLINICAL FEATURES

The common presentation in CP is mostly developmental delay and motor deficits **(Table 2 and Fig. 1)**. Although there are early markers for CP in infancy in the form of developmental delay, neurobehavioral issues, change in posture and tone, and persistence of certain developmental reflexes but the specific CP types are mostly recognized in between 2 and 3 years of age **(Box 1)**. The clinician should be able to differentiate between static insult sequalae

TABLE 1: Etiological risk factors.

Antenatal or prenatal	Perinatal	Postnatal
• Chromosomal/genic disorders • Congenital malformations (Migration disorders such as lissencephaly) • Intrauterine infections • Maternal complications such as chorioamnionitis and eclampsia • Teratogens	• Prematurity/low birth weight • Hypoxia • Sepsis • Birth trauma • Intracranial hemorrhage • Hyperbilirubinemia • Hypoglycemia and other metabolic disorders • CNS infections	• CNS infection • Hypoxic brain injury • Traumatic brain injury • Toxins

(CNS: central nervous system)

TABLE 2: Classification.	
Physiological	**Topographical**
Spastic	Monoplegia (single limb involved)
Dyskinetic	Diplegia (bilateral lower limb predominant involvement)
Ataxic	Triplegia (three limbs affected)
Mixed	Hemiplegia (unilateral upper and lower limb involved)
	Double hemiplegia (bilateral upper and lower limbs involved but one side more than the other and upper limb predominant involvement)
	Quadriplegia (bilateral upper and lower limbs involved)

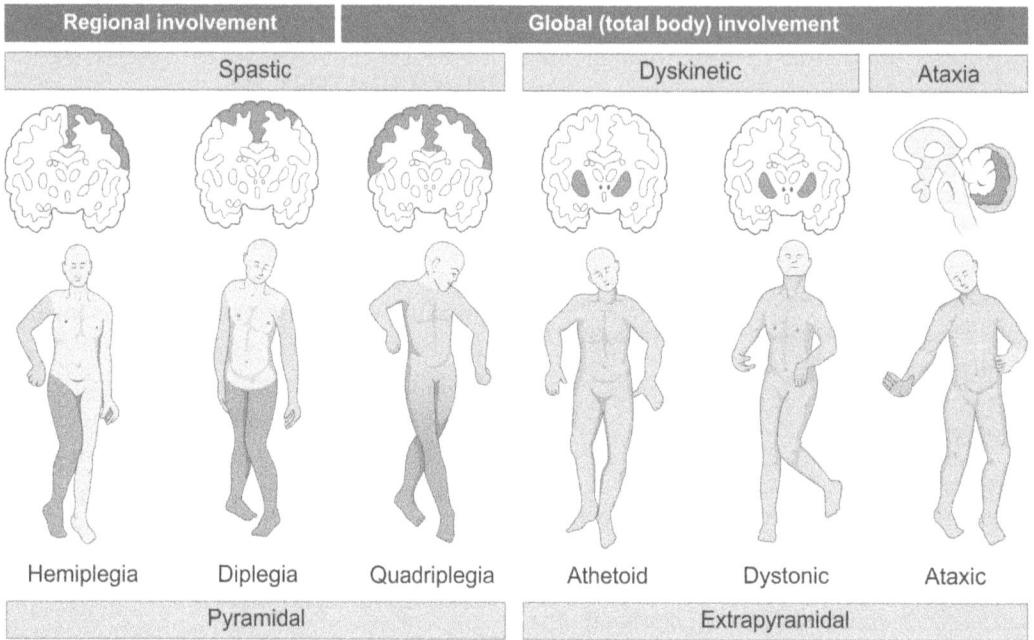

Fig. 1: Types and pattern of involvement in cerebral palsy.

BOX 1: Early signs of cerebral palsy (CP).
- Lack of alertness
- Absence of spontaneous fidgety movements
- Persistent cramped synchronized general movements
- Persistence of obligatory grasp beyond 4 months
- Early and preference
- Persistence of primitive reflexes
- Tone abnormalities
- Persistent asymmetry in posture, movements, and reflexes

and progressive clinical course. One should be able to make out developmental arrest or loss of previously acquired milestones (regression) which can be marker of neurodegenerative disorder (NDD) or metabolic disorders as these can be misdiagnosed as CP. As the CP is an evolving disease, the neurological consequences of CP may be delayed for several months because of the immaturity of the nervous system. The detail clinical features along with imaging findings are discussed in **Table 3**.

DIAGNOSIS/CEREBRAL PALSY MIMICKERS

The diagnosis of CP should be done after detail clinical history and examination as misdiagnoses are not uncommon **(Flowchart 1)**. The clinician should be careful in labeling CP very loosely in children with various chronic neurological disorders. As the CP is a dynamic disease so serial development al evaluations may be necessary in the young child for proper diagnosis and follow-up. The family history of neurological disorders and early or unexplained deaths indicates an undiagnosed inherited neurodegenerative disorder **(Tables 4 to 6)**. Sometimes dystonic CP can be confused with dopa-responsive dystonia (Segawa disease). The early warning signs of CP include developmental delay, toe walking, persistent fisting, microcephaly, epilepsy, irritability, poor sucking, handedness before 2 years of age (indicating hemiparesis), and scissoring of the lower limbs in addition, persistence of primitive reflexes can be an early indicator **(Box 1)**. The clinician should recommend genetic or metabolic tests in case of dysmorphism, positive

TABLE 3: Common types of cerebral palsy with neuroimaging.

Types	Clinical features	Neuroimaging finding
Spastic (50–70%)		
Diplegia (15–25%)	Lower limbs involved more than upper limbs. Usually associated with periventricular leukomalacia (PVL) and periventricular hemorrhagic infarction (PVHI). Some may have associated visual impairment	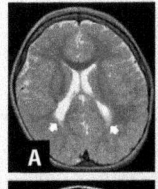 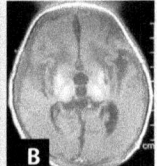 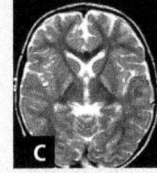 MRI Brain axial section: (A) Bilateral Globus pallidus and thalamus hyperintensity symptom of term HIE, (B) Bilateral irregular ventricular margins with white matter volume loss symptom of PVL, (C) Bilateral Globus pallidus hyperintensity symptom of kernicterus
Hemiplegia (20–40%)	Arms affected more than legs. Most have associated sensory deficits. Associated with intellectual impairment, hemianopia, other visual and behavioral problems	
Quadriplegia (20–40%)	Severe motor impairments. Upper and lower limbs are equally involved. Majority have very little speech and language development, visual impairment, epilepsy and feeding difficulty	
Dyskinetic (10–15%)		
Choreoathetoid	Rapid, disorganized, unpredictable contractions of individual muscles/ muscle groups involving face, bulbar muscles, proximal extremities and digits. There can also be slow writhing movements involving distal muscles. Oropharyngeal difficulties may result from facial grimacing. Primitive reflexes often persist into childhood	
Dystonic	Co-contraction of agonist and antagonist muscles. Can have coexistent pyramidal signs and dysarthria	
Ataxic (5–10%)	Rare. Motor milestones delayed. Ataxia usually improves with time. Should be differentiated from progressive neurodegenerative disorders	

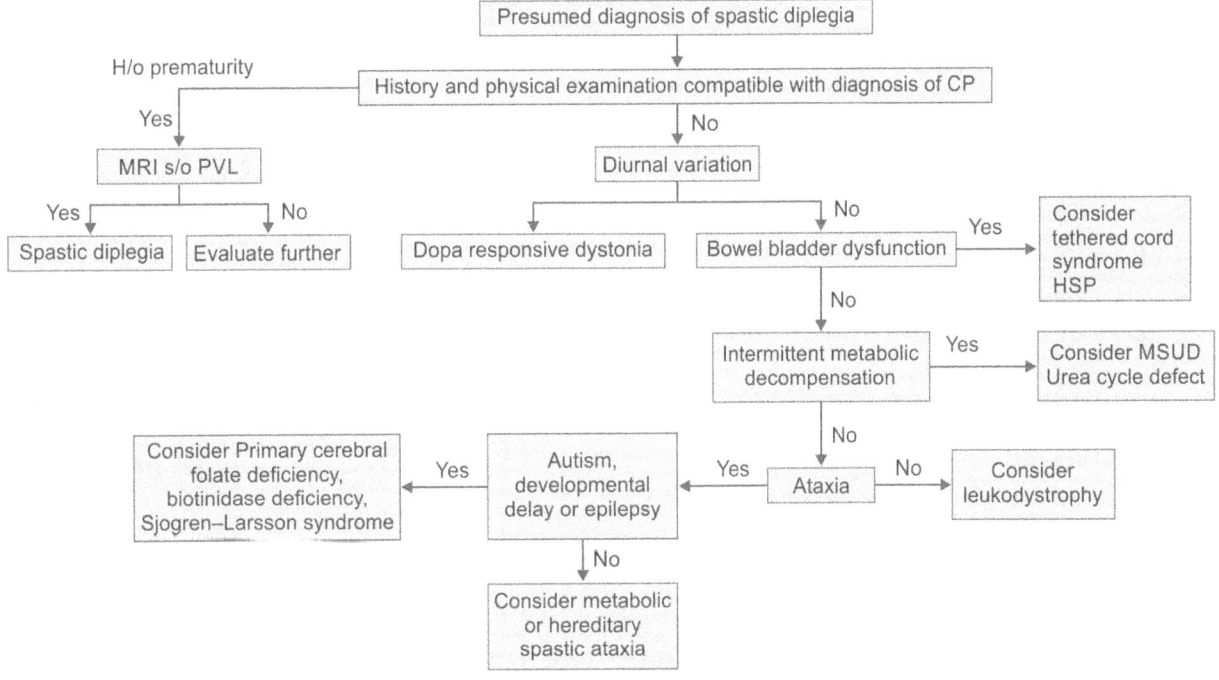

Flowchart 1: Approach to spastic diplegia.

TABLE 4: When should a clinician think beyond cerebral palsy?

History	Examination
No risk factors	Dysmorphic
Regression of skills	Optic atrophy/retinopathy
Fluctuation of symptoms	Pes cavus
Pure neurological signs	Evolving sensory signs
History of consanguinity	
Positive family history	

TABLE 5: Alternative diagnosis in CP by motor type.

Spasticity	Dyskinetic	Ataxia
• Spinal dysraphism	• Dopa-responsive dystonia	• Angelman
• HSP	• Wilsons	• Joubert
• Leukodystrophy	• Glutaric aciduria	• Ataxia telangiectasia
• Biotinidase deficiency	• GLUT 1A	• Friedreich's ataxia
• Arginase deficiency	• Mitochondrial	• Nonketotic hyperglycinemia
	• NBIA	• Maple syrup urine disease

(GLUT 1: glucose transporter 1; HSP: hereditary spastic paraplegia; NBIA: neurodegeneration with brain iron accumulation)

TABLE 6: Common CP mimickers.

Conditions	Clinical features
Hereditary spastic paraparesis (HSP)	Symmetrical spastic weakness of the legs is the main feature. Often accompanied by some urinary urgency and decreased vibration sense in the toes. Commonly autosomal dominant mutation in *Spastin (SPG4), Atoastom (SPG3A) or NIPA1 (SPG6) genes*, X-linked PMOS variants (SPG2)
Arginase deficiency	Children usually present around 3 years of age with progressive spastic paraparesis. Regression of cognitive skills typically follows, with failure to thrive in the context of seizures and tremor. Autosomal recessive disorder of the urea cycle
Biotinidase deficiency	Classical neurological features include seizures, hypotonia, ataxia, developmental delay, disturbed vision and hearing and cutaneous abnormalities (such as alopecia and skin rashes). Older children with profound biotinidase deficiency may exhibit weakness, spastic paresis and optic atopy
Dopa-responsive dystonia (DYT 5)	Characterized by a history of dystonia with diurnal fluctuation, so that gait worsens through the day and is improved by sleep. The dystonia usually shows a dramatic and sustained response to small doses of levodopa
GLUT 1 deficiency	It causes both paroxymal and persistent movement disorders, most often dyskinetic in nature, with dystonic gait or choreoathetosis or ataxia. Diagnosis is confirmed by demonstrating a low CSF to plasma glucose concentration (typically less than 0.4) and mutation in SLC2A1 gene
Worster-Drought syndrome	A supranuclear (pseudobulbar) palsy that presents with sucking and swallowing difficulties, excessive salvation, severe dysarthria, and an exaggerated jaw jerk. Children usually show either a mild spastic diplegia or tetraplegia, variable cognitive and behavioral impairment, and epilepsy

(CP: cerebral palsy; CSF: cerebrospinal fluid; GLUT 1: glucose transporter 1)

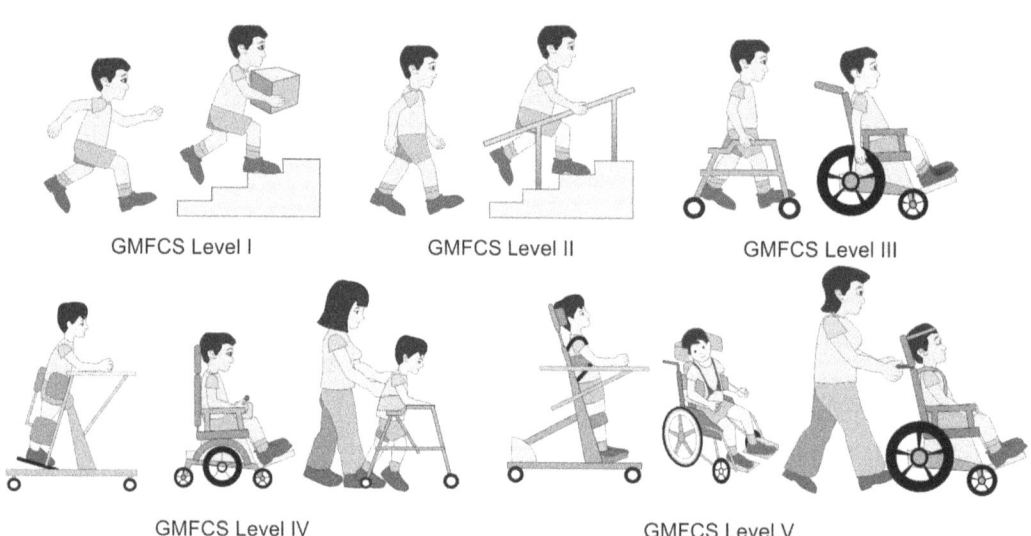

Fig. 2: Gross motor function classification system (GMFCS).

family history of developmental delay, unexplained deaths or any consanguinity. Magnetic resonance imaging (MRI) (brain) is more sensitive than computed tomography (CT), particularly in delineating the extent of white matter changes and posterior fossa changes. The hearing and eye evaluation should be done in all cases of CP. The electroencephalography (EEG) will be done if seizure occurs. Once the diagnosis is established, functional status and associated comorbidities should also be established **(Fig. 2 and Box 2)**. The care givers should be given information in the manner that they are able to cope up with this chronic neurological disorder and will help the multidisciplinary team in improving the outcome of the disease.

TREATMENT

Management of CP requires multidisciplinary approach. Team comprises pediatrician, pediatric neurologist, physiotherapist, ophthalmologist, otorhinolaryngologist, audiologist, orthopedician, psychologist, and dietician. CP has multiple handles **(Fig. 3)**, which need to be addressed for its holistic management. Management of abnormal tone and posture forms the crux in the management of CP. However, various comorbidities **(Box 2)** associated with it require equal attention.

Management plan for children with CP are individualized. Target set for each child depends on baseline functional

BOX 2: Associated comorbidities.

- Malnutrition
- Epilepsy
- Intellectual disability
- Learning impairment
- Behavioral problems
- *Speech*: Aphasia, dysarthria
- Other systemic problems
  - *Vision impairment*: Refractory errors, strabismus, optic nerve hypoplasia, cataract, etc.
  - *Urinary dysfunction*: Urinary incontinence, recurrent urinary tract infections
  - *Respiratory*: Obstructive sleep apnea, pneumonia due to aspiration
  - *Gastrointestinal problems*: Swallowing incoordination, gastroesophageal reflux disease (GERD), constipation
  - Hearing impairment
  - *Orthopedic abnormalities*: Contractures, bony deformities, femur dislocation, osteopenia
- *Pain*: Musculoskeletal, abdominal
- *Sleep disturbances*: Delay in initiation, frequent awakenings

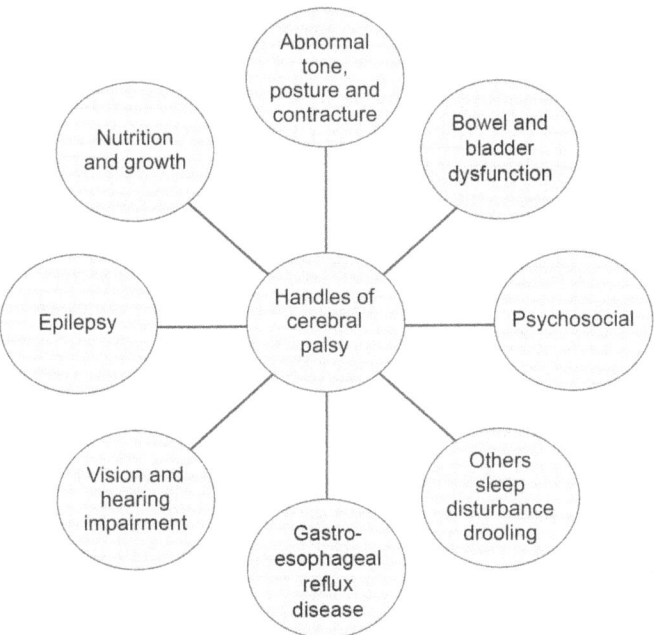

Fig. 3: Management of cerebral palsy (CP).

status, age, and extent of involvement. Parents expectations should also be taken into consideration. For example, a child with spastic paraparesis secondary to preterm sequelae can be expected to sit, stand, achieve independent ambulation and even attend school. However, same is not true for a child with spastic quadriparetic CP whose maximum attained milestone may be neck holding. The systematic review of interventions in CP done by Novak et al. have divided into green light (helpful intervention), yellow light (intervention helpful but with lower level of evidence), and red light (intervention not helpful such as craniosacral therapy, hip bracing, hyperbaric oxygen and sensory integration, stem cells).

Child should be appreciated for every new milestone achieved or new skill learnt. Parents should be appreciated for their efforts too. Goals need revision at each visit depending on the factors mentioned previously.

Nonpharmacological Measures

Physiotherapy forms the backbone of management of CP. It aims to maintain extensibility and prevent joint contractures. Orthotic devices keep muscles stretched and provide necessary support to maximize physical activity. Immobilization should be avoided as spastic muscles get fibrosed and develop fixed contractures. It should be emphasized that drugs cannot replace physiotherapy. Mechanism of spasticity includes abnormal peripheral sensory processing so sensory integration should be an integral part of therapy planned for children with CP.

- Early stimulation should be initiated in high-risk neonates and infants. With simple maneuvers, it reinforces positive developmental patterns.
- Occupational therapy In selected children with CP (hemiplegic CP, spastic diplegic CP), improvement of fine movements enable them to carry out their daily activities and improve their quality of life. Vocational training enables them to have independent living.

Nutrition and growth: Constant increased tone significantly increases the metabolic rate. Increased demand and decreased supply due to oromotor incoordination, dependence on others for feeding and recurrent infections lead to growth faltering. Child should have diet chart prepared by dietician. The diet planned should take into account the affordability, availability, and local feeding culture of the family. At every visit, weight gain should be documented. Problems faced by caregivers while feeding the child should be assessed. Physiotherapy helps in improving oromotor coordination. Motor deficits as well abnormal sensory processing need to be addressed to improve the act of chewing and swallowing and adequate calorie intake should be ensured. Assistive devices are available, which are designed especially for children with CP (**Fig. 4**).

Micronutrient supplementation are given when required. When oral intake is inadequate, nasogastric tube feeding is an alternative. Gastroesophageal reflux commonly

TABLE 7: Drugs for the treatment of spasticity.

Drugs	MOA	Maintenance dose	Guidelines	Side effects	Comments
Diazepam	GABAergic facilitation		0.1–0.8 mg/kg/d (max—10 mg)	Sedation, weakness, memory abnormality, hypersalivation, dependence	
Gabapentin	Inhibits glutaminergic excitatory synapses		Day 1–3: 2 mg/kg TID Day 4–6: 4 mg/kg TID Day 7–9: 6 mg/kg TID Day 10–12: 8 mg/kg TID <5 yrs: 30% higher doses		
Baclofen	GABAergic, GABAb R agonist	Oral- 5–60 mg/day (TID) IT- 50–100 mcg/day	Start with 5–10 mg/d. Slow titration weekly 2.5 OD to 2.5 TID → subsequent titration (<2 years)	Nausea, sedation Sudden withdrawal- Seizures	IT- After resistance to other treatment options
Tizanidine	Alpha 2 adrenergic agonist	0.3–0.5 mg/kg/day (3–4 divided doses)	2–10 years: Start 1 mg HS >10 yrs: Start 2 mg HS		Gradual tapering by 2–4 mg daily

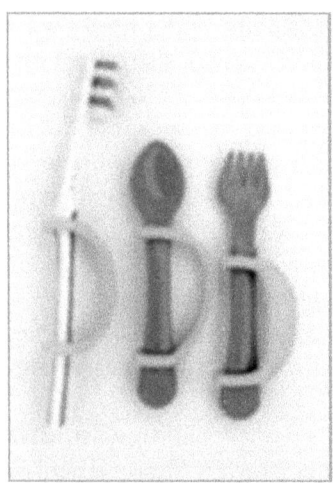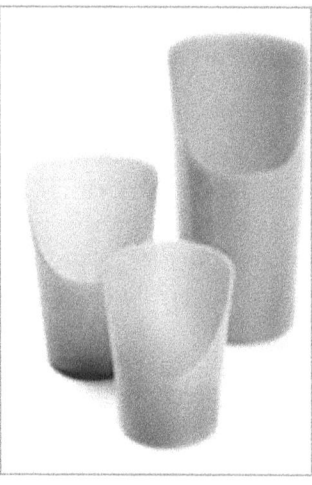

Fig. 4: Assistive feeding devices for children with cerebral palsy.

complicates children with CP, especially spastic quadriplegic infants.
- *Vision and hearing rehabilitation*: Refractive error, cataract, and squint require early intervention. Besides the corrective measures, visual rehabilitation is important for developing orientation, fixation, hand-eye coordination, etc. Hearing assessment, rehabilitation, and speech therapy are important too.
- *Gastrointestinal*: Constipation remains a common accompanying comorbidity. Ambulation and correct diet aid to minimize constipation; however, in severe cases glycerine enema, lactulose, peglec may be required to avoid complications of constipation. Pain and discomfort secondary to constipation are important ongoing stimuli for aggravating spasticity and dystonia.
- Sleep disturbances can be due to pain secondary to ongoing muscle contraction. It needs to be adequately addressed.

- For nonambulatory patients screening and management of bed sores, hip dislocation and scoliosis are important.
- Children with CP should be given the opportunity to read and write. Special educators and benefits should be provided to them.
- Children with CP have behavioral issues such as anxiety, aggression, and oppositional defiant behavior need referral to child psychologist. Parents should also be enquired regarding emotional exhaustion and given psychological support so that they can take best possible care of the child.
- Regular immunization as per universal immunization program is to be ensured as well as additional vaccines such as pneumococcal and annual influenza vaccine to be advised.

Pharmacological and Surgical Intervention

Spasticity
- *Generalized*: Oral drugs—benzodiazepines, baclofen, tizanidine, gabapentin, cannabis
- *Segmental/focal*: Botulinum toxin
- *Spastic diplegia*: Selective dorsal rhizotomy
- *Severe disability*: Intrahecal baclofen pump/deep brain stimulation
- *Surgical*: Tendon lengthening.

Osteotomies
SEMLS (Single event multilevel surgery)

According to the "AAN guideline regarding pharmacological treatment of spasticity in children and adolescents with cerebral palsy," diazepam has the best level of evidence (Level B) among all the oral preparations. Botulinum toxin has Level A evidence for management of segmental or focal spasticity (**Table 7**). However, it has not received the Food and Drug Administration (FDA) approval for use in children with cerebral palsy.

SUGGESTED READING

1. Ashwal S, Russman BS, Blasco PA, Miller G, Sandler A, Shevell M, et al. Practice parameter: diagnostic assessment of the child with cerebral palsy: report of the Quality Standards Subcommittee of the American Academy of Neurology and the Practice Committee of the Child Neurology Society. Neurology. 2004;62(6):851-63.
2. Himmelmann K, Horber V, De La Cruz J, Horridge K, Mejaski-Bosnjak V, Hollody K, et al. MRI classification system (MRICS) for children with cerebral palsy: development, reliability, and recommendations. Dev Med Child Neurol. 2017;59(1):57-64.
3. Surveillance of Cerebral Palsy in Europe. Surveillance of cerebral palsy in Europe: a collaboration of cerebral palsy surveys and registers. Surveillance of Cerebral Palsy in Europe (SCPE). Dev Med Child Neurol. 2000;42(12):816-24.
4. The Definition and Classification of Cerebral Palsy. Dev Med Child Neurol. 2007;49(s109):1-44.

100 CHAPTER

Autism Spectrum Disorder

Alka Srivastava

INTRODUCTION

Autism spectrum disorders (ASDs) are a group of neurodevelopmental disorders that are characterized by difficulty in reciprocal social communication and interaction along with restricted interests, rigid and repetitive behavior. Males are four times more affected than females. It was once thought to be uncommon with reported prevalence rate of 4 per 10,000 in the mid-1960s. The prevalence rates have gone up substantially in the last few decades with recent estimates of up to 1 in 59. The reasons for this rise in prevalence are not entirely clear but they are at least partly due to changing concepts of autism, improved awareness, expansion of diagnostic criteria, better diagnostic tools, and improved reporting. In this chapter, the terms Autism and ASD have been used interchangeably.

CLINICAL PRESENTATION

Symptoms of Autism

These are best explained keeping the DSM-5 (Diagnostic and Statistical Manual of Mental Disorders, 5th edition) criteria in context as below:

- Persistent deficit in social communication and interaction across multiple contexts as manifested by following, currently or by history; must have all three symptoms in this domain:
    1. *Deficits in social emotional reciprocity*, ranging from abnormal social approach and failure of back and forth conversation to reduced sharing of interest and emotions; to failure to initiate or to respond to social interaction.
    2. *Deficits in nonverbal communication* used for social interaction like poor eye contact, gestures or facial expressions.
    3. *Deficits in developing, maintaining, and understanding relationships*, e.g., absence or little interest in peers.
- Restricted, repetitive pattern of behavior, interest, or activities as manifested by at least two of the following, currently or by history; must have two of the four symptoms:
    1. *Stereotyped or repetitive motor movements*, use of objects or speech, e.g., flapping of hands, lining up toys, flipping objects, or echolalia.
    2. *Insistence on sameness*, inflexible adherence to routine or ritualized pattern of verbal or nonverbal behavior, e.g., extreme distress with small changes, difficulties with transition, greeting rituals, need to take the same route or eat same food every day.
    3. *Highly restricted, fixated interests* that are abnormal in intensity or focus
    4. *Hyper- or hyporeactivity to sensory input* or unusual interest in sensory aspects of environment, e.g., apparent indifference to pain and temperature, adverse response to specific sound or texture, excessive smelling or touching of objects, visual fascination with light or movement.
- Symptoms must be present in the early development period.
- Symptoms cause clinically significant impairment in social, occupational, or other important areas of current functioning.

Early Indicators of Autism

Some of the signs and symptoms of autism begin to show in the first year of life but are often missed or dismissed as not significant. Their sensitivity and specificity in terms of predicting diagnosis of autism and differentiating from other developmental disorders is uncertain. While symptoms are typically recognized between 12 and 24 months of age, subtle symptoms may not clearly manifest before 24 months. Some of the early indicators of autism at specific ages are as below:

Age 12 Months

- Poor response to name despite normal hearing
- Poor social smile
- Poor eye contact
- Poor pointing

- Poor imitation skills
- Poor interest in people or other children
- Poor use of gestures such as waving, nodding, or shaking.

Age 18 Months

All of the above-mentioned along with the following:
- Inability to follow pointing (e.g., instead of looking where the other person points to, the child may look at the hand)
- Poor interest in showing things to others to express interest
- Poor understanding of spoken words despite normal hearing
- No use of single words despite normal hearing.

Age 24 Months

All of the above-mentioned along with the following:
- Inability to follow simple commands
- Little or absent pretend play
- Loss of skills (regression).

Autistic Regression

A significant subgroup of children with autism (20–49%) experience developmental regression mostly in the first 2 years of life, which affects language, behavior and social skills. It is therefore important to screen high-risk children at multiple points such as 12, 18, 24, 30 months to account for this. Autism is associated with a high frequency of epileptiform electroencephalography (EEG) abnormalities (prevalence range 10.3–72.4%) and epilepsy (prevalence range 0–44.5%) which may be associated with regression.

ASSESSMENT

Autism is a clinical diagnosis based on the DSM-5 criteria as described above. Assessment of autism should be done by a multidisciplinary team consisting of a developmental pediatrician/pediatric neurologist/child psychiatrist along with speech and language pathologist, occupational therapist, and psychologist. All children should have a detailed developmental, medical and family history. See **Box 1** for specific factors and conditions that are known to increase risk of autism and therefore need to be properly assessed in history.

While an experienced clinician may only need an informal clinical assessment to arrive at a diagnosis, it is always better to use structured tools as described below to make the process as objective as possible.

Screening Tools

There are several screening tools available such as M-CHAT-R/F, Social communication questionnaire (SCQ), Autism behavior checklist (ABC), Social responsiveness scale (SRS) and Childhood Autism screening test (CAST).

> **BOX 1:** Increased risk factors for ASD (adapted from the NICE guidelines).
>
> - *Family history*:
>   - A sibling with autism
>   - Symptoms of autism in parents
> - *Antenatal*:
>   - Advancing paternal and maternal age (>40)
>   - Use of valproate, alcohol in mother
>   - Maternal infections such as rubella
> - *Perinatal*:
>   - Low birth weight and prematurity
>   - Nonspecific birth complications
>   - Birth defects associated with CNS malformation or dysfunction including cerebral palsy
>   - History of threatened abortion
> - *Genetic/medical/psychiatric*:
>   - Fragile-X syndrome
>   - Tuberous sclerosis
>   - Neurofibromatosis
>   - Muscular dystrophy
>   - Epilepsy, especially epileptic spasms
>   - Encephalopathies including epileptic encephalopathy
>   - Certain metabolic disorders such as PKU
>   - Learning (intellectual) disability
>   - ADHD
>
> (ADHD: attention deficit hyperactivity disorder; ASD: autism spectrum disorder; CNS: central nervous system; NICE: National Institute for Health and Care Excellence; PKU: phenylketonuria)

M-CHAT-R/F is the most accepted tool for screening and is available in different languages, e.g., Hindi, Bengali, Kannada, Tamil and Punjabi. The M-CHAT-R can be administered and scored as part of well-baby clinics, and can be used by most professionals to assess risk for ASD. It is a highly sensitive tool but has poor specificity. To address this, they have a follow-up tool called M-CHAT-R/F but it too has a significant number of false positives. However, given the high risk of other developmental disorders and delays in any child who screens positive, an evaluation is warranted on all of them.

Modified checklist for autism in toddlers revised scoring:

1. If you point at something across the room, does your child look at it? (for example, if you point at a toy or an animal, does your child look at the toy or animal?)	Yes/No
2. Have you ever wondered if your child might be deaf?	Yes/No
3. Does your child play pretend or make-believe? (for example, pretend to drink from an empty cup, pretend to talk on a phone, or pretend to feed a doll or stuffed animal?)	Yes/No
4. Does your child like climbing on things? (for example, furniture, play ground equipment, or stairs)	Yes/No

Contd...

Contd...

5. Does your child make unusual finger movements near his or her eyes? (for example, does your child wiggle his or her fingers close to his or her eyes?)	Yes/No
6. Does your child point with one finger to ask for something or to get help? (for example, pointing to a snack or toy that is out of reach)	Yes/No
7. Does your child point with one finger to show you something interesting? (for example, pointing to an airplane in the sky or a big truck in the road)	Yes/No
8. Is your child interested in other children? (for example, does your child watch other children, smile at them, or go to them?)	Yes/No
9. Does your child show you things by bringing them to you or holding them up for you to see not to get help, but just to share? (for example, showing you a flower, a stuffed animal, or a toy truck)	Yes/No
10. Does your child respond when you call his or her name? (for example, does he or she look up, talk or babble, or stop what he or she is doing when you call his or her name?)	Yes/No
11. When you smile at your child, does he or she smile back at you?	Yes/No
12. Does your child get upset by everyday noises? (for example, does your child scream or cry to noise such as a vacuum cleaner or loud music?)	Yes/No
13. Does your child walk?	Yes/No
14. Does your child look you in the eye when you are talking to him or her, playing with him or her, or dressing him or her?	Yes/No
15. Does your child try to copy what you do? (for example, wave bye-bye, clap, or make a funny noise when you do)	Yes/No
16. If you turn your head to look at something, does your child look around to see what you are looking at?	Yes/No
17. Does your child try to get you to watch him or her? (for example, does your child look at you for praise, or say "look" or "watch me"?)	Yes/No
18. Does your child understand when you tell him or her to do something? (for example, if you don't point, can your child understand "put the book on the chair" or " bring me the blanket"?)	Yes/No
19. If something new happens, does your child look at your face to see how you feel about it? (for example, if he or she hears a strange or funny noise, or sees a new toy, will he or she look at your face?)	Yes/No
20. Does your child like movement activities? (for example, being swung or bounced on your knee)	Yes/No

Scoring Algorithm

All questions carry a score of 1 to indicate risk of autism. For all items, except 2, 5, and 12, the response "NO" indicates ASD risk. Based on the scores, risk of autism can be assessed as below:

Low-risk (score < 2): If the child is younger than 24 months, screen again after the second birthday. No further action required unless surveillance indicates risk for ASD.

Medium-risk (score = 3–7): Administer M-CHAT-R/F to get additional information about at-risk responses. If the M-CHAT-R/F score remains at 2 or higher, the child should be referred for detailed diagnostic evaluation. Otherwise, the child should be rescreened at future well-baby clinics.

High-risk (score = 8–20): Refer immediately for diagnostic evaluation.

DIAGNOSTIC TOOLS

These can be divided into interview tools and observational tools although some tools rely on both interview with informants and observation of the child. Autism Diagnostic Interview–Revised (ADI-R), Developmental Dimensional and Diagnostic Interview (3 Di), Diagnostic Interview for Social and Communication disorder (DISCO) are various international interview-based tools used for ASD diagnosis. Autism Diagnostic Observational Schedule (ADOS) is the gold standard observational tool. Since autism is a clinical diagnosis, internationally developed tools would have some limitations when applied on Indian children. To overcome these limitations and to standardize the diagnosis of autism in Indian population, two Indian tools have been developed, i.e., INCLEN Diagnostic tool for autism spectrum disorder (INDI-ASD) and Indian scale for assessment of autism (ISAA), both of which rely on interview and observations of the child's behavior.

Investigations

- *Audiology*: Any child with speech delay should have a hearing test done to rule out hearing loss as a cause.
- *Visual assessment*: It is recommended in any visually inattentive child or child not making eye contact to rule out any refraction error as a cause.
- *Magnetic resonance imaging (MRI) brain*: It is recommended if there is history of regression, seizures or any focal neurological sign on examination.
- *EEG*: It is recommended if there is history of regression or seizures.
- *Genetic testing*: It is recommended in case of a positive family history of developmental disorders or dysmorphic features in the child. Karyotyping and Comparative genomic hybridization (CGH) array are recommended tests. If there are indications to look for syndromes such as Fragile-X or Rett syndrome, point mutations in *FMR1* or *MECP2* can be specifically tested for.
- *Metabolic screening*: It is indicated if there are coarse facial features, organomegaly or other clinical features suggestive of metabolic conditions.

MANAGEMENT

Autism is a lifelong diagnosis and often a level of support is needed for most individuals with autism except for a small minority with high functioning skills. There is no cure for autism. However, early intervention can potentially improve

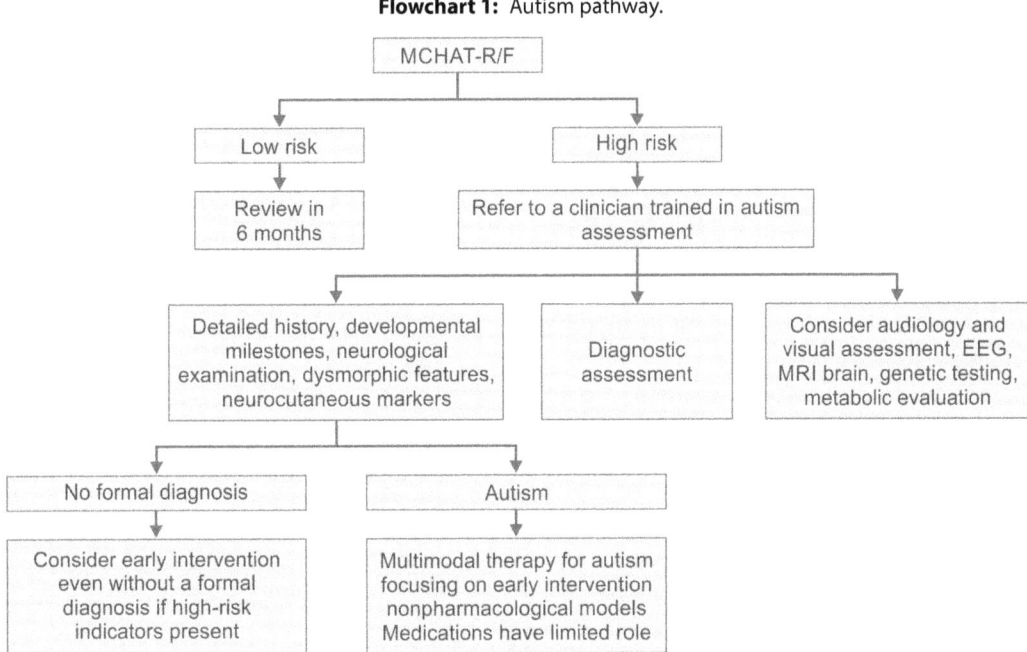

Flowchart 1: Autism pathway.

core symptoms of autism. Ideally, nonpharmacological early interventions can start even without a formal diagnosis of autism provided there are early indicators. Management involves a multidisciplinary team (MDT) similar to the one described under assessment. The management approaches can generally be divided into nonpharmacological and pharmacological as described below.

Nonpharmacological Approaches

Early interventions that are multimodal, intensive, regular, and aim to be at least 20 hours per week of therapy are recommended. In practice achieving 20 hours of therapeutic time per week is not always possible. Hence, parent training becomes extremely important so that therapy can continue at home too where parents can act as therapists. The approaches include principles based on speech therapy, occupational therapy, sensory integration, behavior modification and special education. Various models of structured interventions exist including Early Start Denver Model (ESDM), Applied Behavior Analysis (ABA), Treatment and Education of Autistic and Related Communication Handicapped Children (TEACCH), Social Communication Emotional Regulation and Transactional Support (SCERTS), Picture Exchange Communication System (PECS), Sensory Integration Therapy and CommDEALL (Communication Developmental Eclectic Approach to Language Learning) early interventions program. There are a lot of overlapping strategies used in all of these programs. CommDEALL has the advantage of having been developed in India and is therefore more likely to be applicable to our population.

Pharmacological Management

There is no specific pharmacological treatment for the core symptoms of autism. However, medications can help in the management of specific behaviors discussed below, for which nonpharmacological means are not proving to be satisfactory.

- *Irritability, aggression, and self-injurious behaviors*: Low-dose antipsychotics such as risperidone and aripiprazole may be used but remember to always use the nonpharmacological methods first, either alone or with medications.
- *Restricted and repetitive behaviors*: Risperidone and aripiprazole may be tried, especially if accompanied by irritability, aggression and self-injurious behaviors.
- *Poor sleep*: Melatonin is a commonly used medicine for this indication.
- *Hyperactivity*: Stimulants such as methylphenidate and atomoxetine can be used for hyperactivity but their effects are variable.

PROGNOSIS

Autism spectrum disorders are a group of heterogeneous disorders and prognosis for every case needs to be individualized based on a number of factors. Specifically, presence of a known genetic syndrome, intellectual disability, and poor language skills by age of 5 years indicate poor prognosis. However, even in those individuals who have a good prognosis, some level of support may be needed lifelong (**Flowchart 1**).

KEY MESSAGES

- ASDs are a group of related neurodevelopmental disorders with onset in early childhood with a significant percentage needing lifelong support.
- Autism is a clinical diagnosis based on the DSM-5 criteria and no specific investigation is required to make a diagnosis.

- Investigations may be needed for specific indications such as poor hearing and vision, epilepsy, and genetic conditions.
- Early identification and intervention is the key in management.
- The American Academy of Pediatrics recommends that all children should be screened for developmental delays and disabilities at 9 months, 18 months, and 30 months and specifically for autism at 18 and 24 months.
- There is no cure for ASD and management involves multimodal therapy involving a team.
- Pharmacological treatments may be considered for challenging and repetitive behaviors and for the treatment of comorbid conditions.

SUGGESTED READING

1. American Psychiatric Association. Diagnostic and Statistical Manual of Mental Disorders, 5th edition (copyright 2013).
2. Barbaro J, Dissanayake C. Early markers of autism spectrum disorders in infants and toddlers prospectively identified in the Social Attention and Communication Study. Autism. 2013;17(1):64-86.
3. Hrdlicka M. EEG abnormalities, epilepsy and regression in autism: a review. Neuro Endocrinol Lett. 2008;29(4):405-9.
4. Hyman SL, Levy SE, Myers SM. Identification, Evaluation, and Management of Children with autism spectrum disorder. American Academy of Pediatrics. 2020;145(1):e20193447.
5. Inclentrust.org/INDI-ASD
6. Kanner L. Autistic disturbances of affective contact. Nerv Child. 1943;2:217-50.
7. Robins D, Fein D, Barton M. Modified Checklist for Autism in Toddlers, Revised with Follow-Up. M-CHAT-R/Fhttps://www.m-chat.org/about.php,
8. www.nice.org.uk/guidance/cg128
9. www.Autismspeaks.org
10. www.communicationdeall.com
11. www.thenationaltrust.gov.in/ISAA

101 CHAPTER

Febrile Seizure

Anoop Verma, Vasant Khalatkar

INTRODUCTION

"A febrile seizure (FS) is defined as a seizure associated with fever seen in infants between 6 and 60 months; there is absence of intracranial infections or any known cause or any metabolic disturbance or previous afebrile seizure." [The American Academy of Pediatrics (AAP) Clinical Practice Guideline, 2008]. The highest temperature may be >38.4°C, but temperature is not always practical to measure before a seizure. FS is common between 6 months and 3 years; the peak is seen around 18 months.

International League Against Epilepsy (ILAE) classification:	
Simple FS	Common, 70–80%
Complex FS	Less common, 20–30%
Febrile status epilepticus	5%

- *Simple FS*: Occurring once in a single febrile episode, usually <10-15 minutes, seizure may be generalized, tonic-clonic, or tonic, normal pre- and postseizure neurodevelopment, mostly viral [Human herpesvirus 6 (HHV-6), influenza, adenovirus, and parainfluenza] around 90%, and occurs in first 48 hours of fever in 60% cases.
- *Complex febrile seizure*: The criteria are—focal seizure, persisting more than 10-15 minutes and multiple seizures within the same febrile episode (The presence of one or more of the above features).
- *Febrile status epilepticus*: <30 minutes.

RISK FACTORS FOR FIRST FEBRILE SEIZURES

- Family history of one parent with FS, the risk is 10–25%, one parent and one sibling with FS, the risk is 50%
- Temperature > 38°C
- Delay in development
- Stay in neonatal intensive care unit (NICU) > 28 days
- Attending daycare center (if there is presence of two risk factors, then the probability of FS is 30%).

The history and neurological examination is very important to rule out any evidence of central nervous system (CNS) infection.

INVESTIGATIONS

Simple FS usually does not require investigations for diagnosis. The tests are individualized. Laboratory assistance is required to determine the cause of fever, such as urinary tract infection (UTI), acute respiratory infection (ARI), and malaria, and to rule out presence of intracranial infection. Electroencephalography (EEG) and neuroimaging may be required to analyze seizure in selected case.

- *Complete blood count*: Neutrophilia suggests bacterial infection. Lymphocytosis indicates viral infection. Leukopenia and thrombocytopenia indicate rickettsial infection and viral infections. Blood glucose estimation allows interpretation of cerebrospinal fluid (CSF) glucose. Thick and thin smear, rapid diagnostic test (RDT) in suspected malaria case, and urine routine and microscopic in suspected UTI are performed.
- *Lumbar puncture* is not required in simple febrile seizure; however, the indication of CSF analysis are: (1) Clinical signs and symptoms of meningitis; (2) child between 6 and 12 months who is unimmunized for *Haemophilus influenzae* type b (HiB) and *Streptococcus pneumoniae* vaccination or with unknown vaccination status; (3) in children pretreated with antibiotics for better evaluation.
- *EEG and neuroimaging* is not required in simple FS, but is required in complex FS.

MANAGEMENT

- *Convulsing stage*:
  - Take *care of ABC* of resuscitation.
  - *Control of seizure*: The early, the better. *Lorazepam* is the drug of choice, 0.1 mg/kg, at the rate of 2 mg/min, (maximum up to 4 mg) action last up to 12–24 hours. *Midazolam* 0.2 mg/kg IV over 1–2 minutes, can be given IM/intranasal/buccal in the dose of 0.15–0.3 mg/kg, when IV access in not possible. *Diazepam* in

PRESCRIPTION ASSISTANCE

Pharmacological salt	Market preparation	Availability (drops/syrup/tablets/injection)	Dosages
Acetaminophen	Crocin, Pyrigesic Metacin, T 98	• Drops 100 mg/mL • Syrup (120 mg/5 mL) • DS Suspension (240 mg/mL) • Tablet 325, 500, 650	• 10–15 mg/kg/dose • 6 hourly PO/PR
Clobazam	Frisium/Lobazam/Clozam	Tablets 5, 10, 15, 20 mg	0.75 mg–1 mg/kg/d, BD × 48 hours
Sodium valproate	Valprol, Valparin	• Syrup 200 mg/5 mL • Tablet 200, 500 • Chrono-CR-200, 300, 500	• 30–60 mg/kg/day • Start with 10 mg/kg/day, increase weekly
Midazolam spray	Midaspray (Intas)	Midaspray nasal 50 metered spray	0.2 mg/kg body weight. Dose should be equally divided and administered

dose of 0.3 mg/kg IV, action lasts up to 1 hour, take care of respiratory depression and hypotension. Rectal diazepam can be given 0.5 mg/kg (maximum 10 mg) when no IV access is established.
- *Antipyretics*: Paracetamol 15–20 mg/kg/dose oral or IV. Ibuprofen 5 mg/kg/dose can be tried. (Avoid mefenamic acid, and nimesulide). Tepid sponging is done. Antibiotics are given in bacterial etiology.

RISK FACTORS FOR RECURRENCE OF FEBRILE SEIZURES

- Age < 1 year at the time of first FS
- First-degree family member with history of FS
- Low degree of fever precipitating FS
- If the time duration of onset of fever and seizure is brief.

The risk of recurrence is 70% when all four factors are present, and <20% when no risk factors are present. If the patient is not given any prophylaxis after first FS, the risk of recurrence is 30–40%. If there are two recurrences, about 50% of patients will have further recurrences.

PROPHYLAXIS

- *Intermittent prophylaxis*: *Clobazam* 0.75 mg to 1 mg/kg/day and *Paracetamol* 15–10 mg/kg/dose, 8 hourly, both to be given for 48 hours. Considering the risk–benefit ratio and cost-effectiveness in Indian children, it is always beneficial to give clobazam and paracetamol prophylaxis to every child with FS for 48 hours up to the age of 5 years.
- *Continuous prophylaxis* is only recommended when intermittent prophylaxis fails and the seizures are very frequent. Sodium valproate ranks first to phenobarbitone. Avoid other antiepileptic drugs.

FEBRILE SEIZURES AND EPILEPSY

Febrile seizures are benign with excellent prognosis. Risk of epilepsy in a case of FS is slightly more than general population 2–7%. There is an association of *Mesial Temporal Sclerosis* to prolong febrile status, but there is a paucity of literature in support. Following risk factors contributes for developing epilepsy in a case of FS:
- Complex FS
- History of FS in family
- Pre-existing neurologic impairment.

There are 10% chances of developing epilepsy in the presence of two risk factors.

PROGNOSIS AND CONCLUSION

Febrile seizure are benign with excellent prognosis. Minority develops epilepsy. Complex FS and febrile status epileptics have high chance of developing epilepsy and may require investigations and follow-up. Mortality and morbidity in FS are very low and least effect the cognition. Prophylaxis in FS helps prevent recurrences but not epilepsy.

SUGGESTED READING

1. Steering Committee on Quality Improvement and Management, Subcommittee on Febrile Seizures American Academy of Pediatrics. Febrile seizures: Clinical practice guideline for long term management of the child with simple febrile seizures.. Pediatrics. 2008;121(6):1281-6.
2. Verma A, Kunju PAM. Approach to febrile seizures and fever-related epilepsies. In: Kanhere S, Anandakeshavan TM (eds). IAP Textbook of Pediatric Neurology, 2nd edition. New Delhi: Jaypee Brothers Medical Publishers (P) Ltd., 2019. pp. 183-91.

Childhood Absence Epilepsy

Sanjeev Joshi

INTRODUCTION

This is a common benign epilepsy syndrome starting in early childhood, previously called petit mal epilepsy. The incidence being 1-8 per 100,000 below the age of 15 years. The onset ranges from 3 to 13 years, with a peak at ages 6-7 years. Girls represent 60-76% of patients.

Childhood absence epilepsy (CAE) is classified as an epilepsy syndrome with presumed genetic cause according to the current International League Against Epilepsy (ILAE) classification.

GENETICS

A positive family history of epilepsy is present in about one third of patients. History of febrile seizures can be there. Although an autosomal dominant pattern of inheritance with age-dependent penetrance has been suggested, a multifactorial pattern that involves a combination of genetic and environmental factors is more likely to be associated. Family studies indicate a 17% risk of having typical absence seizures (TAS) in first-degree relatives of patients with CAE.

SEIZURE CHARACTERISTICS

- Absence seizures occur in developmentally normal children. Seizures are brief, most commonly lasting 5-10 seconds (or 5-30 seconds). Seizures start and end abruptly, frequently occurring 10-100 times a day.
- Child complaints that "she cannot attend the class and realizes that she is sitting in the class only when somebody touches and calls her" or else teacher may compliant that he or she is inattentive in class, she is always day dreaming. Seizures occur spontaneously, but may be precipitated by multiple factors, including emotional, intellectual, or metabolic [e.g., hypoglycemia, hyperventilation (HV)]. Absence status can occur in 10% of cases.
- The main feature of absence seizures is loss of responsiveness with cessation of ongoing activity. Automatisms, brief clonic jerks, and loss of postural tone can also be seen.
- *Seizure duration*: The average seizure duration is 9-10 seconds. Approximately, 25% of seizures last less than 4 seconds and approximately 10% are longer than 20 seconds.
- Depending on the associated symptoms, six types of absence seizures can be identified, with six different seizure semiologies:
    1. Simple absence, as impaired consciousness (10%)
    2. Absence with mild clonic components, involving the eyelids (50%)
    3. Absence with atonic components (gradual lowering of the head or arms 20%)
    4. Absence with tonic components (rotating the eyes upward)
    5. Absence with automatisms that are either perseverative (i.e., the patient persists in what he is doing) or de novo, such as lip smacking or swallowing (60%)
    6. Absence with autonomic components (e.g., pupillary dilatation, flushing, tachycardia).

ELECTROENCEPHALOGRAPHY

Electroencephalography (EEG) in patients with suspected CAE should be a sleep-deprived, video-EEG study that includes both intermittent photic stimulation (IPS) and HV, in order to maximize the chance of recording an absence seizure **(Fig. 1)**.

During the ictal period, absence seizures are associated with bilaterally synchronous and symmetrical slow wave discharges that begin abruptly and synchronously in both hemispheres but endless abruptly. The slow wave discharges occur at a frequency of 3 Hz, may slow to 2-2.5 Hz toward the end, and have the highest amplitude in the frontocentral regions.

NEUROIMAGING

Brain magnetic resonance imaging (MRI) is by definition normal in patients with CAE, and structural imaging is not necessary for the diagnosis if patients have typical clinical and EEG findings.

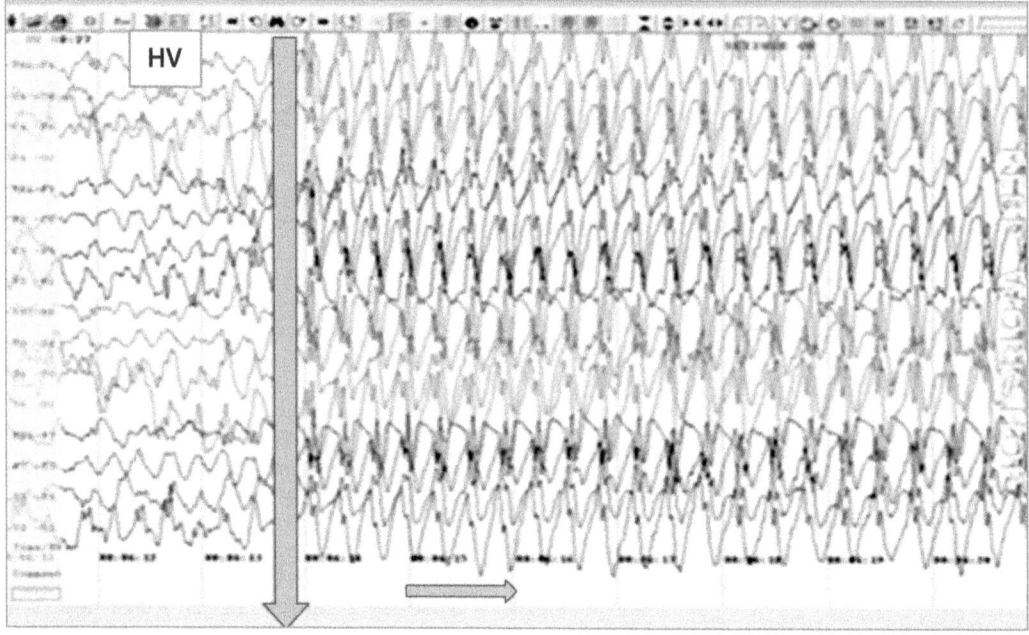

Fig. 1: Electroencephalography tracing depicting abrupt onset of 3 Hz/s, generalized spike and wave induced by hyperventilation (HV).

PROGNOSIS AND EVOLUTION

- Prognostic parameters need to include the seizure and the psychosocial prognosis. The reported percentage of patients who become seizure free varies widely, ranging from 33 to 79.3%.
- Many patients develop generalized tonic-clonic seizures later in the course of the epilepsy. About 40% and generally occur 5-10 years after the onset of absences.
- Absence seizures persist in about 6% of cases. Juvenile myoclonic epilepsy is reported to occur in 44% of patients who do not have remission of their seizures.

Psychiatric comorbidities are common in children with CAE. In a study that included 69 children with CAE, 61% had a psychiatric diagnosis [mostly attention deficit and hyperactivity disorder (ADHD) or anxiety], and 33% had behavioral or social problems. Problems with cognition, learning disabilities may occur in one third of patients.

DIFFERENTIAL DIAGNOSIS

Childhood absence epilepsy must be differentiated from the following conditions:
- Absence seizures with late adolescent onset
- Symptomatic absence epilepsy (e.g., Sturge-Weber syndrome, lipidosis, brain tumors, and moyamoya disease)
- Epilepsy with other seizure types preceding absences (implying a worse prognosis)
- Myoclonic absences
- Nonepileptic staring spells can occur in normal children as well as in association with ADHD, autism, and mental retardation. Unlike typical absence, staring spells can be interrupted by tactile or vocal stimulation, rarely occur during physical activity
- *Glucose transporter type 1 deficiency syndrome*: In patients with early-onset absences, i.e., below 4 years of onset. Genetic disorder with impaired glucose transfer across blood–brain barrier (BBB), associated with low cerebrospinal fluid (CSF) sugar.

TREATMENT

Goals of therapy: Typical absence seizures are characteristically extremely frequent, occurring multiple times each day. Once they are recognized, they should be treated to improve quality of life, school performance, and social acceptance, and possibly to reduce the risk of (rarely) associated convulsive seizures. Complete seizure freedom can often be attained by pharmacologic treatment.
- Both ethosuximide and valproate suppress absence seizures in >80% of patients.
- *Ethosuximide*: Doses start with 5-10 mg/kg in two divided doses, maintenance dose, 15-40 mg/kg/day in two divided doses. Side effect—vomiting, sleep disturbance, drowsiness, and hyperactivity.
- *Valproate*: Dose starts with 10 mg/kg and maintain with 20-40 mg/kg in divided doses. It has the advantage of also controlling generalized tonic-clonic seizures. For the refractory seizures, both medications can be used in combination.
- Lamotrigine may also be effective as monotherapy.

Drugs to Avoid

Several antiseizure drugs have the potential to aggravate absence seizures in patients with CAE and should be avoided.

These include carbamazepine, vigabatrin, gabapentin, and tiagabine. Phenytoin and phenobarbital are known for their ineffectiveness in treating absences and should also be avoided.

Duration of Therapy

In most cases, seizures respond well to first-line drug therapy and remit before puberty. Antiseizure drug therapy should be continued for a minimum of years of seizure freedom. After this period, progressive tapering of antiseizure drugs can be considered.

SUGGESTED READING

1. Berg AT, Levy SR, Testa FM, Shinnar S. Classification of childhood epilepsy syndromes in newly diagnosed epilepsy: interrater agreement and reasons for disagreement. Epilepsia. 1999;40(4):439-44.
2. Berg AT, Shinnar S, Levy SR, Testa FM, Smith-Rapaport S, Beckerman B. How well can epilepsy syndromes be identified at diagnosis? A reassessment 2 years after initial diagnosis. Epilepsia. 2000;41(10):1269-75.
3. Korff MC. (2021). Childhood absence epilepsy. [Online] Avaialble from: https://www.uptodate.com/contents/childhood-absence-epilepsy. [Last acccessed May, 2021].
4. Olsson I. Epidemiology of absence epilepsy. I. Concept and incidence. Acta Paediatr Scand. 1988;77(6):860-6.

CHAPTER 103: Childhood Epilepsy with Centrotemporal Spikes

Sanjeev Joshi

INTRODUCTION

Childhood epilepsy with centrotemporal spikes (CTS) [formerly known as benign childhood epilepsy with centrotemporal spikes (BCECTS) or Rolandic epilepsy] is a self-limiting epilepsy seen in children in their early school years. It is the most common epilepsy syndrome in childhood. It accounts to 13–23% of all epilepsies of childhood. The seizures are brief, hemifacial and may lead to secondary focal to generalized tonic-clonic seizure if they occur nocturnally. In this epilepsy, the neurology and cognition are normal and the neuroimaging is noncontributory. The age of onset is 3–13 years with peak at 7–8 years; the condition resolves by 16 years.

It is seen more commonly in boys; the boy-to-girl ratio is 6:4. 10–20% patients will have single seizure, 20% will have frequent seizure, and <2% will continue to have seizure into adulthood. The syndrome is termed Rolandic epilepsy because of the characteristic features of partial seizures involving the region around the lower portion of the central gyrus of Rolando.

CLINICAL MANIFESTATION

- Seizures occur soon after falling sleep or before awakening. These nocturnal seizures can present in the following ways **(Fig. 1)**:
  - Typical brief hemifacial seizures associated with speech arrest, drooling, and preservation of consciousness (identical to diurnal seizures).
  - Seizures similar to those described above but with gurgling/grunting noises, loss of consciousness, and, at times, vomiting at the termination of the seizure.
  - Generalized convulsions (often secondarily generalized).
- Occurrence of seizures in clusters is common.
- Status epilepticus may occur in as many as 11% of patients.
- Postictal paralysis may occur in 7–21% patients.
- Headache and migraine occur commonly in patients with BECCT in 67% patients.

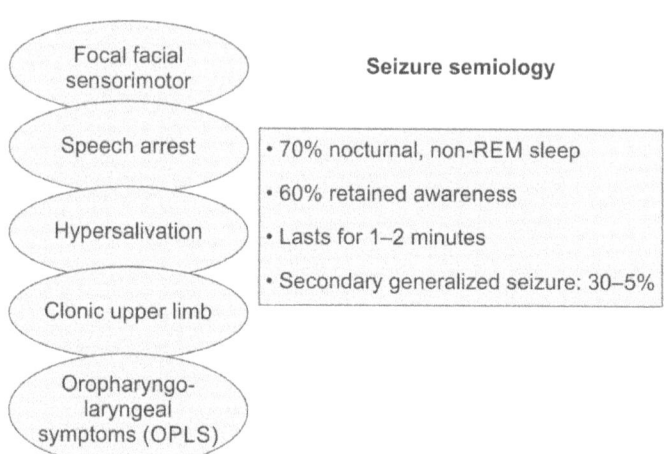

Fig. 1: Seizure semiology: Childhood epilepsy with CT spike.

- Neuropsychological abnormalities are usually transient. They may have problems with visuomotor skills, visuospatial memory and skills, language, and attention.

GENETICS

It is considered to be of genetic in origin. Some patients have significant family history of epilepsy or centrotemporal spikes, although the exact frequency varies, with a range of 9–59%. Isolated electroencephalography (EEG) abnormalities (including Rolandic spikes) are common in families of patients with BECCT.

ETIOLOGY

It arises from the lower portion of the central gyrus of Rolando. Because BECCT is age dependent, it has a strong genetic predisposition with an excellent prognosis, and occurs in structurally normal brain, it most likely represents hereditary brain maturation.

ELECTROENCEPHALOGRAPHY

- Centrotemporal spikes are the hallmark of this condition. These spikes are seen localized in C3, C4, and C5, C6

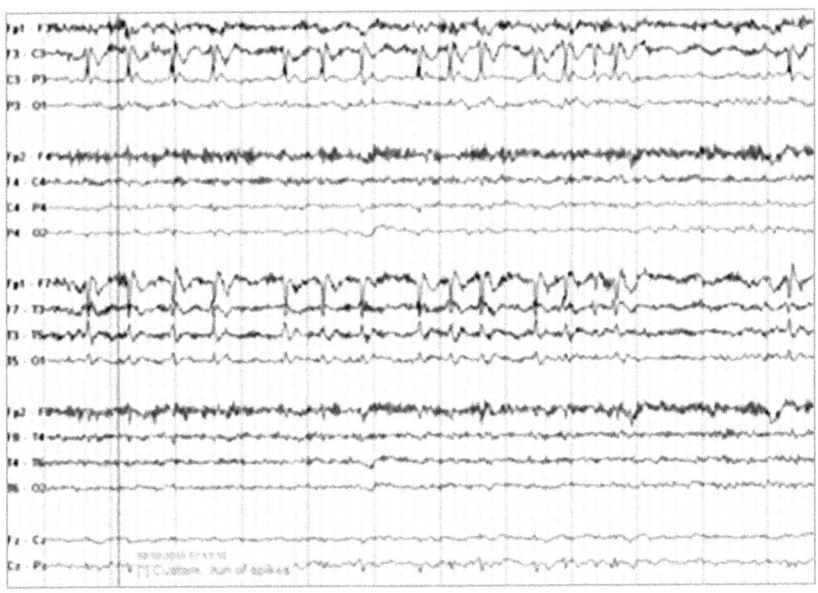

Fig. 2: Electroencephalography showing left centrotemporal discharges.

electrodes and in midtemporal electrodes **(Fig. 2)**; CTS are often bilateral and typically activated by drowsiness and slow [non-rapid eye movement (non-REM)] sleep.
- The spikes are usually slow, high voltage, and diphasic. Typical findings include a negative SW with a blunted peak preceded by a small positive wave and followed by a prominent positive wave with amplitude frequently up to 50% of the preceding negative SW.
- Sleep and drowsiness activate the spikes. Obtain a sleep recording if BECCT is suspected on clinical grounds when the awake EEG is not revealing.
- CTS are diagnostic markers of benign Rolandic epilepsy only in a suggestive clinical presentation. Their frequency location and persistence do not determine the clinical manifestation, severity, and frequency.

Differential Diagnosis on Electroencephalography

Benign Rolandic epilepsy must be differentiated from the following:
- Rolandic spikes and no seizures (often with behavior problems, headaches, or autonomic dysfunction).
- Central spikes occurring commonly in Rett syndrome and fragile X syndrome.
- Malignant Rolandic epilepsy.
- Psychomotor seizures and evolving temporal lobe epilepsy.
- The aphasia-convulsion (Landau-Kleffner) syndrome and massive midtemporal spikes.

NEUROIMAGING

If the case history is typical with normal neurological examination and characteristic EEG findings, then magnetic resonance imaging (MRI) is not needed. If the clinical presentation is a typical and an abnormal EEG, MRI scan should be considered.

TREATMENT

- No treatment is necessary in patients within frequent, nocturnal, partial seizures.
- If seizures are frequent (20%) and disturbing to patient and family, treatment with *carbamazepine, oxcarbamazepine valproate, levetiracetam* and other drugs used in focal seizures can all be used successfully.

Doses of Carbamazepine and Oxcarbamazepine:
- *<12 years*: Initial—10-20 mg/kg/24 hours oral BD; maximum—35 mg/kg/24 hours.
- *>12 years*: Initial—200 mg PO, BD; maximum—dose in children.
- 12-15 years, 1,000 mg/24 hours and in children > 15 years 12,000 mg/24 hours.
- *Duration of treatment*: 2 years.
- *Side effects*: Apart from the well-known side effect, sedation, dizziness, diplopia, aplastic, rash, neutropenia, Stevens-Johnson syndrome, carbamazepine and oxcarbamazepine may aggravate the epileptiform discharges with a continuous spike and wave pattern during slow sleep causing neuropsychological deterioration.
- *Sulthiame* is an excellent drug for childhood epilepsy with CTSe but has limited availability in the market.
- Limited availability in the market.

EVOLUTION AND PROGNOSIS

- Excellent prognosis.
- Spontaneous remission occurs by age 14-16, often much earlier, within 2-4 years of onset.

- Majority of patients have fewer than 10 seizures.
- Some children may develop language, cognitive, or behavioral deficits which improve after remission.

A meta-analysis study on the course of BECCT found that 50% of patients were in remission by age 6 years; by age 18 years, 99.8% of the patients were in remission. Rarely, BECCT can relapse in adulthood; about 2% of patients in BECCT remission experience other seizure types.

SUGGESTED READING

1. Freeman JM, Tibbles J, Camfield C, Camfield P. Benign epilepsy of childhood: a speculation and its ramifications. Pediatrics. 1987;79(6):864-8.
2. Schneebaum-Sender N, Goldberg-Stern H, Fattal-Valevski A, Kramer U. Does a normalizing electroencephalogram in benign childhood epilepsy with centrotemporal spikes abort attention deficit hyperactivity disorder? Pediatr Neurol. 2012;47(4):279-83.
3. Tan HJ, Singh J, Gupta R, deGoede C. Comparison of antiepileptic drugs, no treatment, or placebo for children with benign epilepsy with centrotemporal spikes. Cochrane Database Syst Rev. 2014;9:CD006779.

CHAPTER 104: Juvenile Myoclonic Epilepsy

Anoop Kumar

INTRODUCTION

Juvenile myoclonic epilepsy (JME) is also known as *"Janz syndrome."* It is the most important idiopathic generalized epilepsy (IGE) that is genetically determined. Common age of presentation is between 8 and 26 years. It is quite common, accounting for 26% of IGE. Prevalence is 8–10% in adolescent and adults with epilepsies. Slight female predominance is seen in JME. Some children with childhood absence epilepsy (CAE) may evolve into syndrome of JME.

This syndrome is consists of *triad of absences, jerks, and generalized tonic clonic seizures (GTCS)* with age-related onset for each symptom. The common age of onset for absences is between 5 and 16 years, for myoclonic jerks, 1–9 years later than *absences* (usually around 14–15 years) then GTCS few months later than myoclonic jerks.

SEIZURE SEMIOLOGY

Juvenile myoclonic epilepsy is characterized by:
- *Typical absences*: In more than third of the patients, there is brief subtle impairment of consciousness. Sometimes, it may be associated with mild impairment of cognition or eyelid flickering or both. These absences are distinct with CAE or juvenile absence epilepsy (JAE) in that they are usually shorter and milder.
- *Myoclonic jerks on awakening*: Usually occur within 30 minutes to 1 hour of awakening, shock-like irregular and arrhythmic clonic movements of proximal and distal muscles, mainly of upper extremities. It may be severe enough to cause fall.
- *GTCS*: Follow the onset of myoclonic jerks, especially when they are in clusters and with accelerating frequency and severity and may precede a GTCS-clonic-tonic-clonic generalized seizure. They may also be purely nocturnal or random.
- *Myoclonic status epilepticus* is more common than usual, often precipitated by sleep deprivation or missing medications.
- Pure *absence status epilepticus* is very rare. *GTCS status epilepticus* is infrequent.
- Behavioral, personality, cognitive, and psychological changes may also be seen.

Seizures precipitating factors:
- Sleep deprivation
- Fatigue
- Excessive alcohol intake
- Photic stimulation
- Mental stress and emotions—excitement, concentration, mental psychological arousal, failed expectations, or frustration.

ETIOLOGY

- Genetically determined syndrome
- First- and second-degree relatives were also involved in 50–60% of families of proband
- Polygenic inheritance
- Autosomal dominant with variable penetrance
- Dominant gene on 6p11-12 or 15q14
- Mutation in calcium, potassium, and chloride channels linked to seven different loci.

INVESTIGATIONS

All tests, except magnetic resonance imaging (MRI) and electroencephalography (EEG), are normal.
- *MRI*: In some patients of JME, abnormalities involving mesiofrontal cortical structure with increase in cortical gray matter can also be seen.
- *EEG*: EEG abnormalities were seen in 80% of patients.
  - 3-6-Hz generalized spike-wave discharges (GSWD) with intermittent fragmentation with normal background (4-6-Hz GSWD in 61% and 3-Hz GSWD in 14%).
  - 1/3rd shows photo paroxysmal response.
  - 1/3rd shows focal findings.
  - Sleep-deprived EEG with awakening to be done to increase yield.
  - Myoclonic jerk EEG correlate shows generalized burst of polyspikes of 0.5–2 seconds. Polyspikes consisted of 8–10 spikes with characteristic worm-like appearance.
  - Brief discharges (1–4 seconds) are more common.

DIAGNOSTIC TIPS

- Revealing myoclonic jerks is an essential part of diagnosing JME.
- GTCS usually preceded by myoclonic jerks are nearly pathognomonic of JME if they occur in the morning.

MANAGEMENT

Principles:
- Lifestyle improvement
- Avoidance of precipitating factors
- Avoidance of alcohol indulgence
- Compensating sleep deprivation
- Long-term medication

Antiepileptic drugs (AEDs):
- *Valproate* is the most effective AED in the treatment of JME with up to 86% of patients becoming seizure-free for at least 1 year (possible long-term cognitive effect on fetus).
- *Levetiracetam* is the preferred alternative to valproate in teenager girls and childbearing women. This is only newer AED licensed for treatment of myoclonic seizures in JME.
- *Lamotrigine* should be used as combination with valproate. Monotherapy with lamotrigine has promyoclonic effect. Seizure-free rates of lamotrigine is between 40 and 83%.
- *Clonazepam* is the most effective treatment for myoclonic jerks (can control up to 88% cases) as addon therapy. It should be administered in small doses (0.5–2 mg) as additional drug.
- *Phenobarbitone* is the best option if cost is a concern. It is effective in 60% patient.
- *Topiramate* when used as polytherapy, it is equally effective as valproate and *lamotrigine* but tolerability may be inferior.
- *Zonisamide* is second option, especially in women.
- *Contraindicated AEDs*: Vigabatrin, tiagabine, gabapentin, pregabalin, phenytoin, oxcarbazepine, and carbamazepine
- *Lifelong treatment*: In mild JME, drugs may be tapered over years.

PROGNOSIS

- All seizures are probably lifelong but improved after fourth decade of life.
- Varies in severity from mild myoclonic jerks to frequent and severe falls and GTCS.
- Well controlled with appropriate medications in up to 90% patients.
- If all three types of seizures are present, then it is more likely resistant to treatment.

OUTCOMES

- Lifelong condition with high rate of relapse if weaned off AED therapy (91% remaining on treatment and only 9% seizure free off medication).
- Prognosis is worse in patients of CAE evolving in to JME.
- The decision of discontinuing treatment should be individualized for every patient.

SUGGESTED READING

1. Bureau M, Genton P, Thomas P, Dravet C. Juvenile myoclonic epilepsy In: Dravet C, Bureau M, Genton P, Thomas P (eds). Epileptic Syndromes in Infancy, Childhood, and Adolescence, 5th edition. France: John Libbey Eurotext; 2012.
2. Gourie RP. Juvenile myoclonic epilepsy. In: Epilepsy in Children, 1st edition. New Delhi: Jaypee Brothers Medical Publishers (P) Ltd.; 2014.
3. Panayiotopoulos CP. Juvenile myoclonic epilepsy. In: A Clinical Guide to Epileptic syndromes and their Treatment, 2nd edition. London: Springer-Verlag; 2010.
4. Swaiman KF, Ashwal S, Ferriero DM, Schor NF, Finkel RS, Gropman AL, et al. Myoclonic seizures and infantile spasms. In: Gropman AL, Ferriero DM, Swaiman KF, Shevell M, Schor NF, Pearl PL, Finkel RS, Ashwal S (eds). Swaiman's Textbook of Pediatric Neurology, 6th edition. US: Elsevier Health Sciences; 2017.

CHAPTER 105: West Syndrome

Anoop Kumar

INTRODUCTION

- It is age-related epileptic encephalopathy characterized by triad of presence of unique type of seizures called epileptic (infantile) spasms, cognitive decline, and gross electroencephalography (EEG) abnormality of hypsarrhythmia.
- Onset is between 3 and 12 months (peak at 5 months) in 90% of cases and nearly always before 2 years of age.
- Males (60-70%) predominate.
- Incidence is 3-5 per 10,000 live births.
- Seizure semiology:
  - West syndrome usually starts insidiously with mild epileptic spasm two to three times a day. These symptoms develop over few weeks with spasms typically occurring in clusters of 1-30 per day with each cluster having 20-150 attacks. Onset of spasm is often accompanied by psychomotor deterioration, thus meeting the criterion of epileptic encephalopathy.
- *Epileptic spasms*:
  - Epileptic spasms are the clusters of sudden, brief (0.2-2 seconds), bilateral tonic contractions of axial and limb muscles with a 5-30-second interval between successive spells.
  - They are slower than myoclonic jerks and faster than tonic seizures.
  - They can involve widespread muscle groups or be fragmented involving flexion of the neck only (bobbing of the head), abdomen (mild bending), or just the shoulders (a shrug-like movement).
  - Spasms often followed by motionless or diminished responsiveness lasting up to 90 seconds.
  - Alteration and pauses of respiration during the spasms are common (60%), whereas changes in heart rate are rare.
  - A cry and sometimes laughter often follows the end of the attack.
  - Eye movements consisting of deviation alone or followed by rhythmic nystagmoid movements are also commonly seen during spasms.
- Spasms may be flexor, more often flexor extensor and less frequently extensor.
- *Flexor spasms*: Common (40% of all). Also known as salaam spasms and Jack knife spasms, etc.
- *Extensor spasms*: Less frequent, around 20% of all.
- *Flexor extensor spasms*: Most common (40-50%). Combined sudden con-traction of both flexor and extensor muscles with flexion of neck, trunk, and arms but extension of legs.
- Spasms are usually symmetrical. But 1-30% cases have lateralizing features such as head and eyes turned to one side or one limb consistently moving more vigorously (highly correlating with contralateral cerebral lesion of symptomatic West syndrome).
- Subtle epileptic spasms may present as episodes of yawning, gasping, facial grimacing, isolated eye movements, and transient focal motor activity.
- Spasms predominately occur on arousal and in alert state, less often during Nonrapid eye movement (NREM) sleep (3%) and rarely during REM sleep.
- The twilight state just before sleep or just after awakening acts as precipitating factor.
- In late-onset west syndrome, drop attacks (tonic, atonic or both) may be the first symptom.
- Cognitive decline and developmental delay may occur before or with epileptic spasms.
- Axial hypotonia, lack of hand grasping or eye contact may have negative prognostic significance.

ETIOLOGY

- West syndrome is classified into *symptomatic (80%), cryptogenic (10-15%) or idiopathic (5-30%)*.
- *Symptomatic West syndrome*: Most common. Significant developmental delay is present before the onset of epileptic spasm. Clinical, EEG and radiological features suggest the presence of underlying disorder.
  Causes:
  - Pre-, peri- and postnatal brain ischemia.
  - Traumatic brain injuries.
  - Late hemorrhagic disease of newborn.

- Brain congenital anomalies such as disorders of cortical development and hypothalamic hamartoma.
- Neurocutaneous syndrome such as Tuberous sclerosis.
- Chromosomal abnormalities such as Down syndrome (better prognosis in regards to seizures).
- Congenital or acquired brain infection such as viral, bacterial, protozoan, e.g., TORCH [Toxoplasmosis, Other (syphilis, varicella-zoster, parvovirus B19), Rubella, Cytomegalovirus (CMV), and Herpes infections infection and cerebral abscess].
- Brain neoplasms.
- *Inborn error of metabolism*: Hypoglycemia, Phenylketonuria (PKU), OA, aminoacidurias, pyridoxine deficiency, and mitochondrial disorders.
- *Cryptogenic (probably symptomatic) West syndrome*: When an underlying cause is suspected but it remains unidentified. Prevalence is 10–15%.
- Idiopathic West syndrome has pure genetic predisposition to epilepsy. Normal premorbid development occurs and it carries good prognosis.
- *Reversible causes for epileptic spasms*: Drugs—theophylline and ketotifen—and pyridoxine dependency.
- Familial occurrence is low at 4 or 5%, except tuberous sclerosis or twin pregnancy.
- Rarely X-linked recessive Xp21.3-Xp22.

Inclusion criterion for idiopathic west syndrome:
- Normal development before, during and after the active seizure period, with preservation of visual function
- Normal functional and structural brain imaging or other symptomatic causes
- Symmetrical epileptic spasms and EEG hypsarrhythmia.

Additional criterion:
- A family history of other forms of idiopathic epilepsy or febrile seizures
- EEG genetic traits, such as photoparoxysmal responses or spike-wave discharges or Rolandic spikes
- An EEG-identifiable basic activity and sleep spindles, despite a hypsarrhythmic pattern
- Absence of focal interictal EEG slow-wave abnormalities even after intravenous diazepam
- Reappearance of hypsarrhythmia between consecutive spasms of a cluster
- Spontaneous remissions in untreated patients, which occur frequently.

INVESTIGATIONS

Clinically correlated investigation showed high yield such as cerebrospinal fluid (CSF) for infection or metabolic profile to rule out metabolic etiology or chromosomal analysis.

- *Magnetic resonance imaging (MRI)*: Helpful in neurocutaneous syndromes, congenital anomalies, and cortical atrophy due to excessive steroid therapy.
- *Positron emission tomography (PET)*: Highly sensitive in detecting focal cortical abnormalities. Bilateral hypometabolism in temporal lobes even in the absence of normal CT or MRI scan, has a bad prognostic significance.
- EEG:
  - *Interictal EEG*:
    - Hypsarrhythmia—occur in two-third patients.
    - It is a chaotic cerebral activity, characterized by asynchronous, arrhythmic, high-voltage slow waves variably intermingled multifocal spikes.
    - It is the most common EEG pattern-associated with epileptic spasms in first year of life.
    - It is mainly seen in NREM sleep. REM sleep shows relative EEG normalization.
    - This classic pattern is usually seen in the early stages of infantile spasms, and in patients younger than 1 year of age.
    - Symmetrical hypsarrhythmia is most likely to occur in idiopathic and cryptogenic cases.
  - *Modified or asymmetric hypsarrhythmia*:
    - It is one in which the true hypsarrhythmic pattern is observed mostly over one hemisphere or completely lateralized.
    - These patterns include increased interhemispheric synchronization, asymmetrical or unilateral, focal features, slow waves without spikes and generalized background burst suppression.
    - It occurs in up to 40% cases.
    - It always indicate ipsilateral brain structural lesion.
    - Consistently focal slow waves indicate localized lesion.
    - It is more apparent with intravenous diazepam which reduces the amount of hypsarrhythmia.
    - *Burst suppression pattern*: Mostly seen in lissencephaly and Aicardi syndrome.
    - Hypsarrhythmia gradually becomes more organized with age and developed in to a slow GSWD pattern of Lennox-Gastaut Syndrome (LGS).
  - *Ictal EEG*:
    - Duration may vary from 0.5 second to 2 minutes. Ictal EEG of epileptic spasms show diffuse high-amplitude slow waves which may have predominance over one hemisphere. A spindle-like brief beta activity or very fast rhythmic activity has also been described as EEG counterpart of epileptic spasm.
    - The most common and characteristic pattern in 72% of the attacks is a brief duration (1–5 seconds).
  - *It consists of*:
    - A high voltage-generalized slow waves

PHARMACOLOGICAL ASSISTANCE

Pharmacological salt	Market preparation	Availability	Dosage
ACTH	Acton prolongatum	Injection: 60 IU/mL	1–3 IU/kg/day
Vigabatrin	Sabril	Tablet 500 mg	100–150 mg/kg/day
Prednisolone	Omnacortil, wysolone, predone	• Tablet 5, 10, 20, 30, 40 mg • Syrup 5 mg/5 mL	2 mg/kg/day
Zonisamide	Zonegran	Tablet 50, 100, 300, 400, 600 mg	Start with 2 mg/kg/day
Clonazepam	Zapiz, ozepam, clonotril	Tablet 0.25, 0.5, 1, 2 mg	
Levetiracetam	Levera, levipil	• Tablet 250, 500, 750, 1,000 mg, • Syrup 500 mg/5 mL, 100 mg/5 mL	Start with 10 mg/kg/day.

- Episodic, low-amplitude fast activity
- Marked diffuse attenuation of EEG electrical activity (electrodecremental ictal EEG pattern).

DIFFERENTIAL DIAGNOSIS

- Exaggerated startle response
- Infantile colic
- Benign sleep myoclonus
- Benign myoclonic epilepsy of infancy—normal EEG
- Sandifer syndrome of gastroesophageal reflux.

DIAGNOSTIC TIPS

- Ask the parents to imitate the event physically rather than only describing.
- Video recording may be conclusive.
- Epileptic spasms occur in clusters.

MANAGEMENT

- *Goals of treatment*:
  - Complete cessation of seizure
  - Disappearance of Hypsarrhythmia AEDs.
- *Two therapeutic approaches*: Hormonal treatment (ACTH or corticosteroids) and Vigabatrin.
- They control spasms in two-third patients within few days.
- Daily low doses (1–3 IU/kg/day) of ACTH for 2 weeks followed by 2 weeks of rapid tapering may be used. If case of no response then stop early and give other AED.
- Prednisolone (2 mg/kg/day) may also be used in place of ACTH.
- Steroid toxicity features such as infection, hypertension, gastritis, and hyperexcitability must be monitored.
- Vigabatrin at the doses of 100–150 mg/kg/day is also very effective. It should only used for 3–6 months with regular ERG screening for retinal toxicity leading to irreversible visual field defects as side effect (20% cases).
- Despite the higher responders rate on adrenocorticotropin (ACTH) (74%) than vigabatrin (48%), vigabatrin did better in those with tuberous sclerosis and cortical dysplasia and ACTH in those in perinatal ischemia.
- Valproate and clonazepam control about 25–30% cases but relapse rate is very high.
- Levetiracetam and clobazam are most effective antiepileptic drugs (AEDs).
- Lamotrigine, nitrazepam, topiramate, zonisamide, and pyridoxine may also be used.
- Ketogenic diet may also be used.
- Resective neurosurgery is done in cases of localized structural lesions.
- Cases of drop attacks may benefit from total callosotomy.

PROGNOSIS

- 60% of the West syndrome may develop into drug refractory seizures or syndromes such as LGS or complex focal seizures.
- Half patients have permanent motor disabilities.
- Two-third patients have severe cognitive and psychological impairment.
- Only about 5–12% have normal mental and motor development.
- Patients of west syndrome may have autistic behavior, hyperkinetic syndrome, and psychiatric disorders.
- Idiopathic and cryptogenic west syndrome are having better prognosis than symptomatic type.

SUGGESTED READING

1. Bureau M, Genton P, Thomas P, Dravet C. Infantile spasms In: Dravet C, Bureau M, Genton P, Thomas P (eds). Epileptic Syndromes in Infancy, Childhood and Adolescence. France: John Libbey Eurotext Limited; 2012.
2. Panayiotopoulos CP. Epileptic Encephalo-pathies in Infancy and early Childhood. A Clinical Guide to Epileptic Syndromes and their Treatment. London: Springer; 2010.
3. Passi G. Epileptic Encephalopathies in Infancy and Childhood. Epilepsy in Children. New Delhi: Jaypee Brothers Medical Publishers (P) Ltd.; 2014.
4. Swaiman KF, Ashwal S, Ferriero DM, Schor NF, Finkel RS, et al. Myoclonic seizures and infantile spasms. In: Gropman AL, Ferriero DM, Swaiman KF, Shevell M, Schor NF, Pearl PL, Finkel RS, Ashwal S. Swaiman's Textbook of Pediatric Neurology. Philadelphia: Elsevier Health Sciences; 2017.

Breath-holding Spells

Sanjeev Joshi

INTRODUCTION

- Breath-holding spells (BHS) is a psychosomatic disorder, seen commonly in children between 6 months and 6 years.
- The term BHS is actually a misnomer, as these are not self-induced, but result from the immaturity of the autonomic system. While considered by many to be "attention-seeking" behavior, these spells are not intentional; they result from an involuntary reflex, and the child has no ability to control them.
- The spells can be either Pallid or Cyanotic type.
- Commonly seen in developmentally normal child occurring numerous times a day to one episode a year.

ETIOLOGY

- A positive family history is present in 35% of children with spells suggesting some genetic association.
- Studies suggest a maturational delay in myelination of brainstem to have a possible role in etiology. Other studies reported to show altered selenium and antioxidant levels in children with BHS.

PATHOGENESIS

Both types of spells result from reflex changes that reduce cerebral blood flow.

- The first type is the *pallid BHS*, proposed to be due to parasympathetic system-mediated cardiac inhibit ion leading to bradycardia. The primary mechanism is due to increased vagal tone leading to cerebral hypoperfusion.
- The second type is the *cyanotic BHS*, which does not occur during inspiration, but results from prolonged expiratory apnea and intrapulmonary shunting.
- Anemia is believed to have strong association with the disorder. Regardless of the type of spells, iron deficiency anemia is known to prolong the duration of asystole during spells. Low levels of hemoglobin (Hb) result in reduced oxygen-carrying capacity and prolonged cerebral anoxia.

CLINICAL FEATURES

Episodes start between the ages of 6 and 18 months. Attack frequency varies from many per days to only few irregular intervals and may increase during the second year of life.

Typical Characteristics

Cyanotic BHS

- It the most common type. It usually occurs in response to anger and frustrations, leading to vigorous cry, followed by apnea and rapid onset of cyanosis. It may or may not be followed by loss of consciousness.
- It shows abnormal posturing or repeated generalized-clonic jerks. The child usually regains consciousness within a minute, and resumes normal activities.

Pallid BHS

- It is seen in about 25% of children. It usually occurs in response to fright and pain or an unexpected event.
- The child may grasp or cry, stops breathing, becomes hypotonic and loses consciousness.
- Clonic movements may occur, sometimes associated with prolonged asystole. After regaining consciousness, pallid spells occasionally followed by sleep for several hours.

DIAGNOSIS

- Depends only on good and detailed clinical history, describing the entire episodes as and when it occurred. It must also include precipitating event such as emotional stimuli or trauma. Presence of urinary incontinence, uprolling of eyeballs, and deviation of mouth are commonly seen with seizures, especially if not preceded by a cry.
- A complete physical examination including growth and development is essential, especially cardiovascular examination for rhythm disturbances.
- *Long QT syndrome (LQTS) can present as BHS, ECG to be done in atypical case*: Careful attention to BHS is important to distinguish an innocent BHS from a potential LQTS-triggered cardiac event, so that proper treatment is initiated **(Fig. 1)**.

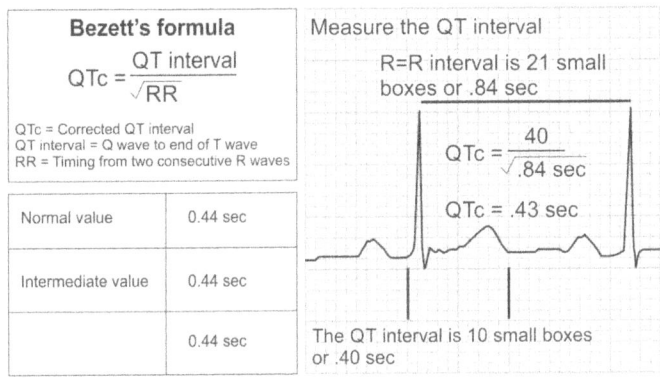

Fig. 1: Long QT syndrome.

Laboratory investigations: Complete blood count (CBC), serum ferritin, and total iron binding capacity (TIBC) for assessment of iron deficiency.

Electroencephalography (EEG) is not required if classical history or video of the event is taken. Neuroimaging is not needed.

MANAGEMENT

- Reassurance to parents regarding the benign nature of BHS is the mainstream of treatment.
- During the episode, parents are requested to place the child in lateral recumbent position as it shortens cerebral anoxia.
- Iron therapy must be initiated in all children with BHS with or without IDA.
- According to Cochrane review published in 2010, iron supplementation at 5 mg/kg/day of elemental iron for 16 weeks appears to reduce the frequency and severity of the spells.
- Atropine (0.01 mg/kg twice or thrice a day) has been shown to be effective in pallid type but in frequent cases.
- The role of piracetam, fluoxetine, levetiracetam, glycopyrrolate, theophylline is not approved by the Food and Drug Administration, needs more trial.

SUGGESTED READING

1. Buckmaster A, Williams K, Wheeler D. Iron supplementation for the treatment of breath-holding attacks in children. Cochrane Database of Systematic Reviews. 2010;5:CD008132.
2. Robinson JA, Bos JM, Etheridge SP, Ackerman MJ. Breath holding spells in children with long QT syndrome. Congenit Heart Dis. 2015; 10(4):354-61.
3. Zehetner AA, Orr N. Congenital heart disease. 2015;10(4): 354-61.

107 CHAPTER: Neurotuberculosis

Vineet Wankhede

INTRODUCTION

Central nervous system (CNS) tuberculosis (TB) accounts for 5–10% of extrapulmonary TB. Though it accounts for 1% of total cases of TB, it is still devastating variant of extrapulmonary syndrome with severe mortality and distressing morbidity. The Revised National TB Control Programme (RNTCP) (Recent 2018) and the Indian Academy of Pediatrics (IAP) (Recent 2012) provide time-to-time guidelines for practicing pediatricians. We will discuss the classification, clinical features, and management strategy with more emphasis on tuberculous meningitis (TBM).

CLASSIFICATION OF CNS TUBERCULOSIS

For all the treatment purpose, CNS TB is considered a single entity. However, for the pathological classification, distinct entities are summarized in **Box 1**.

CLINICAL FEATURES

- *Tuberculous meningitis*:
    - TBM is the most common manifestation of CNS TB and still remains most difficult to manage. Most of the patients may mimic bacterial meningitis in early stage.
    - However, they often have a prodrome of symptoms for 2–8 weeks in the form of failure to thrive, fever anorexia and headache prior to the development of meningeal irritation.
    - Unlike adults, TBM in children presents with nonspecific presentation ranging from persistent unexplained fever to symptomatology of CNS irritation ranging from inconsolable cry to Frank signs of meningism and alteration of sensorium and signs of complications as focal neurodeficits.
    - A history of TB is elicited in only approximately 10% of patients. The presence of active pulmonary tuberculosis (PTB) on chest X-ray ranges from 10 to 15%. Patients coinfected with HIV do not seem to have an altered presentation of TBM.
    - About 10% of cases with TBM have some form of spinal TB.
    - Two or more of the following features, with or without fever, should be present to suggest a clinical diagnosis of TBM—altered sensorium varying from drowsiness to coma, headache, vomiting, history of convulsions (focal or generalized), meningeal signs, bulging fontanel, papilledema, cranial nerve palsy, and motor weakness of the limbs.
- *Tubercular vasculopathy*:
    - Cerebrovascular complications of TBM that occur typically as multiple or bilateral lesions in the territories of the middle cerebral artery perforating vessels manifest in the form of raised intracranial pressure (ICP) with focal neurodeficits based on territory involved.
    - Vessel pathology occurs secondary to focal vasospasms or lumina thrombosis secondary to necrotizing vasculitis and basal exudates around the vessels.
    - A family history of TB can be identified in approximately 50–60% of children, and a positive tuberculin skin test (TST) is found in approximately 30–50%.
    - In children particularly, there appears to be a close association with disseminated (miliary) TB.
- *Tuberculoma*:
    - Tuberculomas are said to develop from the "Rich focus" which consists of tubercular bacilli seeded into the meninges during primary tubercular infection.

BOX 1: Classification of CNS tuberculosis.

- *Intracranial*:
    - Tuberculous meningitis
    - Tuberculous encephalopathy
    - Tuberculous vasculopathy
    - Central nervous system tuberculoma (single or multiple)
    - Tuberculous brain abscess
- *Spinal*:
    - Pott's spine and Pott's paraplegia
    - Nonosseous spinal tuberculoma
    - Spinal meningitis

- Tuberculomas of the brain show a typical granulomatous reaction, comprising epithelioid cells and giant cells around a central area of necrosis.
- Tuberculomas are avascular, granulomatous intracranial space-occupying lesions, with diameters ranging from about 0.1 to 10 cm. They can be single or multiple and may be found anywhere in the brain parenchyma or rarely in the ventricles or along the meninges. The number of identified lesions per patient may range from 1 to 100.
- Clinically, tuberculomas often present with symptoms and signs of focal neurological deficit without evidence of systemic disease specifically focal seizures or neurodeficits depending on site of lesion.
- Tuberculomas are more common in frontal and parietal lobes, usually in parasagittal areas. Intracranial tuberculomas occur in approximately 1% of patients with active tuberculosis and 4.5-28% of cases with tubercular meningitis.
- The radiologic features are also nonspecific ring-enhancing lesions and differential diagnosis includes malignant lesions, sarcoidosis, pyogenic abscess, toxoplasmosis, and cysticercosis.

- *Tubercular abscess*:
  - Tuberculous brain abscess and subdural empyema are extremely rare manifestations of central nervous system tuberculosis account for 4% of total brain abscess of varied etiologies.
  - Most of the cases occur by hematogenous spread from extracranial locations spread of infection to the brain could occur due to active tuberculous infection elsewhere in the body; those that occur following otogenic infection involve the temporal lobe and cerebellum.
  - A tuberculous abscess is characterized by an encapsulated collection of pus-containing viable tubercular bacilli without evidence of the classic tubercular granuloma.
  - Tubercular cerebral abscesses show increased concentrations of lipids and phosphoserine.

Staging of TBM

Clinical signs of patients presenting with TBM can be easily assessed for severity based on modifications of the Medical Research Council staging system, which has been shown to have considerable prognostic value.

- Alert and oriented without focal neurological deficits. Headache and nonspecific symptoms.
- Glasgow Coma Score of 14-11 or 15 with focal neurological deficits/meningismus.
- Glasgow Coma Score of 10 or less, with or without focal neurological deficits: 10% of patients in whom the meningitis is not associated with military involvement.

COMPLICATIONS

- *Pressure of exudates*:
  - Cranial nerve palsies occur in 20-30% of patients and may be the presenting manifestation of TBM. The sixth cranial nerve is most commonly affected.
  - Vision loss due to optic nerve involvement may occasionally be a dominant presenting illness.
  - Optochiasmatic arachnoiditis, third ventricular compression of optic chiasma (if hydrocephalus develops), optic nerve granuloma are possible factors for vision loss in these patients.
  - Ophthalmoscopic examination may reveal papilledema. Fundoscopy may reveal choroid tubercles, yellow lesions with indistinct borders present either singly or in clusters.
- *Hydrocephalus*:
  - Its frequent complication in children leading to raised ICP secondary to basal exudates thereby creating communicating hydrocephalus in 80% cases.
  - Communicating hydrocephalus might be treated with diuretics and serial lumbar punctures. Non-communicating hydrocephalus is treated with ventriculoperitoneal (VP) shunt or endoscopic third ventriculostomy (ETV).
  - A systematic review of procedure in TBM concluded that clinical severity determines the outcome and HIV-1 coinfection had worse prognosis. ETV had higher risk of early recurrence, but lesser long-term complications than VP shunt. However, it is technically difficult to do ETV in acute stage with inflamed, opaque, and thick third ventricle.
  - The contrary viewpoint is that aqueductal stenosis in early-stage TBM should be managed by ETV and VP shunt should be used for chronic burnt out cases or those with communicating hydrocephalus.
  - Ambiguity in selection of one procedure over other for TBM hydrocepha-lus continues in the absence of robust evidence.
- *Occlusive vasculitis and infarction (30-40%)*: Patchy vasculitis with cerebral tissue infarction is known complication of TBM. Depending on site of infarction, the deficit will manifest in the form of cognitive deficit, motor deficit, visual deficit, and psychosocial deficits.
- *Hyponatremia*: It usually develops in initial few days, with or without AKT, which could be due to syndrome of inappropriate antidiuretic hormone secretion (SIADH) or cerebral salt wasting syndrome (CSWS), and it is difficult to differentiate between them clinically. SIADH is managed by fluid restriction while CSW is treated by fluid administration.
- *Paradoxical worsening/immune reconstitution inflammatory syndrome (IRIS)*:
  - Paradoxical enlargement or the development of new intracranial tuberculomas or abscesses in patients

with CNS or extraneural TB on appropriate treatment is well-described.
- Usually occur within the first 6 months after TB treatment initiation but may rarely be delayed for a year or more.
- Paradoxical reactions are often identified when patients present with neurological deterioration during TB treatment, prompting brain imaging. Paradoxical TB reactions are more common in HIV-infected patients (6–29%), particularly in those who commence antiretroviral therapy (ART) after starting TB treatment, in which case it is referred to as paradoxical TB-IRIS.
- The pathogenesis of paradoxical reactions (including IRIS) remains unclear but is likely related to an aberrant immune response to TB antigens rather than failure of TB treatment.
- Anti-inflammatory drugs (corticosteroids and thalidomide) are effective in the prevention and management of paradoxical TB reactions, including tuberculomas.
- *Seizures/epilepsy*:
  - Children with TBM are more likely to experience seizures relative to adults; this may be attributed to the immaturity of CNS, blood-brain barrier, and the immune system of this vulnerable group specifically under the age of 4 years.
  - Predominant seizures are acute symptomatic seizures noted on 35–75% of patients.
  - Early seizures are usually associated with meningeal irritation, cerebral edema, and raised ICP; whereas hydrocephalus, infarction, tuberculoma, and hyponatremia provoke late-onset seizures. However, the probability of getting an epilepsy after brain damage remains in 8–20% of patients with TBM.
  - Phenytoin and levetiracetam are commonly used drugs to control the seizures. Use of valproate should be limited in view of potential hepatotoxicity and drug interaction.
- *Death/permanent disability in up to 50%*: Despite treatment, childhood TBM has very poor outcomes. Poor prognosis and difficult early diagnosis emphasize the importance of preventive therapy for child contacts of patients with tuberculosis and low threshold for empirical treatment of TBM suspects.

INVESTIGATIONS

Lumbar puncture with microbiological testing and radioimaging is cornerstone of evaluation.
- *Laboratory findings*:
  - *Cerebrospinal fluid (CSF) protein elevated*: 100–500 mg/dL (may be higher in spinal block)
  - CSF moderately decreased glucose (~25–50 mg/dL)
  - *CSF pleocytosis*: 100–500/μL
  - Lymphocyte predominant, but can be mixed or neutrophilic early in presentation.
  - GeneXpert is a real-time polymerase chain reaction (PCR)-based assay for detection of *Mycobacterium tuberculosis* in clinical specimens and also detect rifampicin resistance-associated mutations. The assay is approximately 60% sensitive and nearly 100% specific. The test should be used to "rule-in" and not "rule-out" the diagnosis of TBM. GeneXpert Ultra is the second-generation assay works on detection and amplification of a multicopy gene target and is reported by the World Health Organization (WHO) to have 95% sensitivity.
  - CSF adenosine deaminase (ADA) value of 1–4 U/L have a sensitivity of >93% and specificity of <80%, while CSF ADA >8 U/L have a sensitivity of >96% and specificity of <59%. These cutoff values, however, could not consistently differentiate between TBM and bacterial meningitis. TB PCR sensitivity: ~50% (range 40–75%).
  - *AFB smear sensitivity*: ~10%.
  - *AFB culture sensitivity*: 5–50%.
- Radiographic findings in CNS TBM
  - Basal meningeal enhancement (in up to 90%)
  - Hydrocephalus (in ~66%)
  - Infarction (in >50%)
  - Ring-enhancing lesion, i.e., tuberculoma (in ~30%).

Diagnosis of primary infection: Pulmonary disease is diagnosed by doing an X-ray chest and Mantoux test.

TREATMENT

The management of TBM consists of these strategies:
- Killing the TB bacilli with antitubercular treatment (ATT)
- Managing the host immune response and supportive care
- Identifying complication and its management
- Identifying index case and its treatment
- *TB preventive therapy*: TB Prophylaxis.

Definitive Treatment

- The goal of treatment of TB is to ensure high cure rates, prevent emergence of drug resistance, minimize relapses, and cut the chain of transmission through early diagnosis and treatment.
- Treatment of TB is not only a matter of individual health; it is also a matter of public health.

Duration of Treatment

- The WHO recommends that pulmonary and extrapulmonary disease should be treated with the same regimens; however, the experts recommend 9–12 months of treatment for TB meningitis given the serious risk of disability and mortality.
- CNS TB standard treatment is extended to 12 months (2EHRZ/10HR). In cases of TBM, initial hospitalization is recommended.

- *Daily/alternate drug regime*: However, among seriously ill admitted children or those with severe disseminated disease/neurotuberculosis, the likelihood of vomiting or nontolerance of oral drugs is high in the initial phase. Such selected group of seriously ill admitted patients can be given daily supervised therapy during their stay in the hospital using daily drug dosages.
- After discharge they will be taken on thrice weekly DOT regimen (with suitable modification to thrice weekly dosages). Intermittent administration of anti-tuberculosis drugs enables supervision to be provided more efficiently and economically with no reduction in efficacy.

The RNTCP provision:
- Pediatric patient-wise boxes are available with different dosages to be used under four weight bands for children weighing 6–10 kg, 11–17 kg, 18–25 kg, and 26–30 kg.
- *ATT drugs*: Rifampicin 10–12 mg/kg (maximum 600 mg/day), isoniazid 10 mg/kg (max 300 mg/day), ethambutol 20–25 mg/kg (maximum 1,500 mg/day), pyrazinamide (PZA) 30–35 mg/kg (maximum 2,000 mg/day) streptomycin 15 mg/kg (maximum 1 g/day), and pyridoxine 1–2 mg/kg/day. Ethambutol need not be replaced by streptomycin in the intensive phase and continuation phase of the treatment is for 7 months.

Corticosteroids in TB meningitis:
- Dexamethasone 0.4 mg/kg/day split every 6 hours or prednisone 1 mg/kg/day
- Tapered over 6–8 weeks
- Less clear role in tuberculoma or spinal TBM.

Treatment of tubercular abscess: ATT is the mainstay of treatment. Surgical evacuation is advocated depending on the size of the abscess and the neurological condition of the patient. Burr hole aspiration of the abscess is usually sufficient. Craniotomy is advisable in nonhealing and multilocular abscesses.

Tuberculosis Preventive Therapy

- The currently recommended dose of isoniazid (INH) for chemoprophylaxis is 10 mg/kg (instead of earlier dosage of 5 mg/kg) administered daily for 6 months.
- TB preventive therapy should be provided to all asymptomatic contacts (under 6 years of age) of a smear-positive case, after ruling out active disease and irrespective of their Bacillus Calmette–Guérin (BCG), TST, or nutritional status.

Drug-resistant Tubercular Meningitis

- Multidrug resistant tubercular meningitis is resistant to at least isoniazid and rifampicin.
- Extensively drug resistant tubercular meningitis is resistant to isoniazid and rifampicin, as well as any fluoroquinolones and any of the three second-line injectable ATT drugs (amikacin, kanamycin, or capreomycin).
- Drug resistance could be primary (due to the transmission of drug-resistant strain in someone who was not taking ATT) or acquired (resistance developing in someone who was already taking ATT).
- The WHO guidelines for the treatment of multidrug-resistant TBM recommend that initially at least five effective drugs should be used comprising a fluoroquinolone and an injectable second-line agent and duration of treatment should be 18–24 months. It is uncertain regarding the clinical decision point of presumptive treatment failure in TBM. It may not be acceptable to wait for more than 3 months to decide on presumptive treatment failure.

CONCLUSION

- Tubercular bacilli have protean manifestations in CNS secondary to its ability to survive in a dormant state in the body for a long duration.
- It results in diverse pathologies, make its diagnosis and management a Herculean task.
- TBM is a medical emergency associated with high morbidity and mortality. However, the advent of newer microbiological test and radioimaging has helped us to diagnose it early and treat it effectively.
- Early empirical treatment with ATT should be started if clinical suspicion is high. Ensuring compliance with chosen ATT regimen and supportive therapy cannot be overemphasized. Current ATT regimens are extrapolated from PTB regimens and do not consider poor CNS penetration of drugs such as ethambutol, streptomycin, and rifampicin.
- However, constantly changing guidelines provided by the RNTCP and IAP have immensely helped us in management of these devastating disease. Also the improvement in social indicators of a country, namely, malnutrition, poverty, and low income will play an important role in the prevention and control of TB.

SUGGESTED READING

1. Central Tuberculosis Division, Government of India. (2016) Revised National TB Control Programme: Technical and operational guidelines for tuberculosis control in India 2016. [online] Available from: https://tbcindia.gov.in/index1.php?lang=1&level=2&sublinkid=4573&lid=3177. [Last accessed August, 2021].
2. Cherian A, Thomas SV. Central nervous system tuberculosis. Afr Health Sci. 2011;11(1):116-27.
3. Kumar A, Gupta D, Nagaraja SB, Singh V, Sethi GR, Prasad J, Indian Academy of Pediatric. Updated National Guidelines for Pediatric Tuberculosis in India. Indian Pediatr. 2013;50(3):301-6.
4. Tandon PN. Management of tuberculosis of the central nervous system: Our experience. Natl Med J India. 2018;31(3):151-5.
5. Vinny PW, Vishnu VY. Tuberculous meningitis: an narrative review. J Curr Res Scientific Med. 2019;5(1):13-22.

Neurocysticercosis

Anoop Verma, Arun Agrawal, Pranati Sharma

INTRODUCTION

Neurocysticercosis (NCC) is one of the most common helminthic infestations of the brain. It is considered to be the most common cause of acquired epilepsy. The clinical presentation depends on the location, number, and viability of the cysts, as well as the host response. About 60-90% of infested patients have involvement in brain. The common sites are cerebrum and cerebellum, but it may involve brainstem, basal ganglion, thalamus, and lateral sinuses.

CLASSIFICATION OF CYSTS

Cysts are classified as follows:
- Parenchymal
- Extraparenchymal, which includes ventricular, cisternal, ophthalmic, or spinal. Children usually present with solitary degenerating parenchymal cysts.

Parenchymal

Most of the cases of parenchymal involvement is seen usually after the age of 5 years. The live cysts are asymptomatic, but becomes symptomatic once the cyst start degenerating.

Clinical manifestations:
- *Seizure*: Seizure frequency is seen in 70-90% of cases of which partial seizures contributes to 84-87% cases; most of these are complex partial seizures, and about one fourth are simple partial seizures. Status epilepticus has been reported in 1.7-32% of cases.
- *Raised intracranial pressure*: Raised ICT and papilledema are relatively less in children as compared to adults.
- *Focal deficits* in the form of hemiparesis, monoparesis, and oculomotor abnormalities are common.
- *Cysticercal encephalitis* is seen rarely in children and can occur with numerous cysts. They are difficult to treat and have a progressive or recurrent course.

Extraparenchymal

It is rare in children.

Calcification: The incidence of calcification of cysticercus cyst is around 20%.

The antiparasitic therapy does not reduces the calcification rate. The calcification of the lesion is the potential cause of recurrence of seizure and refractory seizures.

DIAGNOSIS

The diagnosis of NCC is dependent upon neuroimaging since the pathological confirmation of the parasite is almost never practically possible in clinical practice.

Computed Tomography Scan

A contrast-enhanced computed tomography (CT) scan is sufficient in majority of the cases. It is cheaper and better at detecting small areas of calcifications. The cysticercal infestation of extraocular muscles can also be picked up. CT scan is also neuroimaging of choice in follow-up visits. In most cases, the lesions are single and <20 mm in size. These are called as "single small enhancing computed tomographic lesions (SSECTL)."

SSECTL Criteria

There are *clinical* and *CT criteria* for the diagnosis of SSECTL.

Clinical criteria: Clinically there should be—
- No feature of *persistent increased intracranial pressure*.
- No evidence of a *progressive neurologic deficit*.
- *No evidence of a systemic illness* such as primary malignancy, tuberculosis and/or focus of pyogenic infections.

Computed Tomography Criteria

- The lesion should be *solitary*.
- The lesion should *enhance* after contrast injection.
- The lesion should *measure <20 mm* in maximum dimension.
- Edema may or may not be present around the lesion and should not cause midline shift.

These criteria are found to have sensitivity of 99.5% and specificity of 98.9%.

TABLE 1: Different stages of parasite, presentation and neuroimaging features.

Stage of parasite	Presentation	Neuroimaging correlation
Vesicular phase (Viable)	• Parasite lies in tiny fluid-filled cyst with thin transparent outer covering • Scolex is eccentric • Asymptomatic	*NCCT*: Circumscribed, rounded hypodense, 10 mm (4–20 mm), no perilesional edema
Colloidal phase (Nonviable)	• Due to by line degeneration, the cyst is filled with gelatinous fluid • Scolex shrinks • Symptomatic	*CECT*: Annular enhancement surrounded by irregular perilesional edema
Nodular phase (Nonviable)	• Degeneration continues the cyst wall becomes nodular and necroses • Scolex gets calcified	*CECT*: Hypodense area with hyperdense rounded nodular image with perilesional edema
Calcified (Dead)	• The collagenous tissue replaces the granulation tissue • Calcification	*NCCT*: Rounded homogeneous hyperdense, no edema

(CECT: contrast-enhanced computed tomography; NCCT: noncontrast computed tomography)

TABLE 2: Neuroimaging differences between NCC and tuberculoma.

Character	NCC	Tuberculoma
Cyst size	<20 mm/single or multiple	>20 mm, often multiple
Associated meningitis	Absent	May be present
Presence in the brain	Gray–white matter junction	Posterior fossa (common)
Site of organ involvement	Eyes, muscle, or subcutaneous tissue	Spread is secondary
Presence of midline shift	Lesser	Greater
Thickness of the ring	Lesser	Greater with shaggy borders
Scolex	Present	Absent
MRI T2W image	Hyperintensity with hypointense scolex	Hyperintensity with midline shift may be present
MR spectroscopy	Multiple amino acid peak	Lipid peak

(MR: magnetic resonance; MRI T2W: magnetic resonance imaging T2 weighted; NCC: neurocysticercosis)

Magnetic Resonance Imaging Scan

- The neuroimaging correlates of various stages and presentation are depicted in **Table 1**.
- Magnetic resonance imaging (MRI) is done *when scolex is not seen* on CT scan.
- MRI is best for *intraventricular cyst/postfossa/brainstem lesion* close to skull and small cyst.
- *Perilesional edema* is much better seen on MRI.
- *MRI protocol* for evaluation of NCC should include high-resolution MR cisternography sequence such as three-dimensional (3D) constructive interference in steady state (CISS) can be instrumental, especially when scolex is not visible in routine MR sequence.
- Magnetic transfer (MT) images and magnetization transfer ratio (MTR) are advised if lesion are not visible on routine MR and to pick up perilesional gliosis. Gliotic area shows low MTR as compared to gray and white matter. Persistent perilesional gliosis surrounding the cysticercus granuloma is associated with *refractory epilepsy.*
- *Magnetic resonance spectroscopy (MRS) scan*: It is done to rule out neurotuberculosis. The presence of lipids on MRS is indicative of tuberculoma whereas low levels of metabolites together with poor signal/noise ratio could indicate NCC.

The neuroimaging features of tuberculoma and NCC has narrow differentiating features **(Table 2)**.

Serological Tests

The seropositivity of test depends on parasite load and also on genotype of *Taenia solium*. A positive test supports the diagnosis of NCC and negative test does not exclude the diagnosis. False positive may be seen in people from epidemic area.

Lentil lectin purified glycoprotein (LLGP)-based enzyme-linked immunoelectrotransfer-blot (EITB) is gold standard for

TABLE 3: Stage-wise treatment approach to neurocysticercosis (NCC).

Stage of NCC	Type of therapy	Recommendation
Viable cysts (vesicular phase)	Antiparasitic therapy	Causes more rapid radiological resolution
1–2 viable cysts (vesicular phase)	Monotherapy with albendazole—15 mg/kg/day, in two divided doses × 10 days	Use monotherapy
>2 viable cysts (vesicular phase)	• Albendazole (as above) + praziquantel 15 mg/kg/day in three daily doses × 10 days • Anti-inflammatory therapy (corticosteroid/decadron) • Antiepileptic therapy	• Combination therapy causes better radiological resolution • Combination of steroid has better seizure control and less side effect • Effective in controlling seizure
Single small enhancing computed tomographic lesions (SSECTL)	• Antiparasitic therapy—albendazole 15 mg/kg/day × 1–2 weeks • Anti-inflammatory therapy—corticosteroid • Antiepileptic drug (AED) monotherapy in all patient	• Short-duration therapy is equally effective than longer in seizure control • Prevent worsening of symptoms due to albendazole therapy • *Can be stopped if no risk factors such as*: Calcification on CT, breakthrough seizure, >2 seizures during the course of disease
Calcified lesion with or without perilesional edema	• Antiparasitic therapy is not recommended. • AED is required • Anti-inflammatory drugs are not recommended	• Since there is no parasite, no cysticidal drug is required • Management guideline similar to other patient with remote symptomatic seizure • Few reports revealed reappearance of perilesional edema after stopping or tapering corticosteroids

serodiagnostic of NCC. The American Academy of Pediatrics (AAP) recommends serologic testing with enzyme-linked immunotransfer blot as a confirmatory test in patients with suspected NCC. It has been reported to be highly specific and nearly 100% sensitive for patients with either multiple active parenchymal cysts or extraparenchymal NCC. For solitary cystic granuloma and calcified lesions EITB has been reported to be positive in 30–70%. Low molecular mass excretory secretary (ES) antigen-based EITB have high sensitivity around 85% and specificity 64% for detection of cysticercus antibody.

Other routine tests are not generally indicated and can be individualized. Garcia et al. proposed a diagnostic criterion for the diagnosis of NCC based upon clinical, radiological, immunological, and epidemiological data but has limited role in routine clinical practice.

TREATMENT

The treatment is discussed under following heads (Table 3):
- Antiepileptic drug (AED) therapy
- Cysticidal drug therapy
- Corticosteroids
- Endoscopy removal.

Antiepileptic Drugs

- Seizures secondary to NCC must be treated as any other symptomatic epilepsy. As most children have partial seizures, carbamazepine should be used as a first choice of AED. Phenytoin and levetiracetam can also be used.
- The seizures seen in active phase of cysticercus are acute symptomatic seizure and should be treated with AEDs for two reasons: (1) *Seizures are likely to recur as long as lesion persists* and (2) *time period for the resolution of CT lesion is quite variable.*
- The seizure which is due to dead parasite and calcified lesions is called as *remote symptomatic epilepsy* and should be considered as unprovoked seizures and should be treated for 2 years seizure-free period.

Recurrence of seizures:
- Recurrence of seizures are seen in 15% of patient with most recurrences is seen since the first 3 months of withdrawal of AED.
- *Risk factor for recurrences are*:
  - More than two seizures during the disease
  - Breakthrough seizures
  - Calcification of the lesion.
- Patient with any of the risk factors are advised to continue AED for at least 2.5 years.

Cysticidal Drugs

Cysticidal drugs **(Table 4)** are required mainly to destroy the live cyst, on the assumption that once the cyst becomes inactive they will cause fewer seizures and other symptoms. Evidence suggests that these drugs hasten the resolution of live parenchymal brain cyst; however, a similar benefit is obtained in the treatment of degenerating cyst is not clear. Recent meta-analysis data revealed that *cysticidal drugs are associated with increase rate of both seizure control and*

TABLE 4: Cysticidal drugs.

Albendazole	Praziquantel
Less expensive	Expensive
Fewer side effect	More
• Better penetration in subarachnoid • Space	Less
Bioavailability of AED (CBZ/PHT) is maintained, with concomitant corticosteroids bioavailability increases	Plasma level decreases with concomitant corticosteroid and AED administration
• *Dose*: 15 mg/kg/day (2–3 divided doses) • *Duration*: 28 days • *Therapy*: Multiple lesions 14–18 days • *Therapy*: Single lesion	• *Dose*: 50 mg/kg/day (single lesion) × 15 days • *Duration*: 15 mg/kg/day × 10 days therapy with • Albendazole-with multiple lesion • 15 days therapy for single lesion

(AED: antiepileptic drug; CBZ: carbamazepine; PHT: phenytoin)

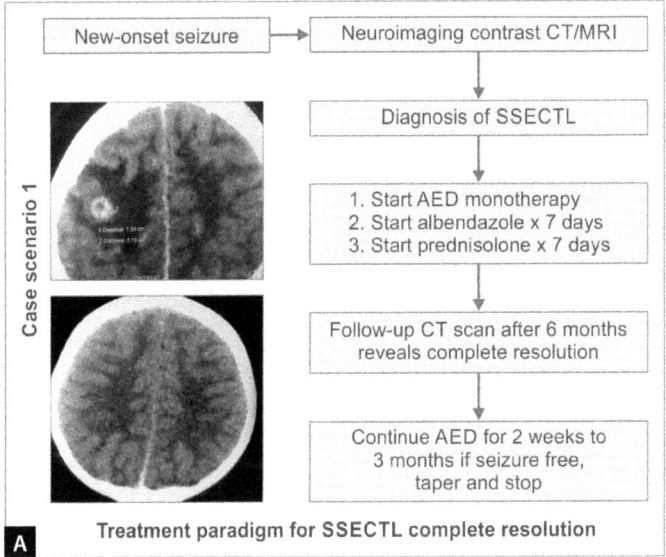

Fig. 1A: Case scenarios depicting various type and stages of presentation of NCC with its treatment paradigm. (A) Case scenario 1: Treatment paradigm for SSECTL (complete resolution).

(AED: antiepileptic drug; CT: computed tomography; MRI: magnetic resonance imaging; SSECTL: single small enhancing computed tomographic lesions)

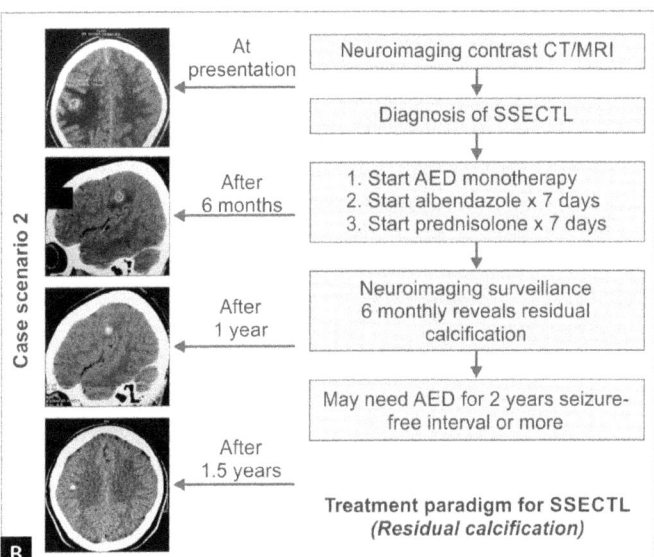

Fig. 1B: Case scenarios depicting various type and stages of presentation of NCC with its treatment paradigm. (B) Case scenario 2: Treatment paradigm for SSECTL (residual calcification).

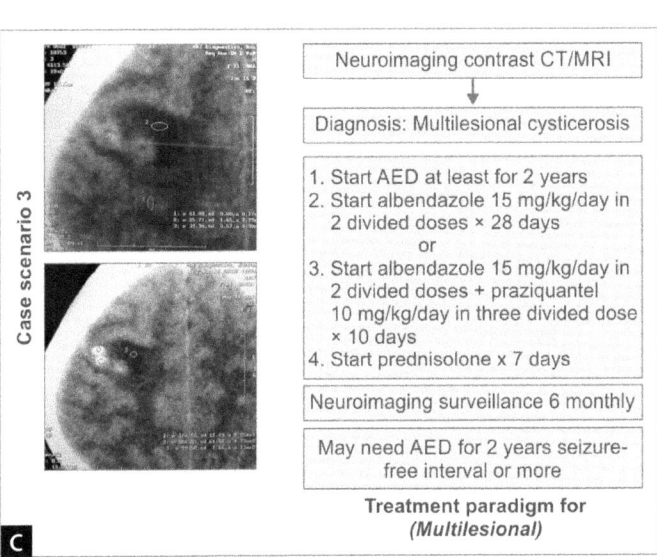

Fig. 1C: Case scenarios depicting various type and stages of presentation of NCC with its treatment paradigm. (C) Case scenario 3: Treatment paradigm for SSECTL (multilesional).

faster resolution in single lesion. The *American Academy of Neurology Guidelines* recommend the use of albendazole and corticosteroid for adult/children with parenchymal NCC, both *to reduce the number of active lesion on neuroimaging and to reduce long-term seizure frequency.*

Combination Therapy

In a recent randomized controlled trial (RCT), *albendazole* 15 mg/kg/day + *praziquantel* 15 mg/kg/day for 10 days was found to be superior to albendazole alone in clearing the cyst from brain. The cyst resolution at 6 months after treatment was noted in 64% of the patients in combined therapy group versus 39% in the standard albendazole therapy. *The combined therapy seems to be a good* option in patient with multilesional NCC.

Corticosteroids

A short course of steroids is commonly used to combat host inflammatory response. Oral prednisolone: 1–2 mg/kg/day must be given 2 days prior to starting the cysticidal drugs and continue for 7 days after initiation of the therapy.

The overall treatment plan of various presentation of neurocystecercosis is given in **Figures 1 A to C**.

PATIENT SURVEILLANCE

Intermittent surveillance is done with imaging until cyst(s) resolve(s), perhaps every 6 months if patient is improving or earlier if patient remains symptomatic. Reimaging of brain should be 2 months after the completion of treatment.

PROGNOSIS

- For single lesion, the prognosis is good.
- The lesion disappears in 6 month in >60% cases and the seizure are well controlled.
- The recurrence of single lesion is around 10–20%.
- The chances of frequent relapses depend on various risk factors.
- Poor prognosis in cysticidal encephalitis

SUGGESTED READING

1. Amudhan S, Gururaj G, Satishchandra P. Epilepsy in India I: Epidemiology and public health. Ann Indian Acad Neurol. 2015; 18(3):286-9.
2. Atluri SR, Singhi P, Khandelwal N, Malla N. Evaluation of Excretory-Secretary and 10-30 kDa antigens of Taenia solium cysticerci by EITB assay for the diagnosis of neurocysticercosis. Parasite Immunol. 2009;31:151-5.
3. Garcia HH. Neurocysticercosis. In: Shorvon SD, Andermann F, Guerrini R (eds). The Causes of Epilepsy. Cambridge: Cambridge University Press; 2011. pp. 495-500.
4. Rodriguez S, Wilkins P, Dorny P. Immunological and molecular diagnosis of cysticercosis. Pathog Glog Health. 2012;106:286-98.

CHAPTER 109: Headache in Children

Anoop Verma

INTRODUCTION

Headache is nonspecific, but is common a symptom causing pain and discomfort in the head and facial structures. It is seen in children of around 3 years of age (3–8%), by 5 years of age (19.5%), at 7 years of age (31–51.5%) and by 7–15 years (26–82%). Brain parenchyma is insensitive to pain whereas dura, large blood vessels, and sinuses are pain-sensitive structures in the cranium and are responsible for primary headache. The extracranial structure which can cause headache is called as secondary headache and have identified etiology. The structures which can give rise to secondary headaches are periosteum, oropharynx, orbit, sinuses, middle ear, teeth, face, neck, and muscle.

PATTERN OF HEADACHE

- *Acute headache* is any single episode of headache without any past history of headache. Common causes are upper respiratory infection (URI) and meningitis but rarely, hypertension, intracranial hemorrhage, or first episode of migraine can also contribute.
- *Acute recurrent headache* are acute episodic stereotyped headache separated from headache-free interval, e.g., migraine.
- *Chronic progressive headache*: There is progressive increase in severity and frequency of headache and is most ominous, seen in various serious conditions, e.g., expanding mass lesion-like brain tumor, abscess, tuberculous, neurocysticercosis, chronic meningitis, subdural hematoma, aneurysm, and others.
- *Chronic nonprogressive headache*: Constant headache occurring frequently without alteration in severity, e.g., chronic tension-type headache, trigeminal neuralgia, sinusitis, dental conditions, benign intracranial hypertension, and chronic posttraumatic headache.
- *Mixed headache*: Appearance of acute recurrent headache like migraine in a patient with preexisting chronic headache.

EVALUATION

Detailed history and examination help in reaching and analyzing the type of headache.

Family History

Patients with secondary headache disorders typically do not possess a family history. Tension-type and cluster headaches may have only minor genetic influences. A family history of headache is very important in migraine; about 50% of patients have a first-degree relative with migraine; some literature support 90% with family history of headache.

MIGRAINE

It is a hereditary disorder with a multifactorial inheritance pattern. *Migraine* is an important primary headache which is intermittent occurring weekly to monthly with asymptomatic interval in between episodes. It is typically unilateral lasting for the duration of 4–72 hours; in children, it may be bifrontal and lasting to <30 minutes.

Children may not able to describe the headache, asking them to draw may help in identifying the aura and pattern. FACES visual scale may help in grading intensity. Prodrome such as mood changes, lethargy, yawning, or pallor may be seen. Migraine headache may be associated with vomiting, sweating, photophobia, photophobia, and flushing.

Headache may be aggravated by sound, light, and smell. Headache is aggravated by bending forward in migraine, whereas headache worsening on lying down is seen in increased intracranial pressure (ICP), and headache worsening on sitting or standing is seen in low ICP.

Classification of migraine with aura (**Table 1**):
- Migraine with aura
- Migraine with brainstem aura
- Hemiplegic migraine [Familial hemiplegic migraine (FHM)]
- Retinal migraine.

TABLE 1: Migraine diagnostic criteria.	
Migraine without aura	**Migraine with aura**

A. At least 5 attacks fulfilling criteria B–D
B. Headache attacks lasting 4–72 hours (untreated or unsuccessfully treated)
C. *Headache has >2 of the following characteristics*:
  1. Unilateral location
  2. Pulsating quality
  3. Moderate or severe pain intensity
  4. Aggravation by or causing avoidance of routine physical activity (e.g., walking, climbing stairs)
D. *During headache >1 of the following*:
  1. Nausea and/or vomiting
  2. Photophobia and phonophobia
E. Not attributed to another disorder
	A. At least two attacks fulfilling criteria B and C
	B. One or more of the following fully reversible aura symptoms:
	  1. Visual
	  2. Sensory
	  3. Speech and/or language motor
	  5. Brainstem
	  6. Retinal
	C. *At least two of the following four characteristics*:
	  1. At least one aura symptom spreads gradually over 5 minutes, and/or two or more symptoms occur in succession
	  2. Each individual aura symptom may lasts for 5–60 minutes
	  3. At least one aura symptoms is unilaterals
	  4. The aura is accompanied, or followed within 60 minutes, by headache

Chronic migraine: Headache persisting for >15 days/month for >3 months. The headache should have a feature of migraine for at least 8 days/month.

Status migrainosus: Severe debilitating migraine attack persisting for >3 days.

Red flags for secondary headache:
- Abnormal neurology first severe headache
- Presentation of atypical features such as vertigo, intractable vomiting
- Headache sufficient to arouse the child from sleep
- Change in headache pattern
- Occipital headache
- Onset subacute bit with progressive severity
- Immunosuppressed child with fresh-onset headache
- Trauma history in recent past
- Detected to have ventriculoperitoneal shunt
- Age < 5 years.

The presence of one or more red flags is the indication for neuroimaging and to fetch neurologist's opinion.

INVESTIGATIONS

- *Blood count*: Complete blood count (CBC), C-reactive protein (CRP), and blood culture may require to rule out infections as the cause of headache, especially considering secondary causes.
- *X-ray sinuses* to rule out sinusitis contributing to headache.
- *Neuroimaging*: Magnetic resonance imaging (MRI) is preferred in nonemergency situation, whereas contrast computed tomography (CT) is imaging of choice in emergency situation. The sensitivity and specificity of MRI are better as compared to CT, for detecting posterior fossa lesion, meningitis, and vascular malformation.

Indications of neuroimaging in children with headache:
- Abnormal neurological signs
- School failure, behavioral change, fall off in linear growth rate recently
- Early morning headache, headache awakens child from sleep
- Focal seizure with headache
- Presence of migraine and seizure occurring in the same episode with vascular symptom precedes the seizure [tumor or arteriovenous (A-V) malformation]
- Focal neurological sign develops during aura with fixed laterality
- Cough headache in a child or adolescent
- *Cerebrospinal fluid (CSF)*: Analysis is indicated in suspected meningitis. CT scan is important before doing lumbar puncture (LP) in the presence of focal features, and raised intracranial pressure.

MANAGEMENT

Headache is a common condition seen in practice. Any patient coming with complaints of headache try to classify which type and pattern of headache we are dealing. Give importance to red flag sign. Rule out presence of any life-threatening conditions.

Secondary Headache

It is utmost important to detect the cause of headache and to treat accordingly. Analgesics in the form of paracetamol and ibuprofen should be used as per **Table 2**.

Primary Headache

Around 25% of children with migraine are free of headache by 25 years of age; boys in a significantly higher percentage than girls and more than half will still have headaches at the age of 50 years.

- *Acute symptomatic treatment*: Mild-to-moderate pain: *Acetaminophen* (15 mg/kg/dose) or Ibuprofen (10 mg/kg/dose)—4-6 hours, total of not more than four doses in 24 hours.

TABLE 2: Drugs used for abortive treatment of migraine.

Medications	Dosages
Simple analgesics	
Acetaminophen	15 mg/kg PO, 4–6 hours
Ibuprofen	10 mg/kg PO 6 hours
Ketorolac	0.5 mg/kg IV (maximum 15 mg/dose)
Dopamine antagonist	
Prochlorperazine	0.15 mg/kg IV (maximum 10 mg/kg/dose)
Metoclopramide	0.1 mg/kg IV (maximum 10 mg/dose)
5HT receptor agonist	
Sumatriptan	5–20 mg IV, 50–100 mg PO, 3–6 mg SC
Almotriptan	6.25 or 12.5 mg PO for ages 12–17 years
Rizatriptan MLT	5 mg PO 6–12 years, 10 mg 12–17 years maximum 30 mg/day
Zolmitriptan	2.5 mg PO for age 12–17 years
Treximet- Sumatriptan + Naproxen	*For age 12–17 years*: 10 mg/ 60 mg PO 85 mg/500 mg PO (maximum dose)

(PO: per oral; IV: intravenous)
Source: Sheridan D, Spiro D, Meckler G. Pediatric migraine: Abortive management in the emergency department. Headache. 2014; 54(2):235-45.

TABLE 3: Drugs for migraine prophylaxis.

Agent	Dose	Side effects
Beta blockers Propranolol	1–3 mg/kg/day	Wheezing, avoids in asthma, cardiac arrhythmia, orthostatic hypotension
Antihistaminic drug Peritol	2–8 mg/day	Increased appetite, weight gain
Tricyclic antidepressant Amitriptyline	1 mg/kg/day	Weight gain, conduction defect, sedation
Antiepileptic drug: • Topiramate • Valproic acid • Divalproate • Levetiracetam	• 2–3 mg/kg/day • 15–40 mg/kg/day • 250–500 mg/day • 250–500 mg/day	Anorexia, weight loss, renal stone, mood changes, weight gain, alopecia, teratogenic effect, hepatic toxicity ovarian cyst
Calcium channel blockers Flunarizine	5–10 mg/kg/day	Weight gain

Source: Freitag FG, Schloemer F, Schumate D. Recent developments in the treatment of migraine in children and adolescents. J Headache Pain Manag. 2016;1:9.

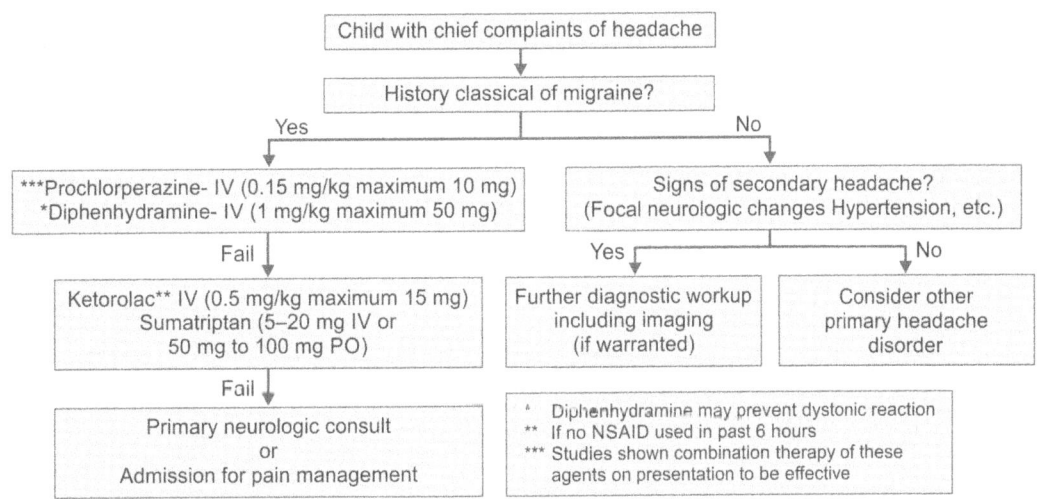

Flowchart 1: Approach to headache.

(NSAID: nonsteroidal anti-inflammatory drug; PO: per oral; IV: intravenous)
Source: Adapted from Sheridan D, Spiro D, Meckler G. Pediatric migraine: Abortive management in the emergency department. Headache. 2014;54(2):235-45.

- *Severe pain*: Sumatriptan tablet (25-50 mg), or nasal spray (5-11 years: 5-10 mg; >12 years: 20 mg) either alone or in combination with naproxen (5-7 mg/kg given 8-12 hours PO).

Promethazine (0.25-0.5 mg/kg PO) if associated with vomiting. It is important to note that the use of these drugs should be limited. For NSAID, no more than 2-3 days/week or less than 15 days/month, and for triptans less than 10 days/month.

- *Lifestyle modification*:
  (SMART):
  - *Sleep*: Regular and adequate sleep
  - *Meals*: Should be adequate and regular including breakfast and water
  - *Activity*: Regular exercise
  - *Relaxation*: Relaxation technique
  - *Trigger avoidance*: Avoiding known triggers

- *Prophylactic medication*: It is indicated if the patient experiences headache for >4 days/month and headache is severe disabling. The goal of treatment is to reduce frequency of headache to <1-2 per month and reducing the disability. The basic principle of prophylactic medication is to start low dose and titrate accordingly, to be continued to 3-6 months and then taper (*see* **Table 3**)
- *Other drugs such as riboflavin*: 25-400 mg/day.

Elemental magnesium: In adolescent, in dose of 350-500 mg/day.

Calcitonin gene-related peptide (CGRP) receptor antagonist (3) BIBN 4096 BS is a 37-amino acid neuropeptide which is potent vasodilator present in perivascular trigeminal nerve fibers that supply the pial arteries, the meningeal arteries and the extracranial cephalic arteries. BIBN4096 BS might be effective in acute migraine treatment.

CONCLUSION

Headache in children is a common problem and >95% headaches are primary in nature. Migraine is more common than other headaches. Do not afford to miss the causes of secondary headaches. Approach to prevention of attacks is to be emphasized. Try to follow a systemic approach as described in **Flowchart 1**. Maintaining headache diary and lifestyle modification are important.

SUGGESTED READING

1. Freitag FG, Schloemer F, Schumate D. Recent developments in the treatment of migraine in children and adolescents. J Headache Pain Manag. 2016;1:9.
2. Headache Classification Committee of the International Headache Society. The International Classification of Headache Disorders, 3rd edition (beta). Cephalgia. 2013;33(9):629-808.
3. Olesen J, Diener HC. Calcitonin gene-related peptide receptor antagonist BIBN 4096 BS for the acute treatment of migraine. New Engl J Med. 2004;350:1104-10.
4. Sheridan D, Spiro D, Meckler G. Pediatric migraine: abortive management in the emergency department. Headache. 2014;54(2):235-45.

CHAPTER 110: Acute Rheumatic Chorea

Anoop Verma, Onkar Khandwal

INTRODUCTION

Sydenham's chorea (SC) is the neurologic manifestation and the most prevalent autoimmune form of chorea in children. SC is a benign and self-limiting condition, lasts for 6 months but usually has a relapsing course for up to 2 years. At worst it may transform to chronic movement disorder.

The *mild features* include difficulty with grooming and feeding. The distortion in handwriting can interfere with daily activities in school or work. The neurological symptoms are motor impersistence, hypometric saccades, hypotonia, tics, clumsiness, dysarthria, and weakness. The *neuropsychiatric* manifestations such as obsessive-compulsive disorder (OCD), personality changes, emotional lability, distractibility, irritability, anxiety, and anorexia are common and may precede the appearance of chorea. *Cardiac presentation* is in the form of mitral valve involvement in about two-thirds and arthritis in about one-third of SC patients.

LABORATORY INVESTIGATIONS

There is no specific laboratory investigation to provide the definite diagnosis of chorea since it is remote manifestation. All patients with chorea need a detailed neurologic and cardiac evaluation as the causes of chorea are many. Test should include complete blood count (CBC), liver function test (LFT), B_{12}, thyroid-stimulating hormone (TSH), and complete metabolic panel (CMP), drug screen, if possible. Anti-DNAse-B titers remain elevated to 1 year after group A streptococcal pharyngitis. Acute phase reactants such as C-reactive protein (CRP), erythrocyte sedimentation rate (ESR), rheumatoid factor, and antistreptolysin O (ASO) titer may not be useful. Echocardiogram is important because 80% of patients with SC have a concurrent cardiac disease.

Brain magnetic resonance imaging (MRI) and computed tomography (CT) scans typically are normal, but there may be reversible hyperintensity in the basal ganglia. In children, obtaining positron emission tomography (PET) scans and single-photon emission computed tomography (SPECT) imaging have demonstrated hypermetabolism and hyperperfusion of the basal ganglia in some case reports, in contrast, to other causes of chorea, which may reveal hypometabolism.

TREATMENT

Treatment consists of four main domain: (1) Elimination of the *Streptococcus*, (2) symptomatic treatment of the involuntary movements, (3) incoordination and psychiatric symptoms, and (4) treatment of the immune and inflammatory response and supportive measures.

Elimination of *Streptococcus*

The treatment to eliminate *Streptococcus* from the throat needs treatment of strep throat and long-term secondary prophylaxis. Secondary prophylaxis with long-term penicillin is primarily given to protect the heart; whether it prevents relapses of SC is still to be proved. Physical activity should be restricted until the acute phase reactants are normalized and then restarted gradually. Adverse outcomes and a chronic relapsing course are more common in children who did not receive 10 days of penicillin, hospitalization, and bed rest **(Table 1)**.

Symptomatic Treatment of Involuntary Movement

The list of drugs for symptomatic therapies is broad and includes drugs like *anticonvulsants* (valproate, carbamazepine) and *dopamine receptor antagonists* (pimozide, haloperidol, and risperidone).

- *Haloperidol* is an effective symptomatic medication "start low and go slow", in a dose of 0.025 mg/kg/day in divided doses going up to a maximum of 0.05 mg/kg/day.
- *Sodium valproate*—20 mg/kg/day in 2 or 3 divided doses, for 12 weeks. It is recommended as the first-line agent in the treatment of SC, especially in severe cases of SC where trials with haloperidol and diazepam have failed.
- *Carbamazepine*—15–20 mg/kg can be used in SC.
- *Risperidone*: In severe chorea (e.g., *chorea paralytica*, in which there is severe hypotonic and the patients are

TABLE 1: Treatment to eliminate Streptococcus.

Drug	Doses	Sore throat treatment	Secondary prophylaxis
Benzathine penicillin, deep IM	1.2 million unit (>27 kg), AST	Single dose	Every 21 day
	0.6 million unit (<27 kg), AST	Single dose	Every 21 day
Penicillin V oral	Children 250 mg QID	10 day	–
Azithromycin oral	12.5 mg/kg/day once	5 day	Not recommended
Cephalexin	15–20 mg/kg/day BD	10 day	Not recommended
Erythromycin	20 mg/kg/dose maximum 500 mg	Not recommended	Twice a day

Note: Patients with no carditis may stop prophylaxis after 5 years or age 18 (whichever is longer), those with mild carditis should continue for 10 years or age 21, and those with moderate to severe carditis should receive lifelong prophylaxis.

bedridden), it acts as a dopamine D2 receptor blocker drug. The doses for *patient <20 kg, the initial dose is* 0.25 mg/day, may increase the dose to 0.5 mg/day, and may further increase by 0.25 mg/day at 2 week intervals. For patient >20 kg, *the initial dose is* 0.5 mg/day, may increase the dose to 1 mg/day after first 4 days of therapy, and may further increase by 0.5 mg/day at 2 week intervals.

Tips:
- Valproate or haloperidol should be considered first, switch to other if no improvement after 2-4 weeks.
- Treatment should be given for *8-12* weeks before considering tapering if child is asymptomatic, but may need to be given longer (*6-9 months*).

Immunological Treatments

Prednisone (2 mg/kg/day) orally for 3-4 weeks with prolonged taper and *methylprednisolone* (25 mg/kg/day) with a prolonged taper are the two most acceptable regimens. Steroids shorten the course of the illness and prevent the complications. Intravenous immunoglobulin (IVIg) and plasmapheresis use has theoretical basis. Plasma exchange acts by removing the antineuronal antibodies. IVIg acts by inactivation of the antineuronal antibodies, the dose of IVIg is 400 mg/kg/day for 5 days.

Supportive Measures

Management of comorbid psychopathologies and supportive psychotherapy and family therapy is recommended. Educational interventions are often needed.

SUGGESTED READING

1. Dean SL, Singer HS. Treatment of Sydenham's Chorea: A Review of the Current Evidence. Tremor Other Hyperkinet Mov (N Y). 2017;7:456.
2. WHO. Rheumatic fever and rheumatic heart disease: report of a WHO expert consultation. WHO Technical Report Series. Geneva: WHO; 2001. p. 923.

CHAPTER 111

Neuro-Wilson's Disease

Vineet Wankhede

INTRODUCTION

Wilson's disease (WD) is an autosomal recessive genetic disorder due to a mutation of the *ATP7B* gene resulting in impaired hepatic copper excretion and copper accumulation.

CLINICAL FEATURES

Classic triad of cirrhosis, neurological manifestations, and Kayser-Fleischer rings constitute the clinical triad of Wilsons. However, it is a multisystemic disease manifest due to excess deposition of copper in different tissues depicted as:

- *Hepatic (50%)*: Asymptomatic hepatomegaly, persistently elevated transaminases, acute hepatitis, chronic hepatitis, cirrhosis (compensated and decompensated), acute liver failure, acute on chronic liver failure, fatty liver, isolated splenomegaly, and cholelithiasis.
- *Neuropsychiatric (40%)*: Neurological: Extrapyramidal syndromes: (A) An akinetic-rigid syndrome similar to Parkinson's disease, (B) Pseudosclerosis dominated by tremor, (C) Ataxia, and (D) A dystonic syndrome. Psychiatric syndromes: Organic dementia, psychosis, psychoneurosis, and behavioral disturbances, deteriorating school performance.
- *Osteomuscular (rare)*: Osteoporosis (24–88%), osteomalacia (14–35%), spontaneous fractures (9–35%), rickets, osteochondritis dissecans, chondromalacia patellae, premature osteopenia, and degenerative arthritis of knees and wrists mostly reported after second decade of life.
- *Hematological*: Coagulopathy Coombs-negative hemolytic anemia thrombocytopenia with or without hemolysis.
- *Ocular*: Kayser-Fleischer (KF) rings, copper accumulates in the Descemet's membrane of the cornea forming the KF ring, which is greenish-brown in color. They are always bilateral and are seen in 50–60% of hepatic and 95–100% cases of neurological WD **(Figs. 1A and B)**. A slit-lamp examination is necessary for confirmation. They appear sequentially at the (Upper > Lower > Medial > Lateral) segment of limbus and on chelation therapy disappear in the reverse direction. Sunflower cataracts are rare.
- *Renal*: Renal stones, renal tubular acidosis, Fanconi syndrome tubular injury (copper deposition in epithelium of proximal and distal convoluted tubules) occurs from WD (8%) but glomerular injury (10%) is

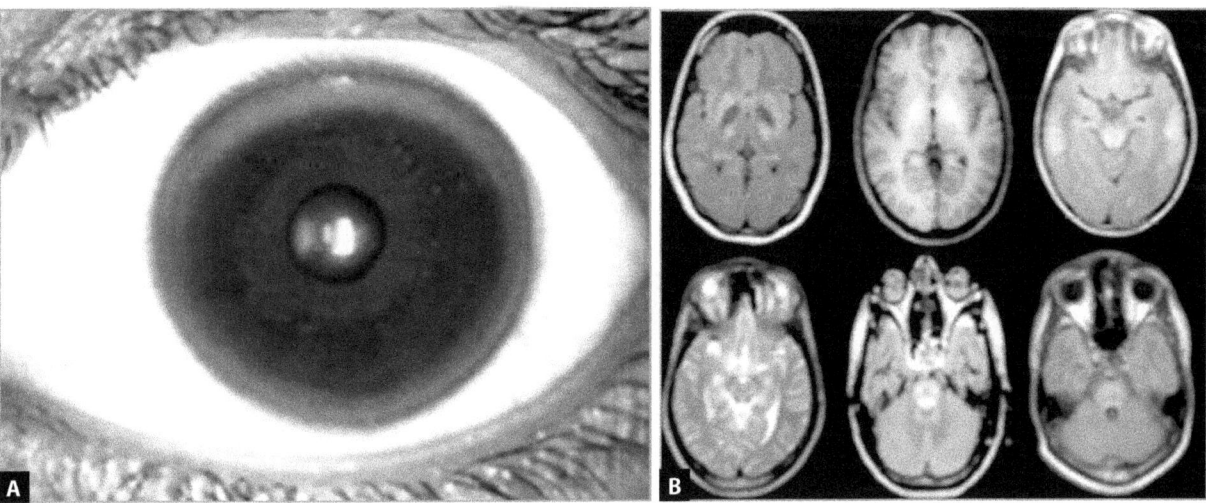

Figs. 1A and B: (A) Kayser Fleischer ring on slit lamp; (B) MRI changes in Wilson. Hyperintensities in basal ganglia/giant panda sign.

usually a complication of chelation therapy. Tubular injury manifests as nephrocalcinosis (microscopic hematuria) and nephrolithiasis (renal colic).

DIAGNOSIS

Diagnosis requires good history, physical examination including slit-lamp examination of KF ring, serum ceruloplasmin, liver function tests, and 24-hour urinary copper.

- *Serum ceruloplasmin*: Two types of assay are available to measure.
  1. Enzymatic assays is superior method than antibody-dependent immunologic assays radioimmunoassay, radial immunodiffusion, or nephelometry.
  2. Normal values range from 20 to 40 mg/dL. Values <10 mg/dL strongly favor the diagnosis of WD. Values between 10 and 20 mg/dL may be seen in both patients and carriers.
- *Twenty-four-hour urinary copper assay*:
  - This is a sensitive test that indirectly reflects the serum-free copper level.
  - Urine sample must be collected in a copper-free container and the test should be done before chelators are started.
  - *Positive test*: A level >100 µg/24-hour is considered virtually diagnostic, but recent studies have shown that lowering the cutoff levels to 40 µg/24-hour for asymptomatic patients increases the sensitivity.
  - D-penicillamine (DP) challenge test (repeat 24-hour sample of urine is collected while the patient is given two 500 mg doses of DP 12 hours apart is not recommended now in view of the high false-positive results).
- *Kayser-Fleischer rings*: KF ring should be sought in all patients suspected to have WD. This test may be negative in asymptomatic siblings or children <10 years of age. These are best seen on conventional slit-lamp examination.
- *Liver copper estimation*: Described as gold-standard test for WD, it is not easily available and may be fraught with logistic and quality issues.
  Biopsy specimens need to be sent in a dry condition in a copper-free container for atomic absorption analysis, although paraffin-embedded specimens can also be analyzed for copper. The normal copper content in liver tissue is <50 µg/g of dry weight, while a level >250 µg/g is commonly encountered even in asymptomatic WD individuals.
- *Genetic test*: WD is associated with over 600 mutations in *ATP7B* gene on chromosome 13. Exon sequencing of *ATP7B* gene is needed to confirm the diagnosis. This will help to pick up same mutations in his/her presymptomatic siblings to differentiate heterozygote carriers.

Ancillary Test

Serum copper: Total serum copper does not reflect tissue levels and therefore unreliable in diagnosis.

Coombs-negative hemolytic anemia: Hemolysis on peripheral smear and a negative Coombs test in a patient with acute liver failure (ALF) makes the diagnosis of WD highly likely.

Liver biopsy: Histopathology reveals steatohepatitis, interface hepatitis, chronic hepatitis with Mallory's hyaline, bridging fibrosis, and cirrhosis, which are nonspecific.

Magnetic resonance imaging brain: Face of giant panda (14.3%), tectal plate hyperintensity (75%), central pontine myelinolysis–like abnormalities (62.5%), and concurrent signal changes in basal ganglia, thalamus, and brainstem (55.3%). These features when present are virtually pathognomonic of WD.

Family Screening

Family screening of first-degree relatives of WD has multiple advantages:

- It allows early detection of disease in presymptomatic phase before a devastating course.
- It makes the family wiser and the physician more prepared.
- It identifies a healthy family member or a heterozygote carrier who can be a potential donor for living-related liver transplantation (LT).

MANAGEMENT

Treatment Phases

- *Initial phase*: This phase aims to reduce the body copper levels to subtoxic threshold. The choice is between chelators (DP or trientine) alone, zinc alone, or a combination of both.
- *Maintenance therapy*: This is a lifelong therapy and prevents copper reaccumulation after the patient has been effectively decoppered. Zinc, in view of its good efficacy, low cost, and toxicity, is the drug of choice. DP in low dose is an alternative but patients should be monitored for side effects.
- *Presymptomatic patients*: An asymptomatic sibling diagnosed to have WD by biochemical or genetic testing should be treated to prevent symptomatic disease. Zinc is the drug of choice. Because of the risk of body copper depletion, it should probably not be started in the first year and could be started at the age of 2 years.

Drugs for Chelation

D-penicillamine

- It is principle chelator used of which every gram promotes urinary excretion of 200 mg of copper. It also induces

hepatic metallothionein, a cytosolic metal-binding protein that sequesters copper, and renders it nontoxic.
- Within an year, clinical and biochemical improvement usually occurs but synthetic functions of liver may take up to 10 years to normalize.
- Despite the serious adverse effects reported in 10–30% of patients on DP therapy, DP is still the primary drug for management of hepatic WD in view of its time-tested efficacy, easy availability, and reasonable cost.
- The dose of DP is 20 mg/kg/day in children, in 2–3 divided doses on an empty stomach. Food reduces its absorption by 50%, and so, food should not be given 1 hour before and 2 hour after the drug.
- Pyridoxine deficiency can occur with therapy because of the inhibit ion of pyridoxine kinase enzyme. Hence, vitamin B_6 should be supplemented at a dose of 20–40 mg in children.
- Treatment with DP results in massive and rapid cupriuresis (>1,000 μg/day) in the initial months of therapy, falling to 200–500 μg/day during the maintenance period.

Trientine
- Trientine (triethylenetetramine-2-hydrochloride) is a chelator with a mechanism of action similar to DP, with fewer adverse reactions.
- The dosage is 20 mg/kg/day for children to be used in selective patients because it is expensive, heat sensitive, and has to be stored in tightly closed containers between 2 and 8°C and can lead to iron deficiency.
- Trientine can also cause paradoxical worsening in neurological WD. Hence, it should be started in low doses and increased slowly similar to DP.

Zinc
- Zinc acts by inducing metallothionein in enterocytes which preferentially binds absorbed Cu, sequesters it in the enterocytes, and prevents its entry into the portal circulation and also induces metallothionein in hepatocytes and protects against Cu toxicity.
- Unlike DP and trientine, Zn acts by increasing the fecal excretion of Cu.
- Zn has a slow action and takes much longer to achieve a negative Cu balance as compared with chelation therapy and hence may be less effective as first-line therapy in symptomatic liver disease.
- Children and those under 50 kg are given only 75 mg/day. Zinc should be taken on empty stomach to ensure better absorption.
- Besides clinical and biochemical improvement, treatment efficacy is determined by a 24-h urinary copper excretion <100 μg.
- Urinary excretion of zinc should be >2,000 μg/day to ensure compliance and also to determine the quality of the zinc preparation used.
- Zinc is used as a first-line drug in presymptomatic patients or symptomatic patients with neurological WD and for long-term maintenance therapy in others after optimal decoppering with chelators owing to its lesser cost and side effect profile.

Ammonium Tetrathiomolybdate
- If ammonium tetrathiomolybdate (TTM) is taken after meals, it binds to the copper in the food, thus preventing its absorption. If taken on empty stomach, it is absorbed into the blood and forms a complex with circulating copper preventing cellular uptake, leading to its excretion in urine.
- The dosage used is 20 mg 3 times a day with meals and 20 mg 3 times a day in between the meals. Owing to its aggressive chelating effects, the reported side effects of ammonium TTM includes paradoxical worsening, bone marrow suppression, and hepatotoxicity.
- However, it has been stated that the potential neurological deterioration and side effects are lesser in comparison to trientine. But currently, ammonium TTM is not available in India.

Management of WD Presenting as ALF
- Patients with encephalopathy should be considered for urgent liver transplantation.
- DP/trientine with or without zinc may be started as an ad hoc measure, but survival is unlikely without transplantation.
- Rapid removal of free copper through molecular absorption recirculating system (MARS) or total plasma exchange (TPE) can benefit patients with fulminant presentation. TPE efficiently removes both ceruloplasmin- and albumin-bound copper, and the fresh-frozen plasma used for exchange can be helpful in treating the associated coagulopathy. MARS is also effective but more expensive and less widely available than TPE **(Table 1)**.

Liver Transplantation for Hepatic Wilson's Disease
- Liver transplantation is indicated in patients with fulminant presentation with hepatic encephalopathy or hemolytic crises.
- New Wilson's index has been used as a predictor of LT (for both acute or chronic present at ion). Rising bilirubin, advanced hepatic encephalopathy, and acute hemolysis have been suggested as better predictors for LT and need validation.
- Living donor liver transplant from heterozygous sibling is effective and safe for both donor and recipient.

TABLE 1: New Wilson's index for predicting survival.

Score	Bilirubin (mg/dL)	INR	AST (IU/L)	WCC (10⁹/L)	Albumin (g/dL)
0	0–5.8	0–1.29	0–100	0–6.7	≥4.5
1	5.9–8.7	1.3–1.6	101–150	6.8–8.3	3.4–4.4
2	8.8–11.6	1.7–1.9	151–200	8.4–10.3	2.5–3.3
3	11.7–17.5	2.0–2.4	201–300	10.4–15.3	2.1–2.4
4	≥17.6	≥2.5	≥300	≥15.4	0–2.0

(AST: aspartate transaminase; INR: international normalized ratio; WCC: white cell count)

TABLE 2: Interpretation of tests used in monitoring drug treatment of Wilson's disease.

	Zinc	D-penicillamine/trientine
Initial treatment	U Cu 100–500 µg/d S free Cu > 25 µg/dL U Zn > 2,000 µg/d	U Cu > 500 µg/d S free Cu > 25 µg/dL
Good control (Maintenance)	U Cu < 75 µg/d S free Cu 10–15 µg/dL	U Cu 200–500 µg/d S free Cu 10–15 µg/dL
Non-compliance/Inadequate dose	U Zn < 2,000 µg/d S free Cu > 15 µg/dL	U Cu < 200 µg/d U Cu > 500 µg/d S free Cu > 15 µg/dL
Overtreatment	U Cu < 25 µg/d S free Cu < 5 µg/dL	U Cu < 200 µg/d S free Cu < 5 µg/dL

(U Cu: 24 h urinary copper; U Zn: 24 h urinary zinc; S free Cu: serum free copper; DP: D-penicillamine)

Liver Transplantation for Neurological Wilson's Disease

- There is evidence that mild-to-moderate neurological involvement may improve after LT, neuropsychiatric disease is a predictor for poor outcome after LT.
- Liver transplantation is not indicated for isolated severe neurological WD. When the liver is also diseased, the decision should be individualized because significant neurological disease is a predictor of poor outcome.

Treatment Monitoring

- Careful clinical monitoring is necessary to determine benefit and adverse effects of the drugs **(Table 2)**.
- Complete blood counts, urine analyses, liver function tests, 24-h urinary copper and protein, and serum-free copper should be monitored frequently at the initial phase of therapy and at least once every 6–12 months thereafter.
- KF ring should be evaluated annually. Serum free copper is calculated by the formula: serum copper – 3 × serum ceruloplasmin.

Clinical Monitoring

In hepatic WD, clinical improvement is characterized by decreasing jaundice, ascites, and portal hypertension. Complete blood counts and liver function tests are performed initially after a week, then at 2 and 4 weeks followed by 3 months, 6 months, and then yearly. Child-Pugh score (based on serum bilirubin, prothrombin time, serum albumin, presence of ascites, and encephalopathy) and MELD score (based on bilirubin, creatinine, and INR) should be documented in those with severe liver disease.

In neurological WD, symptoms on sequential evaluation remain the most critical outcome of therapeutic benefits. Global Assessment Scale for Wilson's disease (GAS for WD) is the preferred scale because it assesses the neuropsychiatric, hepatic, and osteomuscular changes and their impact on quality of life over the observation period. Greater weightage is given to Wilson's facies and KF rings that are characteristic features of WD.

Long-term Outcomes

Wilson's disease is well recognized as one of the treatable genetic disorders and early recognition and institution of therapy holds the key for good outcome. The response to therapy is dependent on various factors including drug compliance and duration/severity of symptoms at the time of institution of therapy.

Overall improvement on therapy was 90% in hepatic presentation and >55% with neurological presentation. Most patients tend to have improvements up to 18–30 months after initiating therapy with good compliance, following which there is a plateau effect.

Poor prognostic factors of patients of clinically severe neurological WD included strong family history and severe MRI brain changes. Despite severe neurological involvement, 50% of patients have good clinical improvement while on treatment. Nonresponders to therapy show progressive, MRI worsening overtime.

Symptomatic Management of Neuro-Wilson Disease

- *Dystonia*: Patients with moderate to significant dystonia need medications such as trihexyphenidyl, tizanidine, baclofen, clonazepam, and tetrabenazine for symptomatic treatment.
- *Tremors*: Mild tremors do not require any specific therapies. In patients who have tremors affecting activities of daily living, drugs including propranolol, clonazepam, anticholinergics, topiramate, and primidone have been used.
- *Parkinsonism*: Levodopa should be tried in all patients with Parkinsonism, which might relieve symptoms. Other drugs of benefit include dopamine agonists, monoamine oxidase inhibitors, and amantadine.
- *Seizures*: Seizures occur in about 6–8% of patients with WD, either at initial present at ion or during the course of the disease. Therapy is on standard lines with antiepileptic medications. In view of associated hepatic dysfunction, antiepileptics with first-pass metabolism in liver should be avoided.

Psychiatric Symptoms

Most of the psychiatric symptoms are managed with behavior modification therapy. However, if medical therapy is needed, use of SSRI, SNRI and atypical antipsychotic is preferred over typical antipsychotics as usually have extrapyramidal side effects. Patients with aggressive manic symptoms or significant psychosis have been treated with electroconvulsive therapies.

Dietary Copper in the Management

- *Low copper food items <1 mg/100 g*: Rice, wheat, maize, millets, barley, legumes, eggs, fish, milk, and dairy products.
- *High copper content > 1 mg/100 g*: Red gram, soybean, all nuts, pepper, cumin, coriander, and liver oyster.

The American Association for the Study of Liver Diseases (AASLD) and European Association for the Study of the Liver (EASL) recommend avoiding foods with high concentration of copper in the first year of treatment <2 mg/day results in protein intake being invariably reduced to 1–1.5 g/kg/day.

Newer Therapies

Newer therapies include hepatocyte transplant, stem cell transplant, and gene therapy, which attempt to restore hepatobiliary copper excretion but still in experimental phase.

SUGGESTED READING

1. Hedera P. Update on the clinical management of Wilson's disease. Appl Clin Genet. 2017;10:9-19.
2. Nagral A, Sarma M, Matthai J, Kukkle PL, Devarbhavi H, Sinha S, et al. Wilson's Disease: Clinical Practice Guidelines of the Indian National Association for Study of the Liver, the Indian Society of Pediatric Gastroenterology, Hepatology and Nutrition, and the Movement Disorders Society of India. J Clin Exp Hepatol. 2019;1;74-98.
3. Palumbo CS, Schilsk ML. Clinical practice guidelines in Wilson disease. Ann Transl Med. 2019;7(Suppl 2):S65.

CHAPTER 112: Ataxia

KP Sarbhai

INTRODUCTION

Ataxia is impaired coordination of voluntary muscle movement. Ataxia is a Greek word, meaning lack of order. There is lack of rate, rhythm, and force of contraction of voluntary muscles.

CAUSES (TABLE 1)

The causes of ataxia are many. The causes according to site of lesion are as follows:
- Dysfunction of cerebellum which produces limb ataxia, unilateral cerebellar lesion cause ipsilateral signs and symptoms, diffuse cerebellar lesions give rise to more generalized symmetric symptoms, vermian lesions cause truncal and gait ataxia with upper limb relatively spared. It presents with dysmetria, dysdiadochokinesia, dyssynergia, dysarthria, rebound phenomena, increased postural sway, hypotonia, asthenia, and nystagmus.
- Vestibular dysfunction causes disequilibrium, vertigo, and gait ataxia with normal speech and normal joint position sense. Impaired proprioceptive afferent input (sensory defect)—peripheral nervous system gathers information about body position in space which is relayed to cerebellum where it is processed to maintain balance.
- *Sensory ataxia*: Ataxia due to posterior column defect is also associated with loss of vibration and position sense. This ataxia worsens with eye closure, and child is comfortable in sitting posture as there is no truncal ataxia.
- Frontal lobe lesion or lesion in frontocerebellar fibers.
- *Congenital ataxia*: Usually associated with cerebellar malformation or acquired. It can be further classified as acute, episodic, or chronic depending upon the rapidity of onset and progression.

HISTORY

A detailed history is the most important and the guidelines for proper history-taking are given as follows:
- *Age of onset*:
  - *Early infancy*: Cerebellar malformations present as developmental delay with hypotonia (floppy baby). Imbalance and dysarthria manifest only later.
  - *Early childhood*: Ataxia-telangiectasia (AT) may manifest in early childhood (autosomal-recessive cerebellar ataxia).
  - *Adolescent*: Friedreich ataxia becomes symptomatic by adolescence.
  - *After 25 years of age*: Spinocerebellar ataxia (SCA) which is dominantly inherited present after 25 years of age. Rarely, SCA2, 3, and 7 may manifest in infancy.

TABLE 1: Differentiating features of important ataxias.

	Cerebellar ataxia	*Sensory ataxia*	*Frontal ataxia*
Base of support	Wide based	Narrow base, looks down	Wide base
Velocity	Variable	Slow	Very slow
Stride	Irregular lurching	Regular with path deviation	Short shuffling
Rombergs	+/−	Unsteady fall	+/−
Heal-shin	Abnormal	+/−	Normal
Initiation	Normal	Normal	Hesitant
Turns	Unsteady	+/−	Hesitant, multistep
Postural instability	+	+++	++++
Falls	Late event	Frequent	Frequent

Type of onset: Acute, recurrent, static, or progressive
- *Acute ataxia*: If ataxia is acute, it raises following possibilities:
  - *Drugs and toxins*: Carbamazepine, phenytoin, antipsychotics, etc.
  - *Cerebrovascular accidents*: Intracranial hemorrhage of infarcts
  - *Acute infections*: Varicella can presents with acute ataxia. It can also be seen with EBV infection.
  - Following seizures in postictal stage or due to the effect of medication used to control the seizures.
  - Acute ataxia can be seen just after seizure activity, i.e., the postictal phase.
  - Intracranial space-occupying lesions (SOL) can present acutely if there is sudden hydrocephalus or hemorrhage into the tumor.
- *Subacute ataxia*:
  - *Postinfectious cerebellar ataxis*:
    - It is a common cause of acute or subacute ataxia in children.
    - There is pure cerebellar dysfunction following, a viral infection such as varicella, Epstein-Barr virus (EBV), measles, and rotavirus
    - Clinically it manifests as truncal and gait ataxia, nystagmus, intention tremor, and ataxia.
    - This condition is usually self-limiting.
    - Neuroimaging is normal in majority.
    - Oral steroids or IV methyl prednisolone hastens the recovery.
  - *Acute cerebellitis*:
    - It is severe form of subacute ataxia due to direct infection of cerebellum by viruses like varicella, EBV, or HSV or due to autoimmunity.
    - There is obstruction of the fourth ventricle due to inflammation of cerebellum may lead to acute hydrocephalus.
    - Hydrocephalus causes herniation of cerebellar tonsil which may lead to brainstem compression and sudden death.
    - *Magnetic resonance imaging (MRI)*: Picture reveals T2 hyperintensity, diffusion restriction and leptomeningeal enhancement over cerebellar folia.
    - *Treatment*: High dose of dexamethasone or surgical decompression may be needed.
  - *Acute disseminated encephalomyelitis (ADEM)*:
    - ADEM may presents with altered sensorium, limping, weakness, optic neuritis, with ataxia
    - *MRI is diagnostic*: The T2-weighted images and fluid-attenuated inversion recovery (FLAIR) sequences typically are bilateral multifocal areas of hyperintensity but may be asymmetric and tend to be poorly marginated. The lesions are multiple in the deep and subcortical white matter while the periventricular white matter is generally spared.
    - *Treatment*: By steroids or immunoglobulin
  - *Intractable SOL*:
    - Infratentorial tumors can produce cerebellar signs and features of hydrocephalus.
    - The tumors responsible are medulloblastoma, astrocytoma, ependymoma, or brainstem glioma.
  - *Opsoclonus myoclonus ataxia syndrome (OMS)*:
    - If subacute-onset ataxia is seen in a toddler with opsoclonus (chaotic multidirectional eye movement), may be myoclonus and tremors of upper, think of OMS.
    - It is associated with neuroblastoma in 25% cases.
    - MRI chest and abdomen, MIBG (metaiodobenzylguanidine) scan, positron emission tomography (PET) scan are diagnostic modalities of choice to detect occult neuroblastoma.
    - Treatment options are adrenocorticotropic hormone (ACTH), high-dose dexamethasone, or IV immunoglobulin. If tumor is found, it has to be removed.
    - Immunosuppression is continued after removal of the tumor. Rituximab is considered in resistant cases.
- *Episodic/recurrent ataxia*:
  - Presents with acute-onset vertigo, vomiting and ataxia, think of basilar migraine. It can occur without headache.
  - Family history of migraine will help in making diagnosis.
  - Repeated exposure to same drug or toxin
  - Metabolic conditions remembered by mnemonic (HUPI)
  - Hartnup disease
  - Urea cycle defect
  - Pyruate dehydrogenase deficiency
  - Intermittent branched chain aminoaciduria
  - *Nonconvulsive status epilepticus (NCS)*: If child walks with unsteady gait and appear confused, with history of seizure in the past. Think of NCS. Confirm the diagnosis by electroencephalography

(EEG) which shows anictal pattern. Patient comes back to normalcy after a prick of lorazepam or phenytoin.
- *Episodic ataxia type 1*: Episode of ataxia lasting for few seconds to minutes with myokymia in between the episodes. The cause is linked to autosomal dominant channelopathy. This is due to mutation in voltage-gated potassium channel (KCNA1). This may respond to phenytoin or carbamazepine.
- *Episodic ataxia type 2*: There are episodes of ataxia, vertigo, and nystagmus. This may respond to acetazolamide. It occurs due to mutation in calcium channel (CACNA1A).
- *Chronic ataxia*:
  - *Joubert syndrome*:
    - Infant presenting with hypotonia, developmental delay, feeding difficulty and speech delay and later shows ataxia and dysarthria speech.
    - There is cerebellar hypoplasia. It is recessively inherited hypoplasia of vermis.
    - There are characteristic facies, oculomotor apraxia, hypotonia, and developmental delay.
    - *MRI brain*: Molar tooth sign is diagnostic.
  - *Neurodegenerative conditions*: If there is insidious onset with slow progression manifesting in late childhood or adolescence is suggestive of neurodegenerative conditions. It manifests as chronic progressive ataxia.

Autosomal Recessive

Ataxia-telangiectasia

- AT is a rare autosomal recessive condition that affects the nervous system, immune system and other systems.
- It is characterized by the presence of, progressive ataxia, oculomotor apraxia (difficulty moving the eyes from side to side), choreoathetosis, telangiectasias. Chances of frequent infections, sensitive to ionizing radiation, increased risk to develop leukemia.
- Serum IgA levels are reduced, serum alpha fetaprotein level is elevated.
- Molecular diagnosis of detecting *ATM* gene is possible.

Friedreich Ataxia

- Friedreich ataxia (FRDA) is an autosomal recessive neurodegenerative disorder characterized by progressive gait and limb ataxia, dysarthria, dysphagia, oculomotor dysfunction, loss of deep tendon reflexes, pyramidal tract signs, scoliosis with cardiomyopathy, diabetes mellitus, visual loss, and defective hearing in some case.
- Molecular diagnosis by testing mutations in the *FXN* gene is confirmatory.
- Motor nerve conduct ion velocity (MNCV) of >40 m/s with absent or reduced sensory nerve action potential.
- *ECG finding*: Inferolateral or widespread T-wave inversion.
- *MRI finding*: Spinal and cerebellar atrophy.
- *Treatment*: There is no cure for FRDA and management is multidisciplinary.

Abetalipoproteinemia

- Abetalipoproteinemia is a rare autosomal-recessive disorder resulting from a microsomal triglyceride transfer protein deficiency.
- There is disrupt ion of cellular fat transport and presents in the first few months. The symptoms of failure to thrive, diarrhea, and steatorrhea are seen win this age group. Fat-soluble vitamins such as A, E, and K are poorly absorbed, leading to dietary deficiency.
- It may present with spastic ataxia, atypical retinitis pigmentosa, and acanthocytosis.
- *Diagnosis*: Lipid analysis, after 12 hours of fasting, measure serum levels of low-density lipoprotein (LDL) (<0.10 g/L), triglycerides (<0.20 g/L), and apolipoprotein B (<0.10 g/L) to be done in patient and their parents.
- Mutations of the *MTTP* or *APOB* genes confirm the diagnosis.

Refsum Disease

- A metabolic disease is characterized by anosmia, cataract, early-onset retinitis pigmentosa, peripheral neuropathy and cerebellar ataxia.
- The other association can be deafness, ichthyosis, skeletal abnormalities, and cardiac arrhythmia.
- There is accumulation of phytanic acid in plasma and tissues, due to deficiency of phytanic acid-alpha-dehydrogenase enzyme.
- There are mutations in the *PHYH* gene (10p13) in >90% of cases, and mutations in the *PEX7* gene (6q21-q22.2) in <10%.
- Treatment needs multidisciplinary approach. Dietary restriction may help to control sensory neuropathy, myopathy, ataxia, and ichthyosis.

X-linked recessive: Pelizaeus–Merzbacher disease.

Autosomal dominant: SCA, which presents after 25 years of age.

APPROACH TO ATAXIA

History:
- Refusal to walk with a wide-based drunken gait
- Vertigo dizziness and vomiting
- Personality and behavior changes
- Abnormal mental status
- History of head or neck trauma
- Recent infection or vaccination or drug intake
- Similar episode of ataxia in the past
- History of ataxia in family members
- Birth history, presence of congenital malformations.

Physical examination includes assessment of alertness, distress, dysmorphism, rashes, ear discharge, papilledema, cardiac murmur, and hepatosplenomegaly.

Complete neurologic examination should be done. Cranial nerves, motor function—tone, power, reflexes, planters, posterior column sensation, focal neurological sign. Look for cerebellar integrity **(Table 2)**.

INVESTIGATIONS

- *Neuroimaging*: MRI of brain or spine
- *Electrodiagnostic tests*: EMG, EEG, ERG, and evoked potential
- *Tests of autonomic dysfunction*: Tilt table test, sympathetic skin response and other tests
- *Ophthalmologic examination*: Pigmentary retinopathy, macular degeneration, cataracts and Kayser–Fleischer ring.

TABLE 2: Assessment of cerebellar integrity.

Classical finding in cerebellar dysfunction	Examination of arms and hand
Hypotonia	Finger to nose
Nystagmus	Finger to finger to nose
Staggering gait	Rapid alternating movement
Titubation	Rebound
Other signs and symptoms	Tone elevation
Action tremor	
Asthenia	Examination of Gait
Ataxia	Assess truncal control
Decompensation of movement	Natural gait and tandem walk
Dysdiadokokinesia	Foot stepping
Dysmetria	Heal-to-shin maneuver
Dyssynergia	Hopping at one place
Impaired rebound	Romberg test*
Pendular deep tendon reflexes	Walk in circle

*Romberg test: Test with Eyes closed, if loss of balance, think of peripheral disease. Test with Eyes open, if loss of balance, think of cerebellum.

- *Genetic tests (available in India)*:
  - *Autosomal dominant ataxias*: SCA1, 2, 3, 6, 7, 8, 10, 11, 12, 14, 17, 23, and 28; DRPLA
  - *Autosomal recessive ataxias*: FRDA, AOA1 and2, AT, ARSACS
  - *X-linked ataxia*: FXTAS
  - *Mitochondrial disorders*: Entire genome sequencing
- *Metabolic workup*: Thyroid function, vitamin B_{12}, E, and B_1, serum cholesterol and plasma lipoprotein profile, urine bile alcohol, phytanic acid, and toxicology screen.
- *Immune function*: Immunoglobulin level, antigliadin antibodies, glutamic acid decarboxylase (GAD) antibodies, and paraneoplastic antibodies.
- *Mitochondrial disorder*: Serum lactate and pyruvate.
- *Heavy metals*: Peripheral smear for acanthocytes, very long-chain fatty acids, hexoseaminidase A/B, alpha-fetoprotein and immunoglobulin, serum ceruloplasmin, and 24-hour urine ceruloplasmin.
- *Tissue studies*: Muscle, skin, and nerve biopsy.
- *Cerebrospinal fluid (CSF) studies*: Cell count, glucose and protein, oligoclonal bands, 14-3-3 protein, GAD antibodies, paraneoplastic antibodies, lactate, and pyruvate.
- *Vitamin levels*: Vitamin B_1, B_{12}, and E levels.

TREATMENT

The treatment of ataxia depends on the cause; however, treatment of the following infections is done as per the case-confirmed varicella zoster virus (VZV), EBV, Bickerstaff's encephalitis, (brainstem, ophthalmoplegia, at ataxia—lower cranial nerve palsy), human immunodeficiency virus (HIV) [lymphoma, progressive multifocal leukoencephalopathy (PML), toxoplasmosis], Creutzfeldt–Jakob disease (CJD), syphilis (tabes dorsalis), and Whipple's disease.

POINTS TO REMEMBER

- Approach to ataxia begins with the knowledge of sign, symptoms, and etiology of ataxia.
- Proper history and thorough clinical examination are must.
- Treatable causes must be identified first and ruled out.
- Autosomal-dominant cerebellar ataxia are more common than recessive ataxias.
- Genetic testing is prudent for providing better insight into the management.

SUGGESTED READING

1. Verma A, Kunju PAM. IAP Textbook of Paediatric Neurology, 2nd edition. New Delhi: Jaypee Brothers Medical Publishers; 2019.

CHAPTER 113

Duchenne Muscular Dystrophy

Kanak Ramnani

DEFINITION

Duchenne muscular dystrophy (DMD) is a lethal X-linked recessive neuromuscular disorder characterized by muscular weakness, motor delay, calf hypertrophy, proliferation of connective tissue within the muscles, finally loss of ambulation and mental retardation due to mutation in *dystrophin* gene causing absence or insufficiency of dystrophin protein.

Incidence: 1:3,500–4,000 male children. The prevalence is estimated as 15.9 per 100,000 population in USA and 19.5 in UK.

GENETICS

It is an X-linked recessive disease. The abnormal gene causing DMD is located on the short arm of the X-chromosome at the Xp21 site. Since it is an X-linked disease, it is seen in males with history of similar illness in the maternal uncle.

However, patients may have DMD because of a de novo mutations (i.e., mother is not a carrier of DMD). Since the female has 2X chromosomes, a carrier female does not show typical features of DMD (however, they do have moderately elevated CPK levels).

A carrier female may demonstrate typical features of DMD in Turner's syndrome and structural variation in X-chromosome or condition causing lyonization.

PATHOGENESIS

Duchenne muscular dystrophy occurs due to mutation in the *DMD* gene that encodes the dystrophin protein and is therefore called as dystrophinopathy. A less severe form also occurs that is better known as Becker's muscular dystrophy (BMD) and rarely the mutation may result in a third form of dystrophinopathy: X-linked dilated cardiomyopathy (XLDC).

The *DMD* gene is the largest known human gene, containing 79 exons. The mutation rate is very high relating with the large variation of mutations that are identified in various patients; DMD is said to be caused by de novo mutation. Nearly, 68% of patients have a deletion and 11% have duplication on one or more exons usually at exons 45–55 and exons 2–10, respectively. Small mutations may be seen in about 20% of the patients. These mutations abolish the dystrophin function by prematurely stopping the protein translation due to either frame-shift mutation or appoint mutation changing a codon to a stop codon. DMD is usually associated with absence of dystrophin expression and BMD with expression of partially functional protein; that at the gene level is explained by "reading frame rule." According to the rule, disease severity is not determined by the number of exons deleted. The "out-of-frame" mutations causing disruption of the open reading frame are responsible for termination of translation; hence, no protein expression causing absence of protein and DMD. The dystrophin protein normally maintains the connection between the actin cytoskeleton and the connecting tissue; thus, preventing its damage during contraction. The absence of dystrophin protein leads to chronic muscle damage that is pathologically evident by degenerative changes and fibrosis of muscle; variation of muscle fiber diameter and endomysial connective tissue proliferation.

CLINICAL FEATURES

Although the disease is present from birth but the babies are apparently normal at birth, delayed motor functions may be evident in some of the infants. By the second year of life, the clumsiness of the toddler is seen which appears to be more prolonged. Symptoms appear by 2–5 years delayed language acquisition is an important clinical feature in these children. Difficulty in climbing stairs or getting up from the floor becomes difficult that can be checked by Gower's sign. At this age, muscle testing by a clinician demonstrates weakness of proximal muscles. By the age of 6–7 years, the strength may improve and the motor function may improve and may plateau for 12–18 months followed by increase in weakness. Cognitive impairment, low IQ (usually seen in patients who have mutations that ablate expression of shorter dystrophin isoforms that are expressed in the brain Dp140, Dp71), and dysarthria due to tongue hypertrophy become evident. The associated symptoms would be autism, attention-deficit/hyperactivity disorder (ADHD), and obsessive compulsive disorder.

Difficulty in walking progresses with age and by 10-12 years of age most of these children are unable to walk. Dependence on wheelchair eventually leads to development of scoliosis. Pseudohypertrophy of calves is a distinctive feature of DMD. The other muscles which may be hypertrophied are brachioradialis, deltoids, gluteus, and muscles of tongue.

By 14-16 years of age, pharyngeal muscles start getting involved causing nasal regurgitation; aspiration of food and respiratory muscles involvement causes breathlessness.

The myopathy is painless; contractures of hip, knees, and ankle are common; severe scoliosis gradually develops gradually. Cardiac muscles are the most common extramuscular muscle involved in DMD.

The DMD care consideration working group identified 11 topics to be considered in DMD:
1. Diagnosis
2. Neuromuscular management
3. Rehabilitation management
4. Gastrointestinal and nutritional management
5. Respiratory management
6. Cardiac management
7. Orthopedic and surgical management
8. Psychosocial management
9. Primary care and emergency management
10. Endocrine management
11. Care across lifespan.

DIAGNOSIS

The diagnostic process begins typically in early childhood after suggestive signs and symptoms are noticed.

When to suspect DMD?
Duchenne muscular dystrophy should be a differential diagnosis if there is any suspicion of abnormal muscle function or if there is a family history of DMD; in the absence of family history, DMD may be expected if the child does not walk by the age of 16-18 months or has Gower's sign or has toe walking or unexplained increase in transaminases level. The next stage would be creatine kinase assessment followed by genetic testing for deletion or duplication. If mutation not found but creatine kinase is high then genetic sequencing should be done. If still mutation not found then muscle biopsy can be done.

LABORATORY FEATURES

Serum creatine kinase (CK) is the first test performed if suspecting a dystrophinopathy; it is increased in both DMD and BMD. CK is also raised during the neonatal time (often >1,000 U/L) and may be used as a screening tool; during childhood, it reaches greater than 20,000 and declines later due to loss of muscle mass. No other blood marker is important in the diagnosis although mild elevation of aspartate aminotransferase (AST) and alanine aminotransferase (ALT) is usually seen.

Molecular Genetic Testing

Detailed mutational analysis is now the standard testing method; with the modern methods, the sensitivity of mutation detection in the peripheral blood-derived genomic DNA sample is 93-96%. These testing are important because they provide prognostic information, facilitate genetic counseling, and determine candidate suitability for specific new therapies. In these methods, all the exons are checked; hence even the complex exon duplication and deletions are detected. It is important that exceptions to the reading frame rule exist and complicate the prognostication. One third of the mutations may be de novo; genetic counseling is essential to address the risk of germline mosaicism in mothers whose DNA analysis is negative.

Muscle Biopsy

Muscle biopsy is only required in patients where there is a high suspicion of dystrophinopathy but there is no detectable mutation on DNA analysis. This allows confirmation of the diagnosis by analysis of dystrophin expression and provides muscle tissue for mRNA extraction necessary for detection of mutations that escape detection by blood-based assays.

Family members of any patient with DMD have to be checked and any carrier should be screened and counseled appropriately. Carrier testing is recommended for the female members of boys suffering from DMD. Preimplant genetic diagnosis or prenatal genetic testing are some of the reproductive choices available for carrier females. These carriers need to be screened for cardiac complications.

As far as the newborn screening is considered; at present, DMD is not currently included in the Recommended Uniform Screening Panel.

NEUROMUSCULAR MANGEMENT

The important step in neuromuscular management is the assessment of passive range of movement, muscle extensibility, posture and alignment, strength, function, quality of life and participation in all the normal activities of life. The North Star Ambulatory Assessment and timed functional test are fundamental to the assessment of function in the ambulatory period and should be repeated 6 monthly. Tests that predict potential upcoming changes may be helpful in deciding the further intervention that is needed and even the future equipment needs. The Bayley-III scale of infant development and Griffith Mental Development Scales can predict early developmental delays in children.

The same test should be used consistently in a particular child to track the changes over time; 4-6 monthly reassessments are recommended.

Interventions

Duchenne muscular dystrophy causes progressive muscle weakness and leads to contractures and deformities. Appropriate and timely management prolongs ambulation and improves the quality of life. A good physiotherapy and occupational therapy along with a multidisciplinary rehabilitation team is a must, which ensues proper and timely assessment of passive ranges of movement, muscle extensibility, chest wall movement and symmetry; can optimize posture, movement, and respiratory functions; and can maintain ambulation and prevent fixed contraction and deformity. Pain needs to be assessed and managed at all ages.

Regular exercises such as swimming and cycling should be advocated; patients should be guided regarding avoidance of eccentric and high-resistance exercises, avoidance of overexertion, proper rest and activities for muscle conservation and the use of assistive technology and adaptive equipment. Passive stretching should be continued to prevent contractures.

Pharmacological Approaches

Glucocorticoids are the mainstay of treatment of DMD; long-term therapies have shown various advantages delay in loss of ambulation by 1–3 years, preserved upper limb and respiratory functions and avoidance of scoliosis surgery. The exact mechanism of action is unknown but it is postulated that steroids act by membrane stabilization, diminished fibrosis, and decreased inflammatory responses. It should be started at early ages. The recommended starting doses are prednisolone 0.75 mg/kg/day or deflazacort 0.9 mg/kg/day. Side effects of steroids need monitoring every 2–3 months. In case of intolerable side effects, the dose should be reduced by 25–33% and reassessed at 1 month. Steroid should not be stopped abruptly.

Newer drugs for DMD that are in pipeline aim at correcting the pathological features of dystrophinopathies include mutation specific therapies including ataluren to be used if DMD is caused by a stop codon in *dystrophin* gene and eteplirsen if the *dystrophin* gene is due to exon 51 skipping. Other drugs in trial include drugs targeting myostatin, certain anti-inflammatory and antioxidant molecules and drugs such as idebenone that inhibit lipid peroxidation that improve mitochondrial functions by mitochondrial electron flux and cellular energy production have shown some improvement in respiratory functions. Researches are being continued to search the molecules that may upregulate dystrophin surrogate utrophin that is seen to be beneficial in mouse model. Another approach is the use of phosphodiesterase inhibitors such as sildenafil and tadalafil to increase neuronal nitric oxide synthase (nNOS) activity in the skeletal muscles.

Gene transfer is directed toward the delivery of a functional version of the gene to the skeletal muscle, heart, and the diaphragm. An initial trial with an early microdystrophin vector version did not prove advantageous in producing significant dystrophin expression. Researches for developing better vectors are in progress.

SUGGESTED READING

1. Birnkrant DJ, Bushby K, Bann CM, Alman BA, Apkon SD, Blackwell A. Diagnosis and management of Duchenne muscular dystrophy, part 2: respiratory, cardiac, bone health, and orthopaedic management. Lancet Neurol. 2018;17(4):347-61.
2. Birnkrant DJ, Bushby K, Bann CM, Apkon SD, Blackwell A, Brumbaugh D, et al. Diagnosis and management of Duchenne muscular dystrophy, part 1: diagnosis, and neuromuscular, rehabilitation, endocrine, and gastrointestinal and nutritional management. Lancet Neurol. 2018;17(3):251-67.

114 CHAPTER

Spinal Muscular Atrophy

Kanak Ramnani

INTRODUCTION

Spinal muscular atrophy (SMA) is the most common monogenetic (usually autosomal recessive) neurodegenerative disorder characterized by degeneration of alpha motor neurons of the spinal cord and in the most severe cases, the bulbar motor neurons and progressive muscular weakness and atrophy.

It is a clinical continuum with a range of phenotypic severity because the rate of progression varies in each patient and is the leading genetic cause of infantile mortality.

EPIDEMIOLOGY

The incidence of SMA has been estimated at 1 in 6,000–11,000 live births. The carrier frequency for the mutation in the *survival motor neuron (SMN1)* gene has been estimated from 1:38 to 1:70. Population studies have indicated that the Asians have the highest carrier frequency.

GENETICS

The most common form of SMA is due to a homozygous deletion or mutation involving the *SMN* gene. Two copies of *SMN* gene (*SMN1* and *SMN2*) are located on each chromosome 5 forming an inverted duplication at to 5q13. In approximately 96% of patients, SMA is caused by homozygous absence of exon 7 and 8 of *SMN1* gene. The majority of patients inherent the SMN1 deletion from their parents, in 2% de-novo deletion in one of the two alleles have been described. In 3–4%, other mutation in SMN1 can be found. The SMN2 copy numbers vary between 0 and 4 per chromosome 5, and it is an important factor affecting the severity of SMA phenotype. In the patients of SMA, small amounts of full-length and fully functional SMN protein can be produced by SMN2, thus higher number of SMN2 copies are associated with milder phenotypes.

PATHOLOGY

Survival motor neuron protein is a 38 kDa intracellular protein that helps in pre-mRNA splicing. It is still unclear whether the splicing defect caused by the deficiency of SMN protein or disruption of additional axonal SMN function causes the disease. The disease is characterized by loss or malpositioning of large number of anterior horn cells; histopathologically these cells appear swollen and chromatolytic. The muscles of the severely affected cases reveal are suggestive of atrophy and signs of denervation.

CLINICAL FEATURES

The range of phenotypic presentations and severity permits the division of this condition in four broad forms as given in **Table 1**.

LABORATORY STUDIES

- *Molecular genetic analysis*: Genetic testing of *SMN1/SMN2* using multiplex ligation-dependent probe amplification (MLPA), quantitative polymerase chain reaction (qPCR) or next-generation sequencing (NGS) is the first-line investigation. If homozygous deletion in the *SMN* gene is identified, no other investigation is required. If clinical picture is highly suggestive but homozygous deletion is not found, then *SMN1* sequencing is done for subtle mutations.
- Serum creatine phosphokinase (CPK) levels may be elevated up to 10 times in SMA III but is typically normal in infantile and intermediate types.
- Electromyography (EMG) may be helpful in diagnosis but is not needed in type I and type II.
  Compound muscle action potentials (CMAPs) may be reduced in amplitude, conduct ion velocity, and sensory nerve conduct ion study results are normal. Needle electrode examination reveals acute denervation along with chronic motor unit remodeling due to a chronic process of denervation and reinnervation. Complex repetitive discharges are a feature of SMA type III.
- Muscle biopsy reveals a highly characteristic pattern called as grouped fascicular atrophy.

TREATMENT

A multidisciplinary approach is the key element in the management of SMA patients. SMA is a complex disorder involving different aspects of care and professionals, and each

TABLE 1: Phenotypic types of SMA.

Type	Age of onset	Life form	Highest motor milestone	Additional findings
Type 1 (Nonsitters)	IA : Prenatal IB : 0–3 months IC : 3–6 months	IA : 6 months IB and IC : <2 years	IA : No ms IB and IC cannot sit without support	Floppy baby, breathing and swallowing difficulty, tongue fasciculations, areflexia, normal cognition, relative facial sparing
Type II (Sitters)	6–8 months	>2 years; 70% are alive at 25 years	Sit independently never walk	Delay in motor development, proximal weakness legs more than arms, hypotonia, areflexia, scoliosis, intercostal muscle weakness
Type III (Walkers) Type IV (Adult)	>21 years	Normal	Normal	

of the aspect should be dealt as a part of multidisciplinary approach.

- *Clinical assessment*: Assessment of musculoskeletal system should include the strength and range of joint movement on regular basis using standard scales.
- *Rehabilitation*: The management objectives are: (1) Maintain active mobility, and independence as long as possible and (2) Prevent the development of contractures and kyphoscoliosis.
  A well-coordinated multidisciplinary approach should be used to optimizing residual functions.
- *Pulmonary care* should be given utmost importance; proper use of antibiotics and chest physiotherapy and positive pressure is essential.
- *Gastrointestinal care and nutrition*: Patients with type I SMA are extremely weak and tired during feeding causing failure to thrive and may cause aspiration and recurrent infections, all of these require proper treatment.
- *Orthopedic*: Close orthopedic follow-up is required for the development of scoliosis and contractures.
- *Drug therapy*: Currently, no definite care for SMA is available. The unique structure of the 5q11.1-13.3 may provide potential therapeutic targets. Research is going on for identifying agents to increase the full-length SMN protein by upregulating the expression of *SMN2* gene or promoting inclusion of exon 7.

SUGGESTED READING

1. Verma A, Kunju PAM. IAP Textbook of Paediatric Neurology, 2nd edition. New Delhi: Jaypee Brothers Medical Publishers; 2019.

CHAPTER 115: Benign Acute Childhood Myositis

Anoop Verma

INTRODUCTION

Benign acute childhood myositis (BACM) is a self-limiting muscle disorder characterized by calf pain, elevated serum creatine kinase, and preceded by an influenza-like illness. The classic clinical presentation, laboratory support may allow for a proper diagnosis. Clinicians may not be familiar with the presentation of BACM, and is often misdiagnosed and interpreted as a more severe disease, and becomes a candidate for unnecessary investigations.

CAUSES

Many viruses are claimed to be responsible for the clinical presentation. Influenza B, influenza A virus, human parainfluenza virus type 1, enterovirus, *Mycoplasma pneumoniae*, dengue virus, H1N1.

BASICS

The exact incidence is not known. Viral infection induces inflammatory process that leads to isolated skeletal muscle degeneration. But still the uncertainty remains as to whether the myositis is caused by a direct viral action or by immune-mediated mechanisms. It can be seen with an epidemic. It affects children 6–8 years of age, boys more than girls.

CLINICAL PRESENTATION

- Symptoms usually occur during early convalescent period of a viral illness. Median time between the onset of fever and the beginning of BACM symptoms is about 3 days.
- Patient presenting with bilateral calf pain, often severe and symmetrical Myalgia is more focal than diffuse.
- Two characteristic gaits were noted in these patient *tip-toe-walking*, and with a *wide-based stiff-legged gait*. The patient refuses to walk or bear weight and presents with limp. The limbs have normal strength and power, with intact tendon reflexes.
- The onset may be mistaken for very severe neurological illness-like Guillain-Barré syndrome or chronic autoimmune diseases occasionally. As a result, unnecessary tests such as radiography, echocardiography, electromyography and magnetic resonance are ordered.
- A different pattern of acute viral myositis is also observed, in which the trapezius muscle rather than the calves was involved. The outbreaks had been recorded under the name *of myalgia nuchae epidemica.*

INVESTIGATIONS

Laboratory testing should be limited to children who will not walk at all. An elevated creatine phosphokinase (CPK) level is one of the most common laboratory findings in BACM. It may rise to a high level of 4,100 U/L. High CPK values are also associated with muscular dystrophy, while in BACM elevated CPK levels will peak after 2 weeks.

Patients can have normal or decreased white blood cell and platelet counts and elevated aminotransferase levels.

In children with a rapidly worsening condition or no symptomatic resolution after a few days, it is advised to perform urine and renal function tests in order to rule out rhabdomyolysis and renal failure. Parents should be encouraged to monitor the child's urine output and the appearance of Coca-Cola-colored urine and swollen legs.

In rare cases, routine complete blood count, C-reactive protein levels, creatine kinase levels, liver function tests, and urine myoglobin measurement are done.

Viral studies and muscle biopsies or myelography are usually not required in BACM.

MANAGEMENT

Children with BACM are managed in outpatients with analgesics and appropriate clinical and laboratory follow-up in 2–3 weeks. Rhabdomyolysis is an infrequently reported complication of BACM, and has to be managed accordingly.

SUGGESTED READING

1. Magee H, Goldman RD. Viral myositis in children. Can Fam Physician. 2017;63(5):365-8.

Bell's Palsy

Anoop Verma

INTRODUCTION

Bell's palsy is an unexplained unilateral isolated facial weakness of unknown cause. It is the most frequent form of facial paralysis in children, and in 70% cases, have a favorable prognosis with spontaneous resolution. The onset is acute and may have additional symptoms of pain in ear, tingling, numbness on the affected side. Hyperacusis and disturbed taste may be associated on ipsilateral anterior part of the tongue.

ETIOLOGY OF FACIAL PALSY

Facial nerve palsy can be *congenital* or *acquired*.

Congenital facial palsy is seen in perinatal trauma, syndromic and nonsyndromic malformations such as Mobius and Goldenhar syndromes. The congenital pseudobulbar palsy (syringobulbia) manifests with facial paralysis, dysphagia, and speech difficulties. Arnold-Chiari syndrome may manifest with congenital facial paralysis along with other cranial nerves paralysis.

Acquired facial palsy may be idiopathic, infectious, inflammatory, neoplastic and traumatic. Viral infect ions are frequently associated with facial palsy. In Ramsay Hunt syndrome, there is reactivation of herpes varicella-zoster which can cause facial palsy (zoster oticus).

Idiopathic facial paralysis is commonly known as *Bell's palsy*, named after the Scottish surgeon, *Sir Charles Bell*, in 1821. In about 50% cases, the etiology is unknown. Incidence of Bell's palsy in children is about 6.1 cases per year per 100,000 between 1 and 15 years of age. It has a favorable prognosis with spontaneous resolution within 3 months, and have no sequelae.

Bilateral facial nerve palsy is seen in infection with Epstein–Barr virus, tuberculosis, *Haemophilus influenzae*, or *Borrelia burgdorferi* infection.

CLINICAL FEATURES

- Facial asymmetry with loss of nasolabial fold, dropping of angle of mouth, drooling of saliva, eyelid widening, and lagophthalmos are classical features of lower motor neuron paralysis of facial nerve.
- Dynamic signs present are inability to whistle, puffing cheeks, frown, inadequate closure of the eyelid. Hyperacusis occurs due to paralysis of the stapedius muscle.
- *Paresthesias and pain of the pinna*: Lacrimal and salivary production can be reduced.
- Metallic taste in the mouth due to the taste alteration of the anterior two thirds of the tongue.
- In very young children and newborns, the unilateral facial paralysis must be differentiated from absence of depressor angular oris muscle, where there is preservation of nasolabial fold, and drooping of angle of mouth toward normal side.

INVESTIGATIONS AND DIAGNOSIS

- History and examination are very important for the diagnosis. Ask about the onset of the course of the paralysis and its eventual progression. A gradual onset of >3 weeks may suggest a neoplastic etiology.
- Inspection of the external auditory canal, the eardrum, and the mastoid region may give the clue.
- Eye and palpebral region, and the lower face are observed at rest and at movement.
- Audiological evaluation to assess the presence of stapedial reflexes.
- Blood pressure is important in recurrent facial nerve palsy.
- Lumbar puncture is performed only when suspecting a meningitis or a Guillain–Barré syndrome.
- Specific laboratory and imaging tests for the diagnosis of Ramsey Hunt syndrome. ELISA serum for IgM and IgG antibody titer against herpes varicella zoster. Serologic tests for Lyme disease when the history of the patient suggests a possible exposure. In suspected neoplastic etiology, computed tomography (CT) and magnetic resonance imaging (MRI) of petrous bone must be performed.
- Electrophysiological studies are not done in pediatric age group.

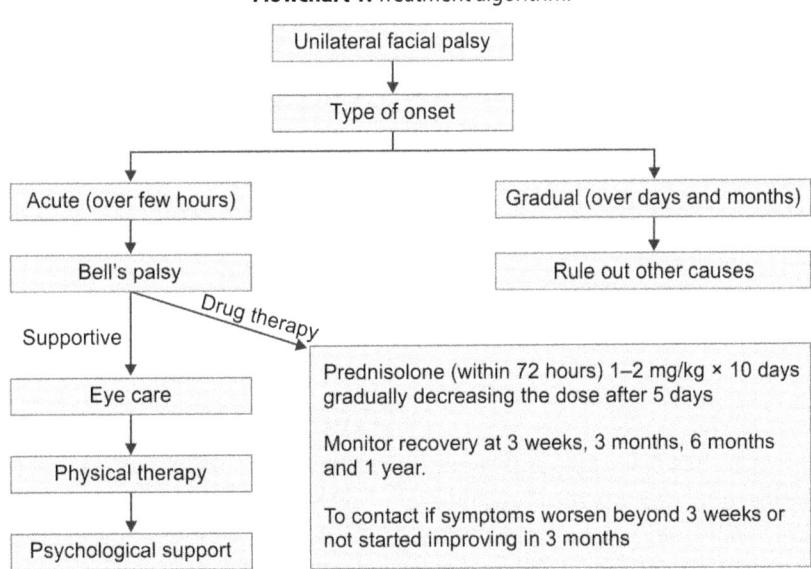

Flowchart 1: Treatment algorithm.

COMPLICATIONS

- Five percent of cases develop contractures, spasms, and synkinesis.
- Synkinesis affects the symmetry and facial expressiveness. It has three possible mechanisms: (1) an aberrant axonal regeneration, (2) an aberrant nerve impulse transmission, and (3) a hyperexcitability of the nucleus of the facial nerve.
- Synkinesis affects the eye and mouth muscles, e.g., smile; there could be an involuntary eye closure and *vice versa*. Though rare, voluntary movements of the mouth or the voluntary eye closure cause involuntary movements of the chin. A similar phenomenon is seen when the autonomic fibers are involved, e.g., the activation of salivation while eating causes lacrimation, the phenomenon is known as "*crocodile tears.*"

TREATMENT

- The treatment of facial palsy is related to the severity and etiology of the palsy. In children, often multidisciplinary approach is needed **(Flowchart 1)**. Bell's palsy in children *recovers spontaneously*, most of the times by 4 weeks. The aim of the drug therapy is to minimize the possibility of incomplete resolutions and reduce the risk of complication, such as synkinesis, autonomic dysfunctions (e.g., crocodile tears), and facial spasms.
- *Oral corticosteroids* in children are recommended to reduce the inflammatory edema of facial nerve, and has to be started within 3 days from onset of symptoms. *Prednisolone* in the dose of 1–2 mg/kg per day for 5 days, gradually decreasing the dose for the next 5 days.
- The *Ramsay Hunt syndrome*, needs quick intravenous steroid with antivirals along in children older than 2 years. Acyclovir 80 mg/kg per day every 6 hours for 5 days or, in children older than 12 years, valacyclovir 20 mg/kg three times per day, up to a maximum of 1,000 mg three times daily. Full recovery is seen in 75% of cases if treated within the first 3 days from onset.
- *Eye care* is very important to protect the cornea from drying and abrasion. Artificial tears are used during the day at least six times a day, and eye ointment to lubricate the eye overnight. It is advised to refer the patient to eye OPD if eye is painful and closure is inadequate.
- Infants with congenital paralysis for perinatal trauma, usually have a good prognosis even without treatment.
- *Antiviral agents*: The combination of steroids with antiviral agents (*acyclovir* or *valacyclovir*) are recommended in severe palsy in adults.
  There is little evidence for the use of antiviral in the absence of any vesicles in children (*Cochrane review 2016*).

PROGNOSIS

- The degree of paralysis depicts the overall prognosis, with partial paralysis the outcome is better, while in severe dysfunctions the possibility of recovery is poor.
- Perinatal trauma usually have a good prognosis, and spontaneous resolution is expected by 4 months.
- Bell's palsy has a functional recovery in a short time represented by a clinical improvement within 3 weeks.
- Ramsey Hunt syndrome has a worse prognosis compared to Bell's palsy; only 10% of the patient with severe paralysis have a full recovery.

SUGGESTED READING

1. Ciorba A, Corazzi V. Facial nerve paralysis in children. World J Clin Cases. 2015;3(12):973-9.
2. Murthy JMK, Saxena AB. Bell's palsy: treatment guidelines. Ann Indian Acad Neurol. 2011;14(Suppl 1):S70-2.

CHAPTER 117

Traumatic Brain Injury

Anil K Goel

INTRODUCTION

Traumatic brain injury (TBI), head injury, and brain trauma are synonymous terms, implying any insult resulted from or by an external force. Fall from height, road traffic accidents (RTA), and sports-related injuries and assaults are common causes in pediatric age group. The causes are different in different ages and in rural and urban areas. The common cause in <5 years is fall, while RTA in school-going children. Boys are more prone to RTA then girls. Fall from a height, unprotected roof, and staircase accounts for the most common mode of TBI in infancy and early childhood. Children with TBI due to RTA are, in fact, pedestrians as observed in several studies other than bicycling and motor bike assaults. The mechanism of injury is crucial to severity of illness. This is different from pediatric stroke, infection of central nervous system, malignancy that can produce brain injuries by different mechanisms. In India, children <15 years constitute 30–40% of the total population and contribute to 20–30% of all head injuries, responsible for one of the important acquired causes of death.

Minor head injury is a common presentation in the pediatric emergency. The challenge is to distinguish it from clinically important traumatic brain injury (ciTBI). Identifying right child for right radiographic investigation is very crucial for early recognition and subsequent management. The key goals should focus on stabilization, timely recognition of clinical deterioration, and early consultation of a neurotrauma team to decrease morbidity and mortality.

SPECTRUM OF PRESENTATION

Briefly, the common spectrum of illness ranges from minor to moderate, severe TBI, concussion, skull fracture, pneumocephalus, intracranial hemorrhage, cerebral edema, diffuse axonal injury (DAI), and cerebral herniation. The injured brain is vulnerable to secondary insults because injury disrupts normal autoregulatory defense mechanisms and disturbances in autoregulation of cerebral blood flow (CBF) can lead to ischemia from hypotension that would otherwise be tolerated by a healthy brain.

DEFINITION

1. *Clinically important traumatic brain injury*: The operational definition ciTBI includes—Presence of a TBI (e.g., epidural hematoma, subdural hematoma, or cerebral contusion) on computed tomography (CT) associated with any of the following:
   - Neurosurgical intervention [either surgery or invasive intracranial pressure (ICP) monitoring].
   - Endotracheal intubation for 24 hours to maintain airway.
   - Hospitalization directly related to the head injury for at least 48 hours.
   - Depressed skull fracture warranting operative elevation (i.e., depressed past the inner table of the skull).
   - Clinical findings of a basilar skull fracture (periorbital ecchymosis, Battle sign, hemotympanum, cerebrospinal fluid (CSF) otorrhea or rhinorrhea).
2. *Concussion*: It is a minor type of TBI caused by a bump, blow, or jolt to the head. Concussions can also occur from a fall or a blow to the body that causes the head and brain to move quickly in successive direction.
3. *Hematoma*: The extradural hematoma is the most common injury pattern, others are epidural, subdural, and intracranial hemorrhage.
4. *DAI*: It is due to shear injuries of axons and blood vessels involving the white matter of the brain. The shear occurs with acceleration and deceleration or rotational forces involving the brain matter. The degree of tissue disruption is indicative of the amount of energy dissipation. DAI may appear normal on CT scan, but as the severity of injury increases, DAI may be associated with multiple intracerebral petechial hemorrhages. Magnetic resonance imaging (MRI) is more sensitive in delineating transient signal changes along white matter tracts.

Severity levels of TBI:
- *Mild*: Glasgow Coma Scale (GCS) score 14–15 (awake). It is also termed as concussion. Presence of spontaneous eye opening with confusion, memory, attention difficulties, headache, and behavioral problems may be there.

- *Moderate*: GCS score 9-13 (lethargic). Eye opening to stimulation. The child might be sleepy, but still arousal.
- *Severe*: GCS score 3-8 (Coma). No opening of eyes even with painful stimulation. It is associated with 20-50% death rate or severe disabilities.

RED FLAGS

The following categories of patients should be given special consideration:

1. Infants and children < 2 years with nonspecific findings, bulging anterior fontanelle, altered mental status as the neuro evaluation is difficult and moreover findings are nonspecific and difficult to interpret
2. Children with in situ shunt—hydrocephalus
3. Bleeding or coagulation disorders such as hemophilia
4. Platelet disorders or platelet dysfunction
5. Arteriovenous malformation
6. Nonaccidental trauma, child abuse
7. Pediatric GCS of ≤14.

CLINICAL FEATURES

It depends upon the severity of injury and involvement of brain and adjoining structure. The usual features include headache, which may be severe, vomiting, confusion, altered mental status defined as a pediatric GCS ≤ 14, seizure, lethargy, focal deficit, obtundation, or signs of a basilar skull fracture, such as Battle sign, periorbital ecchymosis, hemotympanum, and CSF otorrhea or rhinorrheas.

Altered mental status, pupillary changes, bradycardia, hypertension, and respiratory depression are signs of impending cerebral herniation. Children < 2 years of age provide a unique challenge to the emergency department (ED) physician, as they commonly present after minor trauma but may be asymptomatic or clinical assessment may be difficult. Additionally, the clinician must always have a low index of suspicion for nonaccidental trauma, keeping the possibilities of child abuse.

Historical features that may suggest an increased risk of brain injury:
- Abnormal behavior in young children noticed by mother, though not recognized by ED physician
- Seizure, confusion, or loss of consciousness (>5 minutes)
- Severe or worsening headache
- Vomiting more than times after fall
- High-risk mechanism, such as a fall from greater than three times the height of child, significant motor vehicle collision, penetrating, inflicted injury, or unwitnessed fall.

Physical findings that may suggest an increased risk of brain injury:
- Scalp abnormalities, such as hematoma > 3 cm in nonfrontal area, tenderness, or depression
- In infants, bulging anterior fontanel
- Abnormal mental status
- Focal neurologic abnormality
- Signs of basilar skull fracture.

Importance of radioimaging in head trauma:
- ciTBI needs to be recognized and dealt appropriately.
- It is important to not subject patients to unnecessary scans as though less but definite increase in the incidence of malignancy (leukemia) in children subjected to radiation of CT (1 in 1,500).

Indications of CT scan in TBI:
- All ciTBI
- Progressive headache
- Worsening level of consciousness
- Loss of consciousness for >5 minutes
- Focal or abnormal neurological findings
- Signs of a basal or depressed skull fracture
- Persistent seizure or vomiting.

Red flags: The diagnostically challenging patient population are the children in the intermediate-risk category. "Fast MRI" techniques are now being used to assess TBI. MRI utilizing T1, T2, and fluid-attenuated inversion recovery (FLAIR) images is more sensitive allowing delineation of the nature and timing of hemorrhage. Additionally, diffusion-weighted imaging (DWI) are helpful to outline hypoxic–ischemic or DAI. There is no role of X-ray of skull.

Disposition: Minor TBI:
- Cervical spine should be stabilized in cases of RTA.
- Perform neuroimaging only in patients with high-risk signs or symptoms.
- Observation for 6 hours after the injury may offer an alternative to emergent neuroimaging.
- Observation can be done at home by a compliant care giver or in the ER/Clinic itself if condition prevails.

Moderate and severe TBI: Infants and children should receive intensive care unit (ICU) monitoring. Care involves a multidisciplinary team comprising pediatric caregivers from neurologic surgery, critical care medicine, surgery, and rehabilitation, and is directed at preventing secondary insults and managing raised ICP. Initial stabilization of infants and children with severe TBI should follow traditional ABCDE approach. Rapid sequence intubation with spine stabilization along with maintenance of normal extracerebral hemodynamic (e.g., mean arterial pressure) including blood gas values (PaO_2, $PaCO_2$) is crucial for better outcome.

Hypotension is to be treated with fluid boluses and hypotonic fluids should be avoided; normal saline is the fluid of choice. Vasopressors may be needed as guided by monitoring of central venous pressure, with avoidance of both fluid overload and exacerbation of brain edema. A trauma survey should be performed. Once stabilized, the patient should be taken for CT scanning to rule out the need for emergency neurosurgical intervention. If surgery is not required, an ICP monitor should be inserted to guide the treatment of intracranial hypertension. One should be cautious about the herniation (pupillary dilation, systemic hypertension, bradycardia, extensor posturing) during treatment and it should be treated as a medical emergency, with use of hyperventilation, oxygen, sedation and agents to lower the raised ICP, either mannitol (0.25–1.0 g/kg IV) or hypertonic saline (3% solution, 5–10 mL/kg IV).

Intracranial pressure should be maintained at <20 mm Hg. Age-dependent cerebral perfusion pressure (CPP) should be targeted are (approximately 50 mm Hg for children 2–6-years old; 55 mm Hg for those 7–10 years old; and 65 mm Hg for those 11–16 years old).

Primary survey assessment and ongoing management include elevation of the head of the bed, ensuring midline positioning of the head, controlled mechanical ventilation, and analgesia and sedation (i.e., narcotics and benzodiazepines). Neuromuscular blockade may be given under EEG monitoring to check for status epilepticus. This complication will not be recognized in a paralyzed patient and is associated with increased ICP and unfavorable outcome. Besides therapeutic CSF drainage, use of osmolar agents, hypertonic saline (often given as a continuous infusion of 3% saline at 0.1–1.0 mL/kg/h), and mannitol (0.25–1.0 g/kg IV over 20 minutes) can be used to decrease raised ICP. Use of hypertonic saline is more common and has stronger literature support than mannitol, although both are used. It is recommended to avoid serum osmolality > 320 mOsm/L. A urinary catheter should be placed to monitor urine output. Causes of refractory raised ICP to treatment includes unrecognized hypercarbia, hypoxemia, fever, hypotension, hypoglycemia, pain, and seizures, which should be recognized early for better outcome. Repeat imaging should be considered to rule out a surgical lesion. Hyperventilation ($PaCO_2$ 25–30 mm Hg) can be a possible option in some studies. Evidence favoring second-tier therapy is limited. Surgical decompressive craniectomy is a possible option and used in selective centers. Other modalities is using pentobarbital infusion, with a loading dose of 5–10 mg/kg over 30 minutes followed by 5 mg/kg every hour for three doses and then maintenance with an infusion of 1 mg/kg/h. Careful blood pressure monitoring is required because of the possibility of drug-induced hypotension and the frequent need for support with fluids and vasopressors.

Role of hypothermia [32–34°C (89.6–93.2°F)] is controversial but, hyperthermia should be avoided and if present should be treated aggressively. Sedation and neuromuscular blockade are used to prevent shivering, and rewarming should be slow, no faster than 1°C (1.8°F) every 4–6 hours. Hypotension should be prevented during rewarming.

Flowchart 1 is specifically presented for severe TBI, for which the experience with ICP-directed therapy is greatest. Nevertheless, the general approach provided here is relevant to the management of intracranial hypertension in other conditions for which evidence-based data on ICP monitoring and ICP-directed therapy are lacking. The ICP and CPP targets are discussed in the text. (Based on 2012 guidelines for the management of severe TBI, along with minor modifications from later literature).

SUPPORTIVE CARE

Complications of injury or ongoing treatment should be kept in mind and treated. It includes transient cortical

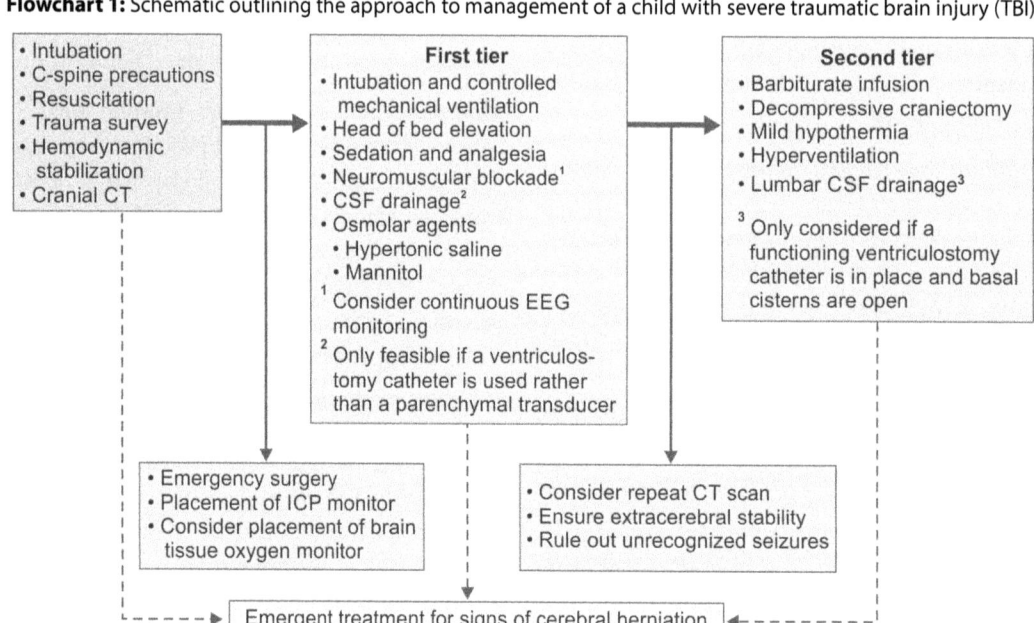

Flowchart 1: Schematic outlining the approach to management of a child with severe traumatic brain injury (TBI).

(CSF: cerebrospinal fluid; CT: computed tomography; EEG: electroencephalography; ICP: intracranial pressure)

blindness, seizures, cranial nerve palsy, diabetes insipidus, syndrome of inappropriate antidiuretic hormone secretion (SIADH), cortical venous occlusion, hemiparesis, SIADH, cerebral salt wasting (CSW), seizures and severe hyperglycemia (to be kept below 200 mg/dL). Prophylaxis anticonvulsant can be stated. Management and care of airway, breathing, circulation should go hand in hand. Early nutrition with enteral feedings is advocated. Corticosteroids should generally not be used unless adrenal insufficiency is documented.

KEY MESSAGES

- Though nonspecific, headache is a common presenting symptom.
- Most injuries are minor that do not necessitate radioimaging and clinical interventions.
- Infants with head injuries may appear to be asymptomatic due to limitations in their neurologic examination.
- TBI in children carries good outcome, if resuscitated and referred early to a neurotrauma center, and managed subsequently on an individualized basis with a well-organized team approach.
- Poor prognosis is noticeable in age group < 4 years, with better outcomes in the age group of 5–15 years.
- Severe TBI in children has a poor outcome.

SUGGESTED READING

1. Gururaj G, Kolluri SV, Chandramouli BA, Subbakrishna DK, Kraus JF. (2005). Traumatic brain injury. [online] Available from: https://nimhans.ac.in/wp-content/uploads/2021/02/Traumatic-Brain-Injury-Report.pdf. [Last accessed November, 2021].
2. Kochanek PM, Bell MJ. Neurologic emergencies and stabilization. In: Kliegman RM, St Geme JW III, Blum NJ, Shah SS, Tasker RC, Wilson KM, Behrman RE (eds). Nelson's Textbook of Pediatrics, 21st edition. Canada: Elsevier; 2020. pp. 557-63.
3. Kochanek PM, Carney N, Adelson PD, Ashwal S, Bell MJ, Bratton S, et al: Guidelines for the acute medical management of severe traumatic brain injury in infants, children, and adolescents-second edition. Pediatr Crit Care Med. 2012;13 Suppl 1:S1-82.
4. Levin HS, Aldrich EF, Saydjari C, Eisenberg HM, Foulkes MA, Bellefleur M, et al. Severe head injury in children: Experience of the traumatic coma data bank. Neurosurgery. 1992;31:435-43.
5. Macmanemy JK, Ji A. Neurotrauma. In: Shaw KN, Bachur RG. Textbook of Pediatric Emergency Medicine, 7th edition. Philadelphia: Wolters Kluwer. pp. 1280-7.
6. Mahapatra AK, Kumar R. Pediatric head injury. In: Mahapatra AK, Kumar R, Kamal R (eds). Textbook of Head Injury. Delhi: Jaypee Brothers Medical Publishers; 2012. pp. 180-90.
7. Satpathy MC, Dash D, Mishra SS, Tripathy SR, Nath PC, Jena SP. Spectrum and outcome of traumatic brain injury in children <15 years: tertiary level experience in India. Int J Crit Illn Inj Sci. 2016;6:16-20.
8. Teasdale G, Jennett B. Assessment of coma and impaired consciousness. A practical scale. Lancet. 1974;2:81.

SECTION 10: Cardiology

118. Approach to a Neonate with Congenital Heart Diseases
119. Approach to a Child with Cyanotic Heart Disease
120. Ventricular Septal Defect
121. Atrial Septal Defect
122. Patent Ductus Arteriosus
123. Endocardial Cushion Defect
124. Tetrology of Fallot
125. Transposition of Great Arteries
126. Complex Congenital Heart Disease
127. Kawasaki Disease (Cardiac Manifestation)
128. Anomalous Left Coronary Artery Originating from Pulmonary Artery
129. Myocardial Disease
130. Pericardial Disease
131. Pulmonary Hypertension
132. Cardiac Failure
133. Cardiomyopathy in Children
134. Cardiac Arrhythmias
135. Infective Endocarditis

CHAPTER 118: Approach to a Neonate with Congenital Heart Diseases

Tapas Som

WHAT ARE CONGENITAL HEART DEFECTS?

Congenital means the disease or the condition exists at or from birth. Congenital heart defects or diseases (CHDs) are heart diseases with which a newborn baby is born. CHDs are the most common congenital birth defects. These can be structural defects or functional defects including rhythm problems. CHDs may be simple or complex and can have mild or severe consequences.

Mild diseases may not need any treatment. Critical CHDs are those heart defects that need surgery or other treatment within the first year of life. Without treatment, critical CHDs may have adverse consequences on the health and survival of infants and children. Sometimes, critical CHDs may need multiple surgeries over the several years.

In the USA, approximately 8 in 1,000 babies are born with CHDs every year, and 25% of them have critical CHD. In India, approximately the incidence is 10-12 per 1,000 live births excluding the small ventricular (VSD) and atrial septal defects (ASD) that close spontaneously within a year of birth.

WHEN DO WE SUSPECT HEART DISEASES IN A NEWBORN BABY?

- At first, we must remember that several diseases of the mother or medications consumed by the mother during pregnancy may increase the risk of CHDs in the fetus.
  - *Maternal lupus*: In mothers with systemic lupus erythematosus (SLE), autoantibodies may pass through the placental barrier and can damage the fetal heart. A large population-based study suggested that neonates born to women with SLE have an increased risk of CHDs with an odds ratio (OR) of 2.62 [95% confidence interval (CI): 1.77-3.88]. Apart from congenital heart block (owing to Anti-SSA/Ro and Anti-SSB/La), offspring of SLE mothers have substantially increased risk of ASD, VSD, and valve anomalies.
  - *Maternal phenylketonuria (PKU)*: A study has described that the babies born to mothers with uncontrolled PKU had an increased risk of CHDs. These are coarctation of the aorta (CoA) and hypoplastic left heart syndrome (HLHS). CHDs have been noticed in mothers with PKU who had PKU level >15 mg/dL by the eighth gestational weeks.
  - *Maternal diabetes mellitus (DM)*: Studies have revealed CHDs in the offspring of mothers with both pregestational and gestational DM. Common defects are atrioventricular septal defects, tetralogy of Fallot (TOF), transposition of great arteries (TGA), CoA, and HLHS. Studies also suggest that interventions achieving glycemic control during pregestational and early gestational periods reduced the burden of occurrence of CHDs. A study mentioned that women with gestational DM might have a similar risk of having fetal CHDs as in women with pregestational DM. This risk is possibly secondary to hyperglycemia, insulin resistance, and undiagnosed pregestational DM.
  - *Maternal rubella*: A meta-analysis has demonstrated a significantly increased risk of CHDs with OR of 3.49 (95% CI: 2.39-5.11) in offspring of mothers with rubella infection in the first half of pregnancy. CHDs are common when the mother is infected during the first 10-12 weeks of gestation, whereas defects are uncommon after 18 weeks of gestation, although fetuses may be infected. Common CHDs in decreasing order of frequency are patent ductus arteriosus (PDA), peripheral pulmonary stenosis (PPS), and septal defects.
  - *Folic acid antagonists*: There are two groups of antagonists. One group is folic acid reductase inhibitors such as trimethoprim and methotrexate. Another group consists of antiepileptics such as phenytoin, valproic acid, carbamazepine, and phenobarbitone. These second group of drugs either degrade or impair absorption from the intestine. An increased risk of CHDs is observed after intrauterine exposure to trimethoprim or methotrexate (HLHS and CoA). All antiepileptics mentioned above are associated with an increased risk of CHDs [Relative

risk (RR): 2.2 with a 95% CI of 1.4–3.5]. Fetal hydantoin syndrome is known to be associated with phenytoin use during pregnancy. Antenatal use of valproic acid is associated with ASD, VSD, and TOF. Recommended daily folate intake is 4 mg to be started before conception to the end of the first trimester to reduce the risk of developing neural tube defects and CHDs.

- *Angiotensin-converting enzyme (ACE) inhibitors*: An increased risk of CHDs is noted following the use of ACE inhibitors in early pregnancy (OR: 2.89; 95% CI: 1.41–5.91) in a recent study.
- Common defects related to the use of ACE inhibitors are VSD, pulmonary stenosis (PS), CoA, and ostium secundum ASD (OS ASD).
- *Lithium*: A systematic review estimated the risk for Ebstein anomaly after exposure to lithium in the first trimester of pregnancy to be 0.05–0.1%. Pregnant women treated with lithium should be monitored for congenital cardiac defects.
- *Drinking alcohol during pregnancy*: A meta-analysis has suggested that maternal alcohol consumption is significantly associated with increased risk of CHDs in the fetus with OR of 1.12 with 95% CI of 1.02–1.22. Specific CHD having a significant correlation was with TOF. Further, the analysis suggested a significant association (OR: 1.48 with 95% CI of 1.22–1.80) between paternal alcohol consumption and CHDs.
- *Smoking*: Women who smoke anytime during the month before pregnancy or during the first 3 months of pregnancy are more likely to have a baby with a CHD than women who do not smoke. The study also supports the dose-dependent nature of the association and augmented risk in older mothers. Common lesions are pulmonary artery anomalies (OR: 1.71), pulmonary valve anomalies (OR: 1.48), and isolated ASDs (OR: 1.22).
- Nowadays, increased use of ultrasonography during pregnancy and increased number of experts in fetal medicine in our country have led to the diagnosis of an increased number of fetuses with CHDs during anomaly scan or fetal echocardiography before 20 weeks or later.

- Several babies are born with birth defects. Approximately 30% of CHDs appears to be related to genetic syndromes. Some of the common syndromes with CHDs are mentioned here.
  - *Down syndrome*: Neonates born with Down syndrome will have characteristic facial dysmorphism. This may be associated with various other congenital anomalies, including cardiac and gastrointestinal defects. All these are attributed to the presence of extra copy of chromosome 21. Conventional karyotyping usually confirms the diagnosis. Common cardiac defects associated with Down syndrome are atrioventricular canal defects, ASDs, VSDs, and TOF.
  - *Turner syndrome*: This is a chromosomal abnormality caused by the absence of or structural anomalies in the X chromosome. This syndrome manifests with different clinical features in girls, including short stature, infertility, and cardiac and renal anomalies. Conventional karyotyping confirms the diagnosis. Cardiovascular malformations are noted in approximately 25–45% live born girls. The most common abnormalities are bicuspid aortic valve (16%) and CoA (14%). Partial anomalous pulmonary venous connection return (PAPVC) and the VSD can also be found.
  - *Noonan syndrome*: This is an autosomal dominant disorder (12q22 qter) manifested with variable features, including short stature, CHD, and facial dysmorphism. Facial dysmorphism includes hypertelorism, downslanting palpebral fissures, ptosis, and low-set posteriorly rotated ears. The most frequent cardiac anomalies are PS with dysplastic valve leaflets (50–65%), hypertrophic cardiomyopathy (20%), and OS ASD (6–10%). DNA sequencing analyses are required to confirm the diagnosis.
  - *Williams syndrome*: This is due to the microdeletion of chromosome 7q11.23. This manifests with characteristic facies that includes depressed nasal bridge, short palpebral fissures, blue eyes, anteverted nares, long philtrum, prominent lips with an open mouth (100%), and CHDs (75–80%) mainly with supravalvular aortic stenosis (AS), CoA, and idiopathic hypercalcemia (15%). This can be diagnosed with the help of the fluorescence in situ hybridization (FISH) technique.
  - *DiGeorge syndrome (CATCH-22)*: This is due to the microdeletion of 22q11.2. Most of the affected children present with CHDs, facial dysmorphism, palatal clefts, hypocalcemia, and immunodeficiency. FISH technique with TUPLE or N25 probes or array comparative genomic hybridization (aCGH) and multiplex ligation-dependent probe amplification (MLPA) can diagnose this condition. The most frequent cardiac anomalies are conotruncal defects, TOF (20%), interrupted aortic arch (IAA) type B (13%), truncus arteriosus (TA) (6%), and VSDs.
  - In addition to those mentioned above, innumerable numbers of genetic syndromes are associated with CHDs. Some of these are Trisomy 18 (VSD), Trisomy 13 (VSD), Kabuki syndrome (CoA), Alagille syndrome (PPS), del 4 p (PS), Holt-Oram syndrome (ASD), CHARGE (TOF, IAA, TA)/VACTERL (vertebral defects, anal atresia, cardiac defects, tracheoesophageal fistula, renal anomalies, and limb abnormalities)

association, Cornelia de Lange syndrome, Carpenter syndrome (PDA, PS), Rubinstein-Taybi, Smith-Lemli-Opitz syndrome.

- Several metabolic diseases (inborn errors of metabolism, known as IEM) are associated with CHDs. Although individual IEM is rare, when considered collectively, the incidence of IEM is approximately 1 in 1,000–3,000. About 5% of all IEMs are associated with CHDs. A few are mentioned here:
  - *Pompe disease*: The common IEMs causing hypertrophic cardiomyopathy (HCM) are glycogen storage disorders. The most common of these is Pompe disease.
  - *PRKAG2*: This is a syndrome of disordered glycogen metabolism characterized by HCM and an electric accessory pathway that may lead to arrhythmia [Wolff-Parkinson-White (WPW) and atrial fibrillation] and sudden death.
  - *Kearns-Sayre syndrome*: This is due to large mitochondrial deletion ± duplications in most of the cases. It is characterized by conduction disturbances in the heart that include prolonged intraventricular conduction time, bundle branch blocks, and complete heart block.
  - Several other IEMs can also lead to different types of cardiomyopathies (dilated cardiomyopathy/HCM), and arrhythmias. These are organic acidemias, fatty acid oxidation disorders, carnitine deficiency, and congenital glycosylation disorders.

HOW CAN WE DIAGNOSE CONGENITAL HEART DISEASES IN AN ASYMPTOMATIC NEWLY BORN BABY?

During Pregnancy

Fetal heart diseases may be suspected on the ground of maternal predisposition to fetal CHDs (diseases, medications during pregnancy, and lifestyle), family and sibling history of CHDs, and based on antenatal findings such as increased nuchal thickness, positive pregnancy markers, or positive anomaly scan. In these situations, if available fetal echocardiography around 20 weeks of gestation may be advised to suggest or refute specific CHDs **(Table 1)**.

After Birth

Once the mother arrives at a hospital for labor/delivery, antenatal records should be checked for pertinent reports of suspected fetal CHD. These include medical diseases in pregnancy, medication records, family history, and health records of the previous child if applicable, antenatal USG, and fetal echocardiography report, if any available.

Suspicion of CHDs while Resuscitating a Newborn Baby

Suspect clinically when a baby appears cyanosed after successful resuscitation. Pulse oximeter saturation is below the target range in room air while the baby is breathing spontaneously. The heart rate is above 100 beats per minute. Oxygen saturation is below 95% despite the administration of free-flow oxygen, and the baby is not showing features of respiratory distress. In this situation, consider to rule out CHD even in the absence of any abnormal findings such as murmur over precordium or back of chest or nonpalpable femoral pulses.

Suspicion of CHD in the Immediate Postnatal Period

Baby should be examined immediately after birth from head to toe for the detection of abnormal findings. Rarely, we may hear murmurs secondary to obstructive lesions such as PS or AS. On subsequent examination within 24 hours after birth, the cardiovascular system should be evaluated thoroughly that includes the following, which may suggest CHD:

- *Inspection*: Cyanosis, edema (rarely, seen in hydropic infants)
- *Palpation*: Palpation of peripheral pulses (rate, rhythm, volume, equality), apex of heart (for determination of situs), liver (situs and hepatomegaly), blood pressure (BP) in four limbs (CoA, IAA)
- *Auscultation*: Auscultation of heart sounds (intensity, murmur), bruit (skull/ liver/back of chest)

TABLE 1: Indications for fetal echocardiography.

Fetus	Maternal-related	Family-related
Suspected CHD on antenatal USG/anomaly scan	*Maternal diseases*: CHD, SLE, diabetes, PKU	Previous child or parent with CHD
Suspected chromosomal anomaly	Mother receiving cardiac teratogenic medications	
Fetal: Extracardiac anomalies	*History maternal*: Alcohol consumption, and smoking	Previous child or parent with genetic diseases associated with CHD
Fetal arrhythmia	Rubella infection	

(CHD: congenital heart disease; PKU: phenylketonuria; SLE: systemic lupus erythematosus; USG: ultrasonography)

Pulse oximetry screening for critical CHDs must be performed in all asymptomatic babies before discharge from the hospital. Four-limb BP should also be measured to rule out CoA or IAA (upper limb BP > lower limb BP by >10 mm Hg).

Pulse Oximetry Screening

Principle: Current evidence suggests that routine clinical examination may miss 25% of newborns with critical CHD. On the other hand, most of the newborns with critical CHD can be treated successfully in a center with optimal facilities upon early diagnosis by echocardiography and subsequent corrective measures to improve overall outcome. Although to date, barring a few centers, optimal facilities have not yet been developed in many cities in India.

Studies have defined reference range for oxygen saturation in healthy newborns during their first 24 hours of life. The median value at 20–24 hours of life (97.8%) is similar to the results for healthy full-term newborns between 2 and 7 days old (97.6 %). However, in duct-dependent (pulmonary or systemic) circulation, saturation will be below 95% in lower limbs or difference between right upper limb (RH) (preductal) and lower limb (RF) (postductal) will be higher than 3%. Generally, the difference in saturation between RH and RF is less than 1%. Echocardiography should be planned for screening positive neonates **(Table 2)**.

Screening Procedure

Methemoglobinemia: It is a clinical condition characterized by the presence of hemoglobin that contains an increased amount of oxidized iron (Fe^{3+}). Methemoglobin cannot carry oxygen and causes varying degrees of cyanosis. Methemoglobinemia can be because of HbM variants or deficiency of the NADH cytb5 reductase enzyme. In this condition, newborns will have cyanosis, and oxygen saturation will be low. However, on arterial blood gas (ABG) analysis, PaO_2 will be high despite cyanosis and calculated oxygen saturation (SaO_2) will be normal. In congenital cyanotic heart diseases, both PaO_2 and oxygen saturation will be low despite supplemental oxygen therapy. Blood containing higher methemoglobin concentration will turn the color of blood into chocolate brown. This can be tested by putting a drop of blood of the baby on a blotting paper beside a drop of normal blood.

Persistent pulmonary hypertension: In this condition, the baby presents with or without differential cyanosis, oxygen saturation on pulse oximeter will be low. An ABG analysis, PaO_2, will be low, and calculated saturation will be low despite supplemental oxygen therapy. The difference in oxygen saturation between the right upper limb and lower limb will be more than 10%.

WHAT ARE THE SIGNS AND SYMPTOMS OF CONGENITAL HEART DISEASES?

Many newborns with CHD will have no signs and symptoms in the beginning.

Signs and symptoms for CHDs depend on the type and severity of the particular defect. Once the pulmonary pressure will decrease, or the ductus will start closing, many newborns with duct-dependent CHDs will develop cyanosis. Significant hypoxemia may result in visible cyanosis. Generally, 3–5 g of deoxygenated hemoglobin is required to produce central cyanosis. Cyanosis will be visible in a newborn baby with hemoglobin of 16 g/dL when arterial oxygen saturation is 75%; similarly, when hemoglobin content is 10 g/dL, the oxygen saturation must be 60% before cyanosis is apparent. With mild hypoxemia, with arterial oxygen saturation of 80–95%, cyanosis will not be apparent. Moreover, the identification of cyanosis is particularly problematic in neonates with pigmented skin.

Sometimes depending on the etiology, the baby might present with features of heart failure. Feeding difficulty is the most prominent symptom of heart failure in a neonate. It will be associated with tachypnea, tachycardia, and perspiration. Respiratory rate will be increased (>60/min), and it is related to lung stiffness secondary to increased interstitial fluids. Depending on the severity, tachypnea may be associated with grunting, nasal flaring, and intercostal retractions. Edema is extremely rare in newborns except in conditions with hydrops fetalis. Do not forget to check the pulse for rate (bradycardia: complete heart block, tachycardia: tachyarrhythmia), rhythm (irregular: ectopics, fibrillation), volume (low: shock), and equality (delay/nonpalpable femorals: CoA, IAA).

Cold extremities, weakly palpable pulses, low blood pressure with narrow pulse pressure may be noted in low output states. Mottling of extremities with increased capillary refill times is seen in severely compromised states.

Neonates with cardiomyopathy will have quiet precordium; on the other hand, neonates with obstructive lesions thrill will be felt. Murmurs will be audible in obstructive (PS, AS) lesions, regurgitating lesions (MR, TR) and lesions with shunts (PDA, VSD).

TABLE 2: List of critical CHDs that can be identified using pulse oximeter screening.

d-TGA	Tetralogy of Fallot
HLHS	Total anomalous pulmonary venous connection
Pulmonary atresia	• Tricuspid atresia • Truncus arteriosus

(d-TGA: dextro-transposition of the great arteries; HLHS: hypoplastic left heart syndrome)

WHAT INVESTIGATIONS DO WE NEED TO PERFORM TO CONFIRM CHDs?

- *Chest X-ray (CXR)*: Radiological features will depend on the type and severity of the lesion. Specific points are to be remembered when exposing a neonate for CXR. CXR should be obtained in anteroposterior (AP) view from a reasonable distance (tube to baby distance at least 45 cm). X-ray tube should be aligned with both planes (horizontal and vertical). Exposure factors should be optimal to obtain a useful X-ray (mAs and KV). Preferably digital radiography be used to decrease radiation exposure. X-ray plate should be marked for side determination (situs). The baby should be positioned correctly to prevent rotation.
    - *Cardiomegaly*: Cardiothoracic ratio should be measured, and it should be >0.6.
- *Features of heart failure*: CXR almost always will demonstrate cardiomegaly except in cases of obstructed TAPVC. Plethoric lung fields will be noted in those with heart failure secondary to a large left-to-right shunt, and a diffuse haziness secondary to pulmonary venous congestion.
    - *Ebstein anomaly*: Enlarged cardiac silhouette with narrow main pulmonary artery segment with oligemic lung fields.
    - *Dextro TGA (d-TGA)*: Enlarged cardiac silhouette with egg on side appearance with plethoric lung fields with a narrow base.
    - *Obstructed TAPVC*: The cardiac silhouette appears normal. However, its margins become obscured owing to lung haziness secondary to pulmonary venous obstruction.
    - *TOF*: Normal cardiac silhouette looks like a boot with oligemic lung fields.
- *Electrocardiogram (also called ECG)*: This is often helpful to arrive at a diagnosis where echocardiography facility is not readily available. However, this is extremely helpful for the diagnosis of arrhythmias. A few diagnostic ECGs are mentioned below.
- *ALCAPA (anomalous left coronary artery from the pulmonary artery)*: It shows abnormal q waves in L1, aVL, V3–V6, and T wave inversion in the same leads.
- *Ebstein anomaly*: Large, bifid P waves with QRS complex suggestive of right bundle branch block (RBBB) with R wave in V1 < 7 mm and widened S in V6.
- *Tricuspid atresia*: Left axis deviation with left ventricular hypertrophy (LVH).
- *Arrhythmias*: These can be of bradyarrhythmias, tachyarrhythmias, and irregular rhythms.
- *Hyperoxia test*: This test may be considered in all newborns with suspected cyanotic CHDs, especially where echocardiography facility is not readily available. PaO_2 should be measured from ABG analysis or using transcutaneous oxygen monitor at both preductal (right hand) and postductal sites. It is to investigate the possibility of a fixed intracardiac right-to-left shunt. PaO_2 is measured in room air and repeated while the newborn is receiving 100% oxygen at least for 10 minutes through hood. In presence of intracardiac mixing, PaO_2 does not exceed 100 mm Hg and rise is not more than 10–30 mm Hg (failed). Whereas a PaO_2 of >250 mm Hg (passed) in both limbs virtually eliminates cyanotic CHDs. For differential cyanosis, right hand PaO_2 will be 10–15 mm higher than that of lower limb. Prostaglandin E1 (PGE1) infusion should be initiated in a neonate who fails the hyperoxia test until an echocardiographic confirmation is made.
- *Echocardiogram*: Echocardiography, including 2D, Doppler, and Color Doppler, is an essential tool in the diagnosis and management of cardiac diseases in the neonate. Entire cardiac anatomy can be delineated through various windows (subcostal, apical, parasternal, suprasternal, and ductal). Functional assessment can be done using M mode and 2D mode. Doppler studies are useful to assess flow in the descending aorta as in CoA. Continuous wave Doppler is used to estimate right ventricular pressure in presence of TR by measuring the gradient between RV and RA. Color Doppler is used to visualize the direction of blood flow through shunts (PDA), regurgitant valves, and septal defects (ASD and VSD).
- *Cardiac catheterization*: Cardiac catheterization is rarely required for anatomic diagnosis now. However, it is used in conditions to elaborate the anatomy of coronary arteries, distal pulmonary arteries, aortopulmonary collaterals in TOF with pulmonary atresia. Increasingly it is performed for therapeutic purposes in CHDs.
- *Magnetic resonance imaging (MRI)*: Cardiac MRI (CMR) is a useful adjunct in diagnosing structures that are difficult to visualize by echocardiography, such as aortic arch and distal pulmonary arteries. This evaluates quantitative ventricular function for different reasons, especially in postoperative cases.

MANAGEMENT OF CHDs

General

Congenital heart diseases in neonates can be classified into four broad groups: (1) Acyanotic CHDs consist of ASD, VSD, PDA, AS, PS, CoA and cardiomyopathies associated with IEMs; (2) Cyanotic CHDs are duct-dependent lesions (IAA, HLHS, TOF), lesions with parallel circulation (TGA), lesions with intracardiac mixing (TA, TAPVC, single ventricle). Fourth group is arrhythmias. Acyanotic group can be suspected owing to the presence of murmur, and diagnosis is confirmed by echocardiography. Rarely neonates become symptomatic as a result of heart failure secondary to these obstructive lesions. Cardiomyopathies usually present with features of heart failure.

119 CHAPTER

Approach to a Child with Cyanotic Heart Disease

Kamirul Islam

INTRODUCTION

Cyanosis or bluish purple discoloration of the skin is an important symptom as well as clinical finding. The blue color is a result of the increased presence of deoxygenated hemoglobin (Hb) or some abnormal Hb variants.

Cyanosis is usually caused by the bluish hue imparted by excessive accumulation of a pigment. Most commonly it is reduced or deoxygenated Hb or abnormal Hb pigments such as methemoglobin and sulfhemoglobin.

Cyanosis can be observed in skin or mucous membrane of any part of the body including mouth, nose, trunk, or extremities. The degree of cyanosis is modified by the racial pigmentation of skin and the thickness of the skin. Most observers can appreciate cyanosis at deoxyhemoglobin levels of 5 g/dL.

The terms cyanosis, hypoxia, and hypoxemia are often used interchangeably but connote distinct clinical entities. Hypoxemia is defined as arterial deoxyhemoglobin level ≥ 2.38 g/dL, corresponding to $SaO_2 \leq 80\%$ and $pO_2 \leq 45$ mm Hg in patients with normal amounts of Hb.

Hypoxia is defined as the failure of oxygenation at the tissue level and usually manifests as metabolic acidosis due to anaerobic metabolism. Though they often coincide, hypoxia is neither necessary nor sufficient to produce cyanosis. Children with congenital cyanotic heart disease may have hypoxemia and cyanosis but no hypoxia in presence of adequate cardiac output and Hb levels. Those with severe anemia may however have tissue hypoxia even without hypoxemia and cyanosis.

Patients with Hb abnormalities such as methemoglobinemia on the other hand may have cyanosis in absence of hypoxemia. Only in the presence of adequate Hb level and normal Hb variants, is the absence of cyanosis reassuring to a clinician.

CENTRAL AND PERIPHERAL CYANOSIS

Cyanosis is classified into central, peripheral, and sometimes mixed variants. Central cyanosis is said to be present if the blood leaving the heart in desaturated form. It may occur either due to defect in oxygenation of the blood or due to venous admixture or shunting. Central cyanosis is reflected in both skin of proximal and distal parts as well as in oral mucosa and tongue. Peripheral cyanosis is due to sluggish flow of blood through peripheral capillary network resulting in abnormally greater oxygen extraction from a normally saturated arterial blood. The resulting cyanosis usually spares oral mucosa and tongue. Mixed cyanosis may occur from conditions such as cor pulmonale or pulmonary edema with heart failure where a desaturated arterial blood is rendered even more deoxygenated by slack circulation. It is the underlying dysfunction which determines the type of cyanosis not the area of distribution.

CARDIAC CAUSES OF CYANOSIS

A myriad of heart diseases can cause cyanosis. Most of them result in central cyanosis, though conditions such as heart failure as well as left-sided obstructive heart diseases can cause peripheral cyanosis by diminishing tissue perfusion. Cardiac mechanisms of central cyanosis include right-to-left shunts either due congenital cyanotic heart with decreased pulmonary blood flow (PBF) (Fallot's physiology) or reversal of a left-to-right shunt (Eisenmenger syndrome), and mixing of venous and systemic blood through anatomical defects [dextro-transposition of the great arteries (dTGA) physiology]. By any means, a significant amount of deoxygenated venous blood must come to the systemic circulation without getting arterialized at the alveolar capillary beds.

Though acquired heart diseases can cause cyanosis-like mitral stenosis or regurgitation causing pulmonary edema and alveolar flooding, a large number of children suffer from anatomical and physiological dispositions toward cyanosis called congenital cyanotic heart diseases (CCHD). Estimated two lacs children are born each year in India with CHD and about a quarter of them suffer from CCHD. These vary wildly in their presentation, severity, management, and outcome. There are multiple ways to subclassify them. The PBF forms the convenient and practically useful criteria. Depending on the amount of blood flowing into the arterializing pulmonary circuit, these disorders can be classified as:

- *CCHD with decreased PBF*:
  - Tetralogy of Fallot (ToF)
  - ToF equivalents (Fallot's physiology):
- *CCHD with increased PBF*:
  - d-TGA
  - Taussig–Bing anomaly
  - Total anomalous pulmonary venous return (TAPVR)
  - Truncus arteriosus
- *CCHD with normal PBF*:
  - Pulmonary arteriovenous fistula
  - Anomalous draining of venacava to left atrium (LA)
  - Unroofing of coronary sinus into LA.

Depending on the hemodynamics of various anatomical lesions, the different patterns can be discerned as:

- *Fallot's physiology*: ToF, pulmonary atresia, tricuspid atresia, Ebstein anomaly, TGA with ventricular septal defect (VSD) with pulmonary stenosis (PS).
- *Transposition physiology*: d-TGA, Taussig–Bing anomaly.
- *Mixing lesions*: Truncus arteriosus, double-outlet right ventricle (DORV), TAPVR.
- *Left-sided obstructive lesions*: Hypoplastic left heart syndrome (HLHS), critical coarctation of aorta or interrupted aortic arch.
- *Near-normal physiology*: Pulmonary arteriovenous fistulae (congenital, acquired, cirrhosis).
- *Reversal of initially left-to-right shunts*: ASD, VSD, PDA with Eisenmengerisation.

The last mechanism required prolonged exposure of pulmonary circulation to excessive blood flow causing gradual onset of pulmonary hypertension and subsequent reversal to a right-to-left shunt. Depending on the site and size of lesion, it may take decades [especially in atrial septal defect (ASD)] to appear and is therefore called cyanosis tardive.

DIFFERENTIAL CYANOSIS

It is a condition in which the cyanosis is limited to the lower part of body with a relatively less affected upper body parts, especially face and upper limbs. This is caused by the location of the aortic end of the ductus just beyond the major branches of the aortic arch that supply the face and upper limbs. A typical example is patent ductus arteriosus (PDA) with Eisenmenger syndrome.

REVERSE DIFFERENTIAL CYANOSIS

As the name suggests, in this condition the cyanosis is deeper in the upper part of the body (preductal) than the lower part (postductal). It is classically seen in d-TGA with pulmonary hypertension or preductal aortic coarctation, and rarely in supracardiac TAPVR.

Assessment

In a child presenting with cyanosis, it is essential to identify the organ system involved. Pulmonary and cardiac causes form the bulk of differentials and are often very difficult to distinguish. Tachypnea, distress, retraction, grunting, and flaring of alae nasi are more likely to occur in pulmonary causes of cyanosis. Cardiac cyanotic disorders may also present with tachypnea and tachypnea but with less severe respiratory adjuncts.

Respiratory disorders may present with characteristic auscultatory findings while significant murmur may point toward cardiac diseases. The fallacy is that many cardiac cyanotic lesions may also predispose and indeed present with their respiratory complications making this distinct clinically difficult and most congenital cyanotic heart diseases have unexceptional precordial findings. Once the needle of suspicion moves firmly toward a possible cardiac cause, these arch for individual lesions must proceed in a stepwise manner.

Symptoms

The age of presentation of various cyanotic heart diseases vary and often provides the first clue toward the eventual diagnosis.

- *At birth*: Apparent cyanosis soon after birth is most commonly due to dTGA. Other causes are PS within tact ventricular septum, HLHS, neonatal Ebstein and obstructed total anomalous pulmonary venous connection (TAPVC).
- *Neonatal period*: Admixture lesions, e.g., TAPVC, single ventricle, DORV (subaortic VSD with PS), truncus arteriosus.
- *Infancy*: Usually CHD, hereditary methemoglobinemia
  - 1–3 months of age: Classical age of presentation for Fallot's physiology. Cyanosis in TOF may be apparent from 4 to 6 months of birth depending on degree of right ventricular outflow tract obstruction (RVOTO).
  - 6 months of age: Due to development or progression of RVOTO in patients with VSD.
- *Childhood*: Usually, CHD due to progressive increase in pulmonary vascular resistance and cyanosis secondary to pulmonary arteriovenous fistula.
  - 2–5 years of age: TOF, Eisenmenger complex due to VSD
  - After 10 years of age: Eisenmenger complex due to VSD.

Another important goal is to assess the status of PBF. Patients with increased PBF will have presenting features of failure (respiratory distress, feeding difficulties with "suck-rest-suck" cycle, failure to thrive), repeated pulmonary infections and relatively less severe cyanosis. Those with diminished PBF have history of varying degree of cyanosis (depending on degree of right ventricular outflow tract obstruction), squatting (in older children) and often may present with characteristic hypercyanotic spells. Cyanotic diseases with duct-dependent systemic circulation may present with severe shock and circulatory failure once the ductus closes.

Antenatal history is vital. TGA is associated with maternal diabetes and maternal alcohol consumption, lithium consumption is associated with Ebstein anomaly and maternal phenylketonuria may predispose to (HLHS).

General Examination

Due to chronic hypoxia and increased basal metabolic rate, failure to thrive may be present. Presence of clubbing indicates the chronicity of cyanosis. Polycythemia is present as a compensatory mechanism to ensure tissue oxygen delivery despite decreased saturation. Absence of polycythemia may point toward functional anemia. Presence of certain syndromic features enhances the possibility of coexisting cyanotic heart disease and merits closer evaluation. ToF is more common in children with Down's syndrome, DiGeorge syndrome, Alagille syndrome. HLHS is common in children in Turner syndrome and CHARGE sequence. All conotruncal anomalies are common in velocardiofacial syndrome and truncus arteriosus can be seen with DiGeorge syndrome. Checking on the vitals pulse volume is diminished in left-sided obstructive lesions whereas high-volume pulse with runoff is seen in truncus arteriosus and severe to for pulmonary atresia with extensive collaterals.

Radiofemoral delay may occur with conditions such as Taussig–Bing anomaly and tricuspid atresia. Elevated jugular venous pressure with prominent a-wave and to an extent, v-waves may be seen in tricuspid atresia and pulmonary atresia. A prominent c-wave may be seen in Ebstein anomaly.

Systemic Examination

Cardiac malpositions should be looked for since conditions such as dextrocardia with situs solitus predispose to conditions such as L-TGA. Usually Fallot's physiology have normal cardiac size with quieter precordium whereas hyperactive precordium is a feature of lesions with high PBF, though exceptions abound. Most cyanotic heart diseases have right ventricular dominance while tricuspid atresia, Ebstein's anomaly with hypoplastic right ventricular and nonrestrictive intra-atrial communication have left ventricular dominance. A loud and split first heart sound is characteristic of Ebstein anomaly with characteristic "multiple heart sounds." Most conditions have single loud S2 (loud A2 in TOF, L-TGA and truncus or loud P2 in high PBF physiology or PAH). Wide split S2 in a cyanotic patient in the absence of right ventricular failure indicates TAPVD or single atrium. Left ventricular third heart sound indicates a high PBF. Pulmonary ejection murmur is heard in TOF physiology—length of murmur being inversely proportional to the severity. As the pulmonary artery is vertically oriented in d-TGA, the PS murmur may be heard well in the upper mid sternal or upper right sternal area. A loud VSD-like murmur can be heard in truncus arteriosus and tricuspid atresia. Mitral mid-diastolic rumbling murmur indicates increased pulmonary flow; in a low PBF group, it may indicate tricuspid atresia or pulmonary atresia with intact IVS. Tricuspid mid-diastolic murmur points to TAPVD, single atrium, AV canal defects or Ebstein. Early diastolic murmur could be of aortic regurgitation in TOF, truncus arteriosus or, pulmonary regurgitation in Eisenmenger syndrome. Continuous murmur occurs in a low PBF group (especially pulmonary atresia)—in second left space due to PDA or over the back due to aortopulmonary collaterals. Venous hum persisting despite occlusion of right jugular vein is characteristic of the classical supracardiac variety of TAPVD due to the increased superior vena caval flow.

INVESTIGATIONS

Arterial Blood Gases

In patients with normal Hb level and variants, the arterial gases taken from patient breathing at room air can confirm or reject central cyanosis. Highly elevated $PaCO_2$ usually points toward respiratory or neurological problems. A low pH with metabolic acidosis may be seen in circulatory shock (left-sided obstructive lesions).

Hyperoxia Test

Designed by Jones in 1976, it is an useful method to differentiate between cardiac and respiratory causes of cyanosis especially in neonates. The baby is given 100% oxygen by hood for 10 minutes and preductal (right radial artery) PaO_2 is measured. A rise beyond 250 mm Hg generally argues in favor of respiratory diseases and failure to rise to even 100 mm Hg goes in favor of cardiac diseases. There are significant caveats though children with severe pulmonary diseases such as hyaline membrane disease (HMD).

May not be able to significantly raise their PaO_2 whereas those with cardiac diseases with increased pulmonary flow like TAPVR may see significant rise. In those patients who "fail" the hyperoxia test, hyperventilation test is done to rule out pulmonary hypertension of the newborn (which improves with hyperventilation) from the cyanotic heart diseases.

Electrocardiography

The ECG can be used to assess cardiac rhythm, atrial situs, ventricular dominance and electrical axis. It is very suggestive in tricuspid atresia (left axis deviation, right atrial hypertrophy and left ventricular hypertrophy) and Ebstein anomaly (RBBB) without increased right precordial voltage, normal or tall and broad P-waves, and a normal or prolonged P-R interval). Dilated atrium and presence of Wolff-Parkinson-White (WPW) may result in tachyarrhythmias in WPW syndrome. Most CCHD will have right ventricular or biventricular hypertrophy. Prominent left-sided forces indicate increased PBF and absence of right ventricular forces indicate tricuspid atresia and pulmonary atresia with intact ventricular septum.

Chest Radiograph

It can be useful to provide information about visceroatrial situs, ventricular dominance, position of great vessels and PBF.

Some CCHDs have characteristically defined appearances; boot-shaped/Coeur en sabot (TOF), egg-on-side/egg-on-string (TGA), massive cardiomegaly/box-shaped heart (Ebstein anomaly), figure of 8/Snowmen appearance (supracardiac TAPVC after a few months of life) and massive pulmonary edema obscuring the cardiac shadow (obstructive variety of TAPVR). Right-sided aortic arch may be seen in case of ToF, pulmonary atresia with VSD and truncus arteriosus.

Echocardiography

It is diagnostic in nearly all CHD and can provide a wide array of information from cardiac structural lesions, functional capacity of both ventricles, degree of PBF, associated anomalies and sometimes, pattern of coronary artery distribution. In children, transthoracic echocardiography is usually sufficient and transesophageal echocardiography is required only in rare instances (such as intraoperative echocardiography). Doppler echocardiography provides additional information on the direction and speed (velocity) of moving blood.

Cardiac Catheterization

Despite diminished diagnostic applications (precise delineation coronary artery anatomy, measuring pulmonary vascular resistance); the therapeutic uses have become frequent. An important indication is to dilate any restricted interatrial communication (Rashkind surgery) in d-TGA, tricuspid atresia or HLHS.

MEDICAL MANAGEMENT

A. In newborn presenting with cyanosis or older children will severe illness, the patient is first stabilized and hypoglycemia, hypocalcemia, and hypothermia should be corrected. Oxygen should be administered because it may help lower pulmonary vascular resistance and improve PBF. If duct-dependent lesions are suspected, PGE1 infusion at 0.05 µg/kg/min may be started to keep the ductus open even before the full diagnostic workup is complete. Significant adverse effects include apnea, seizures, jitteriness and peripheral vasodilation. Once stabilized children should be referred to the nearest center equipped to deal with such cases.

B. Infants and some older children in Fallot's physiology may present with hypercyanotic spells. It is necessary to break the viscous cycle that underlies its pathology. One or more of the following may be needed:
   - Quieting the child and knee–chest positioning
   - Administration of oxygen
   - Morphine sulfate 0.2 mg/kg administered SC or IM
   - Sodium bicarbonate 1 mEq/kg; can be repeated after 10–15 minutes

   Patients not responding may require escalation of therapy including ketamine, propranolol, phenylephrine, and noradrenaline. Decreasing cyanosis and increasing pulmonary ejection murmur portends response to therapy. Oral propranolol therapy (0.5–1.5 mg/kg every 6 hourly) can be used to prevent hypoxic spells.

C. Anticongestive medications may be required if failure develops.

D. Relative iron deficiency state should be detected and treated in these patients. Clinical examination cannot detect the state of relative iron deficiency.

Surgical Management

This includes palliative surgeries to maintain adequate oxygenation of blood till the child can undergo complete repairs and definitive corrective surgeries. The timing of various operations are determined by the underlying defect, associated abnormalities, general health of the child and institutional protocols. Patients with extremely complex heart lesions and those with ischemic cardiomyopathy may require transplant.

Monitoring

Every child with CCHD requires long-term follow-up, even those undergoing corrective surgeries. The child requires general health maintenance, including a well-balanced "heart-healthy" diet, aerobic exercise (within the confines of varying levels of activity limitation). Appropriate immunization with inclusion of pneumococcal and influenza vaccines should be administered. In young infants, prophylaxis against respiratory syncytial virus (RSV) should be considered in RSV seasons. Growth monitoring should be regularly done. Care should be taken to maintain iron sufficiency as well as prevent conditions predisposing to hyperviscosity, especially dehydration. Postoperative patients should be monitored for development of heart failure or late arrhythmias. For patients with residual defects or those with prosthetic materials should be given prophylaxis against subacute bacterial endocarditis (SBE). Those with residual cyanosis after surgery should be monitored for noncardiac manifestations of oxygen insufficiency. Adolescents should be thoroughly counseled about need for avoiding smoking and atherogenic dietary habits. Adequate counseling and parent and peer involvement may be needed to ameliorate any real or perceived notions of inferiority.

Screening

Since many patients become symptomatic only when it is too late, newborns should ideally be screened by pulse oximetry prior to ascertain the possible presence of CCHD. A newborn should have oxyhemoglobin saturation measured in the preductal circulation (right upper arm) and in postductal circulation (any of the legs) at 24 hours of life, and if the saturation is low, or a gradient of saturation is present, an echocardiogram should be obtained prior to discharge.

POINTS TO REMEMBER

- It is important to distinguish child presenting with central cyanosis between those of cardiac and respiratory origin.
- The amount of PBF is the useful distinguishing criteria among congenital cyanotic heart diseases of various hemodynamic physiologies.
- Echocardiography is the most important noninvasive diagnostic tool.
- In newborns suspected of having duct dependent circulations, PGE1 infusion should be started even before completion of specific diagnosis.
- Appropriate identification and timely referral for palliative or definitive surgery determines the outcome.
- Appropriate immunization and required prophylaxis against infective endocarditis.
- Prevention of dehydration and maintenance of iron sufficiency is crucial in long-term monitoring.
- Neonatal screening using pulse oximetry may aid in early identification.

SUGGESTED READING

1. Barnett HB, Holland JG, Josenhans WT. When does central cyanosis become detectable? Clin Invest Med. 1982;5(1):39-43.
2. Lundsgaard C, Van Slyke DD. Cyanosis. Medicine. 1923;2:1-76.
3. Mahle WT, Newburger JW, Matherne GP, Smith FC, Hoke TR, Koppel R, et al. Role of pulse oximetry in examining newborns for congenital heart disease: a scientific statement from the AHA and AAP. Pediatrics. 2009;124(2):823-36.
4. Perloff KJ (Ed). Clinical Recognition of Congenital Heart Diseases, 4th edition. Philadelphia: WB Saunders Co; 1994.
5. Saxena A. Congenital Heart Disease in India: A Status Report. Indian Pediatr. 2018;55(12): 1075-82.
6. Saxena A, Relan J, Agarwal R, Awasthy N, Azad S, Chakrabarty M, et al. Indian guidelines for indications and timing of intervention for common congenital heart diseases: revised and updated consensus statement of the Working group on management of congenital heart diseases. Ann Pediatr Cardiol. 2019;12: 254-86.

120 CHAPTER

Ventricular Septal Defect

Rachita Sarangi

INTRODUCTION

Ventricular septal defect (VSD) is the most common congenital heart disease (CHD) (excluding bicuspid aortic valve) accounting for 20–30% of all CHD. The prevalence varies from 3 to 5/1,000 live births.

Classification according to the site of defect:
- *Perimembranous*: This is the most common type of defect (80%) located in the membranous septum beneath the aortic valve.
- *Outlet (doubly committed)*: Accounts for 5–7% of all VSD located in outlet septum and the rim is formed by aortic and pulmonary annulus.
- *Inlet defects*: Accounts for 5–7% of all VSD located posterior and inferior to perimembranous defect.
- Muscular (Trabecular) defects constitute 5–20% of all VSD. They are frequently multiple when viewing from right side. These could be central (mid-muscular), apical marginal (anterior, septal free wall area) or multiple "Swiss cheese" type.

Classification according to the size of the defect:
- *Small VSD (Restrictive)*:
  - Diameter <one third of size of aortic orifice.
  - Right ventricular (RV) and pulmonary artery (PA) pressures are normal.
  - Left-to-right shunt is <1.5:1.
  - Left-sided cardiac chambers are normal in size.
- *Moderate VSD (Restrictive)*:
  - Diameter of the defect is >one third but less than the size of aortic orifice
  - RV and PA pressures vary from normal to two thirds of systemic pressures
  - Left-to-right shunt is >1.5:1
  - Left-sided cardiac chambers are dilated
- *Large VSD (Nonrestrictive)*:
  - Diameter of the defect ≥ aortic orifice.
  - RV and PA pressures are systemic or near systemic.
  - Left-to-right shunt depends on pulmonary vascular resistance (PVR).
  - The left-sided cardiac chamber is dilated when PVR is normal or mildly elevated.

Hemodynamic

Ventricular septal defect results in shunting of oxygenated blood from left-to-right ventricle. The magnitude of shunt is determined by the size not the location of the defect and degree of PVR. In small VSD, large resistance offered at the defect so it does not depend upon the PVR. But in large VSD, minimal resistance is offered at shunt, so flow is inversely proportional to PVR, so it is called a dependent shunt.

As the pressure difference between both ventricles is very high during systole, the blood flow from left ventricle to right ventricle throughout the systole giving rise to a pansystolic murmur and masking the first heart sound (S1). Toward the end of the systole, the left ventricle pressure becomes less than aortic pressure resulting in early closure of aortic valve (early A2) and masking of A2 by the pansystolic murmur too. Since the flow into the RV and PA is increased the pulmonary valve closure is late and P2 is delayed. Therefore, there is wide but variable split of second heart sound (S2) in patients with large VSD. The left-to-right shunt occurs in systole when the right ventricle is also contracting, so the flow through the shunt goes to the PA directly. The more blood flow through normal pulmonary valve gives rise to ejection systolic murmur at pulmonary area.

The large volume of the blood flows through the lungs resulting in pulmonary vascular congestion giving rise to recurrent chest infection and pulmonary plethora in X-ray chest. The more amount of blood reaching left atrium (LA) gives rise to left atrial enlargement and increased flow through the normal mitral valve produces delayed diastolic murmur at the apex. The intensity and duration of the delayed diastolic murmur are directly proportional to the size of shunt.

When a large VSD is untreated, some irreversible changes occur at pulmonary arterioles giving rise to notably increased PVR approaching to the systemic level and the magnitude of left-to-right shunt decrease. This results in decreased size of left ventricle, overall heart size leaving only PA enlargement and right ventricular hypertrophy (RVH) because of persistence of pulmonary hypertension. The bidirectional shunt may cause cyanosis (Eisenmenger syndrome).

> **BOX 1:** Clinical features of VSD.
>
> - *Small VSD (Restrictive):*
>   - Asymptomatic with normal growth and development
>   - Loud and long pansystolic murmur
>   - LV volume overload minimal
>   - RV pressure and size normal with normal PVR
>   - No cardiomegaly
> - *Moderate VSD (moderate left-to-right shunting):*
>   - Delayed growth, repeated chest infection, decreased exercise tolerance and congestive cardiac failure (CCF)
>   - LV and LA volume overload and dilatation
>   - RV pressure, RV size, and PVR mild-to-moderate increase pansystolic murmur with the mid-diastolic murmur (60%)
>   - Moderate cardiomegaly
> - *Large VSD (degree dependant on ratio of PVR/SVR):*
>   - Failure to thrive, CCF
>   - Shorter and softer pansystolic murmur with mid-diastolic murmur (90%) and wide but variable splitting of S2
>   - LV and LA volume overload and dilatation
>   - RV pressure significantly elevated with RV dilatation and hypertrophy with significantly raised PVR
>   - May lead to Eisenmenger syndrome
>   - Marked cardiomegaly
>
> (LA: left atrium; LV: left ventricular; RV: right ventricular; PVR: pulmonary vascular resistance; SVR: systemic vascular resistance; VSD: ventricular septal defect)

CLINICAL FEATURES (BOX 1)

Patients with VSD become symptomatic at 6–10 weeks of age only after decrease in PVR leading to congestive cardiac failure. The signs and symptoms of the patients depend upon the magnitude of shunt. Small VSD patients may be asymptomatic with normal growth and development. The moderate-to-large VSD patients may have delayed growth, decreased exercise tolerance, frequent respiratory tract infection, palpitation, and signs and symptoms of congestive cardiac failure.

INVESTIGATIONS

X-ray Chest

X-ray chest may be completely normal in small defects. Cardiomegaly involving LA, left ventricular (LV) and RV enlargement may be present with increased pulmonary vascularity with prominent pulmonary artery segment, which is directly related to magnitude of left-to-right shunt. Those with large VSD with significantly elevated PVR shows absence of cardiomegaly, noticeable enlargement of main PA and Hilar pulmonary arteries but peripheral lung fields are ischemic.

Electrocardiography

- Electrocardiography (ECG) may be completely normal in small VSD.
- Patients with significant left-to-right shunt shows signs of LV overload and hypertrophy (tall R waves and tall peaked T waves in inferior and lateral leads with prominent Q waves in V5–V6) and left atrial enlargement (broad-notched P waves in lead I and II with a broad deep P in V1). There may be large equidiphasic RS complexes (Katz-Wachtel pattern) in mid precordial leads.
- In large VSD with pulmonary vascular obstructive disease (PVOD), there is RVH with right axis deviation (RAD) with absence of prominent LV forces (Eisenmenger syndrome).

Echocardiography

Transthoracic echocardiography (ECHO) is the key diagnostic technique providing the diagnosis and assessment of severity. It can provide location, number, size of the defect, severity of chambers overload, PA pressure, aortic cusp prolapse, aortic regurgitation (AR), and about the associated lesions.

Transesophageal ECHO: Occasionally required if the transthoracic ECHO windows are suboptimal. It is very useful during device closure to assess the adequacy of closure of VSD.

Cardiac Magnetic Resonance

Cardiac magnetic resonance (CMR) can serve as an alternative if ECHO is insufficient in assessment of LV volume overload and shunt quantification.

Cardiac Catheterization

Not routinely necessary, it can be performed to know the detailed anatomy, PVR and its response to therapy. It can be also used for interventional purpose in cases undergoing device closure.

Hematology

It is typically normal, except for patients with Eisenmenger syndrome, who may have polycythemia, thrombocytopenia, or coagulopathy.

MANAGEMENT

Management depends upon the size and type of VSD and understanding its natural history. It may be conservative, medical management, or surgical management.

Medical

It depends upon the natural history and clinical symptoms. It mainly aims to control the congestive cardiac failure, treatment of repeated chest infection, treatment of anemia and prevention of infective endocarditis (IE). Patients with signs and symptoms of congestive heart failure (CHF) are treated with diuretics and angiotensin-converting enzyme (ACE) inhibitors.

No restriction of physical activity in absence of LV dysfunction, pulmonary arterial hypertension or arrhythmia.

Antibiotics prophylaxis and good dental hygiene are required to prevent IE. IE prophylaxis is recommended for 6 months after device or surgical closure.

Surgical

Indication for surgery and timing of closure:
- *Small VSD*:
  - Annual follow-up till 10 years of age then every 2–3 years.
  - Closure indicated if child had an episode of IE or develops cusp prolapse with AR or develops progressive significant RV outflow tract obstruction.
- *Moderate VSD*:
  - *Asymptomatic (normal PAP with left heart dilatation)*: Closure of VSD at 2–5 years of age.
  - *Symptomatic*: If controlled with medication, closure at 1–2 years of age.
- *Large VSD*:
  - Poor growth, CHF not controlled with medication (diuretics, enalapril and digoxin) surgery as soon as possible.
  - *Controlled heart failure*: By 6 months of age.
- *VSD with aortic cusp prolapse*: Any VSD with cusp prolapse and directly related AR that is more than trivial, surgery whenever AR detected.

Contraindication for Closure

Severe pulmonary arterial hypertension with irreversible pulmonary vascular disease (PVOD).

Method of Closure: Surgery

Conventionally patch closure is the standard therapy in most cases. Route of closure depends on the location of the defect but left ventriculotomy is avoided.
- *Pulmonary artery banding is a palliative procedure for*:
  - Multiple VSD and inaccessible VSD
  - Patients with contraindication of cardiopulmonary bypass (sepsis)
  - Surgical options for patients with borderline operatively fenestrated VSD patch closure, fenestrated flap valve VSD patch closure or leaving 5 mm atrial septal defect (ASD).

Device closure: Eligibility: Weight >8 kg (5 kg for muscular VSD).

Left-to-right shunt >1.5:1 Indication: Mid-muscular VSD, anterior muscular VSD.

Postoperative Residual VSD

Perimembranous VSD with at least 4 mm from aortic valve.

Contraindication:
- VSD with irreversible pulmonary vascular disease
- Preexisting left bundle branch block (LBBB) or conduction abnormality
- AR
- Associated lesions requiring surgery
- Inlet/subpulmonic VSD.

Device should not be deployed if any degree of AR, complete heart block (CHB)/LBBB, mitral regurgitation or tricuspid regurgitation develop at the time of procedure.

Recommendation for Follow-up

- *Follow-up after surgery*:
  - Clinical, ECG, ECHO in the first year only
  - No further follow-up if no residual defect or pulmonary hypertension
  - Parents explained for reporting only with onset of any cardiac symptoms or arrhythmia.
- *Follow-up protocol for device closure*:
  - Antiplatelet agent (aspirin 3–5 mg/kg/day) for total duration of 6 months.
  - Follow-up visit with ECG/ECHO and clinical evaluation at 1 month, 6 months, 1 year, then annually up to 5 years then every 3–5 years.
  - IE prophylaxis for 6 months with good orodental hygiene.

PROGNOSIS

Patients with isolated VSD have generally good long-term prognosis.

Spontaneous closure occurs in 30–40% cases of small membranous and muscular VSD during first 6 months of life. Inlet or infundibular defect do not become smaller or close spontaneously.
- PVOD may begin as early as 6–12 months of age with large VSD but resulting right-to-left shunt does not develop till teenage.
- Infundibular stenosis may develop with large defect resulting in a cyanotic tetralogy of Fallot (TOF) with decreased left-to-right shunt-and-occasional production of right-to-left shunt.
- Arrhythmia can occur but less frequent than in other form of CHD.
- The incidence of IE in small VSD patients is 1.3 per 1,000 per year.
- A small subset of patients with associated anomalies has poorer outcomes.

A minority will have irreversible pulmonary arterial hypertension, a candidate for heart–lung transplantation.

KEY MESSAGES

- VSD is the most common form of CHD and perimembranous VSD (80%) is most common.
- Clinical features depend upon the size and degree of PVR.
- Muscular VSD are more likely to close but inlet and malaligned VSD almost never close spontaneously.
- Treatment may be conservative, medical, or surgical.
- Long-term prognosis is good in majority of patients.

SUGGESTED READING

1. Allen HD, Driscoll DJ, Shaddy RE, Feltes TF. Moss & Adams' Heart Disease in Infants, Children, and Adolescents Including the Fetus and Young Adult. Philadelphia: Wolters Kluwer Health; 2016.
2. Baumgartner H, Bonhoeffer P, DeGroot NMS. ESC Guidelines for the management of grown-up congenital heart disease (new version 2010). Eur Heart J. 2010;31(23):2915-57.
3. Park MK. Park's Pediatric Cardiology for Practitioners, 6th edition. USA: Elsevier; 2014.
4. Paul VK. Ghai Essential Pediatrics, 9th Edition. New Delhi: CBS Publishers Pvt. Limited; 2019.
5. Rolo V, Walker I, Wilson K. Ventricular septal defects. Paediatric Anaesthesia. 2015;316:1-7.
6. Saxena A, Relan J, Agarwal R, Awasthy N, Azad S, Chakrabarty M, et al. Indian guidelines for indications and timing of intervention for common congenital heart disease: revised and updated consensus statement of the working group on management of congenital heart disease abridged secondary publication. Indian Pediatrics. 2020;57(15):143-57.
7. Working group on management of congenital heart diseases in India. Consensus on timing of intervention for common congenital heart diseases. Indian Pediatrics. 2008;45(17):117-26.

Atrial Septal Defect

Taraknath Ghosh

INTRODUCTION

Atrial septal defect (ASD) is a congenital acyanotic heart disease with left-to-right shunt, where defect found in the interatrial septum. There is an abnormal communication between both atria. Though it is a congenital heart disease (CHD), it usually becomes symptomatic in adult. The defect usually occurs in isolation (ASD is responsible for 10% cases of CHD). About 30% of children with CHD have an ASD as part of other cardiac defect such as total anomalous pulmonary venous connection (TAPVC), pulmonary stenosis (PS), mitral valve prolapse (MVP), mitral regurgitation (MR). It is more common in female than male (M:F = 1:2). Embryologically, both atria develops from a common atrial canal. It is divided into right and left atria by the down growth of septum. Failure of complete closure usually results in defect.

CLASSIFICATION

Depending on the position of defect, ASD can be classified in the following ways: There are three types of defect in ASD: (1) Secundum defect, (2) ostium primum, and (3) sinus venosus defects. Persistent foramen ovale does not produce any intracardiac shunt under ordinary condition.

- *Three types of ASD*:
  1. *Secundum (50–70%)*: It normally occurs in isolation. One third of ostium secundum closes spontaneously by 1–2 years. 10% cases are associated with TAPVC, 20% is with MVP.

Cardiac malformation associated with ASD:
- Partial anomalous pulmonary venous connection, ventricular septal defect, MR, MVP
- Pulmonary valvular stenosis
- Pulmonary arterial branch stenosis
- Persistent left superior vena cava

Common syndromes associated with ASD:
- Holt–Oram, Lutembacher, Ellis–van
- Creveld, Thrombocytopenia-absent radius (TAR), Edward, Patau, Noonan
- Klinefelter, 5 p Deletion syndrome

  2. Ostium primum occurs in 30% of all ASDs including those as a part of complete atrioventricular defects. Isolated ostium primum ASD occurs in 15% of all ASD. Lesions associated with ASD primum are inlet VSD, cleft mitral valve, partial attachment of septal, and leaflet of mitral valve to IV septum.
  3. Sinus venosus type in 10% cases.
- *ASD also may be classified by size*:
  - Small defects had a maximal diameter > 3 mm to < 6 mm
  - Moderate defects measured ≥6 mm to < 12 mm
  - Large defects were ≥12 mm.

HEMODYNAMICS

In normal condition, blood from superior vena cava (SVC) and inferior vena cava (IVC) enters to right atrium (RA) and then flows to the right ventricle (RV). From RV, blood passes to the lungs via pulmonary arteries. Then this blood enters the left atrium through the pulmonary veins immediately after oxygenation in the lungs. In ASD, as there is defect in the atrial septum and the left atrial pressure is higher than the right one, then the blood will flow from left to right atrium. As the difference of pressure between two atria is very little, the flow gradient is low. Hence, no murmur is heard due to shunt. However, increased flow into RA will lead to increased blood flow across normal pulmonary valve (PV) via increase flow through RV. This will produce an ejection systolic murmur **(Fig. 1)**.

CLINICAL FEATURES

Majority of infant and child with ASD are usually asymptomatic and accidentally detected on routine auscultation. Secundum ASD is normally asymptomatic until the third decade of life. On meticulous evaluation, younger children may show features of failure to thrive while older one may present with varying degrees of exercise intolerance. Common symptoms of ASD are palpitation on exercise, fatigability, dyspnea on exertion. Rarely, ASD may present with growth failure, recurrent respiratory tract infection, and congestive heart failure (CHF).

PHYSICAL EXAMINATION

- Relatively thin-built body (Patient not <10th percentile).
- Mild precordial bulge and hyperdynamic right ventricular impulse along the left sternal border with systolic lift may be present.
- A widely split and fixed S2 (If A2–P2 interval is the same in expiration and inspiration, it is called wide and fixed split S2.). In ASD, S2 is wide because the RV volume will increase due to extra flow from left side. This will lead to increase flow in the pulmonary artery. So PV closure will be delayed. At the same time, left ventricle (LV) inflow will be decreased due to shunt across ASD (left to right) resulting in delayed closure of aortic valve. On the other hand, the split is fixed because the difference in the inflow of blood in atrium during inspiration and expiration will not be present in ASD as there is communication between the two atria.
- A grade 2-3/6 systolic ejection murmur is a characteristic finding of the ASD in older infants and children. Murmur is not due to atrial shunt as it is low-pressure shunt. It is functional murmur due to relative pulmonary stenosis.
- With a large left-to-right amid-diastolic rumbling murmur at left lower sternal border (LLSB) may be audible due to increase blood flow across tricuspid valve and it usually indicates a Qp:Qs ratio of at least 2:1.
- Typical auscultatory findings may be absent even in infant with large ASD **(Fig. 2)**.

INVESTIGATIONS

- *X-ray*: It shows varying degrees of enlargement of RA and RV depending upon the shunt. A prominent PA and increased pulmonary vascular markings can be seen. Jug-handle appearance of heart is the classical radiological appearance may be seen in long-standing cases.
- *Electrocardiography (ECG)*: Right axis deviation (RAD) of +90 to +180 and mild right ventricular dominance or right bundle branch block (RBBB) with an rsR' pattern in V1 and typical findings. Presence of left axis (–30°) in primum type of defect
- *Echocardiography (echo)*:
  - A two-dimensional echo study is diagnostic characteristic brightening of the echo image seen at the edge of the defect. In subcostal four-chamber view, echo dropout can be seen at mid atrium for secundum type–at lower atrium in primum type whereas at posterosuperior, aspect in SVC type of sinus venosus ASD.
  - Increase RV and diastolic dimension and flattening and abnormal motion of ventricular septum indicate RV volume overload.
  - Pulsed and color flow Doppler study reveals characteristic flow pattern with maximum left-to-right shunt in diastole. Doppler examination can estimate pressure in the RV and PA.

NATURAL HISTORY

- An ASD of <3 mm spontaneous closure around 100% by 1½ years of age.
- With defects between 3 and 8 mm—80% closure rate.
- ASD with defect >8 mm rarely closer spontaneously.

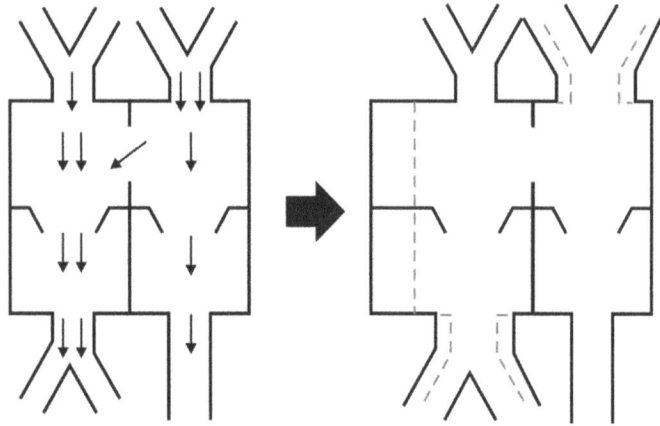

Fig. 1: Hemodynamics and pathophysiology of ASD.

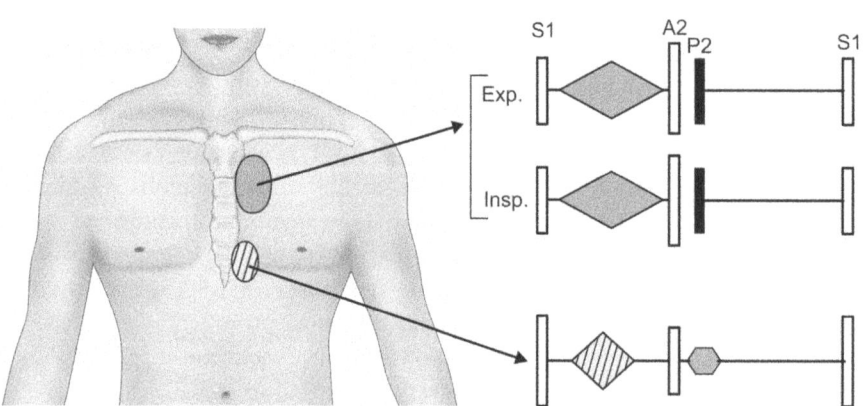

Fig. 2: Auscultatory findings in ASD.

Clinical features at a glance:
- Asymptomatic
- Effort intolerance
- Repeated response to intervention (RTI)
- Parasternal lift
- Wide and fixed split S2
- Ejection systolic murmur and delayed diastolic murmur

PRESCRIPTION ASSISTANCE

Atrial septal defect with CCF:

Pharmacological salt	Market preparation	Availability	Dosage
Furosemide	Lasix (Tablet, injection) Furoped drop	• Tablet 40 mg • Injection 10 mg/mL • Drop 10 mg/mL	1–2 mg/kg/day in two divided doses
Enalapril	Enam Envas	• Tablet 2.5, 5, 10 mg • Injection 1.25 mg/mL	1–5 mg/kg/day in one to two doses

COMPLICATIONS

- If untreated, CHF and pulmonary hypertension develop in adults who are in their 20s and 30s. Rarely, infant may present with CHF.
- With or without surgery, atrial flutter or fibrillation may occur as an adult.
- Infective endocarditis usually does not occur.
- Failure to thrive and recurrent respiratory tract infection may occur rarely, especially in very large ASD.

MEDICAL TREATMENT

- Usually there is no restriction of exercise.
- Prophylaxis of IE is not required unless associated with MVP.
- Infants with CHF medical management is recommended with furosemide and/or angiotensin-converting enzyme (ACE) inhibitor.

CARDIAC INTERVENTION AND SURGICAL CLOSURE INDICATION

- General consensus is that device or surgical closure is not required for patient with small secundum ASD with minimal left-to-right shunts without RV enlargement.
- Surgical or device closure is recommended for all symptomatic patients with Qp:Qs ratio of at least 2:1 with RV enlargement. However, high pulmonary vascular resistance (≥ 10 units/m^2, >7 units/m^2 with vasodilator) is contraindication for surgery.

Timings

- Usually after 1 year of age and before entry into school.
- However, surgery is performed in infants with refractory heart failure and increase O_2 requirement in NICU (neonatal intensive care unit) graduates with bronchopulmonary dysplasia (BPD).

Procedure

- For most children with ASD, percutaneous catheter device closure using an atrial septal occlusive device (Amplatzer or Helex device).
- Open surgery is indicated under cardiopulmonary bypass for the cases only where device closure is not considered. It is usually indicated in primum and sinus venosus type of defect and defect associated with other cardiac defects such as TAPVC and MR.

SUGGESTED READING

1. Park MK. Park's Pediatric Cardiology for Practitioners, 6th edition. USA: Elsevier; 2014.

122 CHAPTER: Patent Ductus Arteriosus

Supratim Datta, Basundhara Bhattacharya, Debapriya Roy

CLINICAL PRESENTATIONS

Case 1: A 1,000-g baby, delivered at 30 weeks of gestation, is admitted to the neonatal intensive care unit (NICU) for preterm care. He does well till day 5 of life and then develops tachypnea and subcostal retractions. There is no cyanosis. A continuous murmur is heard along the left sternal border. Chest radiography reveals pulmonary vascular congestion.

Case 2: A 3-month-old baby, delivered at 39 weeks of gestation and having a birth weight of 2.7 kg, presented to the pediatric emergency room (ER) with complaints of poor feeding, increased respiratory rate and fever for 2 days. On examination, she is found to have tachypnea, tachycardia, chest retractions, tender hepatomegaly, bounding peripheral pulses, and bilateral cataract. A continuous machine-like murmur is heard along the left sternal border, radiating to the left clavicle. The mother gives a history of fever with rash in the first trimester of her pregnancy.

HISTORICAL ASPECTS

- Way back in 1593, Giambattista Carcano in Italy described the "duct us arteriosus."
- In 1852, Karl Von Rokitansky in his illustrated monograph showed the patent ductus arteriosus as a specific congenital malformation.

INTRODUCTION

- *Incidence*: 1 in 2,000 to 1 in 5,000 births
- Predominantly female preponderance, male:female ratio being 2 or 3:1.

DEVELOPMENTAL HISTORY

- The ductus arteriosus is derived from the aortic arch.
- During fetal life, majority of the blood from the pulmonary artery is shunted right to left into the aorta via the ductus arteriosus.
- The aortic end of the ductus is just distal to the origin of the left subclavian artery, and the ductus enters the pulmonary artery to the left of its bifurcation near the origin of the left branch.
- In utero ductal tone is maintained by interplay between the constricting effect of oxygen (relatively weak because of low fetal pO_2) and the dilating effect of endogenous prostaglandin E_2 **(Table 1)**.
- As term approaches, the ductus becomes less responsive to prostaglandin E_2 and more responsive to oxygen.
- Closure consistently begins in the pulmonary arterial end, so duct assumes the shape of a truncated cone, larger at the aortic end.
- Functional closure normally occurs soon after birth as a result of increase in the extrauterine ambient oxygen tension that has a direct constricting effect on the ductal wall.
- Normal functional closure begins within 10–15 hours and gets completed by 2 weeks. Anatomical closure occurs by 2–3 weeks after birth.
- At term, the mature ductus is found to have intimal cushions that protrude into the lumen, which, along with apoptosis and smooth muscle cell proliferation are considered to have a role in anatomical closure. Subendothelial edema occurs which leads to the

TABLE 1: Pathology of the patent ductus arteriosus.

Preterm neonates	Term neonates	Others
Smooth muscle wall of the preterm ductus is less responsive to the increased pO_2, hence closure is delayed	Due to presence of intrauterine subendothelial internal elastic lamina, the intimal cushions cannot approximate and no gross edema occurs, leading to nonocclusion of the ductus	In certain congenital heart lesions (known as "duct us dependent lesions"), the patent ductus plays a life-saving role in providing a source of pulmonary (e.g., in pulmonary atresia) or systemic blood flow (in lesions such as aortic coarctation or interruption)

occlusion. The intimal cushions also contract in response to oxygen and occlude the lumen.
- Spontaneous closure is unlikely beyond 1 year in preterm babies and 3 months in term babies.

Associations:
- Congenital rubella
- Alcohol exposure in utero (fetal alcohol syndrome)
- Birth at high altitude.

Physiological consequences of persistent patent ductus depend on five factors:
1. Size of the ductus
2. Pulmonary vascular resistance
3. Adaptive response of left ventricular volume overload
4. Prematurity
5. Respiratory distress.

CLINICAL FEATURES

The three commonly encountered modes of symptomatic presentations are:
1. Congestive cardiac failure (most common)
2. Infective endocarditis
3. Cerebral steal phenomenon

The presentation of small and large PDA are given in **Table 2**.

INVESTIGATIONS

- *Electrocardiography (ECG):*
  - Moderately restrictive PDA:
    - Prolonged bifid left atrial P
    - PR interval prolonged in 10–20%
    - Normal QRS or right-axis deviation
  - Nonrestrictive PDA:
    - Biatrial P wave
    - Combined ventricular hypertrophy
  - PDA with pulmonary arterial hypertension:
    - Peaked right atrial P waves
    - Right ventricular hypertrophy (RVH) + right-axis deviation.

Echocardiogram (Diagnostic)

- The ductus can be directly visualized.
- Size of the ductus can be estimated, along with ductal flow pattern.
- *In case of large shunts*:
  - Color and pulsed-Doppler examinations can also demonstrate systolic or diastolic (or both) retrograde turbulent flow in the pulmonary artery and aortic retrograde flow during diastole.
  - Left atrial and left ventricular hypertrophy can be detected.
  - Can reveal features of pulmonary over circulation.
- *Chest X-ray (CXR)*:
  - Prominent pulmonary artery with increased pulmonary vascular markings.
  - Cardiac size: Normal or moderate-to-markedly enlarged, depending on the degree of shunting (left atrial and left ventricular hypertrophy).
  - Aortic knob: May be prominent.

TABLE 2: Presentation of small and large PDA.

Small PDA	Large PDA

• Mostly asymptomatic
• Detected incidentally by the presence of the murmur
	• Growth retardation may be present
	• Bounding peripheral arterial pulses, wide-pulse pressure. The pulse may be weak in preterm babies. The typical pulse is brisk, single, or with bisferiens peak and rapid collapse
	• *Cardiological examination*:
	  – The heart is moderately or grossly enlarged
	  – S2 paradoxically or widely split
	  – Apical impulse: Prominent, heaving
	  – A thrill, maximal in the second left interspace, is often present and may radiate toward the left clavicle, down the left sternal border, or toward the apex. It is usually systolic but may also be palpated throughout the cardiac cycle
	  – *Murmur*: Classic murmur described by Gibson Classic continuous murmur, machinery in quality. It begins soon after onset of the first sound, reaches maximal intensity at the end of systole, and wanes in late diastole. It may be localized to the second left intercostal space or radiate down the left sternal border or to the left clavicle. When pulmonary vascular resistance is increased, the diastolic component of the murmur may be less prominent or absent
	The classical murmur may be absent in nonrestrictive patent ductus arteriosus, congestive cardiac failure or right-sided heart failure
	• Eisenmenger ductus (reversal of shunt in case of prolonged pulmonary hypertension):
	  – Isotonic exercise causes leg fatigue without dyspnea
	  – Features of LV failure are absent
	  – The right-to-left shunt does NOT produce a murmur

TABLE 3: Rationale for surgical closure of patent ductus arteriosus (PDA).	
Small PDA	**Large PDA**
To prevent bacterial endarteritis or other late complications (e.g., paradoxical emboli)	• To treat heart failure • To prevent the development of pulmonary vascular disease • Both

TABLE 4: Surgical options.	
Transcatheter PDA closure	**Surgical closure of PDA**
Can be routinely performed in the cardiac catheterization laboratory • *Small PDAs*: Closed with intravascular coils • *Moderate-to-large PDAs*: Closed with an umbrella-like device or with a catheter introduced sac into which several coils are released	• *Video-assisted thoracoscopic surgery (VATS)*: Minimally invasive technique (more popular) • Left thoracotomy

(PDA: patent ductus arteriosus)

TABLE 5: Rationale for surgical closure of patent ductus arteriosus (PDA).	
Small PDA	**Large PDA**

Followed up medically till 6 months of age due to high incidence of spontaneous closure	• *Supportive management*:
	  – Fluid restriction (not more than 120 mL/kg/day)
	  – Anticongestive measures (furosemide)
	• *Medical closure*: Indomethacin (prostaglandin synthetase inhibitor) @ 0.2 mg/kg IV every 12 hours for up to three doses
	• *Surgical closure*: If medical therapy fails/is contraindicated

- Inconspicuous soft convexity between aortic knob and pulmonary artery segment.
- *Cardiac catheterization*:
  - Confirmation of the diagnosis in patients with a typical findings
  - Can demonstrate increased pressure in the right ventricle and pulmonary artery

TREATMENT (TABLES 3 TO 5)

Term Neonates

- Supportive management: Management of congestive cardiac failure (CCF), if present
- Surgical closure: Mainstay of treatment.

Pulmonary hypertension is NOT a contraindication for surgery.

Contraindications for surgery:
- Severe pulmonary arterial disease
- Development of right-to-left shunt.

Ductus-dependent Lesions

The ductus arteriosus is kept patent by prostaglandin E1 (PGE1) infusion till definitive surgical management of the underlying heart lesion can be undertaken.

SUMMARY

- Clinical suspicion of PDA is heightened by premature birth, maternal rubella, or birth at high altitude.
- Arterial pulse is brisk, pulse pressure wide.
- LV impulse is dynamic.
- Auscultation reveals continuous Gibson murmur punctuated by Eddy sounds.
- May present as an asymptomatic case (diagnosed incidentally), cardiac failure, infective endocarditis or Eisenmenger syndrome.
- ECG shows volume overload of LV.
- CXR shows increased pulmonary vascularity with cardiomegaly.
- Echocardiography shows size, flow pattern of PDA, and features of systemic under perfusion and pulmonary overcirculation.
- Treatment can be medical or surgical.

Endocardial Cushion Defect

Kalpana Dutta, Basundhara Bhattacharya, Bonny Sen

CLINICAL PRESENTATION

A 2-month-old baby, a known case of Down syndrome, is rushed to the pediatric emergency with complaints of breathlessness. On examination, she is found to have tachypnea, tachycardia, chest retractions, and wheezes. The liver is palpable 4 cm below the right costal margin. The mother also complains that lately the baby has been sweaty and feeding poorly, and also appears blue around the mouth when she nurses. A more careful examination of the baby after initial stabilization reveals the presence of a systolic as well as a diastolic murmur with splitting of the second heart sound. An emergency electrocardiogram (ECG) shows a superiorly oriented QRS frontal plane axis with counter clockwise depolarization.

EMBRYOLOGY

Development of the Endocardial Cushions

- The primitive heart tube consists of several layers of myocardium and a single layer of endocardium separated by cardiac jelly, an acellular extracellular matrix secreted by the myocardium.
- Cardiac jelly promotes occlusion of endocardial tubular lumen during myocardial contraction.
- It also releases inductive signals that cause endocardial cells lining the AV canal to transform into cardiac mesenchyme.
- Cardiac mesenchymal cells then proliferate between the endocardium and myocardium producing protrusions termed as Endocardial Cushions (ECs) which bulge into the primitive heart tube and provide the valvular mechanism in the AV canal and outflow tract.
- The ECs themselves ultimately fuse forming a wedge that guides the union of internal septal structures, i.e., the atrial and ventricular septum.
- They also provide scaffold for formation of leaflets of the tricuspid valve and the mitral valve.
- Structures developing from the ECs:
  - Atrioventricular (AV) valves with leaflets
  - *Portion of interatrial septum (IAS)*: Foramen primum is occluded in median plane by the merging of the AV cushion fusion and edge of septum primum.
  - *Portion of interventricular septum (IVS)*: Dorsal EC gets ventricular extension and fuses with muscular ventricular septum
- An atrioventricular septal defect (AVSD), also known as an AV canal defect or an EC defect, consists of contiguous atrial and ventricular septal defects with markedly abnormal AV valves.
- The severity of the abnormalities is seen to vary considerably.
- The spectrum of endocardial cushion defects can include **(Figs. 1 and 2)**:
  - A single AV valve common to both ventricles which consists of an anterior and a posterior bridging leaflet related to the ventricular septum, with a lateral leaflet in each ventricle (most severe form, common in children with Down syndrome)
  - Ostium primum defects with clefts in the anterior mitral and septal tricuspid valve leaflets and small VSDs
  - Ostium primum defects with normal AV valves
  - Intact atrial septum but with an inlet VSD is similar to that found in the full AVSD
  - AVSD associated with varying degrees of hypoplasia of either of the ventricles, known as either left- or right-dominant AVSD.

PATHOPHYSIOLOGY (FIG. 3)

Ostium Primum Defects

The basic abnormalities are:
- A left-to-right shunt across the atrial defect (usually moderate to large); and
- Mitral (or occasionally tricuspid) insufficiency (usually mild to moderate)
  - In these cases, the pulmonary arterial pressure is usually normal or only mildly increased
  - Behaves like an ostium secundum atrial septal defect (ASD).

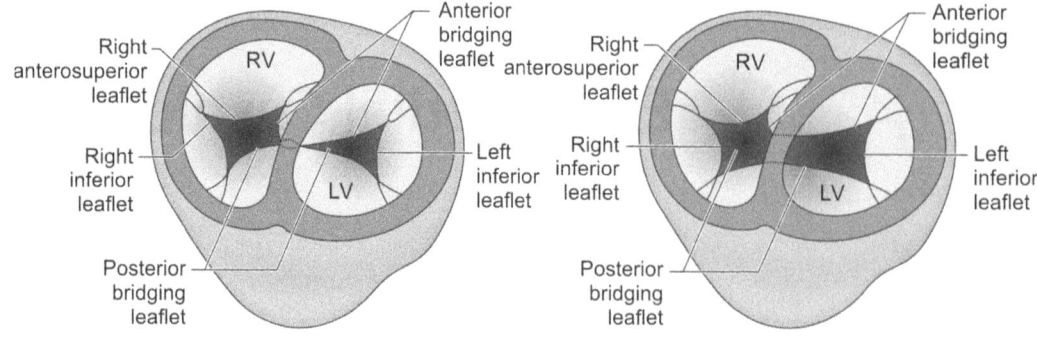

Fig. 1: Leaflet pattern of ECD.
(ECD: endocardial cushion defect)
Source: Perloff J, Marelli A. Perloff's Clinical Recognition of Congenital Heart Disease. 6th edition, USA: Saunders; 2012. p. 255.

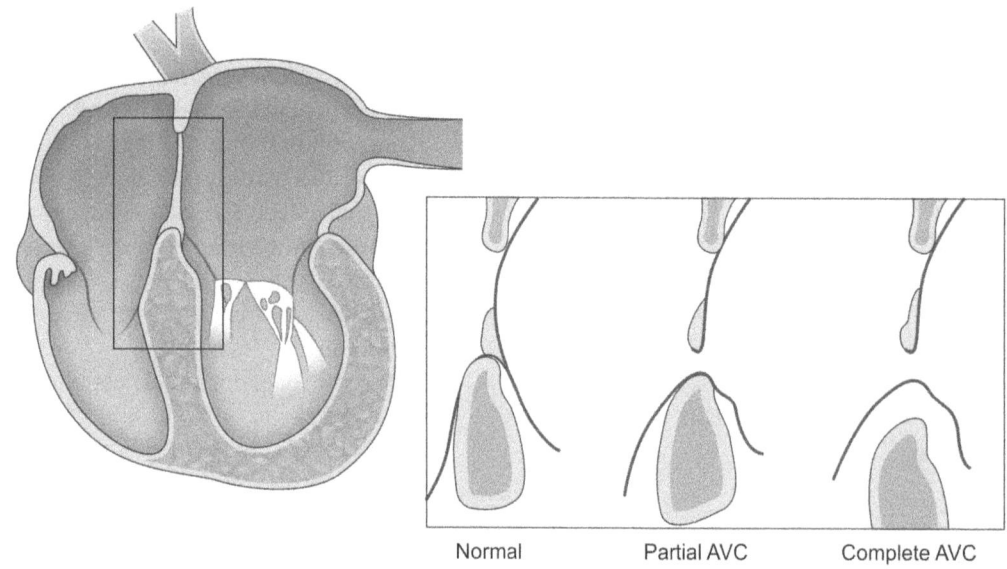

Fig. 2: The internal cardiac crux in AVSD.
(AVSD: atrioventricular septal defect)
Source: Allen HD, Shaddy RE, Penny DJ, Feltes TF, Cetta F. Moss and Adams' Heart Disease in Infants, Children, and Adolescents, 9th edition. Netherlands: Wolters Kluwer; 2016. p. 763

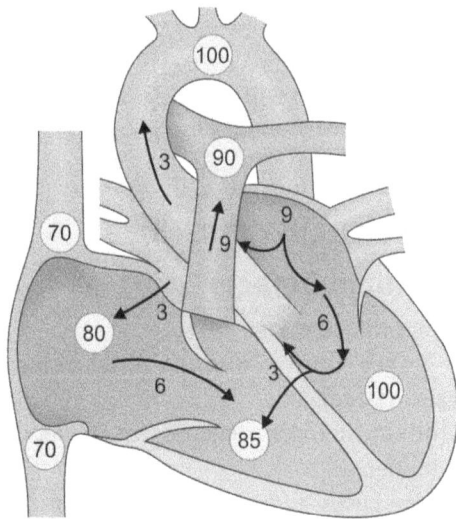

Fig. 3: Physiology of atrioventricular septal defect. The circled numbers represent oxygen saturation values. The numbers next to the arrows represent the volumes of blood flow (in L/min/m^2).
Source: Kliegman RM, St. Geme J. Nelson Textbook of Pediatrics, 21st edition. US: Elsevier; 2020. p. 2376.

Complete Atrioventricular Septal Defects

- The abnormalities here are:
  - The left-to-right shunt occurs at both the atrial and ventricular levels.
  - Additional shunting may occur directly from the left ventricle to the right atrium because of absence of the AV septum.
  - Pulmonary hypertension and an early increase in pulmonary vascular resistance are common.
  - AV valvular insufficiency is present which increases the volume load on one or both ventricles. Thus biventricular hypertrophy is often seen.
  - In case of very large defects, some right-to-left shunting may also occur at bot h the atrial and ventricular levels and lead to mild arterial desaturation.
  - With time, progressive pulmonary vascular disease increases the right- to-left shunt, ultimately resulting in the development of Eisenmenger physiology.

The concept of balance: Both partial and complete AVSDs can be balanced or unbalanced depending on how the AV junction is shared by the ventricles. An AV inlet equally shared by both ventricles is consistent with balanced AVSD, while in unbalanced AVSD one ventricle is hypoplastic; the common AV valve is normal and the larger ventricle is the dominant one.

Associations: Of all patients with complete ECD, about 70% have Down syndrome.

CLINICAL FEATURES

- *Small shunts*: Asymptomatic; the anomaly is discovered during a general physical examination.
- *Moderate shunts and mitral insufficiency*: The physical signs are similar to those of the ostium secundum ASD, but with an additional apical holosystolic murmur caused by mitral insufficiency. The symptoms are more severe in cases of complete AVSDs and appear in early infancy.
- *History*:
  - Poor feeding
  - Exercise intolerance, easy fatigability
  - Recurrent pneumonia
  - Poor weight gain
  - Mild bluish discoloration during feeding or crying
- *Examination*:
  - Moderate or marked cardiac enlargement
  - A systolic thrill is frequently palpable at the lower left sternal border
  - A precordial bulge and lift may be present
  - Hepatomegaly
  - Cyanosis may occur; insignificant at rest but induced by exercise or crying
  - *Auscultatory signs*:
    - Normal or accentuated first heart sound
    - Signs of left-to-right shunt:
      – Wide, fixed splitting of the second sound (in cases with massive pulmonary flow);
      – Pulmonary systolic eject ion murmur sometimes preceded by a click;
      – Low-pitched, mid-diastolic rumbling murmur at the lower left sternal edge or apex, or both, as a result of increased flow through the AV valves.
  - *Signs of mitral insufficiency*: A harsh (occasionally very high-pitched) apical holosystolic murmur that radiates to the left axilla.

INVESTIGATIONS

- *ECG (Fig. 4)*:
  - Superior orientation of the mean frontal QRS axis with left axis deviation to the left upper or right upper quadrant

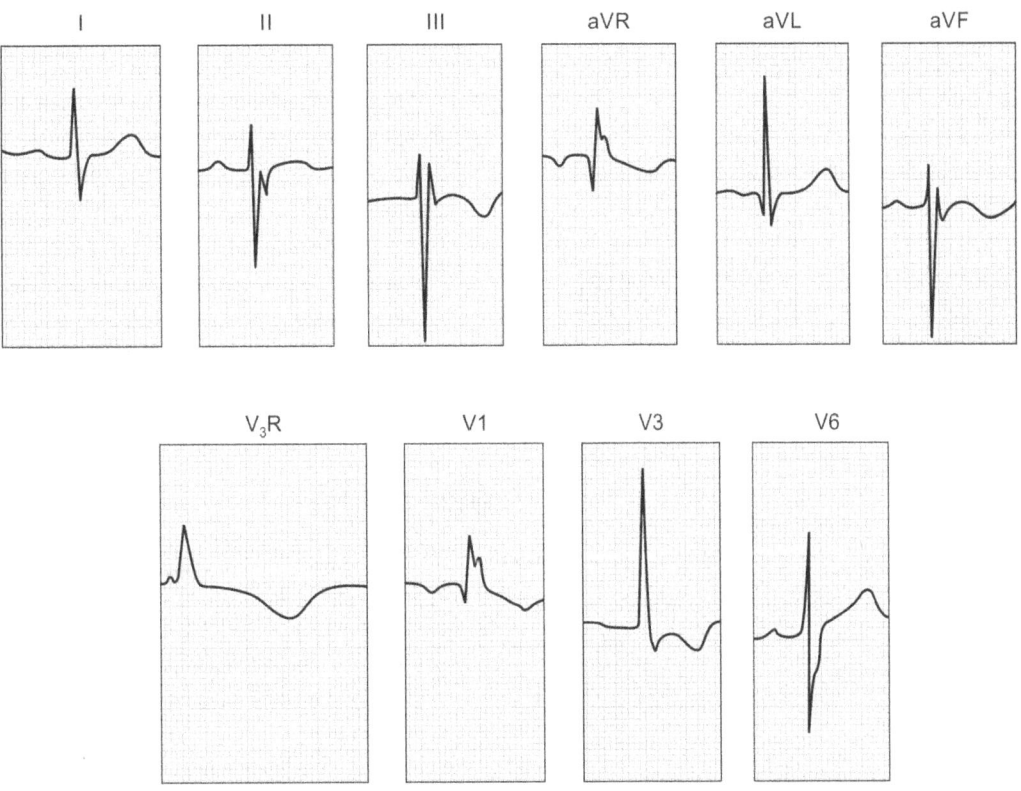

Fig. 4: ECG of a child with ECD. QRS axis of −60° RSR' in V1 and V3.
(ECG: electrocardiogram)
Source: Kliegman RM, St. Geme J. Nelson Textbook of Pediatrics, 21st edition. US: Elsevier; 2020. p. 2378.

- Counterclockwise inscription of the superiorly oriented QRS vector loop (often manifested by a Q wave in leads I and aVL)
- Signs of biventricular hypertrophy or isolated right ventricular hypertrophy
- Right ventricular conduction delay (rSR' pattern in leads V3R and V1)
- Normal or tall P waves
- Occasional prolongation of the P-R interval
  - *Echocardiogram (echo) (diagnostic)*:
    - Right ventricular enlargement
    - Encroachment of the mitral valve echo on the left ventricular outflow tract
    - Abnormally low position of the AV valves which results in a "goose neck" deformity of the left ventricular out flow tract
    - Both aortic and mitral valves insert at the same level because of absence of the AV septum (contrary to what is seen in a normal heart)
    - In complete AV septal defects, the ventricular septum is also deficient and the common AV valve can be readily appreciated
    - Helps in determining the insertion points of the chordae of the common AV valve
    - Evaluating the presence of associated lesions such as patent ductus arteriosus (PDA) or coarctation of the aorta
    - Color and pulsed Doppler examinations:
      - Can demonstrate left-to-right shunting at the atrial, ventricular, or left ventricular to right atrial levels
      - Used to semiquantitate the degree of AV valve insufficiency
  - *Chest X-ray (CXR)* **(Fig. 5)**:
    - Prominent pulmonary artery with increased pulmonary vascular markings.

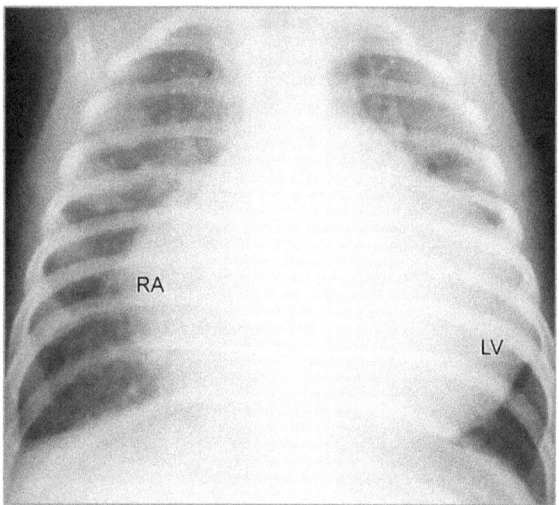

Fig. 5: Chest roentgenogram in ECD.
(ECD: endocardial cushion defect)
Source: Perloff J, Marelli A. Perloff's Clinical Recognition of Congenital Heart Disease. 6th edition, USA: Saunders; 2012. p. 258.

- *Cardiac size*: Moderate-to-markedly enlarged with prominence of both ventricles and atria
- *Cardiac catheterization*:
  - Generally not required for confirmation of the diagnosis
  - Required for confirmation of the diagnosis when:
    - Pulmonary vascular disease is suspected.
    - Patients in whom the development of pulmonary vascular disease may be more rapid, e.g., Down syndrome
  - *Catheterization is useful to demonstrate*:
    - Magnitude of the left-to-right shunt
    - The degree of elevation of pulmonary vascular resistance
    - The severity of insufficiency of the common AV valve
  - By oximetry, the shunt is usually demonstrable at both the atrial and ventricular levels. Arterial oxygen saturation is normal or only mildly reduced unless severe pulmonary vascular disease is present.
  - *Pulmonary arterial pressure*:
    - Children with ostium primum defects generally have normal or only moderately elevated pulmonary arterial pressure.
    - Conversely, complete AV septal defects are associated with right ventricular and pulmonary hypertension and increased pulmonary vascular resistance (in older patients).
- *Selective left ventriculography*:
  - Demonstrates deformity of the mitral or common AV valve and the distortion of the left ventricular outflow tract caused by this valve (goose neck deformity)
  - The abnormal anterior leaflet of the mitral valve is serrated, and mitral insufficiency is noted, usually with regurgitation of blood into both the left and right atria
  - Direct shunting of blood from the left ventricle to the right atrium may also be demonstrated.

TREATMENT

- *Supportive management*: Management of congestive cardiac failure (CCF), if present
- *Surgical closure*: Mainstay of the treatment
  - *Ostium primum defects*:
    - Approached surgically from an incision in the right atrium
    - The cleft in the mitral valve is located through the atrial defect and is repaired by direct suture
    - The defect in the atrial septum is usually closed by insertion of patch prosthesis.

- The surgical mortality rate for ostium primum defects is very low.
- *Complete AV canal defects*:
  - Surgical treatment of complete AV septal defects is technically more difficult.
  - The atrial and ventricular defects are patched and the AV valves reconstructed.
  - Palliative surgery with pulmonary arterial banding is reserved for the patients who have other associated lesions that make early corrective surgery too risky.
  - Because of the risk of early development of pulmonary vascular disease (as early as 6–12 months of age), surgical intervention must be performed during infancy.
  - *Postoperative complications*:
    - Surgically induced heart block (may require placement of a permanent pacemaker)
    - Excessive narrowing of the left ventricular outflow tract (may require surgical revision)
    - Residual tricuspid or mitral regurgitation (may require replacement with a prosthetic valve).

PROGNOSIS

- *Ostium primum defects and minimal AV valve abnormalities*: Asymptomatic/minor, nonprogressive symptoms until they reach the 3rd to 4th decade of life, (similar to the course of patients with ostium secundum ASDs).
- Complete AVSDs
  - Death due to cardiac failure during infancy is often encountered unless an early corrective surgery is undertaken.
  - Pulmonary vascular obstructive disease usually develops in those who survive without surgery.
  - *The prognosis for unrepaired complete AVSDs depends on*:
    - The magnitude of the left-to-right shunt
    - The degree of pulmonary vascular resistance
    - The severity of AV valve insufficiency.

SUMMARY

- Atrioventricular septal defect encompasses a group of anomalies involving specific portions of the atrial and ventricular septa and adjacent AV valves.
- The clinical and laboratory findings reflect the atrial left-to-right shunt and the mitral regurgitation.
- The ECG showing left axis deviation, atrial and ventricular hypertrophy, and incomplete right bundle branch block is quite diagnostic.
- X-ray studies reveal enlargement of each cardiac chamber.

SUGGESTED READING

1. Bernstein D. Atrioventricular Septal Defect (ostium primum and atrioventricular canal or endocardial cushion defect). In: Kliegman RM, Stanton BF, St Geme JW, Schor NF, Behrman RE (eds). Nelson text book of Pediatrics, 21st edition. Philadelphia: Elsevier; 2021. pp. 2376–8.
2. Cetta F, Truong D, Minich LL, Maleszewski JJ, O'Leary PW, Dearani JA, Burkhart HM. Atrioventricular Septal Defects. In: Allen HD, Shaddy RE, Penny DJ, Feltes TF, Cetta F (eds). Moss and Adams' Heart Disease in Infants, Children, and Adolescents, 9th edition. Netherlands: Wolters-Kluwer; 2016, pp. 757-81.
3. Complete & Partial endocardial cushion defect. In: Park MK (ed). Park's Pediatric Cardiology for Practitioners, 6th edition. Philadelphia: Elsevier; 2014. pp. 174–81.
4. Johnson WH, Moller JH. Atrioventricular septal defect. Pediatric Cardiology the Essential Pocket Guide, 3rd edition. Oxford: Wiley Blackwell; 2014. pp. 137-47.
5. Perloff JK, Marelli AJ. Atrial Septal Defect: Simple and Complex. Perloff's Clinical Recognition of Congenital Heart Disease, 6th edition, USA: Saunders; 2012. pp. 254-66.
6. Standring S. Development of thorax. Gray's Anatomy; 41st edition. Philadelphia: Elsevier; 2016. pp. 905-16.

Tetralogy of Fallot

Hemant Kumar

INTRODUCTION

Tetralogy of Fallot (TOF) is one of the conotruncal families of heart lesions in which the primary defect is on anterior deviation of the infundibulum septum (the muscular septum that separates the aortic and pulmonary outflow) **(Fig. 1)**.

The consequences of this deviation are the four components:
1. Obstruction in right ventricular (RV) outflow (pulmonary stenosis)
2. A malalignment type of ventricular septal defect (VSD)
3. Dextroposition of the aorta so that it overrides the ventricular septum
4. Right ventricular hypertrophy (RVH).

It was named after Etienne louis Arthur Fallot, a French physician, who first described the anatomical details in 1888. Obstruction to pulmonary artery (PA) blood flow is usually at both right ventricular infundibulum (subpulmonic area) and pulmonary valve. Complete obstruction of RV outflow (tetralogy with pulmonary atresia) is classified as an extreme form of TOF. The degree of pulmonary outflow obstruction and whether the ducts arteriosus is open or closed determine the degree of patient's cyanosis and the age at first presentation.

PATHOLOGY

- The original description of TOF includes the four abnormalities, a large VSD, right ventricular outflow tract (RVOT) obstruction, RVH, and overriding of the aorta. Actually only two abnormalities are required, a VSD large enough to equal pressure in both ventricle and RVOT obstruction. The RVH is secondary to the RVOT obstruction, and the overriding of the aorta varies.
- The VSD in TOF is a large perimembranous defect with extension into the subpulmonary region.
- The RVOT obstruction is the most frequently in the form of infundibular stenosis (45%). The obstruction is rarely at pulmonary valve (10%). A combination of the two may also occur (30%). The pulmonary valve is atretic in the most severe form of anomaly (15%).
- The pulmonary annulus and main PA are variably hypoplastic in most patient. The PA branches are usually small, although marked hypoplasia is uncommon. Stenosis at the origin of the PA, especially the left PA is common. Occasionally, systemic collateral arteries feed into the lung, especially in severe case of TOF.
- Right aortic arch is present in 25% of cases, with some of them having symptoms of vascular ring.
- In about 5% of TOF patients, abnormal coronary arteries are present.
- Complete AV canal defect occurs in approximately 2% of patient syndrome called, canal tet.

CLINICAL FEATURES

- Infants with mild degree of RV outflow may initially even have symptoms of heart failure caused by a ventricular level left-to-right shunt. In these patients, cyanosis is not present at birth but with increasing hypertrophy of RV infundibulum as the patient grows, cyanosis occurs later in the first few months of life.

RA. Right atrium
RV. Right ventricle
LA. Left atrium
LV. Left ventricle
SVC. Superior vena cava
IVC. Inferior vena cava
MPA. Main pulmonary artery
Ao. Aorta
TV. Tricuspid valve
MV. Mitral valve
PV. Pulmonary valve
AoV. Aortic valve

Fig. 1: Tetralogy of Fallot.

- In contrast, in infant with severe degree of RV outflow obstruction, neonatal cyanosis is noted immediately. In these infants, pulmonary blood flow (PBF) may be partially or almost totally dependent on flow through the duct arteriosus. When the ducts begin to close in the first few hours or days of life, severe cyanosis and circulatory collapse mainly occur. All degrees of variation exist between these two clinical extremes.
- Older children with long-standing cyanosis who have not undergone surgery may have dusky blue skin, gray sclera with engorged blood vessels, and marked clubbing of the fingers and toes.
- In older children with unrepaired tetralogy, dsypnea occurs on exertion.
  They may play actively for a short time and then sit or lay down.
- Characteristically, children assume squatting position for the relief of dyspnea caused by physical effort. Paroxysmal hypercyanotic attacks (hypoxic "blue" or "tet" spells occurs during the first year of life). The infant may become hyperpneic and restless. Cyanosis increases, gasping respiration ensues, and syncope may follow. The spells occur most frequently in the morning on initially awakening or after episodes of vigorous crying.
- Growth and development may be delayed in patient with severe untreated TOF, particularly when SaO_2 is chronically <70%. Puberty may also be delayed.

SIGNS

- The pulse is usually normal, as are venous and arterial pressure.
- In older infants and children, the left anterior hemithorax may bulge anteriorly because of long-standing RVH.
- On palpation, RV impulse can usually be detected. A systolic thrill may be felt along the left sternal border in 3rd and 4th parasternal spaces.
- On auscultation, the systolic murmur is loud and harsh and is heard that may be transmitted widely, especially to the lungs, but is most intense at the left sternal border. The murmur is generally ejection systolic nature at the upper sternal border. It may be preceded by click. The murmur is caused by turbulence through the RVOT. It tends to become louder, longer as severity of pulmonary stenosis increases from mild to moderate. It can actually become less prominent with severe obstruction, especially during a hypercyanotic spell, because of shunting of blood away from RV outflow through the aortic valve. Second heart sound (S2) is single, or the pulmonic component in soft because of the decreased excursion of the stenotic valve. Infrequently, a continuous murmur may be audible, especially if prominent collaterals are present.

INVESTIGATIONS

- *Oxygen saturation*: Typical SPO_2 is in between 65 and 85%.
- *Complete blood count*: Hemoglobin is elevated in proportion to the degree of cyanosis.
- *Coagulation studies*: Severe polycythemia may result in reduced coagulation factors and reduced platelet count.
- Serum iron should be measured as most of the patient with TOF have decreased serum iron.
- *Electrocardiography (ECG)* **(Fig. 2)**:
  - Characteristic finding is right axis derivation and RVH.
  - V4R lead is advisable as lead V1/V2 can show early transition for age.

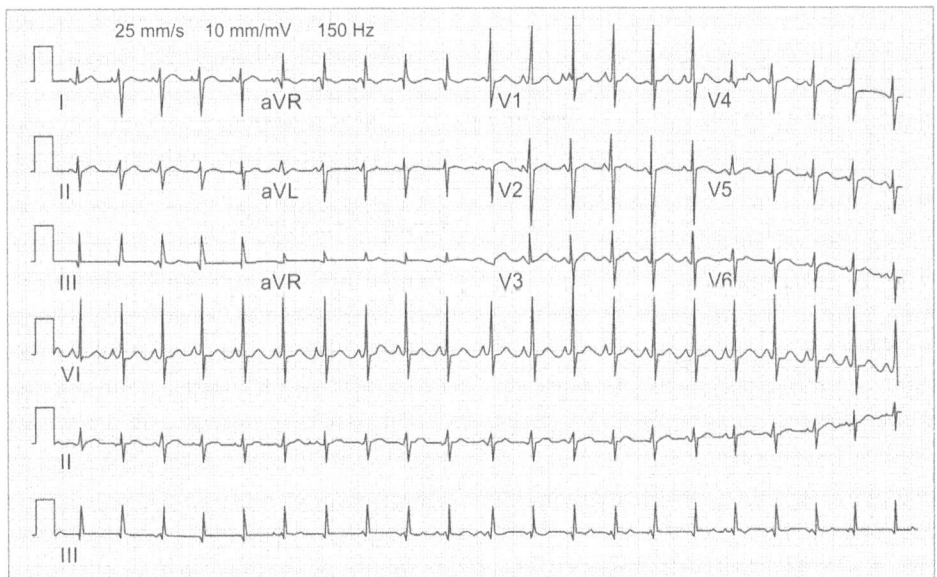

Fig. 2: Electrocardiographic findings in TOF. Right axial deviation and right ventricular hypertrophy.

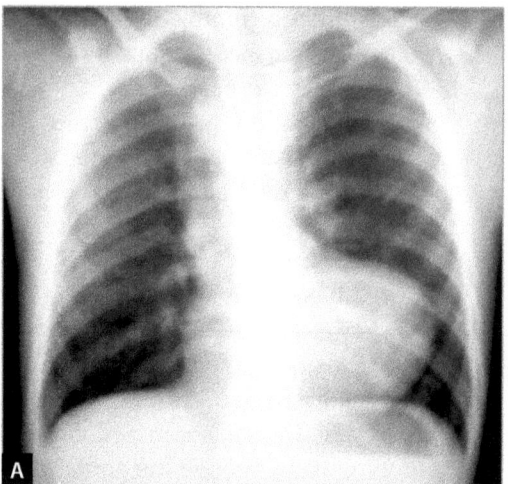 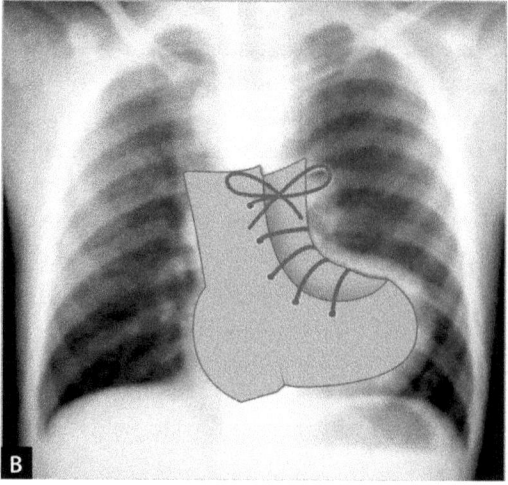

Figs. 3A and B: (A) Cardiac size is normal with upturned apex indicating hypertrophied right ventricle, concavity of PA segment leading to boot-shaped heart, right sided aortic arch, oligemic lung field; (B) Characteristic 'Boot shaped heart" in TOF.

- Wide QRS q with right bundle branch block pattern is sometimes seen after complete repair of TOF.
- *X-ray chest* **(Figs. 3A and B)**:
  - Cardiac size is normal with upturned apex suggestive of hypertrophied right ventricle, along with that there is concavity of PA segment leading to boot-shaped heart.
  - Right-sided aortic arch if present will show indentation on right of tracheal shadow.
  - The lung field is oligemic in cyanotic patients.
  - TOF and absent pulmonary valve may show cardiomegaly with or without pulmonary plethora. The central PA are dilated in these cases.
- *Echocardiography (Echo)*:
  - It is the most important diagnostic tool and must be performed for each case. It establishes the diagnosis and may be able to provide full preoperative information in infants and young children with good acoustic window.
  - The size location of VSD is well defined; the anatomy of right ventricular outflow tract, size of pulmonary annulus, and, main right and left pulmonary arteries can also be adequately assessed by it.
  - Echo is also very useful modality dur-ing cardiac surgery as intraoperative *transesophageal Echo* is able to detect additional VSDs better.
  - It is also useful in long-term follow-up.
- *Cardiac catheterization and angiography*:
  - It is required as a part of preoperative workup of those patients in whom full information is not obtained by Echo.
  - It has additional advantage of providing hemodynamic data, collaterals, and coronary artery details.
  - Filing pressure on right and left side of heart are also obtained.
  - Significant collaterals need to be occluded in the catheterization laboratory prior to surgical repair of TOF.
- *Magnetic resonance imaging (MRI)*:
  - This is rarely performed, except in patients with pulmonary atresia and VSD.
  - It defines aortopulmonary collaterals well, prior to unifocalization surgery.
  - MRI is indispensable for follow-up of postsurgical TOF patients.
  - Right ventricular volume and function, and quantification of pulmonary regurgitation are best estimated serially by MRI.
  - It also helps to determine the timing of pulmonary valve replacement in these patients.
- *Computed tomography (CT) angiography*:
  - CT angiography can be done very fast and with lower doses of radiation.
  - CT angiography is a good preoperative investigation in selected cases where information on Echo is not complete.
  - Also it provides useful information on PA anatomy coronaries and aortopulmonary collaterals.

MANAGEMENT

Hypoxic spell: It is characterized by hyperpnea (that is rapid or deep respiration), increasing cyanosis, irritability, and prolonged crying and decreasing intensity of heart murmur. Peak incidence occurs between 2 and 4 months of age.

Treatment of hypoxic spell aims to break the vicious circle of spell.

Following protocol are generally used:
- Infants should be held in knee–chest position.
- Morphine sulfate, 0.2 mg/kg SC/IM. It suppresses respiratory center and abolishes hyperpnea.

- Correct hydration to avoid hemoconcentration and possible thrombotic episode.
- Oxygen inhalation.
- Sodium bicarbonate ($NaHCO_3$), 1 mEq/kg IV with dilution to overcome acidosis. May be repeated in 10–15 minutes.
- Ketamine, 1–3 mg/kg IV over 60 seconds, works well to increase systemic vascular resistance and sedate infant if hypoxic spell does not respond by above measure.
- Propanol, 0.01–0.25 mg/kg by slow IV push, reduce heart rate and may reverse the spell.
- Neonates with severe RVOT may become cyanosed after birth because ductus arteriosus begin to close and PBF is further compromised. IV administration for prostaglandin E1, (0.01–0.20 µg/kg/min) is useful as it causes dilation of ductus arteriosus and usually provides adequate PBF until a surgical procedure can be performed.
- Normal body temperature to be maintained during transportation because cold increases oxygen consumption.
- Blood glucose level should be monitored because hypoglycemia is more likely to develop in infants with congenital heart defect.

Surgical Therapy

Infant with symptoms and severe cyanosis in the first month life usually has marked obstruction of right ventricular outflow tract. Two options are available in these infants:

- First is corrective open heart surgery performed in early infancy and even in the newborn period in critically ill infants. This approach has widespread acceptance today with excellent short- and long-term results and has supplanted palliative stunt for most cases where corrective surgery is not possible, palliative surgery in form of increasing PBF is required.
- Second infant with less severe cyanosis who can maintain with good growth and absence of hypercyanotic spell. Primary repair is performed electively at between 4 and 6 months of age.

Corrective Surgical Therapy

- It consists of relief of RVOT obstruction by resecting obstructive muscle bundles and by patch closure of VSD.
- If the pulmonary valve is stenotic, as it usually is, a valvectomy is performed.
- If the pulmonary valve annulus is too small or valve is extremely thickened, a valvectomy may be performed, the pulmonary valve annulus split open and a transannular patch placed across the pulmonary valve ring.

Palliative Surgery

- A palliative systemic to PA shunt (Blalock–Taussig shunt) performed to augment PA blood flow to decrease the amount of hypoxia and improve linear growth, as well as augment growth of the branch pulmonary arteries.
- The modified Blalock–Taussig shunt is currently the most common aortopulmonary shunt procedure and consist of a Gore-Tex conduit anastomosed side to side from the subclavian artery to homolateral branch of PA. Sometimes the central shunt is performed which means shunt is directed from ascending aorta to the main PA.

Long-term Follow-up

- Long-term prognosis is generally good for operated patient for TOF (86% survival at 30 years).
- Pulmonary regurgitation is main cause of late reintervention.
- Pulmonary regurgitation may result in dilation of right ventricular which causes exercise intolerance, cardiac arrhythmias, and can cause sudden death.

COMPLICATIONS

- Cerebral thrombosis results, most often in patients younger than 2 years. These patients may have iron deficiency anemia. Therapy consists of adequate hydration and supportive measures. Phlebotomy and volume replacement with albumin or saline are indicated in extreme polycythemia patient who are symptomatic.
- *Brain abscess*: It is less common than cerebral vascular event and occurs usually in older than 2 years. CT scan and MRI confirm the diagnosis. Antibiotic keeps the infection localized, but surgical drainage of abscess is usually necessary.
- *Bacterial endocarditis*: Occurs in right ventricular infundibulum or on the pulmonary, aortic, or tricuspid valves. Endocarditis may complicate palliative shunt or in patient with corrective surgery. Appropriate culture-specific antibiotics for 4–6 weeks are usually recommended.

KEY MESSAGES

- TOF is the most common cyanotic congenital heart disease beyond 1 week of age. It is most common entity grouped under Fallot physiology, which is characterized by decrease or absent pulmonary flow with VSD or single ventricle physiology.
- The degree of pulmonary outflow obstruction and whether the ducts arteriosus is open or closed determine the degree of cyanosis and the age of the presentation.

- Severe cyanosis may progress to cyanotic spell which may be life-threatening.
- The chest X-ray and ECG are quite characteristic. ECHO is investigation of the choice for diagnosis.
- Cardiac catheterization and angiography are required in older children and adults for those in whom full information is not obtained by echocardiography.
- Definite treatment is complete surgical repair.
- Palliative surgery in neonates and young infant is in form of systemic to PA shunt.
- Long-term prognosis is usually good although life-long follow-up is required.
- Pulmonary regurgitation is the major cause of late reintervention. Pulmonary regurgitation results in right ventricular dilatation leading to impaired exercise, tolerance, cardiac arrhythmia, and increased risk of sudden death.

SUGGESTED READING

1. Park MK. Park's Pediatric Cardiology for Practitioners, 6th edition. USA: Elsevier; 2014.

CHAPTER 125: Transposition of Great Arteries

Nurul Islam

INTRODUCTION

Transposition of the great arteries (TGA): It is the most common cyanotic congenital heart disease (CHD) at birth. The disease constitutes 5% of all CHDs.

Male babies are predominantly affected.

- Basic:
- Conotruncal defect occurs during truncal separation at embryonic life of 4–5 weeks; faulty development of conal septum leads to aorta arise from right ventricle (RV) and pulmonary artery (PA) comes from LV instead of RV → results in oxygenated blood from LV to pulmonary circulation and deoxygenated blood from RV to the same systemic circulation → Severe systemic hypoxemia.
- *The classical TGA means dextro TGA (d-TGA)*: Aorta anterior and to the right and PA is posterior and to the left.

In normal situation,

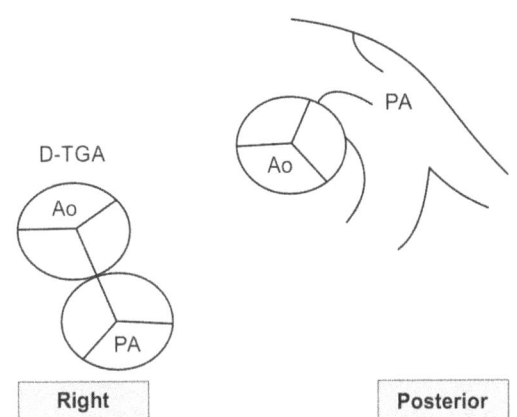

Pulmonary artery is most anterior and to the right of aorta whereas aorta is posterior and to the left.

Basic hemodynamic changes: Normal human circulatory system is in series **(Fig. 1A)** and in TGA, it gets converted into parallel **(Fig. 1B)** system.

In parallel circulation, there needs to be some mixing at atrial or ventricular level [atrial or ventricular septal defect

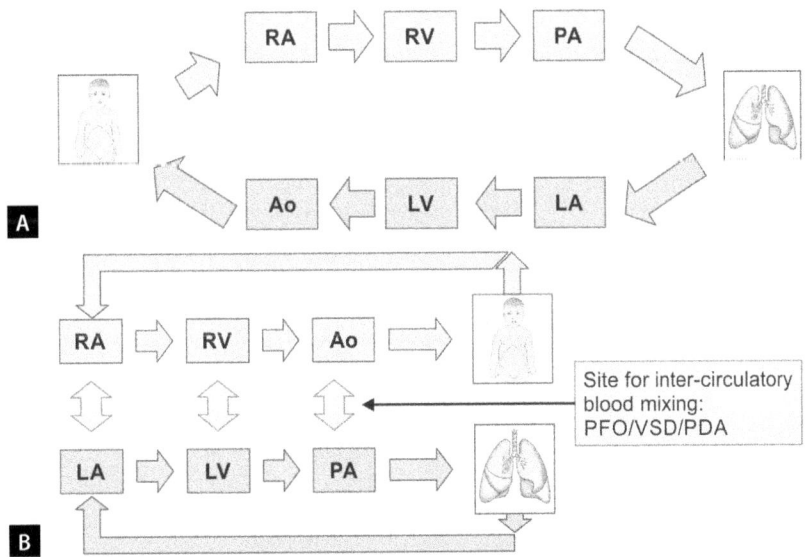

Figs. 1A and B: (A) Normal circulation—in series; (B) TGA circulation—in parallel.
(Ao: aorta; LV: left ventricle; LA: left atrium; PA: pulmonary artery; RA: right atrium; RV: right ventricle; PFO: patent foramen ovale; PDA: patent ductus arteriosus; TGA: transposition of the great arteries; VSD: ventricular septal defect)

(ASD or VSD)] or at the level of great arteries patent ductus arteriosus (PDA), otherwise hypoxemic blood will recirculate in the systemic circulation and will not be compatible to survival.

Common association:
- *Patent foramen oval (PFO) or small ASD or PDA*: 50%
- *VSD*: 40%
- Left ventricular outflow tract [(LVOT) LV to PA path)] obstruction in 5%.
(Management plan changes in this condition, so important to know)

PRENATAL DIAGNOSIS

Risk factors: Gestational diabetes mellitus (GDM), previous baby with cyanotic heart disease, close family members with known congenital heart disease.

How?
By doing fetal echocardiography (Echo) at around 18–22 weeks of gestation.

So all parents will be encouraged to go for fetal Echo during next pregnancy to pick up cardiac abnormality and further planning.

NATURAL COURSE OF DISEASE (FLOWCHART 1)

Classical TGA-with PFO or small ASD or PDA: Sickest group.

- *Circulation in parallel*: Baby survives depending upon number and size of mixing site.
- PFO is tiny, not adequate for good mixing.

PDA: Naturally tends for spontaneous and anatomical closure → results in more hypoxic blood in systemic circulation → Oxygenated blood in left heart (LA-LV-PA) not physiologically helping → hypoxemia manifested by worsening of *cyanosis*—metabolic acidosis and its complications → Early death **(Flowchart 1)**.

Needs urgent procedure balloon atrial septostomy (BAS*)/Medicine prostaglandin E1 (PGE1*) to create place (ASD or Opening PDA) for better mixing and improvement in systemic oxygenation.

- *TGA with VSD or large PDA*: These subsets do not present immediately → VSD is the site for adequate mixing → unless measured SpO_2, cyanosis not picked up clinically → as the baby grows and pulmonary vascular resistance (PVR) drops maximum at 8–10 weeks of life → pulmonary blood flow (PBF) increases → Drop in PVR and increase PBF falsely mimics like large VSD with heart failure (HF) with adequate saturation → clinically treated as VSD with congestive heart failure (CHF) with failure to thrive (FTT).
- *TGA, VSD, and LVOT obstruction*: Clinically mimics as TOF with its ejection systolic murmur (ESM) and cyanosis.

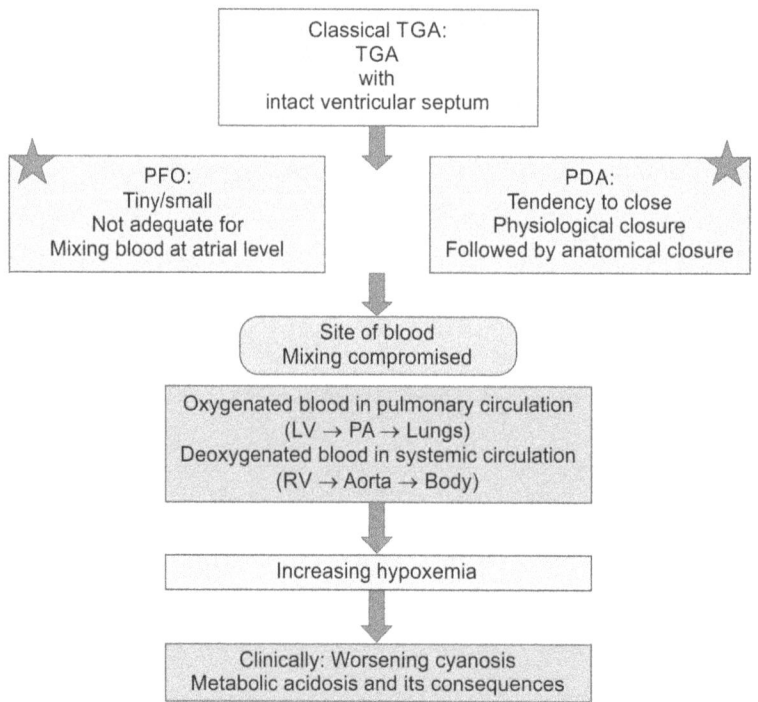

Flowchart 1: Natural course of disease.

(LV: left ventricle; LA: left atrium; PA: pulmonary artery; PFO: patent foramen oval; PDA: patent ductus arteriosus; TGA: transposition of the great arteries)

Sites for intervention: Medical (using prostin) or intervention (BAS).

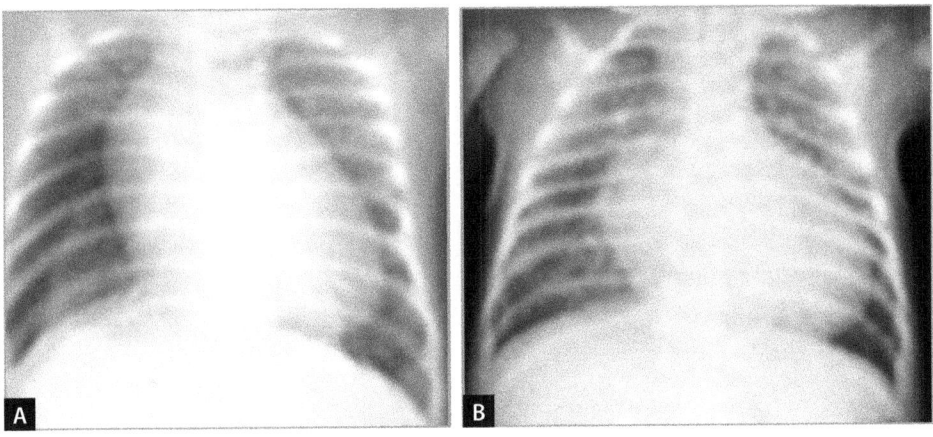

Figs. 2A and B: (A) TGA with intact ventricular septum; (B) TGA with VSD.
(TGA: transposition of great arteries; VSD: ventricular septal defect)

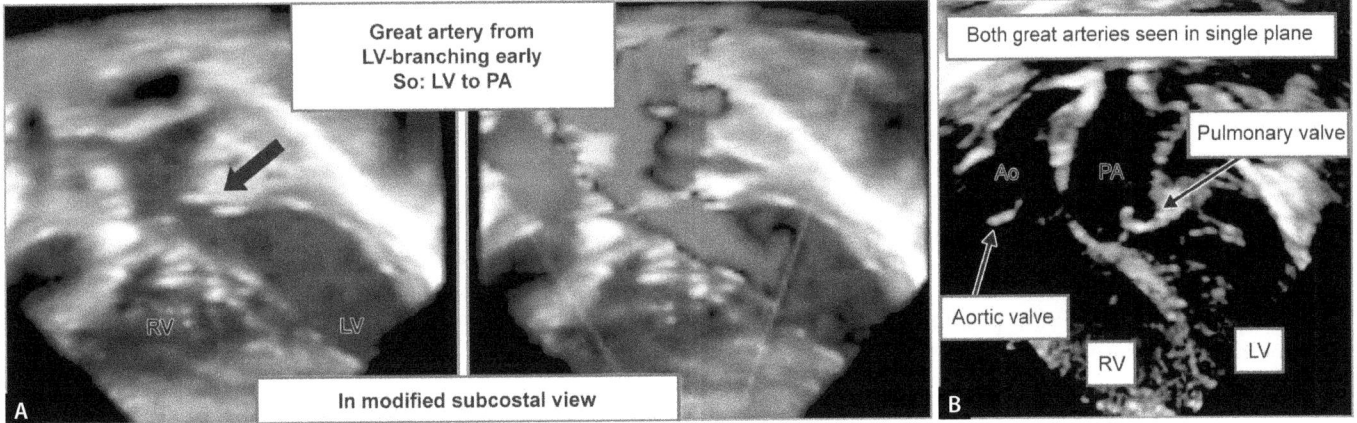

Figs. 3A and B: (A) Modified subcostal view; (B) Second clue: See both the GA in a single plane and parallel.
(LV: left ventricle; PA: pulmonary artery; RV: right ventricle; Ao: aorta; GA: great arteries)

ROLE OF INVESTIGATIONS IN DETAILS

Routine blood tests are not very specific.
- There is association of TGA with large for date baby because of specific flow pattern (containing nutrient-rich blood from placenta) across the celiac trunk.
- Serum calcium—Both total and ionized—CATCH 22 (22q11.2 deletion syndrome) is sometimes associated with TGA.
- Chest X-ray (CXR): In specific clinical setting, CXR is very helpful **(Figs. 2A and B)**.
- Narrow superior pedicle: (Both the great arteries are anterioposterior)
- Cardiac shadow: Egg onside appearance
- Lung parenchyma: Oligemic
- Electrocardiography (ECG) right axis deviation (RAD), right ventricular hypertrophy (RVH)
- Echo: For functional Echo [in neonatal intensive care unit (NICU)].

Consider clinical settings: Newborn; sats: <95%; gradually worsening cyanosis.

Pre- and postductal saturations must be monitored: Almost same because aorta from RV and PDA generally left to right (Ao to PA).

Apart from functional Echo: Try to focus great arteries (GA).

In cases of mixing lesions, aim to maintain SpO_2 >80%. No need to aim higher sats.

First clue:
- GA from LV: Early branching, i.e., PA [ventriculo-arterial (V-A) discordance]
- GA from RV: Late branching, i.e., AO (V-A discordance).

Second clue: See both the GA in a single plane and parallel **(Figs. 3A and B)**.

Third clue:
- Classical short-axis view **(Figs. 4A and B)**
- Normal: Circle and Sausage appearance
- TGA: Double circle sign.

Details Echo preferably by pediatric cardiologist
- Segmental approach: All structures to be identified
- Complete diagnosis to be made

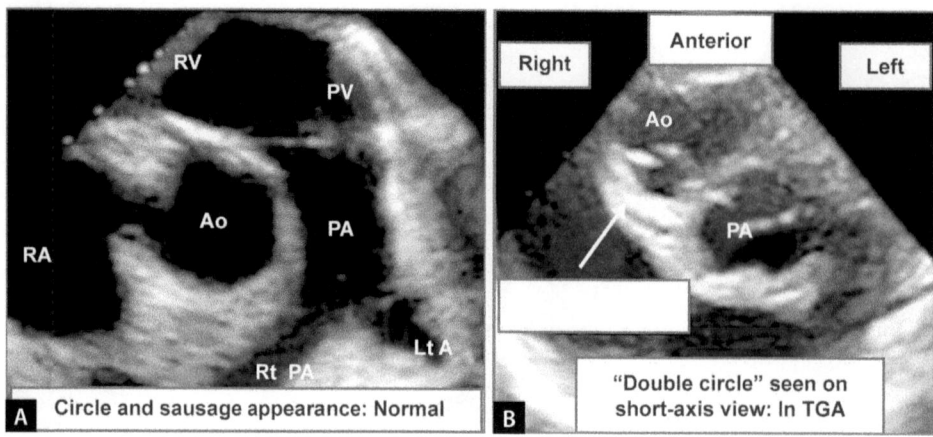

Figs. 4A and B: Classical short-axis view in TGA (A) Normal: Circle and sausage appearance; (B) "Double circle" seen in short-axis view in TGA. (Ao: aorta; Lt: left; LV: left ventricle; Rt: right; RV: right ventricle; PA: pulmonary artery; TGA: transposition of the great arteries)

- Associated lesion to be found (ASD, VSD, PDA, LVOT obstruction)
- *Needs details coronary artery*: Left coronary system and right coronary system—origin from which sinus; course (Coronary system to be reimplanted at original PA end, important for surgery)
- Anticipation of near future problem
- *Proper planning*: *Timing of surgery and *Type of surgery.

In some difficult situation: (To profile associated anomaly, arch anatomy, coronary anatomy)
- CT angiography
- Cardiac catheterization

**Hyperoxia test better not to perform in suspected TGA (TGA with intact septum) presenting at neonatal age—oxygen may accelerate the closure of duct and worsen the situation.

TREATMENT

It starts from the point of diagnosis or there is some possibilities but not confirmed because of lack of support.

Treat other metabolic aspects:
- Acidosis
- Hypocalcemia
- Hypoglycemia
- Rule out sepsis if required.

NOT DIAGNOSED BUT DOUBT RAISED

For all practical purposes—newborn with cyanosis and when it worsen with O_2—probably we are dealing with duct-dependent pulmonary circulation conditions such as:
- TGA with intact ventricular septum (Mixing problem)
- TOF with pulmonary atresia
- Other combination lesions with PDA-dependent circulation.

Target to keep the duct open:
- Call family, explain possibilities of coronary heart disease (CHD), limitations of diagnostic facilities.
- Discuss the plan—medicine, S/E of prostin-like apnea and transport issues.
- Communicate with higher center
- Take a consent for treatment and intubation also.

Preload with caffeine: 20 mg/kg loading: Dissolve in 20 mL NS, run over 30 minutes.

After 24 hours, maintenance dose: 5 mg/kg once a day slow IV.

Start prostin:

Preparing **prostin** solution and dosing

```
One ampoule prostin
(500 μg–1 mL)

NS = (81 ÷ body wt) mL (X mL)

X + 1 mL prostin solution:
If run-
@ 1 mL/h, i.e., 1 μg/kg/min
@ 0.5 mL/h, i.e., 0.05 μg/kg/min
```

Treat other comorbidities:
Advantages of PGE1:
- Overcome the critical period
- Safe transportation
- Get time to solve other issues—sepsis, weight gain.

Disadvantages:
- Fever
- Osteoporosis
- *Tissue fragility*: Difficulty in surgery
- *Chance of apnea*: Intubation—chronic lung disease (CLD), ventilator-induced lung injury (VILI).

Balloon atrial septostomy: (**Fig. 5**)
Indication:
- Tiny PFO or restricted flow—inadequate mixing

**Caffeine will not combat apnea due to prostin in term babies.

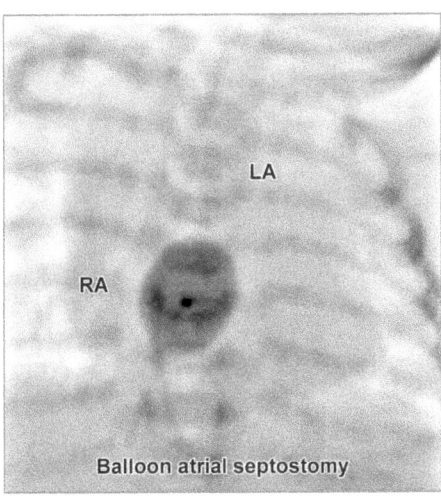

Fig. 5: Balloon atrial septostomy.
(LA: left atrium; RA: right atrium)

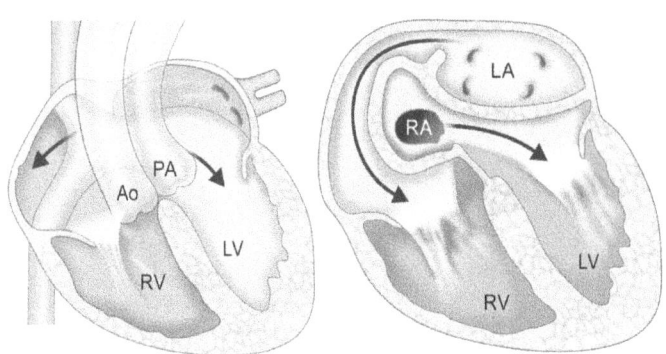

Fig. 6: Senning operation: Physiological correction.
(Ao: aorta; LV: left ventricle; RV: right ventricle; LA: left atrium; RA: right atrium; PA: pulmonary artery)

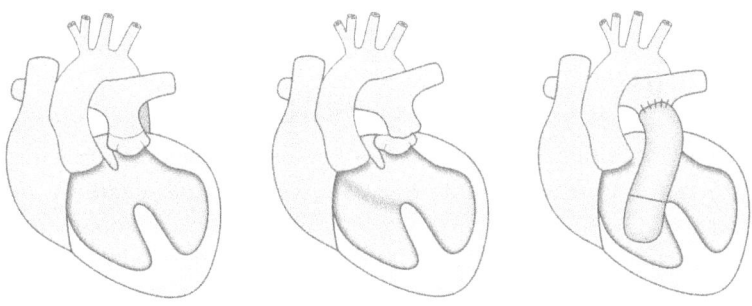

Rastelli operation: LV is rerouted to aorta via VSD
RV connected to PA via artificial tube (Conduit)

Fig. 7: Rastelli operation.
(LV: left ventricle; PA: pulmonary artery; RV: right ventricle; VSD: ventricular septal defect)

- Not ready for the definitive surgery
- *Procedure summary*: BAS is done to create ASD for adequate mixing of oxygenated blood from LA to RA. Procedure is done under sedation in catheterization laboratory under fluoroscopy. The approach is generally through femoral vein. Appropriate size septostomy balloon is taken and inflated within LA and it is pulled back to RA with a jerky hand movement. This force causes tear in atrial septum and create an ASD.
- *If a baby develops features of CHF (TGA with large VSD)*: Diuretics (Digoxin required rarely)
- Rapid volume unload from left side of heart to right side leading to regression of LV muscle mass—LV become flat, thin with less power generation. [normally LV works against high systemic vascular resistance (SVR) but in TGA against low resistance system—lung parenchyma]. So corrective surgery needs to be planned.
- *Specific treatment*: Target to provide oxygenated blood from left side to aorta
 (Atrial switching—Senning operation) **(Fig. 6)**

Atrial level:
- Divert blood from LA → RV → aorta → systemic circulation
- Not routinely performed
- Long-term complication high—arrhythmia from atria.
- Obstruction in pulmonary and systemic venous return path
- Systemic ventricle (RV) failure.

Ventricular level:
- Here pulmonary venous blood-redirected from LV → big VSD → aorta
- Systemic venous blood directed from RV → PA via artificial tube (conduit) **(Fig. 7)**
- This is done in the presence of VSD and pulmonary stenosis (PS) (LVOT obstruction)
- Not very popular
- High surgical mortality (10–30%)
- Late complication high.

Two alternatives:
1. *Réparation à l'ètage ventriculaire (REV) procedure*: In small babies, the conduit is not used rather main

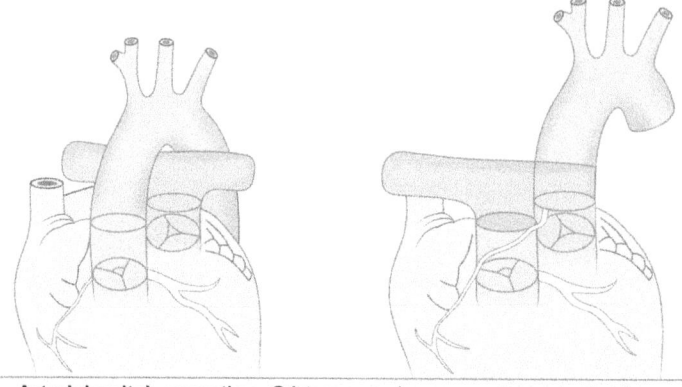

Fig. 8: Arterial switch operation.
(GA: great arteries; MPA: main pulmonary artery; PA: pulmonary artery)

pulmonary artery (MPA) is disconnected from LV and pulled back to RV and attached, blood directly flows into MPA from RV.

2. Arterial switch operation (ASO) **(Fig. 8)**:
   - Procedure of choice
   - It is anatomical correction, less complications
   - Needs coronary translocation from aortic side to neoaortic side (attached to LV)
   - Should be done within 3 weeks otherwise LV regresses.

FOLLOW-UP

- *Immediate post operation*: At 1, 3, 6, 12, weeks postoperatively.
- *Children*: Yearly
- *Adolescent*: Every second yearly
- In each visit
- History
- *Clinical examination*: Any murmur
  - 12-lead (ECG): Any features of rhythm disturbances
- Transthoracic Echo: Look for stenosis—supravalvar aortic stenosis (AS), PS
- Aortic or pulmonary insufficiency, heart function.

PROGNOSIS

- After ASO, expect satisfactory long-term good result with excellent survival rate
- Small chance of reoperation
- Negligible possibilities of arrhythmia
- Good physical growth and development
- *Aortic regurgitation (AR) is the frequent valve complication*: 14–44% mild-to-moderate AR.
- PS is the most common cause of reoperation.
- *Most serious morbidities during long-term follow-up*: Coronary artery obstruction
- Post ASO, children are prone to obesity, need counseling and care.

SUGGESTED READING

1. Park MK. Park's Pediatric Cardiology for Practitioners, 6th edition. USA: Elsevier; 2014.

Complex Congenital Heart Disease

Asok Kumar Datta

TOTAL ANOMALOUS PULMONARY VENOUS RETURN

Here pulmonary veins drain in other areas of heart except left atrium (LA). This abnormal return of pulmonary veins may be in supracardiac region called supracardiac variety, cardiac region called cardiac variety and infracardiac region infracardiac variety.

Hemodynamic Changes

There is development of pulmonary venous congestion with pulmonary edema and respiratory difficulty. This is more common in infracardiac variety. For survival, there must be atrial septal defect (ASD). There is enlargement of right atrium (RA) and right ventricle (RV). Tricuspid regurgitation may be present in some cases.

Clinical Features

- Cyanosis
- Growth retardation
- *Quadruple rhythm*: Right ventricular hypertrophy (RVH).

Investigations

Chest X-ray (CXR): Cardiomegaly, Snowman sign or figure of 8 configuration in supracardiac variety, Scimitar sign in infracardiac variety.

Electrocardiography (ECG): RVH and right axis deviation.
Echocardiography shows the abnormal drainage pattern.

Treatment

- *Medical*: Correction of metabolic acidosis, decongestants in congestive cardiac failure (CCF).
- Surgical correction is the treatment of choice.

TRICUSPID ATRESIA

Hemodynamics

Tricuspid valve is atretic. RV is rudimentary. The blood passes through ASD to LA and then to left ventricle (LV). Ventricular septal defect (VSD) is usually present. LV eject blood in two ways: One through VSD to RV and through aorta to systemic circulation. Pulmonary stenosis is commonly present.

Clinical Features

It presents with Fallot's physiology and clinical picture resembles tetralogy of Fallot. Cyanosis, cyanotic spell, thromboembolic manifestations, etc. are same. Only exception is left ventricular hypertrophy which is prominent here.

Investigations

- *Radiology*: Heart size is normal or slightly increased
- *ECG*: Superior QRS axis
- *Echocardiography*: Establishes the diagnosis.

Management

- *Supportive therapy*: Prostaglandin E1 (PGE1) infusion, balloon atrial septostomy
- *Surgical treatment*: Fontan operation is preceded by palliative procedure if required.

HYPOPLASTIC LEFT HEART SYNDROME

In this condition, the LV and proximal aorta are hypoplastic. The systemic blood supply is solely dependent on patent ductus arteriosus. The newborn may pass on to shock if ductus closes functionally after day two. The left atrial blood passes to the RA, then to RV, and RV takes the load of the circulation.

Chest X-ray shows cardiomegaly, ECG shows RVH, and echocardiography is diagnostic.

Management

- After birth, PGE1 infusion keeps patency of the ductus, and may need supportive therapy
- *Surgery*: Norwood operation.

EBSTEIN ANOMALY

There is downward displacement of septal and posterior tricuspid valve. It is actually arterialization of the ventricle.

The RV is small and its pressure is also low. The right atrial size is large and it is reflected as huge cardiomegaly in CXR.

In neonate, Ebstein presents as cyanosis and cardiac failure. PGE1 infusion is not helpful. The pulmonary vascular resistance is high. Interatrial communication from right to LA is present.

In mild cases, it may present in children with cyanosis, effort intolerance, Quadruple rhythm, palpitation, supra-ventricular tachycardia.

Investigations

- *CXR*: Cardiomegaly, decreased pulmonary vascular markings
- *ECG*: Right atrial hypertrophy (RAH), right bundle branch block (RBBB)
- *Echocardiography*: Diagnostic.

Treatment

- *Treatment*: Symptomatic
- *Surgery*: Palliative surgery to increase pulmonary circulation.

PERSISTENT TRUNCUS ARTERIOSUS

Here, there is a failure of formation of spiral septum and truncus arteriosus fails to divide. As a result, there is mixing of blood and cyanosis results. VSD is present in all cases. The pulmonary trunk takes origin from truncus. There may be increased blood supply to the pulmonary trunk, sometimes causing cyanosis less prominent. CCF is common in this disorder.

Investigations

- CXR shows cardiomegaly
- *ECG*: Biventricular hypertrophy (BVH)
- *Echocardiography*: Diagnostic.

Treatment

- *Medical*: Decongestive therapy
- *Surgical*: Rastelli procedure and VSD closure.

SINGLE VENTRICLE

Here both the atria drain in one ventricle. The ventricle morphology is left ventricular in 80% of cases. The RV is rudimentary and is connected to the LV through bubo ventricular foramen.

Aorta usually takes origin from rudimentary ventricle and pulmonary artery from LV, i.e., dextro-transposition of the great arteries (DTGA) in approximate 70% of cases but the reverse may occur in rest cases. The mitral valve is right sided and the tricuspid valve is left sided.

Presentation depends on the degree of pulmonary circulation. If pulmonary circulation is large, the cyanosis is less and the child may present with features of CCF. If the pulmonary circulation is less due to pulmonary stenosis the cyanosis is increased and the disease follows Fallot's physiology.

Investigations

- *CXR*: Cardiomegaly in CCF and normal in pulmonary stenosis cases.
- *ECG*: Unusual ventricular hypertrophy pattern showing equal QRS complexes in all precordial leads.
- *Echocardiography*: Diagnostic.

Management

- *Medical*: Decongestive therapy, moist O_2, correction of metabolic acidosis, nutrition.
- *Surgical*: Bidirectional Glen operation followed by the Fontan-type operation.

SUGGESTED READING

1. Park MK. Park's Pediatric Cardiology for Practitioners, 6th edition. USA: Elsevier; 2014.

Kawasaki Disease (Cardiac Manifestation)

Asok Kumar Datta

INTRODUCTION

Tomisaki Kawasaki from Japan first reported this disease in a paper with the title "mucocutaneous lymph node syndrome" in 1967. Subsequently other investigators found that coronary arteries abnormalities are associated with this disease and Kawasaki et al. published several cases in literature with coronary artery aneurysm (CAA). The rest of the world subsequently accepted this disease and the name Kawasaki disease became universal. It presents almost all areas of the world though incidence is much more in Asian population.

Kawasaki disease is an acute inflammatory disease of medium-sized blood vessels which leads to affecting all systems with more involvement of coronary arteries often complicated with mostly various cardiac manifestations and also sometimes other systems involvement.

The disease usually affects in <5 years of age but it may occur in older children and adolescents also. It is more common in boys than girls. The cause is not known.

The exact cause of the disease is not known. It resembles viral infections, bacterial infections, rickettsia infections, autoimmune disorders, etc., but none is definitely proved.

Kawasaki disease is the most common acquired heart disease in all part of the world replacing rheumatic fever.

The prevalence of the disease is variable staring from 5–19 per 1 lac population.

The disease is diagnosed when the following clinical pictures are present: Fever for 5 or >5 days along with any four of the following:
1. Nonpurulent bulbar conjunctivitis
2. Cracked lips and/or strawberry tongue
3. Palmer and/or planter edema
4. Perianal and periungual desquamation
5. Skin rashes
6. Unilateral cervical lymph node adenitis with size 1.5 cm. The illness cannot be explained by any other disease process.

Besides other manifestations such as polyarthralgia, polyarthritis (resembling juvenile idiopathic arthritis), accelerated Bacillus Calmette–Guérin (BCG) reaction, diarrhea, features of pneumonia, irritability, etc., may occur.

The important concept for realization is one should not wait for complete diagnostic criteria because chances of complications are much more with increasing the disease duration (e.g., CAA is common after 7 days of duration of the disease) and all the manifestations are not present simultaneously. Early diagnosis and treatment are required.

When along with fever, less than four manifestations are present, then it is called incomplete Kawasaki disease; when all the manifestations requiring for diagnosis are present, then it is called complete Kawasaki disease and when the manifestations are unusual, e.g., nephritis, pneumonia, central nervous system (CNS) manifestations, etc., then it is called atypical. One thing we have to remember that larger blood vessels may also be involved atypically in this disease, e.g., aorta arteritis, involvement of carotid arteries, and subclavian arteries.

The incidence of CAA is common in Kawasaki disease, approximately 25%. We have to diagnose it early.

Along with above features we need investigations: Examination of blood usually shows leukocytosis, normal differential count, and high C-reactive protein (CRP) level and the leukocyte count, CRP, and ESR in first hour are progressively high. These investigations give us a clue to diagnosis of CAA in Kawasaki disease. Platelets count is usually normal in the first week but from 2nd week onward, it is progressively rising.

Other investigations such as urine examination, liver function test—AST level, ALT level, and serum bilirubin level—are required.

Depending on the presentation, other investigations may be needed.

The most important investigation is echocardiography to exclude CAA.

Normally, if the age of the baby is <5 years, the inner diameter of coronary artery should be ≤3 mm; and if it is >3 mm then it is called abnormal. In children >5 years of age, >4 mm of inner diameter of coronary artery is abnormal.

Depending on the internal diameter, the CAA is defined as severe when >8 mm, moderate when >4 to <8 mm and mild when >3 mm. Usually, left anterior descending and right anterior descending coronary arteries are involved.

In addition to that, perivascular brightness is also seen in coronary arteries.

The management should be started as soon as possible preferably before 7 days of duration of the disease otherwise chances of CAA is high.

TREATMENT

- Intravenous immunoglobulin (IVIg) 2 g/kg infusion
- Aspirin 50 mg/kg is given in four equal doses till fever subsides and then 3–5 mg/kg once daily for 6–8 weeks.

Usually patient becomes afebrile within 36 hours after IVIg and if not afebrile within that period or relapse of fever occurs within 7 days of fever then it is called resistant Kawasaki disease.

Treatment of resistant cases are:
- IVIg 2 g/kg infusion
- Infliximab 5 mg/kg infusion over 12 hours.

Usually echocardiography should be repeated at 2 weeks and 6–8-week duration. If no abnormality is there, then the patient should be asked to follow-up after 5 years of age.

Follow-up of the Patient

The patient with no CAA may be followed up after 5 years of age to see lipid profile and to check cardiac status.

- *Patient with mild CAA*: Mild CAA disappears within initial 6–8 weeks—follow-up should be done with echocardiography at 2 weeks and after 6–8 weeks. Cardiac checkup should be done at 3–5 years of age.
- *Patient with moderate CAA*: Aspirin should be continuing till CAA is normal. Serum lipid profile after 1 year and cardiac checkup should be done.
- *Patient with severe CAA*: Aspirin should be continued lifelong. Biannual checkup is required.

Vaccination Following Kawasaki Disease

Vaccination should be stopped 11 months after IVIg therapy. Nonliving vaccine can be given but living vaccine should be avoided. Influenza vaccine should be given. If urgently required, then clopidogrel 1 mg/kg (maximum up to 75 mg) may be an alternative to aspirin.

PRESCRIPTION ADVICES

Drug	Dose	Duration
IVIg	2 g/kg	Over 12 hours infusion (follow the guideline given in pack)
Ecosprin	50 mg/kg	Till fever subsides up to 6–8 weeks
	3–5 mg/kg	Till the echocardiography is normal

CHAPTER 128

Anomalous Left Coronary Artery Originating from Pulmonary Artery

Soutrik Seth

INTRODUCTION

History

Way back in 1886, Brooks described two cases of abnormal coronary artery originating from pulmonary artery (PA). In 1933, Bland, White, and Garland described a case of anomalous left coronary artery (ALCA) originating from pulmonary artery (ALCAPA) in a 60-year-old female.

Anomalous Left Coronary Artery Originating from PA

Anomalous left coronary artery originating from PA is the most common congenital malformation of coronary circulation; incidence is 1 in 3 lac live births.

Rarely other anomalies also occur such as right coronary artery (RCA), left anterior descending artery (LAD), circumflex arteries originating from the pulmonary trunk. ALCAPA is a general designation, does not differentiate right or left pulmonary arteries. The anomalous LCA is a thin-walled vessel, RCA in this case is originating from its normal aortic sinus and is dilated and tortuous. Portion of ventricle supplied by anomalous artery is thinned out, scarred and dilated ultimately forming ventricular aneurysm. Conversely the hypoperfused portion of left ventricle (LV) increases in mass (hypoxic stimuli), the LV endocardium exhibits fibroelastosis and rarely focal calcification.

THEORIES BEHIND ORIGIN OF ANOMALOUS CORONARY ARTERIES

- *Division of embryological truncus arteriosus*: Coronary arteries originate as two endothelial buds; faulty division of truncus can incorporate one or both coronary buds into pulmonary arteries. Incidence of anomalous origin of LCA is higher than RCA due to proximity of left aortic sinus to truncal septum, so small displacement causes LCA originating from PA.
- *Involution and persistence theory*: Originally six coronary artery analgens, three from aorta and three from PA. Anomalous origin results from persistence of PA coronary anlagen together with involution of normally persistent aortic coronary analgen.

PATHOPHYSIOLOGY

Ischemia is a serious sequela of ALCAPA. It does not stem from the fact that only one coronary artery originates from aorta, nor from deoxygenated blood coming from pulmonary trunk.

The answer lies in the direction of blood flow through the coronary bed **(Fig. 1)**.

In fetal and early neonatal life, high pulmonary arterial pressure results in antegrade blood flow into ALCA.

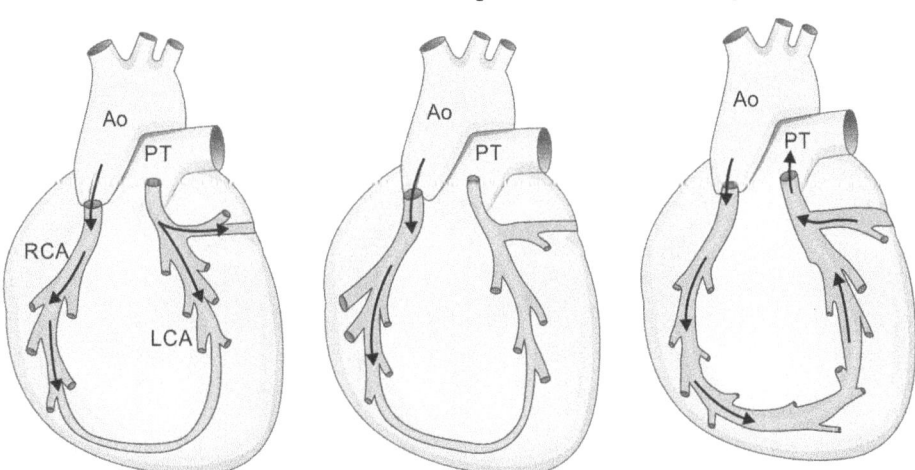

Fig. 1: Direction of blood flow in the coronary bed in ALCA from fetal life to infancy.
(Ao: aorta; LCA: left coronary artery; PT: pulmonary trunk; RCA: right coronary artery)

With subsequent fall in pulmonary pressure, there is parallel fall in blood flow in ALCA, myocardial ischemia is unavoidable unless adequate circulation from right to left coronary arteries is established via intercoronary anastomoses (low-resistance pathways).

Ischemia causes LV to labor under three handicaps:
1. Viable myocardium is compromised, so contractility is depressed.
2. Mitral regurgitation (MR) as a consequence of ischemic papillary muscle dysfunction.
3. Flow via intercoronary anastomosis leading to volume overload on LV ischemia leads to global hypokinesia in infants.

PRESENTATION

Three general patterns of presentation:
1. Serious symptoms in early infancy with death before 1 year (80%)
2. Early symptoms followed by gradual attenuation
3. Asymptomatic

Most babies appear healthy at birth till 2 months, then irritability, dyspnea, wheezing, cough diaphoresis occur (aggravated by feeding, crying or bowel movement).

Sometimes initial symptom may be hoarseness (dilated PA brushing recurrent laryngeal nerve), poor growth and development due to congestive heart failure, and angina delayed until teens. Myocardial ischemia, tachyarrhythmias, atrial fibrillation, or cardiac arrest can also occur.

Pulse: Pulsus alternans mostly, low diastolic pressure due to aortic run off. Left parasternal impulse is noted due to enlarged LA.

Auscultation: It may have no murmur or systolic diastolic or continuous murmur. Holosystolic murmur of MR (ischemic papillary dysfunction).

Continuous murmur is generated by flow through intercoronary anastomoses, located at base of heart or left sterna border.

INVESTIGATIONS

- *Electrocardiogram (ECG)*: Anterolateral myocardial infarction pattern **(Fig. 2)**:
  - Deep and narrow Q waves in lead 1 and aVL, inverted T waves, ST segment shifts in leads 1 and aVL.
- *Left ventricular hypertrophy (LVH)*: Bland, White, Garland described this. Both hypertrophy and hyperplasia occur. Deep S waves and tall R waves are present.
- *LAD*: Mainly due to disproportionate increase in posterobasal LV muscle mass leading to left superior direction of major depolarizing vector.

Normal infants and children do not have q waves; however, in ALCAPA q waves are present though in sharp contrast to shallow broad q waves in adult ischemic heart disease.

- Chest roentgenogram varies between massive cardiomegaly in symptomatic infants to normal or near normal in older children. Increased vascularity occurs due to pulmonary vascular congestion of LV failure **(Fig. 3)**.

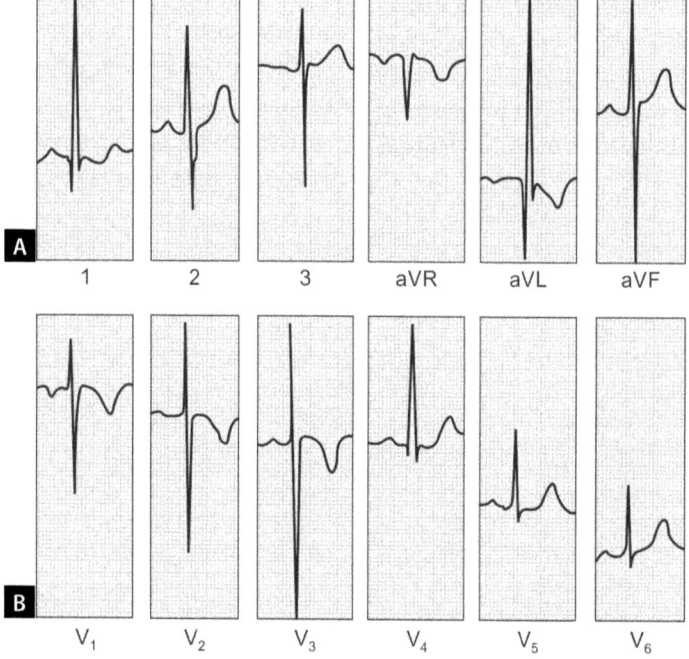

Figs. 2A and B: Electrocardiographic changes seen in ALCAPA including deep Q waves in lead I and aVL, LVH and LAD.

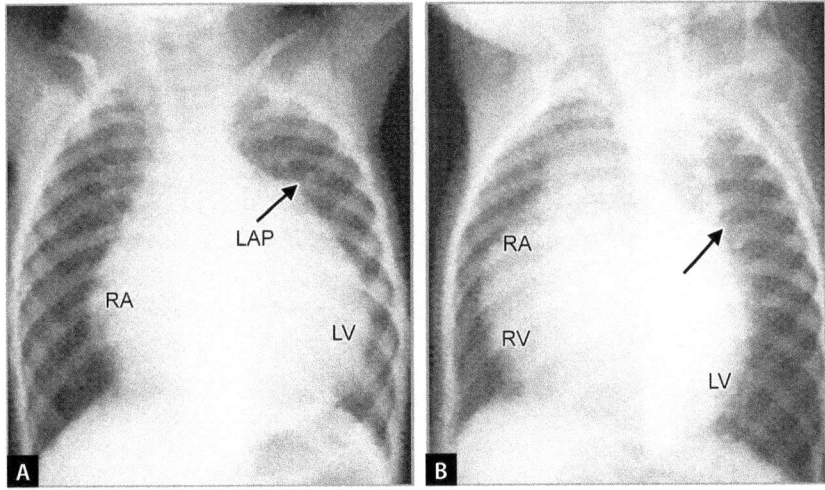

Figs. 3A and B: Increased vascularity occurs due to pulmonary vascular congestion of LV failure (arrows).
(LAP: left atrial pressure; LV: left ventricle; RA: right atrium; RV: right ventricle)

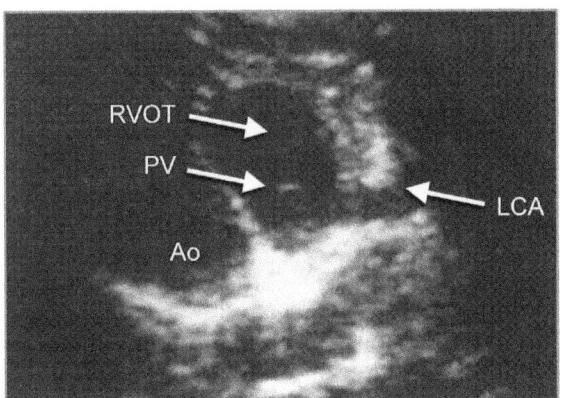

Fig. 4: Echocardiography showing LCA originating from RVOT.
(Ao: aorta; LCA: left coronary artery; PV: pulmonary valve; RVOT: right ventricular outflow tract)

- *Echocardiography*: Diagnostic modality. Aortic origins of LCA and RCA are visualized **(Fig. 4)**. Color flow imaging establishes diastolic or continuous flow entering pulmonary trunk and left ventricle size, motion, ejection fraction, MR quantification, left ventricle myocardial perfusion index for ischemic scarring.
- *Cardiac enzymes*: Relative slow development of myocardial infarction makes it difficult to interpret the changes. Cardiac troponin I may increase.
- Cardiac catheterization **(Figs. 5 and 6)**
- *Cardiac computed tomography*: For coronary artery anatomy.

MANAGEMENT

Medical management alone carries high mortality (80–100%). All patients with diagnosis of ALCAPA need surgery.
- *Palliative surgery*: For critically ill infants. Simple ligation of ALCA prevents steal into LA. Later elective bypass procedure is required.

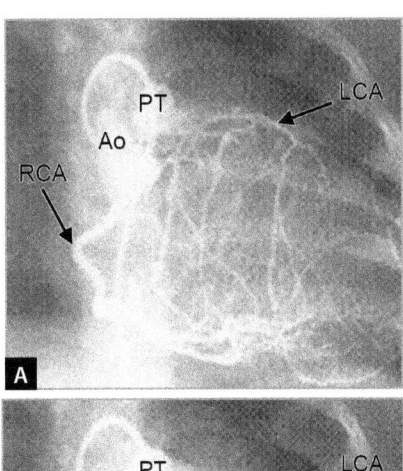
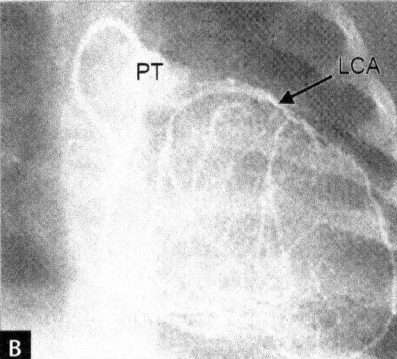

Figs. 5A and B: Coronary arteriogram showing narrowed LCA arising from pulmonary trunk and dilated tortuous RCA arising from aorta.
(Ao: aorta; LCA: left coronary artery; PT: pulmonary trunk; RCA: right coronary artery)

- *Definitive surgery*:
  - *Intrapulmonary tunnel operation (Takeuchi repair)*: Most popular
    An aortopulmonary window is created on anterior wall of PA. Coronary artery is fed by aorta through the AP window while PA opening is closed by flap.
  - LCA implantation (*Tashiro repair* and subclavian to LCA anastomosis).

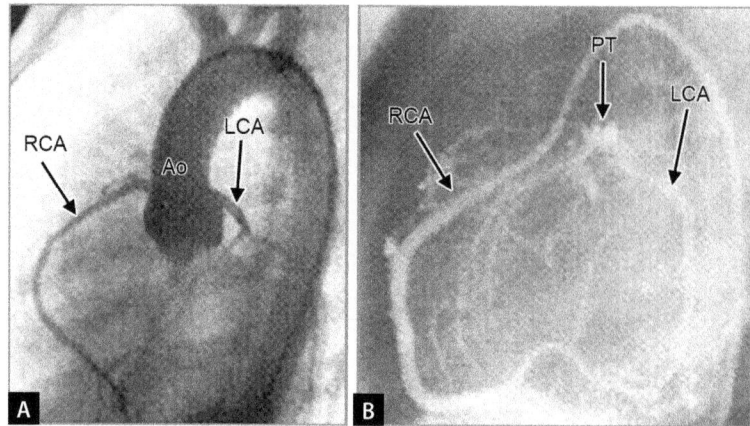

Figs. 6A and B: Coronary arteriogram showing normal LCA originating from aorta in (A) and narrow LCA originating from pulmonary trunk (B).
(Ao: aorta; LCA: left coronary artery; PT: pulmonary trunk; RCA: right coronary artery)

PROGNOSIS

- Most favorable outcome when RCA alone or LAD or circumflex artery alone originates anomalously.
- Both coronary arteries originating anomalously carries poor prognosis.
- There is a wide spectrum of manifestations—death in infancy to asymptomatic adults.

SUGGESTED READING

1. Moss and Adams' Heart Disease in Infants, Children and Adolescents, Vol 1, 9th edition.
2. Neonatal Cardiology, 2nd edition by Michael Artman.
3. Park's Pediatric Cardiology for Practitioners, 7th edition.
4. Perloff's Clinical Recognition of Congenital Heart Disease, 6th editon.

129 CHAPTER

Myocardial Diseases

Asok Kumar Datta

MYOCARDITIS
- It is the inflammation of the myocardium.
- It is caused by virus, bacteria, protozoa, and fungus infections.
- Usual presentations are features suggestive of heart failure, i.e., respiratory difficulty associated with tachycardia, cardiomegaly, gallop rhythm, crepitations in chest, hepatomegaly, edema in dependent areas, etc.
- Sometimes cardiac arrhythmia is associated.
- Chest X-ray shows cardiomegaly, electrocardiography (ECG) shows diminished voltages, nonspecific ST and T changes.

Management is symptomatic; decongestive therapy is done for congestive cardiac failure (CCF); digoxin is better be avoided; angiotensin-converting enzyme (ACE) inhibitor action is good. Management of arrhythmia is done, if present.

CARDIOMYOPATHY
- It is the intrinsic disease of the myocardium.
- It may be primary or secondary to other causes.

There are three types of cardiomyopathy: (1) Dilated cardiomyopathy (DCM), (2) restrictive cardiomyopathy, and (3) obstructive cardiomyopathy.

Of the three, DCM is most common.

Dilated Cardiomyopathy

Secondary causes of DCM:
- The most common is following myocarditis
- Associated with myopathy, muscular dystrophy
- May follow bacterial, viral, fungal, rickettsial disease
- May be a complication of endocrinal disorder, e.g., thyroid disease
- Anomalous origin of left coronary artery from pulmonary artery.

In cases of DCM, we have to exclude secondary causes very carefully. In primary cases, in about half of the cases, a genetic disorder is found.

Here there is no thickening of the wall of the ventricle. There is dilatation of ventricles. Mostly the left ventricle (LV) is affected. Occasionally right ventricle (RV) may also be affected. Due to dilatation, there is cardiomegaly present. The ejection power of LV is reduced and ejection fraction is decreased. Mitral regurgitation is present in some cases. The cardiac output is decreased. There is difficulty of drainage from the left atrium and pulmonary venous pressure is increased. There is chance of coagulopathy due to stagnation of blood in atrium.

Chest X-ray (CXR) will show:
- Cardiomegaly
- Pulmonary edema.

Echocardiography:
Left ventricular hypertrophy (LVH), features of arrhythmia +/−

Management:
- Treatment of CCF, avoid digoxin, cautious diuretics, ACE inhibitor
- Beta blocker, carvedilol may be helpful
- Management of arrhythmia.

Prognosis: Approximate one third of patients improve.

Obstructive Cardiomyopathy

This type of cardiomyopathy causes obstruction to the outflow of the ventricle.

In primary cases, genetic disorder is found in about 50% of cases.

Secondary causes are:
- Infant of diabetic mother
- Glycogen storage disease, e.g., Pompe disease
- Fabry disease.

The cause of obstruction is due to asymmetric hypertrophy of the interventricular septum often associated with malalignment of anterior leaflet of mitral valve. The free wall of the ventricle is not affected. The problem is mainly confined to the LV and sometimes to RV also with improper alignment of tricuspid valve.

When asymmetric septal hypertrophy is associated, it causes ventricular outflow obstruction mainly LV. If pressure gradient is present between ventricle and main artery, it is known as hypertrophic obstructive cardiomyopathy.

Clinical features:
- Easy fatigability
- Angina
- Sharp upstroke of pulse
- Multiple heart sound
- Features of mitral regurgitation
- Variation of murmur with change of posture.

Investigations:
- *CXR*: LV enlargement
- *ECG*: Wave prominent in right precordial leads and deep Q wave in left precordial leads
- *Echocardiogram*: Diagnostic and shows the thickening of the septum.

Management:
- Exercise reduction
- Beta blocker may be helpful
- Ca channel blocker may be helpful
- *Drug refractory cases*: Myotomy
- Management of arrhythmia.

Restrictive Cardiomyopathy

It is uncommon in children.

It is of two types: (1) Endocardial fibroelastosis and (2) endomyocardial fibrosis.

In both the conditions, the capacity of the ventricles is less. So the cardiac output is low because of less amount of end-diastolic volume of the ventricles.

Clinical features:
- Dyspnea
- Embolic manifestation due to stasis of blood in atrium
- Features of mitral regurgitation if there is damage of the papillary and chordae tendineae due to fibrosis.

CXR: Normal

ECG: normal

Echo shows less end-diastolic volume

The most important differential diagnosis is constrictive pericarditis.

Treatment:
- Bed rest
- Decongestive therapy.

SUGGESTED READING

1. Park MK. Park's Pediatric Cardiology for Practitioners, 6th edition. USA: Elsevier; 2014.

130 CHAPTER

Pericardial Disease

Asok Kumar Datta

INTRODUCTION

Pericardial disease is of two types:
1. Acute pericarditis
2. Chronic pericarditis

Acute pericarditis may occur following infection, e.g., bacteria, tuberculous, viral and in some cases of rheumatic fever, collagen vascular diseases, and renal failure. The cause is not known in some cases.

Chronic pericarditis is usually due to tuberculosis but may be following pyogenic infection, trauma, etc. In some cases, cause is not known.

ACUTE PERICARDITIS

Clinical features:
- Chest pain
- Pain may be referred to neck
- Associated with pericardial rub
- Pain disappears after few days with some collection of fluid in pericardial sac
- Sometimes the pericardial effusion may be large enough leading to respiratory difficulty
- Raised jugular venous pressure, hepatomegaly, and edema may develop
- Pulsus paradoxus may be present in large effusion.

Investigations:
- *Chest X-ray*: Obliteration of cardiophrenic angle. The heart is globular.
- *ECG*: ST elevation and T changes.
- Echocardiography shows echo free space in posterior left ventricular wall.

Treatment: Treatment depends on the etiology. Pericardiocentesis may be required in severe cases.

CHRONIC PERICARDITIS

Here the inflow of blood to heart is disturbed due to constriction of the pericardium due to fibrosis.

The common cause is tuberculosis.

Due to difficult drainage in right heart, jugular venous engorgement is seen. Inspiratory filling of neck veins is seen in about half of the cases (Kussmaul's sign). Hepatomegaly, ascites, pedal edema are associated. The lung may show pleural effusion.

Treatment of the cause is essential with keeping in mind the most common cause tuberculosis. Decortication may be needed in some cases.

SUGESTED READING

1. Park MK. Park's Pediatric Cardiology for Practitioners, 6th edition. USA: Elsevier; 2014.

131 CHAPTER: Pulmonary Hypertension

Asok Kumar Datta

INTRODUCTION

Pulmonary hypertension (PH) is defined when the mean pulmonary pressure is >25 mm Hg at rest and >30 mm Hg following exercise.

Pulmonary hypertension may be primary or idiopathic where no cause is known or secondary where there is a definite cause present. In children, idiopathic PH is rare.

CAUSES

- *Large left-to-right shunt*: Here PH due to increase flow of blood is known as hyperkinetic PH and after decongestive therapy and necessary corrective measure, the PH comes down to normal. In long-standing cases, the pulmonary blood vessels may get irreversible changes and known as obstructive PH where after a certain period, the correction is not possible.
- Alveolar hypoxia due to congenital and acquired causes pulmonary hypertension (PH).
- Airway obstruction, e.g., adenoid enlargement causing obstructive sleep apnea causes PH.
- Pulmonary venous hypertension such as mitral stenosis and cor triatriatum.
- Primary pulmonary vascular disease.
- Neonatal persistent PH.
- Other diseases such as collagen vascular diseases, portal hypertension (hepatopulmonary syndrome) and HIV infection.

PATHOLOGY

Six grades of which grades 1 to 3 are reversible and grades 4 to 6 are irreversible.

Grades:
1. Hypertrophy of the media wall of the small muscular arteries
2. Hyperplasia of the intima
3. Hyperplasia and fibrosis with narrowing of the lumen
4. Plexiform lesion
5. Complex plexiform lesion
6. Necrotizing arteritis.

CLINICAL FEATURES

- Exertional dyspnea
- Chest pain
- History of heart defect
- Cyanosis in reversal of shunt
- Features of pulmonary hypertension
- Features of right ventricular failure.

INVESTIGATIONS

- *Chest X-ray (CXR) posteroanterior (PA) view*:
  - Right ventricular enlargement
  - Large pulmonary trunk
  - Cardiomegaly
- Electrocardiography (ECG)
- Right ventricular hypertrophy (RVH), right-axis deviation
- *Echocardiography (ECHO)*: Contributes toward diagnosis
- *Cardiac catheterization*: Presence and severity of pulmonary hypertension.

MANAGEMENT

Treatment of the underlying causes:
- *For chronic cases*:
  - Calcium channel blocker
  - Prostacyclin infusion
  - Endothelin receptor antagonist bosentan
  - Sildenafil
  - Nitric oxide (NO) inhalation
- *For nonresponder*: Cardiac transplantation.

SUGGESTED READING

1. Park MK. Park's Pediatric Cardiology for Practitioners, 6th edition. USA: Elsevier; 2014.

Cardiac Failure

Sibabrata Patnaik

INTRODUCTION

Heart failure is defined by the International Society for Heart and Lung Transplantation (ISHLT) as a clinical and pathological syndrome that results from ventricular dysfunction, volume, or pressure overload, alone or in combination. It leads to characteristic signs and symptoms such as poor growth, feeding difficulties, respiratory distress, exercise intolerance, and fatigue, and is associated with circulatory, neurohormonal, and molecular abnormalities. Heart failure can occur not only due to cardiac disorders, but many noncardiac disorders can also cause heart failure.

PATHOPHYSIOLOGY

In common terms; if heart fails to contract properly during systole, it is *systolic heart failure* and if fails to fill during diastole, it is called *diastolic heart failure*. Common causes of diastolic dysfunction include constrictive pericarditis, restrictive cardiomyopathy, and mitral or tricuspid stenosis. Similarly, heart failure can be only left heart (ventricular) failure or only right heart (ventricular) failure or, may be biventricular failure. As the name implies, there will be congestion in either pulmonary circulation, or systemic circulation or both. If left ventricle fails, then blood will accumulate in left ventricle, which will exert back pressure on left atrium and finally on lungs through the pulmonary veins; leading to pulmonary edema. Similarly in right heart failure, there will be back pressure on right atrium and finally on superior and inferior vena cava, leading to raised jugular venous pressure (JVP), hepatomegaly, and pedal edema.

When the cardiac output starts to decrease, body tries to compensate by two mechanisms (**Flowchart 1**); stimulation of sympathetic nervous system (SNS) and renin-angiotensin-aldosterone system activation. Initially, these two mechanisms will help in increasing the cardiac output, but finally decompensation will occur, leading to florid heart failure. When congestive heart failure progresses, with persistent poor perfusion; the child lands into the state of cardiogenic shock.

Flowchart 1: Pathophysiology of heart failure.

(RAAS: renin–angiotensin–aldosterone system; SNS: sympathetic nervous system)

Very rarely heart failure may be detected with normal or increased cardiac output; but an inadequate amount of oxygen is delivered to meet the demand. This may be found in chronic anemia (reduced systemic oxygen content) or secondary to hyperthyroidism, wet beriberi or hypermetabolism (increased oxygen demands). This condition is known as *high-output failure;* and produces signs and symptoms of heart failure even though the cardiac output is more than normal. It is also seen in large arteriovenous malformations such as vein of Galen malformation. These conditions decrease peripheral vascular resistance and increase myocardial contractility. When the demand for cardiac output exceeds the capacity of heart to pump, heart failure sets in. There is volume overload, which leads to pulmonary edema due to increase in the left ventricular diastolic pressure. On long run, systolic failure also sets in.

Time of presentation of different heart diseases:
- *Fetal period:*
  - Supraventricular tachycardia
  - Severe bradycardia due to complete heart block
  - Severe tricuspid regurgitation due to Ebstein anomaly of the tricuspid valve
  - Mitral regurgitation from atrioventricular canal defect
  - Systemic arteriovenous fistula
  - Myocarditis
- *First day of life:*
  - Hypoglycemia
  - Hypocalcemia
  - Asphyxia
  - Sepsis
- *First week of life:* Critical obstructive lesions such as—
  - Severe aortic stenosis,
  - Coarctation of the aorta (COA)
  - Obstructed total anomalous pulmonary venous connection (TAPVC)
  - Transposition of the great arteries (TGA) with intact ventricular septum
  - Hypoplastic left heart syndrome
- *4-6 weeks of life:*
  - Ventricular septal defect (VSD)
  - Patent ductus arteriosus (PDA)
  - Aortopulmonary window
  - Truncus arteriosus
  - Unobstructed TAPVC
- *Infancy:*
  - *Cardiomyopathy:*
    - Idiopathic
    - Inborn errors of metabolism
    - Syndromic
- *Older children and adolescents:*
  - Rheumatic heart disease
  - Myocarditis
  - Cardiomyopathy
- Palliative congenital heart disease (CHD)
- Rhythm disturbances.

CLINICAL PRESENTATION

Infants with heart failure present with tachypnea, feeding difficulty, excessive sweating, and irritability. Excessive coughing, especially on lying down, is a common finding. Feeding difficulty in infants is a major problem, ranging from prolonged feeding duration along with decreased intake to frank intolerance and vomiting after feeds. Because of poor feeding, the child remains hungry and thus irritable. Persistent heart failure leads to poor weight gain and subsequently failure in linear growth occurs. Muscle wasting and cardiac cachexia may occur due to increased metabolic demand of body and high levels of neurohormones such as tumor necrosis factor. Poor perfusion can lead to bowel wall edema and subsequent malabsorption of nutrients.

The presentation of heart failure in newborn is usually nonspecific. Features of heart failure in older children and adolescents include easy fatigability, dyspnea, orthopnea, effort intolerance, pain abdomen, and pedal edema.

SIGNS

Tachycardia, tachypnea, hepatomegaly, and gallop rhythm are the typical features of heart failure in infants. Left heart failure in infant presents with pulmonary symptoms such as rapid breathing, coughing and on examination, wheeze is usually found. In bigger kids and adolescents, basal crackles are the signs of pulmonary edema. Feature of right heart failure include tender hepatomegaly, pitting edema, and engorged neck veins. Pedal edema is usually not found in infants and young children, but sacral edema is characteristic. Similarly engorged neck veins are difficult to elicit in small babies. Gallop rhythm, cardiomegaly, and cold extremities are features common to both left and right heart failure.

In a child with unexplained heart failure; unequal upper and lower limb pulses, peripheral bruits, high or asymmetric blood pressure, indicate aortic obstruction. Coarctation of aorta in neonates can have normal femoral pulsations if PDA remains open. COA usually causes heart failure in children below 1 year of age. Beyond infancy, the possibility of heart failure is less as many collaterals have developed. If a newborn presents with heart failure along with central cyanosis and a faint or no murmur; possibility of TGA with intact interventricular septum or obstructed TAPVC should be thought of.

If a child presents with heart failure in the first 2 weeks of life, diseases such as TAPVC or COA should be in differential diagnosis. One should be aware that atrial septal defect (ASD) and VSD almost never manifest as heart failure in first 2-3 weeks of life. In infants with newly diagnosed

TABLE 1: Modified Ross classification for pediatric heart failure.	
Class I	Asymptomatic
Class II	• Mild tachypnea or diaphoresis with feeding in infants • Dyspnea on exertion in older children
Class III	• Marked tachypnea or diaphoresis with feeding in infants. Prolonged feeding times with growth failure • Marked dyspnea on exertion in older children
Class IV	Symptoms such as tachypnea, retractions, grunting, or diaphoresis at rest

dilated cardiomyopathy and heart failure, it is mandatory to determine the origins of the coronaries to rule out anomalous left coronary artery from the pulmonary artery (ALCAPA). Congestive heart failure is rare in tetralogy of Fallot. However, heart failure can develop due to complications such as anemia, infective endocarditis, arrhythmia, or increased flow in Blalock-Taussig (BT) shunt.

The modified Ross classification is presently used to assess severity of heart failure in pediatric age group (**Table 1**).

INVESTIGATIONS

Basic investigations such as chest X-ray (CXR), electrocardiography (ECG), and echocardiography are indicated in all patients with suspected heart failure. Some special tests and blood investigations are also required.

Chest X-ray

On chest radiography, the cardiac silhouette is usually enlarged. Cardiomegaly on radiography in children is suggested by a cardiothoracic ratio of >50% in older children. Left-to-right shunt lesions usually present with cardiomegaly, enlarged main and branch pulmonary arteries, and pulmonary plethora. Some cyanotic heart diseases have characteristic radiographic changes; like egg-on-side appearance in TGA, figure of eight appearance in unobstructed TAPVC and snowstorm appearance in obstructed TAPVC. Sometimes large thymus in infants and neonates may mimic cardiomegaly.

Electrocardiography

Most common ECG changes in heart failure in children are sinus tachycardia, left ventricular hypertrophy, ST and T wave changes, myocardial infarction pattern, and conduction abnormalities. Myocardial infarction pattern is suggestive of ALCAPA. ECG is helpful in the diagnosis of arrhythmia like supraventricular tachycardia, atrioventricular block, and ventricular tachycardia.

Echocardiography

Echocardiography is the most useful and widely used low-cost gazette for heart failure patients. It is indicated in all cases of heart failure in children to look for possible anatomical defect and to assess ventricular function. The most frequently used index of cardiac function in children is percent fractional shortening (%FS), which contrasts to adults, where ejection fraction (EF) is the most common functional measurement. %FS is calculated as (LVED−LVES)/LVED, where LVED is left ventricular dimension at end diastole and LVES is left ventricular dimension at end systole. Normal fractional shortening is approximately 28–42%. FS and EF are dependent on preload and afterload. Myocardial performance index and Doppler tissue imaging provide more quantitative assessment of systolic and diastolic functions, and they are less dependent on preload and afterload.

Laboratory Biomarkers

The brain natriuretic peptide (BNP) or amino terminal (NT)-pro BNP are useful to differentiate heart failure from pulmonary causes of respiratory distress. Raised natriuretic peptide levels in heart failure may be associated with bad prognosis. Elevated plasma BNP is a reliable test for recognizing ventricular dysfunction in children with CHD. However, BNP level may be elevated in many noncardiac conditions such as stroke, subarachnoid hemorrhage, renal dysfunction, cirrhosis of liver, severe infection, severe burns, anemia, thyrotoxicosis, and diabetic ketoacidosis. In children with heart failure, serial BNP or NT-pro BNP measurements are helpful for monitoring status of the child.

Blood glucose and *serum electrolytes* such as sodium, potassium, calcium, and phosphorous should be measured in all children with heart failure. *Screening for hypoxia and sepsis* should be done in newborn with heart failure. Both severe hyper- or hypothyroidism can cause heart failure. Thus *thyroid function test* is also required. *Antistreptolysin O* titer and *C-reactive protein* estimation are important if acute rheumatic fever or reactivation of rheumatic heart disease is suspected. In primary cardiomyopathy, *metabolic and genetic testing* is important as genetic cause is implied for >50% of patients with dilated cardiomyopathy (DCM). Creatine phosphokinase-MB (CPK-MB) and troponin I and T are useful if the clinical scenario is suggestive of an ischemic process or myocarditis. *Arterial blood gas and serial lactate measurement* may be helpful in cardiogenic shock.

Special Investigations

Cardiac catheterization: Though noninvasive diagnostic techniques have advanced, cardiac catheterization is still indicated for accurate measurement of pressure gradients in patients with complex valve diseases, evaluation of hemodynamic parameters (pulmonary and systemic vascular resistance, cardiac output, and cardiac index) in Fontan patients or during screening of pretransplant patients.

Endomyocardial biopsy (EMB) and *cardiac magnetic resonance imaging* (CMRI) may be rarely required in heart failure in children.

TREATMENT

The basic principle of management of pediatric heart failure is based on treatment of the cause of heart failure, correction of precipitating factor, and treatment of fluid overload.

In CHDs with prominent left-to-right shunts, early surgery is to be planned once the child is stabilized by conservative management. The CHDs which require early surgical intervention are critical aortic stenosis or COA, obstructed TAPVC, and TGA with intact ventricular septum.

In neonates, if not diagnosed timely, heart failure can lead to acute circulatory collapse. They become very sick once the PDA closes, especially in *duct-dependent circulation*. In this situation, it is required to keep the ductus arteriosus patent by prostaglandin infusion or emergency interventions such as ductal stenting and balloon atrial septostomy (BAS).

Common aggravating factors include anemia, dyselectrolytemia, arrhythmia, reactivation of rheumatic heart disease, infective endocarditis, drug toxicity, or nonadherence to therapy. These factors must be diagnosed and proper corrective measures should be ensured quickly.

General measures:
- Bed rest
- Propped up position
- Humidified oxygen
- Fluid restriction to two thirds
- Control of fever, correction of anemia
- 120–150 kcal/kg/day of caloric intake
- Mild sedation may control the irritability and anxiety, thus reduce catecholamine secretion
- May need mechanical ventilation to reduce the work of breathing.

Pharmacologic Therapy

Medical management is aimed at reducing the preload, increasing the contractility, and reducing the afterload. Reduction of preload is done by use of diuretics thus reducing pulmonary or systemic congestion. Increasing contractility by inotropes, and reducing the afterload by vasodilators improve the cardiac function.

The drugs which are commonly used in the treatment of pediatric heart failure include furosemide, spironolactone, digoxin, angiotensin-converting enzyme inhibitors, β-blockers, and inotropes. Newer agents which are now studied in children include serelaxin, ivabradine, and neprilysin inhibitor.

Diuretics

Diuretics are the first-line drugs for reduction of systemic and pulmonary congestion. Furosemide is given intravenously at a dose of 1–2 mg/kg. For long-term use, 1–4 mg/kg of furosemide or 10–20 mg/kg of chlorothiazide in divided doses are recommended. Continuous infusion of diuretics is recommended in cases of acute decompensated heart failure, as infusion causes less hemodynamic compromise. Addition of spironolactone at a dose of 1 mg/kg to furosemide helps in preventing potassium loss in urine. Spironolactone has also antifibrotic features, thus helpful in heart failure. It is to be avoided in patients with renal failure and hyperkalemia. If male gynecomastia develops with spironolactone, it is required to replace with eplerenone. Over diuresis is sometime dangerous as it can lead to renal insufficiency. This cardiorenal syndrome finally can amplify the end-organ damage.

Angiotensin-converting Enzyme Inhibitors and Angiotensin II Receptor Blockers

In heart failure, compensatory mechanism leads to vasoconstriction in both arteries and veins. Because of arterial constriction, work load on heart increases. Similarly due to venoconstriction, the venous return increases, leading to volume overload. Both of these aggravate the heart failure. Vasodilators like angiotensin-converting enzyme (ACE) inhibitors cause venous and arterial dilatation. Therefore, they decrease the preload and also decrease the workload on heart. They have additional effect of cardiac remodeling by directly influencing cardiac intracellular signaling pathways.

For the management of LV dysfunction in children, ACE inhibitors are routinely recommended. They should be initiated at a lower dose to prevent "first-dose phenomenon" and should be gradually increased to optimum dose. Captopril is more often prescribed in neonates and infants while long acting-agent such as enalapril is used for children above 2 years of age.

Adverse effects of ACE inhibitor include hypotension, renal dysfunction, cough, and angioedema. Angiotensin receptor blockers are required for those, who do not tolerate ACEIs.

Beta-blockers

Previously, beta (β)-blocker use in patients with left ventricular dysfunction was viewed with skepticism. It is now very commonly used along with ACE inhibitor. In children with heart failure, carvedilol is the most commonly studied β-blocker. Carvedilol is started at 0.1 mg/kg/day in two divided doses and increased to 0.5–0.8 mg/kg/day by doubling the dose every 1–2 weeks. Carvedilol has both α and β receptor blocking action along with free-radical scavenging activity. Metoprolol at a dose of 1–2 mg/kg/day in two divided doses or bisoprolol are the alternatives to carvedilol. Metoprolol is also started from low dose to be increased slowly to optimum dose. β-blockers are to be avoided in acute decompensated heart failure.

Digoxin

Despite lack of trial evidence, digoxin is a commonly used agent in pediatric cardiac failure. Rapid digitalization is generally avoided. However, it can be achieved by giving intravenous digoxin. Most of the time, starting with an oral maintenance doses (8–10 µg/kg/day) without loading dose is sufficient. However, if digitalization over 24 hours is required, half of the calculated dose is given first, then one fourth after 12 hours and next one fourth after another 12 hours. Digoxin has a very narrow therapeutic index and it is to be used with caution in preterm babies, acute myocarditis and in renal failure. Hypokalemia and hypomagnesemia and hypercalcemia enhance digoxin toxicity and therefore need prompt correction.

Inotropes

Many inotropes are being used in acute heart failure; the most common agents are the catecholamines such as dobutamine, dopamine, and rarely adrenaline and the phosphodiesterase III inhibitor such as milrinone.

Dosage of commonly used agents are dopamine at 5–20 µg/kg/min and dobutamine at 5–20 µg/kg/min. Epinephrine and norepinephrine are associated with increased myocardial oxygen demand. *Fenoldopam* is a dopamine (DA1) receptor agonist, which when given in low-dose infusion can cause increased renal perfusion and increased urination.

Milrinone is a phosphodiesterase III inhibitor with inotropic and vasodilatory property. It is used in infants and children after cardiac surgery to prevent low cardiac output state. The lusitropic effect of milrinone, causing diastolic relaxation is helpful in heart failure. It does not increase myocardial oxygen consumption. The loading dose of milrinone is 25–75 µg/kg over 15 minutes to 1 hour followed by maintenance dose of 0.25–0.75 µg/kg/min. Because of its vasodilatory property, it can cause hypotension and should be used with caution in children with borderline blood pressure. The hypotension is usually responsive to small fluid bolus or low-dose noradrenalin infusion for a short period. Thrombocytopenia and arrhythmia are rare adverse effects of milrinone.

Levosimendan is a drug with both inotropic with vasodilatory property. It causes calcium sensitization of troponin C, leading to increased cardiac contractility. Its vasodilatory property is by opening up of vascular ATP-dependent K^+ channels. It does not increase myocardial oxygen demand and has cardioprotective effect. It is mostly used in postoperative cardiac patients. The usual dosage of levosimendan is 6–12 µg/kg loading followed by 0.05–0.2 µg/kg/min as infusion.

Serelaxin, recombinant human relaxin-2, has resulted in fewer deaths in acute heart failure.

Ivabradine is a selective inhibitor of I_f current of sinoatrial (SA) node and decreases heart rate without decreasing myocardial contractility. Ivabradine has shown to decrease mortality and decrease hospitalization rate of heart failure cases.

Device Therapy

Device therapy in heart failure mainly includes pacemaker therapy, implantable cardioverter-defibrillator (ICD), cardiac resynchronization therapy (CRT), and mechanical circulatory support. Implantable cardioverter-defibrillator (ICD) is recommended for children with sustained ventricular tachycardia with CHD, in cardiomyopathy with recurrent syncope or with a past history of documented cardiac arrest. CRT restores ventricular synchrony by synchronized biventricular pacing. It is useful for children with a systemic LV with an ejection fraction of <35%, complete left bundle branch block pattern and increased QRS duration. CRT is especially helpful in CHD with intraventricular conduction delay (in TOF and univentricular physiology). Permanent pacemaker implantation is indicated for advanced atrioventricular (AV) block with ventricular dysfunction.

For refractory but reversible heart failure, extracorporeal membrane oxygenation (ECMO) or ventricular assist device (VAD) can be considered as a temporary measure as a bridge therapy. ECMO is also useful as an emergency perioperative salvage therapy. VADs are now frequently used for patients requiring prolonged mechanical support to bridge to heart transplantation.

Heart Transplantation

For children with end-stage heart failure refractory to medical and surgical treatment, heart transplantation is the only modality of therapy left. In present scenario, heart transplantation is an offer only for very limited number of patients because of shortage of donor hearts and specialized centers.

APPROACH TO MANAGING HEART FAILURE

Acute heart failure patients can have symptoms related to fluid overload (wet/dry), underperfusion (warm/cold), or both (**Table 2**). The early management of children with heart failure should address these problems. Four types of scenario will be found. The child may be cold+wet, cold+dry, warm+wet, or warm+dry. "Warm and dry" is the ideal situation and prevention of further damage should be tried in these children. "Warm and wet" children respond dramatically to diuretics. Those who are "cold and wet" will improve from combination of vasodilators and diuretics. "Cold and dry" state is typically a dire situation, which may require aggressive treatment, such as mechanical support.

TABLE 2: Management of heart failure.

	Dry (no congestion)	Wet (congestion)
Adequate perfusion (Warm)	1 "Warm and dry" optimal profile	2 "Warm and wet" Diuretic
Poor perfusion (Cold)	3 "Cold and dry" Limited options for therapy, will require mechanical support	4 "Cold and wet" Vasodilators (milrinone, sodium nitroprusside, nesiritide) with diuretics

Source: Reproduced from Grady KL, Dracup K, Kennedy G, Moser DK, Piano M, Stevenson LW, et al. Team management of patients with heart failure: A statement for health care professionals from The Cardiovascular Nursing Council of American Heart Association. Circulation. 2000;102:2443-56.

SUGGESTED READING

1. Kliegman RM, St. Geme J. Nelson Textbook of Pediatrics, 21st edition. Canada: Elsevier; 2019.
2. Nichols DG, Shaffner DH. Rogers' Textbook of Pediatric Intensive Care, 6th edition. Philadelpjia: Wolters Kluwer; 2015.
3. Masarone D, Valente F, Rubino M, Vastarella R, Gravino R, Rea A, et al. Pediatric heart failure: a practical guide to diagnosis and management. Pediatr Neonatol. 2017;58(4):303-12.
4. Jayaprasad N. Heart failure in children. Heart views. 2016; 17(3):92-9.
5. Kantor PF, Lougheed J, Dancea A, McGillion M, Barbosa N, Chan C, et al. Children's Heart Failure Study Group. Presentation, diagnosis, and medical management of heart failure in children: Canadian Cardiovascular Society guidelines. Can J Cardiol. 2013;29(12):1535-52.
6. Price JF. Congestive heart failure in children. Pediatrics in Review. 2019;40:60 D.
7. Shann F. Drug Doses, 17th Edition. Melbourne: Brand Collective Pty Limited.

Chapter 133: Cardiomyopathy in Children

Sudip Saha

INTRODUCTION

Cardiomyopathy is a disease of the heart muscle characterized by an abnormally large, thick, or stiff heart muscle. The incidence of pediatric cardiomyopathy is ≈1 per 100,000 children.

Cardiomyopathy causes damage to tissue around the heart, as well as heart muscle cells. The heart becomes so weak that it cannot pump blood properly.

This can lead to heart failure or irregular heartbeats (arrhythmias). In some cases, cardiomyopathy also involves a build-up of scar tissue or fat within the heart muscle. In rare cases, the heart muscle cannot relax and blood cannot be filled in the heart properly.

TYPES OF CARDIOMYOPATHY

- Dilated cardiomyopathy (DCMP) is the most common type and occurs when the main pumping chamber of the heart muscle is too stretched out (dilated). Dilated cardiomyopathy makes the heart unable to pump blood effectively.
- Hypertrophic cardiomyopathy (HCMP) makes the heart muscle too thick. Usually, the thickening occurs in the muscle of the left ventricle in the heart, often involving the wall between the heart's two ventricles.
- Restrictive cardiomyopathy is a rare type of cardiomyopathy that causes the heart muscle to become very rigid or stiff. This makes it difficult for the ventricles of the heart to properly fill with blood.
- Arrhythmogenic right ventricular cardiomyopathy (ARVC) is a rare form of cardiomyopathy. It occurs when the muscle of the heart's right ventricle is replaced by thick or fatty scar tissue. The scarring "scrambles" electrical signals within the heart and can make it difficult for the heart to pump blood.

DIAGNOSIS OF CARDIOMYOPATHY

Noninvasive Procedures

- *Chest radiography*: Chest radiographs often reveal cardiomegaly and increased pulmonary vascular markings that are consistent with pulmonary edema.

SYMPTOMS AND CAUSES OF CARDIOMYOPATHY (TABLES 1 AND 2)

TABLE 1: Symptoms of cardiomyopathy.

Dilated	Hypertrophic	Restrictive	Arrhythmogenic right ventricular
Abdominal pain	Abnormal heart rhythm	Fatigue	Abnormal heart rhythm
Chest pain	Chest pain	Persistent coughing	Syncope
Chronic fatigue	Dizziness	Shortness of breath during exercise	Dizziness
Chronic loss of appetite	Syncope	Shortness of breath at night	Swelling in the abdomen
Frequent irritability		Swelling in the abdomen	Swelling in the feet
Frequent vomiting		Swelling in the feet	Rapid or "racing" heartbeat
Pale or clammy skin		Failure to gain weight	Shortness of breath
Rapid breathing			
Rapid/racing heartbeat			
Shortness of breath			
Slow or delayed growth			

TABLE 2: Causes of cardiomyopathy.

Dilated	Hypertrophic	Restrictive	Arrhythmogenic right ventricular
Postviral myocarditis	GSD type II (Pompe disease)	Chemotherapy	Cardiomyopathy caused by channelopathy
Metabolic diseases	GSD type IIb (Danon disease)	Radiation	LQTS
Genetic like muscular dystrophy	PRKAG2	Sarcoidosis	Brugada syndrome
Rheumatoid arthritis	GSD type III (Cori or Forbes disease)	Scleroderma	Catecholaminergic polymorphic VT
Coronary artery disease	Lysosomal storage disorders	Endomyocardial fibrosis	SQTS
Uncontrolled juvenile diabetes	Mucopolysaccharidoses types I and II	Loeffler's syndrome	Lenègre's disease
Obesity	Anderson–Fabry disease	Hemochromatosis	Tachycardia- and pacing-induced cardiomyopathy
Substance abuse	Mucolipidoses (I cell)	Amyloidosis	
Thyroid disease	Noonan syndrome	Tumors in the heart	
Fatty acid Oxidation disorders	Noonan syndrome with multiple lentigines	Buildup of scar tissue in the heart	
Carnitine deficiency	Costello syndrome		
Malonyl coenzyme decarboxylase deficiency	Beckwith–Widemann		
GSDs	Multiple acyl-CoA dehydrogenase (glutaric academia type II)		
GSD type II (Pompe disease)	Long-chain hydroxyacyl-CoA dehydrogenase		
GSD type IV (Andersen disease)	Carnitine acylcarnitine translocase		
Arsenic	Carnitine Palmitoyl transferase II		
Anthracycline	Carnitine-acylcarnitine translocase deficiency		

(CoA: coenzyme A; GSD: glycogen storage disease; LQTS: long QT syndrome; SQTS: short QT syndrome)

- *Electrocardiography*: Sinus tachycardia, ST-T wave changes, Q waves, conduction disease, bundle-branch block, left ventricular (LV) hypertrophy and ectopy, including supraventricular tachycardia, atrial fibrillation, and ventricular arrhythmias in DCMP patients.
- *Echocardiography*: The diagnosis of DCMP is based on the presence of LV enlargement and reduced systolic dysfunction with an ejection fraction <50% or, more stringently, <45%. Echocardiographic findings include LV dilation and systolic dysfunction, with or without mitral regurgitation. In addition, pericardial effusion, especially in myocarditis and heart rhythm irregularities, can be observed.
  Echocardiography in HCMP remains the gold standard for the diagnosis of HCMP in children. LV wall thickness >2 standard deviations above the body surface area-corrected mean (z-score) is sufficient to make a diagnosis. Hypertrophy is defined as >15 mm in adults and >2 z-scores in children. Traditionally, the pattern of hypertrophy is asymmetric, and it affects more than one cardiac segment, preferentially affecting the anterior interventricular septum. Echocardiography is useful in assessing the pattern of hypertrophy, global systolic function, diastolic performance, presence and mechanism of out flow tract obstruction, atrial dimensions, and valvular function.
- *Magnetic resonance imaging (MRI)*: More effective in imaging difficult-to-visualize LV segments, including the LV apex and anterolateral free wall. MRI has been shown to more accurately predict the degree of LVH.
- *Genetic studies*: Genes that cause DCMP generally encode cytoskeletal and sarcomeric proteins, although the disturbance of calcium homeostasis also appears to be important. Familial HCMP is a genetically heterogeneous disorder, which means that a mutation in more than one gene can lead to the same condition.

- *Biomarkers*: An increase in BNP levels is associated with reduced LV systolic function, hypertrophy, raised filling pressures, and myocardial ischemia.

Invasive Procedures

- *Radionuclide ventriculography*: Radionuclide ventriculography may be the best tool to diagnose ARVC. It is used to assess contract ion and filling of the ventricles at rest and with exertion.
- *Cardiac catheterization*: Angiograms may be obtained to determine heart function and check for mitral regurgitation. In addition, endomyocardial biopsy sampling is another method of defining the cause of the disease.

TREATMENT

Medical Therapy

- Angiotensin-converting enzyme inhibitor is recommended for nearly all children with asymptomatic LV dysfunction. Enalapril, (ENAM 2.5/5 mg) @ 0.08 mg/kg/day in one to two divided dosage, is not recommended in children with glomerular filtration rate <30 mL/min, SE hypotension, headache, and cough.
- Diuretics are recommended for children with heart failure to achieve euvolemia and minimize congestive symptoms. Furosemide (LASIX 40 mg) @ 1–2 mg/kg one to two divided dosages. SE tinnitus, hypokalemia.
- Digoxin is recommended if the child remains symptomatic. Digoxin is specifically not recommended for children with asymptomatic LV dysfunction Lanoxin 0.25 mg tablet @ 10–45 µg/kg PO given in three divided doses. Administer one half (50%) the total loading dose initially, then one fourth (25%) the loading dose every 6–8 hours for two doses. Maintenance dose is 3.4–12.9 µg/kg/day once daily. SE-hypo/hyperkalemia, arrythmias, rash
- Beta-blockers and calcium channel blockers are recommended for HCMP.
  - *Propranolol*: Inderal (10/20/40 mg) @ 0.5–2 mg/kg/day
  - *Metoprolol*: Betaloc (25 mg) @ 0.2–0.4 mg/kg/day initially gradually increase up to 1 mg/kg/day in two divided doses
  - *Carvedilol*: Cardace (3.125 mg) @ 0.1 mg/kg/day in two divided doses increase @ 1–2 weekly interval to 1 mg/kg/day maximum of 2 mg/kg/day SE bradycardia, difficulty with breathing, constipation, hyperglycemia.
  - Verapamil-Calaptin 80 mg @ 0.1–0.3 mg/kg IV oral dosage 4–8 mg/kg q8 hr SE constipation, dizziness, increased liver enzymes, hypotension.

Medications such as propranolol and verapamil may be given to reduce the outflow obstruction by slowing the heart rate and relaxing the heart.

Antiarrhythmic medications such as amiodarone and disopyramide may be required to reduce the risk of sudden cardiac death.

Cardiac Resynchronization Therapy

Cardiac resynchronization therapy improves mechanical synchrony, which in turn increases LV filling time, decreases mitral regurgitation, and reduces septal dyskinesis.

Device Implantation

A pacemaker or defibrillator is used when drugs are not effective in alleviating obstruction or when dangerous arrhythmias need to be regulated. Sudden death accounts for 50% of all deaths in children with HCMP.

Hence, defibrillators are often recommended for children with HCMP, RCMP, and ARVC who show evidence of arrhythmias.

Surgical Options

- *Myectomy*: A septal myectomy is sometimes recommended for symptomatic children with obstruct ion associated with HCMP. The purpose of this surgery is to reduce heart failure symptoms related to restricted blood flow from the ventricles or severe mitral regurgitation.
- *Heart transplantation*: Currently, transplants are reserved for patients in the most critical condition, such as those needing inotropes and, most commonly, mechanical ventilatory and mechanical device support. Heart transplantation can eliminate all the symptoms of heart failure and greatly improve the survival of patients.

Additional Treatments

It is strongly recommended that all first-degree relatives of a patient be clinically screened for HCMP. Minimally, this should include a physical examination by a cardiologist, ECG, and transthoracic echocardiography.

SUGGESTED READING

1. Boston's Children Hospital. Cardiomyopathy in children. [online] Available from: https://www.childrenshospital.org/conditions-and-treatments/conditions/c/cardiomyopathy. [Last accessed November, 2021].
2. Hong YM. Cardiomyopathies in children. Korean J Pediatr. 2013;56(2):52-9.
3. Lipshultz SE, Law YM, Asante-Korang A, Austin ED, Dipchand AI, Everitt MD, et al. Cardiomyopathy in children: Classification and diagnosis: a scientific statement from the American Heart Association. Circulation. 2019;140:e9-68.
4. Saxena A, Juneja R, Ramakrishnan S, Working Group on Management of Congenital Heart Diseases in India. Drug therapy of cardiac diseases in children. Indian Pediatr. 2009;46:310-38.

Cardiac Arrhythmias

Soutrik Seth

INTRODUCTION

Normal heart rate varies with age: The younger the child, the faster the heart rate. A child has tachycardia when the heart rate is beyond the upper limit of normal for age, and bradycardia when the heart rate is slower than the lower limit of normal.

THE NORMAL RHYTHM

Normal rhythm originating in the sinus node has two important characteristics:

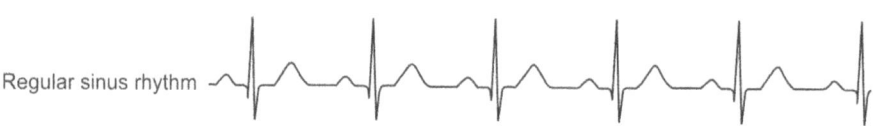

1. P wave is present in front of each QRS complex with a regular PR interval.
2. P axis is between 0 and +90 degrees, often a neglected criterion (produces upright P waves in lead II and inverted P waves in aVR).

Regular sinus rhythm is normal for age with the above characteristics. It is not pathological.

MECHANISM

The normal physiology: Normally, the electrical impulse originates in the sinoatrial (SA) node. The atrioventricular (AV) node, His bundle, and bundle branches transmit the impulses between the atria and ventricles. Conduction through the AV node is usually slowed so that atrial contraction is complete before ventricular contraction occurs **(Fig. 1)**.

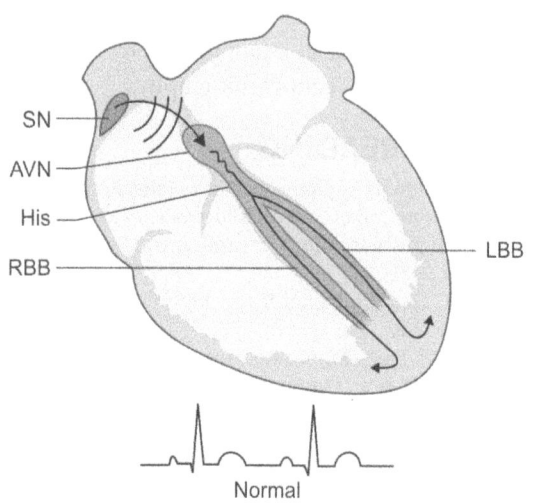

Fig. 1: Mechanism of impulse conduction.
(AVN: atrioventricular node; LBB: left bundle branch; RBB: right bundle branch; SN: sinus node)

Abnormal Impulse Generation

Abnormalities in impulse formation result in sinus bradycardia and tachycardia, premature atrial and ventricular contractions, and ectopic or automatic rhythms from the atria, AV node, or ventricles. Increased automaticity occurs when atrial, nodal, or ventricular cells display autonomous repetitive depolarization at a higher rate than is normal. Onset and termination are often gradual rather than abrupt.

Abnormal Impulse Conduction

Block within the normal conduction system is the most obvious form of abnormal impulse conduction. Block can occur at any point but AV block is most commonly seen. Re-entry, the other form of abnormal impulse conduction, is an important mechanism underlying supraventricular tachycardia (SVT) in infants. Re-entry mechanisms usually cause paroxysmal tachycardias, which may start and stop multiple times in the course of the day **(Flowcharts 1 and 2)**.

TYPES

Rhythms Originating in Sinus Node

Sinus Tachycardia

The characteristics of sinus rhythm are present. A rate above 140 beats/min in children and above 170 beats/min in infants may be significant, usually <200 beats/min.

Flowchart 1: Approach to narrow QRS complex.

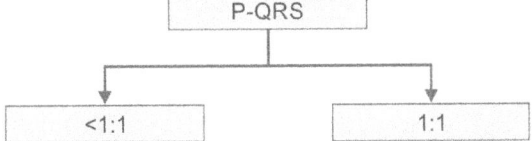

(AVRT: atrioventricular re-entrant tachycardia; AVNRT: atrioventricular nodal re-entrant tachycardia; EAT: ectopic atrial tachycardia; JET: junctional ectopic tachycardia; MAT: multiple atrial tachycardia; PJRT: permanent junctional reciprocating tachycardia)

Flowchart 2: Approach to broad QRS complex.

(AVNRT: atrioventricular nodal re-entrant tachycardia; RBBB: right bundle branch block; SVT: supraventricular tachycardia; VT: ventricular tachycardia)

Causes: Anxiety, fever, hypovolemia, circulatory shock, anemia, chronic heart failure (CHF), catecholamines, thyrotoxicosis, and myocardial disease are possible causes.

Increased cardiac work is well tolerated by the healthy myocardium.

The underlying cause is treated:

Sinus tachycardia

Sinus Bradycardia

Characteristics of sinus rhythm are present. A rate <80 beats/min in newborn infants and <60 beats/min in older children may be significant.

Causes: Vagal stimulation, increased intracranial pressure, hypothyroidism, hypothermia, hypoxia, and drugs such as digitalis and β-adrenergic blockers are possible causes. Some patients with marked bradycardia do not maintain normal cardiac output. The underlying cause is treated.

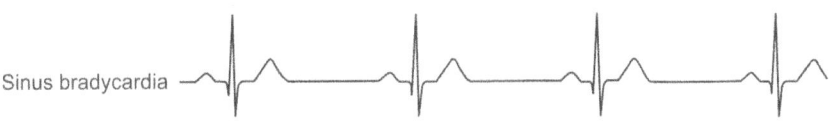

Sinus bradycardia

Sinus Arrhythmia

Sinus arrhythmia is a normal phasic variation in impulse formation from the SA node that is often in cycle with respiration.

The two characteristics of sinus rhythm are maintained.

Sinus arrhythmia is more common at slower heart rates and is therefore more frequent in sleeping infants and in any patient with increased vagal tone.

No treatment is required.

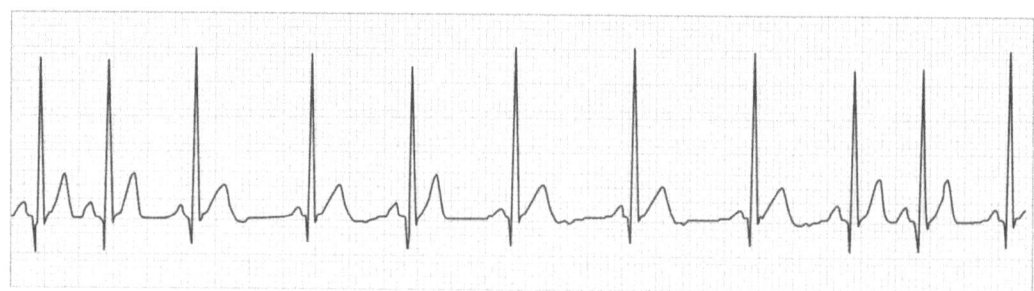

Sinus Pause

In *sinus pause*, there is a momentary cessation of sinus node pacemaker activity, resulting in the absence of the P wave and QRS complex for a relatively short duration. *Sinus arrest* lasts longer and usually results in an escape beat.

Cause: Increased vagal tone, hypoxia, digitalis toxicity, and sick sinus syndrome.

Sinus pause of <2 seconds is normal in young children and adolescents. Treatment rarely needed except for sick sinus syndrome.

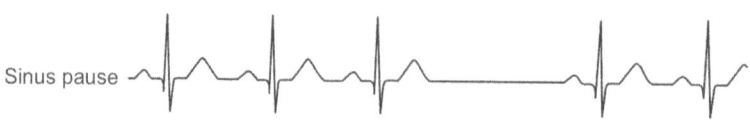

Sinus Node Dysfunction

The sinus node fails to function as the dominant pacemaker of the heart or performs abnormally slowly. It produces a variety of arrhythmias. When these arrhythmias are accompanied by symptoms such as dizziness or syncope, sinus node dysfunction is referred to as sick sinus syndrome.

It requires Holter monitoring for diagnosis.

Bradytachyarrhythmia is the most worrisome rhythm.

Extensive cardiac surgery involves the atria, arteritis, myocarditis, antiarrhythmic drugs, hypothyroidism, and CHD.

Treatment: Severe bradycardia is treated with atropine (0.02–0.04 mg/kg, IV, q2-4 h) or isoproterenol (0.05-0.5 µg/kg, IV) or both.

Temporary transvenous or transesophageal pacing can be used until a permanent pacing system can be implanted.

Permanent pacemaker implantation is the treatment of choice in symptomatic patients. Most patients receive atrial demand pacing. Patients with any degree of AV nodal dysfunction receive dual-chamber pacemakers.

Rhythms Originating in Atrium

Atrial arrhythmias are characterized by the following:
- P waves of unusual contour (abnormal P axis) and/or an abnormal number of P waves per QRS complex
- QRS complexes of normal duration.

Premature Atrial Complex

In premature atrial complex (PAC), the QRS complex occurs prematurely with abnormal P wave morphology. There is an incomplete compensatory pause. An occasional PAC is not followed by a QRS complex (i.e., a nonconducted PAC).

A *nonconducted* PAC is differentiated from a second-degree AV block by the prematurity of the nonconducted P wave (P′) P′ wave occurs earlier than the anticipated normal P rate, and the resulting PP′ interval is shorter than the normal PP interval for that individual. In second-degree AV block, the P wave that is not followed by the QRS complex occurs at the anticipated time, maintaining a regular PP interval.

Premature atrial complex appears in healthy children. No treatment is required.

Ectopic Atrial Tachycardia

There is a narrow QRS complex tachycardia with visible P waves at an inappropriately rapid rate. The P axis is different from that of sinus rhythm. The usual heart rate in older children is between 110 and 160 beats/min, but the tachycardia rate varies substantially during the course of a day, reaching 200 beats/min with sympathetic stimuli.

It represents about 20% of SVT.

Causes: It is believed to be secondary to increased automaticity of nonsinus atrial focus or foci. Myocarditis, cardiomyopathies, atrial dilatation, atrial tumors, and previous cardiac surgery may be the cause.

Treatment: Refractory to medical therapy and cardioversion, radiofrequency ablation may prove to be effective in nearly 90% of cases. Long-term oral antiarrhythmic drugs may be tried.

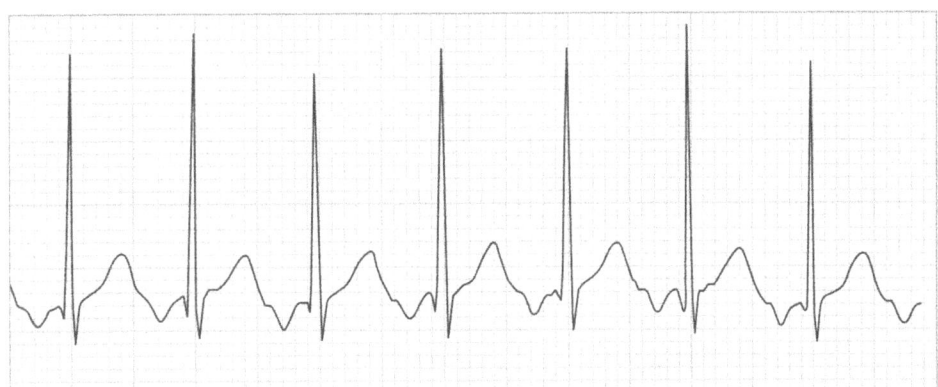

Multifocal or Chaotic Atrial Tachycardia

There are three or more distinct P wave morphologies. The PP and RR intervals are irregular with variable PR intervals. The arrhythmia may be misdiagnosed as atrial fibrillation.

Most patients with this condition are infants; it is very rare after 5 years of age.

It may develop to CHF.

Amiodarone appears to be the current treatment of choice.

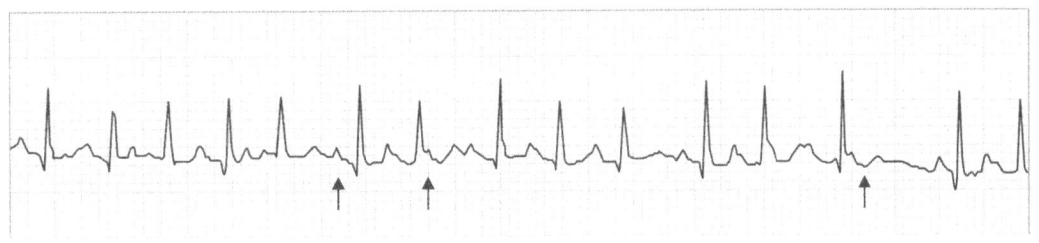

Atrial Flutter

Atrial flutter is characterized by a fast atrial rate (F waves with saw-tooth configuration) of about 300 (ranges 240 to 360) beats/min.

The ventricle responding with varying degrees of block.

Normal QRS complexes

Cause: Structural heart disease with dilated atria, myocarditis, thyrotoxicosis, and previous atrial surgery.

The ventricular rate determines the eventual cardiac output; a too-rapid ventricular rate may decrease the cardiac output.

Uncontrolled atrial flutter may precipitate heart failure.

Treatment: Synchronized cardioversion is the treatment of choice. Adenosine is not effective.

For control of the ventricular rate, calcium channel blockers, propranolol, or digoxin may be used. For prevention of recurrence, class I (quinidine) and class III (amiodarone) antiarrhythmic agents may be effective in some cases.

If a thrombus is found or suspected, anticoagulation with warfarin [with international normalized ratio (INR) 2-3] is started and cardioversion delayed for 2-3 weeks. After conversion to sinus rhythm, warfarin is continued for an additional 3-4 weeks.

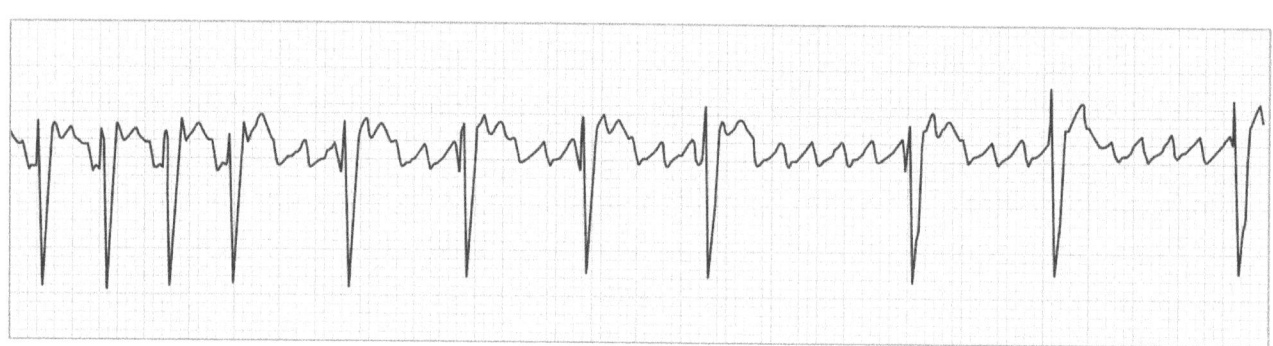

Atrial Fibrillation

Atrial fibrillation is characterized by an extremely fast atrial rate (f wave at 350-600 beats/min) and an irregular ventricular response with narrow QRS complexes.

Structural heart disease with dilated atria, myocarditis, thyrotoxicosis, and previous surgery involving atria.

Rapid ventricular rate and the loss of coordinated contraction of the atria and ventricles decrease cardiac output. Atrial thrombus formation is quite common.

Treatment: If atrial fibrillation has been present for >48 hours, the patient should receive anticoagulation with warfarin for 3-4 weeks to prevent systemic embolization of atrial thrombus, if the conversion can be delayed. Anticoagulation is continued for 4 weeks after restoration of sinus rhythm.

If cardioversion cannot be delayed, heparin should be started, and cardioversion performed when activated partial thromboplastin time (aPTT) reaches 1.5-2.5 times control in 5-10 days.

Propranolol or digoxin may be used to slow the ventricular rate.

In the Cox maze procedure (or the "cut-and-sew-maze"), multiple surgical incisions are made in the right and left atria that are then repaired in an attempt to minimize the formation of a re-entrant loop.

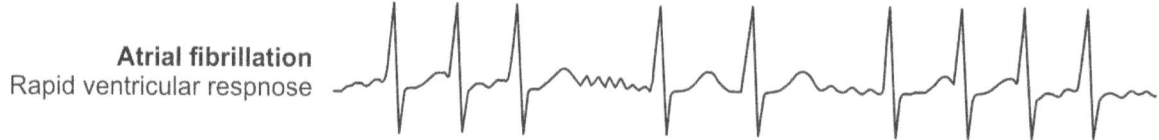

Rhythms Originating in AV Node

Rhythms originating in the AV node are characterized by the following:
- The P wave may be absent, or inverted P waves may follow the QRS complex.
- The QRS complex is usually normal in duration and configuration.

Junctional rhythm describes an abnormal heart rhythm resulting from impulses coming from a locus of tissue in the area of the AV node, the "junction" between atria and ventricles.

Since the nodal-His (NH) region of the AV node is the only part of the AV node with demonstrable ability to pace the heart, some authorities prefer the term "nodal" over "junctional."

Nodal Premature Beats

A normal QRS complex occurs prematurely. P waves are usually absent, but inverted P waves may follow QRS complexes. The compensatory pause may be complete or incomplete.

It is idiopathic; no treatment is required.

Nodal Escape Beats

When the sinus node impulse fails to reach the AV node, the NH region of the AV node will initiate an impulse (nodal or junctional escape beat). The QRS complex occurs later than the anticipated normal beat. The P wave may be absent or an inverted P wave may follow the QRS complex.

No treatment is required.

Nodal Rhythm

In case of persistent failure of the sinus node, the AV node may function as the main pacemaker of the heart with a relatively slow rate (40–60 beats/min).

P waves are absent or inverted P waves follow QRS complexes, may occur post cardiac surgery. No treatment is required.

Accelerated Nodal Rhythm

In the presence of normal sinus rate and AV conduction, if the AV node (NH region) with enhanced automaticity captures the pacemaker function (60–120 beats/min), the rhythm is called accelerated nodal (or AV junctional) rhythm.

P waves are absent or inverted P waves follow the normal QRS complexes.

No treatment is required.

Nodal Ectopic Tachycardia

The ventricular rates vary from 120 to 200 beats/min.

P waves are absent or inverted P waves follow the QRS complexes.

The QRS complex is usually normal.

Arrhythmia is grouped under SVT.

Enhanced automaticity of the junctional area is the suspected mechanism. Two types: (1) Postoperative and (2) congenital.

Postoperative type, a loss of AV synchrony in the presence of a fast rate (nearly 200 beats/min) compromises cardiac output, leading to a fall in BP. Increased catecholamines increase temperature which further aggravates tachycardia.

Treatment: Heart rates < 170 well tolerated, >170 beats/min slowing is necessary either by atrial overdrive pacing, systemic hypothermia, and conservative management.

The drug of choice is amiodarone.

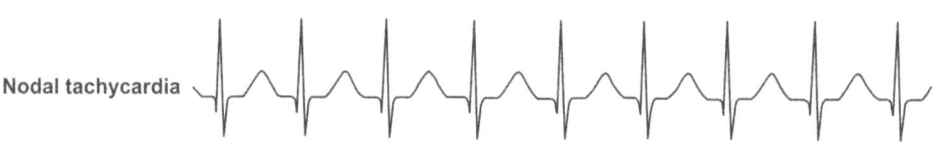

Supraventricular Tachycardia

Supraventricular tachycardia refers to any rapid heart rhythm originating above the ventricular tissue. SVTs are caused by two mechanisms: (1) Re-entry and (2) automaticity.

The heart rate is extremely rapid and regular (usually 240 ± 40 beats/min). The P wave is usually invisible, but when it is visible, it has an abnormal P axis and either precedes or follows the QRS complex. The QRS duration is usually normal.

Most cases are re-entry or reciprocating tachycardia. SVT caused by increased automaticity is infrequent.

Two types: Re-entrant (or reciprocating) AV tachycardia (RAVT):

In SVT due to re-entry, two pathways are involved: (1) AV node (dual pathway nodal RAVT) and (2) accessory pathway (Bundle of Kent), orthodromic and antidromic.

After conversion, both show Wolff-Parkinson-White (WPW) pre-excitation.

Nodal RAVT is more influenced by increased sympathetic tone than accessory RAVT.

Supraventricular tachycardia seen in the first year of life is more likely to have accessory RAVT.

An adolescent who first has SVT is more likely to have nodal RAVT.

Any type of AV block is incompatible with re-entrant tachycardia; AV block would abruptly terminate the tachycardia, at least temporarily **(Fig. 2)**.

Fig. 2: Types of re-entrant AV tachycardia.
(contd: continued; LV: left ventricle; RAVT: re-entrant (or reciprocating) atrioventricular tachycardia; RV: right ventricle)

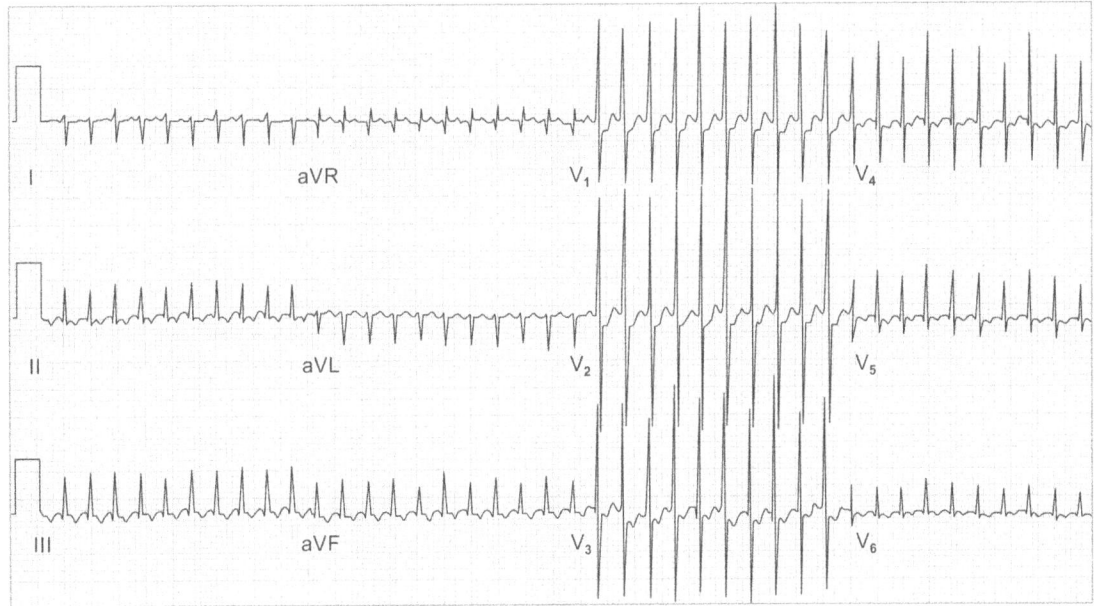

Orthodromic ARAVT: A PAC could initiate the arrhythmia. The PAC may find the accessory bundle refractory, but the AV node may conduct (antegradely), producing a narrow QRS complex. When the impulse reaches the bundle of Kent from the ventricular side, the bundle will have recovered and allows re-entry into the atrium **(Fig. 3)**.

Antidromic ARAVT: Less common is a widened QRS complex with antegrade conduction into the ventricle via the accessory (fast) pathway and retrograde conduction through the (slower) AV node **(Fig. 4)**.

Nodal RAVT: For this type of SVT to occur, the two pathways in the AV node would have to have, at least temporarily, different conduction and recovery rates **(Fig. 5)**.

Orthodromic nodal RAVT: When the normal, slow pathway through the AV node is used in antegrade conduction to the bundle of His; the resulting QRS complex is normal with an abnormal P vector, but the latter is unrecognizable because it is superimposed on the QRS complex.

Antidromic nodal RAVT: In this subtype which is uncommon, the fast tract of the AV node transmits the antegrade impulse to the bundle of His, and the normal, slow pathway of the AV node transmits the impulse retrogradely.

Causes: 50% no cause, cardiac surgeries, WPW pre-excitation.

Significance: Decreased cardiac output, leads to CHF.

Treatment: Vagal stimulatory behaviors—carotid massage, ice-bag over face.

Adenosine is the drug of choice.

Adenosine is given by rapid intravenous bolus followed by a saline flush, starting at 50 µg/kg, increasing in increment of 50 µg/kg, every 1-2 minutes. The usual effective dose is 100-150 µg/kg with maximum dose of 250 µg/kg.

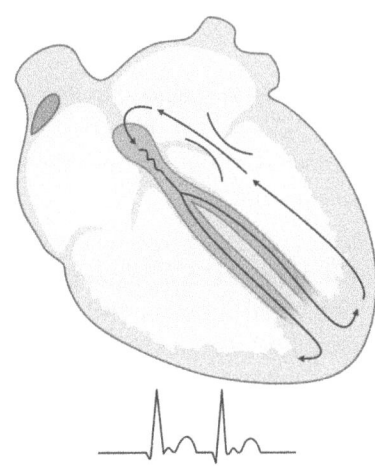

Fig. 3: Orthodromic reciprocating tachycardia.

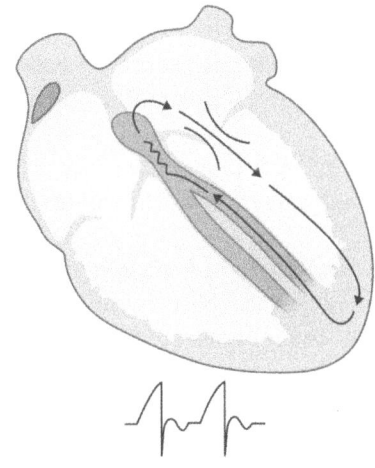

Fig. 4: Antidromic reciprocating tachycardia.

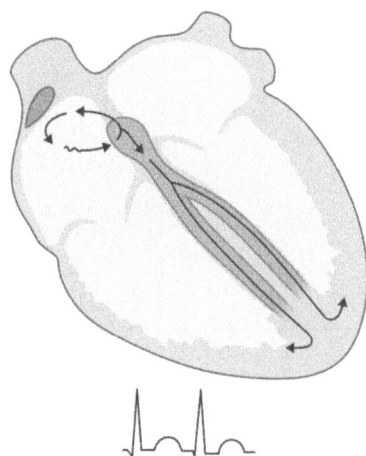

Fig. 5: AV node re-entry tachycardia.
(AV: atrioventricular)

If the infant is in severe CHF, an immediate cardioversion may be carried out. The initial dose of 0.5 J/kg is increased in steps up to 2 J/kg.

Intravenous administration of propranolol is usually successful in treating SVT in the presence of WPW syndrome.

For prevention of recurrence of SVT: In infants without WPW pre-excitation, oral propranolol for 12 months is effective. In children beyond infancy, verapamil can also be used in infants or children with WPW pre-excitation on the electrocardiography (ECG), propranolol or atenolol is used in long-term management. Avoid digoxin and verapamil.

In adolescent patients, catheter ablation may be an effective alternative to long-term drug therapy.

Rhythms Originating in the Ventricle

Ventricular arrhythmias are characterized by the following:
- Bizarre and wide QRS complexes with T waves pointing in the opposite directions
- QRS complexes randomly related to P waves, if visible.

Premature Ventricular Contraction

- Bizarre and wide QRS complexes with T waves pointing in the opposite directions.
- QRS complexes randomly related to P waves, if visible.
- By interrelationship of premature ventricular contractions (PVCs):
  - *Ventricular bigeminy or coupling*: Each abnormal QRS complex alternates with a normal QRS complex regularly.
  - *Ventricular trigeminy*: Each abnormal QRS complex follows two normal QRS complexes regularly.
  - *Couplets*: Two abnormal QRS complexes come in sequence.
  - *Triplets*: Three abnormal QRS complexes come in sequence.

Three or more successive PVCs arbitrarily are termed ventricular tachycardia.

- By similarity among abnormal QRS complexes:
  - *Uniform (monomorphic or unifocal) PVCs*: Abnormal QRS complexes have the same configuration in a single lead, originating from a single focus.
  - *Multiform (polymorphic or multifocal) PVCs*: Abnormal QRS complexes have different configurations in a single lead originating from different foci.
- *Coupling interval*:
  - *Fixed coupling*: PVCs appear at a constant interval after the QRS complex of the previous cardiac cycle. This suggests ventricular *re-entry* within the Purkinje system as the underlying mechanism, most common.
  - *Varying coupling*: When coupling intervals vary by >80 ms, the PVCs may result from parasystole. Ventricular parasystole consists of an impulse-forming focus in the ventricle that is independent of the sinus node-generated impulse and is protected from depolarization by sinus impulses (entrance block).

Causes:
- PVCs may be seen in otherwise healthy children. Up to 50–70% of normal children may show PVCs on 24-hour Holter monitoring.
- Myocarditis, myocardial injury or infarction, cardiomyopathy (dilated or hypertrophic), cardiac tumors, false tendon, and mitral valve prolapse are possible causes.
- Arrhythmogenic right ventricular dysplasia (RV cardiomyopathy), long QT syndrome, and Brugada syndrome may cause PVCs.
- Drugs such as catecholamines, theophylline, caffeine, amphetamines, digitalis toxicity, and some anesthetic agents are possible causes.

Usually benign, unless:
- They are associated with underlying heart disease [e.g., preoperative or postoperative status, mitral valve prolapse (MVP), cardiomyopathy].
- There is a history of syncope or a family history of sudden death.
- They are precipitated by or increase in frequency with activity.
- They are multiform, particularly couplets.
- There are runs of PVC with symptoms.
- There are incessant or frequent episodes of paroxysmal ventricular tachycardia.

Management: Electrocardiography echocardiography (Echo), Holter, exercise testing, cardiac catheterization, electrophysiological studies, and endomyocardial biopsy.

Isolated uniform PVC requires no treatment.

Asymptomatic children with multiform PVCs and ventricular couplets should have 24-hour Holter monitoring.

All babies with symptomatic ventricular arrhythmias and complex PVCs should be treated with beta blocker and class Ia antiarrhythmic drugs.

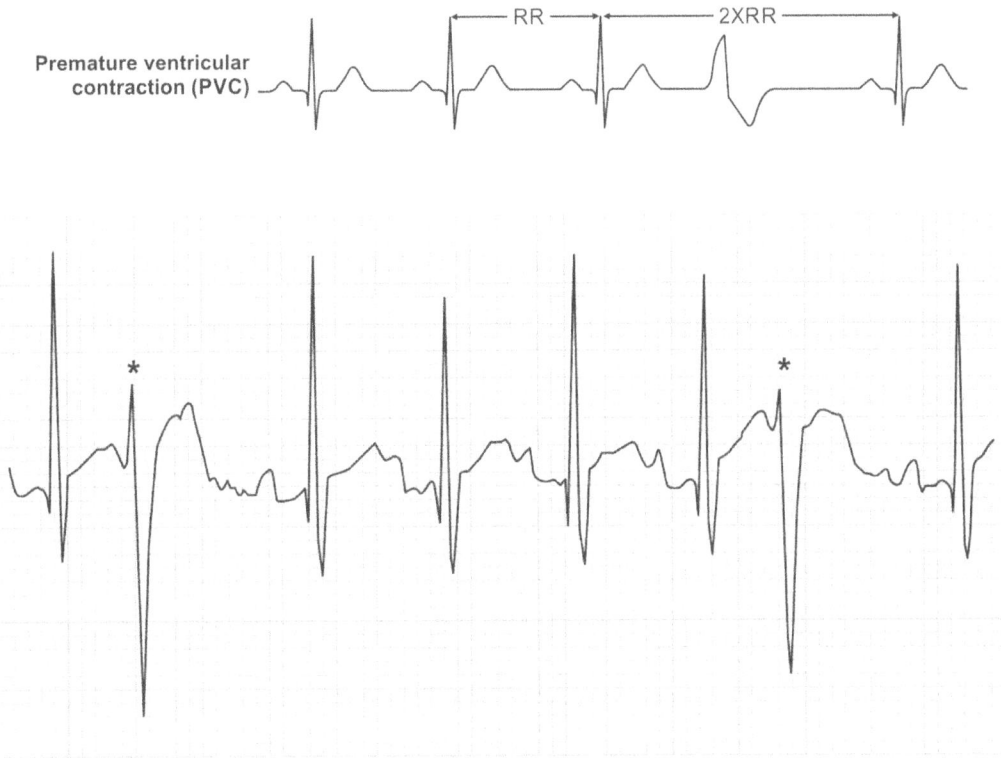

Ventricular Tachycardia

Ventricular tachycardia (VT) is a series of three or more PVCs with a heart rate of 120-200 beats/min. QRS complexes are wide and bizarre, with T waves pointing in opposite directions.

By duration, VT may be classified as: (1) a salvo of VT—a few beats in a row; (2) nonsustained VT—duration of <30 seconds; (3) sustained VT—>30 seconds; and (4) incessant VT—refers to lengthy sustained VT that dominates the cardiac rhythm.

By morphology, VT may be classified as: (1) monomorphic, referring to one dominant QRS form; (2) polymorphic, referring to a beat-to-beat change in the QRS shape; or (3) bidirectional, which is a specific form of polymorphic VT in which the QRS axis shifts across the baseline.

Torsades de pointes (meaning "twisting of the points") is a distinct form of polymorphic VT characterized by a paroxysm of VT during which there are progressive changes in the amplitude and polarity of QRS complexes. Wide QRS tachycardia in an infant or child must be considered VT until proven otherwise.

Causes:
- Structural heart diseases [such as tetralogy of Fallot (TOF), AS, cardiomyopathies, or MVP].
- Postoperative CHDs [such as TOF, dextro-transposition of the great arteries (D-TGA), or double outlet right ventricle (DORV)].
- Myocarditis, myocardial tumors, myocardial ischemia or MI, and pulmonary hypertension.
- Genetic disorders, such as Brugada syndrome or arrhythmogenic RV dysplasia.
- Torsades de pointes may be seen in patients with long QT syndrome.
- Metabolic causes (hypoxia, acidosis, hyperkalemia, hypokalemia, and hypomagnesemia).

Ventricular tachycardia usually signifies a serious myocardial pathology or dysfunction and can cause sudden death. Cardiac output may decrease.

Patients may present with dizziness, syncope, palpitation, or chest pain. ECG, Echo, Holter, exercise testing, cardiac catheterization, electrophysiological studies, and endomyocardial biopsy.

Acute therapy may include the following:
- Prompt synchronized cardioversion (0.5-1.0 J/kg) if the patient is unconscious or if there is evidence of low cardiac output.
- If the patient is conscious, an IV bolus of lidocaine, 1 mg/kg over 1-2 minutes, followed by an IV drip of lidocaine, 20-50 µg/kg/min, may be effective.

Amiodarone for drug refractory VT, beta blockers for long QT syndrome.

Recurrence may be prevented with administration of propranolol, atenolol, diphenylhydantoin, or quinidine.

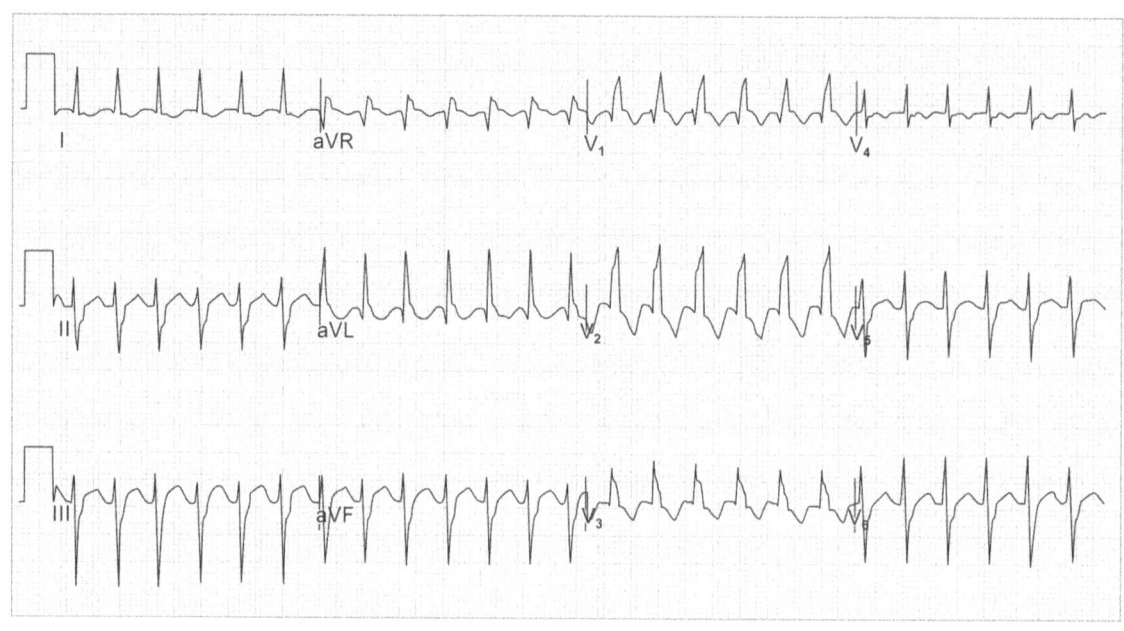

Torsade de pointes

Ventricular Fibrillation

Ventricular fibrillation is characterized by bizarre QRS complexes of varying sizes and configurations. The rate is rapid and irregular, usually fatal.

Causes: Postoperative state, severe hypoxia, hyperkalemia, digitalis or quinidine toxicity, myocarditis, myocardial infarction, and drugs.

Treatment: Immediate cardiopulmonary resuscitation, including electric defibrillation at 2 J/kg, is required. Implantable cardioverter defibrillators (ICDs) are often indicated in patients who survived ventricular fibrillation.

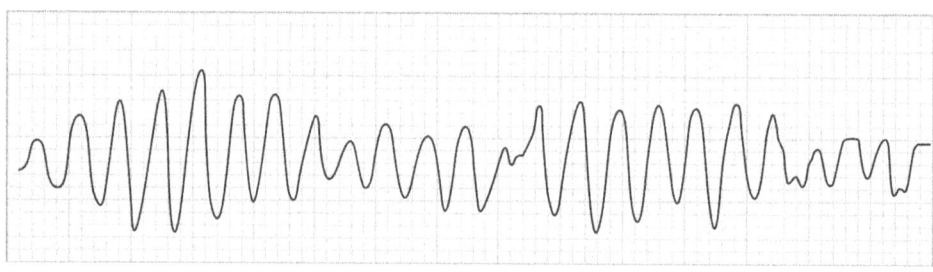

Ventricular fibrillation

LONG QT SYNDROME

Genetic disorder of ventricular repolarization characterized by a prolonged QT interval on the ECG and ventricular arrhythmias, usually torsades.

It may result in sudden death.

Causes

- Congenital—Jervell and Lange-Nielsen syndrome (autosomal recessive mode—prolonged QTc interval + congenital deafness + syncopal spells + family history of sudden death).
  Romano-Ward syndrome (autosomal dominant mode)— prolonged QTc interval + syncopal Spells + family history of sudden death.
  Andersen-Tawil syndrome, the QU interval (rather than QT interval) is prolonged, muscle weakness (periodic paralysis) + ventricular arrhythmias + developmental abnormalities.
  Timothy syndrome is associated with webbed fingers and toes and a prolonged QTc interval.
- *Acquired type*: Drugs, electrolyte disturbances.

Manifestations

Positive family history is present in about 60% and deafness in 5% of patients.

Presenting symptoms may be syncope (26%), seizure (10%), cardiac arrest (9%), presyncope, or palpitation (6%).

It is precipitated by intense adrenergic arousal, intense emotion, and during or following rigorous exercise.

The ECG shows the following:
- The QTc interval is prolonged, usually to >0.46 seconds. The upper limit of normal QTc is 0.44 seconds.
- Abnormal T-wave morphology (bifid, diphasic, or notched) is frequent.
- Bradycardia (20%), second-degree AV block, multiform PVCs, and monomorphic or polymorphic VT may be present.

Holter monitoring and treadmill exercise test give positive results.

Diagnosis

Accurate measurement of the QTc interval is essential in the diagnosis of long QT syndrome.

Lead II (with q waves) and precordial leads (V1, V3, or V5, with well-defined T waves) are good leads in measuring the QT interval.

The diagnosis of long QT syndrome is clear-cut when there is a marked prolongation of the QTc interval with positive family history of the syndrome.

Schwartz diagnostic criteria (ECG, clinical, family history): Defining low probability, intermediate probability, and high probability of LQTS.

Genetic testing may identify different genotypes.

Consider the following risk factors for sudden death before planning management: Bradycardia for age, an extremely long QTc interval (>0.55 seconds), symptoms at presentation, young age at presentation (<1 month), documented torsades de pointes or ventricular fibrillation, T wave alternans.

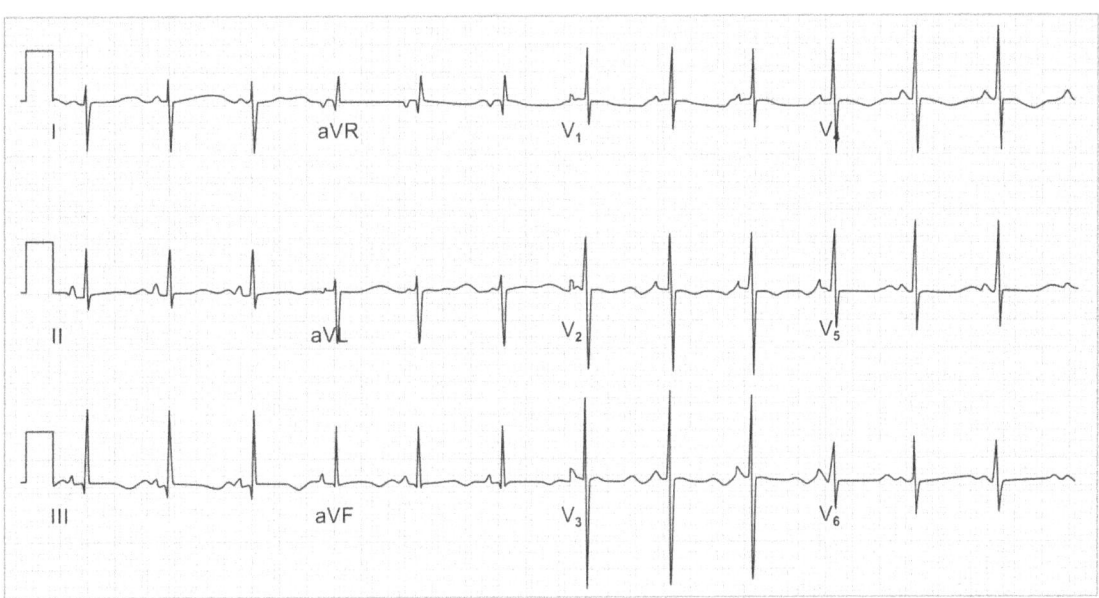

Management
- Avoid drugs that prolong QT interval.
- No competitive sports.
- *Beta blockers*: Current treatment of choice for symptomatic patients reduce syncope and cardiac arrest.
- ICD is the most effective therapy for high-risk patients.
- Sodium channel blocker mexiletine in patients with mutation in the *sodium channel* gene SCN5A.

SHORT QT SYNDROME
- Short QT syndrome is characterized by a very short QTc (≤300 milliseconds), symptoms of palpitation, dizziness or syncope, and family history of sudden death.
- The cause of death is believed to be ventricular fibrillation.
- This syndrome is transmitted in an autosomal dominant manner.
- Suggested use of quinidine to prolong QTc.

BRUGADA SYNDROME

It is an inherited arrhythmogenic disorder.

Sudden cardiac death from ventricular tachyarrhythmia. It is inherited as an autosomal dominant pattern.

Mutations occur in the sodium channel (*SCN5A*) at least in 20% of the patients.

The ECG typically shows concave ST segment elevation (>2 mm) with J point elevation followed by a negative T wave in the right precordial leads (V1-V3) and right bundle branch block (RBBB) appearance.

Most syncope takes place at rest (90%).

β-blockers do not appear to reduce the risk of death in these patients.

In many centers, ICD is the standard practice to prevent sudden cardiac death.

ATRIOVENTRICULAR CONDUCTION DISORDERS

Atrioventricular block is a disturbance in conduction between the normal sinus impulse and the eventual ventricular response.
- First-degree AV block is a simple prolongation of the PR interval but all P waves are conducted to the ventricle.
- In second-degree AV block, some atrial impulses are not conducted into the ventricle.
- In third-degree AV block (or complete heart block), none of the atrial impulses is conducted into the ventricle.

First-degree Block

Prolongation of the PR interval beyond the upper limits of normal, abnormal delay in conduction through the AV node.

Causes: Excessive parasympathetic tone, CHDs, inflammatory conditions (rheumatic fever), cardiac surgery, and certain drugs (such as digitalis, calcium channel blockers).

It has no hemodynamic significance; no treatment is required.

Second-degree Block

Some but not all P waves are followed by QRS complexes (dropped beats).

There are three types: (1) Mobitz type I (Wenckebach phenomenon), (2) Mobitz type II, and (3) high-grade (or advanced).

Mobitz type I (Wenckebach phenomenon): PR interval becomes progressively prolonged until one QRS complex is dropped completely.

Block is at the level of the AV node.

It is caused by myocarditis, cardiomyopathy, myocardial infarction, CHD, cardiac surgery, and digitalis toxicity.

It occurs in individuals with vagal dominance, usually does not progress to complete heart block. Treatment of underlying cause is done.

Mobitz type II: The AV conduction is "all or none." AV conduction is either normal or completely blocked.

Block usually occurs below the AV node (at the level of the bundle of His).

It may progress to complete Adams–Stokes attacks. Underlying cause is treated.

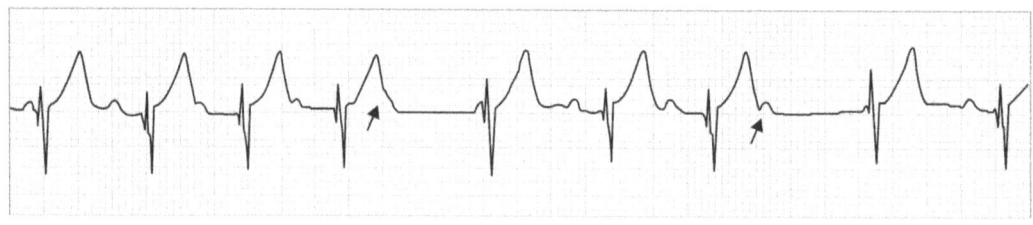

Two to one or higher AV block: A QRS complex follows every second (third or fourth) P wave, resulting in 2:1 (3:1 or 4:1, respectively) AV block.

Some P waves continue to be conducted to the ventricle and the PR interval of conducted beats is constant.

When two or more consecutive P waves are non-conducted, the rhythm is called advanced or high-grade second-degree AV block.

The block is usually at the bundle of His, alone or in combination with the AV nodal block. Occasionally, it progresses to complete heart block.

Higher-grade and second-degree AV block should always be regarded as abnormal.

The underlying cause is treated. Pacemaker therapy is indicated for symptomatic advanced second-degree AV block.

Third-degree AV Block (Complete Heart Block)

The atrial and ventricular activities are entirely independent of each other.

The P waves are regular (with regular PP interval) with a rate comparable to the heart rate of the patient's age. The QRS complexes are also quite regular (with regular RR interval) but with a rate much slower than the P rate.

In AV, dissociation the atrial rate is slower than the ventricular rate.

The third-degree AV block is either congenital or acquired.

Causes: Congenital (lupus, CHDs, neonatal myocarditis, genetic disorders), acquired (post surgeries).

Significance: Asymptomatic, fetal bradycardia, CHF, syncopal attacks, and sudden death.

Treatment: Asymptomatic cases may require only observation; In symptomatic children—atropine or isoproterenol is given until temporary ventricular pacing.

Pacemaker therapy is for the patient if he/she is symptomatic or develops CHF, suffers from dizziness or lightheadedness, with ventricular rate <50-55 beats/min or if the infant has a CHD with a ventricular rate < 70 beats/min, wide QRS escape rhythm, complex ventricular ectopy, or ventricular dysfunction.

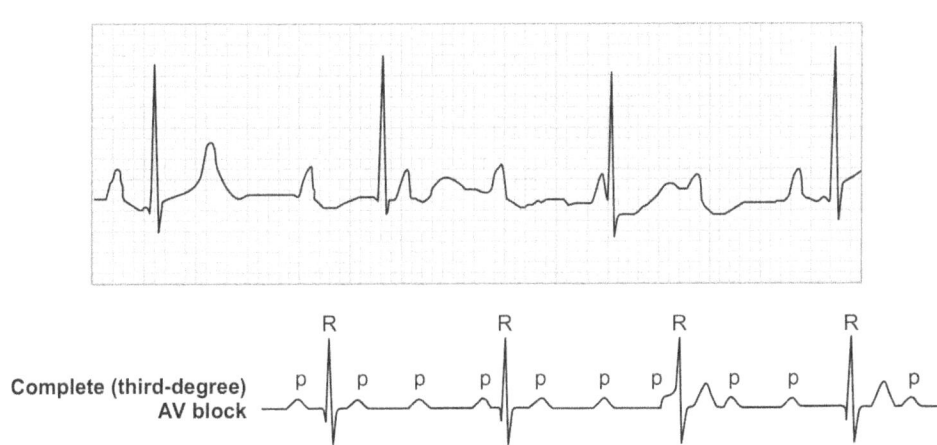

SUGGESTED READING

1. Park MK. Park's Pediatric Cardiology for Practitioners, 6th edition. USA: Elsevier; 2014.

Infective Endocarditis

Asok Kumar Datta

INTRODUCTION

It is infection of the endocardium involving the cardiac valves and the structures associated with it such as chordae tendineae, mural endocardium, and interventricular septum.

It is usually associated with subacute onset when it follows tooth extraction or other dental procedure and there is unexplained fever persisting for >7 days. The fever may be of low grade with subsequent development of other manifestations related to immunological and embolism basis.

The basic pathogenesis of immunological manifestation is the development of antigen–antibody complex which may get deposition at different sites with different manifestations. Embolism occurs following detachment of the vegetations which are formed in the valves.

The damaged endocardium is one contributing factor for the infection. Damage may occur in congenital heart diseases. Bacteremia occurring prior to attachment to the site of damage or on the prosthetic valve and there is accumulation of platelets and fibrous tissue forming vegetation.

In cases of intravenous (IV) drug addict, the organism may rapidly spread and cause acute infection in the endocardium with necrosis of the affected area and formation of new defect. Similar manifestation sometimes occurs following enterobacteria infection or following bacteremia from an abscess or in patients having cardiac operations in the recent past.

The causative organisms vary: In subacute case, it is usually *Streptococcus viridans* which causes the disease. In acute cases, causative organism is *Staphylococcus aureus*. There are other groups of organisms which are detected in infective endocarditis, e.g., HACKEK organism (*Haemophilus* species, *Actinobacillus, Cardiobacterium, Eikenella* and *Kingella*), *Streptococcus pneumoniae,* and *Enterococcus* species.

Other important causative organisms are fungi (particularly in neonate in intensive care with prolonged use of antibiotics, *Coxiella burnetii*, etc.)

REVISED DUKE CLINICAL DIAGNOSTIC CRITERIA FOR INFECTIVE ENDOCARDITIS

Definite clinical diagnosis: 2 major, 1 major and 3 minor, or 5 minor criteria.

Possible clinical diagnosis: 1 major and 1 minor, or 3 minor criteria.

Rejected case: Other diagnosis and disappearance of fever within 4 days of antibiotics.

Major criteria:
- Two positive blood cultures for organisms typical of infectious endocarditis (IE)
- Three positive blood cultures for organisms consistence with IE
- Serologic evidence of *C. burnetii*
- Echocardiographic evidence
- Cardiac abscess
- New valvular regurgitation
- New dehiscence of prosthetic valve.

Minor criteria:
- Predisposing cardiac disorder
- IV drug abuse
- Fever > 38°C
- *Vascular phenomenon*: (a) Arterial embolism, (b) septic pulmonary embolism, (c) mycotic aneurysm, (d) intracranial hemorrhage, (e) conjunctival petechiae, and (f) Janeway lesions
- *Immunological phenomenon*: (a) Glomerulonephritis (b) Osler's nodes (c) Roth's spot (d) Rheumatoid factor
- Morphological evidence of infection consistent with but not meeting major criteria
- Serological evidence of infection consistence with endocarditis.

A typical clinical picture comprises fever, fatigue, irritability, weight loss, arthralgia, and myalgia. Fever may be high in acute cases.

Existing cardiac murmur may change or there might be appearance of new murmur. In some cases, it may present with congestive cardiac failure (CCF).

Spleen may be palpable, clubbing of the finger may be present.

Features related to embolic manifestation in different organs may occur. In kidney, there may be hematuria; mycotic aneurysm of central nervous system (CNS) may be at risk for rupture.

Vascular and immune phenomena may be there. In skin, there may be petechiae which may also be present in conjunctiva; splinter hemorrhage in nail beds and Roth spots (retinal hemorrhages) may be present. Janeway lesions are painless hemorrhages under skin seen mostly on the palms and soles.

Immunocomplex lesions such as small painful subcutaneous nodules on digital fingers (Osler nodes), glomerulonephritis, and splenomegaly may be present.

DIAGNOSIS

- Three successive blood cultures taken within 24-48 hours. At least two should be positive.
- *Blood for complete blood count (CBC)*: Hemoglobin (Hb) reduced, Leukocyte count increased, erythrocyte sedimentation rate (ESR) increased, rheumatoid factor may be positive.
- *Urine routine examination (RE)*: Microscopic hematuria.
- *Echocardiogram*: Show the lesions and damage caused.

MANAGEMENT

- *Empirical therapy*: Penicillin and aminoglycoside. If penicillin allergy or methicillin-resistant case—vancomycin.
- Final selection of antibiotics is dependent on organisms isolated and its sensitivity.
- *Duration of therapy*: 6 weeks.
- *For fungal infection*: Amphotericin B is the drug of choice.

Prophylaxis with dental procedure:

Cardiac causes: Patients with prosthetic valve, previous IE, repaired congenital heart disease (CHD) operated or with valve.

Prophylaxis in other cases:
- Dental procedure involving gum
- Biopsy of respiratory mucosa
- Surgical procedure.

Drugs: Single dose 30-60 minutes before the procedure
- Amoxicillin 50 mg/kg
- Allergy to penicillin cephalexin 50 mg/kg.

SUGGESTED READING

1. Park MK. Park's Pediatric Cardiology for Practitioners, 6th edition. USA: Elsevier; 2014.

SECTION 11: Nephrology

136. Urinary Tract Infection
137. Nephrotic Syndrome
138. Hematuria in Children
139. Renal Stones
140. Hypertension in Pediatrics
141. Voiding Disorders in Children

Urinary Tract Infection

Hemant Kumar, Shashank Kumar

INTRODUCTION

- Urinary tract infection (UTI) is a common bacterial infection in infants and children. The risk of having a UTI before the age of 14 years is 1–3% in boys and 3–10% in girls.
- In girls, the first UTI usually occurs by the age of 5 year, with peaks during infancy and toilet training. In boys, most UTIs occur during the 1st year of life; more common in uncircumcised boys.
- During the 1st year of life, M:F ratio is 2.8–5.4:1; beyond 1–2 years, M:F ratio is 1:10.
- Rapid evaluation and treatment of UTI is important to prevent renal parenchymal damage and renal scarring that can cause hypertension and progressive renal damage.

DEFINITION

- Infection of the urinary tract is identified by growth of a significant number of organisms of a single species in the urine in the presence of symptoms.
- Recurrent UTI is recurrence of symptoms with significant bacteriuria in patients who have recovered clinically following treatment is common in girls.
- *Severe/complicated UTI*: Presence of fever, persistent vomiting, dehydration, fever > 39°C, marked toxicity, and renal angle tenderness suggest complicated UTI.

RISK FACTORS (BOX 1)

BOX 1: Risk factors for urinary tract infection.

- Female gender
- Uncircumcised male
- Vesicoureteral reflux
- Voiding dysfunction
- Obstructive uropathy
- Urethral instrumentation
- Wiping from back to front in females
- Bubble bath
- Tight clothing
- Pinworm infestation
- Constipation
- Anatomic abnormality (labial adhesion)
- Neuropathic bladder

ETIOLOGY

Urinary tract infections are caused mainly by colonic bacteria.
- In girls, 75–90% of all infections are caused by *Escherichia coli*, followed by *Klebsiella* and *Proteus* spp.
- *Proteus*, *Staphylococcus saprophyticus* and *Enterococcus* are pathogens in some cases.

PATHOGENESIS

- Most UTIs are ascending infections.
- The bacteria arise from the fecal flora, colonize the perineum and enter the bladder via urethra.
- In uncircumcised boys, the bacterial pathogens arise from the flora beneath the prepuce.
- In some cases, the bacteria causing cystitis ascends to the kidney to cause pyelonephritis.

Rarely, renal infection occurs by hematogenous spread, as in endocarditis or in some neonates.

CLINICAL MANIFESTATIONS

The three basic forms of UTI:
1. Asymptomatic bacteriuria
2. Cystitis
3. Pyelonephritis

Asymptomatic Bacteriuria

- It refers to a condition that results in a positive urine culture without any manifestations of infection.
- It is most common in girls.
- The incidence is 1–2% in preschool and school-age girls and 0.03% in boys. The incidence declines with increasing age.

Cystitis

- It indicates that there is bladder involvement.
- Symptoms include dysuria, urgency, frequency, suprapubic pain, incontinence, and malodorous urine.
- Cystitis does not cause fever and does not result in renal injury.

Acute Hemorrhagic Cystitis

- It is caused by *Escherichia coli* and adenovirus types 11 and 21.
- Adenovirus cystitis is more common in boys.
- It is self-limiting, with hematuria lasting approximately for 4 days.

Eosinophilic Cystitis

- It is occasionally found in children and is of obscure in origin.
- Children may have been exposed to an allergen.
- Symptoms include cystitis with hematuria and ureteral dilation with hydronephrosis.
- On imaging, typically there are multiple solid bladder masses that consists histologically of inflammatory infiltrates with eosinophils.
- Treatment includes antihistamines.

Pyelonephritis

- *Clinical pyelonephritis is characterized by any or all of the following*: Abdominal or flank pain, fever, malaise, nausea, vomiting, and occasionally, diarrhea.
- Newborns show nonspecific symptoms as poor feeding, irritability, and weight loss.
- Pyelonephritis is the most common serious bacterial infection in infants < 2 years of age who have fever without a focus.

Pyelonephritis may complicate as:

- Acute lobar nephronia (acute lobar nephritis) is a localized renal bacterial infection involving >1 lobe that represents either a complication of pyelonephritis or an early stage in the development of a renal abscess.
- Renal abscess may occur following a pyelonephritis or may be secondary to a primary bacteremia (*Staphylococcus aureus*).
- *Perinephric abscesses*: When pyelonephritis dissects to the renal capsule, it may also be secondary to contagious infection in perirenal area (e.g., vertebral osteomyelitis, psoas abscess).

DIAGNOSIS/LABORATORY INVESTIGATIONS

- The diagnosis of UTI is based on positive culture of a properly collected specimen of urine.
- Urinalysis enables a provisional diagnosis of UTI, a specimen must be obtained for culture prior to therapy with antibiotics:
  - Significant pyuria is defined as >10 leukocytes per mm^3 in a fresh uncentrifuged sample, or >5 leukocytes per high power field in a centrifuged sample.
  - Rapid dipstick-based tests, which detect leukocyte esterase and nitrite, are useful in screening for UTI.
  - Sterile pyuria (positive leukocytes, negative culture) occurs in:
    - Partially treated bacterial UTIs
    - Viral infections
    - Renal tuberculosis
    - Renal abscess
    - UTI in the presence of urinary obstruction
    - Urethritis due to sexually transmitted infection (STI).
- Inflammation near ureter and bladder (appendicitis, Crohn's disease), and interstitial nephritis.
- Collection of specimens for culture **(Table 1)**:
  - A clean-catch midstream specimen is used to minimize contamination by periurethral flora.
  - Contamination can be minimized by washing the genitalia with soap and water.
  - Antiseptic washes and forced retraction of the prepuce are not advised.
  - Catheterized or suprapubic aspiration can be done in non-toilet trained for specimen collection.
  - Application of an adhesive, sealed, sterile collection of bags after disinfection of the skin of genitals can be useful.
  - The urine specimen should be promptly plated within 1 hour of collection. If delay is anticipated, the sample can be stored in a refrigerator at 4°C for up to 12–24 hours.
  - Cultures of specimens collected from urine bags have high false-positive rates, and are not recommended.

TABLE 1: Collection of specimen for culture.

Method of collection	Colony count	Probability of infection
Mid-stream clean catch	>105 CFU/mL	90–95%
Urethral catheterization	>104 CFU/mL	95%
Suprapubic aspiration	Any number of pathogens	99%
Bag specimen	Not recommended	Not recommended

(CFU: colony-forming units)

- A urine culture should be repeated in case contamination is suspected, e.g., mixed growth of two or more pathogens, or growth of organisms that normally constitute the periurethral flora (lactobacilli in healthy girls; enterococci in infants and toddlers).
- The culture should also be repeated in situations where UTI is strongly suspected but colony counts are equivocal.
- The number of bacteria required for defining UTI depends on the method of urine collection.
- With acute renal infection, leukocytosis, neutrophilia, and elevated erythrocyte sedimentation rate (ESR) and c-reactive protein (CRP) are common.
- With a renal abscess, the white blood cell count is markedly elevated to >20,000–25,000/mm^3.
  Because sepsis is common in pyelonephritis, particularly in infants and in any child with obstructive uropathy, blood cultures should be considered.
- *Complete blood count (CBC)*: With acute UTI, especially in complicated UTI there is leukocytosis, neutrophilia, elevated ESR, and CRP.
- *Micturating cystourethrography (MCU)*:
  - MCU is a gold standard for diagnosing vesicoureteral reflux (VUR).
  - In MCU, bladder is filled with radiocontrast agent by transurethral catheterization under fluoroscopic guidance and films taken during voiding.
  - MCU permits grading of VUR, defines urethral and bladder anatomy and function.
- *Radionuclide cystography*:
  - Alternative for diagnosis and evaluation of VUR
  - Higher detection rate than MCU at a lower radiation exposure
  - Useful for follow-up of VUR because of minimal radiation
- *99Tc-DMSA (dimercaptosuccinic acid) scintigraphy*:
  - Sensitive and specific for diagnosis of acute pyelonephritis
  - It demonstrates decrease radiotracer uptake caused by cortical ischemia and tubular dysfunction during acute infection
  - Most reliable investigation for scarring and also assessing renal function
  - For renal scarring, a DMSA scan should be performed preferably after 4-6 months after infection

Further evaluation after the first UTI is done as follows:
- The aim of investigations is to identify patients at high risk of renal damage, chiefly those below 1 year of age, and those with VUR or urinary tract obstruction.
- Evaluation includes ultrasonography, DMSA renal scan and MCU performed.

Flowchart 1: Evaluation after first UTI.

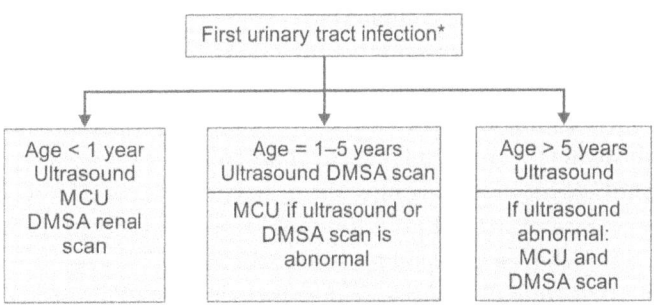

*All patients with recurrent UTI need detailed evaluation with ultrasonography, DMSA scan and MCU.
(DMSA: dimercaptosuccinic acid; MCU: micturating cystourethrography; UTI: urinary tract infection)

- Ultrasonogram provides information on kidney size, number and location, presence of hydronephrosis, urinary bladder anomalies and postvoid residual urine.
- DMSA scintigraphy is a sensitive technique for detecting renal parenchymal infection and cortical scarring.
- MCU detects VUR and provides anatomical details regarding the bladder and the urethra **(Flowchart 1)**.

When to use evaluation tools:
- Ultrasonography—soon after the diagnosis of UTI
- MCU—2-3 weeks after treatment
- DMSA scan—2-3 months after treatment.

TREATMENT

Therapy should be prompt:
- To reduce the morbidity of infection
- Minimize renal damage
- Subsequent complications

Children < 3 months of age and those with complicated UTI should be hospitalized and treated with parenteral antibiotics.
- The choice of antibiotic should be guided by local sensitivity patterns.
- A third-generation cephalosporin is preferred.
- Therapy with a single daily dose of an aminoglycoside may be used in children with normal renal function.
- Intravenous therapy is given for the first 2-3 days followed by oral antibiotics once the clinical condition improves.
- Children with simple UTI and those above 3 months of age are treated with oral antibiotics.
- With adequate therapy, there is resolution of fever and reduction of symptoms by 48-72 hours.
- Failure to respond may be due to presence of resistant pathogens, complicating factors or noncompliance; these patients require reevaluation.

- 14 days for infants and children with complicated UTI.
- 7-10 days for uncomplicated UTI.
- Adolescents with cystitis may be treated with shorter duration of antibiotics, lasting 3 days.

Following the treatment of the UTI, prophylactic antibiotic therapy is initiated in children below 1 year of age, until appropriate imaging of the urinary tract is completed.

- Acute cystitis should be treated promptly to prevent possible progression to pyelonephritis.
- If treatment is initiated before the results of a culture and sensitivities are available, a 3-5-day course of therapy with trimethoprim-sulfamethoxazole (TMP-SMX) or trimethoprim is effective against most strains of E. coli.
- Nitrofurantoin (5-7 mg/kg/24 h in three to five divided doses) also is effective and has the advantage of being active against *Klebsiella* and *Enterobacter* organisms.
- Amoxicillin (50 mg/kg/24 h) also is effective as initial treatment but has a high rate of bacterial resistance.
- In acute febrile infections suggesting clinical pyelonephritis, a 7-14-day course of broad-spectrum antibiotics capable of reaching significant tissue levels is preferable.
- Children who are dehydrated, are vomiting, are unable to drink fluids, are 3 months of age or younger, have complicated infections, or in whom urosepsis is a possibility should be admitted to the hospital for IV rehydration and IV antibiotics therapy.
- Oral third-generation cephalosporins such as cefixime are as effective as parenteral ceftriaxone against a variety of gram-negative organisms other than *Pseudomonas*, and these medications are considered by some authorities to be the treatment of choice for oral outpatient therapy.
- The oral fluoroquinolone ciprofloxacin is an alternative agent for resistant microorganisms.

Parenteral treatment with:
- Ceftriaxone (50-75 mg/kg/24 h)
- Cefotaxime (100 mg/kg/24 h)
- Ampicillin (100 mg/kg/24 h) with an aminoglycoside such as gentamicin (3-5 mg/kg/24 h) is preferable
- Aminoglycosides is particularly effective against *Pseudomonas*.

Urinary Tract Infection in Different Situations

- Children with a renal or perirenal abscess or with infection in obstructed urinary tracts can require surgical or percutaneous drainage in addition to antibiotic therapy and other supportive measures.
- In a child with recurrent UTIs, identification of predisposing factors is beneficial.
- Many school-age girls have bladder bowel dysfunction; treatment of this condition often reduces the likelihood of recurrent UTI.
- Some children with UTIs void infrequently, and many also have severe constipation, in these children behavioral modification with treatment of constipation is often effective.

PREVENTION OF RECURRENT URINARY TRACT INFECTION

General Measures
- Adequate fluid intake and frequent voiding.
- Constipation should be avoided.
- In children with VUR who are toilet trained, regular and volitional low pressure voiding with complete bladder emptying is encouraged.
- Double voiding ensures emptying of the bladder of postvoid residual urine.
- Circumcision reduces the risk of recurrent UTI in infant boys, and might therefore have benefits in patients with high-grade reflux.

Antibiotic prophylaxis (Table 2) is recommended for patients with:
- UTI below 1 year of age, while awaiting imaging studies, VUR.
- Frequent febrile UTI (three or more episodes in a year) even if the urinary tract is normal.
- Long-term, low-dose, antibacterial prophylaxis is used to prevent recurrent, febrile UTI.
- The antibiotic used should be effective, nontoxic with few side effects and should not alter the growth of commensals or induce bacterial resistance.

TABLE 2: Antibiotic prophylaxis.

Medication	Dose, mg/kg/day	Remarks
Co-trimoxazole	1–2*	Avoid in infants < 3 months, glucose-6-phosphate dehydrogenase (G6PD) deficiency
Nitrofurantoin	1–2	May cause vomiting and nausea; avoid in infants <3 months, G6PD deficiency, renal insufficiency
Cephalexin	10	Drug of choice in first 3–6 months of life
Cefadroxil	5	An alternative agent in early infancy

Usually given as a single bedtime dose, *of trimethoprim

KEY MESSAGES

- Urinary tract infection is a common bacterial infection in infants and children.
- Symptoms are to be guiding force for diagnosing UTI rather than chasing only culture reports.
- Evaluation to prevent renal scarring and progressive renal damage is to be kept in mind.
- One third to half of all patients with UTI have VUR; all children with first UTI should be evaluated to rule out VUR/Urinary tract obstruction.

SUGGESTED READING

1. Consensus statement on management of urinary tract infections: Indian Pediatrics. 2001;38:1106-15.

CHAPTER 137

Nephrotic Syndrome

Renu Kale

INTRODUCTION

Nephrotic syndrome is an important chronic disorder in children. It is common in age group of 2-6 years with male preponderance in a ratio of 2:1. Most common type of nephrotic syndrome encountered in general practice is minimal change (idiopathic) in 85-90% patients <6 years of age which responds promptly to steroids. Approximately three fourths have one or more relapses requiring treatment and are prone to steroid toxicity.

DEFINITION

Nephrotic syndrome is a condition characterized by heavy proteinuria, hypoalbuminemia (serum albumin < 2.5 g/dL), hyperlipidemia (serum cholesterol > 250 mg/dL) and edema.

Types:
- *Primary nephrotic* syndrome is categorized as minimal change, membranous and focal segmental glomerulonephritis. Primary *nephrotic syndrome* is more common in pediatric population below 16 years of age.
- *Secondary nephrotic* syndrome is due to systemic diseases such as systemic lupus erythematosus (SLE), diabetes, hepatitis B or C infections, etc.

Signs and symptoms:
- Edema is most common presenting symptom in 95% of children. Edema is typically found in lower extremities, face, periorbital region, scrotum or labia, and abdomen. Early morning periorbital edema is an earliest sign of nephrotic syndrome.
- Abdominal discomfort may be due to ascites, but persistent abdominal pain may be due to primary bacterial peritonitis (potentially life-threatening complication), relative gut ischemia due to hypoperfusion secondary to intravascular volume depletion.
- Some children may present with acute kidney injury (AKI) due to severe intravascular volume depletion leading to oliguria or anuria.
- Seizures may be presenting symptom of cerebral thrombosis.
- Pulmonary edema is rare in nephrotic patients.
- Physical examination should include blood pressure measurement as patient may be in shock due to hypotension or hypertension may be present due to fluid overload.

DIFFERENTIAL DIAGNOSIS IN CHILD WITH EDEMA

- Protein losing enteropathy
- Hepatic failure
- Acute or chronic glomerulonephritis
- Protein malnutrition.

INVESTIGATIONS

First episode of nephrotic syndrome should be investigated in detail before starting treatment with steroids.

Complete blood count: A complete blood count with hemoglobin (Hb), total leukocyte count (TLC), differential leukocyte count (DLC), and platelet count should be done. This helps to rule out any underlying infection which has to be treated before starting treatment with steroid. Thrombocytosis is commonly seen in patient with nephrotic syndrome.

Serum proteins (total) and serum albumin: Total proteins are decreased with alteration in A/G ratio. Serum albumin level of <2.5 mg/dL is diagnostic of nephrotic syndrome.

Blood urea nitrogen (BUN) and serum creatinine: Baseline kidney function test (KFT) is important to rule out any underlying kidney abnormality.

Serum electrolytes: Sodium, potassium, and chloride to rule out dilutional hyponatremia

Serum cholesterol: Serum cholesterol > 200 mg/dL helps in diagnosis of nephrotic syndrome.

Serum complements: Investigation of C3, C4 levels is required if the patient has gross or persistent microscopic hematuria.

Urine: Fresh urine sample is examined for presence of microscopic hematuria, leukocytosis, casts or crystals.

TABLE 1: Quantification of proteinuria in children.

Method	Abnormal proteinuria	Precautions
Urine dipstick	1+ or more in concentrated urine (specific gravity > 1.020)	False positive if urine pH > 8 or specific gravity > 1.025 or tested within 24 hours of radiocontrast study
Sulfosalicylic acid test	1+ or more	False positive with iodinated radiocontrast agent
Urine protein/creatinine ratio (Up/Uc) ratio in spot urine	>0.2 mg/mg in children > 2 years >0.06 mg/mg in 6 months to 2 years *Nephrotic range:* > 2 mg/mg	Protein excretion varies with child's age
Timed urine protein excretion rate	>150 mg/1.73 m^2/24 h nephrotic range >40 mg/m^2/h or >3 g/1.73 m^2/24 h	Inaccurately collected 24-hour specimen urine creatine should be in the range of 16–24 mg/kg in females and 21–27 mg/kg in males

TABLE 2: Sulfosalicyclic acid test.

Grade	Appearance	Protein concentration (g/L)
0	No turbidity	0
Trace	Slight turbidity	0.01–0.1
1+	Turbidity through which print can be read	0.15–0.3
2+	White cloud without precipitation through which heavy black lines or white background can be seen	0.4–1
3+	White cloud with precipitation through which heavy black lines cannot be seen	1.5–3.5
4+	Flocculent precipitate	5

Urine protein: Freshly voided first morning sample is required to test for albuminuria. Quantification of proteinuria is given in **Table 1**. In children, spot urine protein creatinine ratio is preferred as easier to perform. In older children, 24-hour urine sample can be collected for quantification of proteinuria. Parents can be taught to do dipstick or sulfosalicylic test at home **(Table 2)** in order to know if the child is going into relapse.

Urine culture: If UTI is suspected, following additional investigations are done:

Autoimmune markers: Antinuclear antibody (ANA), ds-DNA, Antineutrophil cytoplasmic antibody (ANCA) if any underlying illness is suspected (e.g., SLE)
- Thyroid function test
- Hepatitis B antigen
- X-ray chest and Mantoux test are done only if there is suspicion of tuberculosis, not required before starting steroids in otherwise healthy children.

TREATMENT

Treatment of initial episode: Adequate treatment of initial episode is extremely important. Current evidence suggests that initial episode influences the subsequent course of illness. Proper dosage and duration of treatment may help in decreasing rate of subsequent relapses. It is imperative to treat infections before starting treatment with steroids. Record of patients' weight and height should be maintained for growth monitoring.

Medication

Prednisolone is the drug of choice. Other drugs such as hydrocortisone, and betamethasone should not be used. Deflazacort is a steroid analog is as effective as prednisolone with fewer side effects but still not widely used due to fewer studies supporting its long-term usage in children.

Treatment Regime

Various treatment regimes have been formulated over a period of years. The recommendation given by *Expert Group of Indian Academy of Pediatrics (IAP) and by International Study of Kidney Diseases in Children* favors use of prednisolone over long period of time. Prednisolone is given in dosage of 2 mg/kg (60 mg^2/kg) up to a maximum of 60 mg for 6 weeks daily in two to three divided doses. This is followed by 1.5 mg/kg (40 mg^2/kg) in single morning dose on alternate day for 6 weeks. Treatment with corticosteroids should preferably be given after meals. Corticosteroids are discontinued after 12 weeks. Some meta-analysis have suggested that prolonging alternate-day therapy to 3–6 months is associated

TABLE 3: Definitions to define course of disease.

Remission	Urine albumin nil or trace (or proteinuria < 4 mg/m²/h) for three consecutive days
Relapse	Urine albumin 3+ or 4+ (proteinuria > 40 mg/m²/h) for 3 consecutive days
Frequent relapse	Two or more relapses in 6 months of initial response or more than three relapses in any 12 months
Steroid dependence	Two consecutive relapses when on alternate-day steroids or within 14 days of its discontinuation
Steroid resistance	Absence of remission despite 4 weeks of daily steroid therapy in dose of 2 mg/kg/day

with prolonged remission and reduced number of relapses, but steroid toxicity develops with long-term use. One should adhere to the standard definition which define the course of disease **(Table 3)**.

Treatment of Relapse

Patient who comes with relapse should first be evaluated for underlying infection and treated for these before starting treatment with steroids. Prednisolone is given in dose of 2 mg/kg (in single or two divided doses) until urine protein is trace or nil for 3 consecutive days or 2 weeks. Patient is then put on alternate day regime of 1.5 mg/kg for 4 weeks and then discontinued. Usual duration of treatment is 5–6 weeks. Prolongation of therapy is usually not required in infrequent relapser. In case patient does not acquire remission in 2 weeks treatment can be prolonged for another 2 weeks. If there is still no response, patient should be referred to pediatric nephrologist for further evaluation.

Infrequent Relapser

Patients who have three or less relapses in 1 year can be treated with above regime for each relapse. Evidence of steroid toxicity is low in these patients.

Frequent Relapser or Steroid Dependence

Patient is started on treatment of relapse with prednisolone and steroid is gradually tapered to maintain patient in remission on alternate day dose of 0.5–0.7 mg/kg over 9–18 months. A close watch on growth and blood pressure is kept to monitor for steroid toxicity. If threshold of prednisolone to maintain remission is higher than 0.5 mg/kg or features of steroid toxicity develops, additional immunomodulators can be added. Renal biopsy is not needed in this group of patients but it is important to treat such patients with consultation with pediatric nephrologist.

Immunomodulators

- *Levamisole*: It is administered in dose of 2–2.5 mg/kg on alternate days for 12–24 months. Prednisolone is co-administered in dose of 1.5 mg/kg alternate day for 2–4 weeks and then gradually tapered to maintenance dose of 0.25–0.5 mg/kg, which can be continued for 6 or more months. Major side effects of levamisole are leukopenia, liver toxicity, convulsions, and rarely skin rash. Leukocyte count should be monitored every 12–16 weeks.
- Cyclophosphamide is administered in dose of 2–2.5 mg/kg for 12 weeks, preferably when patient is in remission. Prednisolone is coadministered in alternate day regime of 1.5 mg/kg for 4 weeks, 1 mg/kg for 8 weeks and then steroid is tapered over 2–3 months and then stopped. Leukocyte count is monitored over 2 weeks, if count falls below 4,000/mm³ drug should be temporarily discontinued. Major side effects are alopecia, leukopenia, nausea, vomiting, hemorraghic cystitis, and gonadal toxicity.
- *Calcineurin inhibitors*: Cyclosporine (CsA) and tacrolimus are agents which should be employed after kidney biopsy. CsA is given in dose of *4–5 mg/kg daily for 12–24 months*. Prednisolone is coadministered in dose of 1.5 mg/kg alternate day for 2–4 weeks then tapered every 4 weeks to *maintenance dose of 0.25–0.5 mg/kg for 6 months*. Trough levels of CsA should be maintained between 80–120 ηg/mL. Side effects are hypertension, gum hypertrophy, hirsutism, nephrotoxicity, *hypercholesterolemia, and elevated transaminase*. Therapy should not be given beyond 2 years.
- *Tacrolimus* is given in dose of 0.1–0.2 mg/kg daily over 12–24 months. It is preferred in adolescents due to lack of cosmetic side effects. The side effects are hyperglycemia, headache, diarrhea, and rarely neurotoxicity (seizures). Blood sugar and creatinine should be estimated every 2–3 months.
- *Mycophenolate mofetil* is given in dose of 800–1,200 mg/m² along with *tapering dose of prednisolone*. Side effects are gastrointestinal discomfort, diarrhea, and leukopenia. Leukocyte count should be monitored every 1–2 months and if count falls below 4,000/mm³ treatment should be withheld.
- *Rituximab is a chimeric anti*-CD20 monoclonal antibody that targets CD20 B cells resulting in its significant depletion. It is given in dose of 375 mg/m² as infusion in hospital setting. Side effects include anaphylaxis, fever, chills, rigors, headache, flushing, etc. Should be given with consultation of pediatric nephrologist.

Supportive Care

Diet: A balanced diet with adequate proteins (1.5–2 g/kg) and calories is recommended. Patient with persistent proteinuria should receive 2–2.5 g/kg of protein daily. Not more than 30% calories should be received from fat and saturated fats should be avoided. Salt restriction is not necessary in most patients, but reduction in salt intake (1–2 g/day) is advised if there is persistent deem.

Edema: Control of edema is an integral part of supportive care. Corticosteroid treatment will lead to diuresis in

5–10 days. Diuretics should be avoided unless absolutely essential. Patient with persistent edema and weight gain of (7–10%) should be treated with IV diuretics and be treated in hospital **(Flowchart 1)**.

Other Medications

- *Use of Antacids or histamine (H2) antagonists* is not required unless there are long-term upper gastrointestinal side effects.
- *Calcium supplement at ion (calcium carbonate 250–500 mg)* is given to patient receiving steroid for >3 months.
- *Immunization*:
  - Primary vaccinations should be completed. Immunocompromised patients should not receive live attenuated vaccine; killed or inactivated vaccines are safe (any patient receiving 2 mg/kg or greater or total of 20 mg/day if weighing >10 kg and received treatment for >14 days is considered immunocompromised)
  - Live vaccine can be administered once child is off steroid for 6 weeks but if required can be given to patient on alternate-day dose or <0.5 mg/kg.
  - Vaccines recommended are:
    - *Pneumococcal vaccine*: It should be given to all children, especially those with previous episode of peritonitis. It is given when patient is in remission or when not receiving daily steroids.
    - Booster dose is given every 5 years to those who have received vaccine before 5 years of age.
    - Hib (*Haemophilus influenzae* type b) vaccine.
    - Hepatitis B vaccine.
    - Influenza vaccine annually.
    - *Varicella vaccine*: Patients in remission and not on corticosteroid therapy should receive two doses of vaccine 4 weeks apart.

PATIENT AND PARENT EDUCATION

Parental motivation and involvement is essential in long-term management of these children. Adequate information about disease, complication, and course of disease should be provided. Reassurance regarding long-term outcome should be provided.

What parents should do?
- Maintain diary showing proteinuria, medications received and intercurrent infections.
- Urine examination at home with dipstick or boiling test to find out if patient is going into relapse.
- Ensure normal activity and school.
- Prompt treatment of infections are done as these are associated with morbidity; insist on vaccinations and measures to prevent serious infections.

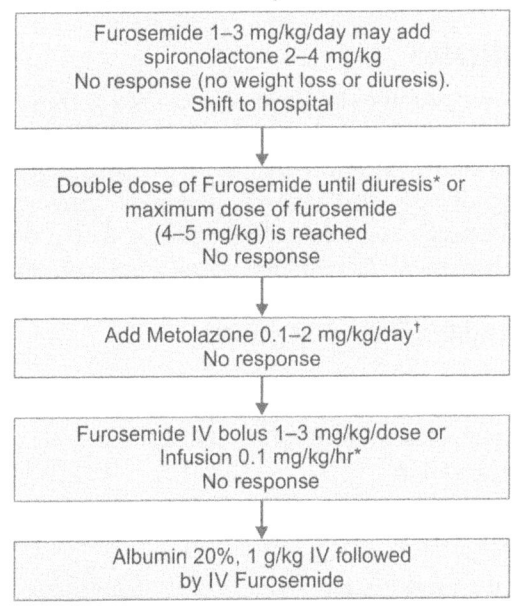

Flowchart 1: Management of edema.

*Reduce stepwise as diuresis sets in.
†Monitor hypovolemia add spironolactone or potassium-sparing diuretic.

COMPLICATIONS

Infections (Table 4)

TABLE 4: Clinical features and management of common infections.

Infection	Clinical features	Common organisms	Antibiotics	Duration of treatment
Peritonitis	Pain abdominal, tenderness, diarrhea, and vomiting. Fever may or may not be present	*Streptococcus pneumoniae* *S. pyogenes Escherichia coli*	Penicillin/ampicillin and aminoglycoside, ceftriaxone	10–14 days*
Pneumonia	Fever, cough	*S. pneumoniae* *H. influenzae*	Oral amoxicillin, cephalexin, IV ceftriaxone	7–10 days*
Urinary infection	Frequency, dysuria, fever	*E. coli, Klebsiella* spp, *Proteus*	Amoxicillin, cephalexin, amikacin	7–10 days*
Cellulitis	Redness, induration, tenderness	Group A streptococci, *Haemophilus influenzae*	Ampicillin and aminoglycoside or, ceftriaxone	7–10 days*
Fungal infections	Pulmonary infiltrates, persistent fever unresponsive to antibiotics	*Candida, Aspergillus* spp	Skin, mucosa: Fluconazole Systemic infection: Amphotericin	7–10 days* 14–21 days

*Initial therapy is parental for 5 days, once patient accepts orally can be shifted to oral antibiotic.
(IV: intravenous)

PHARMACOLOGICAL ASSISTANCE

Pharmacological salt	Market preparation	Availability	Dosage
Prednisolone	Wysolone, Predone, Kidpred, Omnacortil	Tablet: 5, 10, 20, 40 mg, syrup 5 mg/5 mL, 15 mg/5 mL	2 mg/kg
Furosemide	Lasix, Frusenex, Salinex	Tablet: 40 mg, 100 mg, 500 mg, Syrup: 10 mg/mL, Injection: – 10 mg/mL	Oral: 2–6 mg/kg/day q12h IV dose: 1–2 mg/kg/dose IV

(IV: intravenous)

Hypertension

It occurs due to steroid toxicity. Therapy can be initiated with angiotensin-converting enzyme (ACE) inhibitors or calcium channel blockers.

Thrombosis

Children are at risk of venous thrombosis and rarely arterial thrombosis. Reduced intravascular volume, aggressive diuretics, immobilization are few causes for thrombosis. Deep vein thrombosis of calf vein is common sagittal sinus thrombosis following diarrhea, may present with convulsion, altered sensorium. Ultrasonography, Doppler, and MRI is used to confirm diagnosis. Treatment includes correction of dehydration, and other complications, and use of heparin (IV) or low molecular weight heparin followed by oral anticoagulants for long time. There is no role of long-term prophylaxis.

Hypovolemic Shock

Unsupervised use of diuretics, especially in children with sepsis, diarrhea and vomiting will lead to hypovolemic stress. Presenting features are severe abdominal pain, hypotension, tachycardia, cold extremities, and poor capillary refill. Rapid infusion of IV normal saline in dose of 15–20 mL/kg over 20–30 minutes is treatment of choice. This is repeated if hypovolemia persists. Infusion of albumin 5% (10–15 mL/kg) or 20% albumin (0.5–1 g/kg) is used if there is no response to normal saline infusion.

Corticosteroid Side Effects

Prolonged treatment with steroid is associated with increased appetite, cushingoid features, impaired growth, behavorial changes, gastritis, salt and water retention and bone and mineral demineralization.

Steroid during Stress

Patients who have received steroid for >2 weeks in past 1 year show suppression of hypothalamic–pituitary–adrenal axis. These children require supplementation of steroid during surgery, anesthesia, or serious infections. Treatment with corticosteroid should not be stopped during serious infections. Parenteral Hydrocortisone in dose of 2–5 mg/kg/day is given during period of stress, followed by oral Prednisolone in dose of 0.5–1 mg/kg/day once child can accept orally. The dose is administered for duration of stress and then daily by 50%.

Indications for referral to pediatric nephrologist:
- Onset < 1 year of age
- Nephrotic syndrome presenting with hypertension, persistent microscopic or gross hematuria, or impaired renal function
- Complications such as refractory edema, thrombosis, severe infections, and steroid toxicity
- Steroid dependant or frequently relapsing nephrotic syndrome.

PROGNOSIS

Nephrotic syndrome (minimal change) is a chronic disease associated with long-term morbidity. It has a long and relapsing course, but progression to end-stage renal failure requiring dialysis and transplantation is extremely rare. Parenteral and patient motivation is important in treatment and management of patients. Steroid-resistant nephrotic syndrome, especially FSGS has 50% risk of end-stage renal disease within 5 years of diagnosis.

KEY MESSAGES

- Adequate doses and duration of treatment as per protocol
- Immunization
- Parental involvement
- Timely referral.

SUGGESTED READING

1. Bagga A; Indian Pediatric Nephrology Group. Revised Guidelines for management of steroid sensitive nephrotic syndrome. Indian Journal of Nephrology. 2008;18(1):31-9s.
2. Boyer O, Baudouin V, Berard E, Biebuyck-Gouge N. Vaccine recommendations for children with idiopathic nephrotic syndrome. Nephrol Ther. 2020;S1789-7255(20):300004-3.
3. Carter SA, Mistry S, Fitzpatric J, Banh T, Hebert D, Langlois V, Prarl RJ. Prediction of short- and long-term outcomes in childhood nephrotic syndrome. Kidney Int Rep. 2019;5(4):426-34.
4. Hodson E, Knight JF, Willis NS, Craig JC. Corticosteroid therapy in nephrotic syndrome: meta-analysis of randomised control trails. Arch Dis Child. 2000;83(1):45-51.
5. Hodson EM, Willis NS, Craig JC. Corticosteroid therapy for nephrotic syndrome in children. Cochrane Database System Rev. 2005;(1): CD001533.
6. Indian Pediatric Nephrology Group, Indian Academy of Pediatric. Consensus statement on management of steroid sensitive nephrotic syndrome. Indian Pediatr. 2001;38(9):975-86.
7. Kan JA, Alhasan KA, Albana AS. Rituximab versus cyclophosphamide as first steroid-sparing agent in childhood frequently relapsing and steroid dependant nephrotic syndrome. Pediatr Nephrol. 2020;35(8):1445-53.
8. KDIGO. Steroid-sensitive nephrotic syndrome in children. KDIGO Clinical Practice Guidelines and Glomerulonephritis, 2012.
9. Larkin NG, Liu ID, Willis NS, Craig NS, Hodson EM. Noncorticosteroid immunosuppressive medication for steroid sensitive nephrotic syndrome. Cochrane Database Sys Rev. 2020; 4:CD002290.

CHAPTER 138: Hematuria in Children

Seema Jain

INTRODUCTION

Hematuria is a manifestation of disorders of the kidney and the urinary tract. It may be an isolated microscopic hematuria or a gross. When it manifests with either episodes of gross hematuria or persistent microscopic hematuria with significant proteinuria; it might signify a serious underlying illness. A detailed evaluation is therefore necessary.

DEFINITION

Hematuria is presence of RBC in urine. It is gross, when frankly visible to naked eyes and looks rusty, tea colored or as frank blood. Microscopic hematuria is defined as presence of 5 or more RBCs/HPF (red blood cells per high power field) in a centrifuged urine specimen. It is considered to be persistent if present in two to three urine analyses over 2–3-week period. Transient hematuria may be seen in fever, exercise, infections, and trauma. Causes of red-colored urine are given in **Table 1**.

CONFIRMATION OF RBC IN URINE

Microscopic analysis and documentation of red blood cells in the urinary sediment specifically differentiate hematuria from pigmenturias. Dipstick is positive in both as it detects heme. It has 100% sensitivity and 99% specificity. A false-positive dipstick occur if urine sample is very concentrated, alkaline urine with pH > 9, when contaminated with cleaning agents such as povidone iodine, hypochlorite or with microbial peroxidase. It is falsely negative in the presence of formalin or ascorbic acid.

The need for evaluation of hematuria is to determine if it is glomerular or nonglomerular **(Table 2)**. **Flowcharts 1 and 2** show the evaluation of gross hematuria and microscopic hematuria respectively.

ETIOLOGY

Etiology of hematuria is extensive. Patient manifest with edema, oliguria, gross hematuria, and hypertension. These patients may present with respiratory distress and at times misdiagnosed as bronchopneumonia or myocarditis unless blood pressure is recorded and urinalysis is done. IgA nephropathy is associated with synpharyngitic hematuria which ranges from microscopic to gross hematuria systemic symptoms inform of fever, rash, arthritis favors systemic lupus erythematosus (SLE), Henoch-Schönlein purpura (HSP), and vasculitis. Other causes include benign familial hematuria and hemolytic uremic syndrome. A detailed family history of deafness, eye abnormalities such as anterior lenticonus, retinal flakes assisting diagnosis of Alport syndrome.

Nonglomerular causes include urinary tract infection, cystitis (adenovirus infection, schistosomiasis, and drug cyclophosphamide), calculi, Wilms tumor, urinary tract tumor such as hemangiomas, rhabdomyosarcoma, trauma, acute tubular necrosis, hypercalciuria, sickle cell disease. Urologic cases present as initial or terminal hematuria. Initial is due to penile lesions and terminal represents bladder pathology.

TABLE 1: Causes of red-colored urine.

Dark yellow	Concentrated urine, rifampicin
Dark brown, black urine	Bile pigments, methemoglobinemia, alkaptonuria, melanin, tyrosinosis
Red or pink color	Hematuria, hemoglobinuria, myoglobinuria, porphyrins, urates *Food*: Beetroot, blackberries, red dye *Drugs*: Benzene, chloroquine, desferoxamine, and phenolphthalein

TABLE 2: Evaluation of gross hematuria.

Glomerular	Nonglomerular
Tea- or cola-colored urine	Bright red blood
Painless	Painful usually
Normally site is upper tract	Lower tract
Dysmorphic (>20% RBC)	Eumorphic RBC
Associated with cast, proteinuria	No cast or proteinuria
Clots absent	Clots present

(RBC: red blood cell)

Other causes include hematological abnormalities and renal vein thrombosis. Nutcracker syndrome is a condition caused by compression of left renal vein between abdominal aorta and superior mesenteric artery leading to intermittent gross hematuria and left flank pain.

Poststreptococcal Glomerulonephritis

Postinfectious glomerulonephritis occurs frequently in children. It is caused by group A beta-hemolytic streptococci.

The syndrome is a result of glomerular injury with glomerular inflammation and pathologic correlation is of proliferative glomerulonephritis.

CLINICAL FEATURES

It develops in children aged 5–10 years. Clinical presentation varies from mild illness to oligoanuria with severe hypertension. The latent period after infection is usually 10–14 days after pharyngitis and 2–3 weeks after pyoderma. Early presentation is mild periorbital puffiness in morning, due to fluid retention. Hypertension can manifest with headache, confusion, and seizures. Posterior reversible encephalopathy syndrome (PRES) is characterized by occipital blindness, confusion, headache, lethargy, transient motor deficit, and generalized seizures; all is reversible. Respiratory distress occurs due to pulmonary edema.

Loss of appetite, tiredness, itching and nausea may occur due to uremia. There is decreased volume and frequency of urine. Gross or microscopic hematuria is seen.

Presentation can be from only hematuria, encephalopathy, bronchopneumonia to acute renal failure which can mislead to other diagnosis.

INVESTIGATIONS

- *Complete blood count*: Low hemoglobin may reflect mild dilutional anemia in poststreptococcal glomerulonephritis (PSGN), low platelets is seen in hemolytic uremic syndrome (HUS).
- *Urinalysis*: Proteinuria and hematuria are found in almost all patients of PSGN. Cast is best seen in uncentrifuged

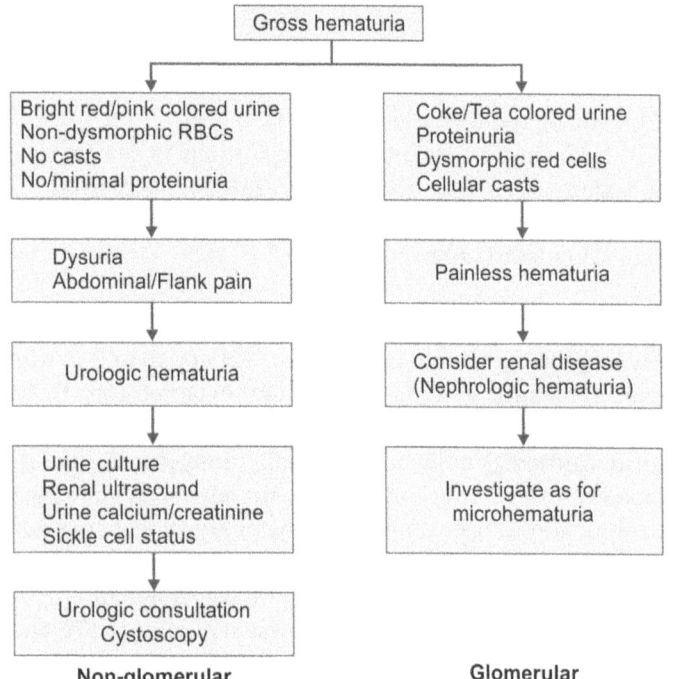

Flowchart 1: Evaluation of gross hematuria.

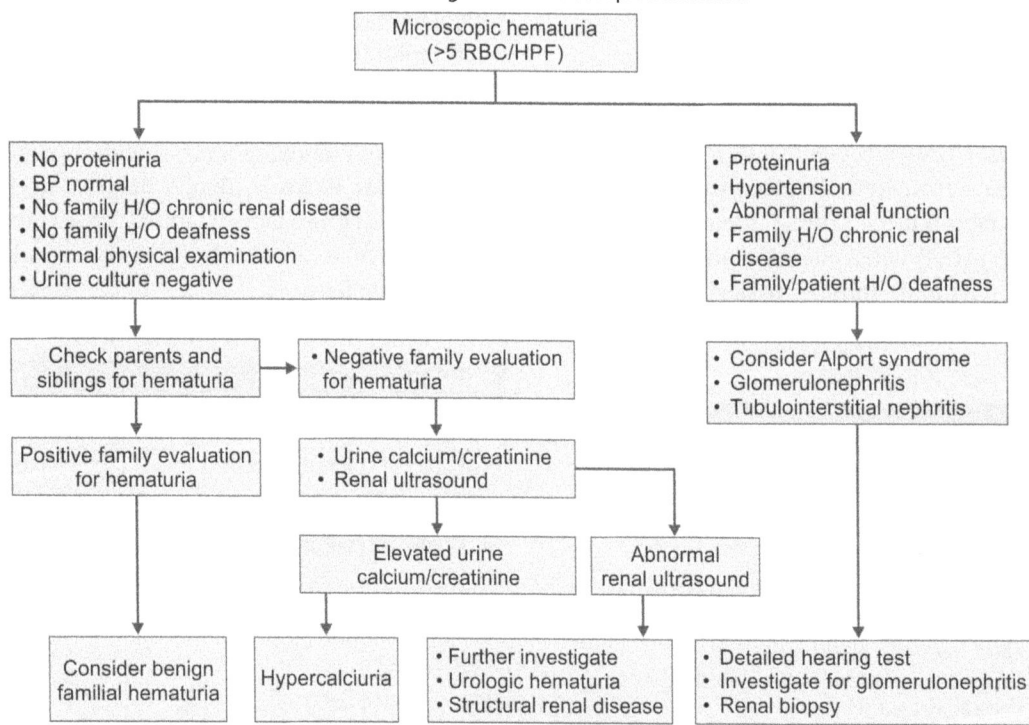

Flowchart 2: Diagnosis of microscopic hematuria.

(BP: blood pressure; H/O: history of; RBC/HPF: red blood cells per high power field)

urine sample, dysmorphic RBC is best seen by phase-contrast microscopy.

- *Serology*: C3 is low in PSGN and C4 may be slightly low. C3 normalizes by 6-8 weeks. IgA nephropathy has normal complements. Antistreptolysin O (ASO) titer is elevated in PSGN while Anti-DNAse B titers are more sensitive in skin lesions. Other test includes antinuclear antibody (ANA), perinuclear/nuclear-staining antineutrophil cytoplasmic antibodies p-ANCA, and cytoplasmic-staining antineutrophil cytoplasmic antibodies (c-ANCA).
- *Kidney function test*: Blood urea, serum creatinine to pickup acute kidney injury (AKI). Urine culture and sensitivity, urinary calcium-to-creatinine ratio for other causes.
- Chest X-ray (CXR) helps to reveal pulmonary edema and cardiomegaly.
- Ultrasonography of kidneys, ureter, bladder, prostrate (adults) helps to rule out congenital anomalies, calculi, and tumors.
- Renal Doppler, abdominal computed tomography (CT), angiography, cystoscopy, X-ray kidneys, ureters, bladder (KUB), magnetic resonance imaging (MRI) brain wherever required.
- *Renal biopsy*: It is indicated whenever there is significant proteinuria, persistent low-serum complement C3, unexplained azotemia, systemic disease, significant familial renal disease or gross hematuria of unknown etiology.

MANAGEMENT

- Patient is advised rest and limited activity.
- *Fluid and salt restriction*: Fluid intake is calculated on basis of urine output and insensible losses. Salt is restricted to 1 g/day.
- Diuretics are given to relieve edema and to control volume. Furosemide is commonly used. Dose is 0.5-2 mg/kg/day up to 5 mg/kg/day. It is a high ceiling diuretic and infusions or higher dose administered is more effective than small divided doses to induce diuresis. It relieves edema and controls volume-related elevation of blood pressure. It causes hypokalemia, hyponatremia, and metabolic alkalosis. Potential caution is necessary for patients with severe azotemia because of potential furosemide ototoxicity.
- Antihypertensives are given to control hypertension.
  - *Amlodepine at dose*: 0.05-0.5 mg/kg/day is administered. It is relatively safe.
  - *Enalapril*: 0.1-0.5 mg/kg/day can be used but it causes hyperkalemia so it should be used cautiously in renal failure. It induces dry cough and should be avoided in renal artery stenosis.
  - *In hypertensive emergency*:
    - Drug of choice is labetalol (0.5-1 mg/kg/h) intravenous (IV) infusion or sodium nitroprusside (0.5-2 µg/kg/min) IV infusion may be used. Caution should be exercised with later when used in patients with severe renal impairment.
    - Nifedipine short acting 0.25-0.5 mg/kg/dose by oral route can also be used.
    - IV mannitol for reducing intracranial pressures 0.5-1 g/kg. Head elevation 30° help in reducing edema.
    - IV lorazepam 0.1 mg/kg, 4 mg maximum or IV levetiracetam 15-30 mg/kg or IV phenytoin sodium 10-15 mg/kg loading then 3-8 mg/kg/day whichever is available for controlling acute seizures.
  - *Dialysis*: If renal failure occurs, dialysis is required in cases of intractable hyperkalemia, fluid overload unresponsive to diuretics, azotemia, acidosis, uncontrolled hypertension, and pulmonary edema.
  - Monitor blood pressure, weight, urine output and kidney functions on regular basis. If clinical condition deteriorates, other causes should be considered and renal biopsy is planned. A pediatric nephrology call can be considered.
  - Antibiotic therapy is given when signs of streptococcal infection persist or throat or skin cultures are positive. Oral penicillin V 250 mg twice daily for 10 days or injection benzathine penicillin G as single dose, 60,000 IU for <27 kg and 1,20,000 IU for >27 kg after sensitivity test is given. Antibiotic treatment does not alter the course of disease but prevents spread of nephritogenic strains to close contacts.

PREVENTION

Early antibiotic therapy of streptococcal infection (within 36 hours of onset) may prevent development of PSGN. Antibiotic treatment of a case may prevent spread of streptococci to close contacts.

PROGNOSIS

In majority of cases, the course of disease is typical with favorable outcome. Immunity to type M protein is type specific, long lasting, and protective; repeated episodes of PSGN are unlikely. Within a week or so, most patients with PSGN experiences spontaneous resolution.

CONCLUSION

Hematuria is uncommon condition in childhood. An episode of gross hematuria and symptomatic microscopic hematuria should be evaluated. One should be concerned about long-term impact on kidneys and progression to chronic kidney disease.

PRESCRIPTION ASSISTANCE

Pharmacological salt	Market preparation	Availability	Dosage
Furosemide	Lasix	Injection lasix (1 mL = 10 mg) Tablet lasix 40 mg	1–2 mg/kg/day, up to 5 mg/kg/day 0.05–0.5 mg/kg/day
Amlodipine	Amlo	Tablet Amlo 2.5, 5 mg	0.05–0.5 mg/kg/day
Enalapril	Enam	Tablet Enam 2.5, 5 mg	0.1–0.6 mg/kg/day
Labetalol	Lobet 100 mg	Injection 20 mg/4 mL and Tablet 100 mg	0.5–1 mg/kg/h infusion and Tablet 10–40 mg/kg/day bid
Mannitol	Mannitol (Alkem)	Injection mannitol 20% as 100 mL, 300 mL	5 mL/kg IV
Lorazepam	Ativan (Wyeth)	Injection	0.05 mg/kg maximum 4 mg
Phenytoin sodium	Eptoin	Tablet/injection Eptoin 100 mg, Injection Epsolin 100 mg/2 mL	
Benzathine Penicillin	Injection Penidure	Injection Penidure 6 lac, 12 lac	<27 kg to 6 lac unit >27 kg to 12 lac unit
Azithromycin	Azithral, Zathrin	Syrup/Tablet Azithral 100, 200 mg	10 mg/kg/day

SUGGESTED READING

1. Avner ED, Harmon WE, Niaudet P, Yoshikawa N, Emma F, Goldstein SL. Pediatric Nephrology, 7th edition. USA: Springer; 2019.
2. Geary DF, Schaefer F. Nephritic syndrome. Comprehensive Pediatric Nephrology. China: Mosby Elsevier; 2008. pp. 194-203.
3. Geary DF, Schaefer F. Postinfectious glomerulonephritis. Comprehensive Pediatric Nephrology. China: Mosby Elsevier; 2008. pp. 309-17.
4. Vasudev AS, Ugra D, Mehta K, Banerjee S, Saha A. In: Banerjee S (Ed). IAP Specialty series on Pediatric Nephrology. New Delhi: Jaypee Brothers medical Publishers (P) Ltd.; 2019.

Renal Stone

Nilam Thaker

INTRODUCTION

Nephrolithiasis is increasingly recognized in children. Factors such as variable clinical presentation, high recurrence of kidney stones associated with abnormalities of metabolism and the urinary tract, and the possible presence of rare genetic kidney stone diseases would require physicians to comprehensively evaluate children presenting with kidney stones.

Urolithiasis: Presence of calculi in the urinary tract.

Nephrocalcinosis: Generalized deposition of calcium throughout the renal parenchyma (usually in medullary region).

ETIOLOGY (BOX 1)

Renal stones occur as a result of the following three factors:
1. Supersaturation of stone forming compounds in urine
2. Presence of chemical or physical stimuli in urine that promote stone formation
3. Inadequate amount of compounds in urine that inhibit stone formation (e.g., magnesium, citrate).

Urinary tract infection (20–25%): Urinary tract infection with urea-splitting organisms such as *Proteus, Pseudomonas,* and *Klebsiella* favors precipitation of magnesium ammonium phosphate stone (struvite stone). Struvite stones tend to produce a stag-horn appearance.

Drugs: Steroids, loop diuretics, and carbonic anhydrase inhibitors such as topiramate, zonisamide, acetazolamide (hypercalciuria) allopurinol (Xanthine stone).

Cancer chemotherapy: Tumor lysis syndrome (uric acid stone).

Dietary consideration:
- Excessive vitamin D
- Ketogenic diet
- Melamine-contaminated milk powder
- Enhanced enteric absorption
- Enhanced absorption of oxalate (enteric hyperoxaluria) related to fat malabsorption, bile salt injury to colonic epithelium or absence of oxalate degrading bacteria following antibiotic treatment
- Inflammatory bowel disease
- Extensive bowel resection
- Pancreatitis, cystic fibrosis
- Idiopathic.

Frequency of kidney stones:
- Calcium with phosphate or oxalate (57%)
- Struvite (24%)
- Uric acid (8%)
- Cysteine (6%)
- Endemic (2%)
- Mixed (2%)
- Other types (1%).

BOX 1: Various causes of stone formation.

Structural abnormalities (10–25%):
- Pelviureteric junction obstruction, vesicoureteric reflux (stasis of urine)
- Autosomal dominant polycystic kidney disease
- Medullary sponge kidney

Metabolic abnormalities/genetic mutation (50–75%):
- *Common abnormalities:* Hypercalciuria, distal renal tubular acidosis (RTA) and hyperoxaluria
  - Hypercalciuria is the most common abnormality **(Box 2)**. Few patients with hypercalciuria may have an incomplete form of distal RTA that is only revealed when acidification mechanism is stressed, as during the furosemide–fludrocortisone test.
  - *Other abnormalities:* Cystinuria, xanthinuria, and hyperuricosuria

---

BOX 2: Metabolic abnormalities causing nephrolithiasis.

- Hypercalciuria **(Table 1)**
- Hyperoxaluria
  - Enteric hyperoxaluria
  - Primary hyperoxaluria, types I and II
- Hyperuricosuria:
  - Lesch–Nyhan syndrome
  - Partial HGPRT deficiency
  - Glycogenosis type 1a, 1b
- Cystinuria
- Xanthinuria
- Hypocitraturia

(HGPRT: hypoxanthine guanine-phosphoribosyltransferase)

TABLE 1: Causes of hypercalciuria.

Hypercalciuria with normal serum calcium	Hypercalciuria with hypercalcemia
• Idiopathic hypercalciuria (most common) • Distal RTA (associated hypocitraturia) • Bartter syndrome • Dent's disease • Lowe syndrome • FHHNC • *Drugs*: Furosemide, corticosteroids • Prolonged immobilization	• Vitamin D overdose • Primary hyperparathyroidism • Sarcoidosis • Malignancy (production of PTH-related peptide) • Williams–Beuren syndrome • Hyperthyroidism

(FHHNC: familial hypomagnesemia with hypercalciuria and nephrocalcinosis; PTH: parathyroid hormone; RTA: renal tubular acidosis)

DIAGNOSTIC EVALUATION

Clinical Evaluation

- *Classical presentation of stone disease in children*:
  - Sudden intense loin pain radiating toward groin
  - Gross hematuria with or without pain
  - Dysuria and urgency
  - Asymptomatic with incidental finding on abdominal imaging
  - Sometimes presents with anuria with acute kidney injury in case of stone in urethra or bilateral ureter. Large number of patients of nephrocalcinosis are asymptomatic. Abnormality is picked up incidentally on an imaging study. Diagnosis may be delayed and patient may present with tubular dysfunction manifested as polyuria, poor growth, rickets, or uremia.
- *History*: Aspects to be enquired are—
  - Dysuria, hematuria, abdominal pain
  - Polyuria, polydipsia, failure to thrive
  - Passage of previous calculus or gravel
  - Recurrent urinary tract infection (UTI)
  - Structural abnormalities of urinary tract
  - Intake of vitamin D
  - Drugs, e.g., frusemide, steroid, anticonvulsant (topiramate)
  - Family history of renal stones.
- *Physical examination*: Examine for—
  - Height and weight for growth
  - Dysmorphic features or rickets suggestive of associated metabolic disorder
  - Genitals for phimosis and vulval adhesion.

Investigations

Radiologic Evaluation

Ultrasonography:
- Satisfactory for detect ion of urolithiasis because of high diagnostic yield, easy availability, avoidance of ionizing radiation and detection of hydronephrosis, hydroureter.
- Can detect radiolucent stone.
- Nephrocalcinosis on USG is seen as increased echogenicity in medullary pyramids. In early neonatal period deposits of Tamm–Horsfall protein (TMP) are mistaken for medullary nephrocalcinosis. TMP deposition, however, disappears within 1–2 weeks, so in such case, evaluation should be repeated after few weeks.
- *Limitation*: Unable to detect small stone < 3 mm, ureteral stones.

Plain X-ray kidney, ureter, and bladder (KUB):
- It reveals radiopaque stones, but misses small stones and provides no information about possible obstruction
- Radiolucent stone (uric acid, xanthine) is missed on plain X-ray.

Noncontrast helical computed tomography (CT): Most sensitive to detect any stone including ureteric stone, radiolucent stone and small stone (1–2 mm).

Other contrast studies: Intravenous pyelography (IVP), CT urography, retrograde ureteroscopy or pyelography are indicated if suspecting (1) obstruction, (2) anatomical abnormality of urinary tract, (3) radiolucent stone.

Metabolic Evaluation

- Metabolic abnormalities occur in 42–84% of children with urolithiasis. Therefore, every child with urinary stone disease should have a complete metabolic evaluation.
- Metabolic evaluation is performed when the patient is consuming a regular diet and free of infection to avoid erroneous results. Urine biochemistry should be done at least 2–3 weeks after stone removal or expulsion.
- 24-hour urine solute estimation is preferred. In very young children, collect first or second void for spot urine solute-to-creatinine ratio **(Table 2)**.

Evaluation of a Patient with Nephrolithiasis/Nephrocalcinosis

Step 1:
- *Blood*: Creatinine, calcium, phosphorus, uric acid, electrolyte, blood gas

TABLE 2: Normal values of urinary solutes.

Constituent	24-hour excretion	Solute/creatinine ratio (mg/mg)
Calcium	<4 mg/kg/d	• 0–6 months: <0.8 • 6–12 months: <0.6 • 1–3 years: <0.53 • 3–5 years: <0.39 • >5 years: <0.2
Oxalate	• <45 mg/1.73 m^2 • <2 mg/kg/d	• 0–6 months: <0.26 • 7–24 months: <0.11 • 2–5 years: <0.08 • 5–14 years: <0.06 • >16 years: <0.03
Uric acid	• <35 mg/kg/d • 815 mg/1.73 m^2	• <1 year: <2.2 • 1–3 years: <1.9 • 3–5 years: <1.5 • 5–10 years: <0.9 • >10 years: <0.6
Citrate	>320 mg/1.73 m^2	• 0–5 years: >0.42 • >5 years: >0.25
Cystine	• <10 years <13 mg/1.73 m^2 • >10 years 30–50 mg/1.73 m^2	<0.07
Creatinine	• Newborn: 8–10 mg/kg/d • Children: 15–20 mg/kg/d	–
Magnesium	>0.8 mg/kg/d	>0.13

- *Urine analysis*:
  - pH (in fresh urine) by pH meter
  - Microscopy for crystals, casts
  - 24-hour urine calcium, oxalate, uric acid, citrate, creatine or spot morning specimen
- Stone analysis

Step 2:

Hypercalcemia	Hypercalciuria with normal serum calcium	Normal urine calcium
• Blood parathyroid hormone • 25-hydroxy vitamin D • Evaluate for sarcoidosis	• *Blood*: Blood gas, electrolyte, magnesium, thyroid-stimulating hormone, T3, T4 • *Urine*: Glucosuria, aminoacidogram, beta 2 microglobulin, phosphaturia • *Furosemide*: Fludrocortisone test in incomplete distal renal tubular acidosis	• Nitroprusside test for cystinuria • Urine oxalate excretion • Urine cystine excretion • Aminoacidogram

Key Points: Evaluation of Renal Stone

- A high proportion (>70%) of children with kidney stones have an underlying etiology.
- Unexplained pyuria and recurrent UTI should raise the suspicion for urolithiasis
- Nephrocalcinosis is usually asymptomatic.
- Calyceal deposits of TMP are harmless, but mimic nephrocalcinosis in preterm neonates.
- Metabolic evaluation is performed when patient is consuming a regular diet and free of infection to avoid erroneous results.

MANAGEMENT

- Increase fluid intake (2–2.5 L/1.73 m^2).
- Decrease salt intake as high sodium increases calcium excretion.
- Decrease animal protein intake as this is associated with increased production of acids.
- Ensure adequate potassium intake, e.g., fruits, vegetables. Low potassium intake enhances urine calcium excretion.
- Maintain normal dietary calcium. Low calcium intake increases oxalate absorption and secondary hyperoxaluria.

- *Potassium citrate*:
  - 2 mEq/kg/day
  - Citrate binds to urinary calcium forming a soluble complex and reducing precipitation of calcium with other anions.

Specific Treatment for Metabolic Abnormality

Hypercalciuria
- All above measures
- If hypercalciuria persists, use thiazide diuretics
- *Hydrochlorothiazide*: 1–1.5 mg/kg/day
- It increases calcium reabsorption in distal renal tubule, thereby reduces its excretion.

Hyperoxaluria
- Avoid oxalate-rich food (spinach, beans, potato, grapes, kiwi, nuts, cocoa, etc.)
- Normal dietary calcium intake and all above written measures
- Pyridoxine supplementation 1–2 mg/kg/day, maximum 5 mg/kg/day for patients identified as pyridoxine responsive (p.Gly170 Arg mutation).

Hyperuricosuria
- Alkalinization of urine with potassium citrate
- Allopurinol and rasburicase if high serum uric acid.

Cystinuria
- Urine alkalinization (pH 7.5–8)
- *Drugs*: Penicillamine, tiopronin.

Xanthinuria
High fluid intake, low-purine diet.

Medical Expulsive Therapy
- Majority of the stones <5 mm in diameter will pass spontaneously.
- Stones >9–10 mm have little chance of spontaneous passage.
- Ureteral stone is present in 20% of all the cases with urinary stone disease and 70% of them are localized to distal ureter. Medical expulsive therapy (MET) is targeted to distal ureteric stones having size of 4–8 mm.
- *Drugs used for MET are*:
  - Calcium channel blocker (*Nifedipine* 0.3–0.5 mg/kg/d)
  - Alpha blocker (*Tamsulosin* dose > 4 years 0.4 mg, <4 years 0.2 mg).

Mechanism of action of these two drug groups involves prevention of uncoordinated contraction induced by the stone without eliminating peristaltic activity of ureter.

Surgical Treatment
Stones >9–10 mm requires surgical intervention. Various surgical procedures including *extracorporeal shock wave lithotripsy, percutaneous nephrolithotomy, ureteroscopy, open surgery, etc.,* are done depending on size and location of stones.

Key Points: Management of Urolithiasis
- Restriction of salt and animal protein intake are effective in reducing hypercalciuria.
- Dietary calcium restriction is not recommended as may cause reduced bone mineralization and increases oxalate absorption and secondary hyperoxaluria.
- Therapy with potassium citrate results in decreased stone formation by reducing precipitation of calcium with other anions.
- MET is effective in lower ureteric stones.

SUGGESTED READING
1. Atan A, Balci M. Medical expulsive treatment in pediatric urolithiasis. Turk J Urol. 2015;41(1):39-42.
2. Habbig S, Beck BB. Nephrocalcinosis and urolithiasis in children. Kidney Int. 2011;80:1278-91.
3. Hoppe B, Kemper MJ. Diagnostic examination of the child with urolithiasis or nephrocalcinosis. Pediatr Nephrol. 2010;25:403-13.
4. Jackson E, Reeber M. Urolithiasis in children—treatment and prevention. Curr Treat Options Peds. 2016;2:10-22.
5. Marra G, Taroni F Berrettini A, Montanari E, Manzoni G, Montini G. Pediatric nephrolithiasis: a systemic approach from diagnosis to treatment. J Nephrol. 2019;32(2):199-210.
6. Velazqez N, Daniel Zapata. Medical expulsive therapy for pediatric urolithiasis: systemic review and meta-analysis. J Pediatr Urol. 2015;11(6): 321-7.

CHAPTER 140: Hypertension in Pediatrics

Amish Udani

INTRODUCTION

Blood pressure (BP) is regulated by neurohumoral and autonomic nervous systems which interact locally and systemically to maintain this cardiovascular function. The net effect of vasoconstrictors and vasodilators, which keeps changing from fetal to adult life, helps to maintain BP. The factors important in children are renin–angiotensin–aldosterone system, kallikrein–kinin system, endothelin-derived vasoactive factors, glucocorticoids, birth weight, maternal nutrition, vasopressin, urotensin II, and renalase.

Definition and classification of hypertension are given in **Table 1**.

- Infection-related glomerulonephritis (IRG) and raised intracranial pressure (ICP) are usually transient causes of secondary hypertension.
- Abnormal function of various sodium channels in renal tubules leads to monogenic cause of persistent secondary hypertension apart from chronic kidney disease (CKD), renal parenchymal and renovascular abnormality.
- Coarctation of aorta (COA) and endocrine diseases also contribute to secondary causes of persistent hypertension.
- Withdrawal of drugs causing hypertension if possible is only needed in medication or substance abuse-induced hypertension.

Technique for monitoring BP is given in **Table 2**. Cuff bladder should be at least 40% of arm circumference measured midway between olecranon and accordion while length should cover 80–100% of the arm in all four limbs in comfortable sitting position after 5 minutes with instrument at heart level preferably except in an infant or symptomatic

TABLE 1: Definition, classification*, nonpharmacologic and indications to start drug therapy.

	Systolic or diastolic BP percentile†	Therapeutic lifestyle changes	Pharmacologic therapy
Normal	<90th	Healthy diet, regular sleep, exercise	–
Prehypertension	90th to <95th or >120/80 in adolescents	Weight reduction or prevent further gain if obese, dietary sodium restrict ion 2–3 g/day, decrease consumption of sugar-containing beverages and energy-dense snacks, portion size control, increase intake of fresh fruits, vegetables, low fat dairy, physical activity for 30–60 minutes every day. Restriction of sedentary activity (television watching, video or computer games <2 hours per day), stress reduction	If CKD, diabetes, heart failure, left ventricular hypertrophy (LVH)
Stage 1 hypertension	95th to 99th + 5 mm Hg		If symptomatic or secondary hypertension or end-organ damage or coexisting diabetes or failure of therapeutic lifestyle changes
Stage 2	>99th + 5 mm Hg		Initiate drug therapy

*Hypertensive urgency if impending end-organ damage, hypertensive emergency if apparent end-organ damage;
†Age, sex, height measured on at least three separate occasions if asymptomatic.

TABLE 2: Technique for blood pressure measurement.	
Technique	Comments
Mercury sphygmomanometry	• *Advantages*: Evidence-based; quick to perform; low cost; noninvasive • *Disadvantages*: Observer bias; mercury spillage environmental hazard
Aneroid manometry	• *Advantages*: Portable; mercury free; noninvasive • *Disadvantages*: Needs frequent calibration
Oscillometric devices	• *Advantages*: Easy to use in infants; no observer bias; noninvasive; • *Disadvantages*: Values of diastolic blood pressure often derived from mean arterial pressure (except Dinamap); requires repeated validation; higher cost; 5–10 mm higher reading than by auscultation; patient not in standardized position; patient cooperation needed
Ambulatory blood pressure monitoring	• *Advantages*: Diagnosis of white coat, masked hypertension; data on diurnal variability; reliable normative data available • *Disadvantages*: Expensive; regular maintenance of equipment; requires patient cooperation; anxiety in children

child (supine position) if hypertension is detected. Percentiles of BP for age, gender, height, in infants has to be correlated with standard.

RISK FACTORS

- Dysregulation of total cardiac output or total systemic vascular resistance, hyperuricemia, insulin resistance or genetic factors can cause systemic essential hypertension (EH).
- Maternal malnutrition, placental diseases, gestational age determining nephron number and glucocorticoid exposure, birth weight, associated maternal diabetes, stress, admission in neonatal intensive care unit (NICU), nephrotoxic drugs in perinatal period plays an important role in determining risk of developing hypertension.
- High sensitivity to sodium or high-sodium and low-potassium diet, obesity, gender, race, physical activity, dyslipidemia, sleep disorders in young children are also considered to be a risk factor for developing hypertension in later life.
- Children who are at risk of having hypertension and mandates BP check during clinic visit have a history of prematurity, very low birth weight, admission in NICU or pediatric intensive care unit (PICU), congenital heart disease (CHD), recurrent urinary tract infection, hematuria or proteinuria, known renal disease or urologic malformations, family history of renal disease, malignancy or organ transplant, systemic illness-like systemic lupus erythematosus (SLE), neurofibromatosis, tuberous sclerosis, and treatment with drugs known to raise BP.

INVESTIGATIONS

Step 1: Differences in BP in upper and lower extremities or feeble pulse or murmur—echocardiography, computed tomography (CT) or magnetic resonance (MR) angiography → CHD, COA, large-vessel vasculitis.

Step 2: Failure to thrive, bony deformities—high serum urea, creatinine → CKD.

Step 3: Edema or oliguria or hematuria or proteinuria or rash, etc.,—urine routine, microscopy, spot urine protein-creatinine ratio, serum creatinine, electrolytes, albumin, C3, C4 levels, antinuclear antibody (ANA), anti-ds-DNA, complete blood count (CBC), erythrocyte sedimentation rate (ESR), cytoplasmic antineutrophil cytoplasmic antibody (c-ANCA), perinuclear ANCA (p-ANCA), renal biopsy → IRG or nephrotic syndrome or acute kidney injury (AKI) or SLE or hemolytic uremic syndrome or Henoch–Schönlein purpura or chronic glomerulonephritis or small-vessel vasculitis.

Step 4: Abnormal ultrasonography (USG) or Doppler-DMSA (dimercaptosuccinic acid) renal scan, micturating cystourethrogram (MCU), CT angiography → congenital renal anomaly or renovascular hypertension or reflux nephropathy or obstructive uropathy or intra-abdominal malignancy.

Step 5: Electrolyte abnormality ± acid–base disorder, normal serum creatinine—serum renin, aldosterone, deoxycortisol levels → congenital adrenal hyperplasia (CAH) or liddle syndrome or apparent mineralocorticoid excess (AME) or Gordon syndrome or glucocorticoid-responsive aldosteronism (GRA) or familial glucocorticoid resistance (FGR).

Step 6: Endocrine disease—thyroid function test, plasma metanephrines, MIBG (meta-iodobenzylguanidine) scan, serum cortisol, adrenocorticotropic hormone (ACTH) levels, random blood sugar (RBS), urine routine → hyperthyroidism or pheochromocytoma or Cushing's syndrome or diabetes mellitus.

Step 7: Overweight, no drug history, no secondary cause—serum uric acid, lipid profile → EH.

MANAGEMENT

- Nonpharmacologic measures.
- Indications of starting antihypertensive drugs are mentioned in **Table 1**.
- Identification and treatment of underlying cause with appropriate antihypertensive treatment is important to control BP **(Table 3)**.
- Hypertensive urgency and emergency in the form of headache, seizures, encephalopathy, and loss of vision, hemiparesis, vomiting, congestive heart failure, pulmonary edema, breathlessness or AKI should be identified and treated in PICU. In first 2–3 hours, BP should be lowered by 20–30% and maintained around 95th percentile over next 24–48 hours. Oral drugs should be started for better control of hypertension to 50th percentile over days to weeks and IV drugs should be tapered and stopped. Commonly used oral and IV antihypertensive drug doses are given in **Table 4**.
- Intervention or surgery may be needed in vascular or renovascular cause of hypertension to control BP. In unilateral RAS, preservation of renal function can be achieved if differential function of affected kidney is >20%. Rarely in unilateral renal parenchymal disease, nephrectomy is advised to achieve better control of BP if differential function is <20%.

FOLLOW-UP

End-organ damage to heart, eyes, and kidneys should be done periodically.

- Left ventricular hypertrophy (LVH) in form of left ventricular mass index and vascular evaluation of carotid intima media thickness on echocardiography should be done once a year if normal or once in 6 months if mild-to-moderate or once in 3 months in presence of moderate-to-severe LVH.
- Ophthalmological assessment for hypertensive retinopathy should be done once in 1–2 years if normal or once in 6–12 months in stage I–II and once in 3 months in stage III–IV.
- Microalbuminuria is an early marker of renal damage and important risk predictor of CKD, especially if coexisting diabetes; hence it should be monitored once in 6–12 months.
- Ambulatory blood pressure monitoring (ABPM) should be done once a year in children with secondary hypertension to optimize therapy and target BP control between 50th and 75th percentiles.

PROGNOSIS

Acute neurological events, cardiovascular complications, loss of vision and AKI are associated with morbidity and mortality. Hypertensive crisis can be avoided with good adherence to life style changes, compliance with drugs, and regular follow-up.

KEY MESSAGES

- At-risk children should be identified and BP should be checked with appropriate cuff and use of BP percentile charts.

TABLE 3: Drug of choice based on underlying etiology.

Diagnosis	First-line drugs	Second-line drugs
IRG, AKI, CKD with edema or oliguria, CHD	Salt-restricted diet, fluid restriction in severe edema 400 mL/m²/day, frusemide	CCB or β-blocker
CKD without edema, renal anomalies, bilateral RAS, COA, hyperthyroidism	CCB or β-blocker	α-blocker or clonidine
Proteinuric renal diseases without AKI, unilateral RAS, coexisting diabetes, CHD	ACEI or ARB	CCB or β-blocker
Liddle syndrome	Amiloride	Triamterene
Gordon syndrome	Hydrochlorothiazide	
AME, CAH, FGR, Conn syndrome	Spironolactone or eplerenone	–
GRA	Glucocorticoids	Amiloride
Pheochromocytoma	Labetalol or α-blocker followed by β-blocker	CCB
EH	Nonpharmacologic measures, treat hyperuricemia and dyslipidemia if present	CCB or ACEI or ARB

[ACEI: angiotensin-converting enzyme inhibitor; AKI: acute kidney injury; ARB: angiotensin receptor blocker; AME: apparent mineralocorticoid excess; CCB: calcium channel blocker; RAS: renal artery stenosis; CAH: congenital adrenal hyperplasia (11β-Hydroxylase deficiency or 17α-Hydroxylase deficiency); EH: essential hypertension; FGR: familial glucocorticoid resistance; GRA: glucocorticoid remediable aldosteronism or familial hyperaldosteronism type 1; IRG: infection-related glomerulonephritis; CKD: chronic kidney disease]

TABLE 4: List of oral and intravenous (IV antihypertensive drugs).

Agents	Dose; frequency	Comments
Calcium channel blockers	–	• Extended-release nifedipine must be swallowed whole • *Side effects*: Headache, flushing, dizziness, tachycardia; lower extremity edema, erythema, hypotension
Amlodepine	0.05–0.5 mg/kg/day; qd-bid	–
Nifedipine tablet (extended release)	0.25–3 mg/kg/day; bid	–
Capsule nifedipine	0.2–0.5 mg/kg sublingual or oral	–
Beta-blockers	–	Reduce dose by 50% at GFR < 50 mL/min/1.73 m^2; alternate day at GFR < 10 mL/min/1.73 m^2; sleep disturbances with metoprolol; hyperlipidemia; avoid in asthma, heart failure; blunt symptoms of hypoglycemia
Atenolol	0.5–2 mg/kg/day; qd or bid	–
Metoprolol	1–6 mg/kg/day; bid	–
Labetalol (α and β blocker)	1–3 mg/kg/day; bid or tid or IV 0.5–3 mg/kg/h infusion or bolus 0.25–4 mg/kg q 30 min	–
Diuretics	–	• Monitor electrolytes, fluid status • *Thiazides*: Dyslipidemia, hyperglycemia, hyperuricemia, hypokalemia, hypomagnesemia • *Frusemide*: Metabolic alkalosis, hypokalemia, hypercalciuria, ototoxicity, interstitial nephritis
Frusemide	0.5–6 mg/kg/day; qd or bid or IV 0.1–0.5 mg/kg/min infusion or bolus 0.5–2 mg/kg q 6–24 hours	–
Spironolactone*	1–3 mg/kg/day; qd or bid	–
Metolazone	0.2–0.4 mg/kg/day; qd	–
Hydrochlorothiazide	1–3 mg/kg/day; qd	–
Amiloride*	0.4–0.6 mg/kg/day; qd	–
Central alpha agonists	–	–
Clonidine	5–25 µg/kg/day; tid	Rebound hypertension if abruptly stopped; sedation
Methyl dopa	20–40 mg/kg/day, tid	Postural hypotension and hemolytic anemia
Vasodilators	–	–
Hydralazine	1–8 mg/kg/day; qid IV 0.1–0.5 mg/kg/dose	Headache, palpitation; fluid retention/pericardial effusions, hypertrichosis with minoxidil; usually used in refractory hypertension
Minoxidil	0.1–0.5 mg/kg/day; bid	–
Sodium nitroprusside	0.3–8 µg/kg/min IV infusion	May increase ICP, risk of cyanide and toxicity
Fenoldopam	0.1–2 µg/kg/min IV	Selective dopamine agonist, limited experience
Nitroglycerin α-blocker	1–3 µg/kg/min IV	Methemoglobinemia, headache, tachycardia
Prazosin	0.1–0.5 mg/kg/day; qd or bid	First dose hypotension, syncope
Phentolamine	0.1–0.2 mg/kg IV maximum 5 mg/dose q 2–4 hours	Tachycardia, abdominal pain
Angiotensin converting enzyme inhibitors (ACEI)	–	• Small dose in neonates, use with caution in GFR < 30 mL/min/1.73 m^2, • RAS. Monitor serum creatinine and potassium at regular intervals • Neutropenia, dry cough with ACEI
Enalapril	0.1–0.6 mg/kg/day qd or bid	–
Enalaprilat	5–10 µg/kg/dose IV tid	–
Angiotensin receptor blocker (ARB)	–	–
Losartan	0.7–1.4 mg/kg/day qd	–

(GFR: glomerular filtration rate; ICP: intracranial pressure)
*Use cautiously with ACEI and ARB

- Identify the cause and appropriate treatment should be initiated.
- Timely referral should be done to prevent hypertension-related complication.

SUGGESTED READING

1. Flynn JT, Ingelfinger JR, Redwine KM (eds). Pediatric Hypertension, 4th edition. Switzerland: Springer International Publishing AG; 2018.

CHAPTER 141: Voiding Disorders in Children

Mahipal Khandelwal

INTRODUCTION

Urinary incontinence is a normal transitional phase between infantile and adult lower urinary tract function. Consequently, wetting disorders often are considered a necessary nuisance associated with the growing years. It usually is tolerated until the child begins to lag behind his or her peers in achieving a state of dryness. Parental concerns about voiding are common and often supersede the child's anxiety.

DEFINITION

The current definition of dysfunctional voiding given by the International Children's Continence Society (ICCS):

"The child with dysfunctional voiding habitually contracts the urethral sphincter or pelvic floor during voiding and demonstrates a staccato pattern with or without an interrupted flow on repeat uroflow when electromyograhic (EMG) activity is concomitantly recorded. This is a term associated with neurologically intact patient."

The ICCS has standardized the terminology used in children with lower urinary tract symptoms.

The symptoms in the storage phase of the bladder are:
- *Daytime frequency*: Applicable in children >5 years of age. Frequency >8 times during the day is considered increased and <3 times per day decreased.
- *Incontinence*: Uncontrollable leakage of urine; intermittent or continuous.
- *Enuresis*: Intermittent incontinence during sleep.
- *Urgency*: The sudden unexpected urge to void—applicable after 5 years of age.
- *Nocturia*: Child has to wake up at night to void.

The symptoms in the voiding phase are:
- *Hesitancy*: Difficulty in initiating the stream of urine. Used in children older than 5 years of age.
- *Straining*: The child needs to use abdominal wall muscles to void. Relevant at all ages.
- *Weak stream*: Urine stream which has no force. Applicable after infancy.
- *Intermittency*: Interruption in the stream of urine.

Other symptoms:
- *Holding maneuvers*: Standing on tiptoes, crossing legs, and squatting with the heel pressing on the perineum to hold urine (Vincent's curtsy sign)
- Feeling of incomplete emptying
- *Postmicturition dribble*: Involuntary leakage of urine after voiding
- Pain while passing urine.

HOW DOES THE BLADDER "NORMALLY" WORK?

The normal bladder stores urine at very low pressure. When the bladder becomes full, it sends a signal of "fullness" to the brain (start looking for a restroom). After 5 minutes to an hour, the bladder sends another signal of "urgency" (you would better have a restroom nearby). Most people can put off voiding as long as they want without leaking urine. These signals are not pressure spikes or spasms within the bladder. The signals are sent from the bladder to the brain without a change in bladder pressure.

When a child decides to void, he/she purposely relaxes the urethral "sphincter" (valve) and the bladder contracts on its own. We cannot directly control our bladder. We can control our bladder indirectly by opening or closing the sphincter. When we open our sphincter, the bladder contracts by reflex.

Likewise, when we close our sphincter, the bladder stops contracting (this takes a few seconds, so there is a short rise in bladder pressure).

The coordination between the sphincter and bladder is very important for normal voiding. Discoordination will lead to increases in bladder pressure.

There are four components of normal bladder emptying—a cycle of events **(Fig. 1)**. When the bladder is full, it sends a signal to the brain. The child has a sensation or perception of fullness, then he/she takes action by going to the restroom and relaxing the sphincter. The relaxation of the sphincter leads to a spontaneous contraction of the bladder. The four components of this cycle are— (1) signal, (2) perception, (3) action, and (4) bladder.

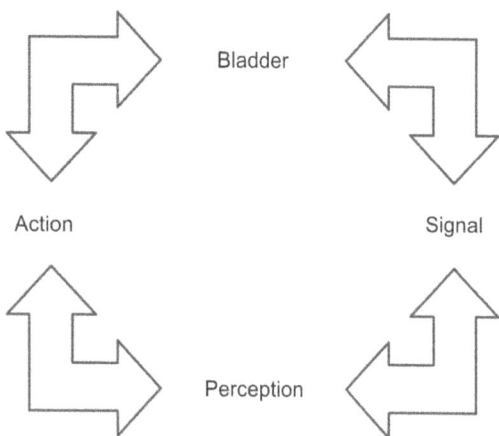

Fig. 1: Components of normal bladder emptying.

WHAT HAPPENS DURING VOIDING DYSFUNCTION?

There are many causes of voiding dysfunction. An abnormality in one component of the voiding cycle can cause abnormalities in other components and perpetuate itself. Thus, voiding dysfunction is a cyclical problem that may worsen without treatment.

Signal Problems

Abnormal bladders can send late signals, no signals, or false signals.
- *Late signals*: Children will complain that the time period between the sensation of fullness and urgency was too short to allow for a restroom break. It is impossible to say whether this is a signal problem or a perception problem.
- *No signals*: This unusual problem is associated with the *lazy bladder syndrome* (large bladder).
- *False signals*: If child has an unstable bladder, then it may be sending false signals. These may be associated with pressure spikes or spasms.

One element of diagnosing and treating voiding dysfunction is teaching your child to recognize these signals and/or suppressing false signals (pressure spikes) with medications.

Perception Problems

This aspect is very difficult to study or explain. Perception abnormalities can be behavioral (under the child's control) or developmental (a skill not yet acquired). Have you ever yelled at your child and received no response? It is amazing! We can all hear what we want to hear. Similarly, a child can subconsciously affect his/her perception of bladder signals.

Children must learn to recognize the signals from the bladder. Even if child has been properly potty trained, he/she can regress and learn abnormal voiding.

One of the tenets of treating voiding dysfunction is to teach the child how to sense the bladder.

Action Problems

- *No action* or *delayed action*: The mind of a child is fascinating. Some children will purposely delay voiding because they are "too busy" playing or watching television. Or they do not want to leave the classroom. A common sign of fighting bladder spasms is the child crossing the legs or kneeling down upon the foot. These postures are performed in an attempt to suppress the bladder spasm or signal.
- *Frequent action*: Some children act upon every bladder signal and void small amounts.
- *Discoordination between the bladder and sphincter*: Some children, consciously or subconsciously, close their urethral sphincter while the bladder is contracting. This is a learned behavior that arises in response to pain, leakage, or a bladder spasm. When the bladder is not coordinated with the sphincter, the bladder will squeeze urine out when the sphincter is closed. This increased workload makes the bladder become muscular and thickened. This leads to an unstable bladder and infections, which can lead to more infections and more pain, and again more discoordination. This again is an example of a vicious cycle.

Bladder Problems

The final component of voiding dysfunction is the bladder. A "bad" bladder becomes thickened (muscular) and has involuntary contractions (spasms) that can lead to leakage or pain. All the above problems—signal, perception, and action—can be caused by a bad bladder. More importantly, these problems also cause the bad bladder, thus, the vicious cycle. Occasionally, we treat the bladder with relaxant medications, such as *ditropan*, to suppress spasms.

Urinary Tract Infections

Many children with voiding dysfunction have a history of urinary tract infections (UTIs). Quite often, UTIs are difficult to treat in children with dysfunctional voiding.

How does the normal bladder prevent infection?
- *Frequent emptying*: If there is no urine in the bladder, the bacteria have nowhere to grow.
- *Complete emptying*: Residual urine provides a home for bacteria.
- *Barrier to bacteria*: The lining of the bladder usually prevents penetration by bacteria.
- Antibodies.
- *Prevent entry of bacteria*: Girls and uncircumcised boys are at risk for UTI due to more bacteria around the urethral opening; proper hygiene is very important.

How does voiding dysfunction lead to infection?
Many children with voiding dysfunction do not empty their bladders completely, which leads to residual urine.

Incomplete emptying can be due to "rushing" out of the restroom or due to discoordination.

Does a UTI change the workup or treatment of voiding dysfunction?

Absolutely. Any child who has had a UTI needs radiologic imaging of the bladder and kidneys to rule out anatomical causes of infection.

Bowel Dysfunction: Constipation

Most children with voiding dysfunction have problems with constipation and/or stool incontinence. The function and control of the bowel is very similar to the bladder. The sphincter of the bowel and urethra are connected and share the same nerves. Quite often, we use the term "dysfunctional elimination syndrome" instead of "dysfunctional voiding", because it more accurately describes the combined problems of the bowel and bladder.

Note: If child is constipated, this must be relieved before treating voiding dysfunction.

Various Presentations of "Voiding Dysfunction"

- *Overactive bladder/urge incontinence*: Usually present with urgency or incontinence associated with urgency.
- *Voiding postponement*: Habitually postpone micturition and use holding maneuvers frequently. They may have incontinence due to full bladder.
- *Under active bladder/lazy bladder*: Have a low voiding frequency and use abdominal muscles and strain to achieve bladder emptying.
- *Dysfunctional voiding*: Habitually contracts the urethral sphincter during voiding—leads to a staccato pattern on uroflow study.
- *Stress incontinence*: Leakage of small amount of urine due to rise in intra-abdominal pressure.
- *Vaginal reflux*: Leakage of small amounts of urine about 20 minutes after voiding.
- *Giggle incontinence*: Leakage of small amounts of urine during laughing.

Associated symptoms:
- Constipation and encopresis
- Recurrent UTIs
- Sleep disorders.

WORKUP OF VOIDING DYSFUNCTION

Elimination Diary

The following details must be recorded. It is relevant in children aged >5 years.
- *Voiding*: Timing and volumes for at least 48 hours, including nighttime voids
- Nocturia episodes, daytime incontinence, enuresis episodes, enuresis volumes, bedtime and wake-up time, other symptoms, bowel movements, and encopresis for at least 14 days
- Fluid intake for 48 hours
- Record of bowel habits
- Questions regarding UTI, hygiene, and school restrooms.

Medical History

- Obtain information about UTI occurrence.
- Inquire about comorbidities and other medical issues.
- Elicit storage and emptying function and associated symptoms suggestive of bladder and bowel dysfunction (BBD).
- Inquire about observed neurologic symptoms.
- Glean information on gastrointestinal symptoms.
- Identify presence of other associated symptoms, behavioral, or psychological issues.
- Family history.

Physical Examination

- Genital examination
- Perineal examination
- Digital rectal examination, if indicated
- *Neurologic examination (especially spine examination)*: Gait, back (meningomyelocele or other spinal abnormality, dimple, lipoma tuft of hair, sacrum), deep tendon reflexes, strength of the lower limbs, focused neurourological examination including the bulbocavernosus reflex, anal tone and perineal sensation, facial expression.

BBD or LUTD Questionnaires

- Several validated questionnaires available for assessment and follow-up of BBD: Bristol stool form and Rome IV criteria of constipation
- 7-day bowel diary with description of stool forms.

Ultrasound (Transabdominal)

- Imaging kidneys and urinary bladder
- Transverse rectal diameter.

Bladder Calculations

- *Expected bladder capacity (EBC)*: This is calculated using the following formula up to 12 years of age.
- EBC = 30 + (age in years × 30) mL.
- The maximum voided volume is considered increased or decreased if it is >150% or <65% of the EBC, respectively.
- *Residual urine*: >20 mL on repeated evaluation is considered significant.

Abdominal Scout Film Radiograph

- For fecal loading
  Spinal bony abnormality

Urinalysis and/or urine culture uroflowmetry and postvoid residual (PVR)
- Uroflowmetry and PVR in toilet-trained children.

Invasive Study

- Voiding cystourethrography for febrile UTI-VUR (vesicoureteral reflux) and dysfunctional voiding
- Urodynamics or videourodynamics for detailed bladder/sphincter function.

CONSERVATIVE TREATMENT (TABLE 1)

- *Time voids*: A voiding schedule of every 2 hours during the day and marked on the voiding diary. Child should be sent to the bathroom at the appointed times without regard to perception of need to void.
- *Double voiding*: Have child void at a specific time, then again a few seconds later.
- *Bladder retraining*: Taking all the pressure off the bladder requires frequent and complete voiding.
- *PVRs*: Used to assess amount of urine in bladder after voiding.

TABLE 1: Conservative treatment.

Methods	Details	Indications
Urotherapy	• Education and demystification • Behavioral modification instruction • *Motivational therapy*: Positive reinforcement (age appropriate) charts, stickers/stars on a calendar, rewards when symptoms improve • Lifestyle advice • Registration of symptoms and voiding habits • Improvement in elimination habits • Support and encouragement to patients and caregivers	All children
Early toilet training	Parental-oriented toilet training method	May be beneficial in infants with elevated postvoid residual
Bowel management	Education, fecal disimpaction, stool softeners, and fiber	All children with constipation
Biofeedback relaxation of pelvic floor	Using biological signals to enhance pelvic floor relaxation and facilitate micturition and defecation emptying	Children with discoordinated sphincter and/or pelvic floor muscles during voiding
Electroneurostimulation	Involving regulation of the cerebral cortex, spinal pathway and the target organ of pelvic floor muscles	Children refractory to conservation or pharmacological treatments
Clean intermittent catheterizations	Drain the bladder intermittently with clear urethral catheter	Children who fall conservative management and pharmacologic treatment

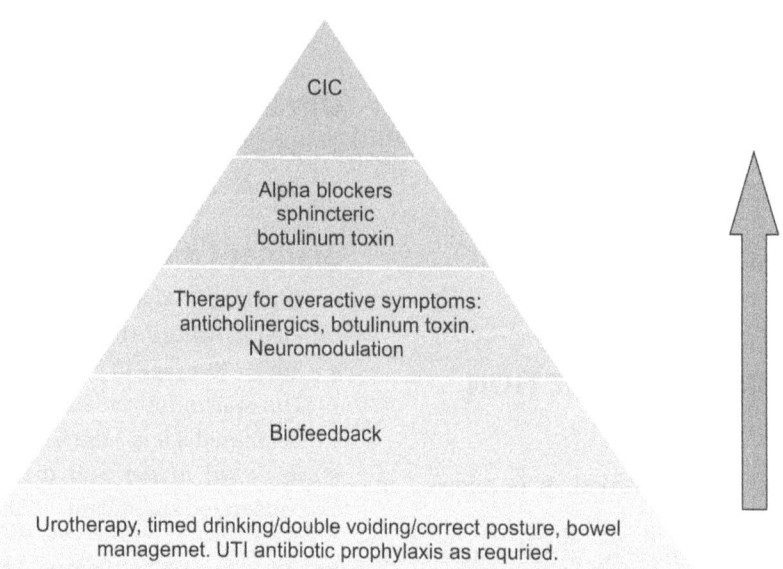

Fig. 2: Suggested treatment escalation for dysfunctional voiding in childhood.
(CIC: clean intermittent catheterization; UTI: urinary tract infection)

PHARMACOLOGICAL TREATMENT

- Treating UTI with appropriate antibiotic and prophylaxis if required.
- Drugs are selected depending on the pattern of urodynamic study (UDS).
- *Detrusor antispasmodics*: Oxybutynin may be used to relax the detrusor during filling. Slow-release oxybutynin may be more effective in some than the conventional preparation. Tolterodine is another option.
- *Alpha-adrenergic blockers*: To relax the external sphincter during voiding.
- *Nonconventional therapies*: Botulinum toxin injections are given into the bladder.

Suggested treatment escalation for dysfunctional voiding in childhood is shown in **Figure 2**.

SUMMARY

Clinician can no longer ignore the effect of altered bladder function on the upper urinary tract, especially in children who have urinary infection and reflux. Wetting should not be viewed as nuisance symptom but rather as a sign of potentially disordered bladder and sphincter functions which may have important current and future implications. Patient will be benefit from being categorized according to severity of symptoms of bladder dysfunction: Inappropriate diagnostic tests will be avoided and patient management will be enhanced.

SECTION 12: Endocrinology

142. Childhood Hypothyroidism
143. Childhood Obesity
144. Type 1 Diabetes
145. Precocious Puberty
146. Disorders of Sex Development

Chapter 142: Childhood Hypothyroidism

Saurabh Uppal, Neeraj Sehgal

INTRODUCTION

Hypothyroidism is one of the most common endocrinopathies in childhood. Primary hypothyroidism is the most prevalent form of hypothyroidism that occurs due to deficient functioning of the thyroid gland. It can be either congenital or acquired. Secondary or central hypothyroidism results from deficient functioning of the pituitary gland and results from a lower central drive to the thyroid gland. Central hypothyroidism may commonly be associated with other pituitary hormone deficiencies. Tertiary hypothyroidism is a term used to describe the disorder arising due to defective hypothalamic stimulation of the pituitary thyroid-stimulating hormone (TSH) levels.

Hypothyroidism presenting in childhood is mostly primary in nature and autoimmune thyroiditis is the most common etiology in this cohort. Rarely congenital hypothyroidism resulting from ectopic/hypoplastic thyroid gland or dyshormonogenesis may present in childhood. The common causes of hypothyroidism are given in **Box 1**.

CLINICAL FEATURES

Childhood hypothyroidism usually has an insidious onset and gradual progression resulting in a significant delay in diagnosis. The clinical presentation is diverse. As the symptoms are often mild and nonspecific, the predictive value of clinical diagnosis is often low, except in the classic presentations. Besides, the nondistressing nature of symptoms in many children leads to the diagnosis being unfortunately delayed. The common clinical symptoms and signs of childhood hypothyroidism are tabulated in **Table 1**. Contrary to commonly held beliefs, isolated hypothyroidism in childhood does not cause cognitive impairment in children nor is it associated with, or causative for obesity in a child who is otherwise growing normally. TSH levels may be slightly higher in obese children but these reflect a physiologic adaptation to obesity rather than its cause. In overweight children with primary hypothyroidism, the body mass index (BMI) values after treatment has been found to be no different from BMI values before treatment if lifestyle changes are not instituted hence ruling out hypothyroidism as a cause for obesity in childhood.

DIAGNOSTIC EVALUATION

The clinical history and physical examination provide vital clues to the diagnosis of hypothyroidism. In addition to the symptoms and signs described in **Table 1**, a family history of

BOX 1: Common causes of childhood hypothyroidism.

- Autoimmune thyroid disease (AITD) (Hashimoto thyroiditis/chronic lymphocytic thyroiditis)
- Hypothalamic–pituitary dysfunction (Central hypothyroidism: Congenital, neoplasia, postsurgical, postirradiation)
- Iodine exposure (Drugs, I^{131} therapy)
- Acute and subacute thyroiditis
- Exogenous goitrogens
- Thyroid irradiation
- Post thyroidectomy
- Syndromic associations (Down syndrome, Klinefelter syndrome, Turner syndrome)
- Secondary hemochromatosis (repeated blood transfusions)
- Cystinosis

TABLE 1: Clinical symptoms and signs of childhood hypothyroidism.

Growth retardation with weight gain	Bradycardia
Lethargy	Delayed deep tendon reflexes
Constipation	Muscle pseudohypertrophy (Kocher–Debre–Semelaigne syndrome)
Easy fatigability	Hypercholesterolemia
Goiter	Pallor (unexplained anemia)
Cold intolerance	Delayed skeletal maturation
Dry, sallow, and puffy (myxedematous) skin	Visual symptoms
Brittle or sparse hair	Facial puffiness
Delayed puberty	Hoarseness of voice
Early pseudopuberty (Van Wyk–Grumbach syndrome)	Diffuse aches and pains
Galactorrhea	Headache and vomiting (secondary pituitary hypertrophy

thyroid disease points toward autoimmune hypothyroidism. Similar complaints in the siblings without a typical familial transmission may point toward dyshormonogenesis causing a delayed presentation of congenital hypothyroidism.

LABORATORY INVESTIGATIONS

In contrast to many other endocrine disorders, the diagnosis of thyroid dysfunction can be reliably made by basal hormone concentrations and is independent of significant circadian variations. In almost all cases of thyroid dysfunction, measurement of TSH, thyroxine (T4), or free T4 and triiodothyronine (T3) are sufficient to reach a diagnosis. Raised TSH with low levels of T4 establish the diagnosis of primary hypothyroidism. T3 may be normal in the initial stages as the levels do not decline until T4 is very low. However, a low normal or low T4, a low T3 and a normal or raised TSH point toward the diagnosis of central hypothyroidism. Free T4 (FT4) levels are usually low in central hypothyroidism. It is important to note that a low T4 and a low T3 with normal TSH in healthy children with no symptoms of hypothyroidism may also be found in cases of thyroid-binding globulin (TBG) deficiency. In doubtful cases, it is often helpful to measure free T4 levels. Raised TSH with normal T4 is suggestive of subclinical hypothyroidism **(Table 2)**.

Raised titers of anti-thyroperoxidase (TPO) antibodies and anti-thyroglobulin antibodies are suggestive of autoimmune etiology. In children with borderline TSH values and low titers of antibodies, it is reasonable to reassess thyroid function every 6–12 months and initiate therapy only if TSH is above the normal range for childhood. However, if the antibody titers are high, treatment should not be delayed.

Ultrasonography

Ultrasonography (USG) examination is not required in all cases of primary hypothyroidism However in patients of AITD, USG may reveal an enlarged thyroid gland with diffuse echo pattern, reduced echogenicity, and increased vascularity.

Radiography of the Hand

Examination of an X-ray of the hand and wrist may reveal significant delay in skeletal maturation. It can serve to date the approximate onset of the disease. Follow-up X-rays may be useful as a guide to dose titration during monitoring therapy to guard against a disproportionate acceleration in skeletal age and hence the corresponding loss in final adult height.

Radionuclide Imaging

Radioactive iodine uptake and technetium-99m (99mTc) scintigraphy scan are not routinely needed for the diagnosis of childhood hypothyroidism, except in very selected cases of late-onset congenital hypothyroidism to document dyshormonogenesis or hypoplastic/ectopic thyroid.

Magnetic Resonance Imaging

Magnetic resonance imaging (MRI) brain is essential in cases of central hypothyroidism to investigate for any structural lesions. In long-standing untreated primary hypothyroidism, pituitary thyrotroph hypertrophy may be erroneously labeled as pituitary adenoma. This hypertrophy regresses after institution of L-thyroxine replacement.

TREATMENT

Replacement therapy with L-thyroxine (levothyroxine) is started immediately at diagnosis. The doses recommended in children are different from those recommended in adults **(Table 3)** and also vary by respective age groups because of varying body surface area-to-weight ratios and increased clearance rate of thyroid hormones from the body. L-thyroxine replacement is maintained by a once daily dosing schedule. Weekly replacement regimen in adolescents is no longer recommended as it leads to high levels of T4 just after the dose is taken and low levels by the week's end. The standard recommendation has been to take the medication on an "empty stomach". However, the timing of medication is a subject of active research as recent

TABLE 2: Changes with age in serum concentrations of TSH, T4, T3, and Free T4.

Age	TSH µU/mL	T4 µg/dL	T3 ng/dL	Free T4 ng/dL
Cord blood	1–20	6.6–15	14–86	1.2–2.2
1–7 days	1–39	11–22	36–316	2.2–5.3
1–4 weeks	0.5–6.5	8.2–17	105–345	0.9–2.3
1–12 months	0.5–6.5	5.9–16	104–245	0.8–2.1
1–5 years	0.6–8	7.3–15	105–269	0.8–2
6–10 years	0.6–8	6.4–13	94–241	0.8–2
11–15 years	0.6–8	5.5–12	83–213	0.8–2
16–20 years	0.5–6	4.2–12	80–210	0.8–2

(T3: triiodothyronine; T4: thyroxine; TSH: thyroid-stimulating hormone)

TABLE 3: Recommended doses for treatment of primary hypothyroidism in childhood.	
Age: 1–5 years	5–6 µg/kg/day
Age: 6–12 years	4–5 µg/kg/day
Age: 12–15 years (pre- and peripubertal)	2–3 µg/kg/day
Postpubertal children	1.6–1.8 µg/kg/day

studies have shown higher blood levels of T4 in subjects who received medication at bedtime. However, the medication should be taken at almost the same time every day.

Different L-thyroxine preparations have different oral bioavailability but the differences are minor from a practical standpoint. Concomitant intake of iron preparations, soy, and high fiber can interfere with the absorption of L-thyroxine.

Children with modestly depressed T4 levels can be initiated on the full replacement dose right at the outset. It is important to note that in children diagnosed with severe forms of long-standing hypothyroidism, treatment should be started with lower doses of L-thyroxine and the replacement dose should be increased slowly over weeks or months. The rapid replacement could rarely lead to symptoms suggestive of pseudotumor cerebri. More commonly, rapid replacement of L-thyroxine may lead to hyperactivity, insomnia, irritability, and deterioration in school performance. The rapid escalation of therapy may disproportionately accelerate the delayed skeletal maturation in the children and compromise final adult height. In children with pseudopuberty secondary to hypothyroidism (von Wyk–Grumbach syndrome), true central puberty may be triggered within 1 or 2 years of starting therapy. Children with central hypothyroidism require lower doses of L-thyroxine in comparison to those with primary hypothyroidism. L-thyroxine is usually well tolerated with minimal adverse effects once steady-state and stable thyroid biochemistry is achieved.

FOLLOW-UP

Once replacement therapy is started, TSH and T4 levels should be re-evaluated at an interval of 6–8 weeks. Once the L-thyroxine dose and thyroid biochemistry stabilize, these children should be followed up at 4–6 monthly intervals. In addition to biochemical evaluation, they should be evaluated for growth as well as symptoms of hypothyroidism. Monitoring may be done more frequently if changes in dose are required. It is important to monitor for associated autoimmune disorders like celiac disease, vitiligo, alopecia, autoimmune hepatitis, adrenal insufficiency, type-1 diabetes and pernicious anemia. Repeated testing for anti-thyroperoxidase and anti-thyroglobulin antibody levels is usually not required.

PROGNOSIS

Childhood hypothyroidism if diagnosed early and treated with adequate replacement therapy and regular monitoring has a good overall prognosis. Children with long-standing untreated hypothyroidism suffer from a significant bone age delay may end up with a significant adult height deficit. Except in very mild cases, most children with autoimmune thyroid disease require lifelong therapy.

SUGGETSED READING

1. IAP Textbook on Pediatric Endocrinology. New Delhi: Jaypee Brothers Medical Publishers (P) Ltd.; 2019.

Childhood Obesity

Ruchi Parikh

INTRODUCTION

Childhood obesity is a persistent, public health problem worldwide, with rising prevalence in developing countries. In India, the prevalence is increasing not only in the bigger cities but also in smaller towns due to the rapidly changing nutritional milieu and habits. According to the World Health Organization (WHO) analysis, prevalence of childhood overweight and obesity has significantly increased from 16.3% in 2001–2005 to 19.3% after 2010. India has the second highest number of obese children in the world after China. Deaths due to noncommunicating diseases are rising alarmingly in our country. Childhood obesity and the related comorbidities can track into adulthood. Hence, preventing pediatric obesity and its comorbidities is of paramount importance.

Definition: Obesity is defined as an excess in fat mass great enough to increase the risk of morbidity, altered physical, psychological, or social well-being and/or mortality *(WHO).*

Methods for determining fat content in body are not feasible in clinical practice. Body mass index (BMI) shows a good correlation with body fat percentage.

ETIOLOGY

Etiology for childhood obesity is broadly classified into **(Table 1)**:
- Exogenous (90%)
- Endogenous (10%)

TABLE 1: Etiology of childhood obesity.

Exogenous	
Chronic imbalance between energy intake and expenditure	• Sedentary lifestyle • Lack of physical activity • Consumption of sugar, sweetened beverages, and junk food
Medications expenditure	High-dose chronic glucocorticoids • Atypical antipsychotics • Tricyclic antidepressants • Consumption of sugar sweetened beverages, and junk food

Medications	• High-dose chronic glucocorticoids
	• Atypical antipsychotics
	• Tricyclic antidepressants
	• Antiepileptics
	• Monoamine oxidase inhibitors
	  – Lithium
	  – Oral contraceptives

Adverse metabolic programming	• SGA • LGA
Endogenous	
Monogenetic disorders	• Leptin deficiency • Leptin receptor deficiency • *POMC* mutation • *MC3R* mutation • *MC4R* mutation

Contd...

Contd...

Syndromic disorders	• Prader–Willi syndrome (PWS) • Bardet–Biedl syndrome • Carpenter syndrome • Cohen syndrome • Alström syndrome
Classic endocrine disorders (short stature and growth failure prominent)	• Hypothyroidism • Cushing syndrome • Growth hormone deficiency • Pseudohypoparathyroidism 1a (PHP1a)
Insulin dynamic disorders	• Hypothalamic obesity (Insulin hypersecretion) • Insulin resistance • Leptin resistance
Other disorders	Rapid-onset obesity with hypoventilation, hypothalamic, autonomic dysregulation, often with neural crest tumor syndrome (ROHHAD NET)

(MCR: melanocortin receptor mutation, POMC: proopiomelanocortin)

EVALUATION OF OBESE CHILDREN

Body mass index is used for measuring obesity. In children, BMI is age, gender, and puberty dependent. In India, there was a need to redefine BMI in children. The 85th and 95th percentile that are used as cutoff points for overweight and obesity in children are arbitrary and are not linked to obesity-related health risks.

Body Mass Index = Wt in kg/Ht in m² (1 m = 100 cm). It is plotted on a graph against a child's age. In children <5 years, the WHO Multicentre Growth Reference Study (MGRS) BMI charts are recommended. Weight for length/height > + 2SD is defined as overweight and weight for length/height >+3SD (97.7th percentile) as obesity. The Indian Academy of Pediatrics (IAP) Growth Chart Committee recommends the IAP 2015 revised growth charts for height, weight, and BMI for assessment of growth of 5–18-year-old Indian children. Adult equivalent of 23 and 27 cutoff lines as presented in BMI charts are used to define overweight and obesity in children from 5–18 years of age, as Asians are more prone to adiposity and central obesity at a lower BMI than their western counterparts.

HEALTH CONSEQUENCES OF OBESITY

- Insulin resistance and type 2 diabetes mellitus
- *Ovarian hyperandrogenism*: Polycystic ovary syndrome (PCOS)
- Dyslipidemia
- Nonalcoholic fatty liver disease (NAFLD)
- Hypertension
- Pseudotumor cerebri
- Sleep apnea
- *Orthopedic disorders*: Slipped capital femoral epiphyses (SCFE), Blount's disease
- Psychosocial problems
- Accelerated growth and bone maturation, gynecomastia
- Cholecystitis
- Pancreatitis
- Stress incontinence
- Proteinuria and focal segmental glomerulosclerosis
- Early subclinical atherosclerosis, cardiovascular disease (CVD) morbidity, and premature mortality in adulthood.

METABOLIC SYNDROME

Definition: Metabolic syndrome is defined as constellation of metabolic abnormalities that confer increased risk of CVD and diabetes mellitus.

As BMI is dependent on weight, it cannot differentiate between muscular from fatty individuals. Up to 25% of children with normal BMIs have excess amount of fat when measured by other means. Abdominal obesity is associated with increased risk of cardiovascular morbidity whereas this was not associated with measures of generalized obesity such as BMI. Hence, additional parameters beside BMI are required for diagnosing metabolic syndrome.

The International Diabetes Federation (IDF) has proposed the following criteria for metabolic syndrome in pediatric population (For children older than 16 years):

Abdominal obesity (Waist circumference >90th centile for age, gender, and ethnicity) plus two or more of following:
1. *Triglycerides > 150 mg/dL*
2. *HDL < 40 mg/dL*
3. *Blood pressure ≥ 95th percentile adjusted for height, age, and gender*
4. *Fasting glucose ≥ 100 mg/dL or type 2 diabetes mellitus.*

However, metabolic syndrome should not be defined in children younger than 10 years. It is suggested that cutoff of 70th percentile should be used in Asian children instead of 90th percentile. Waist circumference normative data of Indian children has been published. The suggestion of using lower cutoffs needs to be validated in different regions to be accepted as a guideline.

CLINICAL SIGNS (TABLE 2)

- Detailed history regarding onset, duration, progression of obesity, weight gain in relation to the stature, drug

TABLE 2: Clinical pointers toward the etiology of childhood obesity.

Clinical features	Etiology
Early onset (<5 years)	Monogenic or syndromic, rarely endocrine (adrenal tumor, or exogenous Cushing syndrome)
Hyperphagia, food foraging behavior	Monogenic syndrome, PWS
Dysmorphism, intellectual impairment, significant behavioral problems	Syndromic
Low birth weight, hypotonia, feeding difficulties	PWS
History of cranial irradiation, chemotherapy, CNS pathology	Endocrine obesity
Dry skin, constipation, cold intolerance	Hypothyroidism
Hirsutism, irregular menses in a girl, acne	Polycystic ovarian syndrome
Polyuria/polydipsia, blurry vision, fungal vaginitis/discharge in girls, and unexplained weight loss	Hyperglycemia
Unexplained headaches	Hypertension
Habitual snoring, restless sleep, morning headaches, generalized tiredness, and/or excessive daytime sleepiness, hyperactive inattentive behavior	Sleep apnea
Gastrointestinal discomfort	Non-alcoholic fatty liver disease
Knee or hip pain, limitation of motion	Slipped capital femoral epiphyses
Physical examination	
Obesity in a short child	Endocrine or syndromic (PWS, ROHHADNET, PHP1a)
Hypogonadism (Buried)	Syndromic, monogenic, endocrine (exogenous)
Hypertension	Cushing syndrome, exogenous
Violaceous striae, fat deposition over nape of neck	Cushing syndrome
Acanthosis nigricans, skin tags	Insulin resistance

TABLE 3: Diagnostic evaluation for the etiology and comorbidities of childhood obesity.

Etiology/Comorbidities	Lab tests
Hypothyroidism	Free T4, TSH
Growth hormone deficiency	GH stimulation test
Cushing disease	Blood and urine cortisol profile
CNS lesion	MRI brain and pituitary
Genetic syndrome	PWS: DNA methylation
Monogenic obesity	MC4R gene, leptin levels
Hepatic steatosis	ALT, hepatic ultrasound
• Glucose intolerance • Type 2 diabetes mellitus	• Fasting glucose > 100 mg/dL or 2-hour glucose > 140 mg/dL • Fasting glucose >125 mg/dL or 2-hour glucose >200 mg/dL, random blood glucose >200 mg/dL, HbA1c > 6.5%
Dyslipidemia	Fasting triglycerides, cholesterol, LDL cholesterol, HDL cholesterol

LABORATORY INVESTIGATIONS (TABLE 3)

Investigations include evaluation and obesity-related morbidity. Fasting lipids, HbA1c, ALT, Fasting glucose should be measured in all children with overweight and obesity, especially after 3 years of age.

MANAGEMENT

The IAP guidelines for growth monitoring recommend:
- Weight, length/height to be assessed at every immunization contact and every 6 months for children < 6 years of age.
- *BMI assessment yearly after 6 years of age*: Intervention includes a combination of diet modification, physical activity, and behavioral therapy in most cases as 90% of these children have exogenous obesity. Family, school, and community play a very important role. Following are the recommendations:
  - Promote and participate in an ongoing healthy dietary and activity education for children and adolescents, parents, and communities, and encourage schools to provide adequate education about healthy eating.
  - Avoid calorie-dense, nutrient-poor foods (beverages, sports drinks, fruit drinks, most "fast foods," high-fat or high-sodium processed foods, and calorie-dense snacks). Encourage whole fruits rather than fruit juices.
  - Eating breakfast and regular timely meals.
  - Reduce unhealthy portions and in-between meal snacking.
  - At least 20 minutes optimally 60 minutes, of vigorous physical activity at least 5 days per week.
  - Increasing incorporation of physical activities.
  - Foster healthy sleep patterns.

history, developmental milestones, antenatal history, and birth weight, family history of obesity, dyslipidemia, type 2 diabetes mellitus, hypertension, dietary history for the type and quantity of beverage intake, the frequency of dining out and the frequency and type of snacks, history of sedentary behaviors such as hours spent on screen activities, and physical activity (e.g., duration, frequency, in school and at home, sports participation).
- *Anthropometry*: Weight, height, waist circumference (in standing position, a nonstretchable tape applied horizontally just above the upper lateral border of the right ileum).
- *Examination*: Vitals, dysmorphism, skeleton, skin, digits and Tanner staging.

- Limit nonacademic screen time to <2 hours/day, none for children less than 2 years.
- Enlist the entire family rather than only the individual patient.
- Prepare more meals at home and eat together as a family.
- Increasing participation of parents in physical recreation as role models for their children.
- Use positive reinforcement (reward) techniques.
- Identify maladaptive rearing patterns related to diet and activity and educate families about healthy food and exercise habits.
- As psychosocial issues are highly prevalent, its pertinent to know about the following:
  - School absences/refusal
  - Teasing by peers regarding weight/appearance
  - Eating disorders—purging, anorexia, binge eating
  - Persistent anxiety, depression/self-harm, anger outbursts
  - Sexual activity, alcohol, drug use
  - Family functioning/family attitudes about weight
- *Bariatric surgery*:

Prerequisites:
- Adolescent who has achieved Tanner Stage 4 or 5 with final or near final height (>16 years of age)
- BMI > 40 kg/m² or > 35 kg/m² with significant comorbidities. Failed 6–12 months of intensive management.
- Competent and stable family, continued healthy diet and activity habits.
- A multidisciplinary team with experienced surgeon, medical, nutritional, and psychological expertise.

Procedures:
- *Purely restrictive*: Reduce stomach to decrease the volume of food ingested, e.g., laparoscopic-adjustable gastric band (LAGB), sleeve gastrectomy.
- *Purely malabsorptive*: Anatomic rearrangement of intestine, e.g., jejunoileal bypass. Not recommended.
- *Combination*: Roux-en-Y gastric bypass (RYGB).
- *Pharmacotherapy*:

Prerequisites:
- BMI > 27 kg/m² with comorbidity
- BMI > 30 kg/m², not improved on intense lifestyle modification
- BMI worsening over 6–12 months.

It is approved for children > 10 years of age. Limited safety and efficacy data are available for children. Use of medication should be in conjunction with lifestyle modification:
- Metformin, approved for >10 years for type 2 diabetes mellitus or insulin resistance, 250–1,000 mg twice a day orally (Not FDA-approved treatment for obesity).
- Orlistat, approved for >12 years, 120 mg twice a day orally (adverse effects of concern: flatus, fecal incontinence, oily spotting, vitamin malabsorption
- *Newer therapy*: Phase III trial of liraglutide, a glucagon-like peptide 1 (GLP-1) analog (12–17 years): Greater reduction in BMI but with gastrointestinal adverse effects.
  - *Specific therapy*:
    - Endocrine:
      - *Growth hormone deficiency*: Growth hormone therapy
      - *Hypothyroidism*: Thyroxine
      - *Cushing syndrome*: Surgery, steroid replacement
      - *Pseudohypoparathyroidism 1a (PHP1a)*: Calcium, calcitriol
    - Syndromic:
      - *Prader–Willi syndrome (PWS)*: Growth hormone therapy
    - Monogenic
  - *Leptin deficiency*: Recombinant leptin
    - *Hypothalamic obesity*: Octreotide.

Follow-up:
Intense follow-up 3–6 monthly recommended.

Long-term complication:
Increased risk of obesity and comorbidities in adulthood:
- Diabetes
- *CVD*:
  - Atherosclerosis
  - Heart (structural changes, functional changes)
- Nonalcoholic fatty liver disease (NASH).

CONCLUSION

Prevention of obesity is easier than management due to limited therapeutic options. Early and continuous tracking should be done by pediatrician, encouraging exclusive breastfeeding till 6 months of age, lowered saturated fat intake for children <2 years of age, healthy complementary food introduction, inculcating physical activity and discouraging screen usage. It is vital to involve the parents and grandparents to enable healthy eating, sleeping and activity habits. Hereditary component with unhealthy lifestyle changes are responsible for early onset of overweight and obesity, which can track into adulthood and harbor a vicious circle of obesity and metabolic syndrome.

KEY MESSAGES

- Childhood obesity has its basis in genetic susceptibilities influenced by a permissive environment starting in utero and extending through childhood and adolescence.

- Endocrine etiologies are rare, usually accompanied by attenuated growth patterns.
- Genetic screening for rare syndromes in presence of specific historical or physical features.
- BMI is the simplest method to identify excess adiposity in clinic setting.
  - *5–18 years*: Revised IAP 2015
    - BMI >23 kg/m² adult equivalent—overweight
    - BMI >27 kg/m² adult equivalent—obesity
  - *0–5 years*: WHO MGRS
    - Weight for length/height > +2SD—overweight
    - Weight for length/height > +3SD—obese
  - Waist circumference provides additional information about metabolic and cardiovascular risk.
  - Pediatric co-morbidities are common; screening for early identification before more serious complications result.
  - The psychological toll necessitates screening for mental health issues and counseling as indicated.
  - The prevention of pediatric obesity is done by promoting healthy diet, activity, and environment.

SUGGESTED READING

1. Dayal AA, Chugh V, Khadilkar V, Lohiya N. Childhood obesity and metabolic syndrome. In: Khadilkar V, Bajpai A, Prasad HK (eds). IAP Textbook on Pediatric Endocrinology. New Delhi: Jaypee Brothers Medical Publishers (P) Ltd.; 2019. pp. 479-503.
2. Indian Academy of Pediatrics Growth Charts Committee; Khadilkar V, Yadav S, Agrawal KK, Tamboli S, Banerjee M, Cherian A, et al. Revised IAP growth charts for height, weight and body mass index for 5-18 year old Indian children. Indian Pediatr. 2015;52(1):47-55.
3. Multicentre Growth Reference Study WHO Group. WHO Child Growth Standards based on length/height, weight and age. Acta Pediatr. 2006;450;76-85.
4. Sriram U. Childhood Obesity. In: Desai MP, Bhatia V, Menon PSN (eds). Pediatric Endocrine Disorders, 3rd edition. University Press;2014. pp. 381-93.
5. Styne DM, Arslanian SA, Connor EL, Farooqi IS, Murad MH, Silverstein JH, et al. Pediatric obesity—assessment, treatment, and prevention: an Endocrine Society Clinical Practice Guideline. J Clin Endocrinol Metab. 2017; 102(3):709-57.
6. Weiss R, Lustig RH. Obesity, metabolic syndrome and disorders of energy balance. In: Sperling MA (ed). Pediatric Endocrinology, 4th edition. Elsevier Saunders; 2014. pp. 956-1014.

Type 1 Diabetes

Saurabh Uppal

INTRODUCTION AND ETIOPATHOGENESIS

Type 1 diabetes is a common chronic disease of childhood. It is the most common form of diabetes in children and accounts for about 5% of all cases of diabetes in the world. It results from deficiency and subsequent absence of insulin secretion by islet cells of the pancreas arising due to autoimmune destruction of pancreatic beta cells in genetically susceptible individuals when exposed to postulated environmental and/or immunological triggers.

When to suspect type 1 diabetes?

The diagnosis of type 1 diabetes is seldom missed by a trained pediatrician. The presentation is usually acute or subacute with the onset of polyuria, nocturia, polydipsia, polyphagia, weight loss and progresses, in absence of timely intervention to a ketoacidotic state characterized by lethargy, drowsiness, tachypnea, pain abdomen, vomiting, and in severe cases such as coma.

INVESTIGATIONS AT DIAGNOSIS

- Outpatient setting in a stable child
  - Random blood glucose to document high blood glucose
  - Urine routine examination for glycosuria and ketonuria
  - Glycosylated hemoglobin (HbA1c)
- Emergency setting in a clinically unstable child (additional investigations to guide the course of management in the intensive care setting)
  - Blood gas (venous)
  - Serum electrolytes
  - Renal function tests
  - Investigations to rule out an underlying infectious disease trigger
- Testing for associated conditions
  - Antitissue transglutaminase (for celiac disease)
  - Thyroid function tests
  - Relevant investigations if clinical features of other autoimmune diseases present:
    - Maturity-onset diabetes of the young (MODY)
    - Type 1 diabetes (T1D)
    - Type 2 diabetes (T2D)

In cases where distinction between T1D and T2D is not clear, specific autoantibody titers may be needed. The commonly tested antibodies are glutamic acid decarboxylase (GAD-65), insulinoma antigen-2 (IA2), and anti-insulin antibodies. Zinc transporter 8 antibodies are not widely available. C-peptide levels can also be helpful in differentiating the types of diabetes after the initial glucotoxic phase is over. The measurement of insulin levels has no role in diagnosis of T1D.

AMBULATORY MANAGEMENT

Clinically stable patients may not be admitted to the hospital and management of diabetes with subcutaneous insulin injections may be started along with ongoing diabetes education.

Diabetes Education

Well-structured yet customizable education at diagnosis is very important to enable the panic-stricken family to adopt the correct approach toward managing the child's condition. Misinformation by society and lack of empathic diabetes education just after diagnosis is one of the most important factors impacting adoption and adherence to the recommended treatment approach. The key aspects of education to be covered at diagnosis are:

- A simple explanation of the disease state and the difference between T1D and T2DM.
- The rationale behind the indispensability of insulin therapy with special emphasis on the lack of "noninsulin" alternatives.
- The dangers of alternative experimental approaches.

Diabetes education and training at diagnosis must include:

- Insulins to rage, handling, and injection technique
- The usage of glucose and ketone testing equipment
- Clear and consistent instructions about treatment goals, glycemic targets and long-term follow-up plan

- Preliminary knowledge of food groups and preferred diet regimens
- Proper technique for sharps and other medical waste disposals
- Home management of hypoglycemia

Insulin

Insulin therapy is the mainstay of pharmacological management of T1D. Children are not small adults. The insulin requirements and challenges faced by children are different from those of adults hence the insulin regimens and recommendations from adult diabetes practice cannot be extrapolated to children without the much-needed modifications. The various insulins approved for children are tabulated in **Table 1**.

The objective of insulin therapy in TID is to try and replicate the physiological pattern of insulin secretion. Intensive insulin therapy with multiple daily injections as a basal-bolus regimen enables us to match the physiological pattern most closely and is the standard of care in children with T1D. Long-acting insulin is administered once or twice a day as basal insulin and additional injections of rapid/short-acting insulin are administered for meals and/or glycemic excursions. Important points to remember while planning and titrating insulin therapy are:

- Insulin may be started at 0.7–11 µ/kg/day. About 30–50% of this dose should be as basal insulin and the rest of it in three divided doses before meals. It is worth remembering that a body weight calculated insulin dosage may only serve as a good starting point. Regular dosage is ultimately dictated by the child's stage of diabetes, diet and lifestyle.
- Fasting blood glucose and premeal blood glucose readings are used to titrate the basal insulin.
- Postprandial blood glucose and to a certain extent the premeal glucose readings are used to titrate the bolus insulin dose.
- Bolus insulin dosage should be titrated once adequate basal levels are achieved.
- Any change in the bolus recommendations may necessitate further fine tuning of the basal insulin dose.
- The recommended ratio of basal and bolus insulin doses as 1:1 is not applicable to children in most situations. The ratio keeps changing during different stages of childhood and it is advisable to follow the blood glucose readings and lifestyle of the child to titrate the respective insulins.
- Evaluation of related lifestyle, diet or behavioral changes, injection site integrity and symptoms related to associated comorbidities must precede any major changes in insulin dose.
- Premixed insulins (coformulation of short- and intermediate/long-acting insulin in ratio of 30:70, 50:50, 25:75, etc.) are generally not recommended for children, except in very selective circumstances. Their use in pediatric T1D should be discouraged.

Traditionally insulin given through syringe, which is considered cumbersome and error prone, particularly when using small doses in children and technically demanding, has been largely replaced by pen devices which are easy to use, relatively less painful and almost free of dosing error. Insulin administration by way of continuous subcutaneous insulin infusion (CSII) also known as insulin pump therapy provides greater flexibility in insulin delivery and improved quality of life for children and their families. Advances in CSII including sensor-augmented therapy and predictive low glucose suspension in insulin delivery are very helpful in T1D. These technologies have found widespread acceptance around the world. Their use has increased in India although the high cost of these therapies makes it unaffordable for the vast majority of Indian patients.

Nutrition

Efficient and effective management of nutrition in childhood diabetes assumes center stage both from the standpoint of glycemic control and provision of adequate nutrition in this chronic disease. The widespread acceptance of basal-bolus insulin regimens has enabled us to match food intake with calculated insulin dosage thereby imparting unprecedented

TABLE 1: Types of insulin preparation and comparative action profiles for subcutaneous administration.

Insulin type	Onset of action (h)	Duration of action (h)	Minimal peak
Bolus therapy			
Ultrarapid-acting analog (faster aspart)	0.1–0.2	1–3	
Rapid-acting analogs (Aspart, Glulisine, Lispro)	0.15–0.35	1–3	
Regular/soluble (short-acting)	0.5–1	2–4	
NPH	2–4	4–12	12–24
Basal therapy			
Glargine	2–4	8–12	22–24
Detemir	1–2	4–7	20–24
Glargine U 300	2–6	Minimal peak	30–36
Degludec	0.5–1.5	Minimal peak	>42

freedom in food choices to families and clinicians to meet the irrespective goals. Dietary requirements of children with diabetes are similar to those of any growing child. Thereby it is advisable that the label of a "diabetic diet" recommendation for children with diabetes be discouraged. The focus should shift to a healthy and wholesome childhood nutrition plan with adequate provision of insulin dose and dose titration.

What are the goals for medical nutrition therapy in childhood diabetes?

- Ensure requisite energy intake for good health as well as normal growth and development.
- Ensure the intake of diverse food items with high nutritional value from every food group to provide all essential nutrients.
- To attain a balance between the dosage of insulin and dietary intake of the child, metabolic requirements and energy expenditure to ensure more regulated blood glucose levels.
- Realize and sustain the requisite body mass index (BMI) as per the age.
- Prevent and treat acute complications of diabetes such as hypoglycemia, hyperglycemia, and appropriately cover for illness and exercise-related problems.
- Inculcate healthy lifelong-term eating habits and encourage the appropriate eating behavior.
- Ensure the involvement of the child and family in dietary decision-making to enhance compliance and prevent diet-related behavioral problems.

The traditional approach of restrictive dietary practices, fixed diet charts and predecided insulin doses indirectly encourages arbitrary increase/decrease of dosage as per blood glucose levels done by caregivers who usually lack any formal training in dose adjustment and are driven by their own bias. The modern-day approach requires an effort to estimate the total carbohydrate content in the diet and administrating the dose accordingly. Modern basal-bolus regimes with thrice a day short/rapid-acting analogs enable flexible meal timings and food compositions rather than compulsive and presumptive eating schedules.

MONITORING ON TREATMENT

Clinical Monitoring

Clinical follow-up is recommended at least once every 3 months. The diabetes follow-up visit should include a comprehensive review of the glycemic status of the child as well as the overall well-being of the child and the environment around the clinical condition. The recommended parameters to be evaluated are tabulated in **Table 2**.

Laboratory Monitoring

The parents are expected to check the blood glucose at home and record it. The blood glucose target recommendations are given in **Table 3**. Measurement of HbA1c is the most widely accepted tool for monitoring a child with T1D and currently

TABLE 2: The recommended parameters to be evaluated during clinical visit.

Self-maintained blood glucose (SMBG) log	• Adequacy of recordings • Outlier readings • Pattern disturbances • Adherence to good practices of SMBG
Insulin therapy	• Dosage • Injection technique • Injection site rotation • Lipodystrophy/lipoatrophy • Insulin storage
Diet review	Quality, quantity, timing, consistency in carbohydrate estimation, food fads if any
Exercise	Adequacy, type timing, effect on blood glucose
Hypoglycemia	Probable cause, corrective action taken, preventive measures instituted
Growth	Adequacy of weight and height gain
Blood pressure	Maintenance less than 95th centile for height
Pubertal status	Onset and progression
Clinical features of associated conditions	Hypothyroidism, celiac disease, adrenal insufficiency, vitiligo, and other autoimmune disorders
Clinical features suggestive of long-term complications	• Neuropathy nephropathy • Cataract/refractive error/retinopathy
Psychosocial well-being of the child and the family	• Coping behavior • Child-care giver conflict • High-risk behaviors, if any

TABLE 3: Blood glucose target recommendations.

Glycemic targets	NICE	ISPAD	ADA
Premeal	70–126 mg/dL	70–130 mg/dL	90–130 mg/dL
Postmeal	90–162 mg/dL	90–180 mg/dL	
Prebed	70–126 mg/dL	80–140 mg/dL	90–150 mg/dL

(ADA: American Diabetes Association; ISPAD: International Society of Pediatric and Adolescent Diabetes; NICE: National Institute of Healthcare Excellence)

TABLE 4: Screening protocol for vascular complications.

	When to start screening	How to screen	Potential interventions
Retinopathy	Annually from age 11 or at the onset of puberty if this is earlier, after 2 to 5 years' diabetes duration	Fundal photography or mydriaticophthalmoscopy (less sensitive)	Improved glycemic control, VEGF, Laser therapy
Nephropathy	Annually from age 11 or at the onset of puberty if this is earlier, after 2 to 5 years' diabetes duration	Urinary albumin/creatinine ratio	Improved glycemic control ACEI or ARBs Blood pressure lowering
Neuropathy	Annually from 11 years with 2–5 years diabetes duration	History and physical examination	Improved glycemic control
Macrovascular disease	After age 11 yr with 2–5 years diabetes duration	Lipid profile every 2 year, blood pressure annually	Improved glycemic control, exercise, ACE inhibitors or ARB, statins

the only measure of long-term control with a strong evidence base. It provides a measure of insulin adequacy, gives a broad estimate of the level of control of blood glucose, and is useful for assessing risk of long-term complications. The goals of HbA1c recommended are based on the Diabetes Control and Complications Trial (DCCT) results and other studies and the general goal is to keep the HbA1c in all patients below 7.5% (<7% if they have access to technology and analog insulins). A better HbA1c in childhood and adolescence is associated with a reduced risk of microvascular as well as macrovascular complications in subsequent years. Hence, an effort to achieve lower HbA1c targets should be made in the early years of diabetes that children spend in pediatric care. The traditional mindset of being liberal with HbA1c goals in children out of a fear of aggravating hypoglycemia has been challenged by recent evidence that lowering HbA1c goals to 7% in children leads to better glycemic control and a lower achieved HbA1c without increasing the frequency of severe hypoglycemia.

Continuous glucose monitoring (CGM) in the interstitial space by means of sensors applied on the skin has revealed unprecedented insights into glycemic variations in individuals. This has led to development of newer metrics to assess glucose patterns and compare glycemic control with standard parameters. Time in range (TIR) is such an emerging metric that quantifies the duration of time in 24 hours that the individual spends in euglycemia, hypoglycemia, or hyperglycemia. Early evidence is emerging that assessment of TIR by CGM may be a better measure to access glucose exposure and glycemic variability than HbA1c.

Monitoring for Complications

Uncontrolled diabetes mellitus can often lead to a number of microvascular and macrovascular complications in children and adults with T1D. The suggested protocol for screening and intervention the respective complications is as in **Table 4**.

Vascular complications are a critical contributor to mortality in patients with diabetes onset during childhood. However, intensive management from an early age can reduce the risk of microvascular complications and the positive effects of intensive intervention continue much beyond the intervention period in the form of a legacy effect.

Management in Special Situations

Sick Day Management

Sick days pose a unique challenge in day-to-day management as an increased insulin requirement due to insulin resistance combines with an inability to eat and parental fears of hypoglycemia resulting in underdosing of insulin.

General principles in management of sick days:
- More frequent blood glucose and ketone (urine or blood) monitoring (2–4 hourly).
- Strict advice against insulin omission. Provision of sugary drinks to maintain hydration and adequate blood glucose levels to enable adequate insulin administration.
- Monitor and maintain salt and water balance.
- Treat the underlying precipitating illness.

- Written instruction to spot warning signs of ketoacidosis at home.
- Guidelines including insulin adjustment should be taught soon after diagnosis and reviewed at least annually.

DIABETES IN SCHOOL

Children spend a lot of time in school without the supervision of parents. The knowledge of school personnel in general in our country regarding childhood diabetes is not up to the required standards. In this situation, the role of the primary physician caring for the child becomes very important and it becomes the responsibility of the parents and the primary physician to provide a detailed management plan for the child to be followed in school in any challenging scenario.

The written detailed management plan should include:
- A basic knowledge of the condition and the unique challenges faced at school
- Glycemic targets in school (similar to other settings)
- The knowledge of signs and symptoms of hypoglycemia and hyperglycemia. A first aid hypoglycemia management kit should be available both with the school as well as with the child
- Clear instructions on administration of carbohydrate in case of hypoglycemia and administration of insulin during instances of severe hyperglycemia
- Detailed instructions for management in special situations such as exercise, school examinations and picnics
- Understanding and knowledge of the diabetes technology device if being used by the child.

CONCLUSION

Management of childhood diabetes is a challenging task both for the family and the treating physician. Constant vigilance on the part of all stakeholders is paramount in ensuring a good long-term outcome. The role of pediatrician is extremely important as the quality of care in the early years determines the patterns of health and morbidity in the long run. The ultimate goal of diabetes management is to provide a good quality of life to the child and the family by facilitating stable glycemic control, normal growth and development, early detection and management of complications and ensuring psychosocial well-being. With the advancement in our understanding of blood glucose management, the overall care and long-term outcomes in childhood diabetes have improved. Consistent efforts by the treating physician during the early years of diagnosis can go a long way in ensuring a healthier lifespan for these patients.

SUGGESTED READING

1. Danne T, Phillip M, Buckingham BA, Jarosz-Chobot P, Saboo B, Urakami T, et al. ISPAD Clinical Practice Consensus Guidelines 2018. Insulin treatment in children and adolescents with diabetes. Pediatric Diabetes. 2018;19 (Suppl 27):115-35.
2. Gabbay MAL, Rodacki M, Calliari LE Vianna DAG, Krakauer M, Pinto MS, et al. Time in range: a new parameter to evaluate blood glucose control in patients with diabetes. Diabetol Metab Syndr. 2020;12:22.
3. Phelan H, Lange K, Cengiz E, Gallego P, Majaliwa E, Pelicand J, et al. ISPAD Clinical Practice Consensus Guidelines 2018: Diabetes education in children and adolescents. Pediatr Diabetes. 2018;19(Suppl 27):75-83.
4. Pihoker C, Forsander G, Fantahun B, Virmani A, Corathers S, Benitez-Aguirre P, et al. ISPAD Clinical Practice Consensus Guidelines 2018: The delivery of ambulatory diabetes care to children and adolescents with diabetes. Pediatric Diabetes. 2018;19(Suppl 27):84-104.
5. Reinehr T. Type 2 diabetes mellitus in children and adolescents. World J Diabetes. 2013;4(6):270-81.
6. The effect of intensive treatment of diabetes on the development and progression of long-term complications in insulin-dependent diabetes mellitus. The Diabetes Control and Complications Trial Research Group. N Engl J Med. 1993;329:977-86.
7. Uppal S. Dietary management of childhood diabetes. In: Khadilkar V, Bajpai A, Prasas HK (eds). IAP Textbook on Pediatric Endocrinology, 1st edition. New Delhi: Japyee Brothers Medical Publishers (P) Ltd; 2019.
8. White NH, Sun W, Cleary PA, Tamborlane WV, Danis RP, Hainsworth DP, et al. Effect of prior intensive therapy in type 1 diabetes on 10-year progression of retinopathy in the DCCT/EDIC: comparison of adults and adolescents. Diabetes. 2010;59(5):1244-53.

Precocious Puberty

Swati Kanodia

INTRODUCTION

Precocious puberty is traditionally defined as the onset of secondary sexual characteristics before the age of 8 years in girls and 9 years in boys. These limits are chosen to be 2–2.5 standard deviations (SD) below the mean age of onset of puberty.

NORMAL PUBERTAL DEVELOPMENT

Gonadotropin-releasing hormone-(GnRH) secreting neurons in the hypothalamus are considered the chief regulator of pubertal onset. Puberty is triggered by increased pulsatile GnRH secretion from hypothala-mus, which stimulates production of gonadotropins (Gn)-luteinizing hormone (LH) and follicle-stimulating hormone (FSH). LH stimulates the ovaries to secrete estradiol (E2) and the testes to secrete testosterone, and FSH promotes the development of the oocytes or spermatozoa and increases the size of the gonads. This phenomenon is termed as activation of hypothalamic–pituitary–gonadal axis (HPG axis).

E2 is responsible for progressive breast enlargement, the pubertal growth spurt, and concomitant bone age advancement in girls, while Testosterone causes penile enlargement and pubic hair growth in boys and, by conversion to E2, causes the male growth spurt.

It is important to note that pubic hair in girls and adult axillary odor in boys and girls is related to the increase in secretion of weak adrenal androgens (primarily dehydroepiandrosterone-sulfate [DHEA-S]), referred to as adrenarche, and is unrelated to activation of the HPG axis.

The earliest clinical manifestation of central puberty in girls is usually breast development (thelarche), followed by pubic hair (pubarche). The pubertal growth spurt typically occurs during Tanner stage II–III, with the first menstrual period, known as menarche, usually occurring at Tanner stage IV. In boys, testicular enlargement (>4 mL) is an early sign of puberty followed by genital growth and development of sexual hairs. The pubertal growth spurt occurs somewhat later during Tanner stage III-IV.

Precocious puberty can be divided into two types:
1. GnRH-dependent/central precocious puberty (CPP)/true precocious puberty
2. GnRH-independent/peripheral precocious puberty (PPP)/precocious pseudopuberty

Central precocious puberty is the result of activation of the HPG axis, activation and secretion of gonadal sex steroids and presents clinically as development of secondary sexual characteristics.

Peripheral precocious puberty is much less common. Development of secondary sexual characteristics results from increased sex hormone production by the gonads, without activation of the hypothalamic–pituitary axis.

PATHOPHYSIOLOGY

Specific genetic causes of CPP have been described relatively recently. The expression of KISS-1mRNA and GPR54 receptor has been correlated with the onset of puberty. GPR54 receptors have been identified in the GnRH-secreting neurons and activating *GPR54* mutation has been postulated as a cause of precocious puberty. The synapses of central regulatory neurons with kisspeptin neurons and ghrelin and leptin receptors in KISS-1 neurons have confirmed the role of kisspeptin in pubertal regulation. Thus KISS-1-kisspeptin-GPR54 system is said to be the gatekeeper of puberty and central to the regulation of pubertal onset and progression.

In children with a family history of CPP, *MKRN3*, and *DLK1* gene mutations have been found to be the most common monogenetic cause of precocious puberty. As both are maternally imprinted genes that are expressed only from the paternal allele, a family history of CPP on the father's side should increase the index of suspicion for a mutation in one of these genes.

ETIOLOGY (FLOWCHART 1)

Precocious puberty represents increased sex hormone production by the gonads either independently—Gn-independent precocious puberty (GIPP) or under the effect of gonadotropins—Gn-dependent precocious puberty (GDPP). GIPP can be heterosexual (development of secondary sexual characteristics of the opposite sex) or isosexual. However, GDPP is always isosexual.

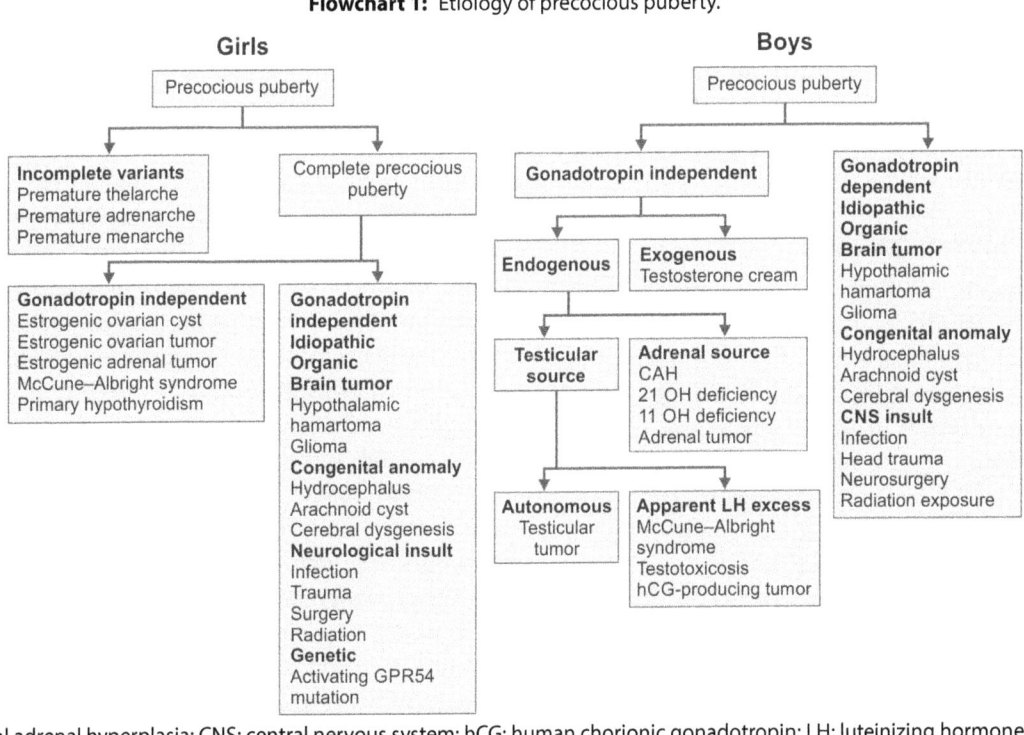

Flowchart 1: Etiology of precocious puberty.

(CAH: congenital adrenal hyperplasia; CNS: central nervous system; hCG: human chorionic gonadotropin; LH: luteinizing hormone)

Source: Adapted from: Bajpai A, Sharma J, Kabra M, Gupta A, Menon PS. Precocious puberty: Clinical and endocrine profile and factors indicating neurogenic precocity in Indian children. J Pediatr Endocrinol Metab. 2002;15:1173-81.

Most girls with precocious puberty have Gn-dependent etiology, while GIPP is commoner in boys. Over 90% girls with GDPP have nonidentifiable neurological cause. However, boys are more likely to have an underlying cause for central precocious puberty.

Incomplete variants: These are more commonly encountered in day-to-day practice and should be ruled out to prevent erroneous diagnosis of precocious puberty **(Table 1)**.

EVALUATION

Precocious puberty is 5–10 times more common in girls than in boys. Detailed history and examination are imperative and might give a clue of possible etiology. Enquiry about onset, duration, and rate of progression of puberty can point toward likely pathology. A family history of precocious puberty is important as it is occasionally inherited. One must enquire about the possible exposure to exogenous sex steroids, including ingestion of oral contraceptive pills or exposure to transdermal estrogen creams or testosterone gels. Presence of central nervous system (CNS) symptoms, including severe frequent headaches or recent visual deficits, or a history of disorders affecting the CNS, such as brain tumor, meningitis, CNS trauma, and cranial irradiation makes GDPP as a more likely etiology.

Physical Examination

Measure height, weight, and height velocity (cm/year). The physical examination should include assessment of visual fields (for CNS pathology) and examination for café-au-lait spots (to rule out McCune-Albright syndrome). Look for signs of hypothyroidism (dull child, dry skin, constipation, and weight gain), especially if child is short

TABLE 1: Incomplete variants of puberty.

Isolated thelarche	• Isolated nonprogressive breast development in a girl, usually a toddler (<2 years age) • Characterized by normal growth, isolated FSH elevation with prepubertal LH levels and age-appropriate bone age
Premature adrenarche	• Appearance of pubic hair, axillary hair, and odor and sometimes mild acne, in girls before 8 years of age and in boys before 9 years of age • Associated with a normal growth rate. Breast development is absent, and skeletal maturation may be mildly advanced • DHEA-S are typically increased for age, but FSH, LH, and estradiol or testosterone concentrations are at prepubertal levels
Premature menarche	• Young girl with one or two brief episodes of vaginal bleeding but no other signs of puberty, it is unlikely an endocrine cause • Isolated menarche should be considered once local trauma, foreign body, infection, sexual abuse, or a vaginal or uterine tumor as a cause of vaginal bleeding is ruled out

(DHEA-S: dehydroepiandrosterone sulfate FSH: follicle-stimulating hormone; LH: luteinizing hormone)

with poor growth velocity. Secondary sexual development is assessed to determine the sexual maturity rating (Tanner stage) of pubertal development, which means staging breast development in girls, genital development in boys, and pubic hair development in both sexes. An orchidometer is useful to measure the testicular volume in boys.

Laboratory Investigations

Baseline laboratory testing includes measuring the gonadotropins (LH, FSH) levels along with either E2 or testosterone. LH is a better indicator of pubertal status compared to FSH. A basal LH of >0.6 IU/L and LH-to-FSH ratio of >1 suggests GDPP. In case of inconclusive Gn levels, a GnRH-stimulation test remains the gold standard for differentiating GDPP from GIPP. Pubertal LH levels (>5 U/L), post GnRH administration, are diagnostic of CPP. A blunted response to GnRH is pathognomonic of PPP.

Adrenal androgens [DHEAS, 17(OH) progesterone] are done in case of isosexual PPP in boys or heterosexual precocious puberty in girls and in precocious pubarche to rule out a pathological cause, like CAH or adrenal tumor. Thyroid-stimulating hormone (TSH) levels should be checked, if height velocity is slow and bone age is delayed.

Imaging

A radiograph for bone age assessment for evaluation of skeletal maturation help with both the differential diagnosis and assessment of whether there may be an impact on final height. A significant advance in the bone age [greater than approximately 2 standard deviations (SD) beyond chronologic age] is more likely to be indicative of pubertal precocity rather than a benign pubertal variant. A pelvic ultrasound has been found to be a useful adjunct to support the diagnosis of CPP over other forms of puberty in girls. Girls with CPP have greater uterine and ovarian volumes compared with girls who are prepubertal or those with premature thelarche. An ovarian mass can be detected in case of PPP in girls. Similarly, an ultrasound of testicles is useful to evaluate cause of PPP in boys. Contrast-enhanced brain magnetic resonance imaging (MRI) is recommended in those diagnosed to have true precocious puberty. In rare cases of isosexual PPP in boys or heterosexual precocious puberty in girls, a CT image of the adrenal can bring forth the likely etiology.

TREATMENT

The aims of management include treatment of the underlying cause, attainment of target height, and amelioration of psychological distress.

The major concern is compromised final height due to advanced skeletal maturation. Although these children appear tall for age, the height for bone age is compromised. An increased risk of aggressive or sexual behavior, substance abuse, and worse academic achievement has been identified in a subset of children with precocious puberty. GnRH analogs are well established as a standard of care for the treatment of CPP worldwide. GnRH agonists work by providing continuous stimulation to the pituitary gonadotrophs instead of physiologic pulsatile stimulation from hypothalamic GnRH. Continuous stimulation leads to desensitization of the gonadotroph cells and suppression of gonadotropins, thus reducing the gonadal stimulation and resulting in decreased sex steroid production and reversal of pubertal changes. It should be recognized, however, some patients will have a nonprogressive or slowly progressive form of CPP, and these patients can achieve normal adult height without any intervention. Therefore, a period of observation and monitoring the progression is usually appropriate prior to starting treatment.

While numerous delivery systems and routes of administration exist, depot intramuscular injections (leuprolide, triptorelin) or sustained-release preparations (histrelin) have been most widely used. GnRH has an admirable safety profile. The most commonly reported adverse events are injection-site reactions which are typically mild and self-limited.

Patients on GnRH analogs should be followed up 3-monthly for pubertal status and growth parameters. Clinical indicators that the medication is working include slowing of the growth velocity along with shrinkage or softening of the glandular breast tissue or the testes. GnRH analog treatment has no effect on pubic hair development as it is controlled by adrenal androgens. Discontinuation of treatment incorporates numerous patient-specific characteristics including absolute and predicted height, chronological age, psychosocial factors, pubertal stage, and family preferences. Most endocrinologists end therapy at bone age of ~10 years in girls and ~12 years in boys. Discontinuation of treatment results in gradual reappearance of secondary sexual characters.

Gonadotropin-independent Precocious Puberty

Treatment of GIPP is directed toward correction of the underlying cause and suppression of sex steroid production or action **(Table 2)**.

CONCLUSION

Precocious puberty is much more common in daily pediatric practice and timely diagnosis and intervention can have favorable results. CPP is seen most often in girls and is associated with a multitude of conditions. CPP in boys is almost always pathological. A substantial proportion (over a quarter) of cases is familial; and genetic causes have begun to be elucidated. The diagnosis is based on a combination of clinical and biochemical factors. Treatment with a GnRH

TABLE 2: Causes of gonadotropin independent precocious puberty.	
McCune–Albright syndrome	• Treatment strategies include the use of medroxyprogesterone acetate, ketoconazole, and spironolactone. Third-generation aromatase inhibitors such as letrozole and anastrozole have been increasingly used in the condition • GnRH analog treatment is indicated in girls with triggered gonadotropin-dependent precocious puberty (GDPP)
Functional ovarian cyst	• Most ovarian cysts regress spontaneously and do not require surgical intervention • Thyroid functions should be assessed in all girls with ovarian cysts
Congenital adrenal hyperplasia	• Physiological glucocorticoid therapy is effective in retarding the pubertal progress • Diagnosis is often delayed in most patients, resulting in triggered GDPP
Testotoxicosis	• Treatment with aromatase inhibitor, testolactone, and ketoconazole has been disappointing • Combination of anastrozole and anti-androgen bicalutamide has recently been shown to be effective

(GnRH: gonadotropin-releasing hormone)

analogs provides the greatest potential benefit for patients who are younger at the time of onset of CPP. Biochemical markers, bone age, and growth velocity should be followed during treatment to ensure efficacy. The available evidence shows that GnRH analogs are safe and effective, and long-term data suggest that reproductive function is satisfactory after the discontinuation of treatment.

SUGGESTED READING

1. Bajpai A, Menon P. Contemporary issues in precocious puberty. Indian J Endocr Metab. 2011;15,SupplS3:172-9.
2. Calabria qA. (2020). Precocious puberty. [online] Available from: https://www.msdmanuals.com/en-in/professional/pediatrics/endocrine-disorders-in-children/precocious-puberty. [Last accessed May, 2021].
3. Chen M, Eugster EA. Central precocious puberty: update on diagnosis and treatment. Paediatr Drugs. 2015;17(4):273-81.
4. Eugster EA. Treatment of central precocious puberty. J Endocr Soc. 2019;3(5):965-72.
5. Fuqua JS. Treatment and outcomes of precocious puberty: an update. J Clin Endocrinol Metab. . 2013;98(6):2198-2207.
6. Harrington J, Palmert MR. (2020). Definition, etiology, and evaluation of precocious puberty. [online] Available from: https://www.uptodate.com/contents/definition-etiology-and-evaluation-of-precocious-puberty. [Last accessed May, 2021].
7. Harrington J, Palmert MR. (2021). Treatment of precocious puberty. [online] Available from: https://www.uptodate.com/contents/treatment-of-precocious-puberty. [Last accessed May, 2021].
8. Kaplowitz P, Bloch C, Section on Endocrinology, American Academy of Pediatrics. Evaluation and referral of children with signs of early puberty. Pediatrics. 2016;137(1):e20153732.

CHAPTER 146: Disorders of Sex Development

Ruchi Parikh

INTRODUCTION

A neonate or a child with atypical genitalia prompts a detailed surveillance based on long-term management strategy. It involves a multidisciplinary team for diagnosis, surgical intervention, understanding psychosocial issues, and recognizing and accepting the place of patient advocacy. In 2006, under the auspices of The Lawson Wilkins Pediatric Endocrine Society and the European Society for Pediatric Endocrinology proposed the term *"Disorders of Sex Development" (DSD)* and recommended a revised classification of the medical terminology to avoid controversial gender-based diagnostic labels as intersex, pseudohermaphroditism, hermaphroditism, or sex reversal **(Table 1)**.

Definition: DSD is a congenital condition characterized by atypical development of chromosomal, gonadal, hormonal or anatomic aspects of sex.

Hence, its a path different from that of typical female or typical male. Incidence of DSD is 1:4,000 live births. The most common etiology is congenital adrenal hyperplasia (CAH).

Normal gonadal differentiation and sex development depend on actions and interactions of specific genes, transcription factors, and hormones **(Fig. 1)**.

CLINICAL APPROACH

History:
- *Maternal virilization*: Acne, hirsutism, clitoromegaly
- *Maternal drug exposure*: Androgens, estrogens, endocrine disruptors
- *Family history*: Infertility, consanguinity, unexplained infant deaths, child with atypical genitalia or unexpected puberty changes.

TABLE 1: Revised Classification of Disorder of Sex Development (DSD), 2006.

Sex chromosome DSD	46XY DSD	46XX DSD

• 45, X (Turner syndrome and variants)
• 47, XXY (Klinefelter syndrome and variants)
• 45, X/46, XY (MGD, ovtesticular DSD)
• 46, XX/46 XY (chimeric, ovtesticular DSD)
	• *Disorders of gonadal (testicular) development*:
	  – Complete gonadal dysgenesis (Swyer syndrome)
	  – Partial gonadal dysgenesis
	  – Gonadal regression
	  – Ovotesticular DSD
	• *Disorders in androgen synthesis or action*:
	  – Androgen biosynthesis defect (e.g., 17-hydroxysteroid dehydrogenase deficiency, 5 alpha reductase deficiency, StAR mutations)
	  – Defect in androgen action (e.g., CAIS, PAIS)
	  – Luteinizing hormone receptor defects (e.g., Leydig cell hypoplasia, aplasia)
	  – Disorders of anti-Müllerian hormone and anti-Müllerian hormone receptor (persistent Müllerian duct syndrome)
		• *Disorders of gonadal (ovarian) development*:
		  – Ovotesticular DSD
		  – Testicular DSD (e.g., SRY+, duplicate SOX9)
		  – Gonadal dysgenesis
		• *Androgen excess*:
		  – Fetal (e.g., 21-hydroxylase deficiency, 11-hydroxylase deficiency)
		  – Fetoplacental (aromatase deficiency, POR (P450 oxidoreductase)
		  – Maternal (luteoma, exogenous, etc.)
		• Other (e.g., cloacal exstrophy, vaginal atresia, MURCS: Müllerian, renal, cervicot horacic somite abnormalities, other syndromes)

(CAIS: complete androgen insensitivity syndrome; DSD: disorder of sex development; MGD: mixed gonadal dysgenesis; PAIS: partial androgen insensitivity syndrome)

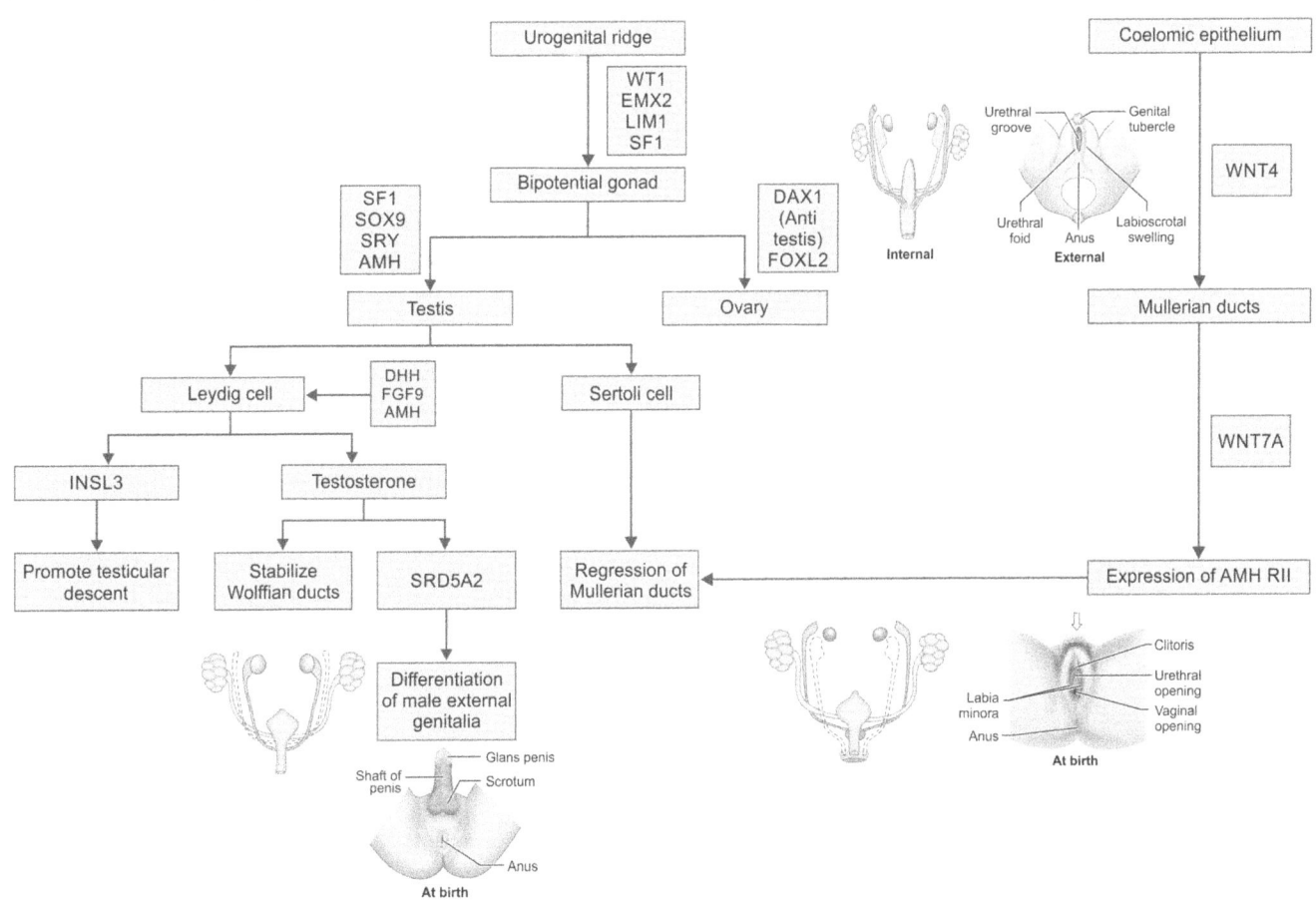

Fig. 1: Normal gonadal differentiation and sex development.

Suggested terminology when dealing with children with atypical genitalia:
- Your baby, instead of him or her
- Phallus, instead of penis or clitoris
- Folds, instead of scrotum or labia
- Gonads, instead of testis or ovaries.

Physical examination:
- Vitals
- Anthropometry
- Associated anomalies: Facial, skeletal, ear, digital.

Genital examination:
- Presence and location of palpable gonad from inguinal region to the folds
- Position of urethral orifice
- Presence of vaginal opening
- Number of perineal openings
- Phallic size from pubic ramus to the tip and diameter, Chordee
- Symmetry of external genitalia
- Degree and extent of labioscrotal fold fusion
- Pigmentation of nipple and genital.

DSDs involve the following elements:
- *In the neonatal period*:
  - Apparent female genitalia with an enlarged clitoris, posterior labial fusion or inguinal/labial mass
  - Apparent male genitalia with bilateral undescended testes, micropenis, isolated perineal hypospadias, or mild hypospadias with undescended testis
  - Overt genital ambiguity (e.g., cloacal exstrophy)
  - Discordance between genital appearance and a prenatal karyotype.
- *In older children and young adults*:
  - Previously unrecognized genital ambiguity
  - Virilization or inguinal hernia in a female
  - Primary amenorrhea
  - Delayed or incomplete puberty
  - Breast development or gross and occasionally cyclic hematuria in a male.

DIAGNOSTIC EVALUATION (FIG. 2)

Diagnostic algorithms exist, but with the spectrum of findings and diagnoses, no single evaluation protocol can be recommended in all circumstances.
- Abdominal/pelvic ultrasonography (USG)/magnetic resonance imaging (MRI): To assess the morphology of adrenal gland and Müllerian structure or morphology and location of gonads.
- Karyotype or fluorescent in-situ hybridization (FISH) for *SRY* gene.
- In a suspected congenital adrenal hyperplasia (CAH)—serum electrolytes, plasma renin activity, 8-AM 17-OH

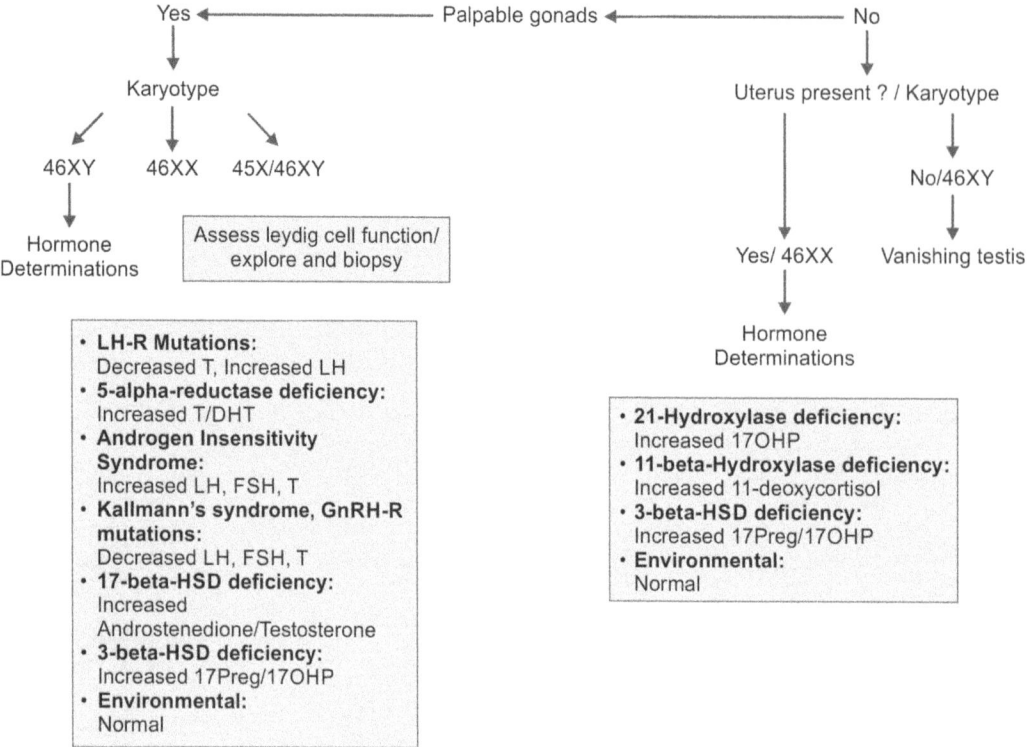

Fig 2: Symmetrical external genitalia.

progesterone (17-OHP), 8-AM serum cortisol, adrenal androgens.
- Determine adequacy of androgen synthesis/androgen action in undervirilized male: 8-AM luteinizing hormone (LH), follicle-stimulating hormone (FSH), testosterone (T), dihydrotestosterone (DHT).
- Determine adequacy of Leydig/Sertoli cell function in undervirilized male—human chorionic gonadotrophin (hCG) stimulation test, anti-Müllerian hormone (AMH), inhibin B.
- Determine adrenal steroidogenesis for milder forms of CAH—adrenocorticotropic hormone (ACTH) stimulation test.
- Genitogram to locate the vaginal–urethral confluence in relation to the bladder neck and the single opening of the urogenital sinus.
- Molecular genetic analysis to confirm the molecular basis of genital ambiguity.

MANAGEMENT

Optimal clinical management comprises the following:
- Gender assignment avoided before expert evaluation
- Evaluation and long-term management at a center with an experienced multidisciplinary team
- Open communication with patients and families
- Patient and family concerns addressed in strict confidence

In an ideal situation, a DSD team comprised of pediatric endocrinologist, pediatric surgeon or urologist, neonatologist/pediatrician, geneticist and a child psychiatrist/psychologist should be enabled, lead by the treating neonatologists/pediatricians. The parents need to participate in the discussions, especially where decisions regarding the options for gender of rearing and possible surgical interventions are to be made.

Medical Management

- Initial goal is to determine any life-threatening condition. Most DSDs in infancy do not require specific medical therapy except those with CAH.
- *Hormonal replacement therapy*: At the time of expected puberty, in children with hypogonadism.
- *CAH*: The goal of medical management is to suppress excess adrenal androgens, maintain replacement therapy for glucocorticoid and mineralocorticoid based on age, growth, and laboratory investigations and also avoid the adverse outcomes of adrenal crisis, stunted growth, pubertal disorders and obesity-related morbidities.

Surgical Management

- Genital reconstruction surgery (Emphasis is on functional outcome rather than a strictly cosmetic appearance. Surgical reconstruction in infancy may need a revision at the time of puberty.)
- Gonadectomy is based on patient's phenotype, karyotype, gender of rearing, psychosocial factors, and gonadal histology **(Table 2)**.

TABLE 2: Risk of gonadal tumors: Carcinoma-in-situ (CIS) or gonadoblastoma (15–30%).

Risk group	Disorders
High	Y (+) Gonadal dysgenesis, intra-abdominal gonads PAIS, nonscrotal gonads Frasier syndrome Denys–Drash syndrome
Intermediate	Y (+) Turner syndrome 17 beta-hydroxysteroid dehydrogenase deficiency Y (+) Gonadal dysgenesis, scrotal gonads PAIS, scrotal gonad
Low	CAIS Ovotesticular DSD Turner syndrome Y (−) gonads
No (?)	5-alpha reductase-2-deficiency Leydig cell hypoplasia

(CAIS: complete androgen insensitivity syndrome; DSD: disorders of sexual development; PAIS: partial androgen insensitivity syndrome)

Psychological Support

Psychosocial care can facilitate team decisions about gender assignment/reassignment, timing of surgery, and sex hormone replacement. Medical education and counseling for children is a recurrent gradual process.

Genetic Counseling

To confirm the diagnosis, explain prognosis, and assess the risk of recurrence in future pregnancies.

Talking to Parents

To explain in detail regarding the development of genital structures from same primordial tissues and there are no exclusive male or female hormones but the environments are characterized by differing relative amounts of these hormones. Discussion of concerns related to gender identity, pubertal development, sexual orientation, sexual function, and fertility.

Gender Assignment

Initial gender uncertainty is stressful for families. Gender assignment is to be done only when evaluation is complete: Diagnosis, surgical options, need for long-term hormone therapy, potential fertility and family and cultural factors.

Outcome

The outcome cannot be generalized across all DSDs due to the complexities involved in the diagnosis and management of different types of DSD. Also information across a range of assessment is insufficient in DSD. Some evidence is available based on long-term studies on outcome of children with CAH, complete androgen insensitivity syndrome (CAIS), and partial androgen insensitivity syndrome (PAIS), disorders of androgen biosynthesis, gonadal dysgenesis, and micropenis. Long-term outcome in DSD include external and internal genital phenotype, physical health including fertility, sexual function, and social and psychosexual adjustment, mental health, quality of life and social participation. It is also based on how smoothly these patients are transitioned from Pediatrics to adult care. It is generally agreed that timely diagnosis and management are important as they potentially prevent adverse health outcomes. The peer and parent support groups for chronic condition such as DSD is valuable and plays an important role in improving long-term health-related quality of life.

KEY MESSAGES

- The Lawson Wilkins Pediatric Endocrine Society and the European Society for Pediatric Endocrinology proposed the term *"Disorders of Sex Development" (DSD)* for children with atypical genitalia in 2006.
- DSD is a congenital condition characterized by atypical development of chromosomal, gonadal, hormonal, or anatomic aspects of sex.
- CAH is the most common etiology. Boys can be missed due to normal looking external genitalia.
- Diagnostic evaluation includes family history, prenatal history, a general physical examination for any associated dysmorphic features, an assessment of the genital anatomy along with hormone measurements, imaging, cytogenetic and molecular studies and in some cases endoscopic, laparoscopic, and gonadal biopsy.
- It is important to rule out life-threatening salt-wasting CAH. Presence of uterus, hyperpigmentation, and absence of palpable gonads suggests 46XX CAH, 21 hydroxylase deficiency.
- Symmetric external genitalia, palpable gonads, and absent uterus indicate toward undervirilized male.
- Management involves a multidisciplinary team for diagnosis, optimal timing for surgical intervention, need for long-term hormone therapy, potential fertility and psychosocial factors.

PRESCRIPTION ASSISTANCE: CONGENITAL ADRENAL HYPERPLASIA

- *Fluids*: Dehydration correction
- Intravenous (IV) hydrocortisone 25 mg/50 mg (infant/child) st at followed by
- 50–100 mg/m² 6 hourly
- Correction for hyperkalemia
- Tablet fludrocortisone 100–300 µg in two divided doses
- Taper hydrocortisone to 8–20 mg/m² in divided doses (three to four times a day)
- Salt 2 g/day till 1 year of age
- Emphasize the need for increased dose during illness, surgery, and stress
- Correction of genital abnormalities.

SUGGESTED READING

2. Dey S, Dey S. Disorders of Sexual Development. In: Khadilkar V, Bajpai A, Hemchand K Prasad (eds). IAP Text book on Pediatric Endocrinology. New Delhi: Jaypee Brothers Medical Publishers (P) Ltd.; 2019. pp. 267-72.
5. Lee MM. Molecular genetic control of sex differentiation. In: Pescovitz Oh, Eugster EA (eds). Pediatric Endocrinology, 1st edition. Philadelphia: Lippincott Williams and Wilkins; 2004. pp. 231-42.
1. Lee PA, Houk CP, Ahmed SF, Hughes IA; International Consensus Conference on Intersex organized by the Lawson Wilkins Pediatric Endocrine Society and the European Society for Paediatric Endocrinology. Consensus statement on management of intersex disorders. International Consensus Conference on Intersex Pediatrics. 2006;118:e488-500.
3. Warne GL, Greggio NA. Evaluation of a child with ambiguous genitalia: diagnosis and management. In: Desai MP, Bhatia V, Menon PSN (eds). Pediatric Endocrine Disorders, 3rd edition. Hyderabad: University Press; 2014. pp. 271-84.
4. Witchel SF, Lee PA. Ambiguous genitalia. In: Sperling MA (ed). Pediatric Endocrinology, 4th edition. Philadelphia: Elsevier Saunders; 2014. pp. 108-56.

SECTION 13: Rheumatology

147. Laboratory Tests in Pediatric Rheumatology
148. Juvenile Idiopathic Arthritis
149. Pediatric Systemic Lupus Erythematosus
150. Lupus Nephritis
151. Rheumatic Fever
152. Juvenile Dermatomyositis
153. Henoch–Schönlein Purpura
154. Kawasaki Disease

Laboratory Tests in Pediatric Rheumatology

Reena Karkhele, Vijay Kamale

INTRODUCTION

Pediatric rheumatic disorders are basically diagnosed with thorough history and physical examination. Laboratory studies are important adjuncts in management of such disorders. Laboratory evaluations help in the screening, confirming, and monitoring of rheumatic diseases. Investigations should be directed by provisional diagnosis in mind and to be used judiciously considering false positives and negatives and resources available.

Commonly done tests in pediatric rheumatology and their importance are illustrated in the following text.

HEMOGLOBIN

Hemoglobin (Hb) is moderately reduced in most rheumatologic conditions. The reason for low Hb is usually anemia of chronic disease. Iron deficiency anemia and anemia of chronic disease can be differentiated by measurement of serum transferrin, transferrin saturation, and ferritin.

Autoimmune hemolytic anemia (AIHA) may be seen in systemic lupus erythematosus (SLE) and related conditions [i.e., Sjögren syndrome, antiphospholipid antibody syndrome (APS) and mixed connective tissue disease (MCTD)]. It requires a positive direct Coombs test (mandatory) and evidence of hemolysis [increased reticulocyte count, increased lactate dehydrogenase (LDH), increased unconjugated bilirubin, and decreased haptoglobin].

Other causes are B_{12} deficiency, blood loss, pure red cell aplasia, macrophage activation syndrome, diffuse alveolar hemorrhage, thrombotic thrombocytopenic purpura (TTP), and drug-induced myelosuppression.

WHITE BLOOD CELL

Increased white blood cell (WBC) counts can be seen in systemic juvenile idiopathic arthritis (sJIA) and vasculitis. SLE and related conditions and drugs such as azathioprine and mycophenolate can cause leukopenia. Malignancies can cause either increased or decreased WBC counts, and is considered in any patient who presents with WBC abnormalities.

PLATELET

Platelets are frequently increased in the rheumatic diseases as one of the acute phase reactants (APR). Significant increases may be seen in sJIA, Kawasaki disease, or other vasculitis. SLE and related conditions, TTP, and APS often cause thrombocytopenia.

Macrophage activation syndrome (MAS) is a potentially life-threatening complication of sJIA, Kawasaki disease, and SLE. Either WBC, red blood cell (RBC), or platelets may decrease. Normalization of previously increased WBC or platelets in the face of a clinically worsening patient should alert to the possibility of MAS requiring urgent intervention. Possibility of MAS can be confirmed by other laboratory parameters including ferritin, LDH, fibrinogen, liver function test (LFT), and hemophagocytosis on bone marrow.

ACUTE PHASE REACTANTS

They include positive APR—erythrocyte sedimentation rate (ESR), C-reactive protein (CRP), ferritin, platelet count, haptoglobin (increased in inflammation) and negative APR—albumin, transferrin (decreased in inflammation) but they are not specific.

Erythrocyte Sedimentation Rate

Although not specific for inflammatory diseases, it is a valuable tool to monitor disease activity. ESR is affected by many factors including age, sex, Hb level, and immunoglobulin level. Persistent increase is associated with active synovitis and predicts more aggressive course in JIA. However, raised ESR is not always associated with disease activity.

Likewise, a normal ESR does not invariably suggest inactive disease. Decreasing ESR in an unwell child with sJIA and features of active inflammation should suggest MAS.

C-Reactive Protein

C-reactive protein has several advantages over the ESR.

It rises and falls early and is not affected by Hb levels. Persistent elevation of the CRP is a risk for amyloidosis, especially in systemic-onset JIA. It also has an important role in distinguishing between SLE disease flare versus an infection: A rise of CRP is uncommon in a disease flare (except with serositis) but increases in infections. Serum procalcitonin is more specific for infection but can be elevated in sJIA.

Both the ESR and the CRP JADAS (juvenile arthritis disease activity score) have been shown to be comparable and are useful markers of disease activity.

Ferritin

It is used to monitor disease activity in sJIA. It is not specific to rheumatologic diseases and can increase in iron overload, malignancies, and infections. In MAS, the ferritin level is frequently more than 10,000 ng/mL.

Liver Function Test and Renal Function Test

They are done in children with rheumatic disease at baseline and then every 3–6 months as indicated whenever they are on disease-modifying antirheumatic drugs (DMARDS).

MUSCLE ENZYMES

Serum levels of muscle enzymes are com-monly used for the diagnosis and monitoring of juvenile dermatomyositis (JDM). Individual patients may have increases in any of the commonly tested enzymes throughout their disease course, and, therefore, serial measurement of creatine kinase (CPK), alanine aminotransferase (ALT), aspartate aminotransferase (AST), LDH, and aldolase is recommended. 10% of children with myositis have normal enzymes.

ANTISTREPTOCOCCAL ANTIBODY

It is used in the diagnosis of acute rheumatic fever (ARF) and poststreptococcal reactive arthritis (PSRA). The most commonly used ones are the antistreptolysin O (ASO), anti-DNase B (ADB). ASO test to be repeated after 2–4 weeks and rising titers are more specific for diagnosis of ARF. After treatment of ARF, ASO levels may begin to normalize after 2 months but can stay increased for 6–12 months (longer if reinfection occurs). The ASO should be interpreted with care in the absence of a clear history of rheumatic fever or glomerulonephritis. In this context, it is likely to be a false positive, because of an unrelated polyclonal B-cell activation.

URINE ANALYSIS

Renal involvement is common in SLE, antineutrophil cytoplasmic antibody (ANCA), vasculitis, and IgA vasculitis which can be screened, diagnosed, and monitored with simple urine analysis. It should be done at every clinic visit. The urine sample should be examined for casts, RBCs, and proteinuria. Hematuria, proteinuria, and presence of cellular casts are indicative of disease activity. 24-hour urine protein estimation is better than urine spot protein/creatinine ratio (UP/UC) though latter is feasible in younger children.

TESTS SPECIFIC TO RHEUMATOLOGIC DISEASES

Rheumatoid Factor

Rheumatoid factor (RF) is useful in differentiating between two subtypes of polyarticular JIA: RF positive and RF negative. Testing for RF is generally not helpful in establishing or ruling out a diagnosis of JIA.

It is nonspecific test that can be seen in SLE, sarcoidosis and Sjögren syndrome. Since transient RF positivity can be seen in children related to infection, it needs to be reconfirmed after 12 weeks.

Anticyclic Citrullinated Peptide Antibodies

Anticyclic citrullinated peptide antibodies (anti-CCP) are highly specific for RA in adults. These antibodies are found primarily in children with polyarticular, and rarely other subsets of JIA. Anti-CCP antibodies have been associated with more aggressive disease. Patients with polyarthritis who are RF or anti-CCP positive, the course tends to be more aggressive.

Antinuclear Antibody

Antinuclear antibody (ANA) aids in diagnosis of various rheumatological conditions but should be used cautiously only when there is clinical suspicion as ANA positivity is seen in up to 20% of children who are either healthy or have benign musculoskeletal complaints also patients on drugs such as sulfasalazine or isoniazid. Conversely, a negative ANA has a strong (0.96–1) negative predictive value for SLE, MCTD, and other overlap disorders.

The gold standard method is indirect immunofluorescence (IIF). IIF provides information about the pattern and intensity of staining. Positive IIF should be followed by specific antibody testing by enzyme-linked immunosorbent assay (ELISA) which is guided by the ANA pattern, e.g., homogeneous pattern is seen in SLE, drug-induced lupus so should test for dsDNA and anti-histone antibody respectively, if there is speckled pattern considering clinical correlation can tests SSA/SSB for Sjögren or U1RNP for MCTD and so on. Some physicians prefer to do ANA immunoblot or ANA line immunoassay which tests different antigens at same time. ANA positivity more than triples the risk of uveitis in JIA; therefore, patients with JIA and a positive ANA are screened more frequently for chronic uveitis, which is generally asymptomatic and detected only through slit lamp examination by an ophthalmologist.

Anti-dsDNA is helpful in diagnosis and monitoring of disease activity in SLE. SSA/SSB antibodies are associated with neonatal lupus and mothers with these antibody positivity should be monitored antenatally for neonatal heart blocks.

Serum Complement Levels

Complement C3 and C4 levels are frequently measured as an adjunct to the clinical diagnosis and monitoring of patients with SLE. Low C3 and C4 is associated with disease activity. Some SLE patients have congenital deficiency of C4 and in them levels stay low despite control of disease activity. In IgA vasculitis, C4 is normal but C3 is low. Inherited and acquired deficiencies of certain complement components (C1, C2, C3, C4, mannose-binding lectin, and C1 inhibitor) are associated with SLE. CH50 assay is reliable screening test for homozygous deficiencies in the classic pathway components, which have strongest association with lupus.

Antineutrophil Cytoplasmic Antibody

Granulomatous polyangiitis (GPA), microscopic polyangiitis (MPA), and eosinophilic granulomatous polyangiitis (EGPA) are grouped under ANCA vasculitis in view of the antibody positivity. In these conditions, the target of ANCA binding is usually either myeloperoxidase (MPO) or serine protease 3 (PR3). MPO and PR3 to be tested by high-quality ELISA and their levels to be monitored for disease activity and remission.

Angiotensin-converting Enzyme

Its level is frequently increased in sarcoidosis, and the level of increase corresponds to clinical disease activity. A large, multicenter study of patients with sarcoidosis revealed the sensitivity of angiotensin-converting enzyme (ACE) for sarcoidosis to be 57% and specificity of 90%. As a substantial number of patients, especially early-onset sarcoidosis may have a normal ACE, the gold standard remains tissue diagnosis.

Antiphospholipid Antibodies

There are three commonly used tests to assay for APLs: (1) Lupus anticoagulant (LA) tests; (2) ELISA for anticardiolipin (ACL) IgG and IgM; (3) ELISA for anti-β2- glycoprotein- I (anti- β2GPI) IgG and IgM. LA is tested for through either the activated partial thromboplastin time (aPTT) or the dilute Russell viper venom time (DRVVT). Persistently positive LA test is only 72% sensitive but confers a strong risk for thrombotic events, especially in patients with underlying SLE.

Anticardiolipin antibodies have high sensitivity, while antibodies to beta-2 glycoprotein have higher specificity. Tests to be repeated after 12 weeks for confirmation.

MISCELLANEOUS TESTS

Thyroid Function Tests

It is important to do thyroid function tests in children with JIA as it is abnormal in up to 12% of patients.

Human Leukocyte Antigen B27

There is a well-established relationship between human leukocyte antigen B27 (HLA-B27) and enthesitis-related arthritis (ERA). HLA-B27 is present in 65–80% of patients with ERA and in about 60% of children with reactive arthritis. Tests is done either by flow cytometry or polymerase chain reaction (PCR) of which PCR is more specific.

TESTS FOR AUTOINFLAMMATORY DISEASES

Autoinflammatory diseases are monogenic diseases; thus, molecular diagnosis is important but available only at few centers across the world. A normal CRP during an attack almost rules out autoinflammatory disease. Most important clue comes when common diseases are excluded and the patient has multiple self-limiting episodes of fever.

KEY MESSAGES

- Laboratory tests are only adjuncts in diagnosis of rheumatic disorders in children, thorough history and examination are indispensable.
- Targeted testing is the best approach.
- Sensitivity, specificity, and false positivity of the tests are to be considered before arriving at conclusion.
- Newer advances in technology and molecular diagnosis will bring the era of precision and personalized medicine.

SUGGESTED READING

1. Hochberg M, Silman A, Gravallese E, Smolen J, Weinblatt M, Weisman M. Hochberg Textbook of Rheumatology. Philadelphia: Elsevier; 2018.
2. Petty RE, Laxer RM, Lindsley CB, Wedderburn L. Textbook of Pediatric Rheumatology, 7th edition. Philadelphia: Elsevier; 2016.
3. Sawhney S, Aggarwal A. Pediatric Rheumatology: Clinical Viewpoint. Singapore: Springer; 2017.

CHAPTER 148

Juvenile Idiopathic Arthritis

Reena Karkhele, Vijay Kamale

INTRODUCTION

Juvenile idiopathic arthritis (JIA) is one of the most common chronic diseases of childhood, with an estimated prevalence of 1 per 1,000 children. JIA broadly refers to a group of heterogeneous diseases that share the common feature of chronic inflammatory arthritis of unknown cause lasting longer than 6 weeks with onset before 16 years of age.

In the International League of Associations for Rheumatology (ILAR) classification, JIA subtypes are categorized based on predominant clinical and laboratory features presenting during the first 6 months of disease. Principle underlying the ILAR classification is that all categories are mutually exclusive **(Table 1)**.

DIAGNOSIS

The diagnosis of JIA is made from history and physical examination. Symptom of morning stiffness is important to differentiate inflammatory arthritis from that of non-

TABLE 1: General definition of JIA.

Jivenile idiopathic arthritis is arthritis of unknown etiology that begins before the sixteenth birthday and persists for at lease 6 weeks; other known conditions are excluded.

Sucategory	Definition	Exclusions
Oligoarticular JIA Two sucategories are recognized: 1. Persistent oligoarticular JIA: affecting <4 joints throughout the disease course 2. Extended oligoarticular JIA: affecting a total of >4 joints after the first 6 months of disease	Arthritis affecting 1–4 joints during the first 6 months of disease	a. Psoriasis or a history of psoriasis in the patient or a first-degree relative b. Arthritis in a human leukocyte antigen (HLA)–B27* male beginning after the sixth birthday c. Ankylosing spondylitis, ERA, sacroilitis with inflammatory bowel disease, Reiter's syndrome, or acute anterior uveitis, or a history of one of these disorders in a first-degree relative d. The presence of IgM RF on at least 2 occasions, at least 3 months apart e. The presence of systemic JIA in the patient
RF - polyarticular JIA	1. Arthritis affecting >5 joints during the first 6 months of disease, and 2. Test for RF is negative	a, b, c, d, e
RF + polyarticular JIA	1. Arthritis affecting >5 joints during the first 6 months of disease, and 2. >2 positive RF tests (as routinely defined in an accredited laoratory), at least 3 months apart during the first 6 months of disease	a, b, c, e

Psoriatic arthritis	1. Arthritis and psoriasis, or
	2. Arthritis and at least 2 of the following:
	  a. Dactylitis
	  b. Nail pitting (minimum of 2 pits on >1 nails at any time) or onycholysis
	  c. Psoriasis in a first-degree relative	

Contd...

Contd...

Sucategory	Definition	Exclusions

Enthesitis-related arthritis	1. Arthritis and enthesitis, or
	2. Arthritis or enthesitis, with at least 2 of the following:
	  a. The presence of or a history of sacroiliac joint tenderness and/or inflammatory lumbosacral pain
	  b. The presence of HIA-B27
	  c. Onset of arthritis in a male >6 years of age
	  d. Acute (symptomatic) anterior uveitis
	  e. History of ankylosing spondylitis, ERA, sacroillitis with inflammatory bowel disease, Reiter's syndrome, or acute anterior uveitis in a first-degree relative
		b, c d, e

Systemic JIA	Arthritis in >1 joints with, or preceded by, fever of at least 2 weeks' duration that is documented to be daily and quotidian (fever that rises to >39°C once a day and returns to <37°C between fever peaks) for at least 3 days, and accompanied >1 of the following:
	  a. Evanescent (nonfixed) erythematous rash
	  b. Generalized lymph node enlargement
	  c. Hepatomegaly and/or splenomegaly
	  d. Serositis
		a, d, e

Undifferentiated arthritis	Arthritis that fulfills criteria in no category or in >2 of the above categories	

(ERA: enthesitis-related arthritis; ILAR: international league of associations for rheumatology; RF: rheumatoid factor)
Source: From Petty RE, Southwood TR, Manners P, et al: International League of Associations for Rheumatology classification of juvenile idiopathic arthritis: second revision, Edmonton, 2001. J Rheumatol. 2004;31(2):390-92.

inflammatory; however, stiffness may be difficult to assess in young children. Joint stiffness is most pronounced in the morning, usually described by parents as an abnormal gait. Older children may report not able to brush or difficulty getting up from bed. Stiffness usually improves throughout the day with increased activity or with warm showers. Similarly, inflammatory back pain is defined when there is early morning stiffness which improves with activity.

Other specific symptom is swelling of joints. Joint pain may be absent, especially in younger children; pain need not be present to diagnose JIA. On physical examination, active arthritis is characterized by joint swelling, warmth, decreased range of motion, and tenderness **(Table 2)**.

OLIGOARTHRITIS

Oligoarthritis is the most common category of JIA. Oligoarthritis is further classified as being either persistent or extended. Disease onset peaks between 1 and 3 years of age; predominant in girls with male-to-female ratio of 1:3. 20–30% of children with oligoarthritis can develop chronic anterior uveitis.

Children with a positive antinuclear antibody (ANA) are at greater risk for the development of uveitis. Serious complications associated with iridocyclitis include posterior synechiae, band keratopathy, cataract, and glaucoma. Since uveitis is asymptomatic at onset, slit-lamp examination every 3 months should be carried out in ANA-positive patients.

POLYARTHRITIS

Polyarthritis accounts for approximately 25% of all JIA diagnoses, and roughly 85% of these patients are rheumatoid factor (RF) negative. RF can be associated with important differences in disease manifestations and response to therapy.

Rheumatoid Factor-negative Polyarthritis

Rheumatoid factor-negative polyarthritis typically presents early between 1 and 3 years of age or later during adolescence. It tends to be limited to articular involvement; however, chronic anterior uveitis occurs in approximately 14%. The temporomandibular joint (TMJ) is commonly affected in patients with polyarthritis, and the risk seems to be higher in the RF-negative category. TMJ arthritis may manifest as micrognathia, retrognathia, asymmetry, and jaw deviation.

Rheumatoid Factor-positive Polyarthritis

This category is often equivalent to typical adult-onset rheumatoid arthritis (RA) in terms of clinical presentation, investigation, and prognosis. It presents with pain and swelling of several joints, including wrists, metacarpophalangeal, proximal interphalangeal, and distal interphalangeal joints of fingers on both hands. Cervical spine arthritis may result in atlantoaxial subluxation. Rheumatoid nodules are reported in about a third of patients.

TABLE 2: Characteristics of the various categories of juvenile idiopathic arthritis.

Category	Age at onset	Affected joints	Systemic features	Major complications
Oligoarticular persistent	Early childhood	Large joints, asymmetric (knee, ankle, wrist, elbow, temporomandibular, cervical spine)	No	Chronic uveitis Local growth disturbances
Oligoarticular extended	Early childhood	Same as above, but more than four joints involved after the first 6 months of disease	No	Chronic uveitis Local growth disturbances
Polyarticular RF negative	Throughout childhood	Any, often symmetric, often small joints	Malaise (sufebrile)	Chronic uveitis Local growth disturbances
Polyarticular RF positive	Teenage years	Any, usually symmetric and involving small joints	Malaise (sufebrile)	Local growth disturbances and articular damage
Systemic	Throughout childhood	Any (not necessarily at disease onset)	High fever, rash, polyserositis, marked acute-phase response	Acute: macrophage activation syndrome Chronic: general growth disturbance, amyloidosis
Psoriatic	Late childhood	Spine, lower extremities, distal interphalangeal joints, dactylitis		Psoriasis Local growth disturbances
Enthesitis related	Late childhood	Spine, sacroiliac, lower extremities, thoracic cage joints	Inflammatory bowel disease	Acute symptomatic uveitis

(RF: rheumatoid factor)

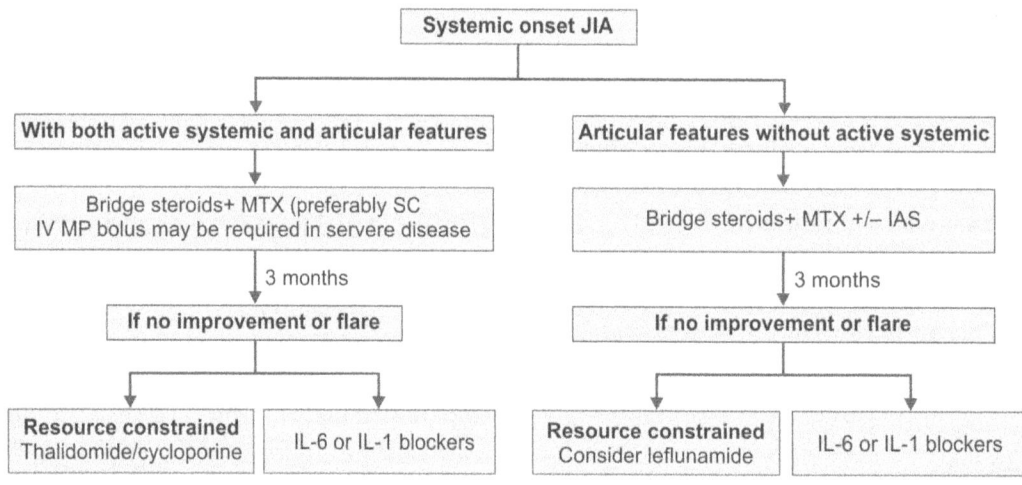

Flowchart 1: Algorithmic approach for systemic onset JIA.

SYSTEMIC ARTHRITIS

It comprises 5% of the total JIA and is defined by its extra-articular features of fever and rash (**Flowchart 1**). Girls and boys are affected equally. The fever typically rises to >39°C daily and returns to <37°C between fever peaks. Fever usually occurs daily or twice daily. Child appears toxic with the fever and can have accompanying shaking chills, but not rigor.

In 90% of cases, a characteristic evanescent salmon-colored macular or maculopapular rash occurs on the trunk, thighs, and upper arms, mostly accompanies fever and can be brought out by scratching of the skin (Köbener phenomenon). Generalized lymphadenopathy and hepatosplenomegaly occur in 50-75% of patients. Liver enzyme levels may be slightly elevated, although fulminant hepatic failure is rare. Polyserositis is common, with about one third of patients having documented pericarditis. Approximately half of the children with systemic JIA develop polyarthritis within 3-12 months of the onset of the fever. The wrists, knees, and ankles are most commonly involved, with the cervical spine, hips, TMJs and hands also being affected.

Macrophage activation syndrome (MAS) is a serious complication that occurs in 5-40% of children with systemic JIA. MAS is characterized by rapid development of fever, rash, and encephalopathy; rapid rise of liver transaminases; disseminated intravascular coagulopathy; neutropenia; thrombocytopenia; increased triglyceride levels; low albumin level; and a low ESR associated with hypofibrinogenemia. The diagnosis is made clinically and is supported by very high ferritin levels (often >10,000 mg/L), high soluble transferrin receptor (sCD25), and demonstration of hemophagocytosis in the bone marrow.

PSORIATIC ARTHRITIS

Dactylitis, nail pitting, distal interphalangeal arthritis, and asymmetric RF-negative peripheral arthritis are typical findings in juvenile PSa. A significant proportion of children may develop inflammatory back disease, including spondyloarthritis and sacroiliitis.

ENTHESITIS-RELATED ARTHRITIS

Enthesitis-related arthritis (ERA) affects boys more than girls and presents most commonly after the age of 6 years. Arthritis typically involves the lower extremities, most commonly the knees and ankles, but the hip can also be affected. Enthesitis, defined as "tenderness at the insertion of the tendon, ligament, joint capsule or fascia to bone," occurs frequently and is commonly seen as plantar fasciitis, Achilles tendinitis, and patellar tendon enthesitis. Inflammatory back pain is often seen. Those with human leukocyte antigen B27 (HLA-B27), a family history of spondyloarthritis, and definite arthritis are more likely to develop spondyloarthritis at follow-up. Iritis is usually acute and symptomatic.

UNDIFFERENTIATED ARTHRITIS

Cases are excluded from the other categories either because they fulfill criteria for two or more categories or because an exclusion criterion did not allow them to be put into any of the other categories. In a Scandinavian study, about 15% of JIA cases could not be classified into any of the other categories.

Growth disturbances are common to all JIA categories and to be looked for. The most common localized growth abnormality is a leg-length discrepancy caused by increased growth from arthritis of the knee.

LABORATORY EVALUATION

There is no single laboratory test that differentiates JIA from other diseases. The main role of laboratory investigations is to exclude other diseases such as leukemia or infection. ANAs, RF, and HLA-B27 are mainly useful in further categorization and prediction of outcome.

Erythrocyte sedimentation rate and C-reactive protein (CRP) are useful tests to differentiate children with JIA from children with noninflammatory disorders. However, normal levels do not rule out JIA.

Anemia can occur in all forms of JIA, Usually the anemia of chronic disease. Serum ferritin level may be elevated. Leukocytosis with a neutrophil predominance is seen in children with systemic JIA. Although thrombocytosis is common, thrombocytopenia is not part of JIA and should prompt a workup for systemic lupus erythematosus or malignancy.

At present, research into new biomarkers of disease activity, such as cytokines and MRP8/14, serum amyloid A, and S100 in addition to immunogenetic markers, is ongoing, but no test has yet been established as a routine clinical tool to help in diagnosis.

IMAGING

Traditional radiography is not able to detect the presence of synovial and soft-tissue inflammation. Ultrasonography and magnetic resonance imaging (MRI) have therefore assumed increasing importance in the diagnostic workup. An increasing range of MRI techniques with different pulse sequences is presently used to improve the visualization of relevant tissue. MRI is expensive and time consuming, and general anesthesia is often necessary in youngest children.

Ultrasonography, which can be done at the bedside, is helpful in visualizing joint effusions, synovitis, and enthesitis. It can be used to guide the needle for intra-articular injections.

TREATMENT

Since systemic arthritis is now considered an auto-inflammatory syndrome, its treatment differs from other JIA class. It will be discussed separately.

The main aims of medications are to achieve complete control of the disease with normalization of physical findings and laboratory markers of inflammation and to prevent any long-term consequences related to the disease.

Since JIA is not a single disease, different therapeutic approaches should be adopted according to the diverse-onset subtypes. Nonetheless, general guiding principles may be considered. Oral nonsteroidal anti-inflammatory drugs (NSAIDs) are the initial treatment for the majority of JIA patients. The approved NSAIDs for use include naproxen, ibuprofen, indomethacin, and meloxicam.

Intra-articular steroid injections are commonly needed at disease onset or during disease course since their quick effectiveness is pivotal in prevention of deformities. The long-acting steroid triamcinolone hexacetonide is used commonly.

Patients who do not respond effectively to these approaches need second-line agents. Methotrexate (MTX) is considered the second-line agent of choice for persistent active arthritis. Its efficacy begins after a lapse of 1–3 months; therefore, especially in patients with severe polyarthritis, a short course of low-dose prednisone might be considered as a bridging agent until MTX is effective. Its most common side effects are nausea, mouth sores, abdominal pain, raised liver enzymes, and less commonly bone marrow suppression.

Monthly blood tests should be performed to monitor liver function and bone marrow abnormalities. To reduce the side effects, supplement at ion with folic acid should be concomitant.

Leflunomide: Although its efficacy in polyarticular JIA has been recently demonstrated in a clinical trial, its use in children is still limited.

Sulfasalazine is more frequently used in ERA and inflammatory bowel disease; however, studies have shown a benefit in both oligoarthritis and polyarthritis. Adverse events include rash and GI upset, sulfa allergy.

For those unresponsive or intolerant to conventional antirheumatic agents, the introduction of biological should be considered. Etanercept, a soluble TNFα (tumor nuclear factor alpha) receptor, is used in polyarthritis/extended oligoarthritis. Adalimumab is anti-TNF of choice in case of JIA-associated uveitis. Other anti-TNFI include infliximab, golimumab, and certolizumab. Abatacept, CTLA-4Ig (cytotoxic T lymphocyte-associated antigen-4-Ig) inhibitor, is an approved therapeutic option for patients with polyarthritis. Interleukin-6 inhibitor, tocilizumab is effective in polyarticular JIA.

The future treatment of oligoarthritis and polyarthritis: Newer therapies that have demonstrated effectiveness in adults with RA are currently being studied in children with JIA. Tofacitinib is a Janus kinase inhibitor has been shown to be effective in polyarticular JIA, PSa, and ERA. Biosimilars are a kintogeneric medication but may not have precise chemical structure of original therapeutic agent because of the slight differences in their manufacture. Biosimilars should help lower the economic costs of biologics.

Physiotherapy and occupational therapy are integrated part of treatment of JIA to avoid contractures and muscle atrophy.

Treatment of Systemic-onset Juvenile Idiopathic Arthritis

For patients with active systemic features (with or without arthritis), a short course of NSAID monotherapy may be indicated in the initial workup of these patients but is not considered appropriate in those with severe disease. The following algorithm explains in brief the approach but will differ for each patient.

The American College of Rheumatology (ACR) recommendations and also a new consensus guideline by the Childhood Arthritis and Rheumatology Research Alliance (CARRA) network have focused heavily on the use of anakinra (IL1 blocker) and tocilizumab for the treatment of the child with systemic JIA.

PROGNOSIS AND OUTCOME

The prognosis of patients with JIA has improved considerably in recent decades. The outcome of JIA is variable, even in the same JIA category, and it is difficult at disease onset to predict. The development of new therapies has markedly increased ability to effectively treat JIA, and future appears promising. However, there is still lack of evidence-based medicine in the treatment of JIA.

KEY MESSAGES

- Juvenile idiopathic arthritis is a diagnosis of exclusion, malignancy, infections and metabolic disorders should be looked for.
- All JIA patients should undergo screening for uveitis as it is asymptomatic.
- Correct diagnosis, prompt referral, and early aggressive therapy are key to success.
- Timely immunization, rehabilitation, psychological and social support are important.

SUGGESTED READING

1. Hochberg M, Silman A, Gravallese E, Smolen J, Weinblatt M, Weisman M. Hochberg Textbook of Rheumatology, 7th edition. Netherlands: Elsevier; 2018.
2. Petty RE, Laxer RM, Lindsley CB, Wedderburn L. Textbook of Pediatric Rheumatology, 7th edition. Philadelphia: Elsevier; 2015.
3. Ringold S, Angeles-Han ST, Beukelman T, Lovell D, Cuello CA, Becker ML, et al. 2019 American College of Rheumatology/Arthritis Foundation Guideline for the treatment of juvenile idiopathic arthritis. Arthritis Care Res (Hoboken). 2019;71(6):717-34.
4. Sawhney Sujata, Aggarwal A. Pediatric Rheumatology: Clinical Viewpoint. Singapore: Springer; 2017.

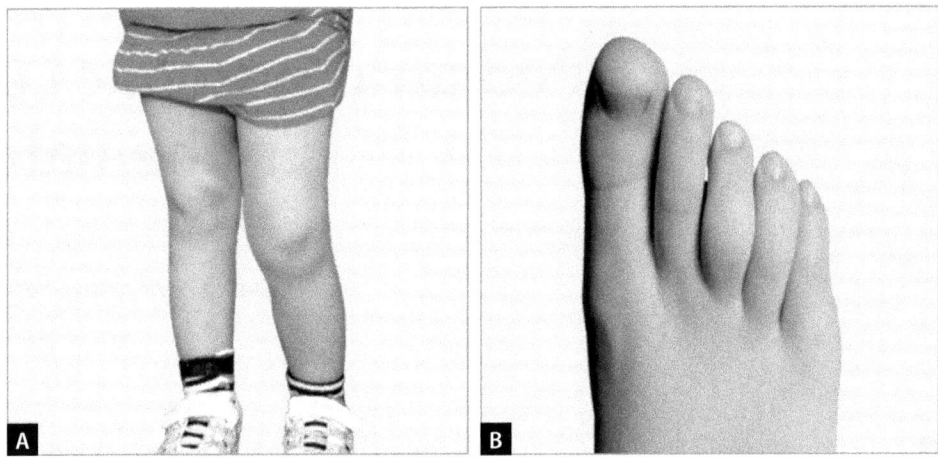

Figs. 1A and B: (A) Oligoarticular jia left knee; (B) Dactylitis of 3rd toe.

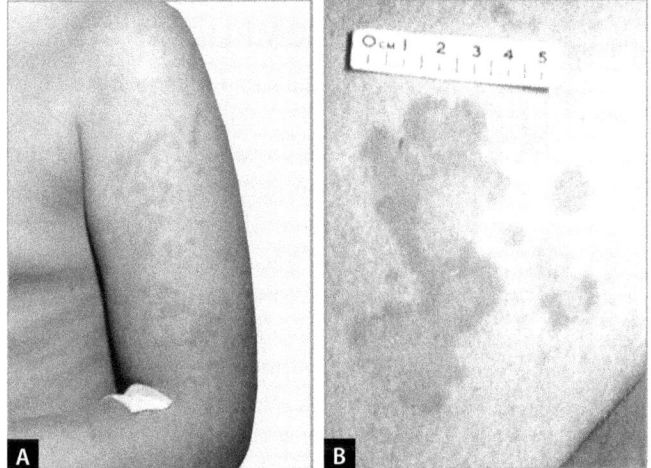

Figs. 2A and B: The rash of systemic juvenile idiopathic arthritis. Larger lesions are becoming confluent (A). This must be differentiated from erythema marginatum (B). Characteristic of the rash seen in rheumatic fever.

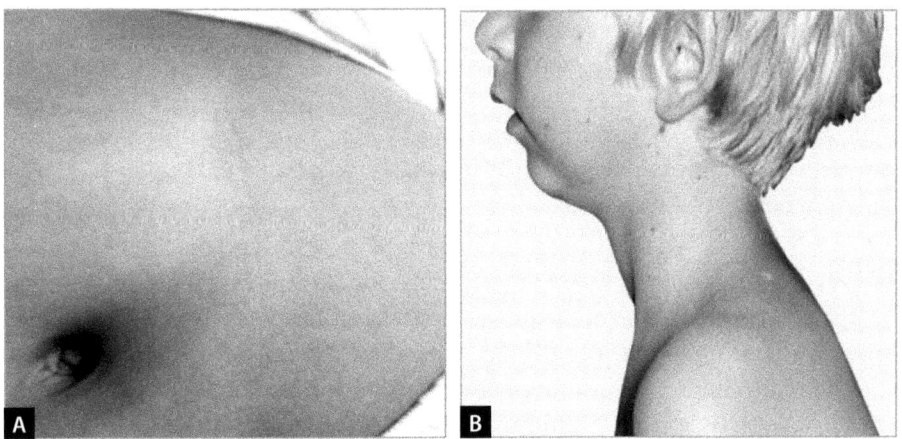

Figs. 3A and B: (A) Koebner phenomenon in a child with SJIA; (B) Retrognathia-TMJ arthritis.

Pediatric Systemic Lupus Erythematosus

Jijo Joseph John, Reny Joseph

INTRODUCTION

Systemic lupus erythematosus (SLE) is a chronic autoimmune disease characterized by multisystem inflammation and the production of antibodies directed against self-antigens. 20% of SLE cases are diagnosed in the first two decades of life. Compared to adults, children with SLE have a more severe disease process and more widespread organ involvement. Reported prevalence of pediatric SLE (pSLE) is 1–6 per 100,000 children. The median age at onset is 11–12 years. There is a female preponderance of the disease with 2–5:1 female-to-male ratio prepuberty and 9:1 female-to-male ratio during reproductive years.

PATHOGENESIS

Systemic lupus erythematosus is caused by loss of tolerance, with the development of antibodies against self-antigens, most commonly nucleic acids. Dysregulation of interferon α is now thought to be an important factor in the loss of self-tolerance, leading to autoimmunity. Autoantibodies form circulating immune complexes and deposit on various tissues, leading to local complement activation, initiation of a pro-inflammatory cascade and tissue damage. Genetic predisposition to SLE is found in individuals with congenital deficiencies of complement factors C1q, C2, and C4. Also, certain human leukocyte antigen (HLA) types such as HLAB8, DR2, and DR3 are found with greater frequency in patients with SLE than in the general population.

There are various other environmental (silica exposure), infectious (Epstein–Barr virus), and hormonal influences that play a role in the pathophysiology of the disease.

CLINICAL FEATURES

Systemic lupus erythematosus is known as one of the great mimickers, as the clinical manifestations are varied and can involve any organ system. In children, constitutional symptoms, hematological abnormalities, and arthritis/arthralgia are the most common presenting features. Pediatric lupus can also develop in children previously diagnosed to have polyarticular/systemic juvenile idiopathic arthritis (JIA). SLE symptoms may not develop at the same time, and new symptoms may develop years after initial presentation, hence longitudinal follow-up of these children is required. The varied presentation of SLE is given in **Table 1**.

COMPLICATIONS

The most common cause of death in the initial few years after diagnosis of SLE is infections, complications from glomerulonephritis, and neuropsychiatric illnesses. Various chronic complications as per the treatment administered should be looked out for such as steroids causing osteoporosis or fractures, and cyclophosphamide causing infertility. These children are at a higher risk of atherosclerosis and myocardial infarction. There is an increased risk of malignancy. A routine eye examination is essential to prevent permanent blindness due to retinal detachment. These children can also have various endocrine problems such as diabetes, obesity, growth failure, and infertility.

Pregnancy during disease flares is associated with an increased risk for spontaneous abortions and hence appropriate contraceptive advice should be given to all teenage girls with SLE.

DIAGNOSIS

The diagnosis of SLE requires detailed clinical and laboratory evaluation to establish the disease as well as to rule out other differentials such as malignancy. Earlier diagnostic criteria included The American College of Rheumatology criteria (ACR-revised 1997), (initially published in 1982 and revised in 1997), and the 2012 Systemic Lupus International Collaborating Clinics (SLICC) classification criteria. However, these classification systems were found to be ideal for long-standing cases and did not classify new cases well. The latest classification criteria are the 2019 European League Against Rheumatism (EULAR)/ACR SLE classification criteria, which uses an entry criterion of antinuclear antibody (ANA) positivity and weighted clinical and immunological features. Children with ANA positivity and a total score of ≥10, with

TABLE 1: Clinical features of SLE.

System involved	Clinical features
Nonspecific constitutional symptoms	Fever, fatigue, anorexia, weight loss, arthralgia, alopecia, generalized lymphadenopathy
Mucocutaneous	• Malar rash, discoid rash, photosensitivity, alopecia, cutaneous vasculitis, Raynaud's phenomenon, vasculitic rash, palmoplantar/periungual erythema, and bullous lesions • Painless ulcers on the hard palate, nasal septal perforation, panniculitis
Musculoskeletal	• Arthralgia and/or non-erosive arthritis,* myositis, tendonitis • Secondary pain amplification, and Avascular necrosis
Hematological	• *Cytopenias*: Leukopenia, lymphopenia, neutropenia, Anemia† • Thrombocytopenia • APLA positivity and thromboembolic phenomenon, thrombotic microangiopathy
Neuropsychiatric	Headache, psychosis, cerebrovascular disease and cognitive dysfunction, seizures, chorea, CVA, transverse myelitis, peripheral neuropathy, cranial nerve palsies, and optic neuritis
Renal	Proteinuria, hematuria††, hypertension, renal failure, nephrotic syndrome
Cardiovascular	Pericarditis, myocarditis, conduction system abnormalities, Libman–Sacks endocarditis
Pulmonary	Pleuritis, interstitial lung disease, pulmonary hemorrhage, pulmonary hypertension
Gastroenterology	Hepatosplenomegaly, pancreatitis, protein-losing enteropathy, peritonitis
Ocular	Retinal vasculitis, scleritis, episcleritis, papilledema, dry eyes, optic neuritis

*Arthritis in SLE is usually symmetrical polyarthritis and involves both large and small joints. One of the most common presenting features in pediatric systemic lupus erythematosus (pSLE).
†Anemia of chronic disease, iron deficiency anemia or Coomb's-positive hemolytic anemia.
††Hematuria can range from microscopic to frank hematuria, similarly, proteinuria can be minimal to nephrotic range proteinuria.
(APLA: antiphospholipid antibodies; CVA: cerebrovascular accident)

at least one clinical criterion are classified as having SLE **(Fig. 1)**.

DIFFERENTIAL DIAGNOSIS

Systemic lupus erythematosus can be a differential diagnosis for a wide variety of clinical scenarios, given its wide array of potential clinical manifestations. The initial diagnosis for children ultimately diagnosed with SLE may include infections [sepsis, Epstein–Barr (EBV), parvovirus B19, endocarditis], malignancies (leukemia and lymphoma), other rheumatological conditions (systemic-onset juvenile idiopathic arthritis, acute rheumatic fever) and drug-induced lupus. Drug-induced lupus refers to SLE manifestations induced by exposure to specific medications such as minocycline, anticonvulsants, sulfonamides, and antiarrhythmic drugs. Drug-induced lupus does not have a female preponderance. Anti-histone antibodies are seen in drug-induced lupus, which is seen only in 20% of individuals with SLE.

INVESTIGATIONS

- *Complete blood counts (CBCs)*: Anemia, leukopenia, lymphopenia, and thrombocytopenia.
- *Metabolic panel*: Liver and renal function tests—to rule out transaminitis, hypoalbuminemia, and elevated creatinine.
- *Inflammatory markers*: Erythrocyte sedimentation rate (ESR) elevated in active disease, while C-reactive protein (CRP) correlates less well with disease activity. Acutely elevated CRP may reflect infection, while mild chronic elevation of CRP may point to increased cardiovascular risk.
- *Urinalysis*: Proteinuria, hematuria.
- *Autoantibody panel*:
  - *Antinuclear antibody*: Good sensitivity as positive ANA is present in 95–99% individuals with SLE; however, 20% of the normal population also has ANA positivity. ANA titers do not correlate well with disease activity.
  - *Anti-double stranded DNA (Anti-dsDNA)*: More specific for SLE, and in some children with significant nephritis, dsDNA levels correlate well with disease activity.
  - *Anti-Smith antibody*: Specific for SLE, no correlation with disease activity.
  - *Anti-ribonuclear protein*: Often indicative of mixed connective tissue disorder (SLE with myositis).
  - *Anti-SSA and SSB*: In neonatal lupus.
- *Complement levels*: Serum levels of total hemolytic complement (CH50), C3, and C4 are decreased inactive disease and improve once disease activity improves.
- *Gamma-globulin*: Hypergammaglobulinemia seen in active disease.

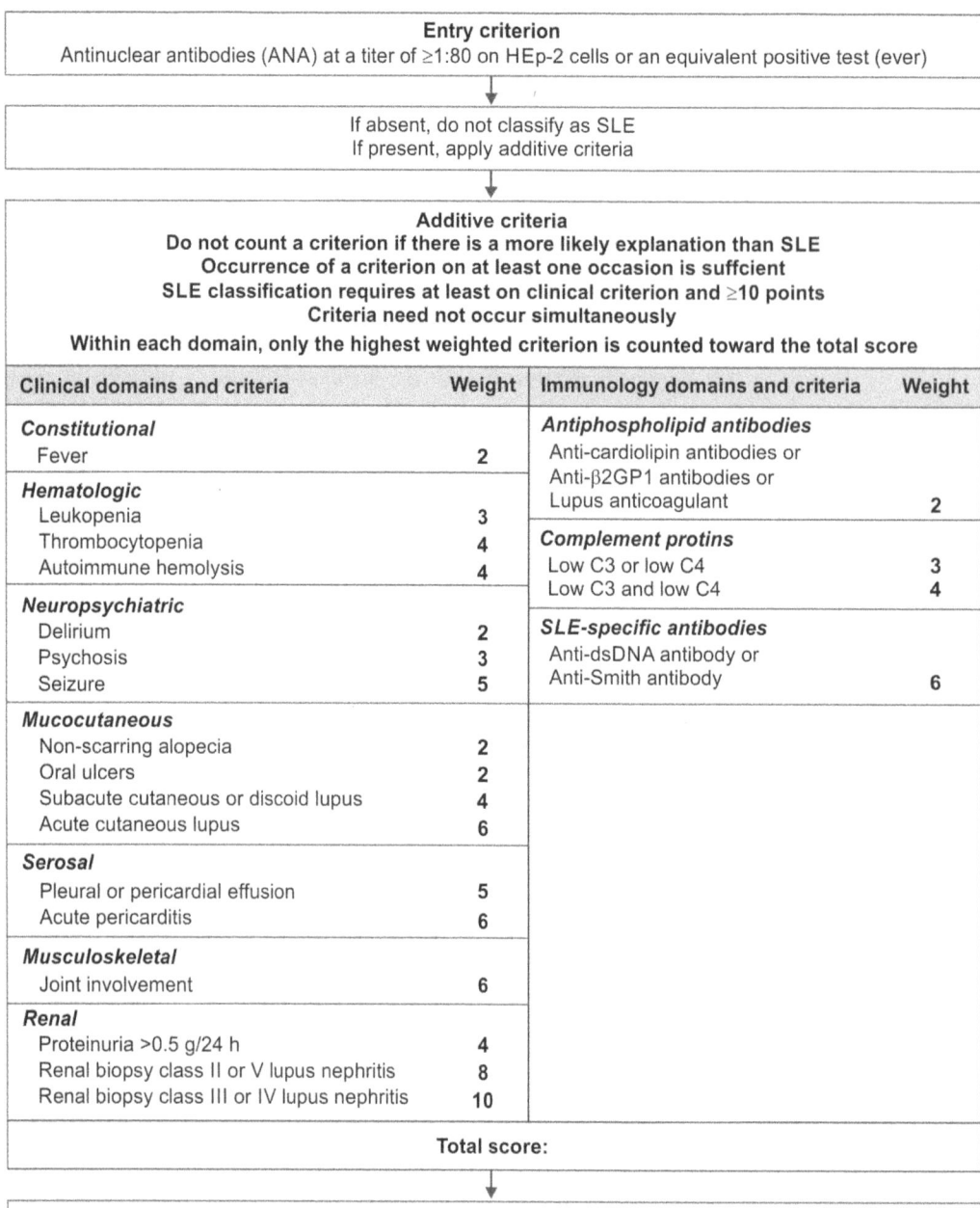

Fig. 1: EULAR/ACR SLE classification criteria 2019.
(ACR: American College of Rheumatology; EULAR: European League Against Rheumatism; SLE: systemic lupus erythematosus)

- *Antiphospholipid antibodies*: Found in up to 66% of children with SLE, denotes an increased clotting risk.
- Direct Coomb's test positivity in the absence of hemolysis.

MANAGEMENT

Treatment is tailored to individuals depending on manifestations. Prolonged sunlight and other UV light exposure avoidance should be stressed at each visit for all patients, along with the use of sunscreen with SPF > 30.

- Hydroxychloroquine (HCQs) (5–7 mg/kg/day up to 400 mg/day) is recommended for all individuals with SLE if tolerated. Potential toxicities include retinal pigmentation and color vision impairment. Ophthalmology consultation is mandatory for all patients for HCQs once every 6–12 months.
- Nonsteroidal anti-inflammatory drugs (NSAIDs) are useful for the management of arthritis and arthralgia. Potential GI, hepatic, and renal side effects should be kept in mind before prescribing long-term NSAIDs.
- *Corticosteroids*: Mainstay of therapy for the treatment of significant manifestations and to treat acute flares. Severe disease is often treated with high-dose methylprednisolone (30 mg/kg/day for 3 days, followed by oral steroids) or high-dose oral prednisolone

(1–2 mg/kg/day). Steroid doses can be gradually tapered over months.
- Steroid-sparing immunosuppressive agents may be needed to prevent cumulative steroid side effects. Commonly used drugs include methotrexate, leflunomide, azathioprine, mycophenolate mofetil, and cyclophosphamide.
- *Biologicals*:
  - *Belimumab*: Belimumab is a human immunoglobulin G1λ monoclonal antibody that inhibits B cell survival by blocking the soluble B-lymphocyte stimulator (BLyS). This was one of the first biologicals to be approved for use in SLE, and the Food and Drug Administration (FDA) approved its use for pSLE in 2019.
  - *Rituximab*: Rituximab is a chimeric monoclonal antibody against CD20 receptors, which binds to CD20-positive B cells and leads to B-cell depletion. It is hypothesized to control disease activity in refractory cases of SLE. Various randomized control trials are underway to demonstrate the significant benefits of Rituximab as a steroid-sparing agent in pSLE.
  - There are various other biological such as T-cell-targeted therapy (Abatacept and Laquinimod), IL-6 targeting therapies (Tocilizumab), Interferon-alpha-targeting therapy (Sifalimumab, Rontalizumab) and anti-tumor nuclear factor-alpha (TNFα) (Etanercept and Infliximab), among various others. Studies are underway to determine clinical efficacy and side-effects of these therapies in pSLE.

MONITORING DISEASE ACTIVITY AND FOLLOW-UP

- *Monitoring disease activity*: CBC, creatinine, urinalysis, CRP, anti-dsDNA, C3/C4, urine protein/urine creatinine ratio. Systemic Lupus Erythematosus Disease Activity Index (SLEDAI) score/systemic lupus international collaborating clinics-American College of Rheumatology (SLICC-ACR) damage index are clinical scores that can be used to monitor disease activity.
- *Monitoring for drug toxicity*: Ophthalmology evaluation, blood pressure (BP) monitoring, CBC, creatinine, liver function test (LFT).
  - *Growth and nutrition*: Weight, height, basal metabolic index (BMI) measurements at each visit
  - Psychological support.
- *Prevention of atherosclerosis*: Cholesterol levels, smoking, BMI, BP, and other cardiovascular risks.
- *Osteoporosis prevention*: Calcium and vitamin D supplementation.
- *Vaccination*: All routine childhood vaccinations along with annual influenza and 23 valent pneumococcal vaccines are recommended.

PROGNOSIS

The severity of the disease is worse in pSLE as compared to adults with SLE. However, modern advances in medicine and monitoring techniques have improved survival rates considerably. Currently, the 5-year survival rate is about 95%, while the 10-year rates are between 80 and 90%. Ensuring good quality of life for the child while dealing with a chronic illness should be the aim of the treatment. Treatment should be done by a multidisciplinary team involving a pediatric rheumatologist.

SUGGESTED READING

1. Aringer M, Costenbader K, Daikh D, Brinks R, Mosca M, Ramsey-Goldman R, et al. 2019 European League Against Rheumatism/American College of Rheumatology classification criteria for systemic lupus erythematosus. Ann Rheum Dis. 2019;78:1151-9.
2. Gladman D, Ginzler E, Goldsmith C, Fortin P, Liang M, Urowitz M, et al. The development and initial validation of the Systemic Lupus International Collaborating Clinics/American College of Rheumatology damage index for systemic lupus erythematosus. Arthritis Rheum. 1996;39(3):363-9.
3. Hochberg MC. Updating the American College of Rheumatology revised criteria for the classification of systemic lupus erythematosus. Arthritis Rheum. 1997;40(9):1725..
4. Kliegman R. Nelson Textbook of Pediatrics, 21st edition. Philadelphia, PA: Elsevier; 2020.
5. Petri M, Orbai A-M, Alarcón GS, Gordon C, Merrill JT, Fortin PR, Bruce IN, et al. Derivation and validation of the Systemic Lupus International Collaborating Clinics classification criteria for systemic lupus erythematosus. Arthritis Rheum. 2012;64(8):2677-86.
6. Thanou A, James JA, Arriens C, et al. Scoring systemic lupus erythematosus (SLE) disease activity with simple, rapid outcome measures. Lupus Science and Medicine. 2019;6:e000365.
7. Weiss JE. Pediatric systemic lupus erythematosus: more than a positive antinuclear antibody. Pediatrics in Review. 2012;33:62.

CHAPTER 150: Lupus Nephritis

Jijo Joseph John, Reny Joseph

INTRODUCTION

Lupus nephritis (LN) is one of the most dreaded complications of systemic lupus erythematosus (SLE) and it is more common in pediatric SLE as compared to adults with SLE. Renal involvement is seen in 50–75% of patients with SLE and most develop nephritis within 2 years of diagnosis. The 5-year renal survival for LN has improved in recent decades to almost 90%. However, mortality rates for children with LN are 19 times higher as compared to a healthy population.

PATHOGENESIS

Pathogenesis of SLE involves a complex interaction of genetic and environmental factors, ultimately resulting in loss of tolerance and chronic autoimmunity. Renal involvement in lupus is a result of the deposition of circulating immune complexes in renal tissues or the formation of immune complexes in situ. This leads to the activation of the classical complement pathway and neutrophil recruitment. Local neutrophil recruitment and activation trigger release of reactive oxygen species, proinflammatory cytokines [interleukin-4 (IL-4), transforming growth factor beta (TGF-β), tumor necrosis factor (TNF), and interferon alpha (IFN-α)] and amplification of inflammatory response in the kidneys. These responses together cause podocyte injury, increase dextracellular matrix synthesis and deposition, and ultimately renal impairment.

CLINICAL FEATURES

Clinical features of LN vary widely and can range from asymptomatic mild proteinuria and hematuria to nephrotic syndrome, acute glomerulonephritis, rapidly progressive glomerulonephritis, hypertension, and acute or chronic kidney injury. Urinalysis may be rarely normal in patients with proliferative LN. Patients with class V nephritis may present with nephrotic syndrome.

DIAGNOSIS

- *Proteinuria*: >0.5 g/day or >3+ by dipstick.
- Urine protein/urine creatinine ratio >0.5.
- *Urinalysis*: Hematuria, red cell casts, leukocyturia in the absence of infection are suggestive of active disease
- *Autoantibodies*: ANA, anti-dsDNA, and other autoantibodies support the diagnosis of SLE, though their role in monitoring LN is unclear.
- *Complement levels*: C3, C4, and total complement (CH50), levels decrease in active disease, particularly in proliferative LN.
- *Creatinine*: Creatinine is a late marker of renal injury; however, it is the easiest and cheapest means of monitoring renal functions. Levels should be monitored at each visit.
- *Urinary biomarkers*: Newer urinary biomarker molecules such as alpha-1 acid glycoprotein, ceruloplasmin, and lipocalin-like prostaglandin D synthase, transferrin have been associated with LN activity. However, their utility in clinical practice needs further clinical trials.
- *Anti-C1q antibody*: Higher titers correlate with active renal disease. Anti-C1q antibody in association with low C3 and C4 can be used to predict renal flares in patients with SLE.
- Renal biopsy is gold standard for diagnosis of renal lupus. *Indications for renal biopsy [American College of Rheumatology (ACR) 2012]*:
  - Increasing serum creatinine without compelling alternative causes (sepsis, hypovolemia, or medications)
  - Confirmed proteinuria of >1 g/24 h
  - Combinations of the following:
    - Proteinuria ≥0.5 g/24 h plus hematuria, or
    - Proteinuria ≥0.5 g/24 h plus cellular casts.

Renal biopsy: Morphological classification
Recommendations from the International Society of Nephrology (ISN) and Renal Pathology Society (RPS): 2018 revisions are used currently as the basis for classification of LN.

The World Health Organization (WHO) Classification of LN differs slightly and is based on light microscopy, electron microscopy, and immunofluorescence (**Fig. 1**).

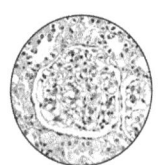
Class I
Minimal mesangial lupus nephritis
- Deposition of imune complexes detectable by immunofluorescence techniques.

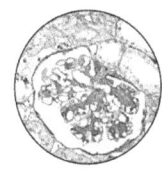
Class II
Mesangial proliferative lupus nephritis
- Mesangial hypercellularity of any degree or mesangial matrix expansion with immune deposits detectable by light microscopy.

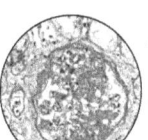
Class III
Focal lupus nephritis
- Active or inactive focal, segmental or global endo/extracapilarry glomerulonephritis involving < 50% of all glomeruli.
- Manifestations include active lesions (A)> chronic inactive lesions (C) or active and chronic lesions (A/C)

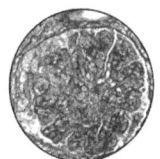
Class IV
Diffuse lupus nephritis
- Active or inactive diffuse, segmental or global endo/extracapilarry glomerulonephritis involving ≥ 50% of all glomeruli. Subendothelial diffuse immune deposits, with or without mesangial alterations, are common.
- This class is also divided in: Diffuse segmental (IV-S), when ≥ 50% of the involved glomeruli have segmental lesions, and diffuse global (IV-G), when ≥ 50% of the involved glomeruli have global lesions.
- It can also manifest A, C or A/C lesions.

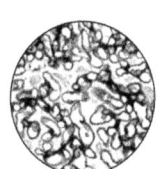
Class V
Membranous lupus nephritis
- Global or segmental subepithelial immune deposition or their morphologic sequelae detectable by light, immunofluorescence or electron microscopy, with or without mesangial alterations.
- It can occur in combination with class III or IV and it can manifest advanced sclerosis.

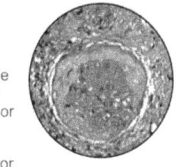
Class VI
Advanced sclerosis lupus nephritis
- Lupus nephritis with terminal prognosis.
- 90% of the glomeruli global sclerosis.

Fig. 1: Histopathological classification of lupus nephritis.

- *Class I*: Minimal mesangial LN—no findings on light microscopy, mesangial immune deposits on immunofluorescence.
- *Class II*: Mesangial proliferative LN—mesangial hypercellularity and increased matrix along with immunoglobulin and complement deposits.
- *Class III and IV*: Interrelated lesions with both mesangial and endocapillary lesions. Class III has <50% glomeruli involved and class IV has more than 50% glomerular involvement. The subclassification scheme helps grade the severity of lesion as segmental (<50% glomerular tuft involved) and global (>50% glomerular tuft involved).
- *Class V*: Membranous nephritis—the lesion is usually seen associated with class III or class IV proliferative nephritis.

Transformation of a histological lesion to more severe forms is commonly seen in poorly treated and controlled LN.

Activity and chronicity index: In addition to pathological classification, activity and chronicity index scoring is done to predict renal prognosis. The activity index reflects a state of active inflammation in the biopsy specimen, while the chronicity index refers to scarring and fibrosis. The activity index may be reversible with medical therapy, while the chronicity index may not. Each item is scored 0-3, and scores for fibrinoid necrosis and cellular crescents are multiplied by 2. The maximum score for activity is 24 while that of chronicity is 12 **(Table 1)**.

TREATMENT (FLOWCHART 1)

Goals of treatment in LN: Produce remission from the disease, while maintaining minimal drug toxicity, prevent chronic kidney impairment, and to improve patient quality of life.

TABLE 1: Activity and chronicity index.

Activity	Chronicity
Endocapillary hypercellularity	Glomerular sclerosis, segmental or global
Neutrophil infiltration	Fibrous adhesions/fibrous crescents
Subendothelial hyaline deposits	Tubular atrophy
Fibrinoid necrosis/karyorrhexis	Interstitial fibrosis
Cellular crescents	
Interstitial inflammation	

The current therapeutic strategy has two phases of treatment:
1. *Induction phase*: To control disease activity, by inducing remission of a disease flare
2. *Maintenance phase*: The target is to avoid relapses.

Class I nephritis usually does not require treatment. Class V is managed with oral steroids with mycophenolate (MMF), and maintenance therapy can be continued with MMF or azathioprine (AZA).

Recurrence or Refractory Cases

- *Mild flare*: Increase the dose of prednisolone and consider changing immunosuppressive medication [hydroxychloroquine (HCQ), azathioprine (AZA), methotrexate (MTX)].
- *Severe flare*:
  - IV methylprednisolone.
  - *High-dose oral prednisolone*: 1-2 mg/kg/day (maximum dose 60 mg/day), followed by tapering, once remission is achieved.
  - Check compliance.

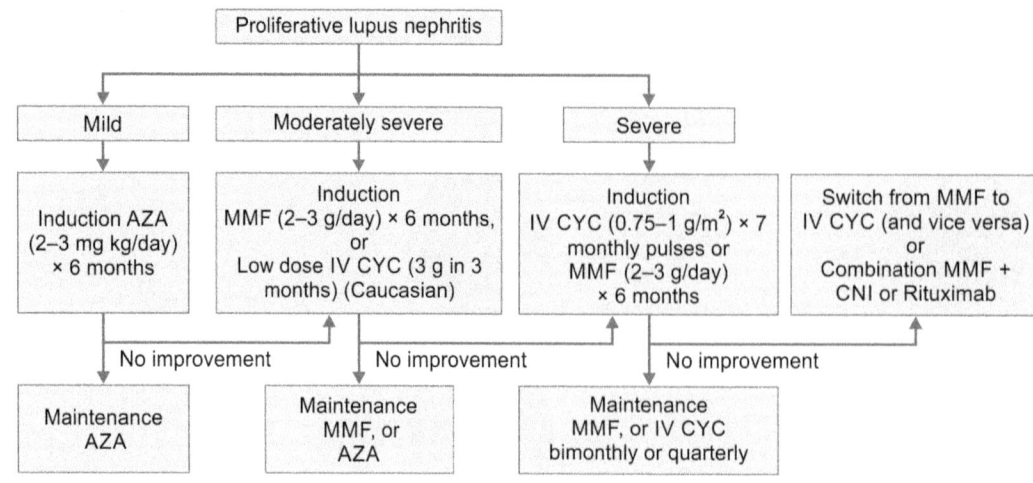

Flowchart 1: Recommended treatment of proliferative lupus nephritis.

Note: Improvement (reduction in proteinuria, stabilization or increase in glomerular filtration rate) is assessed within the first 3–4 months after treatment initiation. All induction regimens include pulse intravenous methylprednisolone (1 g/pulse × 3), followed by oral prednisolone (0.5–0.6 mg/kg for the first 4 weeks of induction, then tapered).
(AZA: azathioprine; CNI: calcineurin inhibitor; IV CYC: intravenous cyclophosphamide, MMF: mycophenolate mofetil)

- *Replace therapeutic agent*: MF, IV cyclophosphamide, or rituximab
- *Consider calcineurin inhibitor*: Cyclosporine or tacrolimus in specific cases

Other Supportive Measures

- Angiotensin-converting enzyme inhibitor (ACEI)/angiotensin receptor blockers (ARBs): For proteinuria
- Treat hypertension and dyslipidemia aggressively.
- *Diet restriction*: According to the degree of hypertension and renal impairment.
- *Calcium and vitamin D supplementation*: Especially in children being treated with steroids. Bisphosphonate may be added.
- Avoid nephrotoxic drugs.
- Contraceptive advise for teenagers to avoid pregnancy.
- Renal transplantation may be considered in patients with end-stage renal disease, sclerosis, and high chronicity index.

Side Effects of Commonly used Medications

- *Glucocorticoids*: Impaired glucose tolerance, cushingoid features, hypertension, growth impairment, and puberty delay, osteoporosis, steroid-induced myopathy, impaired calcium absorption, immunosuppression and increased risk of infections, cataracts, and adrenal insufficiency with prolonged administration and rapid withdrawal.
- *Cyclophosphamide*: Nausea and vomiting, hemorrhagic cystitis, immunosuppression, alopecia, cytopenias, discoloration of skin and nails, infertility, rarely-increased risk of malignancy.
- *Mycophenolate mofetil*: Hyperglycemia, hypertension, hypercholesterolemia, hypomagnesemia, hypocalcemia, hyperkalemia, dyspnea, back pain, increased blood urea nitrogen (BUN), anemia, leukopenia, pleural effusion, peripheral edema, diarrhea, headache, malignancies, pulmonary fibrosis, gastrointestinal (GI) bleeding.
- *HCQ*: Nausea, vomiting, abdominal pain, QT prolongation, bone marrow failure, hemolysis in patients with G6PD deficiency, vertigo, tinnitus, nystagmus, irreversible retinopathy with retinal pigment changes (Bull's eye appearance), visual field defects, acute hepatic failure, angioedema, and bronchospasm, headache, seizures, ataxia, Stevens–Johnson syndrome (SJS), drug rash with eosinophilia and systemic symptoms (DRESS).

PROGNOSIS AND FOLLOW-UP

With newer drugs and treatment protocols, outcomes have improved for patients with LN. Infections and end-stage renal disease are the main contributors to mortality; however, currently the majority of patients attain remission at the end of 12–18 months of treatment and continue to have stable renal functions at 10 years.

SUGGESTED READING

1. Firestein GS, Gabriel SE, Budd RC, McInnes IB, O'Dell JR. Kelley and Firestein's Textbook of Rheumatology, 10th edition. Philadelphia, PA: Elsevier; 2017.
2. Kliegman R. Nelson Textbook of Pediatrics, 21st edition. Philadelphia, PA: Elsevier; 2020.
3. Pinheiro SVB, Dias RF, Fabiano RCG Araujo, Araujo S de A, E Silva ACS. Pediatric lupus nephritis. J Bras Nefrol. 2019;41(2):252-65.
4. Smith EMD, Jorgensen AL, Midgley A, Oni L, Goilav B, Putterman Chaim, et al. International validation of a urinary biomarker panel for identification of active lupus nephritis in children. Pediatr Nephrol. 2017;32(2):283-95.
5. Srivastava RN, Bagga A. Textbook of Pediatric Nephrology, 5th edition. New Delhi: Jaypee Brothers Medical Publishers (P) Ltd.; 2011.

Rheumatic Fever

Vijay Kamale, Nitin Kadam

INTRODUCTION

Rheumatic fever (RF) is a potentially serious infection-related disease, caused by group A beta-hemolytic streptococci (GAS) which can lead to rheumatic heart disease.

EPIDEMIOLOGY

Worldwide, rheumatic heart disease remains the most common form of acquired heart disease in all age groups, accounting for up to 50% of all cardiovascular disease and 50% of all cardiac admissions in many developing countries.

PATHOPHYSIOLOGY

Not all serotypes of GAS can cause RF. The serotypes—M types 1, 3, 5, 6, 18, 29—are more frequently isolated from patients with acute RF than other serotypes. Genetic predisposition is noted in few studies **(Fig. 1)**.

- *The cytotoxicity theory*: GAS produces a number of enzymes such as streptolysin O, which has a direct cytotoxic effect on mammalian cells in tissue culture. However, a major problem with the cytotoxicity hypothesis is its inability to explain the substantial latent period (usually 10–21 days) between GAS pharyngitis and onset of acute RF.
- *An immune-mediated pathogenesis (the most accepted explanation)*: The antigenicity of several GAS cellular and extracellular epitopes and their immunologic cross-reactivity with cardiac antigenic epitopes, lends support to the hypothesis of molecular mimicry.
- Another proposed pathogenetic hypothesis is that the binding of an M-protein N-terminal domain to a region of collagen type IV leads to an antibody response to the collagen, resulting in ground substance inflammation, especially in subendothelial areas such as cardiac valves and myocardium.

CLINICAL MANIFESTATIONS AND DIAGNOSIS

Jones criteria, updated 2015 by the American Heart Association (AHA) **(Table 1)**.

- There are five major and four minor criteria and a requirement of evidence of recent GAS infection. The 2015 revision includes separate criteria for *low-risk populations* (defined as those with incidence ≤2 per 100,000 school-age children per year or all-age rheumatic heart disease prevalence of ≤1 per 1,000 populations) and *moderate/high-risk populations* (defined as those with

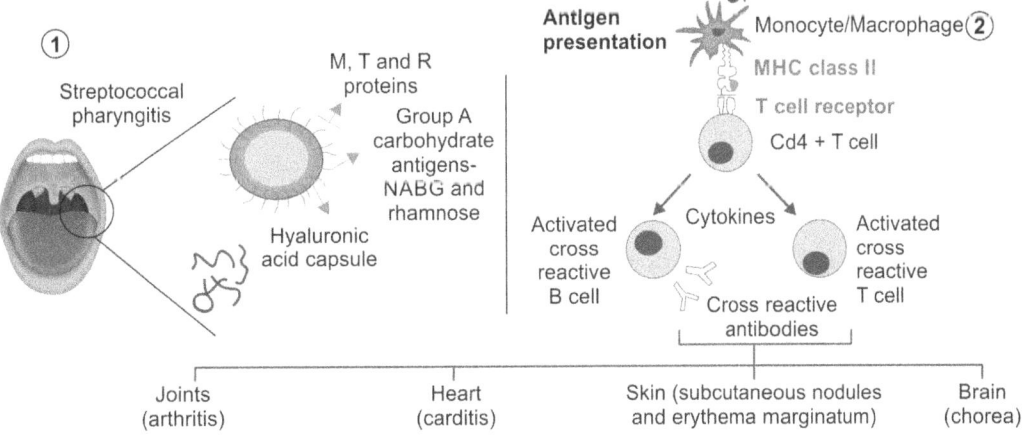

Fig. 1: Pathophysiology of rheumatic fever.
(MHC: major histocompatibility complex; NABG: N-acetyl-beta-D-glucosaminidase)

TABLE 1: Guidelines for the diagnosis of initial or recurrent attack of rheumatic fever (Jones criteria, Updated 2015).

Major criteria	Minor criteria	Supporting evidence of antecedent group A streptococcal infection
• Polyarthritis • Carditis • Chorea • Erythema marginatum • Subcutaneous nodules	*Clinical features:* • Arthralgia • Fever	Positive throat culture or rapid streptococcal antigen test elevated or increasing streptococcal antibody titer
–	*Laboratory features:* • *Elevated acute phase reactants:* Erythrocyte sedimentation rate • C-reactive protein • Prolonged P-R interval	–

higher incidence or prevalence rates) as most developing countries, including India.
- *Initial attack*: Two major manifestations, or one major and two minor manifestations, plus evidence of recent GAS infection.
- *Recurrent attack*: Two major, or one major and two minor, or three minor manifestations (the latter only in the moderate/high-risk population)
   - Carditis is now defined as clinical and/or subclinical (echocardiographic valvulitis).
   - Arthritis (major) refers to polyarthritis as well as monoarthritis or polyarthralgia in *moderate/high-risk populations*.
   - Minor criteria for *moderate/high-risk populations* only include monoarthralgia, fever of >38°C, erythrocyte sedimentation rate (ESR) >30 mm/h.

Major Criteria

Migratory Polyarthritis

- It is seen in almost 75% of patients with acute RF. Larger joints, particularly the knees, ankles, wrists, and elbows are commonly involved.
- Rheumatic joints are classically hot, red, swollen, and exquisitely tender, with even the friction of bedclothes being uncomfortable. The pain can precede and can appear to be disproportionate to the objective findings.
- The joint involvement is migratory in nature, i.e., a severely inflamed joint can become normal within 1–3 days without treatment and many joints are involved, usually sequentially.
- Severe arthritis can persist for several (4–6) weeks in untreated patients and there is often an inverse relationship between the severity of arthritis and the severity of cardiac involvement.
- Monoarthritis in the absence of prior inflammatory therapies, or even polyarthralgia without frank objective signs of arthritis, is a major criterion in *moderate/high-risk populations*. Polyarthralgia as major criteria is new addition in the *moderate/high-risk population*, but other potential causes should be excluded before considering it carefully.
- Synovial fluid in acute RF usually has 10,000–100,000 white blood cells/µL with a predominance of neutrophils, protein level of approximately 4 g/dL, normal glucose level, and forms a good mucin clot.

Carditis

- A major change in the 2015 revision of the Jones criteria is the acceptance of subclinical carditis (defined as echocardiographic evidence of valvulitis, even without a murmur of valvulitis) or clinical carditis (with a valvulitis murmur) as fulfilling the major criterion of carditis in all populations.
- The echocardiographic features of subclinical carditis must distinguish pathologic from physiologic degrees of valve regurgitation. Subclinical (i.e., only echocardiographic) evidence of pathologic mitral regurgitation requires that a jet is seen in at least two views, the jet length is ≥2 cm in at least one view, peak jet velocity is >3 m/s, and the peak systolic jet is in at least one envelope. Subclinical pathologic evidence of aortic regurgitation is similar, except that the jet length is ≥1 cm in at least one view.
- Rheumatic carditis is characterized by pancarditis. Cardiac involvement can be fulminant, potentially fatal exudative pancarditis to mild, transient cardiac involvement.
- Acute rheumatic carditis usually presents as tachycardia, gallop, muffling of heart sounds, and cardiac murmurs. Moderate-to-severe rheumatic carditis can result in cardiomegaly and heart failure with hepatomegaly and peripheral and pulmonary edema (respiratory distress).
- Echocardiographic findings include pericardial effusion, decreased ventricular contractility, and aortic and/or mitral regurgitation (MR).
- MR is characterized typically by a high-pitched apical holosystolic murmur radiating to the axilla. In patients

with significant MR, this may be associated with an apical mid-diastolic murmur of relative mitral stenosis. Aortic insufficiency is characterized by a high-pitched decrescendo diastolic murmur at the left sternal border. Endocarditis (valvulitis) is a universal finding in rheumatic carditis, involvement of pericardium and myocardium is variable. Viral myocarditis or other causes should be ruled out if endocarditis (clinical/echo) is absent in presence of myocarditis or pericarditis.
- Carditis occurs in approximately 50–60% of all cases of acute RF. Approximately 80% of those who develop carditis have it within first 2 weeks of RF. The major consequence of acute rheumatic carditis is chronic, progressive valvular disease, particularly valvular stenosis, which can require valve replacement.

Chorea

- Sydenham chorea occurs in approximately 10–15% of patients with acute RF. It is an isolated movement disorder with emotional lability, incoordination, poor school performance, uncontrollable movements, and facial grimacing are characteristic.
- Abnormal movements are exacerbated and exaggerated by stress and disappear with sleep. Chorea occasionally is unilateral (hemichorea).
- The latent period from acute GAS infection to chorea is usually longer and can be months. It is difficult to recognize for several months due to quasipurposive nature.
- Clinical maneuvers to elicit features of chorea include: (1) demonstration of milk maid's grip (irregular contractions and relaxations of the muscles of the fingers while squeezing the examiner's fingers), (2) pronator sign: spooning and pronation of the hands when the patient's arms are extended, (3) wormian darting movements of the tongue on protrusion, and (4) examination of handwriting to evaluate fine motor movements. The movements can last for many months, without any permanent neurological sequelae.

Erythema Marginatum

Erythema marginatum is a rare (approximately 1% of patients with acute RF) but characteristic rash of acute RF. Rash is erythematous, serpiginous, macular lesion with pale centers and without itching. It occurs primarily on the trunk and extremities, but not on the face, and it can be accentuated by warming the skin.

Subcutaneous Nodules

Subcutaneous nodules are a rare (≤1% of patients with acute RF) finding and consist of firm nodules approximately 0.5–1 cm in diameter along the extensor surfaces of tendons near bony prominences. There is a correlation between the presence of these nodules and significant rheumatic heart disease.

Minor Criteria

- These are more nonspecific than major criteria, and the 2015 revised Jones criteria have included some changes from previous criteria.
- The first of the two clinical minor criteria involve joint manifestations (only if arthritis is not used as a major criterion) and is defined as polyarthralgia in *low-risk* populations and monoarthralgia in *moderate/high-risk* populations.
- The second clinical minor manifestation is fever, defined as at least 38.5°C in *low-risk* populations and at least 38.0°C in *moderate/high-risk* populations.
- The two laboratory minor criteria are:
  - Elevated acute phase reactants, defined as ESR at least 60 mm/h and/or C-reactive protein (CRP) at least 3.0 mg/dL (30 mg/L) in low-risk populations, and ESR at least 30 mm/h and/or CRP at least 3.0 mg/dL (30 mg/L) in *moderate/high-risk populations*
  - Prolonged P-R interval on ECG (unless carditis is a major criterion). However, a prolonged P-R interval alone does not constitute evidence of carditis or predict long-term cardiac sequelae.

Recent Group A *Streptococcus* Infection

An essential requirement for the diagnosis of acute RF is supporting evidence of a recent GAS infection.
- One third of patients with acute RF have no history of an antecedent pharyngitis. The evidence of GAS infection is based on elevated or rising serum anti-streptococcal antibody titers. If only a single antibody is measured (usually antistreptolysin O), only 80–85% of patients with acute RF have an elevated titer; however, 95–100% have an elevation if three different antibodies (anti-streptolysin O, anti-DNase B, anti-hyaluronidase) are measured.
- A slide agglutination test (streptozyme) purports to detect antibodies against five different GAS antigens, but this test is not available in India and is less standardized and less reproducible than other tests. Except for chorea, the clinical findings of acute RF generally coincide with peak anti-streptococcal antibody responses.

Exceptions to Jones Criteria

- Chorea, if it is isolated feature and all possible causes have been ruled out.
- Carditis and its sequel (RHD) in patient presenting long after an probable episode of RF.

DIFFERENTIAL DIAGNOSIS

- *Arthritis*: Rheumatoid, reactive, serum sickness, sickle cell disease, malignancies.
- *Carditis*: Viral, infective endocarditis, Kawasaki disease, congenital mitral or aortic diseases, innocent murmur.
- *Chorea*: Huntington's chorea, Wilson disease, systemic lupus erythematosus (SLE).

TREATMENT

- Bed rest for all patients and monitoring closely for evidence of carditis. The patients with carditis require longer periods of bed rest.
- *Antibiotic therapy*:
  - The patient should receive 10 days of orally administered penicillin or amoxicillin or a single intramuscular injection of benzathine penicillin.
  - If child is allergic to penicillin, 10 days of erythromycin, 5 days of azithromycin, or 10 days of clindamycin is given. Long-term antibiotic prophylaxis for secondary prevention should be instituted afterward.
- *Anti-inflammatory therapy*:
  - Acetaminophen can be used to control pain and fever.
  - Oral salicylates are given to children with typical migratory polyarthritis and in patient with carditis without cardiomegaly or congestive heart failure. The usual dose of aspirin is 50–70 mg/kg/day in four divided doses orally (PO) for 3–5 days, followed by 50 mg/kg/day in four divided doses PO for 2–3 weeks and half that dose for another 2–4 weeks.
- *Prednisolone*: In children with carditis and more than minimal cardiomegaly and/or congestive heart failure. The dose of prednisone is 2 mg/kg/day in four divided doses for 2–3 weeks, followed by half the dose for 2–3 weeks and then tapering of the dose by 5 mg/24 h every 2–3 days. When prednisone is being tapered, aspirin should be started at 50 mg/kg/day in four divided doses for 6 weeks to prevent rebound of inflammation. Supportive therapies for patients with moderate-to-severe carditis include digoxin, fluid and salt restriction, diuretics, and oxygen. The cardiac toxicity of digoxin is enhanced with myocarditis.

Termination of the anti-inflammatory therapy may be followed by the reappearance of clinical manifestations or of elevation in ESR and CRP (rebound). It may be prudent to increase salicylates or corticosteroids until near-normalization of inflammatory markers is achieved.

Treatment of Sydenham Chorea

Anti-inflammatory agents are usually not indicated. Sedatives may be helpful early in the course of chorea. Phenobarbital (16–32 mg every 6–8 hours PO) is the drug of choice. If phenobarbital is ineffective, haloperidol (0.01–0.03 mg/kg/24 h divided twice daily PO) or chlorpromazine (0.5 mg/kg every 4–6 hours PO) should be initiated. Some patients may benefit from a few-week course of corticosteroids.

COMPLICATIONS

The arthritis and chorea of acute RF resolve completely without sequelae. Therefore, the long-term sequelae of RF are essentially limited to the heart.

Actually, characteristic feature of the RF arthritis is a dramatic response to even low doses of salicylates, and the absence of such a response should suggest an alternative diagnosis. If a child with fever and arthritis is suspected to have acute RF, it is advisable to withhold salicylates and observe for migratory progression.

There is no role of routine endocarditis prophylaxis for patients with rheumatic heart disease who are undergoing dental or other procedures. However, the maintenance of optimal oral health care remains an important component of an overall healthcare program. Infective endocarditis prophylaxis remains recommended for children with a prosthetic valve or prosthetic material used in valve repair. Antibiotics other than penicillin are used to prevent infective endocarditis in those receiving penicillin prophylaxis for RF because oral α-hemolytic streptococci are likely to have developed resistance to penicillin.

PROGNOSIS

The prognosis for patients with acute RF depends on the clinical manifestations present at the initial episode, the severity of the initial episode, and the presence of recurrences. Approximately 50–70% of patients with carditis during the initial episode of acute RF recover with no residual heart disease. If the initial cardiac involvement is severe, the risk for residual heart disease is increased. The risk for permanent heart damage increases with each recurrence. Patients without carditis during the initial episode are less likely to have carditis with recurrent attacks, but there is a stepwise increase in cardiac involvement as the number of episodes increases.

RATIONALE FOR PROPHYLAXIS

Patients who have had acute RF are susceptible to recurrent attacks following reinfection of the upper respiratory tract with GAS. Therefore, these patients require long-term continuous chemoprophylaxis.

The risk of recurrence is highest in the first 5 years after the initial episode and decreases with time. Even children with "pure" chorea require long-term antibiotic prophylaxis. It was observed that approximately 20% of patients with

TABLE 2: Secondary prophylaxis—chemoprophylaxis to prevent further gas infection.

Drug	Dose	Route
Penicillin G benzathine	600,000 IU for children weighing ≤27 kg and 1.2 million IU for children >27 kg, every 4 weeks	Intramuscular
Or		
Penicillin V	250 mg, twice daily	Oral
Or		
Sulfadiazine or sulfisoxazole	0.5 g, once daily for patients weighing ≤27 kg 1.0 g, once daily for patients weighing >27 kg	Oral
For people who are allergic to penicillin and sulfonamide drugs macrolide or azalide	Variable	Oral

TABLE 3: Duration of prophylaxis for people who have had acute rheumatic fever: The American Heart Association (AHA).

Category	Duration
Rheumatic fever without carditis	5 years or until 21 years of age, whichever is longer
Rheumatic fever with carditis but without residual heart disease (no valvular disease)	10 years or until 21 years of age, whichever is longer
Rheumatic fever with carditis and residual heart disease (persistent valvular disease)	10 years or until 40 years of age, whichever is longer; sometimes lifelong prophylaxis

"pure" chorea and who were not given secondary prophylaxis developed rheumatic heart disease within 20 years.

Prevention

Prevention of both initial and recurrent episodes of acute RF depends on controlling GAS infections of the upper respiratory tract.

Primary prevention: Appropriate antibiotic therapy instituted before the 9th day of symptoms of acute GAS pharyngitis is highly effective in preventing first attacks of acute RF.

Secondary prevention: It is a continuous antibiotic prophylaxis, which should begin as soon as the diagnosis of acute RF has been made and immediately after a full course of antibiotic therapy has been completed. Because patients who have had carditis with their initial episode of acute RF are at higher risk for having carditis with recurrences and for sustaining additional cardiac damage, they should receive long-term antibiotic prophylaxis well into adulthood and perhaps for life **(Tables 2 and 3)**.

SUGGESTED READING

1. Carapetis JR, McDonald M, Wilson NJ. Acute rheumatic fever. Lancet. 2005;366:155-68.
2. Gerber MA, Baltimore RS, Eaton CB, Gewitz M, Rowley AH, Shulman ST, et al. Prevention of rheumatic fever and diagnosis and treatment of acute streptococcal pharyngitis: a scientific statement from the American Heart Association Rheumatic Fever, Endocarditis, and Kawasaki Disease Committee of the Council on Cardiovascular Disease in the Young. Circulation. 2009;119:1541-51.
4. Gewitz MH, Baltimore RS, Tani LY, Sable CA, Shulman ST, Carapetis J, et al. Revision of the Jones Criteria for the diagnosis of acute rheumatic fever in the era of Doppler echocardiography: a scientific statement from the American Heart Association. Circulation. 2015;131(20):1806-18.
3. Kerdemelidis M, Lennon DR, Arroll B, Peat B, Jarman J. The primary prevention of rheumatic fever. J Paediatr Child Health. 2010;46:534-48.
5. Lennon D, Anderson P, Kerdemelidis M, Farrell E, Mahi SC, Percival T, et al. First presentation acute rheumatic fever is preventable in a community setting: a school-based intervention. Pediatr Infect Dis J. 2017;36(12):1113-8.
6. Tandon R, Sharma M, Chandrashekhar Y, Kotb M, Yacoub MH, Narula J. Revisiting the pathogenesis of rheumatic fever and carditis. Nat Rev Cardiol advanced online publication. 2013;10(3):171-7.
7. Tani LY, Veasy LG, Minich LL, Shaddy RE. Rheumatic fever in children younger than 5 years: is the presentation different? Pediatrics. 2003;112:1065-8.
8. Walker AR, Tani LY, Thompson JA, Firth SD, Veasy LG, Bale Jr JF. Rheumatic chorea: relationship to systemic manifestations and response to corticosteroids. J Pediatr. 2007;151:679-83.
9. Zuhlke LJ, Karthikeyan G. Primary prevention for rheumatic fever. Glob Heart. 2013;8:221-6.

Juvenile Dermatomyositis

TP Yadav, Somdipa Pal

INTRODUCTION

It is one of the most common causes of inflammatory myositis in children. It is a chronic autoimmune disease leading to nonsuppurative inflammation of striated muscle and skin.

EPIDEMIOLOGY

The incidence of juvenile dermatomyositis (JDM) is three cases per 1 million children/year approximately. There is bimodal age distribution, between 4 and 10 years and second peak in late adulthood between 45 and 64 years. The ratio of girls to boys with JDM is 2:1. In 50% cases, one family member is found to have autoimmune disease.

ETIOLOGY

Etiology of JDM is multifactorial; however, no clear theory has emerged. There is interplay between genetic susceptibility and environmental triggers. Human leukocyte antigen (HLA) alleles such as B8, DRB1*0301, DQA1*0501, and DQA1*0301 are associated with increased susceptibility to JDM. Maternal microchimerism has also been reported to play a part in the etiology of JDM.

History of infection is usually respiratory or gastrointestinal; 3-6 months prior to disease onset has also been reported as an environmental trigger. Various organisms are implicated including Group A β-hemolytic *Streptococcus*, toxoplasma, coxsackievirus B, enteroviruses, and parvovirus B19.

PATHOGENESIS

Type 1 interferon pathway is involved in the inflammatory process of JDM and these interferons are secreted by activated plasmacytoid dendritic cells present within the muscles. Inflammation affects microvasculature of skeletal muscles and skin, rarely also lungs, kidney, heart, and eyes. Autoantibodies and genetic factors upregulate the process in the presence of environmental factors.

CLINICAL MANIFESTATIONS

Children with JDM present with insidious-onset fever, fatigue, anorexia, weight loss. Along with constitutional symptoms, 50% cases are heralded by mucocutaneous features; in 25%, muscle weakness can precede and in the rest both can be seen simultaneously.

Mucocutaneous Disease

Periorbital rash (the heliotrope rash) and Gottron papules are pathognomonic of JDM.

The heliotrope rash is a blue-violet discoloration of the eyelids that may be associated with periorbital edema. Violaceous erythema may also be seen in sun-exposed areas, if seen over chest and neck; this erythema is known as the "shawl sign" and over hip, thighs—the holster sign.

Classic Gottron papules are bright pink or pale, shiny, thickened, or atrophic plaques over the proximal and distal interphalangeal joints and occasionally on the knees, elbows, small joints of the toes, and ankle malleoli. Rarely, a thickened erythematous scaly rash develops over palms and soles known as mechanic's hands.

Nailfold telangiectasia, periungual erythema, skin excoriation, pruritus, and interface dermatitis can also be seen.

Musculoskeletal Disease

Symmetric proximal muscle weakness is more typical. Parents may report regression of motor milestones. The shoulder and hip girdle, occasionally anterior neck flexors are involved. Examination reveals Gower sign (use of hands on thigh to stand from sitting position). Dysphonia, dysphagia, and respiratory failure may occur due to palatal, pharyngeal, and respiratory muscle weakness. Nondeforming arthritis and arthralgia may also occur.

Lipodystrophy and calcinosis can be seen in 40% patients and cause serious morbidity. Calcinosis is dystrophic calcification over elbow, knees, digits, or subcutaneous tissue. Lipodystrophy is progressive loss of visceral fat and occasionally associated with metabolic syndrome, i.e., insulin resistance, polycystic ovarian syndrome, hirsutism, acanthosis, hypertriglyceridemia, and abnormal glucose tolerance.

DIAGNOSIS AND LABORATORY TESTS

- Symmetric weakness of the proximal muscle
- Characteristic cutaneous changes consisting of heliotrope rash and/or Gottron papules
- Elevation of the serum level of one or more muscle enzymes (creatine kinase, aldolase, aspartate aminotransferases, and lactate dehydrogenase)
- Electromyographic demonstration of the characteristics of myopathy
- Muscle biopsy documenting histological evidence of necrosis.

The criteria for diagnosis of JDM were formulated in 1977 by Bohan and Peter.

The presence of three of the five findings indicates a probable diagnosis of JDM and at least four of five findings indicates definite JDM.

Other laboratory parameters:

- Erythrocyte sedimentation rate and C-reactive protein elevated, rheumatoid factor negative
- Antinuclear antibody present >80% cases. Anti-NXP2, Anti-Jo-1, Anti-PM-Scl antibody may be associated with calcinosis
- MRI using T2-weighted images noninvasive modality for identification of active site of disease.

TREATMENT

Oral prednisolone at 2 mg/kg is starting dose and slowly tapered over 12 months. Weekly methotrexate (15 mg/m^2) is commonly used as steroid-sparing agent in JDM. Hydroxychloroquine, cyclosporine, and azathioprine are other agents used in refractory cases. Intravenous immunoglobulin and rituximab have shown some promising result in severe cases. Physical and occupational therapy are integral parts of treatment program. All children should avoid sun exposure and apply sun protection cream daily.

Complications

Most complications are related to muscle weakness, i.e., muscle atrophy, contracture, aspiration pneumonia, respiratory failure, etc. Lipodystrophy can lead to hypertension, dyslipidemia, insulin resistance. Children are also prone to complications due to prolong corticosteroid therapy.

PROGNOSIS

Though the mortality have dropped from 33 to 1%, morbidity caused by the disease cannot be overlooked. An early recognition and aggressive treatment and also long-term follow-up are the key to good prognosis. At 7-year follow-up, 75% patients have little residual disability, 25% continue to have chronic weakness.

SUGGESTED READING

1. AM Reed, SR Ytterberg, Genetic and environmental risk factors for idiopathic inflammatory myopathies. Rheum Dis Clin North Am. 2001;28(4):891-916.
2. Artlett CM, Ramos R, Jiminez SA, Patterson K, Miller FW, Rider LG. Chimeric cells of maternal origin in juvenile idiopathic inflammatory myopathies. Childhood Myositis Heterogeneity Collaborative Group. Lancet. 2000;356(9248):2155-6.
3. Bohan A, Peter JB. Polymyositis and dermatomyositis (first of two parts). N Engl J Med. 1975;292(7):344-7.
4. Bohan A, Peter JB. Polymyositis and dermatomyositis (second of two parts). N Engl J Med. 1975;292(8):403-7.
5. Eloranta M-L, Helmers SB, Ulfgren A-K, Rönnblom L, Alm GV, Lundberg IE. A possible mechanism for endogenous activation of the type I interferon system in myositis patients with anti-Jo-1 or anti-Ro52/anti-Ro60 autoantibodies. Arthritis Rheum. 2007;56(9):3112-24.
6. Gunawardena H, Wedderburn LR, Chinoy H, Betteridge ZE, North J, Ollier WER, et al. Autoantibodies to a 140-kd protein in juvenile dermatomyositis are associated with calcinosis. Arthritis Rheum. 2009;60(6):1807-14.
7. McCann LJ, Juggins AD, Maillard SM, Wedderburn LR, Davidson JE, Murray KJ, et al. The Juvenile Dermatomyositis National Registry and Repository (UK and Ireland)–clinical characteristics of children recruited within the first 5 yr. Rheumatology (Oxford). 2006;45(10):1255-60.
8. Medsger Jr TA, Dawson Jr WN, Masi AT. The epidemiology of polymyositis. Am J Med. 1970; 48(6):715-23.
9. Miller LC, Michael AF, Kim Y. Childhood dermatomyositis. Clinical course and long-term follow-up. Clin Pediat (Phila). 1987; 26(11):561-6.
10. Niewold TB, Wu SC, Smith M, Morgan GA, Pachman LM. Familial aggregation of autoimmune disease in juvenile dermatomyositis. Pediatrics. 2011;127(5):e1239-46.
11. Reed AM, Collins EJ, Shock LP, Klapper DG, Frelinger JA. Diminished class II-associated Ii peptide binding to the juvenile dermatomyositis HLA-DQ alpha *0501/DQ beta 1*0301 molecule. J Immunol. 1997;159(12):6260-5.
12. Robinson AB, Hoeltzel MF, Wahezi DM, Becker ML, Kessler EA, Schmeling H, et al. Clinical characteristics of children with juvenile dermatomyositis—the children's arthritis and rheumatology research alliance (CARRA) registry. Arthritis Care Res (Hoboken). 2014; 66(3):404 10.
13. Shah M, Mamyrova G, Targoff IN, Huber AM, Malley JD, Rice MM, et al. The clinical phenotypes of the juvenile idiopathic inflammatory myopathies. Medicine (Baltimore). 2013;92(1):25-41.
14. Symmons DP, Sills JA, Davis SM. The incidence of juvenile dermatomyositis: results from a nation-wide study. Br J Rheumatol. 1995;34(8):732-6.

Henoch–Schönlein Purpura

TP Yadav, Jessica Hlawndo

INTRODUCTION

Henoch–Schönlein purpura (HSP) is one of the most common vasculitides of childhood. It is defined as "small vessel (predominantly capillaries, venules, or arterioles) vasculitis with IgA1-dominant immune deposits; it often involves the skin, gastrointestinal tract, and frequently causes arthritis." The EULAR/PRES/PRINTO (European League against Rheumatism/Pediatric Rheumatology European Society/Pediatric Rheumatology International Trials Organization) criteria for diagnosis is mentioned in **Box 1**.

EPIDEMIOLOGY

Henoch–Schönlein purpura is predominantly childhood disease, frequently affecting children between 3 and 15 years. It is more common in boys than in girls (1.5:1). The disease usually occurs in winter, often (30–50%) preceded by an upper respiratory tract infection.

ETIOPATHOGENESIS

Henoch–Schönlein purpura is a predominantly IgA-mediated dysregulated immune response to antigen and may operate through the alternative complement pathway. The interplay between genetic background and immune dysregulation, which is often triggered by infections, is known. The infections commonly include β-hemolytic streptococci, viral (varicella, rubella, rubeola, hepatitis A and B), *Mycoplasma pneumonia*, *Bartonella henselae*, and *Helicobacter pylori*.

BOX 1: Diagnostic criteria for Henoch–Schönlein purpura.

Palpable purpura (in absence of coagulopathy or thrombocytopenia) and one or more of the following criteria must be present:
- Abdominal pain (acute, diffuse, colicky)
- Arthritis or arthralgia
- Biopsy of affected tissue demonstrating predominant IgA deposition
- Renal involvement (proteinuria or hematuria)

CLINICAL FEATURES

The presentation is often acute; low-grade fever or malaise can be present. The manifestations can be acute or may take weeks.

- *Cutaneous*: Palpable purpura is characteristic, which affects the extensor surfaces and dependent areas in the lower limbs and buttocks. The cutaneous lesions range from small petechiae to large ecchymoses to rare hemorrhagic bullae.
- *Gastrointestinal disease*: It occurs approximately in two thirds of the children, occurs within a week after the onset of rash. The most common feature is intermittent, colicky abdominal pain, followed by vomiting, melena, and hematemesis. Intussusception is a rare complication due to vasculitis of the bowel wall.
- *Renal*: Renal manifestations occurs in up to one third of the children and range from microscopic hematuria and mild proteinuria to nephrotic syndrome, acute nephritis, hypertension, or renal failure. Serious and potentially life-threatening disease occurs in less than 10%. Age of onset of >7 years old, persistent purpuric lesions, severe abdominal symptoms, and decreased factor XIII activity are associated with an increased risk of nephritis. Progression to end-stage renal disease is uncommon (up to 5%).
- *Musculoskeletal*: Arthralgia or arthritis (periarthritis) occurs in up to 50–80% with a predilection for large joints of lower limb. They are transient and nondeforming.

The other features include isolated central nervous system (CNS) vasculitis, headaches, seizure, coma and hemorrhage; Guillain-Barre syndrome; ataxia and neuropathy. Other less common features include orchitis, testicular torsion, carditis, inflammatory eye disease, and pulmonary hemorrhage.

LABORATORY INVESTIGATIONS

Henoch–Schönlein purpura is a clinical diagnosis. The nonspecific findings include leukocytosis, thrombocytosis, mild anemia, elevations of erythrocyte sedimentation rate (ESR) and C-reactive protein. Urinalysis and measurement of blood pressure and serum creatinine are necessary.

BOX 2: Indications for diagnostic renal biopsy.
- Acute nephritic or nephrotic syndrome at presentation
- Raised blood level of creatinine, hypertension, or oliguria
- Heavy proteinuria (early morning urine protein-to-creatinine ratio >100 mg/mmol)
- Persistent proteinuria (not declining) after 4 weeks
- Impaired renal function (glomerular filtration rate <80 mL/min/1.73 m^2)

Biopsy of the skin and kidney characteristically show IgA deposition **(Box 2)**. Bowel wall edema or intussusception can be diagnosed by ultrasound.

TREATMENT

The management is mostly supportive with adequate hydration, nutrition, and analgesia for mild and self-limited HSP. Steroids (prednisolone at 1 mg/kg/day for 1–2 weeks, followed by tapering dose) are used to treat significant gastrointestinal involvement or other life-threatening features. Additional immunosuppressants may be needed for nephritis management depending on the severity of the disease.

PROGNOSIS

Prognosis is excellent for majority in HSP. In most of the children, the entire course lasts for 4 weeks from the onset. One third to half of them have at least one recurrence. Close follow-up for at least 5 years is required for children who had clinical nephritis. Less than 5% of the children progress to end-stage renal failure.

SUGGESTED READING

1. Ardoin SP, Fels E. Henoch-Schonlein Purpura. Kliegman RM, Stanton BF, St Geme III JW, Schor NF (eds). Textbook of Pediatrics. Philadelphia: Elsevier; 2016. pp. 1216-8.
2. Ballinger S. Henoch–Schönlein purpura. Current opinion in rheumatology. 2003;15(5): 591-4.
3. Brogan P, Bagga A. Chronic arthritis in children. In: Petty RE, Laxer RM, Lindsley CB, Wedderbum LR (eds). Textbook of Pediatric Rheumatology, 7th edition. Philadelphia: Elsevier; 2016. pp. 452-8.
4. Emery H, Larter W, Schaller JG. Henoch-Schönlein vasculitis. Arthritis and Rheumatism. 1977;20(2 Suppl):385-8.
5. Gairdner D. The Schönlein-Henoch syndrome (anaphylactoid purpura). QJM: An International Journal of Medicine. 1948;17(2):95-122.
6. Levy M, Broyer M, Arsan A, Levy-Bentolila D, Habib R. Anaphylactoid purpura nephritis in childhood. Natural history and immunopathology. Adv Nephrol Necker Hosp. 1976; 6:183-228.
7. Ozen S, Pistorio A, Iusan SM, Bakkaloglu A, Herlin T, Brik R, et al. EULAR/PRINTO/PRES criteria for Henoch–Schönlein purpura, childhood polyarteritis nodosa, childhood Wegener granulomatosis and childhood Takayasu arteritis: Ankara 2008. Part II: final classification criteria. Ann Rheum Dis. 2010;69 (5):798-806.
8. Rees L, Webb NJA, Brogan PA. Vasculitis. In: Rees L, Webb NJA, Brogan PA, (eds). Paediatric Nephrology (Oxford Handbook). Oxford: Oxford University Press; 2007. pp. 310-3.
9. Rosenblum ND, Winter HS. Steroid effects on the course of abdominal pain in children with Henoch-Schonlein purpura. Pediatrics. 1987;79(6):1018-21.
10. Saulsbury F. Epidemiology of Henoch-Schonlein purpura. Cleveland Clinic Journal of Medicine. 2002;69:SII-87.

Kawasaki Disease

Vijay Kamale, Nimain Mohanty

INTRODUCTION

Kawasaki disease (KD), also known as *mucocutaneous lymph node syndrome* is an acute febrile illness of childhood seen worldwide, with the highest incidence occurring in Japan and to some extent in other Asian children. KD is a vasculitis with a predilection for the coronary arteries. In developed countries, it is the most common cause of acquired heart disease of children, whereas in developing country such as India, acute rheumatic fever still is numero uno. The most common presentation of KD is prolonged fever so prompt recognition of fever in KD is important to avoid severe complications.

ETIOLOGY

The causative factors of KD are still unclear; it is likely to be the result of immune hyperreactivity to a variety of triggers including possible infections in a genetically susceptible host (a polymorphism in the *ITPKC* gene, a negative regulator of T-cell activation on chromosome 19 is strongly associated with susceptibility to the disease). Linkage studies and genome-wide association studies (GWAS) have identified significant potential associations between polymorphisms in the *ITPKC* gene, *CASP3*, *BLK*, and *FCGR2A* and single-nucleotide polymorphisms (SNPs) in the human leukocyte antigen class II region (HLA-DQB2 and HLA-DOB).

EPIDEMIOLOGY

Kawasaki disease commonly affects children under the age of 5 years and results in hospitalization. In countries such as the United Kingdom, South Korea, and Japan, and probably in India the rate of KD seems to be increasing. Several risk stratification models have been constructed to determine which patients with KD are at highest risk for coronary artery disease (CAA). Of these, the Kobayashi score is the most widely used and has high sensitivity and specificity. However, in non-Japanese populations the application of these scoring models does not appear to accurately identify all children at risk for intravenous immunoglobulin (IVIGg) resistance and CAA. Body surface area (BSA)-adjusted coronary artery dimensions on baseline echocardiography in the first 10 days of illness appear to be good predictors of involvement during follow-up. Accordingly, baseline Z-scores may provide a useful imaging biomarker.

PATHOLOGY

Kawasaki disease is a medium-vessel vasculitis with striking predilection for coronary arteries, although other medium-size arteries (e.g., axillary, subclavian, femoral, popliteal, and brachial) can also develop dilation. Arteriopathy usually occurs in three phases. In first week, the first phase of a neutrophilic necrotizing arteritis begins in the endothelium and moves through the coronary wall. Sometimes saccular aneurysms may result from this arteritis. In the second phase, which may last weeks to years, subacute/chronic vasculitis is driven by lymphocytes, plasma cells, and eosinophils, and results in fusiform aneurysms. The third phase is due to development of smooth muscle cell myofibroblasts affected vessels, which cause progressive stenosis. Thrombi may form in the lumen and obstruct blood flow.

The affected vessel may subsequently become ecstatic. Healing of these vessels may, in due course, results in stenosis and thrombosis.

CLINICAL MANIFESTATIONS

Kawasaki disease mainly affects children of 6 months to 5 years old, with a peak at the end of the first year. Affected children are very irritable, have a high-fever (>38.3°C) that is difficult to control by most of the antipyretics. In addition to fever persisting at least 5 days, diagnosis of KD is based on recognition of a constellation of five clinical findings **(Table 1)**.

A typical KD case must have at least 4 out of 5 criteria for diagnosis. KD can be divided into three clinical phases. (1) The acute febrile phase is characterized by fever and the other acute signs of illness and usually lasts 1–2 weeks. (2) The subacute phase is associated with desquamation, thrombocytosis, development of CAA, and the highest risk of sudden death in patients who develop aneurysms; it generally

TABLE 1: Kawasaki disease: Diagnostic criteria.

Criteria	Description
Fever	Duration of 5 days or more PLUS 4 of 5 of following:
1. Conjunctivitis	Bilateral nonexudative conjunctival injection with limbal sparing
2. Lymphadenopathy	Nonsuppurative cervical often >1.5 cm
3. Rash	• Polymorphous, (maculopapular, erythema multiforme, scarlatiniform or less) • Perineal desquamation is common in the acute phase • No vesicles or crust
4. Changes of lips and oral mucosa	Red cracked lips, strawberry tongue, or diffuse erythema of oropharynx
5. Changes in extremities	• *Initial stage*: Edema and erythema of palms and soles • *Convalescent stage*: Peeling/desquamation of finger tips

lasts 3 weeks. (3) The convalescent phase begins when all clinical signs of illness have disappeared and continues until the erythrocyte sedimentation rate (ESR) returns to normal, typically 6-8 weeks after the onset of illness.

There may other nonspecific symptom or signs related to most of the systems. Other findings may be present such as desquamating rash in groin, retropharyngeal phlegmon, anterior uveitis by slit-lamp examination, erythema, induration at bacille Calmette-Guérin (BCG) inoculation site. *However, many patients have some but not all clinical features of KD. These patients are still at risk of CAA. Diagnosis of these "Incomplete KD" cases depends on a high level of suspicion in children presenting with some of the KD features and evidence of systemic inflammation (such as elevated CRP, ESR, or leukocytosis). Early echocardiography may reveal evidence of coronary vasculitis, confirming diagnosis of KD in this patient group. Negative echocardiogram does not exclude diagnosis of KD. In addition, fever of greater than 5 days may also lead to delayed treatment.*

Coronary artery disease occurs in 15-25% of untreated cases, with additional cardiac features including pericardial effusion, pericarditis, myocarditis, valvular incompetence, cardiac failure, and myocardial infarction. Other findings include anterior uveitis, fullness at BCG site, arthritis, aseptic meningitis, pneumonitis, uveitis, gastroenteritis, dysuria, and otitis. Relatively uncommon abnormalities include hydrops of the gallbladder, gastrointestinal ischemia, jaundice, cranial nerve palsy, renal involvement, shock syndrome, febrile convulsions and encephalopathy, and macrophage activation syndrome (Eleftheriou et al, 2014). Occasionally, patients with KD present in cardiogenic shock (KD shock syndrome), with greatly diminished left ventricular function. Almost all the morbidity and mortality in KD occur in patients with large or giant coronary artery aneurysms.

LABORATORY FINDINGS IN ACUTE KAWASAKI DISEASE

Leukocytosis with neutrophilia and immature forms, elevated erythrocyte sedimentation rate, elevated CRP, anemia, abnormal plasma lipids, hypoalbuminemia, hyponatremia, thrombocytosis after week 1, sterile pyuria, elevated serum transaminases, elevated serum γ-glutamyl transpeptidase, pleocytosis of cerebrospinal fluid, and leukocytosis in synovial fluid.

Patients with fever at least 5 days and <4 principal criteria can be diagnosed with Kawasaki disease when coronary artery abnormalities are detected by 2-dimensional echocardiography or angiography. Young infants tend to be more severely affected than older children and are more likely to have "incomplete" cases, in which not all the cardinal features are present.

Clinical features that are *not consistent* with KD include exudative conjunctivitis, exudative pharyngitis, generalized lymphadenopathy, discrete oral lesions (ulceration or exudative pharyngitis), splenomegaly, and bullous, petechial, or vesicular rashes.

Cardiac involvement manifests as tachycardia disproportionate to fever, along with diminished left ventricular systolic function. Occasionally, patients with KD present in cardiogenic shock (KD shock syndrome), with greatly diminished left ventricular function.

Almost all the morbidity and mortality in KD occur in patients with large or giant coronary artery aneurysms, defined by the 2017 American Heart Association (AHA) scientific statement on the diagnosis. Some experts believe that a z-score-based system for classification of aneurysm size may be more discriminating, because it adjusts the coronary dimension for BSA.

DIAGNOSIS

There is no diagnostic test; instead, the diagnosis is made on clinical findings. The diagnosis of KD should be made within 10 days, and ideally within 7 days, of fever onset to improve coronary artery outcomes. In atypical or incomplete KD, laboratory and echocardiographic data can assist in the diagnosis.

Ambiguous cases should be referred to a center with experience in the diagnosis of KD. Establishing the diagnosis with prompt institution of treatment is essential to prevent potentially devastating coronary artery disease. For this reason, *it is recommended that any infant age ≤6 months with fever for ≥7 days* without explanation undergo echocardiography to assess the coronary arteries.

DIFFERENTIAL DIAGNOSIS

Scarlet fever, measles, human herpesvirus (HHV) 6 and HHV-7, toxic shock syndrome, Stevens-Johnson syndrome, drug hypersensitivity, serum sickness, and systemic-onset juvenile idiopathic arthritis (sJIA)

In Indian scenario, measles can be distinguished from KD by exudative conjunctivitis, Koplik spots, rash that begins on the face and hairline and behind the ears, and leukopenia. Scarlet fever and cervical lymphadenitis can be the initial diagnosis in children who are ultimately recognized to have KD. Leptospirosis can also be an illness of considerable severity. sJIA is also characterized by fever and rash, but lymphadenopathy is diffused with hepatosplenomegaly.

TREATMENT

Every child suspected to have KD should be admitted and evaluated. Acute KD should be treated with 2 g/kg of IVIG as a single infusion, usually administered over 10–12 hours within 10 days of disease onset, and ideally as soon as possible after diagnosis.

In addition, moderate (30–50 mg/kg/day divided every 6 hours) to high-dose aspirin (80–100 mg/kg/day divided every 6 hours) should be administered until the patient is afebrile for 48 hours, and then dose of aspirin is usually decreased from anti-inflammatory to antithrombotic doses (3–5 mg/kg/day as a single dose). Aspirin is continued for its antithrombotic effect till follow-up echocardiography is done and found to be normal at 6–8 weeks of illness. If CAAs are found in follow-up echocardiography, aspirin needs to be continued for prolonged periods. Additional anticoagulation (with warfarin or low molecular weight heparin) may be required in children with large aneurysms. While therapy with IVIg and aspirin has dramatically reduced the occurrence of CAAs in KD, a small proportion of patients (approximately 3–5%) still go onto develop CAAs despite appropriate therapy.

The mechanism of action of IVIg in KD is unknown, but treatment results in resolution of clinical signs in approximately 85% of patients. Prevalence of coronary disease, in 20–25% in children treated with aspirin alone, is <5% in those treated with IVIg and aspirin within first 10 days of illness. Other nonsteroidal anti-inflammatory drugs (NSAIDs) should not be given during therapy with aspirin because they may block the action of aspirin.

Strong consideration should be given to treating patients with persistent fever, abnormal dimensions of the coronary arteries, or signs of systemic inflammation who are diagnosed after the 10th day of fever. Patients with CAA continue with aspirin therapy and may require anticoagulation, depending on the degree of coronary dilation. Clopidogrel 1 mg/kg/day (maximum 75 mg/day) may be needed occasionally. For children at particularly high-risk of thrombosis are given warfarin or low molecular weight heparin. Acute coronary thrombosis requires prompt fibrinolytic therapy with tissue plasminogen activator or other thrombolytic agent has to be given under supervision of a pediatric cardiologist. *Corticosteroids* have been used as primary therapy with the first dose of IVIg in hopes of improving coronary outcomes. However, administration of corticosteroids as primary therapy to all children with KD awaits the development of a risk score that identifies high-risk children in a multiracial population.

IVIg-resistant KD: It occurs in approximately 15% of patients and is defined by persistent or recurdescent fever 36 hours after completion of the initial IVIg infusion. Patients with IVIg resistance are at increased risk for CAA. Many scoring systems have been developed to predict IVIg resistance. Of these, Kobayashi score is most widely used with high sensitivity and specificity. These scoring systems do not yield reliable results in populations other than Japanese and therefore may have limited utility.

These children can be given second dose of IVIg (2 g/kg), corticosteroids, and/or infliximab. For serious patients with enlarging coronary aneurysms, additional therapies such as cyclosporine or cyclophosphamide may be administered, with consultation from specialists in pediatric rheumatology and cardiology. In general, mortality is 1–2%.

Long-term follow-up of patients with coronary artery aneurysms is dependent on the past (i.e., worst ever) and current coronary status, with a schedule of testing recommended in the 2017 AHA scientific statement on KD. Testing may include echocardiography, assessment for inducible ischemia, advanced imaging (CT, MRI, or invasive angiography), physical activity counseling, and cardiovascular risk factor assessment and management. Patients with coronary artery stenosis and inducible ischemia may be managed with coronary artery bypass grafting (CABG) or catheter interventions, including percutaneous transluminal coronary rotational ablation, directional coronary atherectomy, and stent implantation.

VACCINATION

Patients undergoing long-term aspirin therapy should receive annual influenza vaccination to reduce the risk of Reye syndrome. IVIg may interfere with the immune response to live-virus vaccines as a result of specific antiviral antibody, so the measles-mumps-rubella and varicella vaccinations should generally be deferred until 11 months after IVIg administration. Nonlive vaccinations should not be delayed.

All children with a history of KD should be counseled regarding a heart-healthy diet, adequate amounts of exercise, tobacco avoidance, and intermittent lipid monitoring.

PROGNOSIS

The majority of patients with KD return to normal health; timely treatment reduces the risk of coronary aneurysms, which is <5% in timely treated children. The prognosis for patients with CCA depends on the severity of coronary disease; therefore, recommendations for follow-up and management are stratified according to coronary artery status. KD can recur in 1–3% treated children. Mortality is 1–3%.

Whether children who have had KD and normal echocardiography findings throughout their course are at higher risk for the development of atherosclerotic heart disease in adulthood remains unclear. All children with a history of KD should be counseled regarding a heart-healthy diet, adequate amounts of exercise, tobacco avoidance, and intermittent lipid monitoring. A landmark study by Kato et al. showed that up to 50% of small-to-medium-sized aneurysms resolve on follow-up. Giant aneurysms (>8 mm size), however, do not resolve and are associated with significant long-term morbidity. Even when the coronary aneurysm appears to have resolved anatomically, functional vessel wall abnormalities are known to persist and may result in myocardial ischemia/infarction later in life.

SUGGESTED READING

1. Chen S, Dong Y, Kiuchi M, Wang J, Li R, Ling Z, et al. Coronary artery complication in Kawasaki disease and the importance of early intervention. JAMA Pediatr. 2016;170(12):1156-63.
2. Gong GWK, McCrindle BW, Ching JC, Yeung RSM. Arthritis presenting during the acute phase of Kawasaki disease. J Pediatr. 2001; 148:800-5.
3. Gorman KM, Gavin PJ, Capra L. Bacillus-Calmette-Guérin scare erythema: "haloing" the diagnosis in Kawasaki disease. J Pediatr. 2015;167:774.
4. Kobayashi T, Saji T, Otani T, Takeuchi K, Nakamura T, Arakawa H, et al. Efficacy of immunoglobulin plus prednisolone for prevention of coronary artery abnormalities in severe Kawasaki disease (RAISE study): a randomized, open label, blinded endpoints trial. Lancet. 2012;379(9826):1613-20.
5. McCrindle BW, Rowley A, Newburger JW, Burns JC, Bolger AF, Gewitz M, et al. Diagnosis, treatment, and long-term management of Kawasaki disease: a scientific statement for health professionals from the American Heart Association. Circulation. 2017;135(17):e927-99.
6. McCrindle BW, Tierney ESS. Acute treatment for Kawasaki disease: challenges for current and future therapies. J Pediatr. 2017;184:7-10.

SECTION 14: Genetic Disorders

155. Genetic Counceling
156. Common Chromosomal Disorders
157. Dysmorphic Child
158. Karyotyping
159. Inborn Errors of Metabolism
160. Prenatal Screening and Diagnosis of Congenital Disorders
161. Lysosomal Storage Diseases in India

Genetic Counseling

Amar Verma, Anita Verma

GENERAL CONSIDERATIONS

- The expanding role of genetics in almost every clinical condition is associated with the increasing development of new genetic and molecular tests, and implementation of these tests is becoming well integrated into medical practice. Therefore, primary care providers, family doctors, pediatricians, and other specialists involved in the care of patients and families affected by genetic conditions will be largely concerned with both genetic tests and genetic counseling.
- It is considered in several stages: Collecting genetic information and pedigree drawing; making or validating the diagnosis; estimating occurrence and recurrence risk; communicating clinical information; and supporting the family to reach a decision and taking appropriate action.
- It is often used to describe the entire approach to patients and families with genetic conditions, sometimes being restricted to the communication and psychotherapeutic process.
- During the last 40 years, the field of genetic counseling has expanded rapidly. Genetic counselors practice in a variety of settings, including hospitals, private offices, laboratories, federal and state government offices, universities, and research units. Patients seeking genetic counseling can be younger, elderly, male or female, pregnant or newly married, affected with a disease or at risk for a disease.
- While on one hand, the counseling provides adequate supportive and essential aid in decision-making for a particular situation that may arise due to the risk of carrying a genetic disorder in an individual; it may raise complex ethical questions on the other hand, which often do not have clear and simple answers.
- It is the process by which patients or relatives, at risk of an inherited disorder, are advised of the consequences and nature of the disorder, the probability of developing or transmitting it, and the options open to them in management and family planning in order to prevent, avoid or ameliorate it.
- It is a communication process which deals with human problems associated with the occurrence/risk of recurrence of a genetic disorder in a family. This approach deals to comprehend medical facts, risk of recurrence, options, choose the course of action.
- It is branched into diagnostic (the actual estimation of risk) and supportive aspects. This process involves appropriately trained persons to help the individual or family to: (1) comprehend the medical facts, including the diagnosis, probable course of the disorder, and the available management; (2) appreciate the way heredity contributes to the disorder, and the risk of recurrence in specified relatives; (3) understand the alternatives for dealing with the risk of occurrence; (4) choose the course of action which seems to them appropriate in view of their risk, their family goals, and their ethical and religious standards, to act in accordance with that decision (5) to make the best possible adjustment to the disorder in an affected family member and/or the risk of recurrence of that disorder.

IMPORTANCE OF COGNITIVE DECISIONS IN PRACTICE OF GENETIC COUNSELING

- Though the counselor discusses the risk factors associated with the ongoing conception in presence of both at-risk spouses, the decision regarding the available options depends solely on the attitude and acceptance of the individuals counseled. No simple correlation has been found between the change in technology to the changes in values and beliefs toward opinion or decision.
- The formulation of an informed, internally evaluated cognitive decision suggests strategies for evaluating the competence of any decision after genetic counseling.
- The value of a cognitive decision against a normative decision rests more on the determination of the quality of counselee-decision and the components tending to improve the process.
- A cognitive decision is a function of attitude (A) modified by others' feeling and sensitivity towards the "taken decision" (E) and the value adjudged to "others"

feeling and opinion shared by the counselee (V0); and is expressed as A + E (V0).
- Enhancing the sensitivity of counseling by approaching to gear up the educational activity related to the counselee's emotional state or by multiple visits, audiovisual aids, communicating the summary for the educational sessions by close interaction has earlier been advocated in Europe and found to be successful in a better implementation of genetic counseling.
- However, in our country these approaches are yet to be considered during the process of genetic counseling. (Despite the fact that we have a greater risk for hemoglobinopathies and associated mortality)

INDICATIONS OF GENETIC COUNSELING

- Congenital malformation in a child, stillbirth, or fetus
- Mental retardation and developmental delay
- Known genetic disease
- Short stature
- Neurodegenerative disorders
- Myopathies
- Chromosomal disorders
- Consanguineous marriages
- Advanced maternal age
- Exposure to teratogens
- Congenital deafness/blindness
- Familial disease
- Familial cancer and cancer-prone disease
- Abnormalities of sexual development and differentiation
- Hemoglobinopathies.

What are components of genetic counseling?
- Information gathering
- Diagnosis
- Risk assessment
- Information giving
- Psychological assessment and counseling
- Decision-making
- Providing support system.

Communication happens in three ways:
1. Body language counts to 55% (facial expression, posture).
2. Paralinguistic communication counts to 38% (intonation, volume, pitch, fluency, timing, etc.).
3. Verbal counts to 7%.

Speech therapist takes note of nonverbal communication that mirror the internal climate of client and becomes richest source of empathy.

METHODS OF GENETIC COUNSELING

- Directive
- Nondirective

Genetic counseling involves couple as a unit rather than the individual. It is not directly related to health of counselees but to their children.

Essential requisites of a good counselor:
- Knowledge in medical genetics.
- Good communication skills
- Capabilities of dealing with related emotional complexities and psychosocial issues
- Command over language
- Sympathetic listener
- Well informed.

Who should be a counselor?
- Clinical geneticist
- Laboratory geneticist
- Genetic nurse
- Genetic counselors
- Social worker
- Psychologists.

REQUIREMENTS OF GENETIC COUNSELING

- Quiet room
- Adequate time
- Both parents
- Local language
- Sensitive manner
- Preparation (test records, review of literature)
- Truthfullness
- Awareness of religious psychosocial background
- Willing to answer questions
- Ability to tackle emotional complexities.

PSYCHOSOCIAL ASPECTS AND NONDIRECTIVENESS IN GENETIC COUNSELING

This must be made clear to the patients and their family members that:
- Genetic disease is not stigma.
- Common misconception about genetic disease has to be well explained.
- Explanation about cause-and-blame phenomenon.
- Interpersonal relationship.

While dealing with prepositus the whole conversation should be in an:
- Unbiased manner
- Dealing with various options and their results
- No personal views and opinions should be offered.

What should be the posture of counselor?
- Sit squarely in relation to client
- Maintain open position
- Lean slightly toward client
- Maintain reasonable eye contact
- Relaxed posture.

Techniques:
- Minimal use of prompts

- Use of calibration (*Calibration*: It is a technology by which a counselor attempts to mirror and empathize with the client).

Responding skills:
- *Funneling*: Moving from general area to more specific
- *Reflection*: Echoing back onto client what counsellor gathers from conversation
- Empathy building
- Clarifying done by summarizing occasionally in order to clarify what is being said.

Mobilizing of body energy: In this, the therapist lets client experience bottled up emotions later release the tension by stretching and breathing out.

Rehearsal/role playing:
- Here the client is coached by the counselor to take roles that he/she is uncomfortable with
- Provides invaluable exercise to face the situation with renewed confidence.

Scheduling:
- It is important to schedule a treatment regimen.
- Most practical sequence is five follow-up sessions over a period of 6 weeks.
- Interesting to note that women abide by most strict regimen suggested by counselor.
- Men are less inclined to do so.

Techniques:
- Attending and hearing skills.
- *Recording*: Advisable to record the happenings in a counseling session. It is helpful for continuity as well as for follow-up.
- *Free-floating attention*: The counselor needs to focus fully outside/himself or herself on client.

He should keep away from internal domain and avoid internal constraints, hunches, and fantasy.
- Cathartic skills.
- *Acknowledging*: Emotions are culture specific; often client needs some assurances from counselor to express them.
- *Reliving*: It is powerful tool to revisiting the past experience.
- *Alter ego*: Client is seated before counselor/freely expresses himself or herself. The seats are exchanged. The counselor mimics the clients expression back onto client.
- *Decision-making skills*: Now that client has experienced catharsis by expressing his or her feelings, client becomes more rational. Counselor assists client in explaining the plausible strategies to solve the problem and thus go toward decision-making.
- *Planning skills*: Planning involves blue print for action, so one has to plan.

SMART:
S: Specific
M: Maintainable
A: Achievable
R: Realistic
T: Time bound

CONCLUSION

- A recent challenge for genetic counselors has been the development of predictive testing for disorders. With modern genetic technology, DNA testing can indicate the relative probability that some individuals will develop a genetic disease but fails to predict the actual outcome. Thus an individual with a 75% chance of developing a particular genetic disease may remain healthy throughout his or her life, while an individual with only 25% probability of disease development may succumb to the disease. In addition, for some diseases (e.g., Alzheimer disease) there are no cures or treatments available, regardless of predictability. In situations such as these, the benefit of predictive testing remains open to debate.
- Pre-Conception and Pre-Natal Diagnostic Techniques (PCPNDT) tests are available at few location in India. The absence of such techniques for prenatal confirmation, the prediction of a fetus at risk and fatality that may become apparent especially in at-risk couples, depends solely on the guess and chance as assumed from laboratory findings and calculation of inherited risk by the genetic counselor.
- Many places of India still are away from the main stream research and diagnostic confirmation facilities. The moral risks associated at individual as well as family and society level have always been in question leading to improper consequences and often refutation. The answers to the queries of the people are generally avoided deliberately and the issues arising thereby are kept unattended.
- Often, it is observed that the introduction of newer facts about the risk associated with one's hemoglobinopathies status at individual level is progressively affected and shaped by a multitude of negative influence and rejection from the family, society, and cultural spheres.
- Consequently, the separation of clinical from supportive process had an important role in most definitions of genetic counseling. Should all those aspects be considered parts of a single process? This is the main question that will be discussed hereafter, under the hypothesis that the synthesis of all those steps should be required to approach any genetic conditions.

In that view, rethinking of genetic counseling from a medical point of view should be seen as an important subject for discussion, and might contribute to bring together clinical and nonmedical aspects.

CHAPTER 156

Common Chromosomal Disorders

Manika Verma, Anita Verma, Amar Verma

INTRODUCTION

As stated very truly by Dr Samuel Johnson, *"A man ought to readjust as inclination leads him; for what he reads as a task will do him little good."* (Quoted from Preface of Emery's Essential of Medical genetics edited by Turnpenny & Sian Allard, 2010). This chapter tries to attract and integrate knowledge of Medical genetics focused in few-to-vast large world of our graduate and postgraduates, who may probably someday assimilate their knowledge in this everchanging world for the benefit of humankind.

- A chromosome disorder results from a change in the *number* or *structure* of chromosomes. Each of our chromosomes has a characteristic structure.
- Scientists have used a staining technique that colors the chromosomes into a *banding pattern*. These banding patterns make each of our individual chromosomes easier to identify like a map.
- A set of chromosomes, as seen under a microscope, is known as a *karyotype*. Any deviation from the normal karyotype is known as a chromosome abnormality.
- Some chromosome abnormalities are harmless; some are associated with clinical disorders. Half of all spontaneous abortions are due to chromosome abnormalities.

Numerical Abnormalities

- The most severe chromosome disorders are caused by the loss or gain of whole chromosomes, which can affect hundreds, or even thousands, of genes and are usually fatal.
- A few numerical abnormalities support development to term, either because the chromosome is small and/or contains relatively few genes or because there is a natural mechanism present to help adjust gene dosage.

Structural Abnormalities

- This is when large sections of DNA are missing from or are added to a chromosome. Structural abnormalities can take several forms. The most common among the major numerical abnormalities that survive to term is Down syndrome.
- The incidence of chromosomal abnormalities among newborn in general is about 6:1,000. If we include stillbirth and perinatal death also, then the incidence may increase up to 50:1,000.

When to suspect chromosomal abnormality?

Chromosomal abnormality of either number or structure has detrimental effect on phenotype of any individual. Aneuploidy of an autosome or nonsex chromosome generally significantly impairs physical or cognitive development.

Usually aneuploidy of sex chromosome does not have much or no significant impairment. A clinician has to look for following points:

- *Clustering of abnormalities* in family members to suggest a problem, although their absence does not rule out a chromosomal abnormality.
- Carriers of an inherited or de-novo reciprocal translocation are usually balanced and subsequently normal. However, their concept uses are likely to be genetically unbalanced and may abort spontaneously or be born with major congenital anomalies.
- *History* of unexplained infertility, multiple spontaneous abortions (three or more) or previous birth of dysmorphic child or child with major congenital anomalies to couple or to a close relative may be an indication that one of the parent carries a balanced chromosomal translocation or rearrangement.

In such situations, advise chromosome study of couple and child both. If translocation is found, an antenatal genetic counseling is indicated. This may also be advisable for extended family members also.

Broadly speaking, there are four types of chromosomal genetic diseases:

1. Disorders inherited through classical Mendelian inheritance—pattern including single gene mutation (Marfan's syndrome, Rett syndrome, Smith Lemli Opitz syndrome, Conradi Hunermann syndrome).

2. Disorders inherited through non-Mendelian inheritance, i.e., teratogenic exposures in utero, disruptions or deformations of previously normal fetal structures.
3. New etiologic mechanism of diseases, i.e., imprinting abnormalities and expansion of trinucleotide repeats in nuclear DNA.
4. Disorders of mitochondrial DNA or mitochondrial functions.

COMMON CHROMOSOMAL DISORDERS OF AUTOSOMAL ABNORMALITY

Down Syndrome

- Incidence of Down syndrome among live born is 1:600–700 but incidence is certainly more than that in Indian subcontinent (pan-India data still unavailable).
- 45% of affected individual born of women older than 35 years. Now even women as young as in early twenties are giving birth to trisomy 21 (Down syndrome).
- The incidence of Down syndrome is far greater in conceptus than live born (on autopsy) but majority of fetuses spontaneously abort.

Etiology

- *Nondisjunction*: Failure of one or more pairs of homologous chromosomes or sister chromatids to separate normally during nuclear division, usually resulting in an abnormal distribution of chromosomes in the daughter nuclei. There are three forms of nondisjunction:
  1. Failure of a pair of homologous chromosomes to separate in meiosis.
  2. Failure of sister chromatids to separate during meiosis II.
  3. Failure of sister chromatids to separate during mitosis.

  Trisomy 21 or part of chromosome 21 fused with another chromosome results from this phenomenon.
- *Translocation*: About 5% of Down syndrome represent centric fusion translocation between the long arms of 21 and those of 13, 14, 15, 21, 22 acrocentric chromosome. Of these, one third inherited from clinically normal-balanced carrier parent. In remaining two thirds of cases, translocation is first time present in the affected child. Fused chromosomes are often Robertsonian translocation or isochromosomes.
- *Mosaicism*: Trisomy 21 cell lines coexist with standard 46 chromosomes as well. Range of phenotype exists from normal to that typical of complete trisomy.

Risk of Recurrence

For straightforward trisomy 21, the recurrence risk is related to maternal age (variable) and the simple fact that trisomy has already occurred (~1%).

The combined recurrence risk is usually between 1:200 and 1:100. In translocation cases, similar figure apply if neither parent is a carrier.

- If a parent carries 21/21 translocation— 100% risk.
- If 21/centric fusion translocation—empiric risk of recurrence—<2%, if the father is a carrier.
- If the mother is a carrier, then risk of recurrence is ~15%. Prenatal diagnosis can be offered based on analysis of chorionic villi or cultured amniotic cells. Prenatal screening programs have been introduced based on the so-called triple or quadruple tests of maternal serum at 16 weeks' gestation.

Clinical diagnosis rests on the findings of recognizable constellation of clinical characteristics, including a combination of following major and minor anomalies:

- Upslanting palpebral fissures
- Small external ears (by length)
- Congenital heart disease (CHD) (45%)—atrioventriular communis, endocardial cushion defect, ventricular septal defect (VSD), etc.
- Gastrointestinal anomaly (5%) most common duodenal atresia, Hirschsprung's disease
- *Thyroid disorder*: Autoimmune thyroiditis
- *Acute and neonatal leukemia*: About 15–20 times more than normal population, transient leukemoid reaction may be seen in newborn
- Shorter than family members and have premature graying of hairs
- Most are infertile but females may reproduce and can have children who will also have Down syndrome approximately one third of the time
- Quantitative abnormalities in many enzyme systems
- *Minor anomalies*:
  - Brachycephaly
  - Inner epicanthal fold
  - Brushfield spots
  - Flat nasal bridge
  - Small mouth with protruding tongue that fissures with age
  - Short neck with redundant skin folds
  - Single transverse palmer creases (Simian crease)
  - Clinodactyly of fifth finger with single digital crease caused by Hypoplasia of middle phalanx
  - Wide spacing between first and second toes (Saddle Toe)
- Cognitive impairment is common but degree of impairment varies with IQ ranging from 20 to 80
- There is mild-to-moderate range of developmental delay. Advent of individualized program of early intervention therapy, education, and sporting activities resulted in improved outcome
- Neuropathologic changes of Alzheimer's disease are seen on autopsy. But only 25% of older Down syndrome patients show Alzheimer's disease

- Progressive loss of cognitive functions after fourth decade of life
- An individual with Down syndrome without CHD may live up to 60's
- The principal cause of death in children with Down syndrome is:
  - Infection
  - CHD
  - Malignancy

COMMON CHROMOSOMAL ABNORMALITIES OF SEX CHROMOSOMES

Turner Syndrome

- It is one of the three most common chromosomal abnormalities found in early spontaneous abortion.
- 1:2,000 live born female has Turner syndrome.

Features

- Primary amenorrhea
- Sterility
- Sparse pubic and axillary hair
- Underdeveloped breast
- Short stature
- Webbing of neck, cubitus valgus, low-set posterior hairline, shield chest and widely spaced nipples, malformed/often protruding ear
- Renal anomaly along with CHD (particularly, bicuspid aortic valve 30%, coarctation of aorta 10%)
- Affected women have infantile uterus; ovaries consist of strands of fibrous connective tissues
- *Newborn*: Lymphedema of feet/hands or both, which may reappear briefly during adolescence
- Mental development—normal
- *Schooling and behavioral*: Same as age specific, although difficulty with Spatial orientation (Map reading). Classic findings in newborn are so less that they may be missed
- First indication of presence of Turner syndrome may be unexplained short stature/failure to develop secondary sexual characteristics by late adolescence

Diagnosis

- Chromosome study or karyotype may be part of workup in such complaints of adolescent girls. In majority, it is 45XO. Turner syndrome unrelated to increase in maternal or paternal age.
- Another 15% of Turner syndrome is mosaic (XO/XX, XO/XX/XXX, or XO/XY). Physical stigma is less marked in mosaics, some of whom may be fertile.
- *Ultrasonography*: Presence/Absence of intra-abdominal gonads (Removal if present).
- *Risk of recurrence*: If karyotype is 45X or mosaic: 1–2%, but may be higher if parent carries a structurally abnormal X chromosome.
- *Antenatal diagnosis*: Discuss possibility with parent if previous birth of any abnormal child. There is relatively good prognosis if detected early.

Clinical Point

Girls with Turner syndrome should receive appropriate hormone therapy during adolescence to enable development of secondary sex characteristics and stimulate menses.

Klinefelter Syndrome

Klinefelter syndrome (KS) (47, XXY) is a chromosomal variation in males in which one extra X-chromosome is present, resulting in XXY sex chromosome karyotype. The extra X-chromosome can affect physical, developmental, behavioral, and cognitive functioning.

- Common physical features may include tall stature, reduced muscle tone, small testes (hypogonadism), delayed pubertal development and lack of secondary male sex characteristics such as decreased facial and body hair and increased breast growth (gynecomastia) in late puberty.
- Common cognitive and behavioral features may include speech and language delays, ADHD (attention deficit hyperactivity disorder), and emotional and social functioning challenges.

The features of 47, XXY (KS) are typically associated with decreased testosterone level and elevated gonadotropin levels.

Symptoms and Signs

- At birth, most neonates with 47, XXY (KS) usually have no dysmorphic or unusual features.
- Infants and young children with 47, XXY (KS) are sometimes initially identified because of an abnormality in the location of the urinary opening in the penis (hypospadias), small penis or testes, or developmental delay (e.g., speech delay).
- Older children and teenagers are sometimes diagnosed with 47, XXY (KS) if secondary sexual characteristics do not develop completely, puberty is delayed, testes are small, or breast development may occur.
- Many males with 47, XXY (KS) are not identified until they have infertility problems as adults. Men with 47, XXY (KS) may have a relatively increased risk to develop breast cancer. Most males with 47, XXY (KS) have normal intelligence but there is an increased risk for language-related learning disorders, dyslexia, and social and

executive functioning challenges. They may exhibit autistic traits.
- Men with 47, XXY (KS) may have an increased risk for endocrine conditions such as diabetes mellitus, hypothyroidism and hypoparathyroidism and autoimmune diseases such as systemic lupus erythematosus, Sjogren syndrome and rheumatoid arthritis.

Clinical Point
Most individuals with 47, XXY (KS) may be identified though prenatal diagnosis or when the child does not progress through puberty completely or adequately.

Affected Populations
47, XXY (KS) is the most common human sex chromosome disorder and occurs in approximately 1 in 500–1,000 males.

Treatment
- One of the hallmarks of Klinefelter syndrome is hypergonadotropic hypogonadism, a condition that results in testosterone deficiency.
  Treatment involves the targeted administration of male hormones (androgens), such as testosterone enanthate, cypionate, or androgel.
  These hormones are given to promote the development of secondary male sexual characteristics (virilization) and alleviate feminization effects that have occurred due to insufficient testosterone levels. Hormone replacement therapy is effective when initiated during early infancy or around pubertal development or even later in life.
- Some men with 47, XXY (KS) who have gynecomastia may require surgical breast reduction for cosmetic purposes. This procedure often may be avoided if proper and timely dosage of testosterone is administered to an individual, although it varies with each individual.
- Speech and language therapy, physical therapy and occupational therapy are often helpful for boys with 47, XXY (KS). These interventions are shown to significantly improve academic, physical, cognitive, and social outcomes in boys with 47, XXY (KS).
- A comprehensive psychoeducational evaluation is recommended to determine what resources may be helpful in the classroom. Social skills training classes can also be beneficial.
- Men with 47, XXY (KS) have low fertility, and with novel assistive and reproductive techniques, more men with 47, XXY (KS) have the opportunity to reproduce a child. Men with mosaic 47, XXY (KS) have higher likelihood of fewer complications with reproduction.
- Surgical extraction of sperm from the testes and intracytoplasmic sperm injection (ICSI) directly into an ovum is a medical technology available to assist men with 47, XXY (KS) to father and children.

MOLECULAR CYTOGENETIC SYNDROMES
- Higher-resolution analysis of genomic DNA from uncultured cells by microarray platforms containing both array-CGH (comparative genomic hybridization) and SNP (single-nucleotide polymorphism) probes (Combo-chips) are now routinely utilized first-tier test in clinical settings.
- The molecular cytogenetics test identifies copy number variation (CNV) and also detects the regions with long or short stretches of homozygosity (ROH) known as DNA copy number neutral alteration. The clinical implications of CNVs are well recognized in diagnosis and management.
- Chromosomal microarray has been extensively shown to provide 10–15 times higher diagnostic yield than conventional cytogenetics methods.

Fragile X Syndrome (Marker X Syndrome, Martin-Bell Syndrome)
- This is mostly due to altered X-linked recessive genes. These may represent new mutation or inheritance of abnormal gene from normal heterozygous (carrier) mothers.
- About 1:150 individuals, usually male, have some form of X-linked mental retardation. Of these estimated 30–50% have Fragile X syndrome.
- The Fragile X syndrome is first recognized example of a trinucleotide repeat disorder. The gene involved is located at Xq27.3 is called *FMR1* and is active in brain cells and sperm.

Symptoms and Signs
Fragile X syndrome is characterized by:
- Moderate intellectual disability in affected males and mild intellectual disability in affected females. The physical features in affected males are variable and may not be obvious until puberty.
- These symptoms can include a large head, long face, prominent forehead and chin, protruding ears, loose joints and large testes.
- Other symptoms can include flat feet, frequent ear infections, low muscle tone, along narrow face, high-arched palate, dental problems, crossed eyes (strabismus) and heart problems including mitral valve prolapse.
- Delayed motor development, hyperactivity, behavior problems, toe walking, and/or occasional seizures can also occur in some patients.
- Autistic behaviors such as poor eye contact, hand flapping, and/or self-stimulating behaviors are also common.
- Motor and language delays are usually present but become more apparent overtime.

Affected Populations

The Fragile X syndrome affects about 1 in 4,000 males and 1 in 6,000–8,000 females in the USA but incidence is not documented in India yet. It affects about twice as many males as it does females. However, about four times as many females appear to be carriers of the altered gene as do males (1:250 females and 1:1,000 males). Fragile X syndrome has been found in all major ethnic groups and races.

Treatment

- Special education, speech, occupational, and sensory integration training, and behavior-modification programs.
- Other treatment may depend on an affected individual's specific symptoms.

Genetic counseling is recommended for affected individuals and their families.

DISORDERS OF IMPRINTING (EPIGENETIC PHENOMENON)

- Two common examples of this disorder are Prader-Willi syndrome (PWS) and Angelman syndrome. These disorders are caused by abnormalities of imprinted genes.
- The concept of imprinting refers to the fact that function of certain genes is dependent upon their parental origin: Maternal versus Paternal.
- Proper genetic imprinting is necessary for normal development. Imprinted genes tend to be found clustered or grouped together.
- Several imprinted genes are found in region 15q11q-13 of chromosome 15. This region also contains an area known as the Imprinting Center, and this area regulates the imprinted genes in this region.

Current diagnostic testing for these disorders includes the following:

- Karyotype with high-resolution cytogenetic technology.
- Methylation studies of which determines whether gene within 15q11–q13 critical region are functional.
- Appropriate dinucleotide arrays that cover and encompass small nuclear ribonucleoprotein associated Polypeptide N (SNRPN) for PWS and D15S10 for Angelman syndrome.
- In some cases of Angelman syndrome—direct analysis of *UBE3A* gene.

Prader–Willi Syndrome

The symptoms and severity of PWS may vary from one person to another. Many features of the disorder are nonspecific and others may develop slowly overtime or can be subtle.

- Infants will exhibit diminished muscle tone (hypotonia), which can cause a baby to feel "floppy" when held. Infantile hypotonia, which is often severe, is a near-universal feature of the disorder.
- After birth, hypotonia is associated with lethargy, a weak cry, poor responsiveness to stimuli, and poor reflexes including poor sucking ability, which result in feeding difficulties and failure to thrive. Infants are usually unable to breastfeed and may require tube feeding. Hypotonia slowly improves overtime, but some adults with PWS may continue to have some degree of hypotonia.
- Distinctive facial features including almond-shaped eyes, a thin upper lip, a down-turned mouth, a narrow bridge of the nose, a narrow forehead, and a disproportionately long, narrow head (dolichocephaly). Distinctive facial features can be noticeable shortly after birth or may develop slowly overtime.
- Typically, between 2 and 4.5 years of age, their weight increases although there may not be a noticeable change in appetite or caloric intake.
Between 4.5 and 8 years old, appetite and caloric intake usually increases, often thereafter developing a need to eat an extraordinarily large amount of food (hyperphagia) usually because they do not feel satisfied after completing a meal (satiety). In addition, there is a decreased calorie requirement in people with PWS due to low muscle, decreased metabolism and decreased physical activity if not treated with growth hormone replacement.
- Hypogonadism is a common finding in PWS.
- Individuals with PWS have growth hormone (GH) insufficiency.
- Affected individuals may also have abnormally small hands and feet, side-to-side curvature of the spine (scoliosis).
- Some individuals may have lack of color (pigment) known as hypopigmentation affecting the hair, eyes, and skin, particularly in those with the chromosome 15q deletion seen in about 60% of those with PWS. They may appear fair-skinned compared to other family members. Near sightedness (myopia) and misaligned eyes (strabismus) may also occur.
- Affected individuals may also experience recurrent respiratory infections.
- Certain conditions are increased in individuals with PWS including fractures due to decreased bone density (osteopenia), altered temperature sensation, a high vomiting threshold, and swelling (edema), and ulcerations of the legs, especially in obese adults.
- Some individuals may have reduced flow of saliva with abnormally thick, sticky saliva.

Affected Populations

Prader-Willi syndrome affects males and females in equal numbers and occurs in all ethnic groups and geographic regions in the world. Most estimates place the incidence between 1 in 10,000–30,000 individuals in the general population and about 350,000–400,000 individuals worldwide.

Diagnosis

- A detailed patient history, a thorough clinical evaluation and identification of characteristic symptoms. Consensus diagnostic criteria for PWS have been established and are effective for identifying potential cases of PWS.
- Genetic testing is required to confirm the diagnosis and to identify the specific genetic subtype (15q11–q13 deletion, maternal disomy 15, imprinting defect). Hence, all infants and newborns with unexplained hypotonia and poor suck should be tested for PWS.
- Confirmation of diagnosis of PWS by *DNA methylation tests* and fluorescent in situ hybridization (FISH).
- *High-resolution chromosomal microarray* studies are most useful in identifying the typical chromosome *15q11–q13* deletion, smaller rearrangements of this chromosome region, imprinting defects and specific maternal disomy 15 subclasses seen in PWS.
- *Prenatal diagnosis* is possible by methylation analysis following amniocentesis, regardless of the cause.

Treatment

- The treatment of PWS is directed toward the specific symptoms that are apparent in each individual. Early intervention and strict maintenance to treatment can greatly improve the overall health and quality of life for affected individuals and their families.
- Multidisciplinary action like help of clinical geneticists, pediatricians, orthopedists, endocrinologists, speech therapists, psychologists, dieticians, nutritionists, and other healthcare professionals may need to systematically and comprehensively plan an effective program for the child's treatment.
- Genetic counseling may be of benefit for affected individuals and their families.
- Parents are strongly recommended to undergo appropriate parenting techniques for the behavioral and eating issues associated with PWS; such education correlates with better prognosis.
- Evaluation and treatment of sleep disturbance is recommended as well.
- Screened for hypothyroidism (which occurs with increased incidence in PWS) and central adrenal insufficiency.
- Sex hormones can be replaced at puberty as they can stimulate the development of secondary sexual characteristics and improve self-image and bone density.

Angelman Syndrome

- Angelman syndrome was first described in the medical literature in 1965 by Dr Harry Angelman, an English physician. The characteristic findings of this syndrome are not usually apparent at birth and diagnosis of the disorder is usually made between 1 and 4 years of age.
- It is a rare genetic and neurological disorder characterized by severe developmental delay and learning disabilities, absence or near absence of speech, inability to coordinate voluntary movements (ataxia); tremulousness with jerky movements of the arms and legs.
- A distinct behavioral pattern characterized by a happy disposition and unprovoked episodes of laughter and smiling. Although those with the syndrome may be unable to speak, many gradually learn to communicate through other means such as gesturing.
- Receptive language ability is good to understand simple forms of language communication.
- Additional symptoms may occur including seizures, sleep disorders and feeding difficulties.

Causes

- Deficiency of the E3 ubiquitin protein ligase (UBE3A) gene expression. The gene is located in chromosome region 15 (15q11–q13).
- In approximately 70–75% of cases there is a microdeletion of region 15q11-13 of the maternally-derived chromosome 15 that includes deletion of the *UBE3A* gene. This deletion usually occurs sporadically (de novo) and is not inherited. The risk of recurrence for the deletion in a family is estimated to be 1–2% or less.

Diagnosis

A diagnosis of Angelman syndrome may be made based upon:
- Detailed patient history, a thorough clinical evaluation and identification of characteristic findings.
- About 80% of cases can be confirmed through a variety of specialized blood tests such as DNA methylation (detects, but does not discriminate between chromosome deletion, imprinting center defect and paternal uniparental disomy).
- Fluorescent in situ hybridization (FISH) or most commonly, microarray chromosome analysis can detect the characteristic deletion (seen in 70% of cases) of chromosome 15q11-q13 in cells of the body.
- Mutation analysis of the Angelman gene, UBE3A, can detect about 10% of individuals with Angelman syndrome who have negative DNA methylation studies.
- Mutation analysis of UBE3A can be either ordered specifically as a single test but, more often now, UBE3A mutations are identified by use of a whole exome sequencing panel.

Treatment

- Symptomatic and supportive only.
- No genetic therapy or curative medication available. Advances in neuroscience and in gene therapy techniques however hold great potential for providing meaningful treatment and/or cure of the syndrome.

- Anti-seizure medications in seizures.
- Sleep disorders are common and may require behavioral therapy and adherence to strict bedtime routines. At time, sedating medications can be helpful.
- Feeding difficulties may be treated by modified breastfeeding methods and by means such as special nipples to assist infants with a poor ability to suck.
- Gastroesophageal reflux may be treated by upright positioning and drugs that aid the movement of food through the digestive system (motility drugs).
- Ankle braces/supports and physical therapy can help in achievement of walking. Scoliosis can develop in about 10% and may require braces or surgical correction. In some cases, strabismus may require surgical correction.
- Early intervention is important to ensure that children with Angelman syndrome reach their potential.

SUGGESTED READING

1. De Grouchy J, Turleau C. Clinical Atlas of Human Chromosomes, 2nd edition. Chichester: John Wiley. 1984.
2. Donnai D, Karmiloff-Smith A. Williams syndrome. Am J Med Genet (Semin MedGenet). 2000;97:164-71.
3. Penny T, Ellard S (eds). Elements of Medical Genetics, 15th edition. 2010.

Dysmorphic Child

Anoop Verma

INTRODUCTION

"Remember always that in clinical practice normality is more common and more variable than abnormality." The more you learn, the more you are compelled to search. There is no replacement of gaining experience, by examining, as much number of patients as possible, and to increase the width of your clinical acumen. There are thousands of malformation syndromes, but the majority is rare. It is not possible to memorize the features of each syndrome and so a diagnostic approach is essential to unravel the complexities of a child presenting with multiple abnormal features.

DYSMORPHOLOGY

The word dysmorphic comes from the Greek words, "dys" (disordered, abnormal, and painful) and "morph" (shape form). Dysmorphology is a discipline of clinical genetics that studies and attempts to interpret the patterns of human growth and structural defects.

Syndrome recognition and its diagnosis are important for several reasons:

- The pattern of anomalies is specific for each syndrome which may direct the investigation in a specific direction, and so is the management.
- It helps providing long-term prognosis and may also help in identifying options available for treatment.
- It helps in genetic counseling, such as estimation of genetic risks and possible means of prenatal diagnosis.

What are the types of congenital abnormalities seen?

- *Major anomalies*: Major malformations are severe, impair normal body function, and require surgery for management, e.g., duodenal atresia, congenital heart defects and meningomyelocele. The frequency of major malformations at birth is 2–3%. Major malformations may be isolated or multiple. They have different prognoses. Isolated malformations in an otherwise normal person are usually due to multifactorial inheritance, while major malformations in varying combinations mostly constitute a dysmorphic syndrome. They are not considered to be a variation of the normal spectrum.

- *Minor anomalies*: These are commonly seen in normal population but do not cause significant morbidity. Approximately 15% of newborn babies will have at least one minor malformation. The presence of a minor malformation should alert the clinician to look for a major malformation such as a heart defect and kidney problems. Children with one or more minor malformations are more likely to have a major malformation. Approximately 1.4% of the newborns with no minor malformations have a major malformation. If one minor malformation is present, the probability of a major malformation is 3%. If three or more minor malformations are present, the risk of a major malformation is 90%. Minor malformations are primarily of cosmetic significance, e.g., small ear, ear tag, and polydactyly **(Table 1)**.

The presence of both major and minor anomalies may be associated with particular syndromes or, may be an isolated finding in an otherwise healthy individual. For example, a cleft lip or palate may be an isolated finding. It is a fact that what appears to be the same birth defect or congenital anomaly may have completely different etiologies in different individuals. The constellation of major and minor

TABLE 1: List of minor anomalies.	
Face	Synophrys, nose: anteverted nostrils, bifid tip of the nose, palate high arched, Uvula bifid, micrognathia
Eye	Epicanthus, palpebral fissure up or downslanting, short palpebral fissure, hyper- or hypotelorism
Ear	Malformation, asymmetric, low-set, small ears, pre-auricular skin tags, ear lobe creases
Head and neck	Webbing of skin of neck and flat occiput
Hair	Parietal whorls are two or more, abnormal posterior whorl
Hand	Cutaneous syndactyly partial, simian crease, Sydney crease, clinodactyly
Trunk	Café au lait patches, hemangioma, accessory nipple, short trunk
Feet	Broad hallux, partial syndactyly

anomalies points to a specific syndrome diagnosis or known *association.*

SYNDROME

The word "*Syndrome*" is derived from the Greek "*Running together.*" It is generally recognized and defined as a *well-characterized constellation of major and minor anomalies that occur together in a predictable fashion,* presumably due to a single underlying cause, which may be monogenic, chromosomal, mitochondrial, or teratogenic in origin. Consider presence of syndrome in a patient when any of three combinations are present:

(1) Presence of more than three minor anomalies, (2) presence of more than one major anomalies, and (3) presence of one major or few minor anomalies.

Association is a group of anomalies that occur more frequently together than would be expected by chance alone but without predictable pattern of recognition or a suspected unified underlying etiology.

Sequence is a group of related anomalies that generally arise from a single initial major anomaly that alters the development of other surrounding or related tissues or structures, e.g., Potter's sequence.

Field defect is often used to describe related malformations in a particular region and sometimes is used interchangeably with sequence. Pierre-Robin sequence is sometimes referred to as a field defect.

What are the types of defective morphogenesis? (Flowchart 1)

When considering dysmorphic features, it is important to keep in mind the various ways in which structures and tissues may become abnormal or deformed.

Malformation signifies the abnormalities of growth and development due to underlying genetic, epigenetic, or environmental factors that altered the development of a particular structure.

Deformation is caused by an abnormal external force on the fetus in utero, which results in abnormal growth or formation of the fetal structure.

Disruption is where a normal fetal structure growth is disrupted. The disrupted agent can be amniotic band, intrauterine infections and tissue ischemia, and hemorrhage.

Dysplasia: The failure of maintaining the intrinsic cellular architecture of the tissue throughout the growth and development. Only one tissue type is affected throughout the body, e.g., skeletal dysplasia, ectoderm dysplasia.

APPROACH TO DYSMORPHIC DIAGNOSIS (BOX 1)

- There is no universally accepted methodology for accurate diagnosis in dysmorphology.
- The diagnosis can be made instantaneously by "Gestalt," or instant recognition based on past experience.
- Identify the diagnostic "*handles*" (which may be the specific features of a particular syndrome), and identifying the links between them and then recognizing whether they fit in a known pattern or syndrome.
- The diagnosis can be reached with the assistance of clinical experience, good history, physical examination, family evaluation, clinical photographs, specialized centile charts, laboratory investigations, and electronic databases.
- The electronic database search (**Box 1**).

History

The good history includes a detailed pedigree analysis (at least three generations), which is constructed using standardized set of symbols. Direct questions are asked to the family members for similarly affected individuals, miscarriages, early deaths, consanguinity, and major and minor malformations.

Examination

A detailed physical examination with adequate anthropometric measurements is necessary. While examining a dysmorphic patient, note the correct description of facial abnormalities, and minor and major malformations. A photograph album of dysmorphic child and family as well is essential to pick common abnormalities in the family. Do not afford to miss the presence of "diagnostic handles" of Hall (**Box 2**).

Examination of Family Members

A careful clinical examination of parents and family members for mild manifestations can be of great use in a patient with

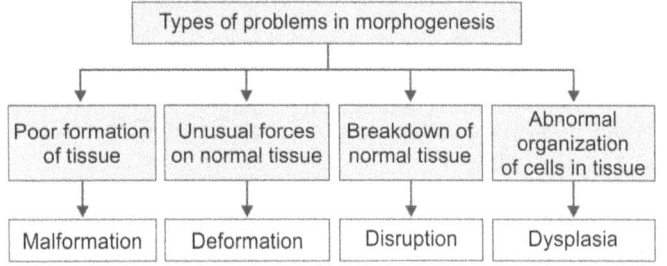

Flowchart 1: Different types of tissue dysmorphogenesis.

BOX 1: Making tentative diagnosis.
Gestalt diagnosis (comes instantaneously by past experience)
Chose a small number of best diagnostic handles (3–5)
Consult dysmorphology text
London Dysmorphology Database (LDDB)
Picture of Standard Syndromes and Undiagnosed Malformation (POSSUM)
Online Mendelian Inheritance in Man (OMIM)
Smith recognizable pattern of human malformations

> **BOX 2:** Pearls of dysmorphology by Hall.
>
> *Pursed up lips:* Whistling face syndrome
> *Broad thumbs/great toes:* Rubinstein–Taybi syndrome, Pfeiffer syndrome, Fanconi anemia
> *Absent clavicles:* Cleidocranial dysostosis
> *Heterochromia iridis:* Waardenburg syndrome
> *Mitten hands:* Apert syndrome
> *Inverted nipples:* Congenital disorder of glycosylation
> *Webbing of the neck:* Turner and Noonan syndromes
> *Eversion of the lateral third of the lower eyelid:* Kabuki make-up syndrome

> **BOX 3:** Skeletal survey (Genetic skeletal survey for suspected dysplasia).
>
> X-ray skull (AP and Lateral)
> X-ray whole spine (AP and Lateral) (from cervical to sacrum)
> X-ray pelvis with both hip joints (AP View)
> X-ray one hand and one foot (AP View)
> X-ray one upper limb (shoulder to elbow; elbow to wrist) (AP View)
> X-ray one leg (knee to ankle) (AP View)
> X-ray wrist and hand (AP view) for (Bone age)
> (AP: anteroposterior)

dysmorphic features, as variable expressions are known in autosomal dominant conditions, e.g., in tuberous sclerosis or neurofibromatosis. The risk of recurrence is 50% when one of the parents is suffering from tuberous sclerosis, while incase both the parents are normal, there is no significantly increased risk of recurrence.

Investigations and Diagnosis

The importance of precise genetic diagnosis cannot be overemphasized. The various investigations which are available for diagnosis includes, e.g., hematological, biochemical, skeletal surveys **(Box 3)**, abdominal sonography, neuroimaging, chromosomal analysis, enzyme assays, amino acid levels, or molecular studies may be needed.

Chromosomal Analysis: *(Table 2)*

Fluorescent in situ hybridization (FISH) is done to detect microdeletion syndromes such as Prader-Willi and Angelman syndromes.

Echocardiography Evaluation

It should be done in all cases of Down syndrome, velocardiofacial syndrome, and in situation where clinical examination is revealing the necessity of Echocardiography.

Metabolic Workup

Metabolic workup is needed especially for *amino acid and organic acid*, when patient presents with cataracts, corneal clouding, delay and regression of milestones, seizures which are resistant to anticonvulsants, hepatosplenomegaly, and unexplained coma.

Other investigations: Liver biopsy, neurophysiological workup [Electromyography (EMG)/NERVE conduction studies (NCV)/brainstem evoked response audiometry (BERA)/visual evoked potential (VEP)]

Clinical Photograph

It is said that clinical photograph and videos are like laboratory test in syndromes. It has to be taken with written

TABLE 2: Approach to dysmorphic diagnosis.

Clinical evaluation	Investigations
History	Chromosomal analysis-Indications:
Pedigree	Presence of typical defined chromosomal disorder, e.g., Downs
Parental age	Presence of four features, MR, Physical retardation, malformation and dysmorphogenesis in a child
Consanguinity	Features of two or more Syndromes in one patient to exclude a contiguous gene syndrome
History of (H/o) abortions/SB/drugs/teratogens	Malformation known to have a high association with a chromosomal disorder, e.g., holoprosencephaly
H/o maternal infections	Karyotyping, FISH, PCR, microarray technology
Examination	Imaging: Conventional and MRI
Major/Minor	Echocardiography
Deformation/Disruption/Malformation/Dysplasia	Metabolic studies
Anthropometry	Amino acid/organic acid
Abnormal genitals	Mucopolysaccharidosis profile
Psychomotor delay, speech delay, MR	Long-chain fatty acid
Hearing assessment/Eye abnormality/Fundus	Cholesterol metabolism
Search for "Pearl of dysmorphology"	Clinical photographs

(FISH: fluorescent in situ hybridization; MR: mental retardation; MRI: magnetic resonance imaging; PCR: polymerase chain reaction)

consent of the patient and parents. The photograph must be taken in bright light or with the use of flash on a contrast background. The focus should be the abnormality seen during examination. The exposure should cover the closeup of face, standing, sitting, lying portion and stripped off (if required). If possible, take the complete family photograph if possible.

Synthesis of Diagnosis

The anomalies picked up is classified as minor or major, single or multiple, presence of major malformations, associations. With an evergrowing list of syndromes, reaching an exact diagnosis may be difficult. Search the available clinical features and clues from the history in electronic database with use of specific *"handles"* and *"prioritization"*. The situation is greatly helped by various computerized databases, namely, London Dysmorphology Database and Pictures of Standard Syndromes and Undiagnosed Malformations (POSSUM) (*see* **Box 1**). Referring to the books, giving detailed descriptions of syndromes, and diagnostic approaches are also of great help.

Limitation

Many times in clinical practice, it becomes difficult to synthesize a diagnosis in spite of literature and database search, in such situation the family is counseled to consult higher center and asked to remain in follow-up, to watch the evolution of the disease and to reevaluate for confirmed diagnosis.

Genetic Counseling

The risk of recurrence will depend on the diagnosis and on the pattern of inheritance. Association, sequences, and complexes have a low chance of recurrence. De novo chromosomal abnormalities have risk of recurrence <1%. In single gene disorder, the risk of recurrence depends on the mode of inheritance.

The fact remains that even the most experienced dysmorphologist in the world have to struggle to make a diagnosis in the majority of the patients.

SUGGESTED READING

1. Aase JM. Diagnostic Dysmorphology, 1st edition. USA: Springer; 1990.
2. Gorlin RJ, Cohen MM, Levin LS. Syndromes of the Head and Neck, 1st edition. UK: Oxford University Press; 1990.
3. Jones KL, Jones MC, del Campo M. Smith's Recognizable Patterns Of Human, Malformations, 7th edition. USA: Saunders; 2013.

Karyotyping

Amar Verma, Anita Verma

INTRODUCTION

Karyotyping in the field of genetics is like complete blood count or CBC for general medical practitioner but the utility and inference drawn from this investigation in field of genetics unlike CBC is limited. However, it is useful for every practitioner in general practice to know some basics of karyotyping, especially when to ask for and what one expects to know from the report?

When *Walther Flemming (1882)* first published the illustration of human chromosome, it took several decades to know its exact numbers by *Tijo and Levan (1956)*. Trisomy was identified by *Lejeune (1959)* from samples of patients of Down's syndrome when he described an extra chromosome in each cell.

- A human cell contains 22 pairs of autosomes numbered 1-22 and a pair of sex chromosome (XX in female and XY in male). Chromosomes are usually harvested from blood lymphocytes stimulated by phytohemagglutinin in a culture bottle. Chromosome can be analyzed from any actively dividing cell. Other common sources are bone marrow, amniocyte, chorionic villi and skin fibroblast cell.
- Divided cells are arrested in metaphase by colchicines (mitotic inhibitor). These cells are then treated with hypotonic solution to destroy the cell membranes and then fixed with fixative made up of methanol and acetic acid. The cell pellet of appropriate quantity is dropped on to glass slide to get metaphase. The chromosomes from a single cell are usually found in groups.
- Chromosomes are then banded using trypsin and stained by Giemsa stain to give G bands, with alternate dark and light bands of various sizes along the length of chromosome.
- Several other banding techniques are used in specific indications. Modification of technique permits high-resolution banding.
- Karyotype refers to an orderly display of chromosomes from the largest chromosome 1 to 22 followed by a pair of sex chromosome. Karyotype is prepared by arranging images by two methods:
  1. Manual method (cut from a photograph)
  2. Using computer software
- Metaphases are then seen under a microscope.
- Imaged individual chromosomes are identified either manually or by software, based on their size and pattern to get the karyotype. The arranged karyotype is called idiogram.

RESULT AND ANALYSIS

Chromosomal abnormalities are either:
- Numerical (aneuploidy)
- Structural
- Numerical (aneuploidy)
  - Most common anomalies are aneuploidies. These include monosomy, 1 copy of a chromosome in otherwise diploid cell, trisomy (3 copies), tetrasomy (4 copies) common examples are: Trisomy-21 (Down syndrome), trisomy-18 (Edwards syndrome), trisomy 13 (Patau syndrome), Turner syndrome (X0), Klinefelter syndrome.
  - In duplication, an extra copy of genomic segments results in partial trisomy.
  - Mosaic contains two or more cell lines with different chromosomal constitution, which are derived from a single zygote.
- Structural
  - Structural chromosomal abnormali-ties are identified by *Band Pattern*. No loss or gain of chromosome material is seen in *Balanced rearrangements*. *Unbalanced rearrangements* have either loss or gain of chromosomal material.
  - *Deletion* refers to either loss or gain of chromosomal segments.
  - *Inversion*, a segment of chromosome, is broken at two places and rejoined in reverse orientation. Inversion may be pericentric, when the breaks are on the either

side of centromere or paracentric when they are on one side.
- *Translocation* involves transfer of a segment of a chromosome to another chromosome. Reciprocal translocations represent one of the most common structural rearrangements in man. It results when two different chromosome sex change segments.
- *Robertsonian translocation* is nonreciprocal and occurs when long arms of any two acrocentric chromosomes join to produce single metacentric or submetacentric chromosome.
- Other structural abnormalities are *isochromosome* (Both arms similar), *ring chromosome, dicentric and acentric* chromosome.

Microdeletions are small deletions that usually escape detection during routine karyotyping due to small size of deletion.

The detection of these need special tests such as FISH (fluorescence in situ hybridization) or MLPA (multiplex ligation-dependent probe amplification). Chromosomal microarray can detect variation in copy number or other small defects.

Types of Banding

Cytogenetics employs several techniques to visualize different aspects of chromosomes:
- G-banding is obtained with Giemsa stain following digestion of chromosomes with trypsin. It yields a series of lightly and darkly stained bands—the dark regions tend to be heterochromatic, late-replicating and adenine–thymine (AT) rich. The light regions tend to be euchromatic, early-replicating and guanine–cytosine (GC) rich. This method will normally produce 300–400 bands in a normal human genome **(Figs. 1 and 2)**.
- R-banding is the reverse of G-banding (the R stands for "reverse"). The dark regions are euchromatic (GC-rich regions) and the bright regions are heterochromatic (thymine–adenine-rich regions).
- *C-banding*: Giemsa binds to constitutive heterochromatin, so it stains centromeres. The name is derived from centromeric or constitutive heterochromatin. The preparations undergo alkaline denaturation prior to staining leading to an almost complete depurination of the DNA. After washing the probe, the remaining DNA is renatured again and stained with Giemsa solution consisting of methylene azure, methylene violet, methylene blue, and eosin. Heterochromatin binds a lot of the dye, while the rest of the chromosomes absorb only little of it. The C-banding proved to be especially well-suited for the characterization of plant chromosomes.
- Q-banding is a fluorescent pattern obtained using quinacrine for staining. The pattern of bands is very similar to that seen in G-banding. They can be recognized by a yellow fluorescence of differing intensities. Most part of the stained DNA is heterochromatin. Quinacrine (Atabrine) binds both regions rich in AT and in GC, but only the AT-quinacrine-complex fluoresces. Since regions rich in AT are more common in heterochromatin than in euchromatin, these regions are labeled preferentially. The different intensities of the single bands mirror the different contents of AT. Other fluorochromes such as DAPI (4′-6-Diamidino-2-phenylindole) or Hoechst 33258 lead also to characteristic reproducible patterns. Each of them produces its specific pattern.

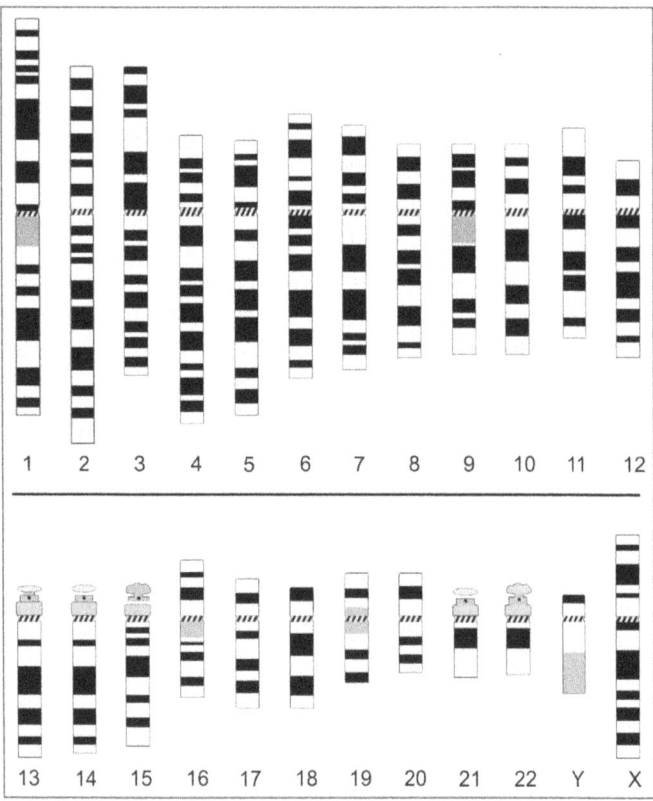

Fig. 2: Schematic presentation of G-banded karyotype (normal male) classic karyotype cytogenetics.

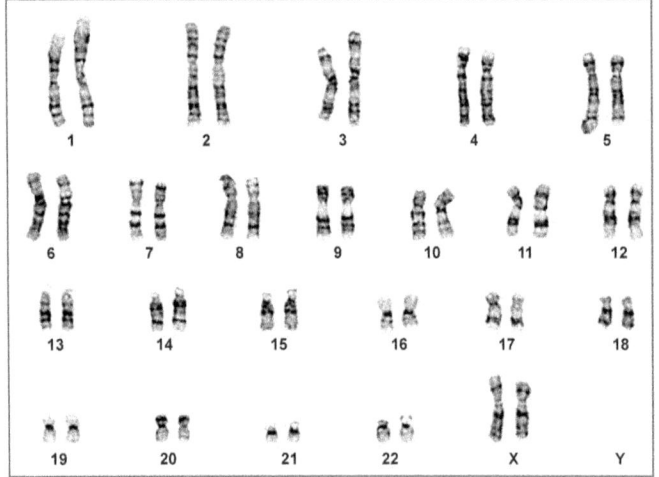

Fig. 1: Arranged karyotype G-banding (normal female).

In other words: The properties of the bonds and the specificity of the fluorochromes are not exclusively based on their affinity to regions rich in AT. Rather, the distribution of AT and the association of AT with other molecules such as histones, e.g., influences the binding properties of the fluorochromes.

- *T-banding*: Visualizes telomeres.
- *Silver staining*: Silver nitrate stains the nucleolar organization region (NOR)-associated protein. This yields a dark region where the silver is deposited, denoting the activity of rRNA genes within the NOR.

Karyogram or Idiogram is depiction of chromosomes on single sheet of photograph.

In the *"classic" (depicted) karyotype*, a dye, often *Giemsa (G-banding)*, less frequently mepacrine (quinacrine), is used to stain bands on the chromosomes. Giemsa is specific for the phosphate groups of DNA. Quinacrine binds to the AT-rich regions. Each chromosome has a characteristic banding pattern that helps to identify them; both chromosomes in a pair will have the same banding pattern.

Karyotypes are arranged with the *short arm [p]* of the chromosome on top, and the *long arm [q]* on the bottom. Some karyotypes call the short and long arms p and q, respectively. In addition, the differently stained regions and subregions are given numerical designations from proximal to distal on the chromosome arms. For example, Cri du chat syndrome involves a deletion on the short arm of chromosome 5. It is written as 46, XX, 5p-. The critical region for this syndrome is deletion of p15.2 (The locus on the chromosome), which is written as 46, XX, del (5) (p15.2).

COMMON INDICATIONS FOR ORDERING A KARYOTYPE

- Dysmorphic features and/or developmental delay
- Fetal or neonatal death with multiple congenital abnormalities
- Indeterminate gender or ambiguous genitalia
- Amenorrhea or primary infertility or other suspected sex chromosome abnormality (e.g., Turner or Klinefelter syndrome)
- Delayed puberty or in appropriate secondary sexual development
- Short stature or unusual growth pattern
- Oligospermia or azoospermia in males
- Parental karyotyping after pregnancy loss of an unkaryotyped fetus with multiple congenital abnormalities or severe intrauterine growth pattern (IUGR)
- Family history of a known chromosome abnormality other than simple aneuploidy due to nondisjunction (normally only first-degree relatives are considered)
- Suspected family history of chromosome abnormality where the karyotype of the affected individual is not known
- Microdeletion/duplication syndromes (Includes FISH testing if probes are available and if diagnosis by known familial chromosome rearrangement)
- *Chromosome breakage syndromes*: Ataxia telangiectasia, Bloom syndrome, Fanconi anemia, etc.
- Terminated fetus (examination of product of conception) for confirmation of an abnormal cytogenetic result diagnosed prenatally or in fetus suspected of having a chromosome abnormality (e.g., multiple markers diagnosed on ultrasound)
- Ultrasound detection of any major structural abnormality including nuchal translucency (NT) > 3 mm before 14-week gestation or a nuchal fold measuring 6 mm or greater between 14 and 20-week gestation (during first-trimester or second-trimester screening) with history of chromosome abnormality indicative of increased risk for future pregnancies
- If there is a family history, karyotyping of the woman or her partner should be undertaken first in order to establish whether prenatal diagnosis is indicated
- Nonroutine cases not fulfilling the above criteria then after discussion and agreement between the referring clinician and the Head of Laboratory
- Sperm and egg donors.

INDICATIONS FOR POSTNATAL CYTOGENETIC TESTING

- Rapid neonatal aneuploidy screening and sex determination by FISH.
- Rapid neonatal screening by FISH for trisomy 13, 18, and 21 and for sex determination can be undertaken if results are needed urgently.

Chromosome analysis and is always followed by a full karyotype.

LIMITATIONS OF KARYOTYPE AS A DIAGNOSTIC TEST

- Numerical chromosomal anomalies and large rearrangements of chromosomes may be detected by karyotype. Submicroscopic changes of below 4–5 Mb are not detected by routine karyotype.
- Single nucleotide mutations of Mendelian disorders are not diagnosed by karyotype.
- The resolution and diagnostic yield of karyotype are limited. The large size and complexities of genome cannot be fully investigated by karyotype.
- Identification of some structural abnormalities may provide a clue for the location of large gene disorders, i.e., Duchenne muscular dystrophy (DMD).
- Addition of molecular cytogenetics along with classical cytogenetics may yield more information.

Inborn Errors of Metabolism

Anupa Prasad

INTRODUCTION

- An inborn error of metabolism (IEM) is a biochemical genetic disorder that causes an altered metabolic profile of patients leading to intoxication, reduced utilization of nutrients, or decreased energy production.
- The prevalence of IEM in India is 1 in 2,497 newborns.
- Single-gene defects are responsible for defective enzymes, cofactors, or transporters in the pathway of amino acids, carbohydrates, or fat metabolism, as well as abnormalities of mitochondrial energy metabolism.
- Most of the IEM have autosomal recessive or X-linked inheritance.
- Clinical suspicion for IEM is given in **Box 1**.

DIAGNOSIS

- It is primarily dependent on *routine* laboratory tests, detailed history, and a high index of suspicion toward a specific IEM.
- The necessary *metabolic investigations* include glucose, electrolytes, lactate, ammonia, arterial blood gas analysis, and ketones (GELAAK) along with plasma amino acids, urinary organic acids, and a plasma acylcarnitine profile.
- *High-performance liquid chromatography (HPLC)* is an acceptable technique to analyze and quantify amino acids, organic acids, and other metabolites from biological fluids.
- Tandem mass spectrometry (TMS) and GC/MS are the advanced techniques for diagnosing metabolic disorders for confirmation.

BOX 1: Clinical suspicion for inborn error of metabolism.
- Acute illness in a neonate or infant after hours or weeks of normalcy
- Intractable seizures, hypotonia, lethargy, and coma
- Persistent or recurrent vomiting
- Failure to thrive
- Unusual odor
- Respiratory distress syndrome or apnea
- Coarse facies
- Jaundice, hepatosplenomegaly
- Family history of neonatal death
- Similar presentation in previous child

Prenatal Diagnosis

- It is offered by direct metabolite assay in the amniotic fluid, enzyme analysis in chorionic villous cells, and DNA analysis in chorionic villus sampling (CVS) or amniotic fluid cells.
- The combination of at least two types of tests enhances the confidence in the diagnosis.

Newborn Screening

- Newborn screening (NBS) is an effective way of reducing morbidity and mortality due to IEM by allowing early intervention.
- TMS helps in the analysis of acylcarnitine and amino acid profiling in the blood of the newborns.
- TMS, traditional enzyme assays, immunoassays, HPLC, and electrophoresis are the mainstay of expanded newborn screening for IEM in India.
- Advancement in the therapeutic intervention of IEM demands an expansion in the NBS strategies.

CLASSIFICATION OF IEM

It based on the size of molecules causing disease symptoms, inborn errors of metabolism are broadly divided into three groups. **Flowchart 1** depicts the different types of disorders in the three broad groups.
1. Large-molecule diseases
2. Small-molecule diseases
3. Others

Large-molecule Diseases

- The large molecule diseases mainly comprise storage diseases, which involve complex molecules.
- They are further subclassified into lysosomal storage diseases, peroxisomal diseases, and disorders of intracellular trafficking and processing.
- The symptoms are insidious, progressive, and independent of intercurrent events.
- The patients present with multisystem involvement leading to growth impairment, coarse facial features, organomegaly, dementia, movement disorders, gradual

Flowchart 1: Classification of IEM based on the size of the molecules.

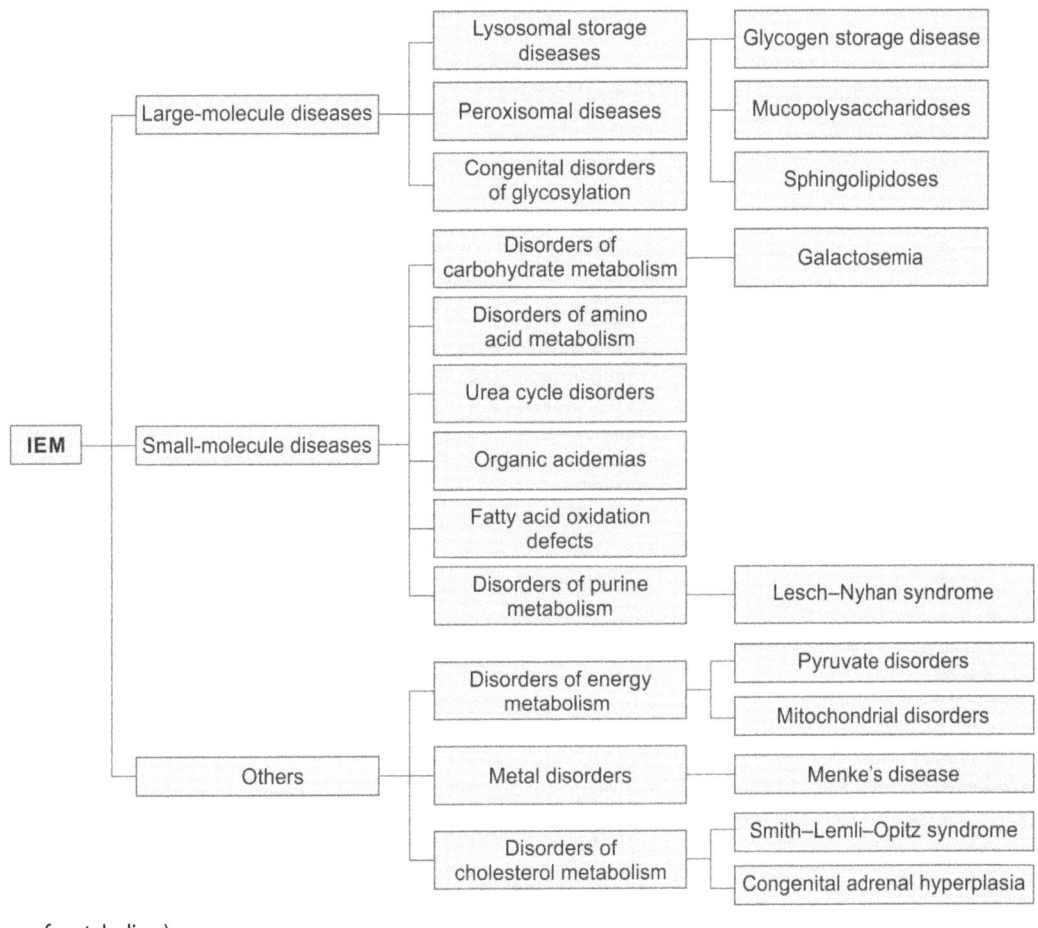

(IEM: inborn errors of metabolism)

loss of vision, spasticity, seizures, and attenuated life span.
- Globally, the most common LSDs are Gaucher disease, Fabry disease, and mucopolysaccharidosis (MPS) type I. **Table 1** demonstrates the list of common lysosomal storage diseases and their clinical features.

Small-molecule Diseases

- Small-molecule diseases are disorders of intermediary metabolism. They include defects of amino acid metabolism, urea cycle disorders, organic acidemias, fatty acid oxidation defects, defects of carbohydrate metabolism, and defects of purine and pyrimidine metabolism.
- Many diseases present acutely and progress to acute encephalopathy if not treated quickly.
- The symptoms are related to food intake and to the intoxication caused by accumulating metabolites.
- **Table 2** presents the biochemical characteristics of major disorders in the group.

Table 3 lists common disorders of intermediary metabolism diseases and their clinical features and the laboratory characteristics.

Diagnostic algorithm for hyperammonemia is given in **Flowchart 2**.

MANAGEMENT OF INBORN ERRORS OF METABOLISM

Immediate Management

Emergency management of suspected IEM should be initiated while awaiting results of initial investigations.
- Airway, Breathing, and Circulation (ABC) should be secured.
- All the protein and lipid intake should be stopped.
- Intravenous glucose infusion should be initiated to provide 6–8 mg glucose/kg/min with or without insulin.
- Proper hydration should be maintained.
- Correction of acid–base and electrolyte disturbances
- Antibiotic cover for infection
- Antiepileptics to control seizures (avoid sodium valproate)
- Transfer to tertiary metabolic center if stable and appropriate

Specific Management

Neonatal hyperammonemia: It is a medical emergency requiring prompt intervention to lower ammonia concentration. Treatment includes (**Table 4**):
- Renal replacement therapy (hemofiltration)
- Sodium benzoate

TABLE 1: Common lysosomal storage diseases and their clinical features.

Group disease	Name of the disease, MIM number	Enzyme/transporter defect	Clinical features	Diagnostic biochemical or lab marker
GSD	Type Ia von gierke disease 232200	Glucose-6-phosphatase	Doll-like facies, hypoglycemia, massive hepatomegaly short stature, seizures.	Enzyme deficiency*, mutational analysis of the gene involved
	Type II Pompe disease 232300	Lysosomal acid α-1,4 glucosidase	Severe hypotonia, hepatosplenomegaly, cardiac defects	Enzyme deficiency*, ECG, echocardiography
MPS	Type I (Hunter's syndrome) 607014	α-L-Iduronidase	Coarse facies, corneal clouding Hepatosplenomegaly Macroglossia, Hoarseness of voice Multiple skeletal abnormalities Spinal stenosis, intellectual disability by three years of age	Enzyme deficiency*, mutational analysis of the gene involved
	Type II (Hunter's syndrome), 309900	Iduronate sulfatase	Coarse facies, corneal clouding, developmental delay. Multiple skeletal abnormalities, cardiopulmonary disease, right blindness, papilledema	
SPL	Gaucher's disease (Type 1) 230800	β-glucocerebrosidase	Hepatosplenomegaly, skeletal dysplasia, anemia, thrombocytopenia, bone infarcts	Enzyme deficiency*, demonstration of gaucher cells in bone marrow
	Tay sach's disease (infantile form) 272800	β-hexosaminidase A	Global developmental delay, cherry-red spot on the macula, neurodegenerative symptoms like ataxia, absent head holding eye movement abnormalities, dysphagia	Enzyme deficiency*, mutational analysis of the gene involved
	Faby's disease 301500	α Galactosidase	Late-onset at age 40–60 years, facial dysmorphism, broad fingertips, corneal opacity, neuropathic pain, anglokeratoma telangiectasia, chronic kidney disease, cardiovascular disease	Proteinuria, enzyme deficiency*, mutational analysis of the gene involved
	Metachromatic leukodystrophy 250100	Arylsulfatase A (ARSA)	Polyneuropathy, ataxia, weakness, areflexia, dysphagia, seizure, thickening of the gall bladder, involvement of liver, pancreas, hepatosplenomegaly and auditory involvement	Increased CSF protein Typical findings on MRI**, enzyme activity*, mutational analysis of the gene involved
	Niemann pick disease type C 257220, 607625	NPC intracellular cholesterol transporter 1	Jaundice, hepatosplenomegaly, mental retardation, dystonia and vertical supranuclear ophthalmoplegia, seizure	Filipin test for cholesterol accumulation in fibroblasts, mutational analysis of NPC genes

(CSF: cerebrospinal fluid; ECG: electrocardiography; GSD: glycogen storage disease; MIM: Mendelian inheritance in man; MPS: mucopolysaccharidoses; MRI: magnetic resonance imaging; SPL: sphingolipidoses)
*Enzyme deficiency is seen in peripheral blood leukocytes or fibroblasts from skin culture.
**The findings of MRI include bilateral symmetrical abnormal T2 signal hyperintensity in corpus callosum and periventricular white matter and the typical "tigroid pattern" in the white matter.

TABLE 2: Biochemical characteristics of the disorders of intermediary metabolism.

Disorders	Hypoglycemia	Hyperammonemia	Lactic acidosis	Metabolic acidosis	Ketosis
Urea cycle disorders	No	+++	No	+	No
Organic acidemia	+	+	++	+++	+++
Fatty acid oxidation disorders	+++	+	+	No	No
MSUD disorders	No	–	No	No	+
Organic acidemia	+	+	++	+++	+++
Fatty acid oxidation disorders	+++	+	+	No	No
MSUD	No	–	No	No	+

(MSUD: maple syrup urine disease)

TABLE 3: Common disorders of intermediary metabolism diseases and their clinical features and the laboratory characteristics.

Disorders of intermediary metabolism	Name of the disease (OMIM number)	Enzyme/ Transport defect	Clinical features	Biochemical or laboratory characteristics
Defects of amino acid metabolism	PKU (261600)	Phenylalanine hydroxylase	Mental retardation, fair complexion, pigmentation	Increased phenylalanine in (B); phenyl pyruvate, phenylacetate and phenylacetate (U)
	MSUD (248600)	Branched-chain keto acid dehydrogenase complex	Lethargy, hypotonia, seizure, coma, vomiting ketosis, brain edema	BC AA (B), BC 2 ketoacid and BC 2 hydroxy acids (U)
	Alkaptonuria	Homogentisate oxidase	Darkening of urine on air exposure, dark pigments in cartilage and joints, arteries	Homogentisic acid (B, U)
	Homocystinuria (236200)	Cystathionine beta-synthase	Mental retardation, ectopia lentis, skeletal abnormalities, marfanoid features	Homogentisic acid (B, U)
	Sulfate oxidase deficiency (272300)	Cystathionine beta-synthase	Mental retardation, ectopia lentis, skeletal abnormalities, marfanoid features	Homocysteine, methionine (B, U)
		Sulfate oxidase	Dysmorphism, mental retardation, ectopia lentis, seizures, hypotonia	Sulfocysteine, taurine (B, U) low cysteine (B, U)

(PKU: phenylketonurea; MSUD: maple syrup urine disease; DC: dicarboxylic acid; B: blood; U: urine; MCAD: medium chain acyl CoA dehydrogenase deficiency; VLCAD: very long chain acyl CoA dehydrogenase)

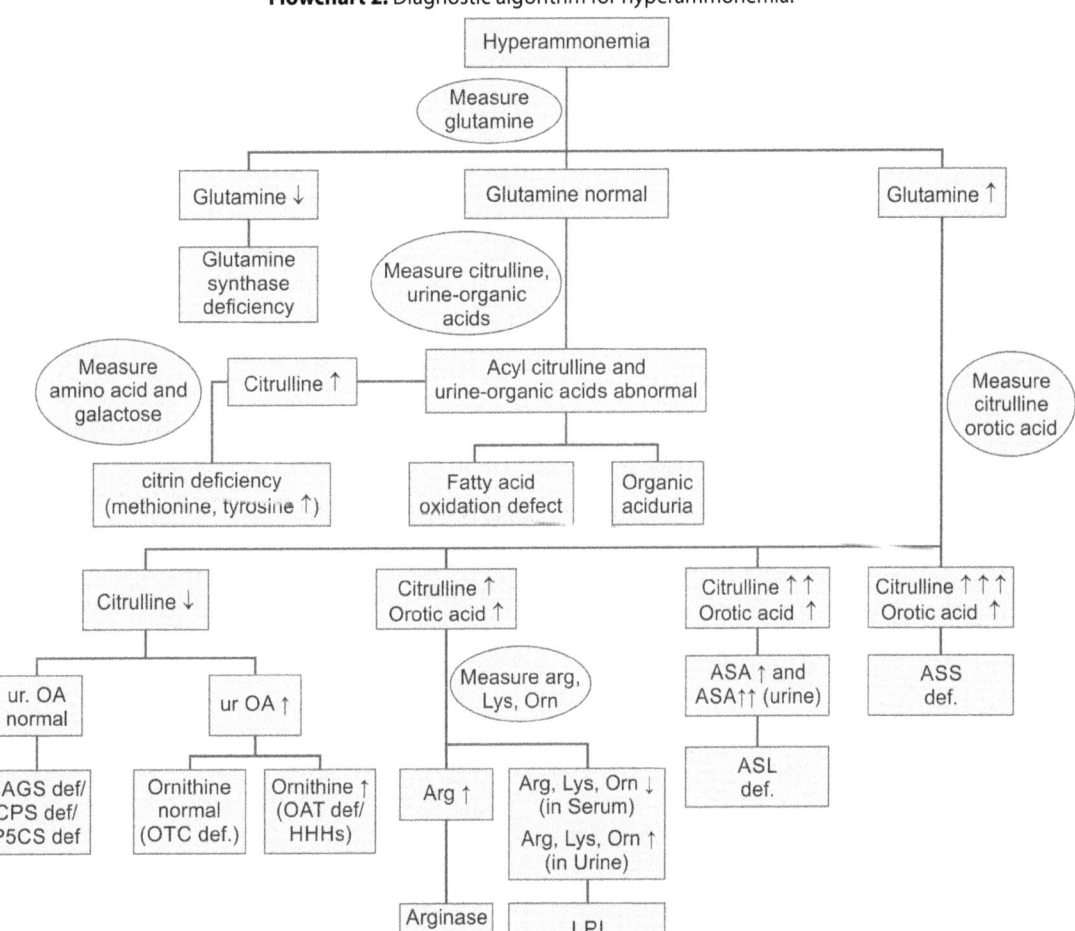

Flowchart 2: Diagnostic algorithm for hyperammonemia.

(OA: orotic acid; Arg: arginine; Lys: lysine; Orn: ornithine; ASA: argininosuccinic acid; ASL Def: argininosiccinate lyase deficiency; ASS Def: argininosuccinate synthase deficiency; CPS1 def: CPS1 deficiency; HHHs: hyperornithinemia-hyperammonemia-homocitrullinemia syndrome; LPI: lysinuric protein intolerance; NAGS def: N-acetyl glutamate synthase deficiency; OTC def: ornithine transcarbamoylase deficiency; OAT def: ornithine aminotransferase deficiency; P5CSD: Δ1-pyrroline-5-carboxylate deficiency)

TABLE 4: Sodium phenylacetate and sodium benzoate dosage and administration in hyperammonemia.

Drugs	Loading dose	Maintenance dose
Sodium benzoate	250 mg/kg IV in 10% dextrose over 90 minutes	250 mg/kg IV in 10% dextrose in 24 hours
Sodium phenylacetate	250 mg/kg IV in 10% dextrose over 90 minutes	250 mg/kg IV in 10% dextrose in 24 hours
*Arginine HCl	200 mg/kg IV in 10% dextrose over 90 hours	200 mg/kg IV in 10% dextrose in 24 hours

*Arginine HCl not to be given in arginase deficiency, L-citrulline should be given in proximal urea cycle disorder (UCD).

(IV: intravenous)

- Sodium phenylacetate
- L-arginine.

Organic acidemias:
- Reduce/stop protein intake
- Hypertonic glucose infusion insulin
- L-carnitine
- Glycine
- Biotin.

SUGGESTED READING

1. ACMG guidelines. Lysosomal storage diseases: diagnostic confirmation and management of presymptomatic individuals.
2. Burtis CA, Ashwood ER, Bruns DE. Teitz Textbook of Clinical Chemistry and Molecular Diagnostics. Philadelphia, Elsevier, 2012.
3. Häberle J, Boddaert N, Burlina A, et al. Suggested guidelines for the diagnosis and management of urea cycle disorders. Orphanet J Rare Dis. 2012;7(32).
4. Scriver CR, Beaudet AL, Sly WS, Valle D, (eds). The Metabolic and Molecular Bases of Inherited Disease. New York, NY: McGraw-Hill Co; 2001.
5. Summar ML, Nicholas Ah Mew. Inborn Errors of Metabolism with Hyperammonemia. Urea Cycle Defects and Related Disorders. 2018;65(2):231-46.

CHAPTER 160: Prenatal Screening and Diagnosis of Congenital Disorders

Sarita Agrawal, Arpana Verma

INTRODUCTION

Congenital anomalies (CAs) are also known as birth defects, congenital disorders, or congenital malformations; defined by the World Health Organization (WHO) as structural or functional anomalies that occur during intrauterine life which are identified prenatally, at birth, or later in life. The prevalence of birth defects in India is 6–7% which translates to around 1.7 million birth defects annually. The objective of prenatal screening and diagnosis is to detect any defect early in pregnancy so as to allow adequate counseling and fully informed decisions about pregnancy management. Despite of tremendous advances in this field over last two decades, all the birth defects and genetic diseases cannot be picked up during prenatal period.

BENEFITS OF PRENATAL DIAGNOSIS

- Malformation incompatible with life or with major handicap can be terminated.
- Certain abnormalities may be correctible in utero.
- It provides opportunity to arrange for corrective measures beforehand.
- It offers a chance to be delivered at a place where the required facilities are available.
- It helps parent's informed decision to continue pregnancy or mentally prepared to have a handicapped child.
- It discovers conditions that may impact future pregnancies.

PRENATAL SCREENING AND DIAGNOSTIC TESTS

The distinction should be made clear between a diagnostic and a screening test. The former confirms or refutes the existence of an actual anomaly in a fetus believed to be at increased risk, whereas the latter identifies an increased likelihood of a fetal abnormality in an apparently normal pregnancy. The value of a screening test is outlined by the fact that most congenital anomalies are found among newborns from pregnancies with low risk factors.

SCREENING TESTS IN FIRST TRIMESTER

Screening for Fetal Aneuploidies

- *Nuchal translucency (NT)*: The maximum width (in mm) of the translucent space at the back of the fetal neck is determined by ultrasound (USG) between 11 and 13 completed weeks (wks) of gestational age (GA) at crown rump length (CRL) between 45 and 85 mm. Accurate measurements as per the criteria by fetal medicine foundation have to be used to avoid wrong interpretation. The risk calculation is based upon the NT measurements and maternal age. NT of ≥3.0 mm or the 95th percentile is associated with significant risk of aneuploidy and cardiac malformations hence warrants for counseling and diagnostic tests.
- *Analyte screening* (double marker) relies upon the levels of maternal serum pregnancy-associated plasma protein-A (PAPP-A), free beta-human chorionic gonadotrophin (free β-hCG) or total hCG combined with maternal age, performed between 9+0 and 13+6 wks of GA.
- *Combined screening*: It combines double marker test together with NT. The blood tests and USG are most commonly performed on approximately the same day between 11+0 and 13+6wks of GA. This is the most commonly used and validated testing for fetal aneuploidies.
- *Integrated test (full)*: The integration of screening tests performed during the first trimester (NT + PAPP-A, hCG) and second trimester (quadruple test) together with maternal age into a single screening test result and the risk is only provided once all tests have been completed.
- *Serum integrated test*: A variation of the full integrated test that does not include the NT.
- *Sequential test*: A variation of the integrated test (full) in which a small proportion of the highest risk women (risk >1:50) are identified as screen positive and results disclosed in the first trimester. The remaining women are provided a risk only after all tests have been completed in the second trimester.

TABLE 1: Detection rate and false-positive rate for Down syndrome screening tests: First and Second Trimester Evaluation of Risk Trial (FASTER) and Serum, Urine and Ultrasound Screening Study (SURUSS).

Test	FASTER trial		SURUSS trial	
	Detection rate (%)	False-positive rate (%)	Detection rate (%)	False-positive rate (%)
Full integrated	85	0.8	85	0.9
	95	5	90	2.1
Serum integrated	85	4.4	85	3.9
	95	17	90	7.4
Combined	85	4.8	85	4.3
	95	21	90	8.4
Quadruple	85	7.3	85	6.2
	95	22	90	10.6

TABLE 2: Biochemical markers and chromosomal abnormalities in first trimester.

	β-hCG	PAPP-A
T21	↑	↓
T18	↓	↓
T13	↓	↓
Triploidy (paternal)	↑↑↑	↓
Triploidy (maternal)	↓↓	↓↓
Sex chromosome abnormality		↓

Note: In normal euploid pregnancies, the average free beta-hCG and PAPPA-A are 1.0 MoM. PAPP-A <0.3 MoM is also associated with high risk for FGR/IUGR.

(β-hCG: beta-human chorionic gonadotropin; FGR: fetal growth restriction; IUGR: intrauterine growth restriction; PAPP-A: pregnancy-associated plasma protein A)

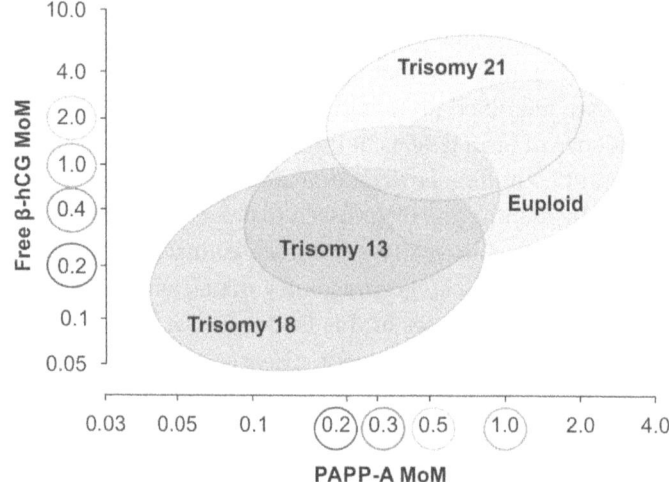

Fig. 1: Biochemical markers and chromosomal abnormalities in first trimester.
(β-hCG: beta human chorionic gonadotropin; PAPP-A: pregnancy-associated plasma protein-A)

The estimated risk in all above screening tests is calculated automatically by computer software. The measured concentration of free β-hCG and PAPPA-A is influenced by the reagents, gestational age (GA), maternal weight, ethnicity, smoking, in vitro fertilization (IVF) pregnancies (PAPP-A is low), multiple pregnancy, hence adjustment according to these are necessary to give calculated risk. The detection rate (DR) and false-positive rate (FPR) of different tests are shown in **Table 1**; the association of various biochemical markers with chromosomal abnormalities is shown in **Table 2** and **Figure 1**.

- *Other first-trimester screening tests*: Although not in clinical use, several studies have shown that a combination of placental growth factor (PlGF), alpha-fetoprotein (AFP) with β-hCG, and PAPP-A between 11+0 and 13+0 wks of GA can detect up to 90% of Down syndrome (DS) but with a FPR of up to 20%. First-trimester combined screening can also be improved by using two or three additional USG markers such as nasal bone, tricuspid regurgitation, ductus venosus, and facial angle. Several other markers such as pregnancy specific B1-glycoprotein (SP1) (7–12 wks) and a disintegrin and metalloproteinase 12 ADAM-12 (8–10 wks) have also been identified as early markers for DS.

Noninvasive Prenatal Testing

This involves isolating cell-free fragments of DNA (cffDNA) from a maternal serum sample which is detectable as early at 32 days. A fraction >4% is required for reliable analysis. Extracted DNA is studied for qualitative or quantitative analysis. Apart from DS, the technique has been tried successfully for X-linked disorders, rhesus (RH) typing, and few single gene disorders. At present, the American College of Obstetricians and Gynecologists (ACOG) recommends noninvasive prenatal testing (NIPT) only for women with high pretest risk of aneuploidy. Due to associated FPR though small, NIPT is regarded as screening test and a positive NIPT is followed by diagnostic testing. NIPT is validated between 10+0 and 21+6 wks GA with a sensitivity of 99%.

TABLE 3: Structural abnormality in first-trimester ultrasound.

Always detectable abnormalities	Undetectable abnormalities (manifest during second or third trimester)	Potentially detectable
Body stalk anomaly (major abdominal wall defect, severe kyphoscoliosis, short umbilical cord and rupture of the amniotic membranes)	*Brain abnormalities*: Microcephaly, hypoplasia of the cerebellum or vermis, hydrocephalus, and agenesis of the corpus callosum	• Potentially detectable with inclusion of detailed examination of relevant structure in the protocol on high index of suspicion (e.g., increased NT and associated defects such as cardiac defects, posterior fossa defects, spina bifida, lethal skeletal dysplasia, and diaphragmatic hernia)
Acrania, anencephaly	Duodenal atresia and bowel obstruction	• Improved training, time and resort to vaginal sonography can detect facial cleft, renal agenesis and multicystic kidneys
Alobar holoprosencephaly		
Exomphalos, gastroschisis	Echogenic lung lesions	
Megacystis	Achondroplasia	
Absent hands or feet and polydactyly mostly	Many renal anomalies including severe hydronephrosis due to ureteric stenosis or vesicoureteric reflux	
	Fetal tumors	

(NT: nuchal translucency)

TABLE 4: Biochemical marker profile in second trimester.

	Aneuploidies				
Marker	T21	T18	T13	Turner	ONTDs
AFP	Low	Unchanged	Increase	Decrease	Increase
hCG	High	Very low	Normal	Very high	Unchanged
uE3	Low	Low	Normal	Decrease	Unchanged
Inhibin A	High	Unchanged	Normal	Very high	Unchanged

(AFP: alpha fetoprotein; hCG: human chorionic gonadotropin; ONTD: open neural tube defects; uE3: unconjugated estriol)

Screening for Fetal Structural Abnormalities (Early Anomaly Scan)

The aim is not just to diagnose trisomies but also the nonenuploidy structural defects, best assessed around 12 weeks of GA. A good way of achieving high performance of screening test for aneuploidies is to carry out serum marker tests at 11 weeks and USG at 12 weeks. The anomalies which can be picked up in first trimester anomaly scan are depicted in **Table 3**.

SCREENING IN SECOND TRIMESTER

Screening for Fetal Aneuploidies

- *The triple screen* consists of maternal serum AFP, hCG (free beta-hCG or intact/total hCG), and unconjugated estriol (uE3) combined with an a priori risk based on maternal age to screen for trisomy 21, 18, and open neural tube defects.
- *Quadruple test (Quad screen)*: It adds diametric inhibin A (DIA) to triple screen which is reported to increase the detection rate for trisomy 21.
- *Penta screen* includes addition of invasive trophoblast antigen (ITA) to the quad screen, although detection rates are not substantially different from the quad screen.
- Second-trimester biomarkers are performed between 15+0 and 21+6 wks GA. They have lower DR as compared to first-trimester screening tests. NIPT may represent a viable alternative for screening with a high DR for eligible patients who present first time in the second trimester. Biochemical marker profile in second trimester is shown in **Table 4**.

Screening for Structural Abnormality

Second-trimester Ultrasound (Targeted Imaging for Fetal Anomalies)

A fetal ultrasound in the second trimester also known as level II scan, in addition to fetal biometry, placental localization, cervical length, and amniotic fluid has also been identified as useful screening tool for aneuploidy by identifying both true structural defects and structural variants, referred to as *"soft markers"*. Presence of one major (omphalocele, endocardial cushion defects, holoprosencephaly, and duodenal atresia) or two minor defects (echogenic focus, choroid plexus cyst, ventriculomegaly, single umbilical artery, and pyelectasis) are indications for further invasive diagnostic tests. Only single minor anomaly does not require invasive testing but further follow-up monitoring is advised. Nyberg and colleagues applied likelihood ratios (LRs) from ultrasound markers to the *a priori* risk on the basis of maternal age describe as age-adjusted ultrasound risk assessment (AAURA). Computerized programs have been developed which permit to estimate the adjusted risk for aneuploidy by combining background risks and biochemical screening together with the above ultrasound features. The optimal time for TIFFA (Targeted Imaging for Fetal Anomalies) is between 18 and 20+6 wks GA. Addition of 3D, 4D, and Doppler studies adds to DR for craniofacial cardiac and renal abnormalities. Fetal middle cerebral artery peak systolic velocity (MCA-PSV) ≥1.5 MoM for the GA is an accurate noninvasive tool for predicting moderate-to-severe fetal anemia of any etiology. Presence of increased nuchal fold thickness (>6 mm), symmetric intrauterine growth restriction (IUGR), poly or oligohydramnios, and one identified anomaly warrants for careful detailed abnormality scan. Most of the structural defects can be picked up in TIFFA scan by experienced sonologist and high-resolution machine except for few which may have late onset (e.g., hydrocephalus, ovarian cyst).

Fetal Echocardiography

The fetal heart can be evaluated at any time during the gestation period. At 11–14-wk scan, presence of a pulsatile ductus venosus or tricuspid regurgitation can be a very strong marker for aneuploidies. The best time to evaluate the fetal heart is between 18 and 22 weeks' gestation. Fetuses with diagnosed extracardiac anomalies, NT >3.5, fetal infections, early IUGR, maternal diabetes, congenital heart defect (CHD), exposure to antiepileptics, systemic lupus erythematosus (SLE) or Sjogren's syndrome should be evaluated with fetal echocardiography. Detection of a cardiac anomaly not only affects the prognosis but also is associated recurrence risk in next child to the extent of 1:20 to 1:100. The basic cardiac examination, four-chamber views and the extended basic cardiac examination, in which ventricular outflow tracts are visualized, must be distinguished from a true fetal echocardiographic examination. The latter in addition 2D includes color-coded Doppler and pulsed Doppler which allows to diagnose most missed cardiac lesions such as outflow tract anomalies (complete transposition, common arterial trunk, aortic coarctation) or minor anomalies such as atrial septal defect (ASD), small ventricular septal defect (VSD), mild pulmonary, or aortic stenosis.

Magnetic Resonance Imaging

Magnetic resonance imaging (MRI) may help to investigate specific anomalies, such as agenesis of corpus callosum, posterior fossa cysts, cerebral cleft, and migrational disorders such as lissencephaly. Use of MRI is being restricted to specific indications only.

PRENATAL INVASIVE DIAGNOSTIC TESTS

Investigations for confirmation of diagnosis can be performed by collecting the required fetal samples by chorionic villus sampling (CVS), amniocentesis, cordocentesis, fetal tissue biopsies for the detection of chromosomal abnormalities, DNA studies, congenital infections, hemolytic disorders and metabolic syndromes, etc. The essentials for any invasive techniques include appropriate indication, adequate counseling, informed consent, experienced operator, continuous USG guidance, sterile technique, local anesthetics and anti-D injection. The patients counseling needs emphasis not only on the procedure-related risks but also the limitations of diagnostic tests in yielding the correct diagnosis.

Indications for invasive testing [ISUOG (International Society of Ultrasound in Obstetrics & Gynecology) 2016]:

- *Increased risk of fetal aneuploidy*: The increased risk may derive from a prenatal screening test, obstetric history (previous fetus or child affected by aneuploidy), or family history (parental carrier of chromosomal balanced translocation or inversion, parental aneuploidy or mosaicism for aneuploidy) and intracytoplasmic sperm injection (ICSI) pregnancy due to oligospermia.
- *Increased risk for a known genetic or biochemical disease of the fetus*: A family hereditary disease with a known mutation or biochemical change, male fetus and carrier status of pregnant woman for a disease with X chromosomal inheritance; carrier status of both parents for an autosomal recessive disorder.
- *Maternal transmittable infectious disease*: Toxoplasma, cytomegalovirus, or rubella to confirm or exclude transmission of the infection to the fetus.
- *Maternal request*: Maternal request is not generally considered a valid indication for invasive prenatal diagnosis except under exceptional circumstances.

DIAGNOSTICS TEST METHODS

Chorionic Villus Sampling

Chorionic villous can represent fetal genetic makeup for accessible prenatal diagnosis; it can be performed early at GA 9–14 wks, ideally at 10 wks. The procedure involves passing a catheter into the uterus under USG guidance transabdominally or transcervically, according to the operator's experience or preference or placental location. Chorionic villi surrounding the sac are aspirated then dissected off the decidual tissue and genetic analysis is carried out from the trophoblastic cells (direct examination or short term culture) or mesenchymal cells (long term culture). The cells are subjected for karyotyping, quantitative fluorescent polymerase chain reaction (QF-PCR) or fluorescence in situ hybridization (FISH) or molecular analysis. A minimum amount of 5 mg villi in each sample is required to achieve a valid result.

Contraindications

- Maternal alloimmunization (A relative contraindication)
- Maternal HIV, hepatitis B, C
- Cervicovaginal infection
- Active bleeding
- Coagulopathy.

Complications

The most serious complications from CVS are fetal loss (0.2-2%), limb-reduction defects, and oromandibular hypogenesis. Others are bleeding (10%), infection, RH sensitization, amniotic fluid leakage, failure to obtain a sample (2.5-4.8%). The limitations are higher rate of maternal cell contamination and confined placental mosaicism (CPM 1-2%) which may result in diagnostic ambiguity requiring amniocentesis to differentiate true fetal mosaicism from CPM.

Amniocentesis

Amniotic fluid is withdrawn from the uterine cavity using a needle, via transabdominal approach under USG guidance. For genetic testing, it is generally performed at GA of 16-20 wks. Amniotic fluid contains *exfoliated fetal cells* which can be cultured, frozen, and stored for genetic analysis. Amniotic fluid *acetylcholinesterase* and AFP level are more sensitive and specific than serum AFP alone in predicting neural tube defects; other tests carried out in amniotic fluid are: *Bilirubin* for fetal hemolytic disease, *L:S ratio* for fetal lung maturity, *amniotic fluid PCR* to exclude specific infections (CMV, parvovirus, etc., in nonimmune hydrops, intracranial calcification) and *enzymes* for rare lysosomal storage diseases in the at-risk patients (consanguinity, previous family history, Ashkenazi Jewish or French, Canadian descent). In twin pregnancies, one needs to obtain amniotic fluid from each sac.

Complications

Most of the complications are similar to that of CVS but to a lesser extent. Rarely needle injuries to the fetus, risk of club foot reported when done at GA <13 weeks. Culture failure occurs in <0.1% and pregnancy loss 0.3-1%. However, these problems are unfolded in experienced hands and new technologies of tissue culture.

Percutaneous Ultrasound-guided Fetal Blood Sampling/Cordocentesis

Percutaneous ultrasound-guided fetal blood sampling (PUFBS) is performed transabdominally after 18+0 weeks, using a 20-22-G needle under ultrasound guidance. The umbilical vein for FBS can be approached at the placental cord insertion site or a free loop, or the intrahepatic portion of the vein.

Indications

- Failed amniocentesis
- Mosaicism in CVS or amniotic fluid cytogenetics
- Rapid karyotyping in late pregnancy
- Red cell alloimmunization
- Hydrops fetalis
- Fetal infections
- Platelets alloimmunization, hemoglobinopathies.

Advantages

- Better and quicker chromosomal preparation than with CVS or amniocentesis.
- Direct estimation of fetal Hb, blood group, hematocrit, platelet, and WBC count for diagnosis of fetal anemia, thrombocytopenia, etc.
- Congenital infections can be diagnosed by serology, identification of viral particles, or culture of blood.
- *Other diagnosis*: Hereditary deficiency of hemostatic system, hemoglobinopathy, metabolic disorders, infections, and Fanconi anemia.

Complications

Bleeding from site of puncture (30%), cord hematoma, fetal bradycardia (5%), fetal loss (1-5%).

Embryoscopy and Fetoscopy: Direct Visualization of Embryo/Fetus

A fine-caliber endoscope is inserted into the amniotic cavity through a small maternal abdominal incision under USG guidance and fetus is visualized to detect subtle external structural abnormalities. It is also used for fetal blood and tissue sampling. It is associated with a 3-5% risk of miscarriage. In modern obstetrics, it is used in the treatment of twin-to-twin transfusion syndrome where laser is used to coagulate anastomotic vessels for Quintero stages II to IV.

Percutaneous Fetal Skin Biopsy

The procedure is performed between 17-20-wk GA to diagnose a number of serious skin disorders (anhidrotic ectodermal dysplasia, epidermolysis bullosa letalis/dystrophica, hypohidrotic ectodermal dysplasia, oculocutaneous albinism and genetic forms of ichthyosis).

Fetal Tissue Sampling

Case reports have described fetal liver biopsy for inborn error of metabolism (ornithine transcarbamylase deficiency, G6PD deficiency, glycogen storage disease type IA, nonketotic hyperglycemia, carbamoyl-phosphate synthetase deficiency) and fetal muscle biopsy (Becker Duchenne muscular dystrophy).

Preimplantation Genetic Diagnosis or Screening

Preimplantation Genetic Diagnosis (PMD) or screening (PMS) refers to testing of an embryo for a specific genetic disorder before implantation performed on polar bodies or, a single blastomere and subjected for cytogenetic techniques.

LABORATORY ASPECTS OF INVASIVE TESTING

Fetal cells obtained by CVS or amniocentesis can be studied directly or after culture by various techniques summarized in **Table 5**. Fetuses with structural abnormalities should undergo microarray as they are at high risk of having

TABLE 5: Tests available for prenatal genetic diagnosis.

Tests	Turnaround time	Resolution	Comments
Conventional karyotype (G-band): Dividing cells are cultured, arrested at metaphase then stained and examined in light microscope	7–14 days	*In blood sample*: 5–10 Mb CVS and amniocytes: 10–20 Mb only sufficient to exclude aneuploidies and larger structural rearrangements	Traditional method for diagnosis of chromosomal abnormalities with highly reliable results; limitations are maternal blood contamination and mosaicism
FISH: Performed in cultured or uncultured cells. Unlike karyotype, it is a targeted approach using fluorescent-labeled DNA probes to identify specific chromosomes or chromosomal regions	• 24–48 hours (uncul-tured cells) • 7–14 days (cultured cells)	• Rapid assessment of major aneuploidies (13, 18, 21 and sex chromosomes) • Specific deletions (e.g., 22q11 for CHD, 12p isochromosomes in DH) • Specific balanced or unbalanced familial translocations	FISH with direct testing cells from CVS is less accurate than with cultured cells from CVS or amniocentesis. Results should be confirmed on cultured cells or CMA, or have additional soft markers before decision-making
• *Quantitative fluorescent polymerase chain reaction (QF-PCR)* • PCR-based copy number analysis	24–48 hours	Rapid assessment of major aneuploidies 13, 18, 21, and sex chromosomes	Does not detect translocations, mosaicism, rearrangements. Abnormal results to be confirmed by karyotype or FISH
• *Chromosomal microarray (CMA)/comparative genome hybridization (microarray CGH)* • Single-standard DNA of patients sample is compared with reference DNA sample when hybridized to complementary sequence, thus array of thousands of oligonucleotides becomes the set of probes each of which is labeled with different fluorophores. Read by high-resolution laser scanner	• 3–5 days (direct testing) • 10–14 days (cultured cells) • 28–56 days when parental follow-up is required	• Copy number variants >50–200 kb • Results vary according to CMA platform used • Average resolution is 60 kb with increased clustering of probes	• Can detect deletions, duplications mosaicisms, with high DR and more accurate for chromosomal abnormalities. • Cannot detect balanced rearrangements and some triploidies • Considered as primary test if fetal structural abnormality detected by USG • Can yield results from nonviable cells that would not grow in culture hence preferred over karyotype for cases of fetal death or still birth
• *Targeted gene sequencing (single gene or multigene)* • *Methods*: Sangers sequencing, multiprobe ligation probe assay (MPLA), pyrosequencing		Single base pair or short sequences 10–20 bases	Designed to detect the specific mutation (to structural anomaly detected) or mutation within the family
• *Next-generation sequencing (NGS)*: Finding mutations in multiple genes by sequencing of millions of small fragments of DNA in parallel hence other name is massive parallel sequencing: – *Whole-genome sequencing*: Sequencing of whole human genome in a single test (each of the three billion bases). Hence, it is nonselective sequencing of coding and noncoding regions – *Exome sequencing*: Sequence only the coding regions of known genes (the exomes known to encode proteins)			• Interpretation of results is complex require consultation medical geneticist • If mutation is identified, confirmation by Sangers sequencing is recommended

(CVS: chorionic villus sampling; CHD: congenital heart defects; FISH: fluorescence in situ hybridization; USG: ultrasound)

genetic abnormalities. In the absence of a structural abnormality, the diagnostic performance of microarray does not appear to be significantly better than with conventional G-band karyotype. If microarray is normal and the phenotypic findings may still suggest a specific genetic disorder; assessing genes for recognized pathogenic variants (genotyping), single gene sequencing, multiple gene sequencing or genotyping through panels, or testing for specific deletions or duplications can be performed as appropriate for the disorder(s) being considered based upon family history or structural abnormalities identified on USG. Some commercial laboratories offer gene panels to analyze a group of genes implicated as per structural abnormality, but the yield of such testing is unclear. Next generation sequencing (NGS) either exome or whole-genome sequencing is to be considered only when a genetic etiology is suspected but standard testing is nondiagnostic. Consultation with a genetic specialist is advised.

CONCLUSION

- All pregnant women should be offered prenatal screening tests for aneuploidy, irrespective of maternal age or other risk factors.
- A first-trimester screen or chromosome result does not obviate the need for second-trimester fetal assessment, including TIFFA and with or without serum AFP.
- A patient with increased risk of having a pregnancy affected by genetic disorder (based upon screening tests or history) should be offered diagnostic tests (CVS or amniocentesis) before pregnancy decisions.
- Genetic counseling with an expert is warranted in all mothers falling in the high-risk group with increased chances of having fetuses with genetic/structural abnormalities.
- Despite of tremendous advances, it needs to be emphasized clearly that all birth defects and genetic diseases cannot be diagnosed by available screening, diagnostic and genetic tests.

SUGGESTED READING

1. Ajao AE, Adeoye IA. Prevalence, risk factors and outcome of congenital anomalies among neonatal admissions in OGBOMOSO, Nigeria. BMC Pediatr. 2019;19(88).
2. Bahado-Singh RO, Oz AU, Kovanci E, Deren O, Copel J, Baumgarten A, et al. New Down syndrome screening algorithm: ultrasonographic biometry and multiple serum markers combined with maternal age. Am J Obstet Gynecol. 1998;179:1627-31.
3. Congenital anomalies overview, [online] Available from: https://www.who.int/health-topics/congenital-anomalies
4. D'Vore G. The aortic and pulmonary outflow tract screening examinations in human fetus. J Ultrasound Med. 1992;11:345-8.
5. Ghi T, Sotiriadis A, Calda P, Da Silva Costa F, Rainen Fenning N, Alfirevic Z, et al. ISUOG Practice Guidelines: Invasive procedures for prenatal diagnosis. Ultrasound Obstet Gynecol. 2016;48: 256-68.
6. Kumar B, Alfirevic Z. Fetal Medicine. Cambridge: Cambridge University Press; 2017. pp. 1-18.
7. Mardy AH, Chetty SP, Norton ME, Sparks TN. A system-based approach to the genetic etiologies of non-immune hydrops fetalis. Prenat Diagn. 2019;39(9):732-50.
8. Pilu G, Perolo A, Falco P, Visentin A, Gabrielli G, Bovicelli L. Ultrasound of the central nervous system. Curr Opin Obstet Gynecol. 2000;12:93-103.
9. Royal College of Obstetricians and Gynae-cologists, Royal College of Paediatrics and Child Health. Fetal abnormalities. Guidelines for screening, diagnosis and management. London, UK: RCPCH, RCOG; 1997.
10. Syngelaki A, Chelemen T, Dagklis T, Allan L, Nicolaides KH. Challenges in the diagnosis of fetal non-chromosomal abnormalities at 11-13 weeks. Prenat Diagn. 2011;31(1):90-102.
11. Wald NJ, Rodeck C, Hackshaw AK, Walters J, Chitty L, Mackinson AM, et al. First and second trimester antenatal screening for Down's syndrome: the results of the Serum, Urine and Ultrasound Screening Study (SURUSS) Health Technol Assess. 2003;7:1.

Chapter 161: Lysosomal Storage Diseases in India

Ravinder Makkar

INTRODUCTION

Lysosomes are membrane-enclosed organelles that function as the digestive system of animal cells. With help of 50 different enzymes present within the lysosome, it hydrolyzes proteins, nucleic acids, polysaccharides, and lipids.

Genetic mutations encoding these enzymes are known to cause more than 50 genetically distinct, but biochemically related, inherited diseases grouped together as *lysosomal storage diseases (LSDs)*.

Epidemiology and Burden of Disease

- They classified as rare genetic diseases.
- The prevalence can range from 1 per 57,000 live births for Gaucher disease (GD) to 1 per 4.2 million live births for sialidosis.
- The rough collective prevalence of an LSD is generally estimated to be 1 in 100,000–200,000 population.
- The overall burden of disease in India is not known; however a retrospective study in 2014 included 1,558 patients with clinical suspicion of various LSDs during 2007 to 2012 suggested 30% of the cases (467) to be affected, with sphingolipidoses as the most common subgroup, followed by mucopolysaccharidoses (MPS) and GD as the most frequently occurring individual.

PATHOPHYSIOLOGY OF LYSOSOMAL STORAGE DISEASES

In LSDs, undegraded material accumulates within the lysosomes of affected individuals due to the deficiency of the catabolizing enzyme. The distribution of accumulating material correlates with which organs are affected. Cells of the mononuclear phagocyte system are especially rich in lysosomes and thus are frequently affected by LSDs. Deficiency of enzyme occurs due to inheritance of specific gene mutation from parents or can occur de novo in some cases.

Inheritance pattern:
- Most LSDs are inherited in an autosomal recessive pattern.
- A few are X-linked (MPSII, Fabry, Danon disease).

CLASSIFICATION OF LYSOSOMAL STORAGE DISEASES

Lysosomal storage diseases are generally classified by the accumulated substrate and include the sphingolipidoses, oligosaccharidoses, mucolipidoses, MPSs, lipoprotein storage disorders, lysosomal transport defects, neuronal ceroid lipofuscinoses, and others **(Table 1)**.

LABORATORY DIAGNOSIS

- The standard initial test for diagnosis of most LSDs is a quantitative enzyme assay. This enzyme assay can be easily performed on *dried blood spot (DBS) sample*.
- Demonstration of glycosaminoglycans *(GAGs) in urine* is a useful screening test for MPS diseases.
- Cultured fibroblasts are required in a few LSDs while cultured amniocytes or chorionic villus cells may be used for prenatal diagnosis.
- The specific *gene mutations* of LSDs can be detected by DNA *analysis* using genome sequencing.
- *Mutation analysis* is used mainly for confirmation or carrier detection and is available in many genetic labs across India.

CLINICAL MANIFESTATIONS OF SOME COMMON LSDs IN INDIA

Mucopolysaccharidoses

- Mucopolysaccharidoses (MPS) are inherited deficiencies of enzymes involved in GAG breakdown.
- Enzyme deficiencies that prevent GAGs breakdown cause accumulation of their fragments in lysosomes and affects bone, soft tissue, and CNS.
- Inheritance of MPS group of diseases is usually autosomal recessive (except for MPS type II).

Clinical Features

Clinical features include coarse facial features, neurodevelopmental regression, joint contracture, organomegaly, progressive airway obstruction and sleep apnea, cardiac

TABLE 1: Classification of lysosomal storage diseases (LSDs).

Type of LSD (based on substrate accumulated)	Subtypes					
Glycogen storage disease type II	Pompe disease (infantile onset/late onset)					
Mucopoly-saccharidoses	MPS type I Hurler or Hurler Scheie syndrome (alpha-L-iduronidase deficiency)	MPS type II A, Hunter syndrome, (duronate sulfatase deficiency)	MPS type III A-D, Sanfilippo syndrome, (heparan N-sulfatase deficiency)	MPS type IV A, Morquio syndrome, classic (galactose 6-sulfatase deficiency)	MPS type VI, Maroteaux-Lamy syndrome (arylsulfatase B deficiency)	MPS type VII, Sly syndrome (beta-glucuronidase deficiency)
Mucolipidoses	Mucolipidosis I (sialodosis)	Mucolipidosis II I-cell disease	Mucolipidosis III (phospho-transferase deficiency)	Mucolipidosis IV (mucolipidin 1 deficiency)		
Oligosacchari-doses	Schindler disease (alpha-N-acetylgalac-tos aminidase deficiency)	Alpha-mannosidosis and beta-mannosidosis	Alpha-fucosidosis	Sialidosis (mucolipido-sis I; alpha-N-acetyl neuramini-dase [sialidase] deficiency)	Aspartylgluc osaminuria (aspartylgluc osaminase deficiency)	
Lipidoses	Niemann-Pick disease types C and D	Neuronal ceroid lipofuscinoses	Wolman disease (acid lipase deficiency)			
Sphingolipi-doses	Niemann-Pick disease type A/B (sphingo-myelinase deficiency)	Gaucher disease (beta-glucosidase deficiency)	Krabbe disease, (galactosyl-ceramidase deficiency)	Fabry disease (alpha-galactosidase)	GM1 gangliodi-dosis; GM2 gangliosido-sis (tay sachs disease)	*Others*: Farber disease. Metachro-matic leukodys-trophy-Galactosiali-dosis, multiple sulfatase deficiency
Lysosomal transport diseases	Cystinosis (cystine transporter deficiency)	Salla disease; sialic acid transporter deficiency				

(MPS: mucopolysaccharidosis)

valvular disease, short stature, and various skeletal deformities.

Diagnosis

- Detailed history, a thorough physical examination, and findings of bone abnormalities (e.g., dysostosis multiplex) during skeletal survey.
- The elevated urinary GAGs can help improve the clinical suspicion.
- Final diagnosis can be confirmed by enzyme analysis and DNA analysis.

Treatment is by enzyme replacement therapy (ERT) is based on type of MPS **(Table 2)**.

Gaucher Disease

- Gaucher disease is the most prevalent sphingolipid LSD.
- The defect in GD is an autosomal recessive inherited deficiency of the lysosomal enzyme glucocerebrosidase caused by a mutation in the *GBA1* gene.
- Deficiency of glucocerebrosidase results in the abnormal accumulation and storage of glucocerebroside within lysosomes of macrophages.

Clinical phenotypes of GD are classified according to the absence or presence of neurological involvement: Type 1 GD is called the non-neuronopathic form; Type 2 GD is the acute neuronopathic form, while type 3 GD is the subacute neuronopathic form.

TABLE 2: Treatments currently approved for LSDs.

LSD	Name of approved drug
Gaucher disease	Cerezyme® (Imiglucerase)
	VPRIV™ (Velaglucerase alfa)
	Elelyso™ (Taliglucerase)
	Cerdelga (Eliglustat tartarate)
	Zavesca (Miglustat)
Pompe disease	Myozyme® (Alglucosidase alfa)
Fabry Disease	Fabrazyme (Agalsidase beta)
	Replagal (Agalsidase alfa)
	Galafold (Migalastat)
MPS I (Hurler, Hurler-Scheie or Scheie)	Aldurazyme® (Laronidase)
MPS II (Hunter disease)	Elaprase® (Idursulfase)
MPS-IVA (Morquio A syndrome)	Vimzim™ (Elosulfase alfa)
MPS VI (Maroteaux-Lamy syndrome)	Naglazyme™ (Galsulfase)
MPS VII (Sly Syndrome)	Mepsevii (Vestronidase alfa)
Niemann Pick Type C (Neurological manifestations both adult and children)	Zavesca (Miglustat)
Lysosomal acid lipase deficiency (LAL-D) – Wolman disease	Kanuma® (Sebelipase alfa)
Late infantile neuronal ceroid lipofuscinosis type 2 (CLN2), also known as tripeptidyl peptidase 1 (TPP1) deficiency.	Brineura® (Cerliponase alfa)

- Type 1 GD is mostly reported in Caucasian population. There is no neurological involvement. The features ranges from mild to severe and may appear anytime from childhood to adulthood. The diagnosis is made only by hematological, visceral, and bone manifestations and, with treatment, the prognosis is good.
- Type 2 GD is characterized by severe and progressive neurological deterioration and it causes death at birth or within 1–2 years of life. These patients are rare to find as most cases die before reaching a diagnosis.
- *Type 3 GD:*
  - It effects the nervous system but it tends to worsen more slowly than type 2.
  - Type 3 GD is the predominant phenotype seen in India.
  - Leu4 83p mutations (preciously classified as L4 44 p) in *GBA* gene renders patients predisposed to develop type 3 or neuronopathic phenotype during their disease.
  - Major signs and symptoms include oculomotor apraxia as the most common a subtle neurological sign suggestive of type 3 disease. Non-neurological features in type 3 GD include moderate-to-severe hepatosplenomegaly, anemia, thrombocytopenia, lung disease, and bone abnormalities such as bone pain, Erlenmeyer flask deformity, fractures, and avascular necrosis of femur. *Any patient with unexplained hepatosplenomegaly in the presence of unexplained anemia and/or* thrombocytopenia should be evaluated to rule out GD.

Diagnosis of GD is established by enzyme assay on DBS (glucocerebrosidase deficient). Mutations diagnosis can be made by sequencing the *GBA* gene, for confirmation.

Treatment of Gaucher Disease

- It is treated with imiglucerase ERT (Cerezyme©, Sanofi Genzyme; Chinese hamster ovarian cell line origin) at a dose of 60 U/kg intravenous infusion every 2 weeks. With the longest safety and efficacy data amongst all ERTs, Cerezyme© is considered the standard of care for type 1 and type3 GD.
- Other ERTs available commercially for GD include velaglucerase (Vpriv©, Takeda; Human fibroblast cell line) and Taliglucerase (Elelyso©, Protalix/Pfizer; carrot plant-based cell line). Oral therapy with Eliglustat tablet (Cerdelga©, Sanofi Genzyme) is approved for adult GD1 cases in US, EU, and some other countries. Indian clinical experience with use of Cerezyme© has been reported that suggests poor efficacy and safety in GD patients from India.

Mucopolysaccharidoses

- Mucopolysaccharidoses are a group of LSDs, each of which is produced by an inherited deficiency of an enzyme involved in the degradation of acid mucopolysaccharides (GAGs).
- These diseases are autosomal recessive, except for MPS type II, which is X-linked. Mucopolysaccharidosis usually manifests during infancy or early childhood.

Clinical Features

Involvement of bone (Dysostosis multiplex, short stature), the viscera (hepatosplenomegaly), connective tissue, and the brain (severe neurologic deficits and mental retardation). Any patient with coarse facies, corneal opacity, deafness, respiratory, neurocognitive and cardiovascular anomalies, and skeletal abnormalities should be evaluated for MPS. Obstructive sleep apnea and obstructive respiratory problems are common in patients with MPS.

Diagnosis

- Diagnosis is based on the clinical picture, radiographic findings, and laboratory results.

- Presence of urinary GAGs can be used as screening test.
- Specific enzyme estimations and mutation testing are required for differential/definite diagnosis of a specific MPS type.
- ERTs effectively slow down the progression and reverse non-CNS complications of the disease.

Treatment

Mucopolysaccharidoses are treated with *ERT*. The ERT available for various MPS are as follows:
- *MPS I*: Aldurazyme (laronidase)
- *MPS II*: Elaprase (idursulfase)
- *MPS IVa*: Vimizim (elosulfase alfa)
- *MPS VI*: Naglazyme (galsulfase)
- *MPS VII*: Mepseii (vestronidase alfa).

Aldurazyme, the only approved ERT for MPS I, is registered in India at present and user experience has been reported with moderate benefits to Indian MPS I patients.

Hematopoietic stem cell transplantation (HSCT) is the treatment of choice for MPS I, for cases < 2.5 years of age; however, this treatment has not been reported from India. Combination of ERT replacement and HSCT as therapy for Hurler syndrome is expected to yield better outcomes.

Pompe Disease

- Pompe disease (PD) is an *autosomal recessive*, inherited enzyme defect that usually manifests in childhood as infantile-onset PD (IOPD) or juvenile-onset PD.
- The deficiency of lysosomal enzyme *alpha-glucosidase* which normally catalyzes reactions that ultimately convert glycogen compounds to monosaccharides, of which glucose is the predominant component, results in glycogen storage in tissues, especially muscles, and impairs muscle strength.

Clinical Features

Symptoms are related to progressive muscle weakness and respiratory involvement. Initial suspicion in infants is based on presences of muscle hypotonia, cardiomegaly, and delayed motor milestones. In adults, it manifests as progressive limb girdle muscle dystrophy leading to wheelchair dependence and need for ventilatory support over time due to progressive respiratory weakness.

Diagnosis

Raised creatine kinase (CK) levels, a biochemical enzyme deficiency on DBS testing confirmed by mutation test provides a definite diagnosis.

All infants presenting with hypotonia, cardiomegaly on chest X-ray (CXR) and raised CK levels in blood should be evaluated for infantile PD.

Treatment

- Enzyme replacement therapy in PD can be lifesaving if patients are diagnosed and treated timely.
- Myzoyme is the only ERT available treatment of PD. It is given at 20 mg/kg intravenous infusion every 2 weeks, and provides benefit in terms of improving muscle function, improved pulmonary function, delays ventilatory support and prolongs life and quality of life (QoL).
- Indian experience in IOPD cases has been reported in a few studies suggesting a delayed diagnosis, late initiation of ERT, and therefore a poorer outcome.
- Newer-generation ERT to improve the efficiency of ERT and various gene therapies are under development to improve long-term outcomes.

Fabry Disease

- Fabry disease (FD) is an X-linked disorder caused by deficiency of the enzyme *α-galactosidase*. It leads to progressive accumulation of globotriaosylceramide (GL-3) in lysosomes.
- *Clinical manifestations* of classic FD in children are angiokeratoma skin lesions, acroparesthesias (burning pain in the limbs), hypohydrosis, corneal opacities (cornea verticillata), and gastrointestinal (GI) pain and discomfort.
- Other presentations include marked fatigue and anxiety. Symptoms appear at a median age of 10–12 years. Later, adults develop progressive kidney disease, cardiac and central nervous system (CNS) complications such as stroke which contribute to morbidity and early mortality. Females typically have milder manifestations; however, they can develop severe complications in some cases.
- FD seems highly underdiagnosed in India. It is prudent that any young patient with unexplained renal disease, unexplained stroke, or unexplained arrhythmia or left ventricular hypertrophy be evaluated to rule out FD. Only few case series, have been described in India in literature so far.

Diagnosis

Diagnosis of FD is established by enzyme assay on DBS (alfa-galactosidase). Mutational diagnosis can be made by sequencing the *GLA* gene for confirmation.

Treatment: Enzyme Replacement Therapy

- Fabrazyme, (agalsidase beta) is available in India for treatment of FD patients. The dose of Fabrazyme is 1 mg/kg every 2 weeks given intravenously. Treatment leads to improvement in renal, cardiac, nervous, and gastrointestinal parameters.

- Replagal (agalsidase alfa), approved in EU and some other countries, is available for treatment of FD at a dose of 0.2 mg/kg dose every fortnightly.
- Migalstat, an oral substrate reduction therapy (SRT), is available in USA and some other countries for treatment of limited number of certain "mutation-specific adult FD patients."

TREATMENT OF LYSOSOMAL STORAGE DISORDERS

- Intravenous ERT has been the standard therapeutic option for treatment of various LSDs. The term "enzyme replacement therapy" refers to therapy with glycoprotein products, intended to augment or replace the activity of a specific endogenous catabolic enzyme within cellular lysosomes.
- All ERT products in LSDs are administered by intravenous infusion, at dosages typically based on patient's body weight, usually weekly or every other week, life long. The infused enzymes are taken up by cells and transported into lysosomes, where they catabolize the specific macromolecule that has been accumulated.
- ERT is now approved for non-neurological or peripheral manifestations in various LSDs (*see* Table 2) such as GD, FD, MPS I, MPS II, MPS IVa, MPS VI, MPS VII, PD, and Baten disease (neuronal ceroid lipofuscinoses, CLN2).
- Advanced research efforts are currently underway to develop ERT options for several other disorders (e.g., Olipudase alfa for Niemann pick B).
- In India, few ERTS are duly approved by Drug controller general of India (DCGI, Indian health regulatory authorities). These ERTs include Cerezyme©, fabrazyme, aldurazyme, and myozyme. Results of their clinical use in India has been reported earlier.
- *Limitation of ERTs*: They cannot cross blood–brain barrier due to their large molecular size and therefore are not effective in improving CNS manifestations of LSDs.

Approved ERTs Available (*see* Table 2)

Substrate Reduction Therapy

In a metabolic or genetic pathway, the lysosomal enzymes catalyze a series of reactions. Each lysosomal enzyme is regulated or mediated by one gene through its RNA and protein products. At each phase in the pathway, enzyme activity catalyzes a reaction in which a precursor molecule (the substrate) is transformed into its next intermediate state. Failure of the metabolic pathway leads to accumulation of the substrate, with possible harmful effects. Substrate reduction therapy addresses this failure by reducing the level of the substrate to a point where residual degradative activity is enough to prevent substrate accumulation. *Eliglustat (GD type 1), Miglustat (GD), Migalastat (FD) are examples of approved SRTs being used as treatment of certain LSDs.*

Newer Therapeutic Approaches

Chaperone therapy, gene therapy, and *gene editing* approaches are experimental at this time and are being tried in various LSDs.

CONCLUSION

- Lysosomal storage disorders are rare disorders caused by genetic mutations that lead to enzyme deficiency.
- Presentations are variable, and diagnosis is difficult and usually delayed.
- There is an urgent need to collect epidemiological data and improve general awareness of these diseases among the medical community.
- ERTs are approved for treating LSDs. They are very expensive.
- By ERTs, progression of disease is slowed down, but they do not improve neurologic features.
- Small-molecule chaperones, HSCT, and gene therapy are newer therapies under development.
- There is no cure for any LSD, and current management remains focused on early diagnosis and treatment.
- Genetic counseling is the only way to reduce the burden in individual families and communities.
- Funding by public health authorities coupled with a public–private partnership with pharmaceutical industries and patient societies is needed to support the treatment of these patients.

SUGGESTED READING

1. Aggarwal S, Lahiri K, Muranjan M, Solanki N. The face of lysosomal storage disorders in India: a need for early diagnosis. Indian J Pediatr. 2015;82(6):525-9.
2. Ferreira CR, Gahl WA. Lysosomal storage diseases. Transl Sci Rare Dis. 2017;2(1-2):1-71.
3. Gupta N, Kazi ZB, Nampoothiri S, Jagdeesh S, Kabra M, Puri RD, et al. Clinical and molecular disease spectrum and outcomes in patients with infantile-onset Pompe Disease. J Pediatr. 2020;216:44-50.e5.
4. Kadali Srilatha, Kolusu A, Gummadi MR, Undamatla J. The relative frequency of lysosomal storage disorders: a medical genetics referral laboratory's experience from India. J Child Neurol. 2014;29(10):1377-82.
5. Kuter DJ, Mehta A, Hollak C, Giraldo P, Hughes D, Belmatoug N, et al. Miglustat therapy in type 1 Gaucher disease: long-term treatment experience from a multicenter, retrospective cohort study. Blood. 2011;118(21):3207.
6. Muranjan M, Karande S. Enzyme replacement therapy in India: lessons and insights. J Postgrad Med. 2018;64(4):195-9.
7. Muranjan M, Patil S. Outcome of Gaucher Disease in India: lessons from prevalent diagnostic and therapeutic practices. Indian Pediatr. 2016;53:685-8.
8. Nagral A. Recombinant macrophage targeted enzyme replacement therapy for Gaucher disease in India. Indian Pediatr. 2011;48(10): 779-84.
9. Nagree MS, Scalia S, McKillop WM, Medin JA. An update on gene therapy for lysosomal storage disorders. Expert Opin Biol Ther. 2019;19(7):655-70.

10. Parenti G. Treating lysosomal storage diseases with pharmacological chaperones: From concept to clinics. EMBO Mol Med. 2009; 1(5):268-79.
11. Phadke S. Lysosomal Storage Disorders: Present and future. Indian Pediatr. 2015;52:1025-6.
12. Puri R, Kapoor S, Kishnani PS, Dalal A, Gupta N, Muranjan M, et al. Diagnosis and Management of Gaucher Disease in India-Consensus Guidelines of the Gaucher Disease Task Force of the Society for Indian Academy of Medical Genetics and the Indian Academy of Pediatrics. Indian Pediatr. 2018;55(2):143-53.
13. Reuser AJ, Verheijen FW, Bali D, van Diggelen OP, Germain DP, Hwu W-L, Lukacs Z, et al. The use of dried blood spot samples in the diagnosis of lysosomal storage disorders-current status and perspectives. Mol Genet Metab. 2011;104(1-2):144-8.
14. Schifmann R Sevigny, Jeff, Rolfs A, Davies EH, Goker-Alpan O, Abdelwahab M, et al. The definition of neuronopathic Gaucher disease. J Inherit Metab Dis. 2020;1-4.
15. Sheth J, Mistri M, Bhaisar R, Sheth F, Kamate M, Shah H, et al. Lysosomal storage disorders in Indian children with neuroregression attending a genetic center. Indian Pediatr. 2015; 52(12):1029-33.
16. Sheth J, Mistri M, Sheth F, Shah R, Bavdekar A, Godbole K, et al. Burden of lysosomal storage disorders in India: Experience of 387 affected children from a single diagnostic facility. JIMD Rep. 2014;12:51-63.
17. Tolar J, Grewal SS, Bjoraker KJ, Whitley CB, Shapiro EG, Charnas L, et al. Combination of enzyme replacement and hematopoietic stem cell transplantation as therapy for Hurler syndrome. Bone Marrow Transplant. 2008; 41(6):531-5.
18. Verma PK, Ranganath P, Dalal AB, Phadke SR. Spectrum of lysosomal storage disorders at a medical genetics center in northern India. Indian Pediatr. 2012;49(10):799-804.
19. Wani MM, Khan I, Bhat RA, Ahmad M. Fabry's disease: Case series and review of literature. Ann Med Health Sci Res. 2016;6:193-7.

SECTION 15: Dermatology

162. Urticaria and Angioedema
163. Papular Urticaria
164. Atopic Dermatitis
165. Pityriasis Versicolor
166. Tinea Infections
167. Scabies
168. Impetigo
169. Acne Vulgaris
170. Stevens–Johnson Syndrome
171. Hand, Foot, and Mouth Disease

Urticaria and Angioedema

Vijay P Makhija

INTRODUCTION

- Urticaria (or hives) is a kind of skin rash notable for pale red, raised, itchy wheals. Hives is often caused by allergic reactions; however, there are many nonallergic causes too. Many different substances in environment can cause urticaria including medications, food, and physical agents.
- It is often associated with degranulation of mast cells mediated by IgE that results in release of histamine. Histamine causes vasodilatation, erythema, leaking of fluid in extravascular compartment and itching. These all are hallmark features of urticaria.
- *Salient features of urticaria*: (1) *Transient, pruritic, erythematous raised wheals with flat tops and edema* that may be tense and painful. (2) Lesions may combine to have a polycyclic serpiginous and annular lesions. (3) Individual *lesions last for 20 minutes to 3 hours* rarely >24 hours. (4) *Lesions disappear later to reappear* at other sites.

CAUSES

Most common causes of urticaria:
- *Drugs*: Medicines responsible for urticaria
  - *Suspect all medications* even nonprescription, ayurvedic, or homeopathic medicines too.
  - Common medicines that can cause urticaria are aspirin, penicillins, sulfa group, nonsteroidal anti-inflammatory drugs (NSAIDs), cephalosporins, clavulanic acid, tetracycline, anticonvulsants, etc.
- *Foods*: Foods often responsible for urticaria.
  - Egg/milk/wheat/peanuts/tree nuts
  - Soy/shellfish/strawberries
  The diagnosis of urticaria caused by foods are by:
- History can be greatly helpful.
- Allergy skin test for foods are helpful.

TYPES

Acute and chronic urticaria:
- Episodes of urticaria lasting <6 weeks—acute
- Lasting on most days for >6 weeks—chronic

Typical hives/urticaria	Atypical urticaria or urticaria associated with SLE/vasculitis or serum sickness
Erythematous, pruritic, raised wheal that blanches with pressure	Lesions burning sensation more than itching
It is transient and resolves without residual lesions	Lasts for >24 hours
	Do not blanch
	Blister heal with scarring and associated with purpura suggest urticarial vasculitis
	Atypical hives/associated symptoms may be manifestation of systemic disease process
Physical urticaria **What are its common causes?**	**Cold urticaria**
Caused by stroking the skin	Cold stimulus—local pruritus/erythema and urticaria/angioedema
Pressure urticaria	Total body exposure—swimming in cold water—massive release of vasoactive mediators—hypotension/loss of consciousness or death if not treated promptly
Solar urticaria or cold urticaria	Diagnosis of cold urticaria by challenge testing for isomorphic cold reaction
Vibratory urticaria	Cold urticaria is associated with presence of cryoproteins as cold agglutinins/cryoglobulins/cryofibrinogen and Donath–Landsteiner antibody
Aquagenic urticaria	In idiopathic cold urticaria, no abnormal circulating plasma proteins are found
May even be caused by light	
Characterized by onset of small punctate pruritic wheals surrounded by a prominent erythematous flaret	Small wheals develop after contact with water irrespective of its temperature

Contd...

Contd...

Cholinergic urticaria	Aquagenic urticaria
Associated with exercise/hot showers or sweating	This feature differentiates it from cold urticaria/cholinergic urticaria
Urticaria subsides in 30–60 minutes as patient's body cools down	Direct water compress over skin used as a test for aquagenic urticaria
Occasionally symptoms of general cholinergic stimulation as lacrimation/salivation/wheezing and as patient's body cools down	In some of these patients, chlorine or other trace contaminants are responsible for it used as a test for aquagenic urticaria
Occasionally symptoms of general cholinergic stimulation as lacrimation/salivation/wheezing and syncope are observed with it	
Cholinergic parasympathetic nerve fibers along with sympathetic fibers innervate sweat glands/musculature-associated symptoms	
Changes in body temperature elevated—histamine—urticaria	

Dermatographism or urticaria factitia	Solar urticaria
Ability to write on skin termed dermatographism	Rare disorder in which urticaria develops within minutes of direct sun exposure
Can be diagnosed by stroking the skin with any blunt object as tongue depressor/reverse side of a pen, etc	Sun light-exposed areas—pruritus—30 seconds later edema follows surrounded by prom erythematous zone
Stroking skin—linear response by reflex vasoconstriction—pruritus/erythema and linear flare caused by secondary dilation of vessels and extravasation of plasma	Lesions disappear in 1–3 hours after cessation of sun exposure
May be isolated or associated with chronic urticaria or other physical urticaria as cold or cholinergic urticaria	Large areas of skin sun exposure—systemic symptoms as hypotension and wheezing can occur

Contd...

Contd...

Pressure urticaria	
Symptoms occur 4–6 hours after pressure has been applied	Diagnosis of pressure urticaria by challenge testing
May present as angioedema or urticaria	Pressure applied perpendicular to skin
Symptoms occur at sites of tight clothing	Sling attached to 5 kg weight placed on patient's arm for 20 minutes
Swelling on feet after walking	
Swelling on buttocks after sitting for few hours	

MANAGEMENT OF ACUTE URTICARIA

- Self-limited illness
- Identification of etiologic factor(s) and subsequent elimination is ideal.
- Requires antihistamines.
- Avoidance of any identified trigger factors.
- H1 antihistamine drugs as hydroxyzine/diphenhydramine—sedating/ effects.
- Fexofenadine/loratadine/desloratadine/cetirizine—nonsedating and longer action.
- Sometimes administration of H2 receptor blocker too helps.
- Antibiotics help if there is an associated bacterial infection.
- Epinephrine 1:1,000 dilution 0.01 mL/kg IM provides rapid relief of acute severe urticaria and angioedema.
- Short-course steroids used only in very severe urticaria/angioedema not responding to antihistamines.

ANGIOEDEMA

Angioedema is a related condition that also occurs from allergic and nonallergic causes though fluid leakage is from much deeper blood vessels in it. It affects 20% persons at some point in their lives. In about 50% cases, chronic urticaria is accompanied by angioedema. The pathology of urticaria/angioedema is edema of superficial dermis occurs in urticaria, while edema of subcutaneous tissue and deep dermis occurs in angioedema. The locations, especially affected are eyelids/lips/tongue/genitals/dorsum of hands and feet, and wall of gastrointestinal tract (GIT).

Pathogenesis of urticaria and angioedema: (1) Often caused by an allergic IgE-mediated reaction, (2) occurs by activation of mast cells by an allergen, and (3) a self-limited process.

Papular Urticaria

Vijay P Makhija

CLINICAL FEATURES

It occurs because of delayed hypersensitivity phenomenon to the insect bite. It usually presents with severe itching and papular eruptions over the exposed parts of body such as face, and upper and lower limbs. Trunk and other parts of body that are covered by clothes are usually spared. Secondary bacterial infection may be associated with it. If puncture marks are present then it confirms the diagnosis of papular urticaria. History is usually negative, as there seems to be a social stigma attached to being a recipient of insect bites.

PROGNOSIS

The recovery is good in this condition as it decreases by itself in next few years (around 7–8 years of age). So, the parents must be reassured regarding overall good prognosis of this condition. But adequate steps must be taken to decrease the morbidity of the child while it is persisting.

TREATMENT

Try to *identify the insect* responsible to prevent the further attacks. Parents are advised to use full sleeves clothes, pyjamas and pants to decrease the exposed skin surface for insect bites. Creams and lotions containing dimethyl phthalate, dibutyl phthalate or diethyl toluamide are extensively used, as insect repellants but are partially effective. Use of mosquito nets, veils, and repellant coils or liquids is useful in preventing skin bites.

Mattresses should be exposed to sun frequently to kill the bedbugs which may cause papular urticaria in some children. Application of insecticides to walls and furniture can help because the bedbugs hide in crevices in walls and joints of furniture during daytime. Infested animals should be treated appropriately.

Oral antihistamines for prolonged periods can significantly help to decrease the itching. Local use of ice and soothing lotions (calamine lotion) can also alleviate the pruritus. If the itching is very severe then local steroid creams can also be used for short periods.

Topical or systemic antibiotics are advised if secondary bacterial infection is present.

If severe systemic reaction is present, systemic steroids or even adrenaline injection may be required.

CASE

A 4-year child presented severe itching of forearms and legs since last 1 year and had taken various consultations and medicines that did not help. No other family members or close ones had similar problem.

Clues: Small 1–2-mm papule seen on face, forearms, and legs of child but trunk is clear. Presence of few pustules

Papular urticaria/insect bite hypersensitivity:
- Presents with severe itching and papular eruptions over exposed parts.
- Presence of puncture marks confirms the diagnosis.

SUGGESTED READING

1. Dhar S. Color Atlas & Synopsis Pediatric Dermatology, 3rd edition. New Delhi: Jaypee Brothers Medical Publishers (P) Ltd.; 2015.

164 CHAPTER

Atopic Dermatitis

Vijay P Makhija

INTRODUCTION

Atopy is a condition of altered reactivity to common and mild environmental stimuli. The word "Atopy" was first used for a group of hereditary disorders in people who had a tendency to develop an urticarial response to foods and inhaled substances.

PATHOGENESIS

There is interplay of various genetic factors, environmental factors and immunological factors results in abnormal reactivity of skin to common environmental stimuli. The antigen attaches to IgE on mast cells and releases various mediators of inflammation in to tissues leading to various features of atopic dermatitis (AD).

Onset and Progress

The onset in 50% patient is seen by first year and 80% presents before 5 years of age. Remissions and relapses are the part of this disease. Many children remit by 2–3 years, some persist with it in childhood, adolescence, and adulthood.

Cardinal features of AD are:
- Intense pruritus
- Cutaneous reactivity in the form of persistent or relapsing eczema
- Present or past, personal, or family history of atopy.

Intense Pruritus

It is a prominent feature of AD. There is *Itch-scratch-itch cycle* which leads to scratching and release of histamine which further promotes itching. Constant Itching often leads to secondary bacterial infection, especially *Staphylococcus aureus*. Constant rubbing and scratching often leads to thickened skin with increased skin markings known as lichenification and seen around flexures.

UK WORKING GROUP: CRITERIA FOR DIAGNOSIS

Atopic dermatitis Itchy skin condition (Obligatory).

PLUS three or more of the following:
1. History of flexural involvement
2. History of asthma/hay fever
3. History of generalized dry skin
4. Onset of rash under the age of 2 years or
5. Visible flexural involvement.

Atopic Dermatitis: Infantile Phase

It is common. And the onset is seen around 3–6 months. It presents bilateral symmetrical papulovesicular, exudative and crusted lesions of acute/subacute eczema, associated with severe itching. More marked on face, scalp, and extensors of extremities. The cheeks are commonly affected but the diaper areas are usually spared because this area is often moist. Secondary infection is common due to profound itching.

Progression: It may remit completely by 2–3 years. In 40% infants, it remits by 18 months and in 60% evolves in childhood AD.

Atopic Dermatitis: Childhood Phase

It may evolve from infantile or may start de novo. There is intense pruritic papules affecting flexures of elbows/knees, popliteal/cubital fossa, but sometimes reversed pattern seen, i.e., in extensors. The face and trunk are uncommonly involved. The involvement is symmetrical; the lesions are usually lichenified and excoriated.

MANAGEMENT OF ATOPIC DERMATITIS

- Identification and avoidance of triggering factors **(Table 1)**
- Hydration of the skin
- Topical therapy **(Table 2)**
- Systemic therapy.

Management

- Lukewarm soaking baths 20 minutes

TABLE 1: Identification and avoidance of triggering factors.

Avoidance of triggers	Which ingestant to avoid?
Dust	40% children with mod/severe AD have food allergy
Cigarette smoke	Severity of AD directly correlated with food allergy
Avoid contact with chemicals	Removal of food allergens helps significantly
Cotton clothing is preferred	Avoid common allergens as milk, egg white, wheat, soy, peanut andoranges
Avoid synthetic/woolen clothings	Increased histamine-containing eatables such as fish, shell fish, cheese, spinach, tomatoes
Second rinse of clothes helps	*Which inhalants to avoid?*
Neomycin preparations as it is a known sensitizer in atopics	Inhalants/aeroallergens, especially avoided in childhood type
Avoid using soap, especially strong ones	Fungi, animal dander, grass or ragweed pollen
Use mild soaps and that too infrequently	Avoidance of dust mite helps significantly
Avoid using too hot/cold water	*How to avoid dust mite?*
Avoid extremes of temperature/humidity	Encasing pillows/mattresses
Avoid emotional stress/tension, especially in adolescents/adults	Remove bedroom carpets
Seasonal changes are primary aggravating factor	Decrease in door humidity with AC

TABLE 2: Role of topical immunomodulators and oral antihistamines.

Topical immunomodulators	Role of antihistamines
Tacrolimus 0.03% and 0.1% ointment	• Oral antihistamines are better
Pimecrolimus 0.1% cream	• Antipruritic and sedative act ion helps
These are useful and serve as steroid-sparing agents	• Decreases severe pruritis, especially in night
• Inhibits activation of key cells involved.	• Antihistamines break itch scratch-itch cycle
• Decreases the pruritis, and inflammation	• Safe and effective
• Proved safe/effective in children	• Hydroxyzine, diphenhydramine, phenothiazine, levocetrizine, Loratidine, fexofenadine
• Sustained efficacy	
• No adverse effects in long term	
• Serves as steroid sparing agent	
• 0.1% approved for > 16 years	

- Apply thick emollients/oil after bath on wet skin, emollient helps by retaining water longer in skin. Petroleum jelly is very good.

Topical Steroids

Topical steroids are the mainstay of therapy which act as anti-inflammatory therapy. The potency of steroids depends on severity of disease, age of the patient and the site affected. Mid potency steroids used topically in chronic AD involving trunk and extremities. High potency is preferably avoided; If used, used for short-term in chronic recalcitrant cases and then switched to lower potency. The preparations of topical steroid used are hydrocortisone, desowen, clobetasol, and mometason.

Toxic effects of steroids:
- *Local adverse effects*: Thinning of skin and striae
- *Systemic adverse effects* related to potency are applied, occlusiveness, and duration of use. The clinical conditions seen are peptic ulcer, hypertension, diabetes, osteoporosis, short stature and cataracts.

Role of oral steroids: Consider short-course oral steroids, and in severe cases.

Association of Atopic Dermatitis with Infection

There is increased tendency of bacterial, viral, and fungal infections with AD. The staphylococcal infection is the most common bacterial infection seen. The drugs such as erythromycin, azithromycin, clarithromycin, cloxacillin, and cephalexin are effective in staphylococcal infection given orally. Locally mupirocin helps. Patients with AD are prone to get secondarily infected with other viral infections such as warts, molluscum contagiosum, and herpes simplex infection. The later has chance of dissemination in AD patient, leading to *Eczema herpeticum*. It is a medical emergency. The topical steroids are temporarily stopped and systemic acyclovir are required.

SUGGESTED READING

1. Dhar S. Color Atlas and Synopsis Pediatric Dermatology, 3rd edition. New Delhi: Jaypee Brothers Medical (P) Ltd; 2015.
2. Williams HC, Burney PG, Pembroke AC, Hay RJ. The U.K. Working Party's Diagnostic Criteria for Atopic Dermatitis. III. Independent hospital validation. Br J Dermatol. 1994;131(3):406-16.

Pityriasis Versicolor

Vijay P Makhija

INTRODUCTION

- The old name tinea versicolor should be discarded as pityriasis versicolor (PV) is not caused by dermatophytes.
- It is caused by *Malassezia furfur* (earlier classified as pityriasis porum ovale) is a commensal yeast. The organisms being lipophilic, inhabit the sebaceous duct and follicular infundibulum and cause lesions in *"seborrheic regions"* of young adults whose sebaceous glands are most active. However, the face is usually spared.
- PV represents a shift in the relationship between the host and the resident yeast flora. The yeast overgrows in hot and humid conditions and releases carboxylic acid which causes hypopigmentation due to reduced tanning of skin. Occasionally lesions may be variously colored as reddish brown, dark brown or black or hypopigmented hence the name versicolor.
- *Morphology*: Perifollicular, hypopigmented, scaly macules on the upper trunk, neck, axilla, and upper arms. Other parts of trunk, groins, proximal extremities and occasionally face and inframammary folds in females are affected.

MANAGEMENT

- *Topical agents*:
  - Topical antifungal agents such as 1% clotrimazole, 2% miconazole, 1% tolnaftate and 2% ketoconazole are applied once daily to the lesions and the surrounding normal skin for 4 weeks.
  - Selenium sulfide (2.5% lotion in a detergent base) is used weekly for 4 weeks. It can cause irritation that can be prevented by diluting the lotion with water.
- *Systemic agents*:
  - *Oral fluconazole* in a single dose of 400 mg provides a convenient therapeutic option. Alternatively, fluconazole 200 mg OD × 2 days or 150 mg OD single dose can be administered. Dose of fluconazole in pediatric patients is 3. It is required in extensive lesions or when the recurrences are frequent.
  - *Oral ketoconazole* 200 mg OD × 10 days are better reserved for persistence or recurrence. Alternatively, ketoconazole 200 mg OD × 3 days, repeat such course for 3–4 months (total 12 tablets).
- Reassurance is important to the patient that the skin color will return to normal after a couple of months even though the fungal infection is controlled within 2 weeks. Thus, hypopigmentation regains color slowly. Color matching of lesions is done with the help of mustard oil/placentrax lotion/vinegar 1:1 dilution local application and exposure to sun for 5 minutes.

SUGGESTED READING

1. Dhar S. Color Atlas and Synopsis Pediatric Dermatology, 3rd edition. New Delhi: Jaypee Medical Brothers (P) Ltd; 2015.

Tinea Infections

Vijay P Makhija

GENERAL CONSIDERATION

- They are mainly caused by dermatophytes as *Trichophyton*, *Epidermophyton*, and *Microsporum* species. Dermatophytes are the fungi that live on keratin.
- Its typical lesion is an itchy, macular, annular/arcuate polycyclic plaque with a clear center and an active periphery with papulovesicles and scaling. It spreads centrifugally.
- Lesions are modified by the site and named accordingly as *Tinea capitis* (scalp), *Tinea faciei* (face), *Tinea corporis* (trunk), *Tinea cruris* (groin), *Tinea pedis* (feet), *Tinea manuum* (hands), and *Tinea unguium* (nails).

Tinea capitis: It is of two types:
1. *Noninflammatory tinea capitis* is caused by anthropophilic organisms (tinea verrucosum).
2. *Inflammatory tinea capitis (kerion)* is caused by zoophilic dermatophytes (*Microsporum canis*) that cause intense inflammation. It is presents as a boggy swelling with pustulation. Often the pus discharges from multiple orifices.

Tinea corporis: It presents with annular arcuate lesions with an active periphery and relative clearing in the center. It affects the glabrous skin of the trunk and limbs.

Tinea cruris: It affects the groin and is a very common condition occurring mainly in summers and rainy season. It affects men more than women. It usually affects thighs and scrotum bilaterally. It is seen as arcuate, sharply, demarcated plaques with peripheral scaling on inner aspects of thighs.

Tinea pedis: It occurs frequently in summers and its development is favored by the hyperhidrosis of soles, occlusive foot wear, sharing of wash places and presence of tinea unguium. It may present as interdigital scaling (athelete's foot) seen most frequently between the lateral two interdigital spaces of the feet or as a well-defined scaly plaque on the sole or as recurrent vesiculation of soles.

Tinea manuum: It is tinea infection of the hands that is usually associated with tinea pedis. Its lesions manifest as unilateral, well-defined plaques or as diffuse erythema of the palms with accumulation of fine scales in the creases.

Tinea unguium is defined as dermatophyte infection of the nail plate. Tinea unguium of toe nail is more common than finger nail infection. It may be associated with tinea pedis. Finger nail infection or tinea pedis may be associated with tinea cruris.

Tinea incognito: It is the dermatophyte infection of the skin that is modified by the use of steroid therapy. It is characterized by atypical lesions with minimal symptoms and signs as scales or papulovesicles.

MANAGEMENT

- *General measures* of management are keeping the area dry, avoiding the use of synthetic clothes. In recurrent infection, one can prophylactically use antifungal talc.
- *Drug therapy*: Antifungal drugs.
- *Local therapy*: Broad-spectrum imidazole derivatives such as miconazole, clotrimazole, and ketoconazole are the mainstay of therapy for localized forms of tinea. They are effective but response is usually slower. Allylamines as terbinafine 2.5% cream have a relatively rapid response so shorter course of therapy is required.
- *Systemic therapy* is recommended in extensive dermatophytic infections, tinea capitis and tinea unguium.
- These days we are frequently finding extensive tinea infections and that are recurring quite frequently. Many studies done have revealed that it is not due to increased resistance to usual antifungals as was thought by many treating personnel.
- *Fluconazole*: It is very much important to give systemic antifungal therapy along with local antifungals in all such patients for prolonged period of 3–6 months. Previously, *fluconazole* was not regarded to be a good drug for tinea infections. But *fluconazole* 3–6 mg/kg is found quite effective in these patients with extensive or recurrent tinea infections. *Itraconazole* can be used in selected cases. It is quite effective drug but is relatively more expensive. Important aspect is that continuing therapy

- for longer period is crucial to get the best results in such patients.
- Griseofulvin was the mainstay of systemic therapy for dermatophytic infections now being replaced by *terbinafine*. It is fungistatic against dermatophytes and is given in a dose of 10 mg/kg daily. Duration of therapy is 4 weeks for tinea corporis, cruris, and faciei, 6 weeks for tinea capitis, manuum, 8 weeks for tinea pedis, 6 months to 1 year for fingernails and 1–2 years for toenails.
- Terbinafine is a newer fungicidal drug. So, its response is rapid. It is recommended for 2 weeks in tinea corporis and 6 weeks in finger nails and 12 weeks in toenail infections. Relapses are also less frequent with it.

SUGGESTED READING

1. Dhar S. Color Atlas and Synopsis Pediatric Dermatology, 3rd edition. New Delhi: Jaypee Brothers Medical Publishers; 2015.

167 CHAPTER

Scabies

Vijay P Makhija

CLINICAL FEATURES

- Scabies is a Latin word, which means "*to scratch*." It is caused by a mite, "*Sarcoptes scabiei.*"
- Scabies is considered in a patient who complains of itching that is *worse at night.*
- Family history of similar itching is quite helpful in diagnosis.
- It is characterized by pruriginous lesions over *interdigital clefts, wrists, elbows, trunk, areola breasts, umbilicus, genitalia, buttocks,* and *ankles.*
- In infants, *palms, soles, face,* and *scalp* are also affected.
- These areas are usually spared in older children and adults.
- Its primary lesions are *burrows and a rash of papules* over specific sites.
- Its secondary lesions are secondary infection, eczema and excoriations.
- Presence of *burrows* is pathognomonic of scabies.
- Itching occurs due to *hypersensitivity to feces of female itch mite* that causes burrows in the skin of the patient.
- Itching is worse at night in scabies.
- *Advantage of itching*: Itching is definitely advantageous to a great extent; it helps to open the burrow of the mite and thus helps to decrease the mite population in patient.
- *Transmission and spread of scabies*:
  - Transient contact does not spread scabies, so doctors and nurses need not be too be afraid.
  - Prolonged physical contact is main way of its spread.
  - Prolonged holding of hands is significant for spread.
  - Though sometimes *sexual contact* is also responsible.

Norwegian Scabies

It is named so, because it was first found in Norwegian lepers. In immunosuppressed patients such as HIV patients, old persons, patients of malignancies or those receiving immunosuppressive therapy or leprosy patients (pruritus sensation lost) or mental retardation or Down syndrome patients (unable to take care of themselves) suffer from its rare severe variant called as *Norwegian or keratotic scabies*.

It is characterized by intensely keratotic and erythematous plaques over trunk, extremities, scalp, and face. These patients are highly infectious.

Infectivity and Management of Norwegian Scabies

- It is highly infectious.
- Patients should be isolated.
- Nurses caring such patients should wear gown and gloves.
- All nursing staff, medical staff, and persons living with them should be treated with topical scabicide.
- It responds to a topical keratolytic as 3% salicyalic acid in addition to repeated applications of scabicidal drugs. Removal of thick scales/repeated permethrin application and ivermectin orally may be repeated after 1 week.

Scabies Incognito

When steroids are applied in a patient with scabies then it becomes fulminant and its classical picture changes. It is difficult to identify this situation and is therefore called *Scabies Incognito*.

COMPLICATIONS

Secondary bacterial infections may lead to *pustules, impetigo,* and *eczematization*. Some patients may develop *poststreptococcal glomerulonephritis* because of secondary infection of scabies lesions with nephritogenic strain of streptococci. Sometimes nodules are formed in scabies called nodular scabies, which are extremely resistant to treatment and may require several months to resolve even after adequate antiscabicidal treatment.

LABORATORY INVESTIGATIONS AND CONFIRMATION OF DIAGNOSIS

- Diagnosis of scabies is mainly clinical.
- It is usually done by demonstration of mite.
- *Microscopic examination*: Slice off the unscratched papule or burrow with No. 15 blade and examine it

microscopically under the oil immersion lens; identification of the female mite, her eggs, and feces are confirmatory clues for the diagnosis of scabies.

MANAGEMENT

General Measures

- Patient and all family members should be treated simultaneously.
- Treatment should be explained in detail.
- All clothes should be washed in hot water, dried, and ironed before use. Undergarments and night clothes should be specially laundered in boiling water and used after drying in sun and ironing. Same treatment should be given to other garments, bedsheets, pillow covers, towels, napkins, and mattresses.

Specific Measures

- *Permethrin* is a safe alternative in children. It is the drug of choice in children. It is relatively nontoxic and can be applied over face or scalp. It is to be applied once only as it is not only miticidal but also ovicidal in action. It has to be reapplied after a period of 7 days.
- *Topical 1% gamma benzene hexachloride lotion (lindane)* is applied from neck to toe for 2 days (no bath on second day of treatment) and repeat it after 7–14 days. It is likely to be concentrated in the central nervous system, especially in infants and thus can cause neurotoxicity restricting its use in infants. Whole family and close contacts are to be treated. It can be applied in adolescent and adult.
- *Crotamiton (Crotorax)* is another safe alternative in children and can be applied over face and scalp. It is scabicidal and has antipruritic effect. It can be applied daily for 7 days.
- Currently orally available *ivermectin* is a breakthrough in the treatment of scabies. Tablets ivermectol, 3 and 6 mg, are available in market. It is recommended in a dose of 200 μg/kg two doses at 1-week interval has been recommended. It is given above the age of 2 years.
- *Control of infection*: Before starting scabicidal treatment, the infection must be controlled either by local or by systemic antibiotics.
- *Control of itching*: Antihistamines such as hydroxyzine, phenothiazine, chlorpheniramine, cetirizine, or loratadine are administered to control the itching. But itching may not resolve immediately. It improves gradually over 2–3 weeks as it occurs because of hypersensitivity to feces of itch mite.
  Superficial epidermis containing allergenic mite feces is shed over this period.

LESSON LEARNED

Case 1

A 9-month-old infant presented with wheals, papules, vesicles, pustules on trunk, back, axillae, groins, buttocks, and extremities.

Clues

- Scratch marks visible
- Itching more severe in night
- History of similar problem in other siblings.

Scabies

- *Presence of burrows is a pathognomonic sign.*
- *Infants may show lesions over face/head/palms and soles that are spared in older children.*

Case 2

A 16-year-girl comes with extremely itchy rash over abdomen, genitals, hands, and legs.

Clues

- Went home for holidays where younger brother had similar rash
- Has trouble sleeping as itching most severe in night
- Papules, vesicles, itch marks, plaques distributed over wrists/axilla/breast/navel and inner thigh
- Dark wavy lines that end in a pearly bleb in between her fingers.

Scabies with Burrow

Drop of mineral oil on a bleb unroof it and examine the scrapings under the microscope.

Case 3

A 1-year-old infant presented with severe itchy rash on face/hands/feet and trunk for 5–7 days.

Clues

- History of similar problem in parents since 1 month
- Parents suffering from HIV infection
- Infant also found HIV positive.

Severe Scabies

- *Hands, feet, face, and head are affected in infants.*
- *Scabies is very severe in immunocompromised patients.*
- *If steroids is applied in scabies, the lesions are temporarily suppressed and may persists as atypical appearance called Scabies incognito.*

SUGGESTED READING

1. Dhar S. Color Atlas and Synopsis Pediatric Dermatology; 3rd edition. New Delhi: Jaypee Brothers Medical Publishers; 2015.

Impetigo

Vijay P Makhija

INTRODUCTION

Impetigo is a superficial pyogenic infection of the skin. This is the most common skin infection of children in world. It is caused by *Staphylococcus aureus* and group A beta hemolytic *Streptococcus*.

Types:
- *Bullous impetigo*: It is seen in infants and young children, caused by *Staphylococcus*. It is a sort of localized staphylococcal scalded skin syndrome (SSSS). There is presence of flaccid transparent bullae on skin of face, buttocks, trunk, perineum, and extremities.
- Nonbullous impetigo accounts for 70% cases seen on face, extremities.

The manifestation starts with the preceding lesions such as insect bite, lacerations, abrasions, varicella, scabies, pediculosis, and burns.

A tiny vesicle, pustule initially rapidly turns into honey-colored crusted plaque generally <2 cm. Usually no pain or erythema is associated with it. Infection spreads to other parts of body by fingers, clothing, and towels. Regional adenopathy is common (>90%) followed by associated leukocytosis (50%).

MANAGEMENT

- *Local therapy*: Ointment mupirocin 2% tid × 10–14 days or ointment retapamulin 1% tid × 10–14 days.
- *Systemic therapy*: Oral cephalexin 25–50 mg/kg/day tid/qid × 7–10 days. There is no evidence that 10-day course is superior than 7-day course.

If MRSA (methicillin-resistant *Staphylococcus aureus*) is suspected then clindamycin/doxycycline or sulfamethoxazole/trimethoprim indicated.

COMPLICATIONS

- Osteomyelitis/septic arthritis, pneumonia, septicemia, cellulitis/scarlet fever (occasionally after streptococcal infection).
- Acute rheumatic fever does not occur after impetigo, infection with nephritogenic strains M groups 2, 49, 53, 55, 56, 57, and 60 of group A beta-hemolytic *Streptococcus pyogenes* (GABHS), and acute poststreptococcal glomerulonephritis (PSGN). It most commonly affects 3–7 years-aged children. Latent period of impetigo is 18–21 days in acute PSGN and in pharyngeal infection is 10 days in acute PSGN.

SUGGESTED READING

1. Dhar S. Color Atlas and Synopsis Pediatric Dermatology; 3rd edition. New Delhi: Jaypee Brothers Medical Publishers; 2015.

Acne Vulgaris

Vijay P Makhija

INTRODUCTION

Acne is a chronic infection and inflammation of pilosebaceous apparatus. It usually manifests as comedones, papules, nodules, and pustules. Its pathogenesis is contributed by many factors due to increased end-organ sensitivity to androgens; there is increased sebum secretion, follicular duct hypercornification, and colonization with *Propionibacterium acnes*.

CLINICAL FEATURES

It is usually seen around 12–14 years of age. The typical lesions are polymorphic eruptions consisting of papules, pustules, nodules, cysts, and comedones. The lesions heal with pitted or hypertrophic scars.

Comedones are small flesh-colored acne papule. The comedones are open and closed.

- *Open comedones (blackheads)*: The obstruction at the opening of the sebaceous follicle mouth is characterized by a lesion with a wide patulous opening filled with a plug of stratum corneum cells which is called an open comedone or blackhead. It is the predominant lesion in adolescent acne. It does not progress to inflammatory acne.
- *Closed comedones (whiteheads)* are caused by obstruction just beneath the follicular opening in the neck of the sebaceous follicle leading to cystic swelling of the follicular duct beneath the epidermis leading to an enlarging sphere just beneath the skin surface. Closed comedones usually progress to inflammatory acne.

Site of acne: Face, upper trunk (chest and back), and deltoid region.

MANAGEMENT

- Acne cannot be cured but early treatment gives best result by reducing the chances of scarring.
- Its management depends on the type of the lesion and the severity.

Mild acne: Comedolytic agents as *retinoic acid (0.025–0.1%)*, *adapalene (0.1%), and benzoyl peroxide* are used. There is no role of systemic drugs.

Moderate acne, i.e., comedogenic acne, a combination of retinoic acid and benzoyl peroxide to be used. Oral antibiotics or topical antibiotics are used, if inflammation is suspected, in addition to topical retinoic acid or benzoyl peroxide.

Severe acne: The drugs used are retinoic acid, glycolic acid, azelaic acid, or mometasone. One can be used once daily sequentially.

It can also be managed by using *retinoic acid or benzoyl peroxide* and *oral antibiotics* or *antiandrogens* (in females) or *oral retinoids*.

Various combinations are successful in managing severe acne. Retinoic acid and benzoyl peroxide gel are most efficacious for the management of acne. Oral retinoids are also very effective. The use of benzoyl peroxide gel in the morning and tretinoin at night is equally effective.

Retinoic acid is a potent keratolytic agent. It is used for the management of acne, scars, pits, postinflammatory marks, and wrinkles. It often causes drying of skin as a side effect. It is applied once daily at night after drying soap-washed skin. It should not be applied in day as sun exposure may cause problem. It can be used for long term without problem. It also works as an antiaging agent.

Benzoyl peroxide 2.5% gel is used once in morning. It is especially used, if lesions are infected. Other drugs that help topically are adapalene, azelaic acid, glycolic acid, and topical antibiotics (erythromycin and clindamycin). Adapalene 1% gel may be more effective than 0.025% tretinoin gel and may have fewer side effects. It is a derivative of naphthoic acid. It is comedolytic and anti-inflammatory. Azelaic acid has antimicrobial and keratolytic properties. A 20% cream is as effective as 0.05% tretinoin cream.

Oral retinoids are quite effective in controlling severe acne. But oral retinoids have severe side effects, so especially used with great caution. It can cause teratogenic effects in fetus. So, it is used in females. They must avoid pregnancy during its use and it should be strictly avoided in pregnant women.

Topical Antibiotics

Topical antibiotics include clindamycin and erythromycin; they may be applied once or twice daily. Although not as effective as orally administered antibiotics or benzoyl peroxide, they serve as a useful therapeutic adjunct by inhibiting growth of *P. acnes*. The effectiveness of atopical antibioticis is enhanced by concurrent use of benzoyl peroxide or tretinoin.

Systemic Antibiotics

Systemic antibiotics: Tetracycline or doxycycline are two commonly used systemic antibiotics in acne. But they should never be used in children below 8 years of age due to toxicity.

Systemic antibiotics especially tetracycline and its derivatives are used if:
- Patients cannot tolerate topical medications.
- Those who have not responded to topical medications.
- Those with moderate-to-severe inflammatory papulopustular or nodulocytic acne and those who have an increased propensity for scarring.

Tetracyclines and erythromycin are especially concentrated in the sebum. So, they are very effective in the management of inflammatory acne. Their usual recommended dose is 0.5–1 g OD or BID on empty stomach with nil orally for next 2 hours. They are advised to be continued for 2–3 months till acne lesions are suppressed.

One commonly used regimen is tetracycline 1 g/24 h divided twice daily for at least 6 weeks followed by a gradual decrease to the minimal effective dose. These drugs are best administered in combination with topical benzoyl peroxide or tretinoin but not topical antibiotics.

Avoid using soaps rather use ingenious packs and then wash off after 5–10 minutes. One must keep on changing the type of packs. Similarly, one must avoid use of oils, creams on face and scalp, or hair sprays.

SUGGESTED READING

1. Dhar S. Color Atlas and Synopsis Pediatric Dermatology; 3rd edition. New Delhi: Jaypee Brothers Medical Publishers; 2015.

Stevens–Johnson Syndrome

Anoop Verma

INTRODUCTION

Stevens–Johnson syndrome (SJS) and toxic epidermal necrolysis (TEN) are potentially life-threatening disorders characterized by widespread epidermal necrosis of skin and mucosa. It is sort of late-onset allergic reaction due to adverse drug reaction of Type IV hypersensitivity. The clinical manifestation of both conditions are same, except the extent of epidermal involvement.

Classification is based on body surface area (BSA) affected:
- If <10% of BSA is involved, it favors SJS.
- If the involvement of BSA is between 10 and 30%, it favors SJS-TEN overlap.
- If the involvement of BSA is >30%, it favors TEN.

Incidences: SJS and TEN are reported to have incidence of 1-7 and 1-2 cases per million, respectively, in general population.

CLINICAL FEATURES

- Prodromal period starts with nonspecific symptoms lasting 1-7 days, may precede the onset of the SJS/TEN disease. It consists of vague discomfort, dysphagia, and itching of eyes, followed by high pyrexia, with respiratory symptoms. There is involvement of mucous member of mouth and genital followed by rashes with blisters over the skin.
- There is fast progression, often within 12 hours, of bullous lesions which develops on skin and mucous membranes.
- Nikolsky's sign may be positive. (An epidermis can be detached by the tangential pressure applied on erythematous, nonblistering skin). Involvement of multiple organ systems is seen. TEN has severe rate of complication than in SJS. The corneal complications are seen in both the conditions equally.

CURRENT CONCEPTS OF MECHANISM OF TISSUE INJURY IN SJS/TEN

- The cause of keratinocyte apoptosis is due to granulysin, which is present in the cytotoxic granules.
- The cause of keratinocyte apoptosis is by the production of intracellular caspases, in the activated cytotoxic T cell inducing cytotoxic signal including Fas–Fas Ligand.
- The cause of keratinocyte apoptosis is by cytotoxic signals in the form of perforin and granzyme B-activating the capsizes.
- Tumor necrosis factor (TNF)-alpha and interferon (IFN)-alpha induce nitric oxide, which may induce caspases.

The injury of keratinocyte and its apoptosis leads to detachment of skin and mucous membranes. There is huge collection of CD8 lymphocyte in the blistering fluid, indicating drug-specific cytotoxicity.

Antiepileptics, antibiotics, and non-steroidal anti-inflammatory drugs (NSAIDs) are the more common triggers **(Table 1)**.

The most common drug in the antiepileptic drug group are carbamazepine, followed by phenytoin, phenobarbital and levetiracetam. The antibiotic includes erythromycin, cefotaxime, trimethoprim–sulfamethoxazole, cloxacillin, and amoxicillin.

Anticold medications and NSAIDs and acetaminophen also contribute as triggering factors.

Infections causing SJS/TEN: Mycoplasma pneumoniae and viruses (influenza, Epstein-Barr, cytomegalovirus,

TABLE 1: Drugs causing Stevens–Johnson syndrome/toxic epidermal necrolysis.

Antiepileptics	Carbamazepine, phenytoin, phenobarbitone, lamotrigine
Antibiotics	Penicillins, cephalosporins, cefotaxime, amoxicillin, quinolones, minocycline, erythromycin, cotrimoxazole, sulfasalazine
Nonsteroidal anti-inflammatory drugs	
Paracetamol/acetaminophen	
Nevirapine	
Allopurinol (>100 mg/day)	
Contrast media	

TABLE 2: Association of HLA type and SJS/TEN.

HLA type	Population	Offending drug	Type of reaction
HLA-B*1508	Han Chinese, Thai, Malaysia, and South Indian	Carbamazepine	SJS/TEN
HLA-B*5801	Han Chinese	Allopurinol	SJS/TEN
HLA-B*5701	European	Abacavir	SJS/TEN
HLA-A*3101	European	Carbamazepine	SJS/TEN
HLA-B*13:01 and HLA-C*14:03, HLA-A*02:06 and HLA-B*44:03	Japanese	Acetaminophen	SJS/TEN/SOC
HLA-B*5701	European	Abacavir	SJS/TEN
HLA-A*3101	European	Carbamazepine	SJS/TEN
HLA-B*13:01 and HLA-C*14:03, HLA-A*02:06 and HLA-B*44:03	Japanese	Acetaminophen	SJS/TEN/SOC

(HLA: human leukocyte antigen; SJS: Stevens–Johnson syndrome; SOC: severe ocular complication; TEN: toxic epidermal necrolysis)

coxsackievirus, herpes, parvovirus), bacteria (*Streptococcus β-haemolyticum*, group A), *Mycobacterium*, and rickettsia are also associated with pediatric SJS/TEN.

There is close association of various types of HLA prevalent in different populations and its adverse response to various drugs are given in **Table 2**.

COMPLICATIONS

Mucocutaneous complications are seen in 90% of cases. Ocular complications are seen in TEN (50–67%) leading to bilateral blinding caused by corneal scarring and vascularization in severe cases. Secondary skin infection, pneumonia, hepatitis, and septicemia are also observed.

DIFFERENTIAL DIAGNOSIS

Drug-induced linear IgA and drug reaction with eosinophilia and systemic symptoms (DRESS), maculopapular exanthema, the staphylococcal scalded skin syndrome (SSSS), and the erythema multiforme.

DIAGNOSIS

- Diagnosis mainly based on clinical signs and symptoms. There is no definitive laboratory test to confirm the role of triggers.
- *Complete blood count (CBC)*: Anemia, lymphopenia, neutropenia, eosinophilia, and atypical lymphocytosis.
- Liver function test (LFT) and renal function test (RFT).
- Chest X-ray (CXR) and cardiac assessment.
- *Skin biopsy*: Full epidermal thickness necrosis is not always required for diagnosis.
- Algorithm of drug causality for epider-mal necrosis (ALDEN) score to identify suspected culprit medications: Algorithm considers five items, i.e., to say index day, half-life, prechallenge/rechallenge, dechallenge, and notoriety.
- Serological tests and polymerase chain reaction (PCR) for diagnosing various viral infections and *M. pneumoniae* should be carried out.
- *Cytokine determination*: For diagnosing SJS before performing a skin biopsy, this is for diagnostic, prognostic, and possible therapeutic target. Granulysin expression in CD4+ cells by flow cytometry, granzyme B production by ELISpot assay, and IFN-γ levels in cell supernatant by cyto-kine bead array have been investigated.
- The lymphocyte transformation test (LTT) is for identifying the offending drug. It is a safe and reproducible test but its reliability is a controversial issue.

MANAGEMENT

Management is conservative and requires multidisciplinary skills.
- Discontinue the offending drug and start supportive care, fluid and electrolytes balance, and respiratory and nutritional support.
- Pain management analgesics and topical aesthetics.
- Admission to a specialized burn unit when skin involvement is >25–30%.
- Systemic antibiotics to control the secondary bacterial infection.
- Use of immunosuppressive treatment with TNF-α inhibitors—infliximab and etanercept—have shown to be effective at halting disease progression; TNF-α antagonist—etanercept—in a randomized trial showed some advantages toward corticosteroids. Cyclosporine (3 mg/kg/day for 7 days followed by 1.5 mg/kg/day).
- *Involvement of other discipline*:
  - Ophthalmologist is involved for continuous monitoring of ocular sequelae in high-risk patient.

- Dermatologist examines biopsy from the border of bullies lesion to rule out other causes of bullous dermatosis and is involved in skincare and wound management.
- Urogynecologist evaluates acute lesion and long-term sequelae.

ALGORITHM

- Take detailed history of possible intake of all medications in last 8 weeks. Make use of ALDEN.
- Immediately stop and withdraw any suspected culprit drug.
- *Role of laboratory diagnosis*: Baseline workup, testing for infective etiology (Conduct various supportive tests to rule out infective etiology, if required in any given case), CXR if needed.
- Monitoring of fluid balance and electrolytes, and respiratory and nutritional support.
- Intravenous (IV) antibiotics, analgesics if needed.
- Wound care includes debridement of broken blisters, removal of necrotic skin, topical antiseptics or antibiotics, bandages, preferably by surgical colleague.
- Clinical photographs to document the disease process with proper consent.
- Since the condition requires multi-disciplinary approach, take opinion of an ophthalmologist, dermatologist, urologist, and gynecologist, as per the need for any individual patient.

SUGGESTED READING

1. Lucia L, Silvia C, Bottau P, Bernardini R, Cardinale F, Saretta F, et al. Clinical features, outcomes and treatment in children with drug induced Stevens-Johnson syndrome and toxic epidermal necrolysis. Acta Biomed. 2019;90(3-S):52-60.
2. Ueta M, Nakamura R, Saito Y, Tokunaga K, Sotozono C, Yabe T, et al. Association of HLA class I and II gene polymorphisms with acetaminophen-related Stevens–Johnson syndrome with severe ocular complications in Japanese individuals. Hum Genome Var. 2019;6:50.

Hand, Foot, and Mouth Disease

Anoop Verma

GENERAL CONSIDERATION

- Hand, foot, and mouth disease (HFMD) is a viral infection, which mainly affects infants and children below 10 years of age.
- It is a contagious disease and spreads via orofecal or respiratory routes. It occurs typically in small epidemics in months of summer and autumn.
- It is caused by enterovirus coxsackievirus (CV) *A16, A5, A10 and enterovirus-71 (EV-71)*. The infection caused by CV-A16 is less severe as compared to that caused by EV-71.
- The World Health Organization (WHO) has published concerns on growing threat of HFMD.
- The disease that kept a low profile for long became a cause for concern in recent times.
- The usual incubation period is 3–7 days.

PATHOGENESIS

- The transmission of virus is horizontal.
- After being implanted in the buccal and ileal mucosa, the virus spreads to the regional lymph nodes within 24 hours. There is appearance of erythematous macules over oral cavity, evolving into 2–3-mm vesicles, on an erythematous base.
- These lesions are seen over palate, buccal mucosa, gingiva, lip and tongue. These vesicles are clinically less apparent, as they transform into ulcers rapidly.
- There is no virus flora in the intestine normally, and only one type of enterovirus multiplies within the intestine of an individual at any given point of time. By virtue of extensive polio vaccine campaign, the polio viruses are eliminated from the gut, thereby increasing the chances of CV and echoviral infections to multiple in intestine. The explanation of the emergence of HFMD in India may be related to the mass polio vaccination.

GENETIC SUSCEPTIBILITY

- There is strong genetic susceptibility of various population in many Asian countries depending on their genetic makeup.
- The presence of human leukocyte antigen *(HLA)-A33* haplotype, glucose-6-phosphate dehydrogenase (G6PD) deficiency, cytotoxic T-lymphocyte antigen haplotype (CTLA-4) and some inflammatory cytokines are contributing factors. Prevalence of *HLA-A33* haplotype in Asian populations is 17–35%, and is significantly higher, as compared to the Caucasian populations. HLA-A33 and HLA-DR17 are linked to the severity of the disease caused by human enterovirus 71 (HEV71) infection.

CLINICAL FEATURES

- Early symptoms start with fever and sore throat and appearance of painful sores, after 1–2 days, in the mouth or throat.
- Rashes are seen on hands, feet, oral cavity, buttocks, knees and elbow. Oral lesions appear as vesicles, turning rapidly into multiple small superficial ulcers with erythematous base.
- Oral ulcers are usually seen on the tongue, palate, buccal mucosa, gums, and lips, producing discomfort.

COMPLICATIONS

- HFMD resolves normally of its own, but is said to be associated with severe complications. There is sharp rise in incidence, severity of complications and even fatal outcomes that were almost unseen before.
- Neurological complications are aseptic meningitis, encephalitis, acute flaccid paralysis (AFP), frequently noted in HFMD associated with HEV71 but is rare in CVA16-associated cases. This is because of existence of a specific HEV71 receptor on neuronal cells which causes neurological damage.
- The mortality in HFMD occurs in children <3 years of age, due to cardiac and neurological complications such as brainstem encephalitis.

DIAGNOSIS

The clinical diagnosis and relative benign nature of the disease contributes much to the diagnosis.

Laboratory Diagnosis

- *Culture*: Sample from stool, throat swab, and vesicle fluid are taken for viral culture.
- Neutralizing antibody detection is done to identify the involved serotypes, especially to detect neutralizing antibody of HEV71.
- *Enzyme-linked immunosorbent assay (ELISA)*: This test is useful from first week till many weeks after infection, with high degree of sensitivity. IgM ELISA is used for rapid diagnosis and for large mass testing.
- Reverse transcriptase-polymerase chain reaction (RT-PCR) is now considered as the primary modality for EV "serotype" identification. It is costly and laboratory confirmation is not possible always.

TREATMENT

- *Strict hygiene protocols*: Cleanliness of the hands and utensils and drinking water and avoiding direct contact with affected people. Avoiding children from attending schools or other outdoor activities is a very simple but effective strategy.
- Local therapy is given in the form of local anesthetics and viscous lidocaine for painful oral ulcers. Antipyretics and analgesics for fever and joint pain. Low-level laser therapy has also shortened the duration of painful oral ulcers.

SUGGESTED READING

1. Sarma N. Hand, foot, and mouth disease: current scenario and Indian perspective. Indian J Dermatol Venereol Leprol. 2013;79(2):165-75.

SECTION 16

Miscellaneous

172. Common Ophthalmic Problems in Children
173. Common Orthopedic Problems in Children
174. Common Pediatric and Neonatal Surgical Problems
175. How to Read X-ray Chest? (Step-by-Step Guide)

Common Ophthalmic Problems in Children

Rajiv Kumar Gupta, Vishal

CONGENITAL DACRYOCYSTITIS

- It is inflammation of lacrimal sac in newborn which may be bilateral.
- It occurs due to imperfect or noncanalization of nasolacrimal duct.

Signs and Symptoms

- Continuous watering from the eye, usually near inner canthus
- The discharge may become purulent.
- There may be regurgitation of discharge when pressure is applied over sac area.

Treatment

- Must be started as soon as the condition is diagnosed, otherwise it becomes chronic and may cause orbital cellulitis and meningitis.
- Repeated massaging is done by giving pressure with thumb downward and medially over lacrimal sac area.
- Instillation of topical antibiotic (Tobramycin).
- Probing of nasolacrimal duct under general anesthesia if there is no relief.

STYE

- Also known as hordeolum externum, is a very common ocular disorder in young children.
- It is an acute suppurative inflammation of gland of Zeis and Moll, which may occur in crops, alternating with other eye.

Etiology

- *Staphylococcus aureus* is the most common causative organism.
- Refractive error and diabetes mellitus are the precipitating factors.

Symptoms

- Very painful condition, more pronounced at the site of affected gland
- Swelling of eyelids.

Signs

- Lid margin is congested and swollen.
- A painful, tender, hard swelling is noticed at the lid margin.
- An abscess may form, which points near the base of eyelash.
- Pain is relieved when the abscess bursts.

Treatment

- Frequent hot fomentation
- Instilling topical antibiotic eye drops
- Systemic broad-spectrum antibiotic and anti-inflammatory drug
- Evacuation of pus by pulling the affected eyelash or incision and drainage of abscess.

Key Points

- Acute suppurative inflammation of gland of Zeis
- Very painful condition
- Refractive error and diabetes mellitus should be ruled out
- Lid margin is congested and swollen where a painful tender swelling can be seen
- Treated by hot fomentation and local/systemic.

BLEPHARITIS

It is a chronic inflammation of eyelid margin, which is frequently seen in those children who are debilitated and live in poor hygienic condition.

Types

- Anterior blepharitis
  - Squamous blepharitis
  - Ulcerative blepharitis
- Posterior blepharitis.

Anterior Blepharitis

Etiology

- It may be continuation of chronic conjunctivitis caused by *S. aureus*.

- Parasites such as *Demodex folliculorum*, crab louse, or head louse may also cause the disease.

Squamous Blepharitis
- Numerous white-colored small scales accumulate on the eye lashes, which readily fall out and get replaced without any distortion.
- On removing the scales, underlying skin is red and congested.
- It is a metabolic disorder like seborrhea and is frequently associated with dandruff of scalp.

Ulcerative Blepharitis
- Yellow crusts are formed on the eyelashes, which are matted together.
- On removing the crusts, the underlying surface is congested and ulcerated, which bleeds easily.
- The eyelashes fallout readily but are replaced by distorted eyelash.

Symptoms:
- Painful condition
- Eyelid margin is congested and swollen
- Lacrimation and photophobia.

Treatment:
- Clean the lid margin with 3% sodabicarbonate lotion.
- Meticulous removal of scales and crusts.
- Weak distorted cilia are plucked out.
- Topical antibiotic drop and ointment are applied over lid margin.
- Systemic administration of broad-spectrum antibiotic and anti-inflammatory drug.
- Accompanying dandruff of scalp must be treated with antidandruff lotion.
- Personal hygiene and general health should be improved.

SUBCONJUNCTIVAL HEMORRHAGE
- It is extravasation of blood in the conjunctiva due to rupture of conjunctival blood vessels.
- The affected conjunctiva becomes bright red, sharply demarcated from the normal conjunctiva.
- It is a very unsightly condition which forces the parents to seek immediate treatment.

Etiology
- Spontaneous hemorrhage without any cause
- Minor injury to eye, e.g., finger nail injury
- Severe bacterial or viral conjunctivitis
- Forced mechanical straining such as whooping cough and vomiting
- Bleeding disorders such as hemophilia and leukemia.

Symptoms
- One of the most common cause of red eye
- Fresh blood is seen beneath the conjunctiva
- It is a self-limiting disease which undergoes spontaneous resolution in 2–3 weeks.

Treatment
- No treatment
- Assurance to parents
- Cold compress
- Treatment of cause.

Key Points
- It is extravasation of blood in the conjunctiva.
- Common cause of red eye
- A very unsightly condition forcing parents to seek immediate redress
- Bleeding disorder should be ruled out.

CONJUNCTIVITIS
It is an acute inflammation of conjunctiva.

Types
- *Infective*:
  - Bacterial conjunctivitis
  - Viral conjunctivitis
- *Noninfective*: Allergic conjunctivitis

Bacterial Conjunctivitis
- In neonates, it is also known as ophthalmia neonatorum.
- In infants and children, it occurs as acute mucopurulent/purulent conjunctivitis.

Ophthalmia Neonatorum
- It is conjunctivitis in newborn within 1 month of life, characterized by mucoid, mucopurulent, or purulent discharge from one or both eyes.
- It is a sight-threatening disease, which if not treated properly may cause visual loss in 50% of cases. This is rare now a days due to improved healthcare facility.

Etiology
- Most common causative organism is *Neisseria gonorrhoeae*.
- The infection is usually contracted at the time of vaginal delivery due to maternal infection or delivery conducted in unhygienic septic condition.

Clinical Features
- The eyelids are profusely swollen, so much that there is difficulty in separating the eyelids.
- There is usually copious purulent discharge.
- The conjunctiva is grossly congested and chemosed.
- Corneal ulcer with its accompanying complications may occur.

Diagnosis

- Any discharge from eye soon after birth or within first month of life, should be properly examined to rule out the disease
- Depending upon the nature and timing of discharge, after birth, the etiological agent can be provisionally diagnosed
- Within 48 hours—*N. gonorrhoeae*
- 48–72 hours—*Streptococcus pneumoniae*
- 5–7 days—herpes simplex virus
- After 7 days—*Chlamydia oculogenitalis.*

Treatment

- Meticulous cleaning of eyelid with normal saline
- Frequent instillation of antibiotic drops till infection subsides
- Intravenous administration of systemic broad-spectrum antibiotic
- Antiviral eye ointment (acyclovir 3%) in case of viral infection.

Complications

Neisseria gonorrhoeae penetrate normal epithelium so it causes serious complications which may result in visual loss if left untreated.

Infective Conjunctivitis

It is a self-limiting bilateral inflammation of conjunctiva. It is highly contagious which spreads by finger, flies or fomites and is the most common cause of red eye.

Causative organism: Bacterial or viral

Clinical Features

- Eyelids are swollen.
- In bacterial etiology, discharge is mucopurulent, leading to sticking of eyelids, especially in the morning while in viral infection discharge is serous.
- Grittiness and foreign body sensation.
- Lacrimation and photophobia.

Signs

- Conjunctival congestion which is fiery red
- Chemosis of conjunctiva
- Subconjunctival hemorrhage
- Follicles in inferior fornix (viral conjunctivitis).

Complication

If left untreated, it may infect cornea causing ulcer and its associated complications.

Treatment

Therapeutic:
- Bacterial conjunctivitis
    - Meticulous cleaning of eyelid with normal saline
    - Frequent instillation of topical antibiotic
    - If no response, systemic antibiotics are administered after culture and sensitivity test
    - Application of eye ointment at night before sleep, which prevents sticking of eyelids in morning
- Viral conjunctivitis
    - No antiviral drug is effective
    - Cold compress
    - Artificial tears four to six times daily
    - In severe, nonresponding cases or associated with keratitis, topical corticosteroid can be used.

Supportive
- Being a contagious disease, it can be prevented by:
    - Isolation of patient till there is no discharge
    - Avoid close contact with other person
    - Segregate articles used by patient such as pillows, towel, soap, handkerchief, bed sheet
    - Avoid contact from infected finger
    - Frequent wash of hands and eyes
    - Separate eye drops for individual patient.

Allergic Conjunctivitis

This is usually an IgE-mediated type1 hypersensitivity reaction of conjunctiva in response to exogenous or endogenous allergens.

Types

- Seasonal allergic conjunctivitis
- Perennial allergic conjunctivitis
- Vernal keratoconjunctivitis
- Atopic keratoconjunctivitis
- Giant papillary conjunctivitis
- Phlyctenular keratoconjunctivitis.

Seasonal Allergic Conjunctivitis

Usually occurs due to exogenous allergens such as pollen, dust, drugs, and pets.

Symptoms:
- Intense itching is the most prominent feature.
- Photophobia and lacrimation
- Conjunctival congestion and chemosis
- Lids are swollen.

Vernal Conjunctivitis (Spring Catarrh)

- It is bilateral recurrent inflammation of conjunctiva which occurs with onset of summer season.
- It is a self-limiting disease which may persist for several years.
- More prevalent in boys during prepubertal age.
- Cornea is involved in majority of patients (vernal keratoconjunctivitis).

- Caused by exogenous allergens and exacerbated by hot weather.

Diagnostic criteria:
- Intense itching
- Thick white ropy discharge
- Cobblestone like appearance in upper palpebral conjunctiva
- Horner-Tranta's spots around limbus.

Phlyctenular Conjunctivitis

- It is an allergic manifestation of conjunctiva, characterized by formation of phlyctens.
- It is usually seen in children between 4 and 15 years, who lives in crowded, unhygienic condition.
- When cornea is involved called as phlyctenular keratoconjunctivitis.
- Endogenous bacterial protein from septic foci such as tonsillitis, adenoiditis caused by *Staphylococcus* or tubercular protein of *Mycobacterium tuberculosis* are the usual causative allergens.
- Sometimes allergens of intestinal parasites may be responsible.

Diagnostic criteria:
- Phlyctens at or near limbus in the bulbar conjunctiva usually in the interpalpebral space
- The phlyctens are grayish or yellow, small, round nodule, which are raised above the surface. They may be solitary or multiple
- Conjunctival congestion is only around the phlycten
- Ciliary congestion and fascicular corneal ulceration when cornea is involved
- May be associated with tonsillitis, adenoids, and enlarged neck glands.

Treatment of Allergic Conjunctivitis

Therapeutic:
- Topical antiallergic eye drops (olopatadine 0.1%, bepotastine 1.5%, alcaftadine 0.25%)
- Topical instillation of corticosteroid drop and ointments
- Topical antibiotics and cycloplegics (1% atropine) when cornea is involved
- Treatment of tuberculosis, tonsillitis, adenoids, and intestinal parasites.

Supportive:
- Cold compresses
- Avoidance of known allergens
- Improve personal hygiene and general health of patients
- Use of dark protective glasses
- Discourage children from frequent rubbing of the eye.

CONGENITAL/DEVELOPMENTAL CATARACT

- Any opacity in lens or its capsule is called cataract.
- Congenital cataract is present at birth, while developmental cataract develops after birth.
- It is usually a bilateral condition.

Etiology

Exact causes is still unknown, but supposed to be due to:
- Maternal malnutrition
- Maternal infection by virus, e.g., Rubella
- Deficient oxygenation due to placental hemorrhage
- Metabolic disorder such as galactosemia.

Diagnosis: Usually noticed by parent as white pupillary reflex.

Symptoms: Depends upon site and extent of cataract.
If opacity is central and large it can cause visual impairment leading to nystagmus, squint, or amblyopia

Signs: White pupillary reflex (Leukocoria)
May be associated with other congenital anomaly as deafness, mental retardation, etc.

Treatment: Depends upon location and extent of opacity
- No treatment if there is no visual defect or lenticular opacity is stationary.
- If vision is compromised, cataract should be removed surgically with intraocular lens implantation. The surgery should be undertaken as early as possible.

Key Points

- Maternal malnutrition/viral infection during pregnancy is the most common cause.
- White pupillary reflex is usually noticed by parents.
- Visual disturbance depends upon location and extent of opacity.
- Surgical intervention is required when vision is compromised.

RETINOPATHY OF PREMATURITY

- Retinopathy of prematurity (ROP) is a bilateral sight-threatening disease which usually occur in preterm baby born before 32 weeks of gestational age, weighing less than 1,500 g and are given high concentration of oxygen for nursing during first few weeks of life.
- It is a fibrovascular disease caused by abnormal growth of blood vessel on retina, which being weak and fragile, bleeds easily.
- Absorption of blood vessel and blood results in retinal scar and detachment, producing visual impairment and loss of vision.

Associated Risk Factors

- Sepsis
- Respiratory distress syndrome

- Anemia
- Cardiac defect
- Blood transfusion.

Diagnosis
- By examining fundus of eye with indirect ophthalmoscope
- Screening
- All premature baby should be screened within first 4 weeks of birth
- Repeated at every 2–4 weeks till retinal vascularization is completed or one/both eye develops ROP.

Treatment
- Nearly 80% of ROP gets spontaneous resolution.
- When ROP is diagnosed, treatment must be started within 48 hours.
- Treatment options are:
  - Laser photocoagulation
  - Surgery for retinal detachment
  - Vitrectomy
  - Intravitreal injection of anti-VEGF (anti-vascular endothelial growth factor) drug such as avastin (bevacizumab).

Complications
- Nystagmus
- Strabismus
- Myopia
- Glaucoma
- Impairment or loss of vision.

Key Points
- ROP is a sight-threatening disease usually occurs in preterm baby <32 weeks or <1500 g requiring oxygen therapy
- Screening should be done within 4 weeks of life repeated every 2–4 weeks
- Fibrovascular disease characterized by proliferation of abnormal retinal blood vessel leading to retinal scars and detachment.

RETINOBLASTOMA
- It is highly malignant most common intraocular tumor of childhood, which manifests either at birth or within 2–3 years of life.
- It develops from neurosensory retina and can grow into vitreous cavity or in subretinal space leading to increased intraocular pressure.
- It may have extraocular extension into orbit and have distant metastasis in brain, bone, liver, and lymph nodes.
- Usually unilateral, but may be bilateral in 25–30% of cases.
- Majority of cases are sporadic, but some of them have family history.

Clinical Presentation
- Most of the cases present with white pupillary reflex (Leukocoria) followed by strabismus.
- Hypopyon/hyphema with strabismus may be another presentation.
- Buphthalmous, proptosis, orbital cellulitis, and severe pain in the eye are infrequent presentations.

Diagnosis
- *Clinical examination*: Indirect ophthalmoscopy
- Ultrasonography (B scan)
- X-ray, computed tomography (CT) scan and magnetic resonance imaging (MRI) of orbit.

Treatment
- Chemotherapy
- *Local therapy*: Radiotherapy, photocoagulation or cryotherapy
- *Surgery*: Enucleation is indicated when the life of child is in danger and there is no scope of visual preservation.

Prognosis
- Very bad if untreated
- Fair if enucleation done before extraocular extension and distant metastasis
- Poor if the optic nerve is involved and tumor cells are undifferentiated.

Key Points
- Most common intraocular tumor of childhood
- Highly malignant, which manifest at birth or within 2–3 years of life
- Majority of the cases presents with white pupillary reflex
- Though enucleation is the standard treatment, chemotherapy.

DRY EYE
- It is an ocular surface disorder, caused by disturbance of natural function and protective mechanism of the tear film, resulting in dry and lusterless conjunctiva and cornea.
- It can be due to deficient production or excessive evaporation of tear.

Computer Vision Syndrome
- It is common ocular disorder of school going children caused by prolonged use of electronic gadgets such as mobile phone, laptop, and computer.
- Dryness of eye occurs due to evaporation of tears.

Symptoms
- Discomfort and burning sensation
- Early fatigueness of eye

- Blurring of vision
- Mild conjunctival congestion and lacrimation.

Treatment
- Frequent instillation of tear substitute in eye
- Correction of refractive error
- To use protective antiglare glasses
- Rest the eye after working for 1–2 hours.

Key Points
- Ocular surface disorder, due to deficient production or excessive evaporation of tear.
- Common in school going children, due to prolonged use of electronic gadgets.
- Irritation, burning sensation, pain, and early tiredness of eye are the prominent symptoms.
- Treated by frequent instillation of tear substitute.

XEROSIS (VITAMIN A DEFICIENCY)
- It is dryness of conjunctiva and cornea due to vitamin A deficiency.
- This is now uncommon due to improvement in healthcare facilities and improvement in standard of living.
- Usually associated with protein–energy malnutrition and is caused by
  - Reduced intake
  - Defective absorption
  - Excessive utilization

Clinical Features
- *Night blindness*: Earliest symptom
- Xerosis of conjunctiva, with the formation of Bitot's spot in both eyes
- Xerosis of cornea, which become dry and lusterless
- Corneal ulceration and keratomalacia
- Scarring of corneal ulcer leading to corneal opacity, anterior staphyloma.

Treatment
Administration of vitamin A: day 0, 1, and 14.

Oral:
- *Children below 6 months*: 50,000 IU
- *Children between 6–12 months*: 1 lakhs IU
- *Children above 1 year*: 2 lakh IU

Parenteral:
- Through intramuscular injection of vitamin A dose: 1 lakh IU
- Treatment of corneal complications
- Supplementation through vitamin A-rich diet.

Key Points
- A systemic disorder due to deficiency of vitamin A
- Xerosis of conjunctiva and cornea, which become dry and lusterless.
- Night blindness and Bitot's sports are diagnostic.

ERRORS OF REFRACTION
- A common ocular disorder of school-going children
- It is an optical error, where parallel rays of light coming from infinity does not focus on retina, when accommodation is at rest.
- Prolonged use of electronic gadgets such as mobile phone, laptop, and computer may be exciting factors.
- *Etiology*: It can be due to abnormality in: *Length of eyeball*
  - *Too long*: Myopia
  - *Too short*: Hypermetropia
- *Curvature of corneal or lenticular surface*
  - *More curved*: Myopia
  - *Less curved*: Hypermetropia
- Refractive index of the media
  - *High*: Myopia
  - *Low*: Hypermetropia.

Types

Myopia or Short Sightedness
It is most common error of refraction, where parallel rays of light coming from infinity focus in front of retina, when accommodation is at rest.

Types
- *Congenital/developmental*
  - Usually stationary
  - May be unilateral or bilateral
  - Bilateral myopia may be associated with strabismus.
- *Simple*:
  - Most common
  - Usually not progresses beyond adolescence
  - Do not progress above -5D/-6D
- *Pathological or progressive*:
  - Myopia is progressive in nature.
  - Usually begins at 5–6 years and progresses till 21–22 years of age
  - Strongly familial
  - Associated with degenerative changes in vitreous and retina
  - Myopia more than -6D, may increase up to -15D to -20D.

Hypermetropia
- It is an error of refraction, where parallel a ray of light coming from infinity focuses behind the retina, when accommodation is atrest.
- Less common
- A newborn is invariably hypermetropic, with average +2.5D, which decreases as the eye advances.

Astigmatism

- It is an error of refraction, where parallel ray of light coming from infinity cannot converge to a point focus on retina.
- It is due to unequal refraction in different meridian of the optical system of the eye.
- It is corrected by cylindrical lens.

Features

- Eye strain
- Frontal headache
- Blurring of vision
- Burning and dryness of eye
- Black floaters in front of eye.

Treatment

- Glasses
  - *Myopia*: Concave glass
  - *Hypermetropia*: Convex glass
  - *Astigmatism*: Cylindrical glass
- Contact lenses
- Refractive surgery
- Prolonged use of electronic gadget should be discouraged.

Key Points

- An optical error, were parallels ray of light coming from infinity do not focus on the retina, when accommodation is at rest.
- Due to abnormality in length of eyeball, curvature of refractive surface, and refractive index of media
- Myopia, hypermetropia, and astigmatism are the common types.
- Myopia is most common, progressive type of which is associated with degenerative changes in eye.
- Eye strain, blurring of vision, and frontal headache are common symptoms.

Common Orthopedic Problems in Children

Raman Shrivastava

INTRODUCTION

It is not uncommon for the Pediatricians to encounter worried parents in OPD with their child having pain/swelling/decreased movement of the limb or some form of limb deformities. Many a times things are straightforward and either you need to refer them to Pediatric Orthopedician or to counsel the parents along with giving some analgesics to the child. Here in this chapter, we will try to make us more familiar with common orthopedic problems in pediatric age group which we see in our day-to-day practice.

Rare diseases and complications and their management are beyond the scope of this chapter and we will be focusing on common conditions and their management.

TOE-IN (PIGEON TOES)

Toe-in (Pigeon toes) or Toeing-in deformities are presented mostly when the child starts walking. This pattern of walking may be associated with one of the following common but mostly autocorrectable conditions.

Metatarsus Adductus

Parents and grandparents raise the concern of foot turned in at neonatal age. On examination, the foot looks curved-like "C" but unlike in clubfoot, heel comes down on ankle dorsiflexion and is in valgus (forefoot in varus but hind foot is in valgus).

Treatment

If the deformity is easily correctable to normal or near-normal position of the foot then stretching exercises by mother with every feed will rectify the problem. If the foot is resistant to passive stretching then serial cast correction followed by splinting will be needed.

Femoral Anteversion

"W" sitting is the most comfortable sitting position for these children. Log-roll test (rotating the thigh in and out by holding the knee with extended hip and knee) shows internal rotation up to 90° but limited external rotation.

Treatment

It usually resolves by 10–12 years of age in most cases, but we should discourage the child from sitting in "W" position. Rarely orthopedic surgery is needed to correct the resistant severe in-toeing cases.

THE FOOT

The common foot problems in children for which they are brought to our OPD are foot pain and foot deformities.

Foot Pain

Foot pain can be caused by following common conditions in pediatric age group:
- *Osteochondritis of navicular or metatarsal head* causes localized pain over the medial border of foot while weight bearing or palpation. X-rays are diagnostic and show an increased density and fragmentation. Treatment requires rest and cast application in some cases.
- *March or stress fracture* are due to overuse or repetitive trauma and usually involve the 2nd metatarsal. X-rays show changes after 2 weeks and treatment involves rest and cast application. Sometimes shoe modification is advised.
- *Accessory navicular* presents with complaints of pain and palpable swelling on medial border of foot just over the arch. X-rays are diagnostic after age of 5–6 years and the child should be referred to orthopedic surgeon for management.
- *Tarsal coalition*: History of repeated ankle sprain and strains in 9–12 year age groups may be caused by talocalcaneal or calcaneonavicular bar, which restricts the subtalar movement. Computed tomography (CT) and magnetic resonance imaging (MRI) are definitive diagnostic tools. Treatment involves walking cast and sometimes excisional arthroplasty or arthrodesis are required.
- *Foreign body* through examination of the skin is a must in toddlers and young children who cannot point the pain properly. X-rays for radiopaque and ultrasonography

(USG) for radio-non-opaque foreign body are diagnostic tools. Puncture wounds of the foot must be treated appropriately as there are high chances of developing cellulitis and abscess in these injuries.

- *Peroneal spastic flat foot* is presented as painful, stiff, flat foot which is externally rotated and occasionally associated with lateral calf pain. It is important to rule out tarsal coalition, fracture, and foreign body, or inflammatory arthritis as a causative factor. Orthopedic referral is required when symptomatic treatment does not work.
- *Flat feet* are painless absence of medial arch of foot. Generally medial arch develops by 5–6 years of age in children. Examination requires making the child sit by the corner of the couch with hanging feet and if a medial arch is seen then the cause of flat foot on weight-bearing is due to flexibility of the ligaments and does not require any treatment. If the flat foot is rigid and painful, then an orthopedician's opinion should be taken.
- *Calcaneal valgus foot* is a common deformity caused by intrauterine positional problem where the top of the forefoot touches the anterior leg. Treatment consists of stretching exercise by mother at every feed. It usually resolves in 4–6 weeks' time. If deformity persists then orthopedician's opinion is required.
- *Congenital vertical talus or rocker bottom foot* is opposite of club foot. Here medial arch of foot is reversed and a palpable head of talus is present. Treatment is by serial casting and surgery.
- *Club foot* is a very common foot deformity diagnosed at birth. Three components of the deformity are: (1) forefoot varus (adductus), (2) midfoot cavus (medial crease), and (3) hind foot equines (it differentiates it from metatarsus adductus). Examination for other anomalies such as hip and spinal problem is a must. Treatment involves serial casting and tenotomy (70–80%) cases by pediatric orthopedician.
- *Toe walking*: After development of independent walking, it is unusual for a child to walk on toes. Usually it is bilateral and a thorough neurological examination is a must to rule out cerebral palsy, muscle disorders, or spinal deformities. Idiopathic toe walking generally resolves by 3–4 years of age and if it persists then a percutaneous tenotomy and cast is corrective in most cases.

KNEE

- *Genu varum or bow legs*: Most of the time up to the age of 2–2.5 years, it is a physiological bowing for which parents and family friends show concern. But pathological conditions such as Blount's disease, rickets, and tibial torsion must be ruled out. Keeping the child in supine position with extended hips and knees and both medial malleoli together, if the distance between the medial sides of knees is >10 cm then treatment is required.
- *Genu valgum or knock knee*: Between the age of 3.5 and 5 years, is considered normal for a growing child who usually gets straight legs by 5–6 years of age. If the intermalleolar distance (measured in a supine child with extended hips and knees and femoral medial condyles together) is >10 cm then pathological causes such as rickets, Morquio's disease, or trauma should be ruled out. Bracing in severe cases is of limited value and child should be referred to pediatric orthopedician.
- *Knee pain*: Many a times referred pain from hip presents as knee pain due to common nerve supply of the both. So X-rays of hip along with knee should always be asked for complete evaluation. Following are the common cause of knee pain in children:
  - *Discoid meniscus* presents as snapping knee or painful instability which is due to the failure of development of the meniscal semilunar cartilage. A "Clunk" upon flexion and extension of the knee can be heard or felt. MRI is confirmatory and arthroscopic debridement is treatment of choice.
  - *Apophysitis of the tibial tubercle (Osgood–Schlatter disease)* presents as "Knobby Knees" with painful localized swelling over tibial tubercle (just below the knee anterior prominence). Mostly it is due to overuse which responds to rest, analgesics and hot fomentation or in few cases knee immobilizer or cylindrical cast is applied.
- *Swelling around knee* are commonly due to two types of benign lesions:
  1. Exostosis (osteochondroma) which is firm painless mass palpable on medial or lateral side, which can be diagnosed with X-rays.
  2. Popliteal cyst (Baker's cyst) is a palpable soft cystic mass on the medial side of the back of the knee. Mostly it heals by itself and sometimes it needs aspiration.

THE HIP

- *Congenital dislocation of hip or developmental dysplasia of the hip (DDH)* (better term as this disorder may occur pre-, peri- or postnatally): Screening in susceptible groups (first-born female child, breech delivery, family history of DDH) can affect the outcome considerably as early treatment can result in a normal healthy hip whereas if left untreated it lend-up into degenerative hip disease. Ortolani and Barlow's test is described to diagnose this condition clinically in neonates (femoral head is attempted to bring in and push out of socket, i.e., acetabulum).

Other useful signs are in equality of limb length (knee level in Galeazzi sign), asymmetrical thigh folds and limitation of abduction, delayed walking, and limping gait are seen in late presenters. If in doubt, these cases should be referred to pediatric orthopedician for further management.

- *Perthes or Legg-Calvé-Perthes disease* is caused by interruption of the blood flow to the femoral head causing avascular necrosis or AVN. Sickle cell disease patients with hip and/or knee pain shall always be looked for hip changes in X-rays. Clinical presentations of this disease are pain and limp which in due course may become painless. Hemophilia and other blood dyscrasias are also susceptible to hip AVN. Treatment involves rest, traction, and splinting in early stage of disease but may need containment surgeries for late advanced stages.
- *Slipped capital femoral epiphysis (SCFE)*: Adolescent male (10–16 years) with obese body built and family history of thyroid disorder coming to OPD with pain in the hip or knee and limp must be examined for restriction of hip rotation and X-ray shall be taken to rule out SCFE. This condition needs an urgent treatment to prevent an acute minor slip of epiphysis of femur head going into complete slip off. Surgical sterilization of the epiphysis is a must otherwise condition may go into chronic stage and any time in future with even trivial trauma can become acute-on-chronic slip.

SPINE

- *Congenital torticollis*: Here the child keeps the head tilted to one side and reluctant to turn head to opposite side. Chin points opposite to involve side. In neonates, a small soft mass may be felt in the sternocleidomastoid muscle which later becomes contracted and stiff. Often it is associated with vertebral anomalies and X-rays of the spine must be taken. Initial treatment starts with encouraging the child to rotate the head by placing bright colored objects on opposite side, manual stretching exercise, physiotherapy and if it fails then surgical release is advised at around 3–4 years of age.
- *Sprengel's deformity* or asymmetrical shoulder height is due to failure of scapula to descent down during fetogenesis. Often associated with Klippel-Feil syndrome and scoliosis, milder forms are of cosmetic concern only but for severe varieties surgical correction is required to improve the shoulder joint's overhead abduction.
- *Low back pain* is not a common complaint in pediatric age group, hence, a child complaining of persistent back pain must always be examined thoroughly to diagnose the course. Low back pain localized to the lumbosacral region may be due to spondylosis or spondylolisthesis (fracture of the pars and slippage of vertebra of L_5 on S_1). Loss of lumbar lordosis, tight hamstring muscle causing inability to bend forward to touch toes, positive "Stork sign" and "Scotty dog" appearance on X-ray are diagnostic of this condition. Treatment requires rest, orthosis, or surgical stabilization.
- *Tuberculosis of the spine (Pott's disease)* is not rare in our region. It involves vertebral end plates and anterior body or pedicles. Night pain or continuous dull aching pain localized to a particular vertebral area, fever, history of contact to TB are indicative to search for the Pott's disease. X-rays and MRI are diagnostic tools and treatment involves antitubercular medicine and high-protein diet. Drainage of the abscess as and when required and bracing till the disease heals.
- *Scoliosis* or curved back (right thoracic single curve is most common) can be nonstructural (which can be corrected on bending film and are due to limb length deficiency or neuromuscular imbalance) or structural (fixed curve which can be idiopathic, congenital, post-trauma or pathological). Adam's Bend test is designed to screen the scoliosis in school going children. Early management depends on the severity of the curve and its progression potential. Treatment varies from observation to brace and surgical stabilization.

UPPER LIMB

- *Brachial plexus injuries* are of Erb's and Klumpke's type which are seen following difficult deliveries causing injury to 5th and 6th cervical nerve roots and 7th, 8th, and T_1 nerve roots, respectively. Association of Horner's syndrome is indicative of more severe lesion. Pseudoparalysis secondary to a clavicle fracture is very common which can be ruled out by an X-ray. Mostly these cases recover at their own but passive stretching is recommended to prevent contractures during nerve regeneration. Some cases may need nerve repair or transplant or muscle release procedure.
- *Clavicle fracture* is quiet common in children after fall, tender on palpation diagnosed on X-rays and treatment mostly requires assurance and conservative treatment in the form of sling and analgesic for few days.
- *Humerus fracture* is a common injury in difficult delivery cases and heals completely over time with conservative management. Newborns with even widely displaced fragments need immobilization for 10–15 days and they do well.
- *Pulled elbow* is a subluxation of proximal radioulnar joint due to sudden pull or due to trapped arm while child is turning on bed. X-rays are unremarkable but many a time therapeutic as while aligning the limb for X-ray the technician turn the child's forearm and the joint get reduced. Otherwise treatment consists of gentle supination and flexion of elbow, which produces a click sound or a feel of reduction to clinician and in few minutes child becomes comfortable and playful. A sling for few days is all that is required.
- *Infection of bone and joints in children* must be treated aggressively. Growing bone and joints can get infection from hematogenous route, external inoculation or direct extension from nearby wound. Most common

causative organisms are *Staphylococcus aureus*, streptococci, *Haemophilus influenzae* and *Mycobacterium tuberculosis*.

- Symptoms such as fever may not be obvious in neonates but swelling and decreased movement of adjacent joint are finding which should definitely raise an alarm for bone and joint infections. In older children, conditions like sickle cell disease and other blood dyscrasias should also be thought of for bone cries. Cellulitis and thrombophlebitis are very uncommon in children and these patients should be considered to have osteomyelitis until it is ruled out. X-rays are positive generally after 10 days from infection starts, and blood cultures are negative in >60% of times. So antibiotic treatment should commence at once, without waiting for blood reports. USG and MRI are very useful tools and confirm the diagnosis in patients with raised c-reactive protein, erythrocyte sedimentation rate, and total leukocyte count blood picture. Treatment involves intravenous antibiotic, joint aspiration, immobilization, and drainage of pus.

SUGGESTED READING

1. Joseph B, Nayagam S, Loder RT, Torode I. Pediatric Orthopaedics: A System of Decision Making.
2. Staheli LT. Practice of Pediatric Orthopaedics.
3. Herring JA. Tachdjian's Pediatric Orthopaedics, 6th edition.

Common Pediatric and Neonatal Surgical Problems

Nitin Sharma

INTRODUCTION

Most of the pediatric clinics deal with a number of conditions that require surgical intervention. Some of the conditions are elective where a surgical procedure can be planned while others require an emergency intervention. For the ease of convenience, we can divide these conditions into two broad categories:
1. Obvious externally visible congenital anomaly
2. *Not visible anomaly*:
   a. Asymptomatic detected on imaging or antenatally diagnosed
   b. Symptomatic anomalies:
      i. The tachypneic baby
      ii. Not taking feeds
      iii. Vomiting
      iv. Distended abdomen
      v. Not passing urine.

The commonly observed surgical conditions are as discussed in the chapter.

BIRTH INJURIES AND CEPHAL HEMATOMA

- These cases present with a palpable flabby swelling in the scalp due to collection of blood in the subcutaneous or subgaleal space or may present with an obvious crepitus.
- Most of these cases are managed conservatively and parental counseling with monitoring of the neonate is required.
- Those which undergo secondary infection or those presenting with high intractable jaundice require drainage.

Hydrocephalous

- It is the collection of cerebrospinal fluid (CSF) in the ventricle which presents with increase in the head circumference, sun set sign, or with features of raised intracranial pressure and failure to thrive. The diagnosis can be made on ultrasound cranium in neonates or with computed tomography (CT) head.
- *Indications of surgery are*:
  - Obvious deformity of the head due to ventriculomegaly or presentation with the features of raised intracranial pressure and failure to thrive.
  - Patients with intractable headache and a history of meningitis may also require intervention.
- Hydrocephalous is managed by shunting of CSF either into the peritoneum (ventriculoperitoneal shunt), pleura (ventriculopleural shunt) or in vein or atrium from where the excess of the CSF is absorbed. It is also managed by endoscopic third ventriculostomy.

CYSTIC HYGROMA/LYMPHANGIOMA

- Hygroma in Greek means water-containing tumor. They are congenital malformations of lymphatic system. Cystic hygroma occurs more frequently as compared to other type of lymphangiomas, and may compose of single or multiple macrocystic lesions.
- *Location*: The common location of these lesions are cervicofacial region (especially posterior cervical triangle), axilla, mediastinum, groin, and below tongue. Occasionally, these malformations occur in liver, spleen, kidney, and intestine.
- *Presentation* of cystic hygroma apparent at birth is a painless mass. The other modes of presentations are related to the complications or effects of cystic hygroma, such as respiratory distress, feeding difficulty, fever, sudden increase in the size, and infection in the lesion.
- *Diagnosis*: Ultrasound—multicystic lesion with internal septations and no blood flow on color Doppler ultrasonographs. Other modalities such as CT scan and magnetic resonance imaging (MRI) can be employed to delineate the lesion, in a better way.
- *Management*: The most preferred modality of treating cystic hygroma is complete surgical excision. Many recent case reports and case series have increasingly documented remarkable results for management of such lesions with sclerosing agents. The other treatment modalities that have been employed with variable results include simple drainage, aspirations, radiation, laser excision, radiofrequency ablation, and cauterization.

Cleft Lip and Palate

- The anomaly is characterized by the lack continuity of tissues forming the lip, alveolus, and soft and hard palate.
- Goals of treatment of the child with a cleft lip and palate should include repairing of the birth defect (lip, palate, and nose), achieving normal speech, language, hearing, functional occlusion, and good dental health.
- Early referral to the infant-feeding specialist or nurses associated with cleft teams can facilitate to solve their problem.
- *Management*: Lip repair is performed at 3 months of age and palate repair at 9-12 months of age (Millard technique). Other schools perform surgery earlier (soft palate repair at 3 months of age and lip and hard palate repair at 6 months of age) as in the case of Malek protocol.

CONGENITAL HERNIA AND HYDROCELE

- Pediatric inguinal hernia is usually a protrusion of intra-abdominal contents through a patent processus vaginalis.
- A pediatric inguinal hernia will not close spontaneously, and it must be repaired. While repair is not a surgical emergency, prompt referral to a pediatric surgeon is always recommended.
- Most inguinal hernia repairs in full term, healthy infants, and older children may be performed electively soon after the diagnosis is made.
- Infants younger than 1 year of age, particularly former preterm infants, are at greater risk for an incarcerated hernia. Repairs in preterm infants should be carried out as soon as it is convenient.

Incarcerated and Strangulated Hernias

- Incarceration of an inguinal hernia is more common in the first year of life. An incarcerated hernia usually presents as firm swelling in the inguinal region (possibly extending to the scrotum). This swelling is tender to palpation and does not reduce readily with pressure.
- The child may be extremely irritable and unwilling to eat. Intestinal obstruction, with abdominal distension and vomiting, may be present.
- *Treatment*: Reduction of an incarcerated hernia should be attempted, and it can be achieved in the majority of cases. Sedation and firm, gentle, and steady pressure over the hernia may help in reduction. If the reduction is successful, the child should be admitted to hospital (because of the high risk of recurrence), and surgical correction should be undertaken after 1-2 days (to allow edema to resolve). If a reduction cannot be achieved, an urgent exploration is required.

Hydrocele

- A hydrocele is a collection of fluid in the scrotum without an obvious inguinal hernia. The typical hydrocele is observed at or shortly after birth as a unilateral or bilateral swelling in the scrotum, which may fluctuate in size.
- *Management*: Better is observation during the first 1-2 years of a child's life, unless the diagnosis of a hernia cannot be excluded. Hydroceles that persist or appear beyond that age are unlikely to resolve spontaneously and should undergo elective surgical repair.

Undescended Testis and Ectopic Testis

- *Definition of undescended testes (UDT)*: Terms such as undescended testis, retentio testis, cryptorchidism, and maldescended testis describe a testis that is not normally located at the bottom of the scrotum. The UDT may be situated along its normal route of descent or in an ectopic position.
  - *Cryptorchid/undescended:* Testis neither resides nor can be manipulated into the scrotum.
  - *Ectopic:* Location is aberrant, viz., femoral, pubopenile, perineal, or crossed scrotal.
  - *Retractile:* Testis can be manipulated into scrotum where it remains without tension.
  - *Gliding:* Testis can be manipulated into upper scrotum but retracts when released.
  - *Acquired:* Testis previously descended or after orchidopexy or other inguinal surgery (hernia), then "ascends" spontaneously.
- *Classification of UDT*: Undescended testis is classified as:
  - Congenital and acquired
  - Palpable and nonpalpable
  - Unilateral or bilateral
- About 80% of UDT are palpable and 20% are nonpalpable. Palpable UDT are located along the inguinoscrotal descent route. The term nonpalpable means that the testis was not found during the patient's examination. It means that we are dealing with an abdominal testis or with lack of testis (anorchia). Anorchia can be a result of testicular agenesis or testicular atrophy.
- *Diagnosis of UDT*:
  - *Medical history:* History of pregnancy, medication used and exposure to environmental toxins, as well as birth weight, position of testes at birth, other defects and diseases of the child and family history.
  - *Physical examination*: Palpation is a basic technique to examine UDT. It is mandatory to assess the appearance of external genitalia to exclude disorders of sexual differentiation (DSD). A patient should be examined in both supine and standing (older boys) position in a warm comfortable room. Gonads should be carefully examined for size, turgor, any palpable paratesticular anomalies, and the presence of hernia or hydrocele. Most of the cases of true undescended testis are characterized by underdeveloped/hypoplastic scrotum.

- *Imaging*: A Prader orchidometer helps the surgeon in proper counseling and assessment of the case. Different imaging techniques have been evaluated for the assessment of UDT.
  - *Ultrasonography (US)*: It is good to assess the size of inguinal testes. It is however less reliable for abdominal testes. In good hands it can be a good imaging tool.
  - *CT*: It may be helpful for bilateral impalpable testes. Due to associated high radiation exposure and less sensitivity it is less recommended.
  - *MRI*: It may be helpful for bilateral impalpable testes; it is performed under general anesthesia in young children; it is more expensive and require long duration.
    - Of the above imaging techniques, US with a high-resolution transducer (> 7.5 MHz) offer the greatest accuracy in assessment of 100% of palpable and of 84% of nonpalpable UDT (with a sensitivity of 76% and a specificity of 100%).
- *Treatment*: There are two basic modes of treatment of UDT used for many years and are accepted all over the world: Hormonal and surgical.
  - *Hormonal treatment:* Hormonal therapy is usually carried out using hCG (human chorionic gonadotropin), gonadotropin-releasing hormone (GnRH), [luteinizing hormone releasing hormone *(LHRH)] or a combination* of both.
  - *Surgical treatment (orchidopexy)*:
    - The surgical therapy for the palpable UDT is orchidopexy with creation of a subdartos pouch. Fixation is achieved by the scarring of the everted tunica vaginalis to the surrounding tissues.
    - When the testis is nonpalpable, diagnostic laparoscopy through an umbilical port is the procedure of choice. If the testicular vessels exit through the internal ring, an inguinal incision allows one to locate the testis (orchidopexy) or its remnants (removal and histopathologic examination).
    - Approximately half of intra-abdominal testes are located close to the internal ring, and the Fowler–Stephens (F-S) maneuver (also called the F-S operation) is recommended then as a routine procedure.
  - *Timing of orchidopexy:* Currently orchidopexy is recommended between 6 and 12–18 months. The main goal of this timing of orchidopexy is to prevent the impairment of spermatogenic function and decrease the risk of testicular germ cell tumors (TGCT) in adult life.

Hypospadias

It is a common type of surgical anomaly and is characterized by abnormal location of the urethral meatus and is associated with incomplete prepuce and occasionally meatal stenosis. It is classified as per the location of the meatus.
- Distal penile hypospadias
- Mid penile hypospadias
- Proximal penile hypospadias
- Scrotal and perineal hypospadias.

Management

- The chordee is managed by elective urethral reconstruction using local tissue called as urethroplasty.
- The recommended age of hypospadias repair is between 1 and 5 years. The long-term outcome in this disease is good.

EPISPADIAS AND EXTROPHY

- Epispadias is opposite to hypospadias which is characterized by a defect in the dorsal aspect of the penis so that the urethral plate is wide open and there is a continuous dribbling of urine. This may be an isolated deformity or may be associated with open bladder plate also known as exstrophy of bladder.
- *It is classified as*:
  - *Continent epispadias*: Where the bladder neck is intact and there is urinary continence so that the problem is mainly of the appearance of the phallus while there is no urinary complains, except for poor stream.
  - *Incontinent epispadias* where the bladder neck is wide open so that there is continuous dribbling of urine and urinary incontinence is there.

  It may also be classified as:
  - Isolated epispadias
  - Epispadias with exstrophy of bladder
  - Cloacal exstrophy
- *Management*:
  - Epispadias is repaired electively between 1 and 5 years of age.
  - The repair of epispadias is done commonly by Cantwell–Ransley epispadias repair.
  - Bladder exstrophy is repaired by three-staged repair. First stage involves closure of the bladder with or without osteotomy before 6 months of age. This is followed by bladder neck reconstruction between 1 and 2 years of age and augmentation with or without ureteric reimplantation later onto increase the bladder size and achieves pseudocontinence.

ANTERIOR ABDOMINAL WALL DEFECTS

Gastroschisis

- Gastroschisis is a common birth defect with an increasing incidence worldwide. Routine ultrasound has allowed

this birth defect to be identified in utero with high specificity and sensitivity.
- *Surgical repair:* Primary abdominal wall closure is preferred and a silo is created only when primary closure is not possible. The success of primary closure is dependent on the amount of visceroabdominal disproportion.
- *Primary closure advantages*: Shorter interval to oral feeding, reduced hospital stay, and decreased surgery.
- Increased abdominal pressures require the use of delayed fascial closure techniques using temporary coverage with silastic/Dacron intra-abdominal pouch (Silo) or the use of mobilized lateral skin flaps.

Omphalocele

Omphalocele is a defect in the ventral abdominal wall characterized by an absence of abdominal muscles, fascia, and skin, which are covered by a membrane consisting of peritoneum and amnion. The umbilical cord inserts into the membrane covering the omphalocele at a location far from the abdominal wall.

Surgical Repair

- Following delivery, newborn care should be directed toward preoperative stabilization, involving airway stabilization and sterile wrapping of the abdominal defect to prevent heat and minimize insensible fluid losses.
- Major effort is made to avoid trauma and contamination of the omphalocele sac. Peripheral vascular access should be established to administer intravenous fluids and antibiotics.
- Mechanical ventilation is frequently necessary due to secondary lung hypoplasia with large omphaloceles. Prompt decompression of the stomach is important initially followed by intermittent gastric suction.
- For the last two decades, the preferred method of omphalocele repair is primary fascial closure. The benefits are a lower incidence of sepsis and biliary obstruction/ fistula as well as reduced operations and mortality.

UMBILICAL GRANULOMA

- Umbilical granuloma (UG) is the most common umbilical abnormalities encountered in neonatal practice. UG is not a true congenital abnormality. It represents ongoing inflammation and granulation tissue formation, of an umbilicus that has yet to epithelialize.
- *Presentation*: Classically they are round, moist, erythematous, pedunculated and usually between 3 and 10 mm in diameter. Bacterial colonization and low-grade infection may play a role in their pathogenesis.
- *Treatment*: Cauterization with 75% silver nitrate is usually preferred, and is repeated two to three times. However, many other forms of chemical cauterizing agents such as copper sulfate and concentrated salt solution have also been tried.
- Rarely, persistent UG need surgical removal/cauterization. If a presumed UG fails to respond to cauterization, alternative diagnosis must be considered. The congenital remnants of the urachus and patent vitellointestinal duct can pose diagnostic difficulties, as their clinical manifestations are often nonspecific and they can resemble UGs.
- Ultrasound imaging may be used to distinguish these lesions by identifying their relationship to, and their continuity with, the umbilicus and the urinary bladder.
- Diagnosis is operator dependent and the final decision ultimately rests on the clinical judgment. A patent vitellointestinal duct (VID)/urachus is managed by umbilical exploration and transfixation of the duct.

SPINA BIFIDA AND MENINGOMYELOCELE

- Spina bifida is a congenital malformation in which the spinal column is split (bifid) as a result of failed closure of the embryonic neural tube. In its most common and most severe form, the spinal cord is open dorsally.
- *Clinical presentation*:
  - Patient often exhibit motor and sensory neurological deficit below the level of the lesion. This may result in lower limb weakness or paralysis that hampers or prevents walking, and lack of sensation that enhances the risk of pressure sores.
  - Urinary and fecal incontinence occur frequently. It is also associated with hind brain herniation (Chiari II malformation), hydrocephalus which often requires shunting.
  - Orthopedic abnormalities including talipes (club foot), contractures, hip dislocation, scoliosis and kyphosis are also frequently observed. There is a strong correlation between the axial level of lesion and the degree of disability experienced by individuals with meningomyelocele (MMC).
- *Diagnosis, screening and prevention*: Prenatal diagnosis of an elevated concentration of alpha-fetoprotein (AFP) and assay of acetyl cholinesterase in amniotic fluid samples from pregnancies with anencephaly or MMC shown to be diagnostic. *(Refer to chapter of Antenatal diagnosis)*.
- *Management*: The management of MMC traditionally involves surgery within 48 hours of birth. The child's back is closed to minimize the risk of ascending infection that can result in meningitis.
- Virtually all neonates with thoracic level lesions need a ventriculoperitoneal shunt, whereas around 85% of patients with a lumbar level lesion, and about 70% with a sacral lesion require shunting.

- Endoscopic third ventriculostomy with choroid plexus coagulation has also become an alternative treatment for hydrocephalus associated with spina bifida.
- Orthopedic deformities are usually treated shortly after birth, with long-term follow-up.
- Bladder and urinary tract management often includes a combination of clean intermittent catheterization, pharmacological agents, and surgery.
- Bowel function is not an issue in neonates, but older children require bowel management including the use of suppositories, enemas or laxatives, and the use of antegrade colonic enemas.

PREPUTIAL ADHESIONS, PHIMOSIS, AND MEATAL STENOSIS

- It is important to distinguish these three entities. At birth, the glans is covered with prepuce, the meatus is not easily visible and the prepuce is not retractable. This nonretractable prepuce is due to normal preputial adhesions that bind preputial skin to glans penis.
- At the end of the first year of life, retraction of the foreskin behind the glandular sulcus is possible in only about 50% of boys; this rises to approximately 90% by the age of 3 years.
- If there is a delay in this process and the child is said to have difficulty/pain during micturition, preputial adhesions release is indicated. Circumcision is not indicated for this condition as such. True phimosis is not common and it occurs as a result of scarring due to recurrent balanoposthitis.
- "Physiological" phimosis is more common and this may go hand in hand with preputial adhesions. Congenital adhesion of the prepuce to the glans penis is more frequent. It is often mistaken for phimosis in a child. Both the congenital preputial adhesions and true phimosis predispose to smegma collection, which in turn can be a cause of recurrent balanoposthitis and result in true phimosis.
- If physiological phimosis is not resolved by 3 years of age and the child has history suggestive of dysuria preputial dilatation is recommended. Preputial dilatation is generally followed with preputial adhesions release.

Meatal Stenosis

- Meatal stenosis can result in urinary tract obstruction. The usual causes are inappropriate instrumentation and ammoniacal meatitis in circumcised boys.
- Congenital meatal stenosis is rare, but boys with hypospadias may have a stenosed meatus.
- The child presents with a thin stream of urine and has to strain at micturition. There may be frequency and dysuria.
- *Treatment* consists of regular meatal dilatation, which can be carried out by the parents at home. If this is not feasible, meatotomy or meatoplasty may be needed. This is, however, often associated with a recurrence and need for repeat intervention.

POSTERIOR URETHRAL VALVES

- Congenital valves in the posterior urethra constitute the most common cause of lower urinary tract obstruction in boys. Posterior urethral valves (PUV) are located just distal to the verumontanum at the junction of the anterior and posterior urethra.
- They have been classified into three types by young and this classification is still applicable currently.
  - *Clinical features*: A case of PUV can present as an antenatally detected bilateral hydrouretro nephrosis or postnatally as an infant with features of *obstruction such as* dribbling of urine, weak stream, straining, retention, and a palpable bladder. Patients may also present with features of recurrent urinary tract infection such as fever, dysuria, hematuria, vomiting and failure to thrive. Varying degrees of renal function impairment may also be present.
- *Diagnosis*: PUV is confirmed by micturating cystourethrogram (MCU), which shows a dilated posterior urethra, poor flow into the distal urethra and abnormalities of the bladder (thickened wall, trabeculations, and sacculations).
- *Management*:
  - *Antenatal management:* The vesicoamniotic shunt has been described to overcome such poor prognosis, to buy some time for prolonging pregnancy and protecting the developing kidneys. The present scientific evidence shows that although shunting is effective in reversing oligohydramnios, it makes no difference to the outcome and long-term results of patients with PUV.
  - *Postnatal treatment*:
    - *Bladder drainage*: If a boy is born with suspected PUV, an MCU and drainage of the bladder at the earliest is indicated. The baby is catheterized and MCU is performed to confirm that the diagnosis is correct. If the baby is stable, endoscopic incision or resection of the valves is done at the earliest.
    - *Valve ablation*: When the medical situation of the neonate has stabilized, the creatinine level decreased/decreasing trend, and there is no gross pyuria; the next step is to remove the obstruction by valve fulguration at 5, 7, and 12 o'clock positions using 4.5–6-Fr cystourethroscope in neonates and a 8-Fr cytsourethroscope in older children. If the facility of cystoscope is not available, a vesicostomy can be done as a temporary measure till definitive fulguration is achieved.

- *High diversion*: The diversion becomes indicated if there are recurrent infections of the upper tract; no improvement in renal function and/or an increase in upper tract dilatation, despite adequate bladder drainage.
- *The step ladder protocol*:
  - This includes assessment of the baby at the time of admission. If the child is stable, then fulguration/incision can be planned.
  - If the baby is sick and acidotic, bladder catheterization is recommended. On catheterization, the condition of the baby is reassessed after 48 hours.
  - After 48 hours, if there is an improvement in the acidosis, the general condition, the child will improve with the fulguration/incision.
  - However, if there is no improvement on catheterization, a high diversion is needed and ureterostomy should be planned.

MEGAURETER

- A ureter is considered as a megaureter if the lumen is dilated. Although the dilation is rarely subtle, for the terms of definition any diameter >8 mm is considered abnormal.
- *Classification*: It can be classified into primary or secondary based on the etiology. Primary mega ureter is usually a functional disorder while secondary mega ureter is secondary to some pathology.
- *Primary obstructive mega ureter* is thought to be due to an aperistaltic juxtavesical (adynamic) segment in the ureter, leading to a lack of propagation of the ureteral peristalsis and therefore urine flow.
- *Secondary obstructive* megaureter represents an obstructive process secondary to elevated intravesical pressure of some other cause.
- *Causes* include spinal dysraphism and neurogenic bladder, which may elevate detrusor pressure to over 40 cmH_2O, causing a physiologic obstruction and hydronephrosis in the collecting system. Nonneurogenic voiding dysfunction, if severe enough to elevate bladder pressure above the safe range, may also be a cause.
- *Clinical feature* includes urinary infection, groin pain, and occasionally hematuria and calculus formation.
- *Investigations*: Intravenous pyelography, diethylenetriaminepentaacetic acid (DTPA) renogram and MCU are performed.
- *Treatment*: Surgery consists of excision of the obstructing lower segment of the ureter and its reimplantation. Satisfactory recovery may occur. Nephroureterectomy is rarely necessary if the split renal function of the same side is very poor.

PELVIURETERIC JUNCTION OBSTRUCTION

- Obstruction of the pelviureteric junction (PUJ) is one of the most frequent causes for hydronephrosis. Koff described two types of PUJ obstructions, viz., intrinsic and extrinsic. The most common type was found to be the intrinsic type due to the dynamic segment.
- *Clinical presentation*:
  - These cases can present as an asymptomatic child with an antenatal hydronephrosis. Some others may present with symptoms such as pain (this may be dull constant pain or severe spasmodic pain), lump or features of pyonephrosis.
  - A characteristic feature may be the occurrence of abdominal pain with the appearance of a mass and both resolving with the passage of a large amount of urine *(Dietl's crisis)*.
- *Diagnosis*: These cases can be antenatally diagnosed or in later age while doing ultrasound for the symptoms. Once the child with an antenatal diagnosis is born the follow-up protocol is as under:

Follow-up protocol for antenatal hydronephrosis:
- *Timing of initial ultrasound*: All newborns with history of antenatal hydronephrosis should have postnatal ultrasound examination done within the first week of life.
- In neonates with suspected posterior urethral valves, oligohydramnios or severe bilateral hydronephrosis, US should be performed within 24-48 hours of birth.
- In all other cases, the ultrasound should be performed preferably within 3-7 days, or before hospital discharge.

Diagnosis and grading of postnatal hydronephrosis: Assessment of severity of postnatal hydronephrosis should be based on the classification proposed by Society for Fetal Urology or anteroposterior diameter of the renal pelvis.

Guidelines for postnatal monitoring:
- Neonates with normal ultrasound examination in the first week of life should undergo a repeat study at 4-6 weeks.
- Infants with isolated mild unilateral or bilateral hydronephrosis [anteroposterior diameter (APD) < 10 mm or SFU grade 1-2] should be followed by sequential ultrasound alone, for resolution or progression of findings.

Guidelines for MCU:
- A MCU should be performed in patients with unilateral or bilateral hydronephrosis with renal pelvic APD > 10 mm, SFU grades 3-4 or ureteric dilatation under proper antibiotic coverage.
- MCU should be performed early, within 24-72 hours of life, in patients with suspected lower urinary tract obstruction. In other cases, the procedure should be done at 4-6 weeks of age.

- MCU should be done for infants with antenatally detected hydronephrosis who develop a urinary tract infection.

Guidelines for diuretic renography:
- Infants with moderate-to-severe unilateral or bilateral hydronephrosis (SFU grades 3-4, APD > 10 mm) who do not show vesicoureteric reflux should undergo diuretic renography.
- Infants with hydronephrosis and dilated ureter(s) and no evidence of vesicoureteric reflux should undergo diuretic renography.
- The preferred radiopharmaceuticals are 99mTc mercaptoa-cetyltriglycine (MAG3), ethylene dicysteine (Tc-EC) or DTPA.
- Diuretic renography should be performed after 6-8 weeks of age. The procedure may be repeated after 3-6 months in infants where ultrasound shows worsening of pelvicalyceal dilatation. However, EC scan can be performed as early as 4 weeks.

Micturating cystourethrogram: It is indicated in cases of bilateral PUJ obstruction to rule out PUJ obstruction secondary to reflux.

Gadolinium DTPA-enhanced magnetic resonance urography (MRU) (Gd MRU): Gd-MRU is the only study that has the capability of providing excellent morphologic details typical of MRI and also functional information that is equivalent to DRS.

- *Management*: Indications of surgical intervention:
  - Reduction in split renal function (<40%) in association with a t½ > 20 minutes 10% fall in the split renal function during the follow-up.
  - Symptomatic child with palpable lump or pain.

Surgical procedures:
- The reconstruction technique is dismembered pyeloplasty that can be performed using an extraperitoneal approach. Success rates in providing drainage are high following surgery.
- Unilateral nephrectomy may rarely be required in patients with extremely poor renal function (<10%), particularly in the presence of systemic hypertension.

ANORECTAL MALFORMATIONS

- Anorectal malformations (ARMs) comprise a wide spectrum of diseases, which can affect boys and girls, and involve the distal anus and rectum as well as the urinary and genital tracts.
- Currently accepted classification of ARM is as described in **Table 1**.
  Important associated anomalies include genitourinary defects, which occur in approximately 50% of all patients with ARMs.
- The presence of a single perineal orifice is clinical evidence of a patient with persistent cloaca. Patients with

TABLE 1: Classification of anorectal malformation.

Males	Rectoperineal fistula
	Rectourethral bulbar fistula
	Rectourethral prostatic fistula
	Rectobladder neck fistula
	Imperforated anus without fistula
	Complex and unusual defects
Females	Rectoperineal fistula
	Rectovestibular fistula
	Cloaca with short common channel (<3 cm)
	Cloaca with long common channel (>3 cm)
	Imperforated anus without fistula
Complex and unusual defects	Cloacal exstrophy, covered cloacal extra
	Posterior cloaca
	Associated to presacral mass
	Rectal atresia

these anomalies also have small genitalia. In patients with cloaca, examination of the abdomen may reveal an abdominal mass which likely represents a distended vagina (hydrocolpos).

- *Perineal fistula*: Perineal fistulas in both male and female have traditionally been called "low" defects. In these cases, the rectum opens in a small orifice, usually stenotic and located anterior to the center of the sphincter. In males, the perineum may exhibit other features that help in recognition of this defect, such as a prominent midline skin bridge (known as "bucket handle") or a subepithelial midline raphe fistula that looks like a black ribbon because it is full of meconium.
- A simple anoplasty enlarges the stenotic orifice and relocates the rectal orifice posteriorly within the limits of the sphincter complex. The operation is called a "minimal posterior sagittal anoplasty".
- *Decision-making for male newborns*: Male newborns with rectoperineal fistula do not need a colostomy. They can undergo a posterior sagittal anoplasty whereas male babies *with evidence of a rectourinary tract* communication should undergo fecal diversion with a colostomy.
- *Decision-making for female newborns*: The decisions involved in managing the female newborn are less complicated. In 90% of patients, a meticulous perineal inspection will demonstrate the anorectal defect. Waiting 16-24 hours for enough abdominal distension to demonstrate the presence of a rectoperineal fistula or rectovestibular fistula applies to females as well. The most common anomaly in females is a rectovestibular fistula.

ESOPHAGEAL ATRESIA WITH OR WITHOUT TRACHEOESOPHAGEAL FISTULA

- Esophageal atresia (EA) is the most common congenital anomaly of the esophagus. Most cases of EA are associated with tracheo-esophageal fistula (TEF).
- Most common variant anomaly (87%) is proximal EA associated with distal TEF. The proximal esophagus is hypertrophied and dilated from amniotic liquid pressure. Impingement on the trachea by the dilated pouch is the cause of faulty cartilaginous ring development also known as tracheomalacia.
- Second most common anomaly is pure EA (8%) associated with a poorly developed distal esophagus.
- *Diagnosis*:
  - Prenatal diagnosis of EA using ultrasound relies on the finding of a small or absent fetal stomach bubble associated with maternal polyhydramnios.
  - Most babies born with EA have symptoms since the first hours of birth. They consist of excessive salivation, first feeding causing reflux, asphyxia, and cough followed by cyanosis, respiratory distress and inability to pass an orogastric tube. The abdomen could be either scaphoid or distended depending on the presence of a distal TEF.
  - The diagnosis of EA is confirmed after watching a coiled orogastric tube in the proximal esophagus in simple chest X-ray films or inability to pass a red rubber catheter beyond 8–10 cm.
  - Abdominal films should be obtained to rule out the occurrence of associated gastrointestinal anomalies. The presence of air in the gastrointestinal tract suggests that a distal TEF is present, whereas absent air makes the diagnosis of pure EA.
  - Associated malformations between 50 and 70% of children born with EA have associated congenital anomalies that affect prognosis and survival. Cardiovascular anomalies are the most commonly found (29%), followed by genitourinary (14%), gastrointestinal (13%), skeletal (10%), and chromosomal defects (4%).
- *Surgical management*:
  - *Preoperative management*: Time should be taken to optimize the physiologic state of the baby before urgent repair. This includes securing the airway, avoiding further aspiration and managing the associated pneumonitis (chest physiotherapy). An orogastric tube (Replogle) set to low intermittent suction can remove secretions from the upper esophageal pouch. The child should be placed in a prone or lateral position to avoid gastric content travel from the stomach to the lungs through the TEF.
  - *Intraoperative management*: Pure EA is managed by primary diversion, i.e., cervical esophagostomy and abdominal esophagostomy. While EA with TEF is managed by thoracotomy with ligation of TEF with end-to-end esophago-esophageal anastomosis whenever possible. In case of long-gap deformity, the primary aim is to divert by cervical esophagostomy and abdominal esophagostomy followed by esophageal replacement using stomach, gastric tubes, colon or small bowel.

SUGGESTED READING

1. Bajpai M, Dave S, Gupta DK. Factors affecting outcome in the management of posteriorurethral valves. Pediatr Surg Int. 2001;17(1):11-5.
2. Boothroyd and R. E. Cudmore, "Ultrasound of the Discharging Umbilicus," Pediatric Radiology, Vol. 26, No. 5, 1996, pp. 362-64.
3. da Silva Filho OG, de Castro Machado FM, de Andrade AC, de Souza Freitas JA, Bishara SE. Upper dental arch morphology of adult unoperated complete bilateral cleft lip and palate. Am J Orthod Dentofacial Orthop. 1998;114(2):154-61.
4. Ferro F, Lais A, Matarazzo E, Capozza N, Caione P. Retractile testis and gliding testis. Two distinct clinical entities. Minerva Urol Nefrol. 1996;48:145-9.
5. Fowler R, Stephens FD. The role of testicular vascular anatomy in the salvage of high undescended testes. Aust NZ J Surg. 1959; 29:92-106.
6. Kanemoto K, Hayashi Y, Kojima Y, Maruyama T, Ito M, Kohri K. Accuracy of ultrasonography and magnetic resonance imaging in the diagnosis of nonpalpable testis. Int J Urol. 2005;12:668-72.
7. Lattimer JK. Scrotal pouch technique for orchiopexy. J Urol. 1957;78:628-32.
8. Mahajan JK, Bharathi V, Chowdhary SK, Samujh R, Menon P, Rao KL. Bleomycin as intralesional sclerosant for cystic hygromas. J Indian Assoc Pediatr Surg. 2004;9(1):3-7.
9. Orford J, Cass DT, Glasson MJ. Advances in the treatment of oesophageal atresia over three decades: The 1970s and the1990s. Pediatr Surg Int. 2004;20(6):402-7.
10. Perez M, Lemelle JL, Barthelme H, Marquand D, Schmitt M. Bowel management with antegrade colonic enema using a Malone or a Monti conduit—clinical results. Eur J Pediatr Surg. 2001;11(5):315-8.
11. Ramareddy RS, Alladi A, Siddappa OS. Ectopic testis in children: Experience with seven cases. J Pediatr Surg. 2013;48:538-41.
12. Sanders RC, Blackmon LR, Hogge WA, Spevak P, Wulfsberg EA. Gastroschisis. Structural Fetal Anomalies: The Total Picture, 2nd edition. St Louis: Mosby; 2002. pp. 209-11.
13. Sheila S, Nazarian-Mobin, Simms K, Urata MM, Tarczy-Hornoch K, Jeffrey A. Misleading presentation of anorbital lymphangioma. Oral Surg Oral Med Oral Pathol Oral Radiol Endod. 2010;109:82-5.
14. Sonnino RE. Hydroceles. In: Reece R (ed). Manual of Emergency Pediatrics, 4th edition. Philadelphia: WB Saunders Company; 1992. pp. 261.
15. Sonnino RE. Inguinal hernias. In: Reece R (ed). Manual of Emergency Pediatrics, 4th edition. Philadelphia: WB Saunders Company; 1992. pp. 261-2.
16. Virtanen HE, Bjerknes R, Cortes D, Jørgensen N, Rajpert-De Meyts E, Thorsson AV, et al. Cryptorchidism: classification, prevalence and long-term consequences. Acta Paediatr. 2007;96(5):611-6.
17. Wang M-H. Surgical management of meatal stenosis with meatoplasty. J Vis Exp. 2010;(45):2213.

CHAPTER 175

How to Read X-ray Chest? (Step-by-step Guide)

Amar Verma, Ravi Kant Narayan, Anita Verma

INTRODUCTION

First put a chest X-ray in view box and stand in front of it, in a well-lit room then start by following these points. Get in the habit of always checking the following items before anything else. It takes a few seconds and is an important legal safe guard as well.

Administrative

- Patient's name
- Date of examination done (very important if comparing prior examinations)
- Check for position markers—right versus left, upright
- Other items to check before commencing with clinical review of the film include following items as a routine:
  - Type of film [although this is a chest program, practice noticing if it is a plain film, computed tomography (CT), angiography, magnetic resonance imaging (MRI), etc.]
  - *Patients position*: Supine, upright, lateral, or decubitus
  - *Technical quality of examination*: Learn what are the acceptable limits for the examination. You cannot find a subtle pneumothorax if there is patient motion or the film is overexposed.

Initial Survey

- A basic principle to adopt is going from general observations to specific details. Sometimes a change may be so major that the old saying about "missing the forest for the trees" comes true. For instance, an absent breast shadow on a film of a patient after a mastectomy.
- After completing your administrative housekeeping, get a general overview of the film before zooming in on tiny detail.
- Notice the following because it may change the baseline normal, you use as reference points, and you may be sensitized to look for specific findings.
  - General body size, shape, and symmetry
  - Male versus female
  - Is this an infant, child, young adult, or an elderly person?
- *Survey for foreign objects*: Tubes, intravenous (IV) lines, electrocardiogram (ECG) leads, surgical drains, prosthesis, etc., as well as nonmedical objects, bullets, shrapnel, glass, etc.

SOFT TISSUES AND SKELETAL STRUCTURES

Focus your attention on specific areas. Teach yourself to concentrate on one thing at a time and ignore everything else on the film. Most radiologists have mental checklists of specific things they look for in each region. Practice that technique until it is automatic. Begin on the frontal view with the left shoulder girdle, follow with the left chest wall, the abdomen, right chest wall, right shoulder girdle, neck, and finish with spine and ribs. On the lateral view, the sternum, spine, and abdomen are examined.

Left Shoulder Girdle

- *Soft tissues*: Look again at overall amount, then check for the following: calcifications, obvious mass effect, abnormal air collections (called subcutaneous emphysema), and soft-tissue companion shadow for the clavicle (this is a normal but variable finding).
- *Bones*: Look at each bone for the following items (notice again the progression from general to increasingly specific detail throughout the review). If your anatomic memory is hazy, refresh with a review of the gross anatomy radiology review program.
  - Overall size, shape, and contour of each bone
  - The density or mineralization
  - Compare cortical thickness to medullary cavity, trabecular pattern; look for erosions, fractures, any lytic, or blastic regions
  - At joints, check whether articular relationships are normal, or look if joint spaces are narrowed, widened, or look for any calcification in the cartilages, air in the joint space, abnormal fat pads, etc.

Left Chest Wall

Look for overall thickness, subcutaneous emphysema, and calcification. Look for sharp, distinct muscle fat planes.

Breast Tissue

In males and females, some asymmetry can occur from standing with unequal pressure against the film holder. Notice how the apparent lung density changes from the lung area covered by the soft tissue of the breast to the lung area inferior to the breast.

Abdomen

The visibility of structures is highly variable but look for the following even if you see very few on any one examination.
- *Gastric and bowel gas*: Is amount and location normal?
- *Check for organ size of liver, spleen, and kidneys if visible.*
- *Check for free peritoneal air*: Remember position of patient will change location of free air.
- *Look for calcifications and masses*: Can they be localized to a specific structure?

Right Chest Wall

Look for overall thickness, subcutaneous emphysema, and calcification. Look for sharp and distinct muscle fat planes.

Right Shoulder Girdle

- *Soft tissues*: Look again at overall amount, then check for the following: Calcifications, obvious mass effect, abnormal air collections (called subcutaneous emphysema), and soft-tissue companion shadow for the clavicle (this is a normal but variable finding).
- *Bones*: Look at each bone for the following items (notice again the progression from general to increasingly specific detail throughout the review). If your anatomic memory is hazy, refresh with a review of the gross anatomy radiology review program.
  - Overall size, shape, and contour of each bone
  - The density or mineralization
  - Compare cortical thickness to medullary cavity, trabecular pattern; look for erosions, fractures, or any lytic or blastic regions.
  - At joints, check whether articular relationships are normal, or look if joint spaces are narrowed, widened, or look for any calcification in the cartilages, air in the joint space, abnormal fat pads, etc.

Neck Soft Tissues and Spine

- Check overall amounts of soft tissue, presence of calcifications, subcutaneous emphysema, and position and size of trachea. For the cervical spine, check alignment and note any major congenital abnormalities.
- Then look at specific parts of the vertebra and disk spaces; check for erosions, lytic or blastic lesions, disk and synovial joint narrowing or other abnormalities.

Thoracic Spine and Rib Cage

Two reminders at this point:
1. Remember the principle of general to more detailed review in each section, concentrate on the skeletal detail—"look through" the mediastinum and lungs.
2. First check overall alignment of the spine and symmetry of the rib cage, double, and check bone density (This is a gross estimate).

Thoracic Spine

Look at specific parts of each vertebra and the disk spaces as far caudally as the image allows, compare frontal and lateral projections.

Some checklist items to watch for are: Height of vertebral bodies and disk spaces, integrity of cortical margins around the bodies, pedicles, and lamina, presence of any lytic or sclerotic areas, normal spacing of synovial joints, versus narrowing or sclerosis.

Ribs

Compare individual ribs side to side, check specific parts, cortical margins, and trabecular patterns. Make a note if the anterior cartilages are calcified, frequently the first one does so irregularly and may obscure or mimic underlying lung lesions.
- Posterior rib
- Anterior rib.

MEDIASTINUM GENERAL AND SUPERIOR

- An enormous amount of information about the mediastinum can be extracted from plain films.
- The key is a thorough knowledge of anatomical relationships and how structures are likely to project on a radiograph.
- Use of cross-sections from CT and MRI will supplement this section.
- Understand on plain films the mediastinum projects as a water density surrounded by the two air-filled lungs and intersected by the air-filled trachea and major bronchi.
- The interfaces of these air-soft tissue margins may be distorted by pathological processes, usually masses, that otherwise would be hidden in the mediastinum.

Mediastinum

- At this time, look at the overall size and shape of the entire mediastinum on the frontal and lateral views and decide if it is normal for the patient's age.
- Also look for obvious masses and calcifications, double check for tubes, electrical leads, a pacemaker or artificial valves.

- Check for evidence of mediastinal shift and if present, is the entire mediastinum shifted, or just a section of it.
- Look at the trachea and major bronchi for size, position, and presence of intraluminal masses.

Superior Mediastinum: Lateral

Although there are several methods of dividing the mediastinum into regions, this program will continue with the system taught in gross anatomy.

- The superior mediastinum begins at the root of the neck and ends caudally at a line drawn between T-4 vertebrae and the sternomanubrial junction. Usually that line skims the top of the aortic arch.
- The area between this line and the diaphragm is further divided into three regions: (1) Anterior, (2) middle, and (3) posterior. Basically, the heart and pericardium form the middle section, everything anterior to the heart is the anterior region, and everything posterior to the heart back to the spine is the posterior mediastinum.

Superior Mediastinum: Posteroanterior

- First, check the overall width for normal size, again look for masses, calcifications, and free air.
- The rest of the superior mediastinum review is a detailed search for subtle distortion of several major plural mediastinal interfaces.
- Not all of the following structures are seen on every film, but try to find them.

Margin of Superior Vena Cava

The superior vena cava (SVC) is seen on the frontal view only, and depending how laterally it projects, its right edge may cast a subtle line on the film. Sometimes the entire edge is seen, often only a portion, but it should not bulge into the lung with a convex border.

Superior Vena Cava

Look at the CT and superior vena cavogram to understand how the edge of the SVC may be seen on the plain frontal film.

Right Paratracheal Stripe

- The normal width is <5 mm, usually it is only 2-3 mm. This is an important marker for otherwise subtle adenopathy.
- The distal end of the stripe is formed by the azygous vein, and if the vein is distended, that portion of the stripe may normally be up to 1 cm wide.
- The medial margin of the stripe is the air-soft tissue interface along the right mucosal surface of the trachea.
- The outer margin of the stripe begins around the level of the medial end of the clavicle and is formed by the plural surface of the right upper lobe (RUL) against the mediastinum.
- The only structures normally at that level to give soft-tissue density between the air-filled trachea and the RUL are the right wall of the trachea, nerves, some fat, lymph nodes, and pleura of the RUL.
- The stripe ends where the RUL bronchus sweeps under the azygous vein as the latter arches anteriorly to empty into the posterior surface of the SVC.

Plain Tomogram of the Right Paratracheal Stripe

On this view, the azygous vein is distended giving a tear drop shape to the terminus of the stripe.

Computed Tomography at the Level of the Mid Trachea

The two accompanying CTs demonstrate why the right paratracheal stripe changes in thickness at the azygous arch.

Left Subclavian Stripe

The normal width is 1.0-1.5 cm. Its inner margin is the air mucosal interface along the left mucosal surface of the trachea, and its outer margin is the interface of the medial aspect of the left upper lobe against the lateral margin of the left subclavian artery. You usually will pick up the outer edge of the stripe at the level of the clavicle and will be able to follow it down to the bulge of the aortic arch.

Left Subclavian Stripe: CT

The accompanying CTs demonstrate why the left subclavian stripe is so wide.

Lateral View of Tracheal Wall

On the lateral view, the posterior tracheal wall, if visible, should measure no more than 4 mm.

ANTERIOR, MIDDLE, AND POSTERIOR MEDIASTINUM

- These regions are superimposed on the frontal view. The major structure is the heart. For all practical purposes, the pericardium will be inseparable from the heart on plain film views.
- Review the heart for overall size and shape. A rough yardstick for size on the frontal film is the ratio of the widest diameter of the heart to the widest width of the thoracic cage as measured from inner aspect of rib to rib. This cardiothoracic ratio should be <50%.
- Look carefully for calcifications, pneumopericardium, pneumomediastinum, sutures, prosthetic valves, etc., that you may have overlooked on the general survey of the entire mediastinum.

Heart

Follow the outline on both frontal and lateral views for specific chamber enlargement.

Computed Tomography at the Level of the Heart

Look at the CT and MR to reinforce heart-chamber relationships. See how these relationships correlate to chamber borders seen on the plain film.

Aorta

- Try tracking it from the root to distal descending aorta. In the young adult, the ascending aorta usually is hidden in the mediastinum; in older people, it may swing to the right enough to cast a soft-tissue bulge.
- The arch should always be seen; make sure it is to the left of the distal trachea and actually pushes the distal trachea slightly to the right.
- Check for aortic calcifications and size.
- The left lateral border of the descending aorta abuts the left lung. On the lateral view, the aorta is usually not seen.

Pulmonary Artery

- On the frontal view, the only part of the main pulmonary artery seen is the left lateral border where it meets the left lung.
- It can be relatively straight or convex (most commonly in young females).
- When convex, it forms a "middle mogul" just above the heart. The upper "mogul" is the aortic knob, the lower mogul is the left ventricle. The left pulmonary artery is directly behind the main pulmonary artery, and is visible on frontal films as a branching structure.

Azygoesophageal Line or Paraesophageal Line

This is seen on the frontal view only and is formed by the right lower lobe where it meets the portion of the mediastinum containing the esophagus and the azygous vein. It usually overlies the thoracic spine, at or near the midline, and is usually fairly straight, vertically. If it bulges convex toward the lung, be suspicious of a mediastinal mass, usually subcarinal lymph nodes or an enlarged left atrium.

Computed tomography of the azygoesophageal line: Use the CT image to understand exactly what structures form the border of the esophageal line. Air in the esophagus changes this edge into a line.

Right and Left Pulmonary Arteries

- On the frontal view, the left pulmonary artery is the soft-tissue density behind the main pulmonary artery, branching into the lung.
- The proximal right pulmonary artery is buried in the mediastinum, and is not seen on the frontal view until it branches as the right hilum.

Pulmonary Arteries: Lateral View

- The right pulmonary artery is seen on the lateral view as an ovoid branching structure, just anterior to the air column of the trachea and main bronchi.
- The left pulmonary artery is never seen as clearly as the right, unless it is markedly enlarged. It is a curved shadow, similar in shape to the aorta, just behind the air column.

Aorticopulmonary Window

- This is another area radiologists double check for subtle mediastinal masses. It is seen on the frontal view (line of white dots) and is formed by a portion of the upper lobe sitting in the space immediately lateral to the area between the aortic arch and left pulmonary artery (remember ligamentum arteriosum and left recurrent laryngeal nerve).
- The aorticopulmonary (AP) window should have a concave or straight border. If there is a mediastinal mass in the AP window region, the lung will be pushed laterally and the border becomes convex.

Paraspinal Edges (Stripes)

Sometimes on the frontal view, the plural edge is seen as a vertical density running parallel to the lateral margins of the vertebral bodies. If visible, this edge should be only a few millimeters beyond the vertebral bodies, and should not be lumpy or bulging. (The paraspinal edges are not visible on this image.)

Miscellaneous

On the lateral view, the anterior mediastinum cephalad to the heart in the adult should be lung-air density, not soft-tissue density. In infants and young children, thymus fills this area. Also check the posterior sternal margin for small masses that might represent internal thoracic lymph node enlargement.

Hila

Frontal View

- As visible on the frontal view, most of the hilar shadows are the left and right pulmonary arteries.
- The bronchi run with the arteries, but are, of course, lucent.
- The pulmonary veins are not clearly seen because they are behind the widest parts of the heart, inferior to the hila, where they converge into the left atrium.
- The left pulmonary artery is always more superior than the right, thus making the left hilum appear higher.
- Calcified lymph nodes may be visible within the hilar shadows.

Lateral View

Because both hila are superimposed on the lateral view, visualizing abnormalities is more difficult. Sometimes the left lower lobe pulmonary artery may present as a fairly discrete oblong density adjacent to the left main stem bronchus. We have already mentioned the variable appearance of the right main pulmonary artery.

Lungs

Compare overall size of one lung to the other, this is also a double check on your earlier look at the rib cage size.

At this time, look for major areas of abnormal lucency or density, and train your eyes to look through the heart and upper abdomen to lung posterior to these areas.

Blood Vessels in the Lungs

Compare the right and left upper lobes and right and left lower lobes for roughly equal distribution side to side.

Compare the size (diameter) of an upper lobe vessel in the middle third of the lung to a lower lobe vessel in the same middle zone of the lung.

In an upright person, the pressure differential is enough that the lower lobe vessel should be wider (i.e., larger) because blood flow is greater to this region. If they are the same size or reversed in size, redistribution of flow has occurred. Be careful, this phenomenon does not apply if the person is semirecumbent or supine.

Parenchyma

Large abnormalities will have already been seen, but now is the time to search carefully for small masses, infiltrates, calcifications, etc. Compare small sections of lung side to side at a time.

Use the same techniques as you used for comparing ribs but now ignore the bone and look at the lung.

There are three areas in which small lung lesions are easily overlooked:
1. Behind the calcified anterior first rib cartilage
2. Behind the heart
3. Behind the diaphragm

Lateral View of the Lung

The lateral view is your great chance to look at the lung in the posterior costophrenic recess and anterior mediastinum.

Pleura

Check the frontal view for minor fissure thickness and location, and on the lateral view, look for minor and major fissures even if you do not see them in their entirety which you rarely will. These are normally fine delicate structures that do not show up on the digitized images.

Anteroposterior View of the Pleura

Follow the pleural surface around the lung periphery making the following observations:
- On the frontal view, the apex of the hemidiaphragms should be in the mid third of each hemithorax with the right hemidiaphragm usually 2–2.5 cm higher than the left. The costophrenic angles laterally should be sharp.
- The lung should abut right up against the inner margins of the rib cage. If the pleural space is widened by fluid or mass, the lung will be pushed away by soft-tissue density.
- Also check for pleural calcifications, and presence of pneumothorax.

Lateral View of the Pleura

On the lateral view, follow the pleura into the posterior costophrenic recess and if possible along the inner aspect of the posterior ribs. Recheck along the posterior sternal margin.

CHECKLIST

- Check patient name, position, and technical quality.
- Soft tissue including breast, chest wall, and companion shadow.
- Review soft tissues and skeletal structures of shoulder girdles and chest wall.
- Review abdomen for bowel gas, organ size, abnormal calcifications, free air, etc.
- Review soft tissues and spine of neck.
- *Review spine and rib cage*: Check alignment, disk space narrowing, lytic or blastic regions, etc.
- Review mediastinum, overall size and shape.
- *Trachea*: position, margins—SVC, ascending aorta, right atrium, left subclavian artery, aortic arch, main.
- Pulmonary artery, left ventricle.
- *Lines and stripes*: Paratracheal, paraspinal, paraesophageal (azygoesophageal), para-aortic retrosternal clear space.
- Review hila.

PRACTICE REPORTING CHEST X-RAY

- Normal relationships
- Size
- Review lungs and pleura
- Compare lung sizes
- *Evaluate pulmonary vascular pattern*: Compare upper to lower lobe, right to left, normal tapering to periphery.
- Pulmonary parenchyma
- Pleural surfaces
- Fissures—major and minor—if seen
- Compare hemidiaphragms
- Follow pleura around rib cage.

This step-by-step guide is for practice for chest X-ray film you encounter. The methodology will not let you forget any significant findings.

Index

Page numbers followed by *b* refer to box, *f* refer to figure, *fc* refer to flowchart, and *t* refer to table

A

Abdomen 657
Abetalipoproteinemia 398
Abortions, recurrent spontaneous 63
Abrasions 626
Absolute neutrophil count 261, 285, 304
Absolute reticulocyte count 261, 285
Acanthocyte 267, 268*f*
Acanthosis 567
Accidental aspiration 344
Acetaminophen 386
    administration of 151
Acetazolamide 505
Acetone-inactivated vaccine 104
Acetylcholinesterase 603
Acid
    base status 244
    fast bacilli 68, 168, 173, 335
    reflux 194
    suppression 208
Acidosis 448, 481
Acne 538
    comedogenic 627
    mild 627
    moderate 627
    neonatal 88
    neonatorum 35
    nodulocytic 628
    severe 627
    site of 627
    vulgaris 627
Acrodermatitis enteropathica 14, 15
Acroparesthesias 609
Acropustulosis, infantile 87-89
Actinobacillus 486
Activated partial thromboplastin time 61, 208, 288, 297, 476, 547
Acute blood transfusion reaction 305
    diagnosis of 305
    management of 305
Acute liver failure 223, 231, 233, 235*ft*, 242, 243, 245, 249
    causes of 233*t*
    management of 235*t*
Acute respiratory distress syndrome 162, 185, 342
Acyclovir 407
    oral 152
    parenteral 152
    prophylaxis 301
Adapalene 627

Adefovir 240
Adenine 592
Adenoids 310
Adenosine
    deaminase 332
    triphosphate 58
Adenovirus 139, 309, 315, 318, 328
    infection 501
Adipose tissue lipolysis releases glycerol 51
Adrenal androgens 536
Adrenocorticotropic hormone 54, 397, 510, 540
Adrenocorticotropin 373
Adriamycin 292
Advisory Committee for Vaccines and Immunization Practices 101, 105, 107, 151
Aggression 359
Airflow limitation 325
Air-fluid level 313
Airway 595
    compression of 326
    disease 80
    maintenance 59
Akinetic-rigid syndrome 391
Alagille syndrome 416, 422
Alanine
    aminotransferase 187, 223, 231, 238, 401, 546
    transaminase 283
Albendazole 27, 28
Albumin, serum 224, 496
Aldurazyme 609
Aliphatic hydrocarbon 342
Alkaline phosphatase 7, 8, 204, 224
Alkaptonuria 92
Allergen immunotherapy 18, 326
Allergenic food 18
Allergic conjunctivitis 638, 639
    treatment of 640
Allergic rhinitis 310, 311
Allergy
    skin prick test 18*f*
    testing for 313
Allogenic hematopoietic stem cell transplantation 289
    types of 300*fc*
All-trans retinoic acid 261
Alpha-1
    acid glycoprotein 558
    antitrypsin deficiency 339

Alpha-adrenergic blockers 517
Alpha-blocker 508
Alpha-chains 281
Alpha-fetoprotein 217, 225, 234, 239, 247, 600, 601, 651
    serum 243
Alpha-glucosidase 609
Alpha-hemolytic streptococci 564
Ambulatory blood pressure monitoring 511
Amebic liver abscess 141
Amenorrhea, primary 582
American Academy of Neurology Guidelines 384
American Academy of Pediatrics 74, 91, 114, 361, 382
American Association for Study of Liver Diseases 395
American College of Chest Physicians 339
American College of Obstetricians and Gynecologists 600
American College of Rheumatology 552, 556-558
American Heart Association 561, 565*t*, 571
Amikacin 171, 379
Amino acid 589
Aminoglycoside 487, 494
Aminotransferase, serum 150
Amitriptyline 194
Amlodepine 503
Ammonia 244, 594
    serum 225
Ammonium tetrathiomolybdate 393
Amniocentesis 603
Amniotic fluid measurement 62
Amoxicillin 40, 141, 154, 172, 270, 313, 331, 494, 629
Amphotericin B 301
Ampicillin 33, 141, 335, 494
Amylase, serum 213
Amylophagia 270
Analgesics 194, 279
Anaphylactic reaction 97
Anaphylaxis, causes of 18
Ancillary test 392
Ancylostoma 27
Andersen-Tawil syndrome 482
Androgen 538
    insensitivity syndrome 538, 541
Anemia 246, 264, 264*t*, 473, 555, 608, 641
    causes of 260*t*
    congenital

dyserythropoietic 269
  sideroblastic 284
  history of 265
  megaloblastic 267, 273
  microangiopathic hemolytic 266
  microcytic 270t
  normocytic 264, 269fc
  physiologic 33, 265
  severe 166
Angelman syndrome 585, 589
Angina 460
Angioedema 17, 615, 616
  pathogenesis of 616
Angiography 442
Angiotensin receptor blocker 466, 511, 560
Angiotensin-converting enzyme 184, 217, 246, 416, 431, 459, 466, 500, 547
  inhibitor 466, 511, 560
Anhidrotic ectodermal dysplasia 603
Anisochromia 267, 267f
Anisocytosis 267
Ann Arbor staging system 292
Anomalous coronary arteries, theories behind origin of 455
Anomalous left coronary artery 419, 455, 465
Anorectal malformation 654
  classification of 654t
Antacids 499
Antegrade continence enema 196
Anterior abdominal wall defects 650
Anthropometry 227, 234, 526, 539
Antiandrogens 627
Antiarrhythmic drugs 474
Antibiotics 40, 193, 214, 280, 289, 629
  choice of 280, 331t
  doses 133t
  oral 154, 627
  prolonged use of 47
  prophylaxis 494, 494t
  systemic 617, 628
  therapy 34, 140, 564
  topical 628
Antibodies, polyclonal 321
Anticardiolipin 547
  antibodies 63
Anticold 629
Anticonvulsants 28, 273, 389, 506, 589
Anticyclic citrullinated peptide antibodies 546
Antidandruff lotion 638
Antidepressants 193
Antidiphtheria serum 132
Antiepileptics 629
  drugs 163, 370, 373, 382, 383
  therapy 382
Antifolate 273
Antifungals 289
  drugs 622
Antigen
  detection assay 27
  presenting cells 101

Antigenic drift 113
Anti-gliadin antibody 201
Antihistamines 625
  oral 617, 619t
Antihistaminic agents 193
Anti-hyaluronidase 563
Antihypertensive drugs 512t
Anti-inflammatory drugs 378, 637
Antimalarials 280
  drug 280
Antimicrobials 289
Anti-Müllerian hormone 538, 540
Antineoplastics 289
Antineutrophil cytoplasmic antibody 192, 497, 546, 547
Antinuclear antibody 234, 497, 503, 510, 546, 549, 554, 555
Antiparasitic drugs 27
Antiphospholipid antibody 547, 556
  syndrome 545
Antipsychotics 397
Antipyretics 144, 316, 362, 633
Antirabies vaccination 116
Antiretroviral 71, 159
  therapy 71, 158, 172, 378
Anti-ribonuclear protein 555
Anti-rickettsial drugs, summary of 164t
Anti-saccharomyces cerevisiae antibody 192
Anti-Smith antibody 555
Antismooth muscle antibody 234
Antispasmodic 193
  drops 44
Antistreptococcal antibody 546
Antistreptolysin O 389, 465, 503, 546, 563
Anti-thyroperoxidase, titers of 522
Anti-tissue transglutaminase 201, 529
  immunoglobulin A 201
Anti-tubercular
  therapy 335
  treatment 68, 69, 171, 378
Antivirals 280
  agents 407
  drug 280
Aorta 445, 447-449, 455, 457, 458
  arch, interrupted 416
  coarctation of 415, 464, 509
Aortic cusp prolapse 427
Aortic regurgitation 426, 450
Aortic stenosis 416, 450
  severe 464
Aphasia-convulsion syndrome 367
Aplastic anemia 284, 285, 287, 300
  acquired 286
  complications of 287
Aplastic crisis 279
Apnea 51
Appetite 334
Arachnoiditis 169
Arginine 597

Argininosiccinate lyase deficiency 597
Argininosuccinic acid 597
Arnold-Chiari syndrome 406
Array comparative genomic hybridization 416
Arrhythmias 419
  cardiac 343, 472
  management of 460
Arrhythmogenic right ventricular cardiomyopathy 469
Artemisinin 28
  combination therapy 166
Arterial blood gas 418, 422, 465
  analysis 594
Arterial embolism 486
Arterial switch operation 450, 450f
Arteriovenous fistula, systemic 464
Arteriovenous malformation 409
Arteritis, necrotizing 462
Arthralgia 176
Arthritis 11, 551
  childhood 552
  enthesitis-related 547, 549, 551
  juvenile idiopathic 286, 548, 550t, 554
  poststreptococcal reactive 546
  rheumatoid 549
  systemic-onset juvenile idiopathic 552, 572
Arthropod-borne disease 161
Articaria, acute 616
Ascaris 27
Ascites 216
  grading of 216t
Ascitic adenosine deaminase 217
Ascitic fluid 216
Ascorbic acid 187
Asparaginase 289
Aspartate
  aminotransferase 223, 231, 283, 401, 546, 567
  transaminase 394
Asphyxia 464
Aspiration
  pneumonitis 332
  simple 340
Asthma 311, 325, 327
  bronchial 326
  control 324
  history of 618
Astrocytoma 397
Ataxia 391, 396, 396t, 399, 568
  acute 397
  chronic 398
  congenital 396
  recurrent 397
  subacute 397
  telangiectasia 396, 398, 593
Atelectasis 343
Atherosclerosis, prevention of 557
Atopic dermatitis 90, 618, 619

itchy skin condition 618
  management of 618
Atrial fibrillation 456, 476
Atrial septal defect 64, 415, 421, 427, 429, 435, 451, 464, 602
Atrial switching 449
Atrioventricular canal defect 464
Atrioventricular conduction disorders 484
Atrioventricular node 472
Atrioventricular re-entrant tachycardia 473
Atrioventricular septal defect 435, 436
  physiology of 436f
Atrioventriular communis 581
Attack, recurrent 562
Attention deficit hyperactivity disorder 357, 364, 400
Auscultation 417, 456
Autism
  behavior checklist 357
  diagnostic observational schedule 358
  early indicators of 356
  pathway 359fc
  red flags for 82t
  spectrum disorder 356-358
Autistic regression 357
Autoantibody 293, 558
  panel 555
Autoimmune diseases, chronic 405
Autoimmune disorders 285, 300
Autoimmune hemolytic anemia 266, 545
Autoimmune thrombocytopenia 262
Autoimmune thyroid disease 521
Autoinflammatory diseases, tests for 547
Automated auditory brainstem response 92
Automated blood culture systems 48
Automated external defibrillator 3
Autonomic dysfunction, tests of 399
Autonomic system abnormalities 60
Autosomal abnormality, common chromosomal disorders of 581
Autosomal dominant 398
  ataxias 399
Autosomal recessive 15, 398
  ataxias 399
Axillary hair 582
Azathioprine 273, 285, 559, 560
Azithromycin 22, 141, 154, 331, 619
Azygoesophageal line 659
  computed tomography of 659

B

Bacillary index 173
Bacillus cereus 20
Bacillus-calmette-guérin 68, 172, 184, 379, 453, 571
Baclofen 354
Bactec method 48
Bacteria
  prevent entry of 514
  shedding of 22

Bacterial foodborne diseases 20fc
Bacterium's ability 170
Bacteriuria, asymptomatic 491
Bag and mask ventilation 3
Balloon atrial septostomy 446, 448, 449f, 466
Band pattern 580, 591
Bar code sign 339
Barker hypothesis 62
Barth syndrome 241
Bartonella henselae 568
Basal ganglia 391f
Basal metabolic index 557
Basophilia, causes of 263b
Basophilic stippling 266, 266f
Basophils 262
Battle sign 408, 409
Bayley scales 79
Becker Duchenne muscular dystrophy 400, 603
Beckwith-Wiedemann syndrome 53
Bedaquiline 172
Behavior, abnormal 47
Belimumab 557
Bell's palsy 406, 407
Bendamustine 292
Benzodiazepines 354
Benzoyl peroxide 627
Berlin-Frankfurt-muenster 289
Beta-2 glycoprotein 547
Beta-adrenergic blockers 473
Beta-blocker 343, 459, 466, 471, 483
Beta-globin 281
Beta-hemolytic streptococci 561
Beta-human chorionic gonadotropin 600
Beta-hydroxybutyrate 51, 53
Beta-ketothiolase 244
Beta-thalassemia 277, 281, 283
Bicarbonate 53
Bile acid 225
  synthesis defect 225, 242, 243
  transport disorders 242
Biliary atresia 220
Biliary sludge 204
Bilirubin 268, 603
  serum 63, 153, 223, 285
Biochemical
  disturbances 63
  markers 600f, 600t
  tests 204
Biochemistry 61
Biopsy 289
Biotin 598
Biotinidase deficiency 92
Birth
  asphyxia 58, 84
    acute management of 59
  injuries 648
Birt-Hogg-Dube syndrome 339
Bitot's spots 12

Black measles 144
Bladder 514
  calculations 515
  drainage 652
  problems 514
  retraining 516
Blalock-Taussig shunt 443
Bleomycin 292
Blepharitis 637
  anterior 637
  posterior 637
  ulcerative 637, 638
Blindness, congenital 578
Blood
  absorption time of 92
  brain barrier 117, 364
  component therapy 303
  count 386
  culture 48
  donor, hematocrit level of 92
  flow, direction of 455f
  gas 53, 60, 529
    values 409
  glucose 465, 531
    target recommendations 532t
  loss 545
  pressure 59, 278, 417, 502, 509, 525, 557
    measurement, technique for 510t
    noninvasive 59
  sample 3
  tests, techniques for 92
  transfusion 279, 280, 282, 289, 641
    reaction, acute 305
  urea nitrogen 198, 207, 496, 560
  vessels 660
Bloody diarrhea 22
Bloom syndrome 593
Blount's disease 525, 645
Blueberry muffin rash 72, 181
B-lymphocyte stimulator 557
Body
  energy, mobilizing of 579
  mass index 251, 521, 524, 525
  surface area 570, 629
Bone 169
  infection of 646
  marrow 274, 300
    aspirate 269
    examinations 244, 285, 294
    transplantation 286, 287, 301
Borderline leprosy 173
Bordetella parapertussis 138
Bordetella pertussis 138
Borrelia burgdorferi 406
Botulinum toxin 354
Bow legs 35, 645
Bowel dysfunction 515
Bowel movement, frequency of 195
Brachial plexus injuries 646
Brachycephaly 581

Bradycardia 483
    severe 464
Brain
    abnormalities 601
    evoked response auditory 83
    iron accumulation 351
    natriuretic peptide 465
Brainstem
    aura 385
    evoked response audiometry 70, 79, 589
    glioma 397
    lesion 381
Breast
    engorgement of 39
    insufficient drainage of 40
    milk diarrhea 37
    nipples, contaminated 34
    tissue 657
        bacterial infection of 40
    underdeveloped 582
Breastfeeding 39, 40, 100, 321
    frequency 41
    proper technique of 42
Breath
    holding spells 374
    shortness of 185
British Thoracic Society 339
Broad-spectrum anthelmintics 28
Bronchiolitis 318, 326, 330
Bronchoalveolar lavage 330, 336
Bronchodilators 320
Bronchopleural fistula 335, 337, 341
Bronchopulmonary dysplasia 319, 324, 327, 431
    development of 62
Bronchoscopy
    fiberoptic 345
    rigid 345
Brown fat, deficiency of 56
Brucellosis 306
Brugada syndrome 481, 483
Brushfield spots 581
Budd-Chiari syndrome 216, 234
Budesonide 311
Bulging fissure sign 336
Bull's eye appearance 560
Bull-neck appearance 131
Bullous impetigo 89, 626
Burr cell 268f
Burst suppression pattern 372
Byler's bile 244

C

Cabot's rings 266, 267f
Café-au-lait spots 535
Calaptin 471
Calaspargase pegol 289
Calcaneal valgus foot 645
Calcification, proximal zone of 8

Calcineurin inhibitors 250, 498, 560
Calcitonin gene-related peptide 388
Calcium 9, 63, 505, 560
    administration 8
    carbonate stones 203
    channel 398
    channel blocker 193, 462, 471, 508, 511
    serum 447
Campylobacter infections 23
Cancer
    antigen 217
    familial 578
    prone disease 578
Cancrum oris 143
Candida albicans 41
Candidal diaper dermatitis 88
Candidiasis, congenital 88
Cannabis 354
Capillary refill time 59
Capreomycin 171, 379
Caput quadratum 7
Caput succedaneum 32, 34, 36
Carbamazepine 28, 367, 383, 389, 397, 415
    doses of 367
Carbamoyl-phosphate synthetase deficiency 603
Carbohydrate-deficient glycoprotein syndrome 248
Carboplatin 292
Carboxypeptidase1 genes 213
Carcinoembryonic antigen 217
Carcinoma-in-situ 541t
Cardiac catheterization 419, 423, 426, 438, 442, 448, 457, 462, 465, 471, 480
Cardiac disease, signs of 63
Cardiac enzymes 58, 457
Cardiac failure 463
    congestive 433, 434, 438, 451, 459, 487
Cardiac magnetic resonance imaging 419, 426, 466
Cardiac resynchronization therapy 467, 471
Cardiac size 433, 438, 442f
Cardiac transplantation 462
Cardiobacterium 486
Cardiology 413
Cardiomegaly 419, 452, 459
Cardiomyopathy 53, 475, 459, 464, 469
    causes of 469, 470t
    dilated 459, 465, 469
    hypertrophic 417, 469
    obstructive 459
    symptoms of 469, 469t
    transient hypertrophic 63
Cardiophrenic angle, obliteration of 461
Cardiovascular disease 164, 525
Cardiovascular system 17, 59, 61, 343
Carditis 562, 563
Caroli disease 248
Caroli syndrome 248
Carpenter syndrome 417

Cartridge-based nucleic acid amplification test 170, 334
Carvedilol 471
Case fatality rate 120
Cataract 148
    congenital 640
    developmental 640
Catchup vaccine 151
Cationic trypsinogen 213
Cefaclor 331
Cefixime 22, 154
Cefotaxime 331, 494
Cefpodoxime 22
Ceftriaxone 280, 331, 335, 494
Cefuroxime 331
Celiac disease 14, 15, 195, 201, 202fc
Cell
    culture vaccines 118
    free fragments 600
    mediated immunity 168
Cellular abscess 337
Centers for Disease Control and Prevention 80, 108, 114
Central nervous system 56, 58, 61, 67, 169, 176, 222, 288, 342, 349, 357, 361, 376, 453, 487, 535, 568, 609
    disease 289
    infection 158
    involvement 153
    tuberculosis 169
        classification of 376, 376b
Central pontine myelinolysis 392
Cephalexin 619
Cephalhematoma 32, 34, 36, 648
Cephalic tetanus 136
Cephalosporins 33, 141
Cerebellar ataxis, postinfectious 397
Cerebellar integrity, assessment of 399t
Cerebellitis, acute 397
Cerebral blood flow 408
Cerebral palsy 349, 350f, 351, 354f
    early signs of 350b
    management of 353f
    mimickers 350
    types of 351t
Cerebral perfusion pressure 410
Cerebral salt wasting syndrome 377, 411
Cerebrospinal fluid 48, 67, 100, 147, 153, 158, 163, 169, 364, 372, 378, 386, 399, 408, 410, 596, 648
    interpretation of 361
    otorrhea 409
    pleocytosis of 378, 571
Cerebrovascular accidents 397
Ceruloplasmin 225, 558
    serum 225, 243, 392
Cervarix 111
Cervical cancer 109
Cervical lymphadenitis 316
Cervicovaginal infection 603

Cestodes 27
Chagas disease 306
Chaotic atrial tachycardia 475
Chaperone therapy 610
Chelation, drugs for 392
Chemoprophylaxis 317, 565t
Chemotherapy 28
Cherry red spot 243f
Chest
    pain 461, 462
    syndrome, acute 279
    X-ray 48, 170, 186, 187, 288, 319, 332, 339, 343-345, 419, 433, 438, 444, 447, 451, 459, 461, 462, 465, 503, 609, 630
        abnormal 68
Chick embryo cell vaccine, purified 118
Chickenpox 66, 117
Childhood autism screening test 357
Childhood hypothyroidism 521
    causes of 521b
    signs of 521t
    symptoms of 521t
Childhood obesity 203, 524
    comorbidities of 526t
    etiology of 524t, 526t
Chimeric vaccine 122
Chlamydia
    oculogenitalis 639
    pneumonia 328, 331
Chloramphenicol 141, 182
Chloroquine 174
Cholangiography, intraoperative 221
Cholecalciferol 8
Cholecystectomy 204
Cholecystitis 204
    acute 204
    chronic 204
Choledocholithiasis 204
Cholelithiasis 54
Cholera 181
    vaccine, oral 181
Cholestasis 220, 232, 244, 246
    chronic 243
    etiologies of 220fc
Cholestatic disease 221t
Cholesterol stones 203
Chondromalacia patellae 391
Chorea 563
    paralytica 389
Chorioamnionitis 47, 71, 349
Chorionic villus sampling 594, 602, 604
Choroid plexus cyst 602
Chromosomal abnormalities 372, 580, 591
Chromosomal analysis 372, 589
Chromosomal disorders 578, 580, 581
Chronic obstructive pulmonary disease 338
Chronicity index 559
Ciclesonide 311
Cilastatin 172

Ciprofloxacin 172, 182
Circulation 595
Circulatory system 60
Cirrhosis 14, 224
Clarithromycin 172, 174, 331, 619
Clavicle fracture 646
Clavulanate 172, 313
Clavulanic acid 336
Cleft
    lip 649
    palate 649
Clindamycin 336, 626
Clobazam 362
Clobetasol 619
Clofazimine 172, 174
Clonazepam 370
Clonorchis 27
Clostridium
    botulinum 20
    tetani 134
Cloxacillin 335, 619, 629
Club foot 645
Coamoxiclav 331
Cochlear implant 102
Coenzyme A 470
Cognitive behavior therapy 193, 194
Colchicine 273
Cold
    common 309
    compresses 640
    environment 56
    linen 56
    stress 56
Colic crying-colic cycle 44
Colichine 174
Colostrum, discarding of 47
Coma 3, 589
Comedones 627
Communication disorder 358
Comparative genomic hybridization 358
Complementation test 269
Complete blood count 22, 25, 49, 61, 69, 140, 157, 178, 198, 208, 211, 221, 243, 259, 265, 270, 279, 288, 293, 297, 329, 335, 361, 375, 306, 405, 441, 487, 493, 502, 555, 630
Complete heart block 427, 464, 485
Computed tomography 58, 69, 81, 83, 186, 192, 198, 204, 228, 246, 253, 332, 334, 336, 352, 383, 386, 389, 406, 408, 410, 442, 503, 510, 641, 644, 648, 656, 658, 659
    angiography 212
    criteria 380
    scan 339, 380
Computer vision syndrome 641
Concomitant serum albumin 232
Congenital adrenal hyperplasia 91, 510, 511, 535, 538, 539, 541
Conjugation, defective 223

Conjunctiva, chemosis of 639
Conjunctival petechiae 486
Conjunctival xerosis 12
Conjunctivitis 638
    bacterial 638
    giant papillary 639
    infective 639
    phlyctenular 640
    seasonal allergic 639
    viral 638
Conradi Hunermann syndrome 580
Consciousness
    impaired 166
    level of 51
Constipation 515
    chronic 195
    severe 194
Continent epispadias 650
Continuous glucose monitoring 532
Continuous positive airway pressure 319, 320
Continuous subcutaneous insulin infusion 530
Contrast-enhanced computed tomography 27, 213, 230, 380, 381
Convulsions 3, 185, 186
    generalized 366
    history of 376
Coombs' test 295, 545, 556
Copper, serum 392
Cor triatriatum 462
Cord care 32
Corneal surface 12
Corneal ulceration 12
Corneal xerosis 12
Cornelia de Lange syndrome 417
Coronary arteriogram 457f, 458f
Coronary artery
    aneurysm 453
    bypass grafting 572
    disease 570
Coronavirus disease-2019 (COVID-19) 182-185
    disease, stages of 185f
Corticosteroids 171, 289, 316, 320, 373, 378, 382, 384, 556, 572
    side effects 500
Corynebacterium diphtheriae 131, 180
Coryza 315
Cotrimoxazole
    preventive therapy 159
    prophylaxis 72, 100
Cow's milk 195
    protein allergy 17
Coxiella burnetii 486
Coxsackievirus 630
    B 566
    infection 151
C-peptide 529
Cradle cap 38

Cranial irradiation 289
Cranial nerve palsy 411
Craniotabes 7, 34
C-reactive protein 13, 25, 47, 163, 186, 192, 271, 278, 329, 335, 386, 389, 453, 465, 493, 545, 551, 563
    levels 405
Creatine kinase 546, 609
    levels 405
Creatine phosphokinase 58, 403, 405, 465
Creatinine 558
    phosphokinase 243
    serum 166, 496
Crepitations, post-tussive increase of 169
Creutzfeldt-Jakob disease 399
Crigler-Najjar syndrome 223242
Crocodile tears 407
Crohn's disease 14, 492
Crossing legs 513
Croup 315
Crown rump length 599
Cryoprecipitate 179, 304
Cryotherapy 641
Cryptogenic West syndrome 372, 373
Crystalloids, dextrose-containing 214
Cubital fossa 618
Culture-negative neutrocytic ascites 217
Cushing's disease 262, 527
Cushing's syndrome 510
Cutis marmorata 88
    alba 89
    telangiectasia congenita 89
Cyanosis 185, 462
    cardiac causes of 420
    central 186, 420
    peripheral 420
Cyanotic spells 51
Cyclophosphamide 289, 292, 501, 560
    intravenous 560
Cycloserine 172
Cyclosporine 194, 250, 498, 630
Cyst
    classification of 380
    intraventricular 381
    popliteal 645
Cysteine 505
Cystic fibrosis 92, 195, 242, 244, 324, 327, 336
    transmembrane generator 213
Cysticercal encephalitis 380
Cysticidal drugs 382, 383*t*
    therapy 382
Cysticidal encephalitis 384
Cystinuria 508
Cystitis 491
    acute hemorrhagic 492
    eosinophilic 492
    hemorrhagic 301
Cytarabine 289
Cytolysis 67

Cytomegalovirus 72, 84, 147, 156, 227, 228, 250, 262, 285, 303, 328, 372, 629
    infection, congenital 72
Cytoplasmic antineutrophil cytoplasmic antibody 503, 510
Cytosine 592
    morphologic analysis 289
Cytotoxic T-lymphocyte antigen haplotype 632
Cytotoxicity theory 561

D

Dacarbazine 292
Dacryocystitis, congenital 637
Dark adaptometry 13
Dark-field microscopy 70
Dasatinib 289
Daunorubicin 289
Daytime incontinence 515
D-dimer 288
    levels 186
Deafness, congenital 578
Deep brain stimulation 354
Dehydration 4
Dehydroepiandrosterone-sulfate 534
Demodex folliculorum 638
Dengue 141, 176, 179, 234
    classification of 177*fc*
    hemorrhagic fever 176
    management 178
    severe 176
    shock syndrome 176
    treatment of 178*fc*, 179*fc*
    virus 176
        isolation of 177
Dental care 75
Denver development screening test 81
Deoxyribonucleic acid 238, 239
Depression 195
Dermatitis
    herpetiformis 151
    neonatal irritant 90
Dermatomal vesicular rash 150
Dermatomyositis, juvenile 546, 566
Dermatosis, neonatal 87
Detrusor antispasmodics 517
Device
    implantation 471
    therapy 467
Dexamethasone 289
Diabetes Control and Complications trial 532
Diabetes insipidus 411
Diabetes mellitus 115, 510
    gestational 53, 63, 446
    maternal 415
    type 1 529
    type 2 529
Diametric inhibin A 601
Diamidino-2-phenylindole 592

Diamond-Blackfan
    anemia 284, 300
    syndrome 285
Diarrhea 15, 15*b*, 33, 227
    acute 23
    chronic 14
    persistent 265
Diazepam 137, 361
Diazoxide 54
Dibutyl phthalate 617
Dicarboxylic acid 597
Diepoxybutane test 269
Diet
    restriction 560
    therapy 25
Dietary copper 395
Dietary interventions 193, 196
Dietary modification 194
Diethyl toluamide 617
Diethylenetriaminepentaacetic acid 653
Dietl's crisis 653
Differential leukocyte count 496
Diffusion-weighted imaging 409
DiGeorge syndrome 416, 422
Digital intelligence 82
Digital rectal examination 210
Digitalis 482
Digoxin 459, 467
Dihydrotestosterone 540
Dilute russell viper venom time 547
Dimercaptosuccinic acid 493, 510
Diphenhydramine 152
Diphenylhydantoin 481
Diphtheria 101, 131, 136, 180
    tetanus toxoids and whole-cell pertussis 43
    toxoid 95
    vaccine against 139
Direct antiglobulin test 269, 293
Direct observation chart 81, 81*t*
Directly observed therapy 175
Disaccharides 193
Discoid meniscus 645
Disease-modifying antirheumatic drugs 546
Disseminated intravascular coagulation 84, 140, 162, 225, 297, 305
Ditropan 514
Diuretics 466
Dopamine
    infusion 306
    receptor antagonists 389
Doppler examinations 438
Double-balloon enteroscopy 212
Double-blind placebo-controlled 18
Double-outlet right ventricle 421, 481
Down's syndrome 372, 416, 422, 438, 580, 581, 591, 600
    screening tests 600*t*
Doxorubicin 289

Doxycycline 22, 154, 182, 626, 628
D-penicillamine 392
Dried blood spot 606
Drug
    rash 560
    reaction 630
    sensitivity test 171
    therapy 404, 622
Dry blood spot 72
Dry pleurisy 332
Dry skin, generalized 618
Dual-energy X-ray absorptiometry 251
Duchenne muscular dystrophy 400, 593
Duck embryo vaccine, purified 118
Duodenal atresia 602
Duodenal ulcers 206
Dysfunctional elimination syndrome 515
Dyshidrotic eczema 87
Dyshormonogenesis 521
Dyskeratosis congenita 285
Dyskinesia, primary ciliary 324
Dyslipidemia 525, 567
Dysmorphism 399
Dysmorphology 587
Dysostosis multiplex 608
Dyspepsia, functional 191
Dysphagia 566
Dysphonia 566
Dyspnea, exertional 462
Dysrhythmia, cardiac 17
Dystonia 395
Dystonic syndrome 391
Dystrophin 400, 402

E

Ebstein anomaly 419, 422, 423, 451, 464
Ebstein-Barr virus 262
Echinocyte 267, 268f
Echocardiogram 289, 419, 433, 438, 487
Echocardiography 58, 278, 405, 423, 430, 442, 446, 451, 457, 457f, 459, 462, 470, 589
    functional 59
    transthoracic 426
Eclampsia 62
Ecosprin 454
Ectoderm dysplasia 588
Ectopic atrial tachycardia 473, 475
Ectopic tachycardia, junctional 473
Ectopic testis 649
Eczema 310
    herpeticum 620
    subacute 618
Edema 615
    management of 499fc
    perilesional 381
    pulmonary 166, 326, 459
Edmonston-Zagreb strain 144
Edwards syndrome 591
Ehlers-Danlos syndrome 339

Eikenella 486
Ejection systolic murmur 446
Elaprase 609
Electric breast pumps 40
Electrocardiogram 419, 437, 456, 656
Electrocardiography 58, 283, 422, 426, 430, 433, 441, 447, 451, 459, 462, 465, 470, 480, 596
Electroencephalography 58, 352, 361, 363, 364f, 366, 367, 367f, 369, 371, 375, 397, 410
    isolated 366
Electrolytes 60, 594
    imbalance 87, 200
    serum 329, 465, 496, 529
Electromyography 403, 589
Electron microscopy 269
Elevated serum transaminases 571
Elispot assay 630
Elixir 196
Elliptocyte 267, 268f
Elliptocytosis, hereditary 267
Embryo, direct visualization of 603
Embryological truncus arteriosus, division of 455
Emicizumab 298
Empirical antibiotic, choice of 49t
Empirical therapy 487
Empyema 335, 337
    thoracis 334
        management of 335fc
Enalapril 503
Encephalitis 120, 141
    causes of 120
    postinfectious 149
    syndrome, acute 120
Encephalomyelitis
    acute disseminated 397
    postinfectious 143
Encephalopathy 58, 140, 198
Encopresis 515
Endemic disease 166
Endocardial cushion
    defect 435, 436, 438, 581
    development of 435
Endocardial fibroelastosis 460
Endocarditis 555
    bacterial 423, 443
    infectious 486
Endocrine
    disruptors 538
    effects 301
    issues 251
    management 401
Endocrinology 519
Endomyocardial biopsy 466, 480
Endomyocardial fibrosis 460
Endomysial antibody 192, 201
Endoscopic retrograde cholangiopancreatography 205, 214

Endoscopic sclerotherapy 208
Endoscopic therapy 212
Endoscopic third ventriculostomy 377
Endoscopic variceal ligation 209
Endoscopy 208
Endothelin receptor antagonist bosentan 462
Energy
    failure, secondary 58
    metabolism disorders 241
    utilization 59
Entecavir 240
Enteric duplication cyst 210
Enteric fever 140
Enterobacter 494
Enterobiasis 27
Enterocolitis, Hirschsprung-associated 210
Enteroscopy 212
Enterovirus 139, 405, 566, 632
    coxsackievirus 632
Enuresis episodes 515
Enzyme 603
    assays 589
    immunoassay 70, 330
    linked immunoelectrotransfer-blot 381
    linked immunosorbent assay 66, 153, 154, 162, 173, 177, 192, 546, 633
    replacement therapy 607, 609
Eosinophilia 560, 630
    causes of 262b
Eosinophils 262, 309
Ependymoma 397
Epicutaneous test 17
Epidermal necrosis 630
Epidermolysis bullosa 89
    letalis 603
Epidermophyton 622
Epigenetic phenomenon 584
Epiglottitis 315, 316
Epilepsy 362, 378
    benign childhood 366
    childhood 363, 366, 366f
    idiopathic generalized 369
    juvenile myoclonic 369
    remote symptomatic 382
Epileptic spasms 371
    reversible causes for 372
Epinephrine 320
Epiphora 37
Episodic ataxia 398
Episodic diseases, diagnostic criteria for 199t
Episodic wheeze 323
Epispadias 650
Epistaxis 206
Epsilon amino caproic acid 298
Epstein-Barr virus 147, 228, 233, 234, 250, 285, 397, 554
Erwinia chrysanthemi 289
Erythema
    marginatum 553f, 563

periumbilical 47
  toxicum 37, 89
Erythematoxicum 34
Erythroblastopenia, transient 284
Erythrocyte
  adenosine deaminase 269
  sedimentation rate 25, 153, 163, 192, 198, 389, 487, 493, 510, 545, 551, 555, 562, 571
Erythromycin 22, 331, 619
Erythropoiesis, ineffective 284
Erythropoietin, serum 269
Escherichia coli 20, 289, 336, 491
E-selectin 48
Esophageal atresia 655
Esophagitis 206
  eosinophilic 17, 253
Estrogens 538
Ethambutol 68, 171
Ethionamide 172
Ethosuximide 364
Ethylene dicysteine 654
Etoposide 292
Euphoria 343
European Association for Study of Liver 216, 395
European League Against Rheumatism 554, 556
European Society for Pediatric Endocrinology 541
European Society for Pediatric Gastroenterology, Hepatology and Nutrition 202
Exfoliated fetal cells 603
Exostosis 645
Expert Group of Indian Academy of Pediatrics 497
Expresses breast milk 66
Extensor spasms 371
Extracorporeal membrane oxygenation 467
Extracorporeal shock wave lithotripsy 508
Extrophy 650
Eye
  care 32, 407
  complications 144
  disease 67, 158

F

Fabrazyme 609
Fabry disease 595, 609
Facial palsy
  acquired 406
  congenital 406
  etiology of 406
Facial structures 385
Failure to thrive 25, 227, 242, 446
Faine's criteria 154
  modified 154, 154t
Fallot's physiology 420, 421
Famciclovir 152

Familial glucocorticoid resistance 510, 511
Famotidine 187
Fanconi anemia 265, 284, 285, 300, 593, 603
Fas-fas ligand 629
Fast foods 526
Fasting glucose 525
Fat
  necrosis, subcutaneous 35
  paucity of 56
Fatty acid oxidation 242, 244
  disorder 53, 228
Febrile 176
  convulsions 143
  seizure 361, 362
    recurrence of 362
  status epilepticus 361
Feeding problem 39
Femoral inter-condylar distance 7
Fenoldopam 467
Ferritin 545, 546
  serum 268
Fertility rate, total 179
Fetal aneuploidy 602
  screening for 599, 601
Fetal blood sampling, percutaneous ultrasound-guided 603
Fetal bradycardia 485
Fetal demise, high-risk of 62
Fetal echocardiography 417t, 602
Fetal growth
  assessment 62
  restriction 600
Fetal infections 603
Fetal period 464
Fetal structural abnormalities, screening for 601
Fetal thrombocytopenia 84
Fetal tissue sampling 603
Fetoscopy 603
Fetus
  biochemical disease of 602
  direct visualization of 603
Fever
  acute rheumatic 546, 565t
  biphasic 176
  flu-like symptoms of 40
Fibrinogen 545
Fibroscan 225
Fibrosis, pulmonary 560
Fine-needle aspiration cytology 170
First contralateral pneumothorax 341
First-line drug therapy 54, 365
Flaccid paralysis, acute 632
Flat feet 645
Flat nasal bridge 581
Flavivirus 176
Flexor spasms 371
Fluconazole 301, 622
  oral 621
Fluctuant swelling 32
Fludrocortisone 541

Fluid 59, 60, 503
  analysis 216
  attenuated inversion recovery 397, 409
  imbalance 87
  management 214
Fluorescence in situ hybridization 285, 288, 539, 585, 589, 603, 604
Fluorescent
  antibody staining 150
  leprosy antibody absorption test 173
  treponemal antibody absorption test 70
Fluoro-2-deoxyglucose 291
Fluoroscopy 345
Fluticasone mometasone 311
Folate 269
  levels 274
  malabsorption of 265
Folic acid
  antagonists 415
  deficiency 265
Folinic acid 69, 70, 157
Follicle-stimulating hormone 534, 540
Food allergies 16
Food and Drug Administration 92, 172, 283, 354
Food
  intolerance 16
  poisoning 20, 21t
    prevention of 23
  reactions, adverse 16fc
Foodborne diseases 20
Forchheimer spots 148
Forefoot varus 645
Foreign body 253, 344, 644
  aspiration 324
  ingestion 253
Fragile X syndrome 583
Free beta-human chorionic gonadotrophin 599
Free erythrocyte protoporphyrin 270
Free fatty acid 51, 53
Free radical-induced injury, suppression of 59
Fresh frozen plasma 60, 164, 179, 208, 304
Friedreich ataxia 398
Fructose intolerance, hereditary 227, 234, 242, 244, 245
Full blood count 63
Functional abdominal pain
  disorders 191
  management of 193
Functional constipation, diagnostic criteria for 195b
Fundus 243f
Furosemide 431
Fusion protein 146

G

Gabapentin 354
Galactogogues, role of 42

Galactosemia 92, 227, 242
Gallbladder 153, 221
Gallstone 203
　　treatment 204fc
Gamma-aminobutyric acid 137
Gamma-globulin 555
Gamma-glutamyl
　　transferase 204, 221, 283
　　transpeptidase 224, 225, 243
Gardasil 111
Gastric aspirate 170
Gastritis 206
Gastrocolic reflex 32
Gastroenteritis 17, 22, 166
Gastroenterology 189
Gastroesophageal disease 192
Gastroesophageal reflux 32, 586
　　disease 37, 44, 198, 324, 336
Gastrointestinal care 404
Gastrointestinal disease 568
Gastrointestinal disorders, functional 191
Gastrointestinal tract 58, 168, 253, 271, 616
　　complication 151
Gastroschisis 650
Gatifloxacin 172
Gaucher disease 228, 242, 606, 607
　　treatment of 608
Gauze granuloma 344
G-band karyotype 605
Gene
　　mutations 606
　　therapy 610
Genetic 363, 366, 400
　　counseling 541, 577, 578, 590
　　　　components of 578
　　　　indications of 578
　　　　requirements of 578
　　disease 578
　　disorders 485, 575
　　mutation analysis 213
　　skeletal survey 589b
　　studies 470
　　test 392, 399, 465
Genital examination 515
Genitalia
　　atypical 53
　　symmetrical external 539, 540f
Genitourinary system 169
Genome-wide association studies 288, 570
Genu valgum 645
Genu varum 7, 645
Genu vulgus 7
Genus rubivirus 148
Geophagia 270
Germ cell tumors 300
Gestational age 599, 600
Giant cell pneumonia 143
Giant panda sign 391f
Giggle incontinence 515
Gilbert syndrome 223

Glasgow coma scale 408
Glaucoma 641
Globotriaosylceramide 609
Glomerulonephritis 175, 486
　　acute 496
　　chronic 496, 510
　　infection-related 509, 511
　　poststreptococcal 502, 624, 626
Glossitis 270, 273
Glucagon-like peptide 1 527
Glucocerebrosidase deficient 608
Glucocorticoids 402, 540, 560
　　responsive aldosteronism 510
Gluconeogenesis 51
Glucose 594
　　6-phosphate dehydrogenase 91, 164, 175, 265, 632
　　delivery rate 54
　　galactose malabsorption 97
　　large quantities of 33
　　tolerance, abnormal 567
　　transporter 1 351
　　　　deficiency syndrome 364
Glutamic acid decarboxylase 399, 529
Glycerine enema 354
Glycine 598
Glycogen storage
　　disease 227, 470, 596, 603
　　disorder 53, 241, 245, 247
Glycogenolysis 51
Glycogenosis 53
Glycoprotein 293
Glycosaminoglycans 606
Glycosylation, congenital disorders of 241
Goldenhar syndromes 406
Golimumab 552
Gonadal tumors, risk of 541t
Gonadoblastoma 541t
Gonadotropin 534, 536
　　independent precocious puberty 536
　　　　causes of 537t
　　releasing hormone 534, 537, 650
Gordon syndrome 510
Gottron papules 566, 567
Gower's sign 400, 401, 566
Graft failure 301
Graft-versus-host disease 286, 287, 301, 303
Gram staining 336
Granulocyte
　　colony stimulating factor 286
　　concentrate 304
　　elastase 217
Granuloma, umbilical 36, 90, 651
Great arteries 447, 450
　　dextro-transposition of 418, 420, 452, 481
　　transposition of 415, , 445-448, 464
Griseofulvin 623
Gross hematuria, evaluation of 501t, 502fc
Gross motor function classification system 81, 352f

Growth hormone 54, 584
　　deficiency 527
Guanine 592
Guillain-Barré syndrome 22, 114, 143, 405, 406, 568
Gum hypertrophy 498

H

H1N1 112
Haemophilus influenzae 72, 100, 127, 295, 301, 312, 313, 316, 327, 361, 406, 499, 647
Haloperidol 389, 390
Hamartoma, mesenchymal 247
Hand, foot, and mouth disease 632
Hansel strain 309
Hansen's disease 173, 175
Haplotype 632
Haptoglobin 545
　　serum 269
Harlequin color change 34
Hartnup disease 397
Head circumference 79, 227
Head deformity 36
Headache 385, 387fc
　　acute 385
　　chronic 385
　　mixed 385
　　pattern of 385
　　primary 386
　　secondary 386
Hearing
　　assessment 79fc, 92
　　rehabilitation 354
Heart
　　defect
　　　　congenital 63, 415, 602, 604
　　　　history of 462
　　disease 64
　　　　complex congenital 451
　　　　congenital 63, 89, 319, 415, 417, 418, 420, 425, 429, 445, 487, 510, 581
　　　　coronary 324, 448
　　　　cyanotic 420
　　　　maternal cyanotic 64
　　　　palliative congenital 464
　　　　rheumatic 464
　　failure 330, 427, 446, 467
　　　　chronic 473
　　　　congestive 301, 319, 343, 426, 429, 446
　　　　diastolic 463
　　　　features of 419
　　　　management of 468t
　　　　pathophysiology of 463fc
　　　　systolic 463
　　rate, normal 472
　　sound, multiple 460
　　transplantation 467, 471

Heavy metals 399
Heinz bodies 266, 267f
Helex device 431
Helicobacter pylori 192, 270, 293, 568
Heliox 320
Helminthiasis 27, 28
Helminths treatment 28
Hemagglutinin 113, 146
Hemangiomata, capillary 34
Hematemesis 206
Hematochezia 207, 210
Hematocrit 259, 260, 264, 270, 274
Hematological system 60
Hematology 426
Hematoma 408
Hemato-oncology 303
Hematopoietic stem cell transplantation 286, 287, 300, 609
Hematuria 501, 510
Hemodynamics 429, 430, 451
Hemoglobin 83, 259, 264, 270, 274, 278, 281, 286, 303, 420, 487, 496, 545
    glycosylated 529
    low levels of 374
Hemoglobinopathy 92, 578, 603
Hemoglobinuria 166, 305
Hemogram 27
Hemolysis, elevated liver enzymes low platelet syndrome 62, 242
Hemolytic anemia, Coombs-negative 392
Hemolytic crisis 279
Hemolytic uremic syndrome 22, 210, 294
Hemophagocytic syndrome 187
Hemophilia 297
Hemorrhage
    conjunctival 138
    diffuse alveolar 545
    intracerebral 81
    intracranial 85, 293, 486
    intraventricular 78, 81
    subconjunctival 32, 34, 638, 639
    subgaleal 36
    subperiosteal 11
Hemorrhagic disease 371
Hemorrhagic skin eruption 144
Hemorrhagic varicella 151
Hemothorax, spontaneous 341
Hemotympanum 408, 409
Henipavirus 182
Henoch-Schönlein purpura 11, 210, 501, 510, 568
    diagnostic criteria for 568b
Hepatic encephalopathy, classification of 234t
Hepatic failure 496
Hepatic fibrosis, congenital 248
Hepatic veno-occlusive disease 301
Hepatitis
    A 106, 107
        vaccine 106
        virus infection 106, 231
    acute 223, 231
    anicteric 231
    autoimmune 234
    B 107, 156, 603
        antigen 497
        chronic 224, 238, 238t, 239, 239fc
        immunoglobulin 65, 240
        surface antigen 65, 285
        virus 65, 228, 231, 238, 239, 240
    B E-antigen 65, 238, 238, 239
    C virus 65, 228, 231, 293
    chronic 224
    E virus 65
        infection 231
    icteric 231
    neonatal 157
    relapsing 232
    viral 154
Hepatobiliary scintigraphy 221
Hepatoblastoma 247
Hepatocellular carcinoma 238, 246, 247
Hepatomegaly 53, 177, 282, 461
Hepatopulmonary syndrome 462
Hepatorenal syndrome 218
Hepatosplenomegaly 69, 148, 157, 242, 589
Hernia
    congenital 649
    umbilical 35, 36
Herpes 234, 630
    infections 228
    simplex
        virus 67, 88, 156
        neonatal 87-89
    zoster 150, 151
Hiccups 33, 38
High soluble transferrin receptor 551
High-efficiency particulate air 301
High-flow nasal cannula 186
High-performance liquid chromatography 92, 271, 594
High-resolution computed tomography 344, 345
Hilar pulmonary arteries 426
Hind foot equines 645
Hip
    congenital dislocation of 645
    developmental dysplasia of 645
Hirschsprung's disease, diagnosis of 38
Hirsutism 498, 538, 567
Histamine 499
Histocompatibility complex 300
Hoarse voice 315
Hodgkin's lymphoma 291, 292, 300, 304
Holoprosencephaly 602
Holotranscobalamine 274
Holt-Oram syndrome 416
Homocitrullinemia 597
Homocystinuria 92, 273
Homozygosity, short stretches of 583

Hookworms 27
Hormonal replacement therapy 540
Horner's syndrome 646
Horner-Tranta's spots 640
Howell-Jolly bodies 266, 266f
Human bocavirus 318
Human chorionic gonadotropin 535, 540, 601
Human diploid cell vaccine 118
Human enterovirus 632
Human herpesvirus 233, 234, 361, 572
Human immunodeficiency virus 71, 78, 172, 262, 285, 293, 312, 399
    infection, perinatal 71, 158
    prevention of 100
Human leukocyte antigen 286, 300, 303, 547, 548, 554, 566, 630
Human metapneumovirus 309, 318, 328
Human milk fortifier 80
Human monoclonal antibody 119
Human papillomavirus 109
    vaccine 109
Human parvovirus B19 269, 306
Human rhinovirus 96, 309
Humerus fracture 646
Hunter's syndrome 596
Huntington's chorea 564
Hydralazine 63
Hydration 316
Hydrocarbon aspiration 342
Hydrocele 36, 649
    congenital 35, 649
Hydrocephalus 89, 169, 377, 648
Hydrochlorothiazide 508
Hydrocortisone 619
Hydropneumothorax 340, 341
Hydrops fetalis 241, 603
Hydroxychloroquine 556, 559
Hydroxylase deficiency 511
Hydroxyprogesterone 92
Hydroxytryptamine 193
Hydroxyurea 273
Hydroxyzine 152
Hygroma, cystic 648
Hyperaldosteronism, familial 511
Hyperammonemia 597, 597fc, 598t
    neonatal 595
Hyperbilirubinemia 242, 265
Hypercalciuria 506, 508
    causes of 506t
Hypercholesterolemia 498, 560
Hyperglycemia 560
    nonketotic 603
Hyperinsulinism, congenital 52
Hyperkalemia 481, 482
Hyperkeratosis 10
Hyperketonemia 51
Hyperkinetic syndrome 373
Hyperlipidemia 251, 496
Hypermetropia 642

Hyperornithinemia 597
Hyperoxaluria 508
Hyperoxia 60
    test 419, 422
Hyperpigmentation 53
Hyperplasia, focal nodular 247
Hypersensitivity 624
Hypersplenism 282
Hypertension 62, 251, 278, 500, 509, 510, 525, 560, 567
    essential 511
    persistent pulmonary 418
    portal 242
    pregnancy-induced 62
    pulmonary 462
Hypertonic glucose infusion insulin 598
Hypertonic saline 320
Hypertriglyceridemia 567
Hypertrophic scars 627
Hypertrophic tonsils 310
Hypertrophy
    biventricular 452
    right atrial 452
Hyperuricosuria 508
Hyperventilation 363, 364f
Hypnotherapy 193
Hypoadrenalism, long-term therapy of 55
Hypoalbuminemia 163, 224fc, 496
Hypocalcemia 63, 448, 464, 560
    symptoms of 7
Hypochondriasis 10
Hypochromia 267
Hypogammaglobulinemia 301
Hypoglycemia 51, 54, 63, 166, 363, 448, 464
    categories of 53fc
    defense mechanism against 51
    disorder, congenital 54
    monitor babies for 63
    persistent 53
    symptoms of 51
    transient 53
Hypohidrotic ectodermal dysplasia 603
Hypohydrosis 609
Hypokalemia 481
Hypomagnesemia 60, 481, 560
    familial 506
Hyponatremia 331, 377
Hypophosphatasia 8
Hypophosphatemic rickets 7
Hypopituitarism
    evidence of 53
    long-term therapy of 55
Hypoplastic left heart syndrome 415, 418, 421, 451, 464
Hypoplastic myelodysplastic syndrome 284
Hypoplastic thyroid gland 521
Hypopyon 641
Hyporesponsiveness 104
Hypospadias 539, 650
Hyposplenism 268

Hypothalamic-pituitary-gonadal axis 534
Hypothermia 52, 56
    mild 56
    moderate 56
    neonatal 56
    role of 410
    severe 56
    whole-body 60
Hypothyroidism 474, 527
    childhood 521
    congenital 91, 92
    primary 523t
Hypotonia 52
Hypoxanthine guanine-phosphoribosyltransferase 505
Hypoxia 56, 481
    screening for 465
    severe 482
Hypoxic spell 442
Hypoxic stimuli 455
Hypoxic-ischemic encephalopathy 58, 78, 349
Hypsarrhythmia 372
    asymmetric 372
    disappearance of 373

I

Ichthyosis, genetic forms of 603
Icterus 37
Idiogram 593
Idiopathic thrombocytopenic purpura 304
Idiopathic west syndrome 372
Ifosfamide 292
IgM dipstick test 141
Imerslund-Gräsbeck syndrome 273
Iminodiacetic acid, hepatobiliary 221
Imipenem 172
Immune deficiency 313, 324
Immune reconstitution inflammatory syndrome 377
Immune thrombocytopenia 207, 293
    chronic 262
    management of 294t
Immune thrombocytopenic purpura 124
Immunization 72, 75, 80, 250, 499
Immunofluorescence 330
Immunofluorescence assay 162
Immunoglobulin 25, 106, 144, 312
    A 201
    G 201, 293
    heavy-chain 288
    M 154, 156
Immunomodulators 498
Immunosuppressive therapy 284, 286, 287
Immunotherapy
    subcutaneous 326
    sublingual 326
Impetigo 624, 626
Implantable cardioverter defibrillators 467, 482

In vitro fertilization 179
Incontinentia pigmenti 89
Indian Academy of Pediatrics 74, 95, 104, 114, 376, 525
    Advisory Committee on Vaccines and Immunization Practices 144
    Committee on Immunization 114
Indian Council of Medical Research 202
Indian Leptospirosis Society's Criteria 153
Indian Scale for Assessment of Autism 358
Indirect antiglobulin test 269
Indirect immunoperoxidase assay 163
Infantile tremor syndrome 273
Infection 301
    asymptomatic 68
    bacterial 40, 150
    control of 625
    neonatal 68
    prevention of 32
    secondary bacterial 151
    viral 492
Infectious Disease Society of America 312
Infective endocarditis 426, 433, 486
    revised Duke clinical diagnostic criteria for 486
Inferior vena cava 59, 280, 429
Inflammatory bowel disease 192, 210
Influenza 139, 141, 328, 629
    A 147
    immunization 115
    vaccination, childhood 113
    vaccine 112
        types of 113
    virus 113
        types of 112
Inhalation method 320
Inhaled corticosteroid 320, 324
Inherited bone marrow failure syndromes 284
    exclusion of 286
Injectable typhoid conjugate vaccine 142
Inotropes 466, 467
Insulin 530
    preparation, types of 530t
    resistance 567
Insulinoma antigen-2 529
Intense pruritus 618
Intensive care unit 84, 278, 409
Intercellular adhesion molecule 1 48
Interdigital clefts 624
Interferon 240
    alpha 240, 558
Interleukin 187, 218, 558
Intermediary metabolism, disorders of 596t
Intermittent photic stimulation 363
International Children's Continence Society 513
International Diabetes Federation 525
International League Against Epilepsy 361, 363

International League of Associations for
    Rheumatology 548, 549
International Society for Heart and Lung
    Transplantation 463
International Society of Nephrology 558
International Society of Ultrasound in
    Obstetrics and Gynecology 602
International Study of Kidney Diseases in
    Children 497
Intertrigo 88
Interventricular septum, portion of 435
Intestinal biopsy, role of 202
Intestinal obstruction 195
Intra-abdominal gonads, absence of 582
Intra-abdominal pressure 35
Intracranial pressure 380, 385, 410, 473, 509
    invasive 408
Intracytoplasmic sperm injection 583, 602
Intradermal rabies vaccination 118
Intradermal skin test 17
Intrahecal baclofen pump 354
Intrahepatic cholestasis, progressive
    familial 221, 225, 241, 242
Intrapartum antibiotic administration 47
Intrauterine growth restriction 52, 53, 62,
    72, 181, 600, 602
Intrauterine hypoxia, chronic 84
Intravenous immunoglobulin 134, 164,
    187, 295, 390, 454, 570
    therapy 85
Intussusception, history of 97
Iron
    chelation 282
    deficiency 75, 267
        anemia 10, 264, 270
        hydroxide polymaltose complex 271
        impaired utilization of 270
        loss of 270
    serum 243, 268
    studies 268
        serum 271
    therapy, oral 271
Irritable bowel syndrome 191
Ischemia, myocardial 456
Ischemic papillary dysfunction 456
Isochromosome 592
Isolated perineal hypospadias 539
Isolation 88, 139, 177
Isoniazid 69, 171, 172, 233, 379
Isonicotinic acid 171
Itching
    advantage of 624
    control of 625
Itch-scratch-itch cycle 618
Itraconazole 622
Ivabradine 467
Ivermectin 28

J

Janeway lesions 486
Janus kinase inhibitors 187
Janz syndrome 369
Japanese encephalitis 120
Jaundice
    neonatal 32
    recurrent 243
    significant 63
Jejunoileitis 201
Joints, infection of 646
Jones criteria 561, 562t, 563
Joubert syndrome 398
Jugular venous pressure 463

K

Kabuki syndrome 416
Kanamycin 171, 379
Kangaroo mother care 31
Karyogram 593
Karyotype 539, 580, 593
    limitations of 593
Kasabach-Merritt syndrome 246
Kasai's portoenterostomy 220, 222
Katz-Wachtel pattern 426
Kawasaki disease 154, 184, 185, 453, 454,
    564, 570, 571, 571t
Kawasaki syndrome 144
Kayser-Fleischer rings 391, 391f, 392, 399
Kearns-Sayre syndrome 417
Keratoconjunctivitis
    atopic 639
    phlyctenular 639
Keratomalacia 12
Keratotic scabies 624
Kernig's sign 169
Ketamine 443
Ketoconazole 172
    oral 621
Ketogenesis 51
Ketones 244, 594
    bodies 53
Kidney
    chronic 509, 511
    function test 496, 503
    injury
        acute 162, 164, 496, 503, 510, 511
        molecule-1 218
King's College Hospital Criteria for Acute
    Liver Failure 237
Klebsiella 491, 494, 505
Klinefelter syndrome 582, 591
Knee
    degenerative arthritis of 391
    pain 645
Knock knee 645
    physiological 35
Koilonychias 270
Koplik spots 143
Kussmaul's sign 461

L

Labioscrotal fold fusion
    degree of 539
    extent of 539
Lacerations 626
Lacks immune memory 104
Lactate 53, 244, 594
    dehydrogenase 62, 225, 268, 285, 288,
        292, 318, 545, 567
    serum 274
Lactic acidosis 198
Lactic dehydrogenase 216
Lactobacillus reuteri 44
Lactulose 354
Lamivudine 240
Lamotrigine 370
    seizures free rates of 370
Landau-Kleffner syndrome 367
Lange-Nielsen syndrome 482
Language
    and speech assessment 81
    evaluation scale Trivandrum 81, 83
Large-molecule diseases 594
L-arginine 598
Laryngoscopy 316
Laryngotracheitis 315
Laryngotracheobronchitis 143, 315
Larynx 344
Laser photocoagulation 641
Lawson Wilkins Pediatric Endocrine
    Society 541
Lazy bladder syndrome 514
L-carnitine 598
Lead poisoning 195
Leflunomide 552
Left atrial pressure 457
Left atrium 421, 425, 426, 445, 446, 449, 451
Left bundle branch block 427, 472
Left coronary artery 455, 457, 458
Left ventricle 430, 445-449, 451, 455, 457,
    459, 478
Left ventricular
    hypertrophy 456, 459, 509, 511
    outflow tract 446
Legg-Calvé-Perthes disease 646
Legionella pneumophila 328
Leishmaniasis, viral 141
Lennox-Gastaut syndrome 372
Lentil lectin purified glycoprotein 381
Lepra reaction 174
    types of 175t
Lepromatous leprosy 173, 175
Lepromin test 173
Leprosy 173
    clinical type of 173, 174t
    intermediate 175
    management of 174
    multidrug therapy in 175t
Leptin deficiency 527
Leptospirosis 141, 153, 234
Lesch Nyhan syndrome 243
Leukemia 286, 288
    acute 581
        lymphoblastic 288, 300

lymphocytic 290
  myelogenous 288, 290
  myeloid 286, 289, 300
 childhood 290
 chronic
  myelogenous 288
  myeloid 261, 263, 289, 300
 juvenile myelomonocytic 261
 neonatal 581
Leukocyte
 adhesion deficiency 300
 buffy-coat of 11
 counts 150
 esterase 217
Leukocytosis 150, 493, 496, 571
Leukoencephalopathy, progressive multifocal 399
Leukomalacia, periventricular 73, 78, 81, 349
Leukopenia 176, 555
Leuko-reduced red cells 303
Leukotriene receptor antagonist 324
Levamisole 498
Levetiracetam 367, 370
Levofloxacin 172
Levosimendan 467
Liddle syndrome 510
Light index 339
Light's criteria, modified 335
Limpness 52
Linezolid 172
Lipoprotein
 low-density 398
 storage disorders 606
Lithium 416
Live attenuated vaccine 107, 114
Liver
 biopsy 221, 244, 392, 589
 cirrhosis of 14
 copper estimation 392
 disease 227, 268
  chronic 224, 242, 245, 249
   complications of 249b
   end-stage 249
   fibropolycystic 248
   pediatric end-stage 224, 249
 failure
  acute 223, 231, 233, 235f, 242, 243, 245, 249
  chronic 232, 243, 249
 fatty acid-binding protein 218
 function test 25, 61, 67, 149, 157, 192, 198, 207, 213, 221, 223, 231, 239, 243, 285, 292, 389, 405, 545, 546, 557, 630
  abnormal 223
 injury, drug-induced 224
 transaminases 551
 transplantation 233, 240, 249, 392-394
  emergency 236
  pediatric 249b, 250

Lockjaw 134, 135
London dysmorphology database 588
Long chain 3 hydroxyacyl coenzyme A dehydrogenase 242
Long QT syndrome 374, 375f, 470, 482
Loose index 324
Low back pain 646
Low birth weight 31, 57, 326, 349
Löwenstein-Jensen culture medium 170
Lower gastrointestinal bleeding 206, 210
 causes of 211t
Lower respiratory tract infection 318
L-thyroxine 522, 523
Lumbar puncture 68, 289, 361, 386
Lung 660
 abscess 331, 336
  primary 336
  secondary 336
 disease
  chronic 80 448
  interstitial 338
 injury
  acute 305
  ventilator-induced 448
 lateral view of 660
 parenchyma 447
Lupus 485
 anticoagulant 63, 547
 nephritis 558
  histopathological classification of 559f
Luteinizing hormone 534, 535, 540
 releasing hormone 650
Lyme's disease 306
Lymph node 169
 tuberculosis 169
Lymphadenopathy 157, 291, 571
Lymphangioleiomyomatosis 338
Lymphangioma 648
Lymphocyte 261
 intraepithelial 202
 transformation test 630
Lymphocytic choriomeningitis virus 156
Lymphocytic inflammatory infiltrate 146
Lymphocytopenia, causes of 262t
Lymphocytosis, causes of 262t
Lymphohistiocytosis, hemophagocytic 184, 228, 286, 300
Lymphoma 291
Lymphopenia 555
Lymphoproliferative disease 141
Lysine 597
Lysosomal storage diseases 227, 596t, 606
 classification of 606, 607t
 pathophysiology of 606
 treatment of 610
Lysosomal transport defects 606

M

Macrocephaly 89
Macrophage activation syndrome 545, 551
Maculopapular rash 157
Magnesium 8, 63, 187
Magnetic resonance 192, 381, 510
 angiography 212
 cholangiopancreatography 204, 214
 imaging 25, 58, 81, 83, 198, 214, 221, 246, 253, 352, 358, 363, 367, 369, 372, 381, 383, 386, 389, 397, 406, 408, 419, 442, 470, 503, 522, 536, 539, 551, 589, 596, 602, 641, 644, 648, 656
  brain 392, 398
  protocol 381
  scan 381
 spectroscopy 381
Main pulmonary artery 449, 450
Major histocompatibility complex 561
Malabsorption syndrome 14
Malaria 15, 166
 classification of 166
 parasite density, patency level of 166
 severe 166
  complicated 166
Malassezia furfur 90, 621
Malnutrition
 maternal 640
 severe acute 3, 170
Mantoux test 68, 69, 170
Manual breast pumps 40
Maple syrup urine disease 92, 596, 597
March fracture 644
Marfan's syndrome 338, 339, 580
Marsh-Oberhuber grading, modified 202t
Martin-Bell syndrome 583
Masseter muscle spasm 135
Massive blood transfusion 304
Mastitis 40
 neonatorum 34, 36
Maternal immune thrombocytopenia 85
Maternal transmittable infectious disease 602
Mature-B all 288
Maturity-onset diabetes of young 529
Maxillary osteitis 313
McCune-Albright syndrome 535
Mean corpuscular hemoglobin concentration 259, 274
Mean corpuscular volume 259, 260, 274, 284
 values 260t
Measles 117, 143
 inclusion body encephalitis 143
 mumps, rubella 108, 144, 149, 293
 vaccine against 147
Meatal stenosis 652
Mebendazole 28
Mechanical ventilation 134, 320
Meckel's diverticulum 210, 212
Meckel's scan 212

Meconium
- nonpassage 33
- passage 195

Mediastinal mass 291

Mediastinum 657
- anterior 658
- posterior 658
- superior 658

Medical expulsive therapy 508
Medical nutrition therapy 531
Medium-chain
- acyl-coenzyme A dehydrogenase 198, 597
- triglycerides 222

Medulloblastoma 397
Megakaryocytes 294
Megaloblastic anemia 267, 273
- diagnosis of 274fc
- hematologic laboratory features of 274t

Melanocortin receptor mutation 525
Melatonin 187
Melena 206, 207, 210
Membranes, preterm premature rupture of 47
Mendelian inheritance 596
Meningitis 313, 637
- signs of 361
- symptoms of 361
- tuberculous 154, 376

Meningococcal infection 128
Meningococcal vaccine 127
Meningoencephalitis 148, 162, 163
Meningomyelocele 651
Mental
- apathy 273
- retardation 195, 578, 589
- status 343

Mesenchymal cells 602
Mesial temporal sclerosis 362
Metabolic disease 92, 227
Metabolic disorders 58, 91, 603
Metabolic liver disease 241, 242, 245
- pathogenesis of 241f

Metabolic syndrome 525, 567
Metabolic tests, advanced 244t
Metabolism, inborn errors of 25, 47, 53, 78, 91, 241, 300, 372, 464, 594, 594b, 595
Metaiodobenzylguanidine 397, 510
Metaphyseal dysplasia 8
Metatarsus adductus 644
Methemoglobinemia 418
Methotrexate 289, 415, 551, 559
Methyldopa 63
Methylmalonic acid, serum 274
Methylmalonic aciduria 273
Methylprednisolone 390
Metoprolol 471
Metronidazole 23, 137
Microcephaly 63, 73, 273
Microcolon 63

Microdeletions 592
Micropenis 53, 539
Microphthalmia 148
Microscopic agglutination test 154
Microscopic hematuria, diagnosis of 502fc
Microsporum canis 622
Micturating cystourethrogram 493, 510, 652, 654
Midazolam 361
Middle cerebral artery peak systolic velocity 602
Midfoot cavus 645
Mid-gut volvulus 210
Migalastat 610
Migraine 385
- abdominal 191, 194
- chronic 386
- classification of 385
- diagnostic criteria 386t
- familial hemiplegic 385
- hemiplegic 385
- prophylaxis 387t, 562
- retinal 385
- treatment of 387t

Miliaria 37, 87
Miliaria crystallina 87, 89
Miliaria pustulosa 87
Miliaria rubra 87
Miliary tuberculosis 168
Milkman pseudofracture 8
Milrinone 467
Mineralocorticoid 540
Minocycline 174
Miscarriage, spontaneous 63
Mitochondrial disorders 399
Mitochondrial myopathy 198
Mitomycin 269
Mitral insufficiency, signs of 437
Mitral regurgitation 427, 429, 456, 464, 562
- features of 460

Mitral stenosis 462
Mitral valve prolapse 429, 480
Mixed connective tissue disease 545
Mixed gonadal dysgenesis 538
Mobius syndromes 406
Molecular absorption recirculating system 393
Molecular cytogenetic syndromes 583
Molecular genetic
- analysis 403
- studies 269
- testing 401

Molluscum contagiosum 620
Mometason 619
Mongolian spot 36
Monoamine oxidase 233
Monoclonal antibodies 321
Monocytes 262
Monocytosis, causes of 262b
Mononucleosis, infectious 306

Monosaccharides 193
Moraxella catarrhalis 312
Morbillivirus 143
Mosaicism 581
Motavizumab 321
Motor neuron 403
Mouse brain-derived inactivated vaccine 121
Mouth disease 67, 158
Moxifloxacin 172
Mucolipidoses 606
Mucopolysaccharidoses 8, 227, 595, 596, 606-609
Mucosal bleeding 177
Mucosal edema 313
Mucositis 301
Multicentre growth reference study 525
Multicystic appearance 247
Multidisciplinary team 359
Multidrug therapy 174, 175
Multidrug-resistant cefixime 141
Multifactorial inheritance pattern 385
Multi-organ dysfunction 185
- evidence of 58

Multiple atrial tachycardia 473
Multiplex ligation-dependent probe amplification 403, 416
Multiplex polymerase chain reaction 48
Multivitamin supplementation 80
Mumps 146
Murmur 450
Muscle
- biopsy 401
- enzymes 546
- relaxants 134
- spasms 134

Muscular dystrophy 459
Musculoskeletal disease 566
Myalgia 176
- nuchae epidemica 405

Mycobacterium 630
- leprae 173
- tuberculosis 68, 168, 330, 332, 334, 378, 640, 647
- demonstration of 170

Mycophenolate 559
- mofetil 250, 498, 560

Mycoplasma 139, 285, 331
- pneumonia 144, 328, 405, 568, 629

Mycotic aneurysm 486
Myectomy 471
Myelitis, transverse 143
Myelodysplastic syndrome 267, 269, 286
Myeloperoxidase 547
Myocardial diseases 459
Myocardial infarction 482
Myocarditis 162, 464, 474, 475, 482
- neonatal 485

Myoclonic jerks 369
Myoclonic status epilepticus 369

Myopathy 578
Myopia 641, 642
Myositis, benign acute childhood 405
Myotomy 460

N

N-acetyl glutamate synthase deficiency 597
N-acetyl-beta-D-glucosaminidase 561
Naglazyme 609
Nailfold telangiectasia 566
Nalidixic acid 141
Napkin rashes 34
Naproxen 194
Nasal cannula 185
Nasal diphtheria 131
Nasal polyp 310, 313
Nasal sumatriptan 194
Nasal zolmitriptan 194
Nasogastric tube 4
Nasolacrimal duct
 blockage 32
 noncanalization of 637
National Institute for Health and Care Excellence 196, 357
National Institute of Allergy and Infectious Diseases 16
National Neonatology Forum 91
National Nutrition Monitoring Bureau 264
National Tuberculosis Control Programme, revised 376
Neck soft tissues and spine 657
Necrotizing enterocolitis 47, 54, 62, 84, 210
Neisseria gonorrhoeae 638, 639
Neisseria meningitidis 127
Neonatal alloimmune thrombocytopenia 84, 85
Neonatal cholestasis syndrome 242, 245
Neonatal hypoglycemia 51
 causes of 52*t*
Neonatal intensive care unit 47, 361, 432, 447, 510
Neonatal resuscitation program 61
Neonatal sepsis 46, 47, 50
 classification of 46*t*
 late-onset 46
Neonatal symptomatic disease 69
Neonatal thrombocytopenia 84
 causes of 84*t*
 early-onset 85
 late-onset 85
Neonatal thyroid-stimulating hormone 92
Nephritis 162
Nephrocalcinosis 505, 506
Nephrolithiasis 505*b*, 506
Nephrolithotomy, percutaneous 508
Nephrology 489
Nephrotic syndrome 496, 500, 510
 primary 496
 secondary 496
Nephrotoxicity 498

Nervous system, sympathetic 463
Neural tube defects 63
Neuraminidase 113
 protein 146
Neuroblastoma 300
Neurocutaneous syndrome 372
Neurocysticercosis 380, 381, 382*t*
 treatment of 27
Neurodegenerative disorder 350, 578
Neurodevelopmental disorder 80
Neuroimaging 81, 386, 399, 589
Neurological complication 132, 143, 151
Neurological disorders 89
Neurological examination 61, 79, 80
Neurological signs 73
 abnormal 386
Neurology 347
Neuronal ceroid lipofuscinoses 606
Neuronal nitric oxide synthase 402
Neurotuberculosis 376
Neuro-Wilson disease 391
 symptomatic management of 395
Neutropenia 284, 551
 causes of 261*t*
 severe congenital 300
Neutrophil 259, 261
 gelatinase-associated lipocalin 218
Neutrophilia 493
 causes of 261*t*
Nevirapine 71, 159
Nevus simplex 34
New Wilson's index 394*t*
New York Heart Association 64
Newborn intensive care unit 57, 78, 79
Newborn screening program 91
Next-generation sequencing 403, 605
Niemann-Pick disease 228, 241, 244
Night blindness 12, 642
Night crying 44
Nikolsky's sign 629
Nipah virus 182
Nipple
 cracked 39
 flat 39
 pigmentation of 539
 retracted 39
 sore 39
Nitric oxide inhalation 462
Nitrofurantoin 494
Nocturia 529
 episodes 515
Nodal ectopic tachycardia 478
Nodal escape beats 477
Nodal premature beats 477
Nodal rhythm 477
Nodular regenerative hyperplasia 247
Nodules, subcutaneous 563
Nonalcoholic fatty liver disease 227, 228, 525, 527
Nonbullous impetigo 626

Noncontrast computed tomography 381, 506
Nonconvulsive status epilepticus 397
Non-Hodgkin lymphoma 291, 292, 300
Noninvasive ventilation 186
Non-rapid eye movement 371
 sleep 367
Nonsteroidal anti-inflammatory drugs 178, 207, 279, 295, 387, 551, 556, 572, 615, 629
 oral 174
Noonan syndrome 416
Normocarbia 60
Norwegian scabies 624
 management of 624
Nosocomial infection 47
Nuchal translucency 593, 599, 601
Nucleic acid testing 159
Nutrition 214, 250, 530
Nutritional diseases 5
Nutritional management 60, 401
Nystagmus 641
Nystatin suspension 41

O

Obesity
 abdominal 525
 childhood 203, 524
 health consequences of 525
 hypothalamic 527
Obsessive-compulsive disorder 389
Obstructive mega ureter, primary 653
Obstructive sleep apnea 325
Occlusive vasculitis 377
Oculocutaneous albinism 603
Ofloxacin 172, 174
Oligoarthritis 549
 future treatment of 552
Oligosaccharides, fermentable 193
Oligosaccharidoses 606
Omphalitis 47
Omphalocele 651
Oncovin 292
Open neural tube defects 601
Ophthalmia neonatorum 638
Ophthalmic zoster 150
Opsoclonus myoclonus ataxia syndrome 397
Optic
 chiasma, third ventricular compression of 377
 neuritis 313
Optochiasmatic arachnoiditis 377
Oral contraceptive pill 175
Oral food challenge test 19
Oral prednisolone, high-dose 559
Oral rehydration solution 23
Oral steroids, role of 619
Orbital cellulitis 637
Orchidopexy, timing of 650

Organic acid 589
Organic acidemia 227
Ornithine 597
    aminotransferase deficiency 597
    transcarbamylase 198, 234
        deficiency 603
Orotic acid 597
Orthopedic disorders 525
Osgood-Schlatter disease 645
Oski's pediatrics principles 318
Osler's nodes 486, 487
Osmotic laxatives 196
Osteitis, frontal 313
Osteochondritis 644
    dissecans 391
Osteomyelitis 11
Osteopenia
    generalized 10
    premature 391
Osteoporosis 448
    prevention 557
Osteotomies 354
Ostium primum 429
    defects 435, 438, 439
Otitis media 100, 143, 316
    serous 310
Otoacoustic emission 69, 79, 83, 92
Ovarian hyperandrogenism 525
Oxalate 505
Oxcarbamazepine 367
    doses of 367
    valproate 367
Oxcarbazepine 370
Oxybutynin 517
Oxygen
    carrying capacity 374
    saturation 185, 441
Oxymetazoline 311

P

P wave 484
Packed red blood cell 282, 303
    transfusion of 271
Pain
    abdomen 177, 191, 191*t*, 192*t*, 210
    management 60, 214
Painful crisis 279
Palliative surgery 443, 457
Palpitation 452
Pancreas, pseudocyst of 214
Pancreatitis 332
    acute 204, 213, 461
        recurrent 213
    chronic nonprogressive 213, 461
Pancytopenia, severe 301
Panencephalitis, subacute sclerosing 143, 149
Papilledema 399
Papules, rash of 624
Para-aminosalicylic acid 172, 273

Paracentesis, large-volume 217
Paracetamol 44, 144, 362
Paradoxical reactions, pathogenesis of 378
Parainfluenza 139, 328
    virus 309, 315
Parapsoriasis 151
Parasite density 166
Paraspinal edges 659
Parathyroid hormone 7, 506
    level 8
Paratyphoid
    A 104
    B 104
Parenchyma 660
Parenchymal inflammation 336
Parenteral iron therapy 271
Paresthesias 406
Parkinson's disease 391
Paroxysmal hypercyanotic attacks 441
Paroxysmal nocturnal hemoglobinuria 269, 286
Partial androgen insensitivity syndrome 538, 541
Partial thromboplastin time 304
Parvovirus B19 156, 227, 228, 372, 555, 566
Patau syndrome 591
Patent ductus arteriosus 148, 415, 432, 434, 434*t*, 438, 445, 446, 464
    pathology of 432*t*
Patent foramen oval 445, 446
Paucibacillary disease 169, 170
Peak expiratory flow 325
Pearson syndrome 284
Pediatric acute liver failure 221, 233
Pediatric heart failure, Modified Ross classification of 465*t*
Pediatric intensive care unit 208, 510
Pediatric Rheumatology European Society 568
Pediatric Rheumatology International Trials Organization 568
Pediculosis 626
Pelkan spur 11
Pelvic ultrasonography 539
Pelviureteric junction 192, 198, 653
    obstruction 653
Penicillin 70, 487, 615
Penta screen 601
Percutaneous fetal skin biopsy 603
Perennial allergic conjunctivitis 639
Pericardial disease 461
Pericarditis 162
Perihilar opacities 343
Perinatal asphyxia 47
    evidence of 59
Perineal fistula 654
Periodic acid-schiff 244
Periorbital cellulitis 313
Periorbital ecchymosis 408, 409
Periorbital rash 566

Peripheral blood 300
    smear 271, 274, 285
Peripheral pulmonary stenosis 415
Peritonitis, spontaneous bacterial 217, 232
Periungual erythema 566
Periventricular calcifications 73
Permethrin 625
Peroneal spastic flat foot 645
Peroxisomal diseases 594
Peroxisomal disorders 227, 241
Personal protective equipment 187
Pertussis 138, 180
    stages of 138*t*
    toxin 138
Pharmacologic therapy 193, 466
Phenobarbitone 221, 370
Phenylephrine 311
Phenylketonurea 357, 372, 417, 597
    maternal 415
Phenytoin 28, 370, 383, 397, 415
Pheochromocytoma 510
Phimosis 652
Phosphate 7, 505
Phosphocreatine 58
Photocoagulation 641
Picture exchange communication system 359
Pigment stones 203
Pimozide 389
Pinna, pain of 406
Pinworm 27
Pityriasis versicolor 621
Pizotifen 194
Placenta previa 71
Placental failure 62
Placental growth factor 600
Placentrax lotion 621
Plague 181
Plasma
    glucose 51
    metanephrines 510
    product 303
    protein-A, pregnancy-associated 599, 600
    renin activity 539
    zinc level, estimation of 14
Plasmodium falciparum 166, 277, 280
    parasite 15
Platelet 262, 274, 545
    alloimmunization 603
    concentrates 304
    count 263, 545
    distribution width 259
    products 303
    transfusion guideline 85, 85*t*
Pleura 660
    anteroposterior view of 660
    fluid lactate dehydrogenase 334, 335
    lateral view of 660
Pleural effusion 332

Pleural fluid
    protein 335
    testing 332
Pleural tear 339
Pleurodesis 341
Plexiform lesion 462
Pneumatocele 331
Pneumococcal conjugate vaccine 101
Pneumococcal disease 100
    invasive 100
    noninvasive 100
Pneumococcal polysaccharide vaccine 101
Pneumococcal vaccination 102
Pneumococcal vaccine 102, 103, 499
Pneumocystis carinii pneumonia 338
Pneumocystis jiroveci 301
    pneumonia 286
Pneumomediastinum 341
Pneumonia 100, 143, 344
    bacterial 154
    childhood community-acquired 328*t*
    community-acquired 162, 327
    incidence of 100
    necrotizing 331
    secondary 143
    vaccine 100
    viral 154
Pneumonic plague 182
Pneumonitis, interstitial 143, 148
Pneumothorax 338
    bilateral 341
    classification of 338*fc*
    encysted 341
    iatrogenic 338
    large 339, 340
    noniatrogenic 338
    primary spontaneous 338
    recurrent 340, 341
    secondary spontaneous 338, 340
    spontaneous 341
    traumatic 338
Polio vaccine, oral 72, 96, 108
Poliomyelitis 22
Polyangiitis
    granulomatous 547
    microscopic 547
Polyarthritis 549
    future treatment of 552
Polycystic ovarian syndrome 525, 567
Polycythemia 63
Polydipsia 529
Polyethylene glycol 194, 196, 240
Polygenic inheritance 369
Polyhydramnios 63, 64
Polymerase chain reaction 66, 88, 139, 141, 144, 147, 149, 150, 154, 162, 170, 173, 177, 182, 285, 318, 330, 547, 589, 630
    quantitative 403, 602
Polymorphonuclear cells 309
Polyneuritic leprosy 173

Polyols 193
Polyphagia 529
Polysaccharide 606
    vaccine 101, 104, 127
        status of 104
Polyuria 529
Pompe disease 417, 609
Port-wine stain 89
Positive bronchodilator reversibility test 325
Positive end-expiratory pressure 164, 186
Positron emission tomography 372, 389, 397
Postchemotherapy 267
Posterior reversible encephalopathy syndrome 502
Postnatal cytogenetic testing 593
Post-transplant lymphoproliferative disease 250
Potassium
    citrate 508
    hydroxide 88
Pott's disease 646
Prader-Willi syndrome 527, 584
Praziquantel 27
Precocious puberty 534
    central 534
    etiology of 535*fc*
    peripheral 534
Pre-Conception and Pre-Natal Diagnostic Techniques 579
Prednisolone 171, 292, 407, 564
    tapering dose of 498
Prednisone 70, 289
Pre-eclampsia 53, 62
Pregnancy 600
    acute fatty liver of 242
    mid trimester loss 64
Premature atrial complex 474
Premature ventricular contraction 480
Prenatal invasive diagnostic tests 602
Preterm labor 63
Prickly heat 87
Probiotics 193
Procaine penicillin G 70
Procalcitonin 47, 50
    serum 329
Proliferative lupus nephritis 560*fc*
Promethazine 387
Propanol 443
Propionibacterium acnes 627
Propranolol 194, 471
Prostacyclin infusion 462
Prostaglandin E1 434, 451
Prosthetic valve 486
Protein
    energy malnutrition 13
    losing enteropathy 496
    serum 496
    total 232

Proteinuria 510, 558
    quantification of 497*t*
Proteus vulgaris 162
Prothionamide 172
Prothrombin time 61, 208, 225, 231, 288, 297, 304
Proton pump inhibitors 44, 208
Pruritus 87
Pseudobulbar palsy, congenital 406
Pseudohypoparathyroidism 1A 527
Pseudo-membranous colitis 211
Pseudomonas 494, 505
    aeruginosa exotoxin A 104
Pseudoparalysis 10
Pseudopuberty, precocious 534
Pseudotumor
    cerebri 525
    inflammatory 247
Psoriatic arthritis 551
Psychiatric disorders 373
Psychiatric syndromes 391
Pubertal development, normal 534
Puberty, incomplete variants of 535*t*
Pulmonary artery 419, 425, 427, 440, 445-450, 455, 465, 659
Pulmonary blood flow 420, 441, 446
Pulmonary hypertension 462
    features of 462
Pulmonary trunk 455, 457, 458
Pulmonary valve 429, 457
Pulmonary vascular
    disease 426, 427
    pattern 660
    resistance 425, 426, 446
Pulse
    oximeter screening 418, 418*t*
    sharp upstroke of 460
Pupillary reflex 13, 641
Pure red cell aplasia 269, 545
Purkinje system 480
Pustules 624
Pyelography 506
    intravenous 506, 653
Pyelonephritis 491, 492
Pyogenic infection 626
Pyrantel pamoate praziquantel 28
Pyrazinamide 68, 171
Pyridoxine 171
Pyrimethamine 70, 157
Pyrimidine 5'-nucleotidase deficiency 266
Pyruate dehydrogenase deficiency 397

Q

Q-banding 592
QT syndrome 481
Quadrivalent flu vaccine 113
Quadruple rhythm 451, 452
Quadruple test 601
Quinidine 481
    toxicity 482

R

Rabies vaccine 116-118
Radiation 31, 56
Radioallergosorbent test 18
Radioimmunoassay 173
Radiolucent stone 506
Radionuclide
　cystography 493
　imaging 522
　ventriculography 471
Radiotherapy 641
Raised intracranial pressure 376, 380
Raised jugular venous pressure 461
Ramsay Hunt syndrome 406, 407
Random blood sugar 510
Randomized controlled trial 15, 384
Rapid diagnostic test 178, 182, 280, 330, 361
　quality-assured 166
Rapid plasma reagin 70
Rarefaction, Trümmerfeld zone of 11
Rash 37
　erythematous 34
Rastelli operation 449f
Real-time amplification systems, quantitative 48
Red blood cell 245, 259, 264, 274, 278, 303, 501, 502, 545
Red cell
　alloimmunization 603
　distribution width 259, 260, 270
　folate 269
Red-colored urine, causes of 501t
Re-entrant atrioventricular tachycardia 478
Reflexes, abnormal neonatal 60
Refraction, errors of 642
Refsum disease 398
Regurgitation 37, 39, 404
Rehabilitation management 401
Renal abscess 492
Renal artery stenosis 511
Renal biopsy 503, 510, 558
Renal disease 62
Renal disorders 64
Renal function test 8, 529, 546, 630
Renal Pathology Society 558
Renal replacement therapy 235, 595
Renal stone 505
　evaluation of 507
Renal system 60
Renal tract anomalies 63
Renal tuberculosis 492
Renal tubular acidosis 7, 506
Renin-angiotensin-aldosterone system 463
Respiratory care 186
Respiratory distress syndrome 63
Respiratory fluoroquinolones 313
Respiratory infection, acute 323, 361
Respiratory sounds 278
Respiratory syncytial virus 139, 309, 315, 318, 319, 323, 328, 423
Respiratory system 15, 17, 60, 307
Respiratory tract 17
　infection, recurrent 429
Restrictive cardiomyopathy 459, 460
Resuscitation, cardiopulmonary 3
Reticulocyte
　count 261, 271
　hemoglobin content 271
Retinal detachment 177, 178
Retinal pigmentation 89
Retinoblastoma 641
Retinoic acid 627
Retinoids, oral 627
Retinol, serum 13
Retinopathy of prematurity 80, 640
　classification of 80
　guidelines, early treatment for 80
Retinopathy, pigmentary 148
Retropharyngeal abscess 143
Rett syndrome 580
Reverse transcriptase-polymerase chain reaction 185, 288, 633
Reye syndrome 143, 572
Rhabdomyolysis 53
Rhesus 600
Rheumatic chorea, acute 389
Rheumatic fever 154, 484, 553f, 561, 562t
　pathophysiology of 561
Rheumatoid factor 389, 486, 546, 549
Rheumatologic diseases 546
Rheumatology 543
　pediatric 545
Rhinitis 325
Rhinorrheas 409
Rhinosinusitis 312, 325
　acute 312, 313
　chronic 312, 314
　predisposing factors for 312t
Rhinovirus 328
Rib resection 335
Ribonucleoprotein 113
Rickets
　etiology of 7t, 13t
　nutritional 7
Rickettsia 161
Rickettsial diseases 161, 162, 459
Rickettsial infections 161, 165
　classification of 161t
Rifampicin 171, 174
Right atrium 445, 449, 451, 457
Right axis deviation 426, 447
Right bundle branch block 419, 430, 452, 473
Right coronary artery 455, 457, 458
Right upper limb 418
Right ventricle 429, 445, 447-449, 451, 457, 478
Right ventricular
　failure, features of 462
　hypertrophy 425, 433, 440, 441f, 447, 451, 462
　outflow tract 421, 440, 457
Ring chromosome 592
Ringer's lactate 4, 214
Risperidone 389
Rituximab 292, 498, 557, 560
Road traffic accidents 408
Robertsonian translocation 592
Rocker bottom foot 645
Rocky mountain spotted fever 163
Rolandic spikes 366
Romano-Ward syndrome 482
Ross classification, modified 465ft
Rotarix 96, 99
Rotasiil 97, 98
Rotateq 96, 98
Rotavac 97, 98
Rotavirus
　disease 98
　gastroenteritis 96
　infection 96
　spread 97
　vaccination 97, 98
　vaccine 96, 97, 99
Roth's spot 486
Roundworm 27
Routine mumps vaccination 147
Roux-en-Y gastric bypass 527
Rubella 148, 227, 228, 328, 372
　syndrome, congenital 148, 149, 157, 180, 433

S

Sacral agenesis 63
Salmon patches 34
Salmonella 20
　enteric
　　fever 23
　　serotype typhi 140
　infection 22
　typhi
　　infection 105
　　vaccine 104
Sarcoidosis 546
Sarcoptes scabiei 624
SARS-CoV-2 182, 184, 187, 328
Scabies 87, 624, 626
　incognito 624, 625
　spread of 624
Scarlet fever 572
Schistocyte 268, 268f
Schistosomes 27
Schistosomiasis 501
Schwartz diagnostic criteria 483
Sclerema neonatorum 89
Scoliosis 646
Scratch 624
　marks 625
Scrub typhus 161
Scurvy 10
Sebaceous gland hyperplasia 89
Seborrheic dermatitis 88, 90

Secundum defect 429
Segawa disease 350
Seizures 52, 369, 378, 382, 395
    complete cessation of 373
    complex febrile 361, 362
    control of 361
    frequency 384
    multiple 166
    recurrence of 382
    semiology 366*f*
    typical absence 363
Senning operation 449*f*
Sensorineural deafness 148
Sensory ataxia 396
Sensory disorder 79
Sepsis 464, 465
    antibiotic use for 49*fc*
    classification of 46
    early-onset 47, 48*t*
    late-onset 47
    screen 47
Septal deviation 310
Septic pulmonary embolism 486
Septicemia 337
Septicemic plague 181
Sequential test 599
Serelaxin 467
Serial lactate measurement 465
Serological tests 153, 178, 381, 630
Serotonin antagonists 193
Serum alanine aminotransferase 67
Serum alkaline phosphatase 224
Serum ascitic albumin gradient 216
Serum glutamic
    oxaloacetic transaminase 223
    pyruvic transaminase 223
Serum integrated test 599
Severe attack 325
Sex chromosome
    abnormalities of 582
    karyotype 582
Sex development, disorders of 538, 538*t*, 541, 584
Sexually transmitted infection 492
Shallow breaths 334
Shawl sign 566
Shigella 20
Shock
    anaphylactic 17
    circulatory 473
    compensated 179
    hypotensive 179
    hypovolemic 500
Short QT syndrome 470
Short sightedness 642
Short stature 578, 582
Short-acting beta-agonist 319, 324
Shwachman-Diamond syndrome 285, 300
Sick day management 532
Sickle cell 268, 268*f*
    anemia 92, 300
    crisis 280
        types of 278*t*
    disease 102, 277, 327
    disorders 277
    trait 277
Siderocytes 266, 267*f*
Sildenafil 462
Single-nucleotide polymorphisms 570
Single-photon emission computed tomography 389
Sinus
    arrhythmia 474
    aspiration 313
    bradycardia 473
    node 472
        dysfunction 474
    tachycardia 472
    venosus defects 429
Sinusitis 310, 312
Sjögren syndrome 545, 546, 602
Skeletal dysplasia 588
Skeletal survey 589, 589*b*
Skin
    biopsy 630
    disease 67, 158
    excoriation 566
    flushing of 17
    hydration of 618
    integrity breach 47
    prick test 17
    sensitivity test 117
    smears 173
    temperature 56
    tests 170
    to-skin contact 57
Sleep apnea 525
Sleepiness, excessive 34
Slide agglutination test 154
Slipped capital femoral epiphyses 525, 646
Small intestinal biopsy 25
Small molecule diseases 595
Small nuclear ribonucleoprotein associated polypeptide N 584
Smith-Lemli opitz syndrome 417, 580
Sneezes 38
Social responsiveness scale 357
Sodium 526
    benzoate 595
    bicarbonate 443
    channel 483
    phenylacetate 598, 598*t*
    picosulfate 196
    valproate 389
Soft tissue 656
    malignancies 11
Sore buttocks 34
Sparse pubic hair 582
Spasmodic croup 316
Spastic diplegia 351*fc*, 354
Spastic paraplegia, hereditary 351
Spasticity, treatment of 354*t*
Spatula test 136
Spherocyte 268, 269*f*
Sphincter 514
Sphingolipidoses 596, 606
Spina bifida 195, 651
Spinal muscular atrophy 403
Spinal tuberculosis 169, 646
Spinocerebellar ataxia 396
Splenectomy 282
Split-virion vaccine 113
Spot protein 546
Sprengel's deformity 646
Spur cell 268*f*
Squamous blepharitis 637, 638
Standard agglutination test 154
Staphylococcal folliculitis 87, 88
Staphylococcal scalded skin syndrome 626, 630
Staphylococcus aureus 20, 147, 316, 328, 334, 336, 486, 492, 618, 626, 637, 647
Staphylococcus saprophyticus 491
Status epilepticus, pure absence 369
Status migrainosus 386
Steatosis 244
Steinherz-Bleyer algorithm 289
Stem cells, infusion of 301
Stenosis, pulmonary 416, 429, 449
Sterile pyuria 492, 571
Sterility 582
Steroids 28
    role of 164
    systemic 320
    topical 619
Stevens-Johnson syndrome 367, 560, 572, 629, 629*t*, 630
Stimulation test 540
Stone formation, causes of 505*b*
Stork bites 34
Strabismus 641
Stratosphere sign 339
Streptococcus beta-haemolyticum 630
Streptococcus infection 563
Streptococcus pneumoniae 100, 127, 312, 328, 334, 486, 639
    vaccination 361
Streptococcus pyogenes 316, 626
    infection 88
Streptococcus viridans 486
Streptomycin 171
Stress
    hyperinsulinism, perinatal 52
    incontinence 515
Stroke 198
Strongyloides 27
    stercoralis 27
Sturge-Weber syndrome 89
Subperiosteal abscesses 313
Substrate reduction therapy 610
Subunit virion vaccine 113

Succinyl-CoA transferase 244
Suckling blister 89
Sudden infant death syndrome 75
Sulfadiazine 69, 70, 157
Sulfamethoxazole 22, 23, 139, 141, 233, 286, 494, 626, 629
Sulfasalazine 273
Sulfonamides 273
Sulfosalicyclic acid test 497t
Sulthiame 367
Sumatriptan 194
Superior mesenteric artery 62, 198
Superior vena cava 60, 429, 658
    margin of 658
Supraventricular tachycardia 452, 464, 465, 472, 473, 478
Surgery 214
    indications of 648
Swelling around knee 645
Sydenham's chorea 389
    treatment of 564
Syncopal attacks 485
Syndrome of inappropriate antidiuretic hormone secretion 335, 377, 411
Synovial fluid 571
Synthesis, disorders of 241
Syphilis 11, 227
    congenital 70, 71, 158, 159fc
    diagnosis of 70
    infection 70
    serologic tests for 70
Systemic disorder, chronic 62
Systemic inflammatory response syndrome 185
Systemic juvenile idiopathic arthritis 545
    rash of 553f
Systemic lupus erythematosus 11, 63, 262, 285, 415, 417, 496, 501, 510, 545, 554, 556, 558, 564, 602
    activity index 557
    pediatric 554
Systemic lupus international collaborating clinics 554, 557
Systemic therapy 618, 622, 626
Systemic vascular resistance 236, 426, 449

T

Tachyarrhythmias 456
Tachycardia 17
    antidromic reciprocating 479f
    orthodromic reciprocating 479f
Tachyphylaxis 54
Tachypnea, transient 63
Tachyzoites 68
Tacrolimus 250, 498
Taenia solium 381
Tamm-Horsfall protein 506
Tandem mass spectrometry 54, 92, 234, 594
Taper hydrocortisone 541
Tapeworm 27

Target cell 268, 269f
Tarsal coalition 644
Tashiro repair 457
Taussig-Bing anomaly 421
T-banding 593
T-cell
    dependent response 101, 104
    dysfunction 301
    lymphoma, enteropathy-associated 201
    receptor 288
Tectal plate hyperintensity 392
Teeth, congenital 35
Telbivudine 240
Temporomandibular joint 549
Tension pneumothorax 339, 341
Terbinafine 623
Testicular germ cell tumors 650
Testicular torsion, neonatal 36
Testis, undescended 53, 649
Tetanus 101, 134, 136, 180
    generalized 135
    immunoglobulin 134, 136, 137
    mild 137
    neonatal 136
    severe 137
    toxoid-conjugated vaccine 104
    vaccine 134
Tetracycline 628
Tetralogy of Fallot 64, 415, 421, 427, 440, 440f, 481
Tetrathiomolybdate 393
Thalassemia 281, 301
    major 281, 300, 303
    nontransfusion-dependent 281
    syndromes, spectrum of 281f
    transfusion dependent 281
Thalidomide 378
Therapeutic hypothermia 58, 60, 61
    mechanism of action of 59
    side effects of 61
    technique of 60
    use of 59
Thioacetazone 172
Third-generation cephalosporin 335
Thoracic plombage 344
Thoracic spine 657
Thrombocytopenia 62, 86, 148, 176, 284, 429, 551, 555
    amegakaryocytic 294
    causes of 84
    risk of 85
Thromboelastography 236
Thrombopoietin receptor agonists 295
Thrombosis 500
Thrombotic thrombocytopenic purpura 294, 545
Thumb sign 316
Thymine 592
    serum 14

Thyroid
    binding globulin 522
    disorder 581
    function test 465, 497, 510, 529, 547
    stimulating hormone 283, 389, 521, 522, 536
Thyroxine 283, 522, 336
Tibial tubercle, apophysitis of 645
Tinea
    capitis 622
        inflammatory 622
        noninflammatory 622
    corporis 622
    cruris 88, 622
    faciei 622
    incognito 622
    infections 622
    manuum 622
    pedis 622
    unguium 622
    verrucosum 622
Tinidazoles 23
Tip-toe-walking 405
Tissue
    cysts containing bradyzoites 68
    dysmorphogenesis, types of 588fc
    fragility 448
    injury, mechanism of 629
    studies 399
    transglutaminase 192
Tizanidine 354
Tobramycin 637
Toe walking 645
Toluidine red unheated serum test 70
Tone abnormalities 60
Tongue tie 35
Tonic clonic seizures, generalized 369
Tonsillopharyngeal diphtheria 131
Tonsils 291
Topical antiallergic eye drops 640
Topical antibacterial cream 89
Topical gamma benzene hexachloride lotion 625
Topical immunomodulators, role of 619t
Topiramate 370, 505
Torsade de pointes 482
Torticollis, congenital 646
Total anomalous pulmonary venous connection 421, 429, 464
    return 421, 451
Total iron binding capacity 221, 268, 270, 271, 375
Total leukocyte count 496
Total parenteral nutrition 47, 60
Total plasma exchange 393
Toxic epidermal necrolysis 629, 629t, 630
Toxic metabolites, production of 55
Toxic shock syndrome 572
Toxoplasma 566
    gondii 68

Toxoplasmosis 68, 84, 141, 156, 228, 306, 372, 399
   congenital 157
Toxoplasmosis, other agents, rubella, cytomegalovirus, and herpes simplex 84, 349
   infections 156, 157, 157*t*
      general principles of 156
      titers 157
Trachea 660
Tracheal wall, lateral view of 658
Tracheoesophageal fistula 78, 336, 655
Tracheomalacia 324
Transcobalamin
   deficiency 273
   receptor defects 273
Transesophageal echo 426, 442
Transfusion
   monitoring chart 306
   transmitted infections 306
Transient neonatal pustular melanosis 88, 89
Transjugular intrahepatic portosystemic shunt 208, 217
Traumatic brain injury 371, 408, 410*fc*
Trematodes 27
Tremors 52, 395
Trichinella 27
Trichophyton 622
Trichuriasis 27
Tricuspid
   atresia 419, 451
   regurgitation 303, 464
   valve 451
      Ebstein anomaly of 464
Trientine 393
Triglycerides 525, 551
Triiodothyronine 522
Trimethoprim 22, 23, 139, 141, 233, 286, 289, 415, 494, 626, 629
Trismus 135
Trisomy 416, 591
Trivandrum development screening chart 81
Trophoblastic cells 602
Truncus arteriosus 416, 421, 464
   persistent 452
Tube thoracostomy 340
Tubercular abscess 377
   treatment of 379
Tubercular infection, primary spontaneous 376
Tubercular meningitis, drug-resistant 379
Tubercular vasculopathy 376
Tuberculin skin test 170, 376
Tuberculoid leprosy 173
Tuberculoma 376, 381*t*
Tuberculosis 68, 69, 168, 263, 324, 338, 376
   abdominal 169
   coinfection 172
   congenital 68
   control of 379
   gastrointestinal 169
   prevention of 379
   preventive therapy 378, 379
   pulmonary 169, 376
   Wallgren's timetable of 168, 168*t*
Tuberous sclerosis 372
Tucson's Children Respiratory Study 324
Tumor
   benign epithelial 247
   necrosis factor 558, 629
   nuclear factor alpha 552
Turner syndrome 416, 582, 591
T-wave 456
   morphology, abnormal 483
Twin-twin transfusion 265
Typhidot test 141
Typhoid 104
   conjugate vaccine 104
   polysaccharide vaccine 105
   severe 142*t*
   uncomplicated 141*t*
   vaccine 104, 142
Tyrosinemia 242
Tzanck smear 88, 89

U

Ultrasonography 48, 83, 192, 198, 221, 244, 253, 278, 283, 289, 332, 334, 339, 417, 493, 522, 551, 582, 641, 650
   abnormal 510
Ultrasound 204, 515, 599, 604
   abdominal 207
Umbilical artery, single 602
Umbilical polyp 90
Umbilical swelling 36
Unconsciousness 185
United States Food and Drug Administration 97, 144
Upper esophageal stricture 253
Upper gastrointestinal
   bleeding 206, 208
   endoscopy 197, 207
Upper respiratory tract 169
   infection 312, 323, 385
Urea cycle defect 397
Ureteroscopy 508
   retrograde 506
Urethral orifice, position of 539
Urethral valves, posterior 652
Uric acid 505
   level 288
   serum 243
Urinalysis 502, 555, 558
Urinary biomarkers 558
Urinary culture 48
Urinary ketone levels 54
Urinary solutes, normal values of 507*t*
Urinary tract infection 47, 192, 198, 361, 491, 491*b*, 493, 494, 505, 514, 516
   recurrent 494, 506
Urine
   alkalinization 508
   analysis 507, 546
   culture 497, 516
   myoglobin measurement 405
   output 41
   protein 497
   routine examination 487
Urolithiasis 505
   management of 508
Ursodeoxycholic acid 205, 221, 222, 232
Urticaria 615
   papular 151, 617
   pathogenesis of 616
   rash 17

V

Vaccination 106, 557, 572
Vagal stimulation 473
Vaginal bleeding 32, 34, 37
Vaginal discharge 32
Vaginal reflux 515
Valacyclovir 152, 407
Valganciclovir 158
Valproate 364, 389, 390
Valproic acid 415
Valve ablation 652
Valvulitis, echocardiographic 562
Van Wyk-Grumbach syndrome 521, 523
Varicella 123, 125, 150, 151, 626
   causative agent of 66
   congenital 160
   infection 66
   perinatal 160
   unusual complications of 151
   vaccine 123, 124, 126, 499
      contraindication of 151
   zoster 227, 372, 406
      immunoglobulin 160
      virus 66, 123, 150, 156, 233, 328, 399
Vascular ring 324
Vasculitis 546
   large-vessel 510
Venereal disease research laboratory test 70, 158
Ventricular assist device 467
Ventricular bigeminy 480
Ventricular cells 472
Ventricular fibrillation 482
Ventricular septal defect 148, 421, 425, 426, 440, 445, 447, 451, 464, 581, 602
Ventricular tachycardia 465, 473, 481
Verapamil 471
Vernal conjunctivitis 639
Vernal keratoconjunctivitis 639
Verocell rabies vaccine, purified 118
Very low birth weight 72, 102

Vesicoureteral reflux 493, 516
Vesicular fluid
    culture of 66
    Wright stain of 89
Vessel vasculitis 510
Vibrio cholerae 181
Vibrio parahaemolyticus 20
Video fluoroscopy 345
Video-assisted thoracoscopic surgery 333, 335, 340
Vimizim 609
Vincent's curtsy sign 513
Vincristine 289, 292
Viomycin 171
Viremia, maternal 66
Virilization, maternal 538
Vision 354
    blurring of 642
    loss of 641
    screening 80
Vitamin
    A
        deficiency 12, 13
        prophylaxis program 13
        supplementation 144
    A D capsules 9
    B1 399
    B12 265, 266, 399
        deficiency, biochemical diagnosis of 275t
    C
        overdoses of 11
        plasma level of 11
        supplementation 11
        urinary excretion of 11
    D 7, 8
        deficiency 7
        dependent rickets 7
        drops 9
        injection 9
        preparations 9
        supplementation 560
    K 59
    levels 399
    supplementation 245
Vitellointestinal duct 651
Voiding disorders 513
Voiding dysfunction 514, 515
    treatment of 515
Volt age-gated potassium channel 398
Vomiting 197t
    causes of 198t
    persistent 177
    recurrent 197
    symptomatic treatment for 200, 200t
von Meyenburg complexes 248
von Willebrand disease 294
Voriconazole 301

W

Waldeyer's ring 291
Warm chain, concept of 56
Watery diarrhea, acute 15
Weak stream 513
Weil-Felix test 162, 163t
West syndrome 371
    symptomatic 371
Wheezing 323
Whipple's triad 51
White blood cell 49, 259, 261, 274, 545
White cell count 394
White line of Frenkel 11
White pupillary reflex 640
Whole-virion vaccine 113
Widal test 141
    modified 141
Williams syndrome 416
Wilson's disease 225, 227, 234, 241, 391, 394, 394t, 564
    global assessment scale for 394
    hepatic 393
    neurological 394
Wilson's facies 394
Wimberger ring sign 11
Wiskott-Aldrich syndrome 300
Wolff-Parkinson-White 422, 478
Wolman disease 227, 242, 243f
World Health Organization 14, 180, 238, 264, 270, 323, 330t, 524, 558, 599, 632
Worm infestation 27
Wright stain 88, 89, 266, 266f, 267f

X

Xanthine stone 505
Xanthinuria 508
X-chromosome 400, 582
Xerophthalmic fundus 13
Xerosis 642
X-linked ataxia 399
X-linked dilated cardiomyopathy 400
X-linked disorders 600
X-ray 430
    abdomen adrenal calcification 243f
    chest 426, 442
    kidneys, ureters, bladder 503, 506
    knee joint 8
    sinuses 386
    wrist 8

Y

Yawns 38
Yersinia 20, 22
    enterocolitica 20, 22
    pestis 181

Z

Zagreb schedule 118
Zellweger syndrome 227, 243
Zidovudine 71, 285
    therapy 273
Ziehl-Neelsen staining 173
Zinc 174, 393
    deficiency 14
        causes of 14
        clinical manifestation of 14
    dose schedule of 15b
    preparations, overdoses of 15
    role of 15
    status, assessment of 14
    sulfate 15
    supplementation 100
Zonisamide 370, 505
Z-scores 570

EU GSPR Authorised Reprsentative
Logos Europe, 9 rue Nicolas Poussin
1700, La Rochelle, France
Phone: +33 (0) 6 67 93 73 78
E-mail: contact@logoseurope.eu

www.ingramcontent.com/pod-product-compliance
Ingram Content Group UK Ltd.
Pitfield, Milton Keynes, MK11 3LW, UK
UKHW050458150426
5217IPUK00025B/1742